THE OXFORD HANDBOOK OF

VOICE
PERCEPTION

THE OXFORD HANDBOOK OF

VOICE PERCEPTION

Edited by

SASCHA FRÜHHOLZ

and

PASCAL BELIN

OXFORD
UNIVERSITY PRESS

OXFORD

UNIVERSITY PRESS

Great Clarendon Street, Oxford, OX2 6DP,
United Kingdom

Oxford University Press is a department of the University of Oxford.
It furthers the University's objective of excellence in research, scholarship,
and education by publishing worldwide. Oxford is a registered trade mark of
Oxford University Press in the UK and in certain other countries

© Oxford University Press 2019

The moral rights of the authors have been asserted

First Edition published in 2019

Impression: 1

Published in the United States of America by Oxford University Press
198 Madison Avenue, New York, NY 10016, United States of America

British Library Cataloguing in Publication Data

Data available

Library of Congress Control Number: 2018962508

ISBN 978–0–19–874318–7

Printed and bound by
CPI Group (UK) Ltd, Croydon, CR0 4YY

To Wiebke and Elia
To Marie-Hélène, Jules, Mathilde, and Félix

PREFACE

THE past decades have seen an explosion of research into the psychological, cognitive, neural, biological, and computational mechanisms of voice perception. These mechanisms refer to the general ability to extract information from voices produced by other living beings or by technological systems. Voice perception research is now a lively area of research studied from many different perspectives ranging from basic research on the acoustical analysis of vocalizations, to its neural and cognitive mechanisms, to comparative research across ages, species, and cultures, to clinical work including neurology and psychiatry, up to applied research in the field of machine-based generation and decoding of voices, telecommunication, etc. This handbook provides a comprehensive and, we hope, authoritative overview of the major research fields related to voice perception, in an accessible form, for a broad readership of students, scholars, and researchers. The handbook is divided into seven major parts, each dealing with a central perspective on voice perception, and covering: what makes the voice special compared to other acoustic signals; the evolutionary and ontogenetic roots of voice perception; emotional and motivational vocal expression; the social cues extracted from voice signals; machine-based recognition of voices; and the clinical disorders that affect voice perception.

From conception to publication of this handbook took several years, and it would have been impossible without the help of many people. We are extremely thankful to all who provided continued support throughout its preparation and publication. First and foremost, we give our heartfelt thanks to all the authors for their excellent chapter contributions, which make this handbook one of the most valuable resources for those interested in past and current research on voice perception. From Oxford University Press, we gratefully thank Martin Baum (Senior Commissioning Editor), Charlotte Holloway (Senior Assistant Commissioning Editor), and April Peak (Assistant Commissioning Editor) for their indispensable and continued support. We also thank Carole Sunderland, Sai Sarath Ram, and Anula Griffiths from the book production team. Finally, we acknowledge the help and support of many colleagues throughout all the years of our scientific endeavours: Patrik Vuilleumier, Didier Grandjean, Stefan Schweinberger, Manfred Herrmann, Yves Samson, Robert Zatorre, and Guillaume Masson.

We gratefully acknowledge the long-term financial support from the Swiss National Science Foundation (SF), from the British Biotechnology and Biological Sciences Research Council (PB), and from the French Fondation pour la Recherche Médicale and Agence Nationale de la Recherche (PB).

Sascha Frühholz (Zurich, Switzerland)
Pascal Belin (Marseille, France)
2018

CONTENTS

PART IV: EMOTIONAL AND MOTIVATIONAL VOCAL EXPRESSION

PART V: VOCAL IDENTITY, PERSONALITY, AND THE SOCIAL CONTEXT

PART VI: MACHINE-BASED GENERATION AND DECODING OF VOICES

PART VII: CLINICAL DISORDERS

Audios

The following audio files can be found at http://neuralbasesofcommunication.eu/projects/oxford_handbook_of_voice_perception/

1.1   'Buzzing' produced by periodic oscillations of the vocal folds in the larynx.

1.2   Different phonemes in human speech.

2.1   Frogs, Leipzig, Germany.

2.2   Sarcastic/sincere utterances: (a) American English; (b) Korean

2.3   Word accent contrasts: (a) American English: noun, noun phrase (green house, yellow jacket); noun, verb (import, convict); (b) Swedish: duck, spirit.

2.4   Ditropic utterances: (a) American English: idiomatic, literal; (b) Korean: idiomatic, literal; (c) French: idiomatic, literal.

2.5   Sentence focus.

3.1   Voice without speech.

3.2   Example of vocal block in the voice localizer.

3.3   Example of non-vocal block in the voice localizer.

3.4   Male voice average.

3.5   Female voice average.

5.1   Infant-directed speech, showing prosodic modifications: (a) English, 3 months old; (b) English, 9 months old; (c) English, 12 months old; (d) English, 15 months old; (e) English, 18 months old; (f) Mandarin, 21 months old.

5.2   Adult-directed speech, showing prosodic modifications: (a) English, 3 months old; (b) English, 9 months old; (c) English, 12 months old; (d) English, 15 months old; (e) English, 18 months old; (f) Mandarin, 21 months old.

6.1   Example of the voice source of a real voice, derived by eliminating the effects of the vocal tract on the sound.

6.2   Stimuli that received the highest and the lowest mean ratings of pressedness in the study by Millgård et al. (2015).

6.3   Typical example of a register break in a male voice.

6.4   Synthesized tone, first presented without, and then with, vibrato.

6.5   Synthesized vowel with vibrato rates of 7, 6, and 5 Hz, presented twice, first with an extent of ±0.5 semitone, then with an extent of ±1 semitone.

6.6   Timbral effect of clustering formants so as to create a singer's formant cluster in a synthesized vowel. First, formants 3, 4, 5, and 6 are at 2500 Hz, 3700 Hz, 4900 Hz, and 5500 Hz. Then, the fourth is changed to 2700 Hz; then the fifth is changed to 2900 Hz; and finally the sixth is changed to 3500 Hz.

16.3   Sounds from different mammal species, all negative state, varying in intensity: wild boar (a) low pitch (b) high pitch; tree shrew (c) low-pitch squeak, close distance (d) low-pitch squeak, long distance; pig (e) low pitch (f) high pitch; kitten (g) low pitch, isolated state (h) low pitch, handling state; horse (i) low pitch (j) high pitch; cattle (k) low pitch (l) high pitch; silver fox (m) low pitch (n) high pitch.

17.1   Tamarin mobbing call: (a) at normal speed; (b) slowed to human auditory range. Note the noisy dissonant structure.

17.2   Tamarin confident threat: (a) at normal speed; (b) slowed to human auditory range. Note the harmonic structure of the call.

17.3   Chorused tamarin long call, used to bring group members together. Note the long harmonic notes and antiphonal calling.

17.4   Calming music for tamarins. (Copyright: David Teie)

17.5   Arousing music for tamarins. (Copyright: David Teie)

18.1   Vocalizations of rhesus macaques (to accompany Figure 18.1A): (a) archscream; (b) coo; (c) growl; (d) tonal scream; (e) harmonic arch; (f) bark. (Original description of species-specific vocalizations in the macaque by Hauser, 1996.)

18.2   Band-passed noise bursts (to accompany Figure 18.2A): (a) pure-tone burst; (b) 0.333 octaves; (c) 0.5 octaves; (d) 1 octave; (e) 2 octaves; (f) white-noise burst.

20.1   Successively building fragments of a pseudo-sentence conveying anger, as used in a typical emotional prosody gating study, together with the full sentence: (a) gate 1; (b) gate 2; (c) gate 3; (d) gate 4; (e) gate 5; (f) gate 6; (g) full sentence.

20.2   Successively building fragments of a pseudo-sentence conveying fear, as used in a typical emotional prosody gating study, together with the full sentence: (a) gate 1; (b) gate 2; (c) gate 3; (d) gate 4; (e) gate 5; (f) gate 6; (g) full sentence.

20.3   Successively building fragments of a pseudo-sentence conveying happiness, as used in a typical emotional prosody gating study, together with the full sentence: (a) gate 1; (b) gate 2; (c) gate 3; (d) gate 4; (e) gate 5; (f) gate 6; (g) full sentence.

21.1   Non-linguistic vocalizations: (a) sadness, male; (b) sadness, female; (c) pleasure, male; (d) pleasure, female; (e) neutral, male; (f) neutral, female; (g) happiness, male; (h) happiness, female; (i) fear, male; (j) fear, female.

21.2   Pseudospeech: (a) surprise, male; (b) surprise, female; (c) sad, male; (d) sad, female; (e) neutral, male; (f) neutral, female; (g) happy, male; (h) happy, female; (i) fear, male; (j) fear, female; (k) disgust, male; (l) disgust, female; (m) anger, male; (n) anger, female.

22.1   Different types of laughter: (a) tickling; (b) taunting; (c) sniffing; (d) schadenfreude; (e) through nasal cavity; (f) nasal cavity open; (g) laughter phrases; (h) joyful/friendly; (i) inhalation and voiced; (j) inhalation and exhalation; (k) fricative; (l) cough-like.

24.1   Parameter-specific voice morphing: examples of adaptor types used in Skuk et al. (2015). Adaptor types differ with respect to the acoustic parameters that have been morphed along a male–female gender continuum: (a) Fo adaptor type with male/androgynous/female Fo contour and with androgynous timbre; (b) timbre adaptor type with male/androgynous/female timbre and with androgynous Fo contour; (c) full adaptor type with male/androgynous/female Fo contour and timbre; (d) voice gender continuum of full morphs (Fo and timbre) spanning from male to female in steps of 10%.

24.2   Voice samples of male and female, young and old speakers uttering the German sentence 'Die nachfrage bestimmt den preis'. [Demand determines the price.] Stimuli for young speakers are taken from Zäske et al. (2014), and all samples are taken from the Jena Speaker Set Database: (a) male, 75 years old; (b) male, 68 years old; (c) male, 65 years old; (d) male, 25 years old; (e) male, 23 years old; (f) male, 21 years old; (g) female, 71 years old; (h) female, 65 years old; (i) female, 64 years old; (j) female, 23 years old; (k) female, 19 years old; (l) female, 18 years old.

25.1   Acoustic cues for identity perception: (a)–(d) four different, natural, female voices uttering the same syllable; (e) female voice prototype, corresponding to the average of thirty-two voices.

26.1   A trustworthy male voice demonstrates a slightly higher pitch than average: compare (a) trustworthy male, with (b) untrustworthy male. For females, trustworthiness relates to the glide of the voice: compare (c) rising intonation of untrustworthy female voice, with (d) dropping intonation of trustworthy female voice.

26.2   Dominance is a strong influence of formant dispersion, with lower dispersion associated with higher dominance: compare (a) male, dominant, with (b) male, non-dominant; and (c) female, dominant, with (d) female, non-dominant.

26.3   (a) Male Trustworthiness (PC1) Continuum, from Low To High; (b) Female Trustworthiness (PC1) Continuum, from Low To High; (c) Male Dominance (PC2) Continuum, from Low To High; (d) Female Dominance (PC2) Continuum, from Low To High.

30.1   Three sample accents used in the neuroimaging study by Bestelmeyer et al. (2015): Scottish accent; Southern English accent; and General American accent.

31.1(a–e)   Morphed voices of a German sentence 'Keine antwort ist auch eine antwort' ['No answer is an answer as well'] resulting from the interpolation of a 22-year-old male speaker with a 71-year-old male speaker.

31.2   Parameter morph continua between a male and a female /aba/: (a) full morph continuum; (b) Fo morph continuum; and (c) timbre morph continuum.

Videos

Tables

....

Boxes

Abbreviations

2AFC	two-alternative forced-choice
A1	primary auditory cortex
AB	accessory basal
AC	auditory cortex
ACC	anterior cingulate cortex
AD	Alzheimer's disease
ADS	adult-directed speech
AFP	anterior forebrain pathway
AG	angular gyrus
AL	anterolateral area
ALSP	audio-linguistic signal processing
AM	acoustic model
ANN	artificial neural network
ASD	autism spectrum disorder
ASM	auditory sensory memory
ASR	automatic speech recognition
AST	asymmetric sampling time
AST	anterior superior temporal
ATL	anterior temporal lobe
AVH	auditory verbal hallucination
AVI	audiovisual integration
AVQI	Acoustic Voice Quality Index
B	basal
BA	Brodmann area
BBD	bilateral brain-damaged
BBW	best bandwidth
BG	basal ganglia
BoAW	bag-of-audio-words
BOLD	blood oxygen level dependency
BoW	bag-of-words
BP	band-passed
BPN	band-passed noise
CL	caudo-lateral area
CM	centromedian
CNN	convolutional neural network
CPP	cepstral peak prominence
CS	combination sensitivity

CS	conditional stimulus
CSD	Caesarean section delivery
CSID	Cepstral Spectral Index of Dysphonia
DBS	deep brain stimulation
DFT	discrete Fourier transform
DLPFC	dorso-lateral prefrontal cortex
DMN	default mode network
DSI	Dysphonia Severity Index
DTI	diffusion tensor imaging
EEG	electrophysiology
EM	expectation maximization
EMG	electromyography
EPI	Eysenck Personality Inventory
ERP	event-related potential
ESG	ectosylvian gyrus
FFA	fusiform face area
FFT	fast Fourier transform
FG	fusiform gyrus
FTLD	fronto-temporal lobar degeneration
FM	frequency-modulated
fMRI	functional magnetic resonance imaging
fNIRS	functional near-infrared spectroscopy
FTPV	fronto-temporal positivity to voice
GEMAPS	Geneva Minimalistic Acoustic Parameter Set
GEMEP	Geneva Multimodal Emotion Portrayal
GMM	Gaussian mixture model
GUI	graphical user interface
GVMT	Glasgow Voice Memory Test
HG	Heschl's gyrus
HLA	human leukocyte antigens
HMM	hidden Markov model
HNR	harmonics-to-noise ratio
HSMM	hidden semi-Markov model
IDF	inverse document frequency
IDS	infant-directed speech
IFC	inferior frontal cortex
IFG	inferior frontal gyrus
LB	laterobasal
LB	lateral and medial belt
LBD	left brain-damaged
LFP	local field potential
LLD	low-level descriptor
LM	language model
LMAN	lateral magnocellular nucleus of the anterior neostriatum
LP	linear prediction
LPC	linear prediction coefficient

LPC	late positive complex
LSTM-RNN	long short-term memory recurrent neural network
LTAS	long-term average spectrum
LTP	long-term potentiation
M	median
M1	primary motor cortex
MANOVA	multivariate analysis of variance
MAP	maximum a posteriori
MAV	Montreal Affective Voices
MDL	minimum description length
MEG	magnetoencephalography
MFC	medial frontal cortex
MFCC	Mel-frequency cepstral coefficient
MGB	medial geniculate body
MHC	major histocompatibility complex
ML	maximum likelihood
ML	middle lateral area
MMN	mismatch negativity
MMR	mismatch response
MMST	maternal mental state talk
MS	multidimensional scaling
MTG	middle temporal gyrus
MTL	middle temporal lobe
MUC	memory, unification, and control
MVP	Multidimensional Voice Program
MVPA	multivoxel pattern analysis
NAQ	normalized amplitude quotient
NLP	non-linear phenomena
NLP	natural language processing
OFA	occipital face area
OFC	orbitofrontal cortex
OGB	own-gender bias
OT	oxytocin
PAG	periaqueductal grey
PANSS	Positive and Negative Syndrome Scale
PARC	preferential auditory-related cortex
PARCOR	partial correlation
PCA	principal component analysis
PDD	pervasive developmental disorder
PDF	probability density function
PET	positron emission tomography
PFC	prefrontal cortex
PIN	posterior intralaminar nucleus
PLP	perceptual linear prediction
(d)(v)PMC	(dorsal) (ventral) premotor cortex
PND	postnatal depression

PNN	prosody neural network
PPC	posterior parietal cortex
PPI	psychophysiological interaction
PR	perisylvian regions
PSOLA	pitch synchronous overlap and add
PT	planum temporale
PTSD	post-traumatic stress disorder
R	rostral area
RAM	Realistic Accuracy Model
RBD	right brain-damaged
RBM	restricted Boltzmann machine
REL	resting expiratory level
ROI	region of interest
rTMS	repetitive transcranial magnetic stimulation
SEM	standard errors of the mean
SF	superficial
SFA	spectral facilitation
SFG	superior frontal gyrus
SGL	socially guided learning
SIT	social identity theory
SLF	superior longitudinal fasciculus
SLI	specific language impairment
(pre) SMA	(pre)supplementary motor area
SMG	supramarginal gyrus
SMP	song motor pathway
SPL	sound pressure level
SPM	Statistical Parametric Mapping
SSP	social signal processing
STG	superior temporal gyrus
STN	subthalamic nucleus
STP	supratemporal plane
(a)(p)ST	(anterior) (posterior) superior temporal cortex
STS	superior temporal sulcus
SVM	support vector machine
SVR	support vector regression
tACS	transcranial alternating current stimulation
TD-PSOLA	time-domain pitch synchronous overlap add
tDCS	transcranial direct current stimulation
TEEP	Tripartite Emotion Expression and Perception
TFA	temporal facilitation
TF-IDF	term frequency inverse document frequency
TMS	transcranial magnetic stimulation
ToBI	Tone and Break Indices
TTS	text-to-speech
TVA	temporal voice area
US	unconditional stimulus

V1	primary visual cortex
VAAE	vocal-age after-effect
VBM	voxel-based morphometry
VD	vaginal delivery
VENEC	Vocal Expressions of Nineteen Emotions across Cultures
VGAE	voice-gender after-effect
VLPFC	ventrolateral prefrontal cortex
VLSM	voxel-based lesion-symptom mapping
VOT	voice onset time
VPAS	Vocal Profiles Analysis Scheme
VTA	ventral tegmental area
WM	working memory

Contributors

Jennifer L. Agustus Dementia Research Centre, UCL Institute of Neurology, University College London, UK

Kai Alter Language and Brain Laboratory, Faculty of Linguistics, Philology and Phonetics, University of Oxford, UK and Institute of Neuroscience, Faculty of Medical Sciences, Newcastle University, UK

Attila Andics MTA-ELTE 'Lendület' Neuroethology of Communication Research Group, Department of Ethology, Eötvös Loránd University, Budapest, Hungary and Hungarian Academy of Sciences, Budapest, Hungary

Jorge L. Armony Department of Psychiatry, McGill University, Canada

Pascal Belin Institut de Neurosciences de la Timone, CNRS & Aix-Marseille Université, Marseille, France and Département de Psychologie, Université de Montréal, Québec, Canada

Mireille Besson CNRS & Aix-Marseille Université, Laboratoire de Neurosciences Cognitives, Marseille, France

Patricia E.G. Bestelmeyer School of Psychology, Bangor University, UK

Samantha Carouso-Peck Department of Psychology, Cornell University, USA

Leonardo Ceravolo Faculty of Psychology and Educational Sciences, Swiss Center for Affective Sciences, University of Geneva, Switzerland

Michelle G. Craske Department of Psychology, UCLA, Los Angeles, USA

Volker Dellwo Department of Computational Linguistics, University of Zurich, Switzerland

Emmanuelle Dionne-Dostie Sainte-Justine University Hospital Research Centre, Montreal, Canada and Centre de Recherche en Neuropsychologie et Cognition, University of Montreal, Canada

Eva Dittinger CNRS & Aix-Marseille Université, Laboratoire de Neurosciences Cognitives and Laboratoire Parole et Langage, Marseille, France

Stefan Elmer Auditory Research Group Zurich (ARGZ), Division Neuropsychology, Institute of Psychology, University of Zurich, Switzerland

Thomas Ethofer Department for Biomedical Magnetic Resonance, University of Tübingen, Germany and Clinic for Psychiatry and Psychotherapy, University of Tübingen, Germany

Tamás Faragó Eötvös Loránd University, Institute of Biology, Department of Ethology, Budapest, Hungary

David R. Feinberg Department of Psychology, Neuroscience, and Behaviour, McMaster University, Canada

Peter French The University of York, UK

Sascha Frühholz Department of Psychology, University of Zürich, Switzerland, Neuroscience Center Zurich, University of Zurich and ETH Zurich, Switzerland, and Center for Integrative Human Physiology (ZIHP), University of Zurich, Switzerland

Anne Gallagher Sainte-Justine University Hospital Research Centre, Montreal, Canada and Centre de Recherche en Neuropsychologie et Cognition, University of Montreal, Canada.

Bruce R. Gerratt Department of Head and Neck Surgery, School of Medicine at UCLA, USA

Nathalie Giroud Institute of Psychology, University of Zurich, Switzerland

Michael H. Goldstein Department of Psychology, Cornell University, USA

Sarah M. Haigh Clinical Neurophysiological Research Laboratory, Department of Psychiatry, Western Psychiatric Institute and Clinic, University of Pittsburgh, USA

Julia C. Hailstone Dementia Research Centre, UCL Institute of Neurology, University College London, UK

Lei He Phonetics and Speech Sciences, Department of Computational Linguistics, University of Zurich, Switzerland

Keikichi Hirose Professor Emeritus, National Institute of Informatics, University of Tokyo, Japan

Derek M. Houston Department of Otolaryngology—Head and Neck Surgery, Ohio State University, USA and Nationwide Children's Hospital, Columbus, USA

Kenneth Hugdahl Department of Biological and Medical Psychology, University of Bergen, Norway, Division of Psychiatry and Department of Radiology, Haukeland University Hospital, Bergen, Norway, and NORMENT Center of Excellence, University of Bergen, Norway

Hideki Kawahara Center for Innovation and Joint Research, Wakayama University, Japan

Matthias Keller Institute of Psychology, University of Zurich, Switzerland

Laura Kischkel Great Ormond Street Institute of Child Health, University College London, UK

Kristiina Kompus Department of Biological and Medical Psychology, University of Bergen, Norway and NORMENT Center of Excellence, University of Bergen, Norway

Sonja A. Kotz Faculty of Psychology and Neuroscience, Department of Neuropsychology and Psychopharmacology, Maastricht University, The Netherlands and Department of

Neuropsychology, Max-Planck Institute for Human Cognitive and Brain Sciences, Leipzig, Germany

Benjamin Kreifelts Department of Psychiatry and Psychotherapy, University of Tübingen, Germany

Jody Kreiman Department of Head and Neck Surgery, UCLA, USA

Morten L. Kringelbach Department of Psychiatry, University of Oxford, UK, Center of Functionally Integrative Neuroscience (CFIN), Aarhus University & The Royal Academy of Music, Aarhus/Aalborg, Denmark, and Center for Music in the Brain (MIB), Department of Clinical Medicine, Aarhus University, Denmark

Bernd J. Kröger Department of Phoniatrics, Pedaudiology, and Communication Disorders, Medical School, RWTH Aachen University, Germany

Maryse Lassonde Sainte-Justine University Hospital Research Centre, Montreal, Canada and Centre de Recherche en Neuropsychologie et Cognition, University of Montreal, Canada

Marianne Latinus U1253, iBrain, Université de Tours, INSERM, Tours, France

David I. Leitman PSYR2—Psychiatric disorders: from Resistance to Response, Centre de Recherche en Neurosciences de Lyon (CRNL) INSERM-CNRS, Centre Hospitalier Le Vinatier, France

Corrina Maguinness Max Planck Institute for Human Cognitive and Brain Sciences, Leipzig, Germany

Phil McAleer School of Psychology, University of Glasgow, UK

Evelyne Mercure Institute of Cognitive Neuroscience, University College London, UK

Martin Meyer Institute of Psychology, University of Zurich, Switzerland and Cognitive Psychology Unit (CPU), University of Klagenfurt, Austria

Alan K.S. Nielsen Center for Language Evolution, School of Philosophy, Psychology, and Language Sciences, University of Edinburgh, UK

Natacha Paquette Sainte-Justine University Hospital Research Centre, Montreal, Canada and Centre de Recherche en Neuropsychologie et Cognition, University of Montreal, Canada

Christine E. Parsons Department of Psychiatry, University of Oxford, UK and Department of Clinical Medicine, Aarhus University, Denmark

Silke Paulmann Department of Psychology and Centre for Brain Science, University of Essex, Colchester, UK

Tyler K. Perrachione Department of Speech, Language, and Hearing Sciences, College of Health and Rehabilitation Sciences, Sargent College, Boston University, USA

Catherine Perrodin Institute of Behavioural Neuroscience, University College London, UK

Christopher I. Petkov Institute of Neuroscience, Newcastle University Medical School, UK

Katarzyna Pisanski School of Psychology, University of Sussex, UK and Institute of Psychology, University of Wroclaw, Poland

Josef P. Rauschecker Laboratory of Integrative Neuroscience and Cognition, Department of Neuroscience, Georgetown University Medical Center, Washington, USA and Institute for Advanced Study, TUM, Munich, Germany

Drew Rendall Departments of Biology and Psychology, University of New Brunswick, Canada

Claudia Roswandowitz Max Planck Institute for Human Cognitive and Brain Sciences, Leipzig, Germany

Klaus R. Scherer University of Geneva, Switzerland and University of Munich, Germany

Maximilian Schmitt Chair of Complex and Intelligent Systems, University of Passau, Germany

Björn Schuller Chair of Complex and Intelligent Systems, University of Passau, Germany and Department of Computing, Imperial College London, UK

Stefan R. Schweinberger Department of General Psychology and Cognitive Neuroscience, DFG Research Unit Person Perception, and Voice Research Unit, Friedrich Schiller University, Jena, Germany

Amanda Seidl Department of Speech, Language and Hearing Sciences, Purdue University, USA

Verena G. Skuk Department of General Psychology and Cognitive Neuroscience, DFG Research Unit Person Perception, and Voice Research Unit, Friedrich Schiller University, Jena, Germany and Department of Otorhinolaryngology, Jena University Hospital, Germany

Charles T. Snowdon Department of Psychology, University of Wisconsin, Madison, USA

Alan Stein Department of Psychiatry, University of Oxford, UK

Sarah Stevenage Department of Psychology, University of Southampton, UK

Johan Sundberg Department of Speech, Music and Hearing, School of Electrical Engineering and Computer Science, KTH Royal Institute of Technology, Sweden

Diana Van Lancker Sidtis Department of Communicative Sciences and Disorders, New York University, USA and Nathan Kline Institute for Psychiatric Research, Orangeburg, New York, USA

Alessandro Vinciarelli School of Computing Science and Institute of Neuroscience and Psychology, University of Glasgow, UK

Katharina von Kriegstein Max Planck Institute for Human Cognitive and Brain Sciences, Leipzig, Germany, Humboldt University zu Berlin, Germany, and Technische Universität Dresden, Faculty of Psychology, Dresden, Germany

Peter Vuust Center of Functionally Integrative Neuroscience (CFIN), Aarhus University & The Royal Academy of Music, Aarhus/Aalborg, Denmark and Center for Music in the Brain (MIB), Department of Clinical Medicine, Aarhus University, Denmark

Yuanyuan Wang Department of Otolaryngology—Head and Neck Surgery, Ohio State University, USA and Nationwide Children's Hospital, Columbus, USA

Jason D. Warren Dementia Research Centre, UCL Institute of Neurology, University College London, UK

Jocelyne C. Whitehead Integrated Program in Neuroscience, McGill University, Canada

Dirk Wildgruber Department of Psychiatry and Psychotherapy, University of Tübingen, Germany

Katherine S. Young Department of Psychology, UCLA, Los Angeles, USA and Department of Psychiatry, University of Oxford, UK

Romi Zäske Department of General Psychology and Cognitive Neuroscience, DFG Research Unit Person Perception, and Voice Research Unit, Friedrich Schiller University, Jena, Germany and Department of Otorhinolaryngology, Jena University Hospital, Germany

PART I

THE VOICE IS SPECIAL

CHAPTER 1

··

THE SCIENCE OF
VOICE PERCEPTION

··

SASCHA FRÜHHOLZ AND PASCAL BELIN

1.1 INTRODUCTION

VOICES are omnipresent in our daily natural and social environments (Belin et al., 2004; Belin, 2006). We hear voices of other people talking, babbling, singing, whispering, laughing, crying, screaming, coughing, harrumphing, humming, or acting. We hear vocalizations of animals, like a dog barking, a frog croaking, a bird chirping, a whale singing, a lion roaring, a monkey chattering, a cat meowing, a horse whinnying, an owl hooting, or a duck quacking. Not only do we hear natural voices and vocalizations, but also vocalizations produced by technical systems, such as train announcements at stations, the computer voice in customer service calls, the digital voice of a text-to-speech synthesizer, the vocal instructions at ATM machines, or the friendly voice of GPS navigation systems. Sometimes we even hear voices in the absence or the confusion of an external source, such as vocal illusion or delusion.

However, it is not only the daily perception of voices in general that makes them an important auditory object that regulates and adapts social behaviour. The wealth of socially relevant information portrayed and conveyed by voices (Schweinberger & Burton, 2011; Frühholz et al., 2016) provides speakers with a powerful tool for voluntarily and involuntarily expressing such information in the voice, and allows listeners to also voluntarily and involuntarily perceive and to make use of such information (see Parts IV and V). The importance of accurately extracting information from voices in our environment, to orientate ourselves and adapt our behaviour, is seen not only in healthy living beings but also especially in the social and behavioural deficits of patients who fail to recognize voices or important voice features (see Part VII).

For the normal human listener, voices are most obviously used for supporting one of the most evolved psychological and cognitive functions for interpersonal communication—speech and language. However, in addition to speech, voices carry a wealth of socially relevant information, and individuals can encode such information in different levels of vocal expression ranging from verbal messages to non-verbal communication (Frühholz & Grandjean, 2013). This non-verbal communication conveys speaker information about such as their identity (e.g. gender, age), their emotional and motivational states (e.g. happy, sad), or their personality. Evidence covered in this book suggests that human listeners have developed exquisite perceptual mechanisms to extract all sorts of non-verbal, paraverbal (i.e. vocal intonations superimposed on speech), or verbal vocal information in far greater detail than for other sound categories, akin to a 'perceptual zooming' on a particular sound category of high evolutionary relevance and overwhelming presence (Kreiman & Sidtis, 2011).

Besides speech, socially relevant information in voices, vocalizations, and voice perception is thus one of the major sources of non-verbal and paraverbal auditory communication (see Part I). Furthermore, these more basic channels of vocal communication, unlike the uniquely human speech, are shared among many species (see Part III). This arguably makes the non-verbal channel of vocalizations an even more powerful medium of social communication—one with the potential of conveying 'honest signals', not easy to consciously modify, upon which reliable impressions and predictions are often formed. Many species have developed exquisite abilities to control their vocal tract for producing sophisticated vocalizations (Fitch, 2000; Fitch et al., 2016) and, in parallel, cognitive and neural abilities to decode the useful information contained in non-verbal vocal messages of conspecifics as well as of heterospecifics (Belin et al., 2000; Petkov et al., 2008; Andics et al., 2014). The latter is a new important topic in voice research, pointing to the ability that non-verbal voice information cannot only be recognized by conspecifics but also across species (Andics et al., 2016; see Andics & Faragó, this volume).

Voices and vocalizations thus have a very specific and important role for social interactions and communication for a broad variety of species, and many behaviours and social dynamics cannot be understood without investigating vocal behaviour across different vertebrate species, especially mammalian species. Given the importance of vocalizations for social behaviour, the scientific investigation of vocalizations and voice perception has attracted attention since ancient days.

Modern investigations into this topic started in the nineteenth century, with an important landmark given by Darwin's investigations on the evolutionary continuity of the manifestation and perception of social expressions between man and animals (Darwin, 1899). Newer scientific methods and tools of investigation across several disciplines in the late nineteenth and twentieth centuries finally led to an explosion of empirical investigations on the mechanisms of voice perception. Technological advancements such as the possibility for electroacoustic analysis of voices, the invention of telephone and radio, new auditory recordings and storage technologies, medical vocal tract examination techniques, and experimental paradigms and approaches in a diversity of scientific disciplines, were the pacemakers for the flourishing field of voice perception research towards the end of the twentieth century.

1.2 WHAT IS A VOICE?

Again, voice and vocalizations are omnipresent in the natural and the social world, and given the obvious ease with which voices are perceived and distinguished from other auditory objects, it should be an easy endeavour to give a straightforward definition of what a voice really is. However, any attempt at a definition needs to deal with the fact that every voice has usually two sides to its existence, which makes that definition of a voice a juggling between perspectives. The two sides are the production of a voice on one side, and the perception of a voice on the other side. Any definition can focus on one of these sides, but a complete definition of a voice needs certainly to take both sides into account.

1.2.1 The Voice from the Viewpoint of Voice Production

Let us start by looking at the voice production side first. To be able to perceive a voice it needs to be produced by an organic or by a technical system. The most common case is that a voice is produced by the organic vocal tract of a living being. The anatomical and neural voice production system has undergone some changes in evolution (Figure 1.1) but most mammalian species, like humans, produce voices and vocalizations with a collection of anatomical structures, not all of which have roles solely for producing vocalizations (Figure 1.2). In

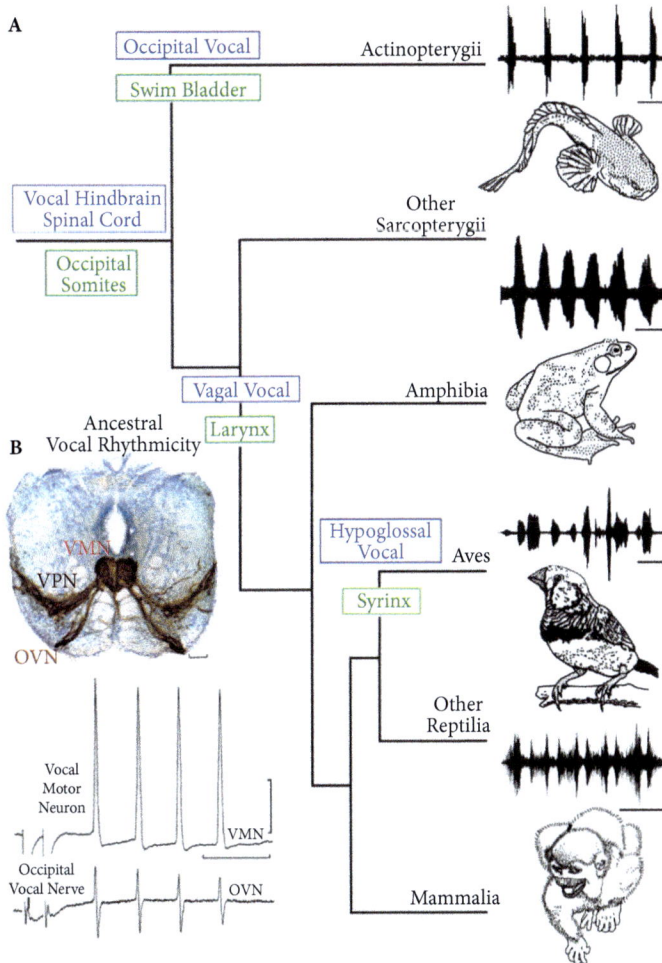

FIGURE 1.1 Evolution of vocal behaviours across different species of vertebrates. (A) Evolutionary hierarchy of vocalizations and neural control of vocalizations across vertebrate species. For each species, an amplitude waveform is shown for a typical voice call. (B) The neural circuit to produce vocalizations in batrachoidid fish shows a translation of neural motor activity into vocal patterns generated by the occipital vocal nerve.

From Bass A.H., Gilland E.H., & Baker R., 'Evolutionary Origins for Social Vocalization in a Vertebrate Hindbrain–Spinal Compartment', *Science*, Volume 321, Issue 5887, pp. 417–21, Copyright © 2008, doi: 10.1126/science.1157632. Reprinted with permission from AAAS.

primates, voices and vocal modulations are produced by a three-partite system comprising a power source (lungs, trachea), a sound source (larynx, vocal folds), and a sound modifier or filter system (pharynx, oral cavity, nasal cavity). Note that the voice production mechanisms are largely conserved in evolution and highly similar across many species (see Van Lancker Sidtis; Nielsen & Rendall; Rauschecker; this volume).

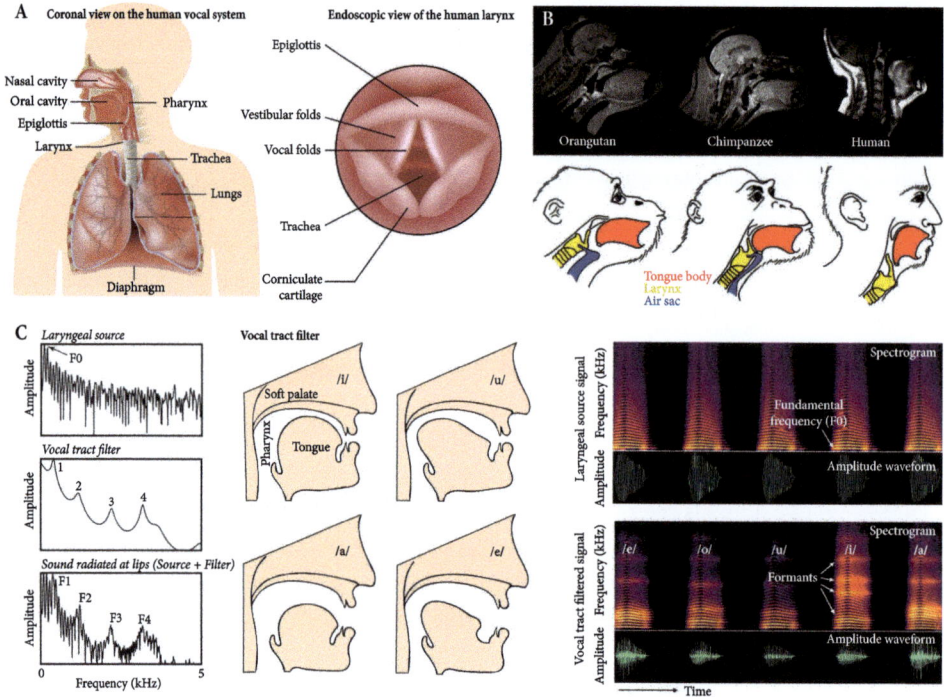

FIGURE 1.2 Source and filter mechanism of voice production. **(A)** Coronal and endoscopic view in the human vocal system. The human vocal system consists (left panel) of a power source (lungs, trachea), sound source (larynx), and a sound modifier or vocal tract filter system (pharynx, oral cavity, nasal cavity). The sound source is generated by the larynx, and periodic oscillations of the vocal folds in the larynx (right panel) produce a 'buzzing' sound with a highly harmonic structure called glottal pulses (Audio 1.1). **(B)** The shape of the vocal system shows a variable anatomical structure across species, and the image shows the differences especially for different primate species. **(C)** The left panel shows the spectral profile of sound generated by the laryngeal source; depending on the shape of the vocal tract filter, certain frequencies of the laryngeal sound are enhanced or decreased. The sound radiated at the lips is the combination of the sound source filtered by the vocal tract. Thus, depending on the configuration of the articulators, different frequency bands (called formants) are modulated, which we, for example, perceive as different phonemes in human speech (the vowels /e/, /o/, /u/, /i/, /a/; Audio 1.2) (middle panel). The right panel shows, on the top, the spectrogram and amplitude waveform of five glottal pulses that, after filtering by five different articulator configurations, result in different vocalized and perceived vowels.

(B) Adapted from *Trends in Cognitive Sciences*, Volume 4, Issue 7, Fitch W.T., 'The evolution of speech: a comparative review', pp. 258–67, Copyright © 2000 Elsevier Ltd., with permission from Elsevier, http://www.sciencedirect.com/science/article/pii/S1364661300014947.

(C) Reprinted with permission from *Current Biology*, Volume 18, Issue 11, Ghazanfar A.A. & Rendall D., 'Evolution of human vocal production' pp. 457–60, Copyright © 2008 Elsevier Ltd., doi: 10.1016/j.cub.2008.03.030, with permission from Elsevier.

The most common vocal sounds (i.e. 'voiced sounds') correspond to a periodic oscillation of the vocal folds with a generally well-defined fundamental frequency (Fo). The range of Fo values a given organism can achieve during normal phonation or singing (i.e. the 'register') is fairly extended, but the average Fo of an individual is largely a function of the size of his or her vocal folds. The mean body size of males is usually larger than that of females, resulting in larger vocal folds in males than females or children, and generally lower Fo values (although there are certain exceptions, e.g. males with a high vocal pitch or females with a low pitch). The vocal tract above the larynx acts as an acoustic filter reinforcing certain frequencies of the source, which are called 'formants'. Formant frequencies depend on the particular configuration of the articulators during speech and also on the individual's vocal tract size. Thus, when pronouncing the same vowel, males have lower formant frequencies than females or children.

An important characteristic of most vocal sounds is that they are generally highly harmonic, which means that they are more spectro-temporally regular than the majority of sound categories, apart from many instrumental sounds. This regularity can be captured by acoustical measures such as the harmonic-to-noise ratio (HNR), or jitter and shimmer as measures of short-term perturbation of fundamental frequency and amplitude, respectively. Yet in addition to the 'normal' mode of phonation, the larynx is frequently used in other modes such as the 'falsetto' register, the 'fry' register, or during whispering (Belin et al., 2004; Latinus & Belin, 2011; Deng et al., 2016, 2017; Frühholz et al., 2016), contributing to a greater diversity of possible vocal sounds. This diversity is an important part of a certain type of vocalizations such as in the field of singing (see Sundberg, this volume). Highly trained singers and also certain animals can use a broad variety of vocal registers during vocal expressions in singing.

Linguistic information is essentially conveyed by changes in formant frequencies, with the notable exception of tone languages such as Mandarin in which the Fo pattern can discriminate different speech sounds. Whispered speech, where the sound source is replaced by turbulent expiration noise, remains intelligible as formant frequencies are clearly perceptible (Frühholz et al., 2016; Deng et al., 2017). Fo variations, on the other hand, tend to carry information concerning linguistic and affective prosody (see Meyer et al.; Frühholz & Ceravolo; this volume), as well as on perceived personality impression (see McAleer & Belin; Pisanski & Feinberg; this volume).

Other acoustical features of voices are loosely regrouped under the general category of 'timbre', which is the auditory equivalent of visual 'colour', and include widely different aspects of phonation such as an individual's particular division of acoustical energy across frequency (i.e. the long-term average spectrum, LTAS) or the amount of phonation noise. These voice features together span a multidimensional acoustic space. Within this space, certain voice features can be used to distinguish voice sounds along certain dimensions that are relevant for social interactions. For example, the distinction of a female from a male voice can be done based on the Fo and/or formant frequencies (Pernet & Belin, 2012) (Figure 1.3).

This definition of voice from the viewpoint of its production is certainly a valid definition, and many features of what characterizes a voice are based on the acoustic properties resulting from that voice's production mechanisms. We thus say a voice has a fundamental frequency (Fo), harmonics as multiples of the Fo, formants caused by vocal tract filtering, and several other features describing vocal timbre. This definition of voice is also the basis for its standard visual representation and illustration based on spectral analysis. Voices, as many other types of sound, are travelling air waves, which oscillate at different frequencies. The power of these oscillations over time, at different frequencies, is commonly depicted in a spectrogram (see Figure 1.2c).

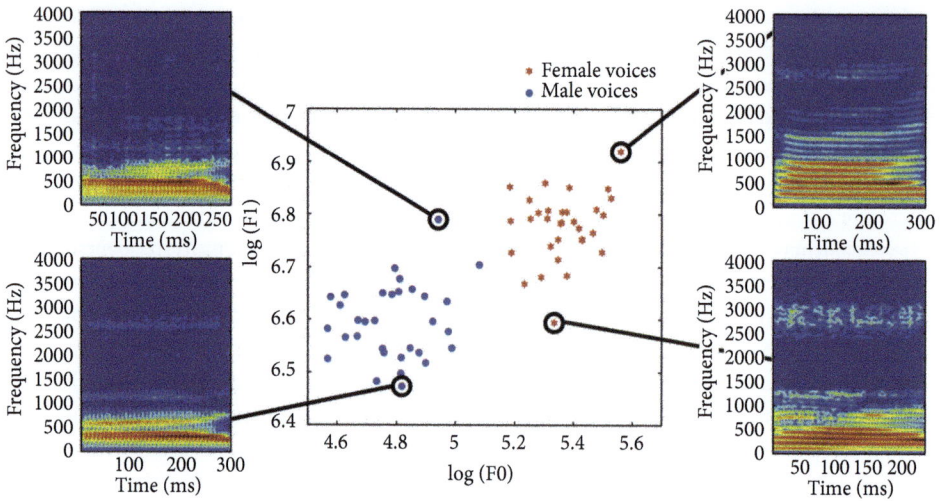

FIGURE 1.3 An acoustical voice space. Shown are two examples of spectrograms for human male voices (left panel) and two examples of human female voices (right panel). For each voice the mean level of the fundamental frequency (F0) and its first formant (F1) can be scored and plotted in a two-dimensional space (mid panel). Male and female voices differ considerably along the dimension of F0, but far less along the dimension of the F1.

Reprinted with permission from *Current Biology*, Volume 21, Issue 4, Latinus M. & Belin P., 'Human voice perception', Figure 1, pp. 143-5, Copyright © 2011 Elsevier Ltd., with permission from Elsevier, http://www.sciencedirect.com/science/article/pii/S096098221001701X.

1.2.2 The Voice from the Viewpoint of Voice Perception

However, external sensory information is not always perceived as it seems to exist in the outside world. Voices, once produced, are not passively registered by the neural and cognitive system of listeners. Thus, the production of voices is a necessary condition for their perception, but including only the production perspective in a definition of voice is not sufficient to describe the processes of recognizing voices in listeners. Thus, a second and extended definition of what a voice is needs also consider the perceptual mechanisms in listeners. We might thus say that a voice is the perceptual recognition of a sound, based on the perceptual impression of listeners of having classified a sound as being a voice. This perceptual impression of a voice needs not be based on an external vocal sound, although in most cases it probably does, since other non-vocal sounds or even internal signals might also induce the impression of having heard a voice. If we take this second perspective seriously, we obviously need to be able to describe what a vocal sound impression really is. How does a voice sound for listeners? What is the perceptual quality that also distinguishes this impression from other sound impressions?

The issue about perceptual voice impressions revolves around the much-discussed topic of 'voice quality'. The major problem of determining voice quality is to find a finite list of terms that essentially characterize the perceptual quality of voice as a specific type of sound. Different approaches have been taken to create such a list of acoustic descriptors of voice, ranging from theoretical descriptors about scholars have traditionally thought a voice is, to voice-synthesis approaches based on perceptual impressions, to statistical approaches aimed at reducing a large variety of terms to the most common descriptors that explain empirical ratings by listeners to a large degree of variance.

Besides these approaches taken from the perspective of voice production in healthy humans, several important approaches also come from the field of clinical voice disorders for the purpose of describing the disturbed voice quality in certain neurological and psychiatric disorders. A major example of the latter perspective is the GRBAS scale (Hirano, 1981)—its abbreviation referring to the central voice quality features of dysphonia *grade, roughness* (i.e. irregularity of vocal fold vibrations), *breathiness* (i.e. vocal turbulences), *asthenia* (i.e. vocal weakness and loss of vocal power), and *strain* (i.e. vocal tension).

Except for the recurring feature of the pitch of voice, directly related to the F0, no definitive description, from all these different approaches, of what perceptual features define a voice has emerged. This points to the potential fact that perceptual impressions of voices are largely subjective for each specific listener, and that it seems difficult for listeners to attribute the complex impression of a voice to isolated descriptive features.

Besides these subjective ways of processing voices, it has also been proposed that different strategies or sets of voice features are used for different purposes. For example, while discrimination of unfamiliar voices seems to be based on specific features that discriminate well between two voices, recognition of familiar voices seems to rely more on a 'gestalt' that combines multiple features (Sidtis & Kreiman, 2012). The scientific study of voice perception not only relies on the voice production of the speaker but also indispensably needs to take into account the perceptual and partly subjective processes induced in listeners by these voices.

Given these difficulties of finally defining what a voice or a vocalization is, one can probably offer at least a minimalistic definition that takes into account both the perceptive of how a voice is produced and how a voice is perceived by listeners. We might thus define a *voice* as follows:

> *A voice is an acoustic signal produced by the anatomical and physiological vocal tract system in a variety of vertebrate species or equivalently modelled and simulated in technical systems. This signal is acoustically registered and auditorily perceived mainly by conspecifics, and is detected, rated, and potentially classified as a distinctive vocal auditory object or as a distinctive voice feature depending on its specific voice quality compared to other auditory objects.*

This minimalistic definition of a voice, sometimes enriched by individual- or discipline-specific viewpoints and perspectives, might have guided scientific research throughout the nearly last two centuries of voice research, which we quickly outline in the following sections.

1.3 THE VOICE AS A TOPIC OF SCIENTIFIC RESEARCH

During the last decades, there has been an explosion of research into the biological, cognitive, and cerebral mechanisms of voice perception, and on the ability to extract and process information in voices. In particular, the emergence of tools such as computerized voice analysis and synthesis techniques (see Vinciarelli; Schmitt & Schuller; Kröger; Hirose; Dellwo et al.; this volume) and, more recently, voice morphing techniques (see Kawahara & Skuk, this volume), have permitted novel, better controlled experimental designs of the kind that were until recently only achievable with much simpler tonal sound.

Voice perception research is now a lively area of research, which is studied from different, complementary perspectives by many disciplines: acousticians and phoneticians study the acoustical structure of voice and vocalizations; voice pathologists measure disordered voice quality; neuroscientists examine the neural substrate of voice processing; psychologists dissect voice perception mechanisms and build cognitive models of voice perception; biologists compare voice perception across species; engineers work on automated voice synthesis and analysis and on more intelligent hearing aids and cochlear implants; psychiatrists examine voice hallucinations in schizophrenic patients; and neurologists study voice emotion and identity perception deficits. This list comprises the most important disciplines working in the field of voice perception, but it is far from exhaustive.

Although the scientific works on the topic of voice perception belong to different scientific domains, they nevertheless converge onto a novel, emerging field of research into voice perception. The general aim of this handbook is to provide the first general overview of this emerging field of research in a form accessible to a broad readership.

1.4 The Structure of this Handbook

Given the multitude of scientific disciplines representing the great number of scientists and scholars that deal with the processes and mechanisms of voice perception, and the enormous body of empirical evidence that has now accumulated, we think that the entire research field has come to a stage which necessitates a scientific handbook that summarizes and edits the research, providing overview chapters for central research topics. We especially hope that interested scholars and students that are new to this research field will find this handbook a useful first orientation to this flourishing field.

The overall goal of this handbook is to bring together the different research areas and approaches from biology, psychology, neuroscience, computer science, clinical science, phonetics, and linguistics to illustrate the contemporary and comparative research in the field of *voice perception* and integrate this into a comprehensive and authoritative resource. The handbook is intended to be a contemporary scientific guide to this topic and aims at providing a broad and extensive review of the current literature and the research approaches in the different fields and disciplines concerned with voice perception. The chapters in this handbook are intended to be written in an accessible form for scholars, researchers, and students working and studying in the specific field of vocal communication.

The handbook is divided into seven major sections. Part I is entitled 'The Voice is Special' and deals with the very notion of what makes voices special, in its basic sense. On a fundamental acoustic level, one might argue that voices are not different from any other type of acoustic signal in natural and social environments, and thus not so special as we claim. This notion is certainly true and raises a level of scientifically analysing voices that makes them comparable to other natural and unnatural acoustic signals in the outside world. However, beyond the basic acoustic level, voices are nonetheless special regarding the important role that they play in social interactions, not only for humans but also for a broad variety of other species. The possibility for auditory communication using voices and vocalizations has evolved not only for individuals to express and transfer meaning and information, but also to specifically convey this meaning and information to other conspecifics.

Thus, the voice is special. Firstly, because it is an important and essential means of general communication across a broad variety of species. Secondly, because it is the carrier of what is assumed to be the most elaborate system for communication that appears in human primates and is referred to as speech and language. Thirdly, because the rules and mechanisms of vocal communication are special compared to other channels of communication, such as the visual channel. Concerning the latter point, we of course know that social communication involves common mechanisms of how information is exchanged between social partners, but since voice is an acoustic signal that evolves in time, vocal communication has also its own specific rules that are determined by this temporal perspective. Part I includes chapters that highlight the special role and status of voices from an evolutionary, psychological, neuroscientific, and linguistic perspective.

Voice perception, or some basic mechanisms of it, is an ability that seems partly inherited by nature, with more fine-grained perceptual abilities developing during the early periods of a living being. This does not mean that voices cannot be physically heard by infants, which they certainly can, even *in utero*. However, the ability to distinguish that a voice is an auditory object that is different from other kinds of natural and unnatural auditory objects seems partly a developmental achievement. Part II, accordingly, is entitled 'Ontogenetic Development of Voice Perception' and includes chapters on the perceptual and neural mechanisms that develop in infancy for voice perception. It also follows the complementary question of how adults perceive vocalizations in infants based on the assumptions that early voice perception abilities develop in line with the close relationship of infants with caregivers.

Complementary to this ontogenetic perspective, Part III introduces a phylogenetic perceptive on how voice perception abilities might have evolved alongside natural evolution. This part is entitled 'Evolution and Comparative Perspective' and includes chapters on voice perception and voice learning abilities across a variety of species. Voice perception abilities are shared across a broad variety of species and are not unique to a certain species. Human primates share the cognitive and neural mechanisms of voice perception with other primate species, and voice communication seems even possible across species and call types. Based on the notion that voice perception abilities have evolved on a phylogenetic scale, the neural hardwiring of these abilities might have done so accordingly. Some chapters in Part III outline the comparative neural machinery of these abilities.

Part IV deals with the variety of socially important information that is voluntarily and involuntarily contained in the acoustic quality of voices, and is entitled 'Emotional and Motivational Vocal Expression'. This ability to express emotion and motivation in the tone of voice is not only characteristic of humans but is shared with many other species. One might also think that the tone of the voice is one of the best channels for such information to be expressed, given the vast modulatory possibility in how voices and voice quality can be produced, but given also the dramatic impact that such voices can have on listeners, even across spatial distances. This might also be a major reason why vocalizations appeared in the evolutionary lineage as a means of communication with impact and with survival benefits. Part IV thus includes chapters that outline the social function of emotional and motivational vocal expressions and the neural mechanisms of their perception.

The voice cannot only be used to express emotional and motivational information, but also to convey many physical features about the speaker— both simpler features of familiarity, identity, age, and gender, and also socially more complex features, such as personality and attractiveness. Part V is entitled 'Vocal Identity, Personality, and the Social Context' and deals with the cognitive and neural mechanisms of perceiving such information in voices. The wealth of such information that listeners perceive from the acoustic quality of voice is actually enormous, and this part only deals with a selection of voice information for which a broad amount of empirical evidence is available right now.

In modern societies and cultures, voices and vocalization are not only produced and perceived by humans and other animals, but also by a variety of technical systems. Humans interact almost daily with human computer interfaces, and these devices have become very sophisticated in recent years, not only for detecting and recognizing voice signals, but also in terms of autonomously learning and improving their abilities. Part VI is entitled 'Machine-based Generation and Decoding of Voices' and includes chapters on how certain non-verbal voice features can today be generated with technical systems, but more importantly how voices and important voice features can be detected and classified in such technical systems.

The final part of the handbook, Part VII, is entitled 'Clinical Disorders'. Many of the previous parts in this handbook describe how voice recognition abilities evolved on an ontogenetic, phylogenetic, and machine-learning level. However, these abilities can also get lost again in some patients suffering from psychiatric and neurological disorders. Part VII thus includes chapters describing some of these disorders and how voice perception abilities are either impaired or have completely vanished in these patients. Since voice perception abilities can be differentially impaired across many different disorders, these differential pictures contribute to the notion that voice perception abilities are a cognitive function that is dependent on a variety of processing components. The latter can be selectively impaired in specific disorders.

1.5 Additional Information on this Handbook

We would like to finish this introductory chapter to the handbook by mentioning some of its general and novel features. First, although scientific illustrations can, as in all such handbooks, be used to illustrate the features of the voice and vocalizations, there is an inevitable limit to how well they can do this. Thus, this handbook is complemented by a wealth of sound examples, in the form of audio files, that accompany many of the chapters. These can be accessed at http://neuralbasesofcommunication.eu/projects/oxford_handbook_of_voice_perception/. Second, although this handbook is a cohesive scientific piece of work, with each chapter contributing to the overall quality and general compendium of the current state of voice perception research, each individual chapter is also available in digital form from the Oxford University Press website (https://global.oup.com/).

Finally, as editors of this handbook, we hope it will be viewed as a representative book on the topic of voice perception for scholars and students across many disciplines—and prove to be an enjoyable read!

REFERENCES

Andics, A., Gabor, A., Gacsi, M., Farago, T., Szabo, D., & Miklosi, A. (2016). Neural mechanisms for lexical processing in dogs. *Science*, 353(6303), 1030–1032. doi: 10.1126/science.aaf3777

Andics, A., Gácsi, M., Faragó, T., Kis, A., & Miklósi, Á. (2014). Voice-sensitive regions in the dog and human brain are revealed by comparative fMRI. *Current Biology*, 24(5), 574–578. doi: 10.1016/j.cub.2014.01.058

Bass, A. H., Gilland, E. H., & Baker, R. (2008). Evolutionary origins for social vocalization in a vertebrate hindbrain–spinal compartment. *Science*, 321(5887), 417 LP-421. Available at: http://science.sciencemag.org/content/321/5887/417.abstract.

Belin, P. (2006). Voice processing in human and non-human primates. *Philosophical Transactions of the Royal Society of London B Biological Sciences*, 361(1476), 2091–2107. Available at: http://www.ncbi.nlm.nih.gov/entrez/query.fcgi?cmd=Retrieve&db=PubMed&dopt=Citation&list_uids=17118926.

Belin, P., Fecteau, S., & Bedard, C. (2004). Thinking the voice: neural correlates of voice perception. *Trends in Cognitive Sciences*, 8(3), 129–135. doi: 10.1016/j.tics.2004.01.008S1364661304000257 [pii]. Available at: http://linkinghub.elsevier.com/retrieve.

Belin, P., Zatorre, R. J., Lafaille, P., Ahad, P., & Pike, B. (2000). Voice-selective areas in human auditory cortex. *Nature*, 403(6767), 309–312.

Darwin, C. (1899). *The Expression of the Emotions in Man and Animals*. New York: D. Appleton & Co.

Deng, J., Frühholz, S., Zhang, Z., & Schuller, B. (2017). Recognizing emotions from whispered speech based on acoustic feature transfer learning. *IEEE Access*, 5, 5235–5246. doi: 10.1109/ACCESS.2017.2672722

Deng, J., Xu, X., Zhang, Z., Frühholz, S., & Schuller, B. (2016). Exploitation of phase-based features for whispered speech emotion recognition. *IEEE Access*, 4299–4309. doi: 10.1109/ACCESS.2016.2591442

Fitch, W. T. (2000). The evolution of speech: a comparative review. *Trends in Cognitive Sciences*, 258–267. doi: 10.1016/S1364-6613(00)01494-7

Fitch, W. T., de Boer, B., Mathur, N., & Ghazanfar, A. A. (2016). Monkey vocal tracts are speech-ready. *Science Advances*, 2(12). doi: 10.1126/sciadv.1600723

Frühholz, S. & Grandjean, D. (2013). Multiple subregions in superior temporal cortex are differentially sensitive to vocal expressions: a quantitative meta-analysis. *Neuroscience & Biobehavioral Reviews*, 37(1), 24–35. doi: 10.1016/j.neubiorev.2012.11.002

Frühholz, S., Trost, W., & Grandjean, D. (2016). Whispering—the hidden side of auditory communication. *NeuroImage*, 142, 602–612. doi: 10.1016/j.neuroimage.2016.08.023

Frühholz, S., Trost, W., & Kotz, S. A. (2016). The sound of emotions—towards a unifying neural network perspective of affective sound processing. *Neuroscience & Biobehavioral Reviews*, 68, 96–110. doi: 10.1016/j.neubiorev.2016.05.002

Ghazanfar, A. A. & Rendall, D. (2008). Evolution of human vocal production. *Current Biology*, 18(11), R457–460. doi: 10.1016/j.cub.2008.03.030

Hirano, M. (1981). *Clinical Examination of Voice*. Wien: Springer-Verlag.

Kreiman, J. & Sidtis, D. (2011). *Foundations of Voice Studies: An Interdisciplinary Approach to Voice Production and Perception*. Oxford, UK: Wiley-Blackwell.

Latinus, M. & Belin, P. (2011). Human voice perception. *Current Biology*, 21(4), R143–5. doi: 10.1016/j.cub.2010.12.033

Pernet, C. R. & Belin, P. (2012). The role of pitch and timbre in voice gender categorization. *Frontiers in Psychology*, 3(FEB). doi: 10.3389/fpsyg.2012.00023

Petkov, C. I., Kayser, C., Steudel, T., Whittingstall, K., Augath, M., & Logothetis, N. K. (2008). A voice region in the monkey brain. *Nature Neuroscience*, 11(3), 367–374. Available at: http://www.ncbi.nlm.nih.gov/pubmed/18264095.

Schweinberger, S. R. & Burton, A. M. (2011). Person perception 25 years after Bruce and Young (1986): an introduction. *British Journal of Psychology*, 102(4), 695–703695–703. doi: 10.1111/j.2044-8295.2011.02070.x

Sidtis, D. & Kreiman, J. (2012). In the beginning was the familiar voice: personally familiar voices in the evolutionary and contemporary biology of communication. *Integrative Psychological & Behavioral Science*, 46(2), 146–159. doi: 10.1007/s12124-011-9177-4

CHAPTER 2

ANCIENT OF DAYS
The Vocal Pattern as Primordial Big Bang of Communication

DIANA VAN LANCKER SIDTIS

2.1 THE VERY BEGINNING: VOCALIZATION

IT is a charming notion, and roughly true considering geologic time, that the rudiments of familiar voice recognition appeared on the earth at about the same time as flowers— 250 million years ago. This period heralded the advent of amphibians, which have been observed in contemporary studies to recognize the vocal patterns of their conspecifics, and we dare to assume that they have always done so (Bee, 2004; Simmons, 2004). Although vocalizing occurs in time, the various kinds of acoustic material manifest quickly and are densely integrated, yielding a veridical perceptual pattern, which can be mapped and stored to serve various biological functions. As humans, we tend to view our behaviours as special and unique, but, stated simply, 'A frog possesses a capacity for individual voice recognition' (Bee & Gerhardt, 2002, p. 1443), and frog structure and function have remained stable through the millennia, with some species showing direct descent from their earliest appearance (Cannatella, 2007). Vocalization, a social imperative in the lives of frogs and toads, is governed by sensory motor structures centred in the midbrain. Frog neighbour–stranger recognition abilities discriminate very small feature differences in the signal and/or utilize whole patterns (Gasser et al., 2009), as is assumed for mammalian (Ehret & Kurt, 2010) and for human familiar voice recognition (Kreiman & Sidtis, 2011).

Still more impressive are reports that between eight hundred and one thousand types of fish, the most evolutionarily ancient of vertebrates with a 400-million-year history, produce a wide variety of sounds with modulated frequencies, temporal characteristics, and amplitudes (Bass et al., 2015; Chagnaud & Bass, 2014; Roundtree et al., 2002; Than, 2008), performing a variety of survival-related functions, such as courtship, defence of territory, and fright response (Connoughton et al., 2002). The female midshipman fish will mate only with a partner who is humming, leading to up to an hour of constant humming by the male (National Science Foundation/NSF, 2008). In a further home run for animal neuropsychology, the cichlid, a fish popular in home fish tanks and belonging to a large vertebrate family, has been reported to recognize familiar faces (Kohda et al., 2015). Can familiar fish-voice recognition be far behind?

Interest in familiarity recognition in non-human animals, based on voice, has exploded in the past few decades. Studies have documented innate voice recognition abilities in the social rodent (degu or brush-tailed rat) (Fuchs et al., 2010), in deer (Charlton et al., 2007; Torriani et al., 2006), in goats (Terrazas et al., 2003), in dogs (Adachi et al., 2007), in sheep (Sèbe et al., 2010; Searby & Jouventin, 2003), in African elephants (McComb et al., 2002), in Australian sea lions (Pitcher et al., 2010), in wolves (Goldman et al., 1995), in mares (Wolskia et al., 1980), in seals (Aubin et al., 2015; Charrier et al., 2001, 2003; Insley, 2001), and in parrots (Berg et al., 2011). Individual vocal recognition skills of numerous non-human primates have come to light: macaques (Fischer, 2004; Masataka, 1985), rhesus monkeys (Hansen, 1976; Rendall et al., 1996), vervet monkeys (Cheney & Seyfarth, 1980), and baboons (Cheney & Seyfarth, 1999).

Penguins and bats win this year's prize for prodigious vocal recognition skills. The enormity of penguins' vocal prowess has justifiably received much attention, given their successful personal identity recognition in the ambient cacophony generated by tens of thousands of milling parents and offspring, sometimes augmented by whirling snow and wind (Aubin et al., 2000; Jouventin et al., 1999; Searby et al., 2004). Additionally, their use of vocal information has adapted to their reproductive behaviour (Jouventin & Aubin, 2002). Bats, which recognize individual contact calls (Arnold & Wilkinson, 2011; Balcombe, 1990; Boughman & Wilkinson, 1998; Guo et al., 2015) as well as signature echolocation signalling (Voigt-Heucke et al., 2010; Yovel et al., 2009), have raised the ante even higher by exploiting genetically inherited vocal signatures mutually in place—before hearing or vocalizing anything—in mother and offspring (Scherrer & Wilkinson, 1993).

The extensive research on amphibians is of particular interest. Frogs represent the evolutionarily earliest of individual vocal pattern recognizers (Bee & Gerhardt, 2002; Bee et al., 2001; Feng et al., 2009). Anuran (amphibian) researchers state that ' … acoustic communication forms the foundation for their reproductive social behavior' (Wilczynski & Endepols, 2007, p. 242) (see Figure 2.1). Frog vocalizations are individualized and they are dynamic, plastic, and graded in acoustic form (Burke & Murphy, 2007; Gerhardt & Bee, 2007) (Audio 2.1). Amphibian calls may increase in rate and duration, signal-to-noise ratio, frequency, or overall spectral energy in response to social conditions (Wells & Schwartz, 2007). Túngera frogs have been reported to honour the size code for voice, in that females prefer larger larynges and lower frequency calls (Ryan & Guerra, 2014). An intricate interrelationship between anuran sites in the midbrain for vocalization and auditory behaviours often has been described (Narins & Feng, 2007), leading to a proposal of a 'sound communication' system with associations to 'motor, endocrine, motivational, and mnemonic processes linked to social interactions' (Wilczynski & Endepols, 2007, p. 242). For mammalian vocalization, a cortical–subcortical network has been demonstrated, integrated by motivational and emotional impulses from the midbrain periaqueductal grey area (Hage, 2010). A comparable proposal is the polyvagal hypothesis for mammals, whereby coordinated activity in audition and vocalization permit expression and perception of emotional states (Porges & Lewis, 2010).

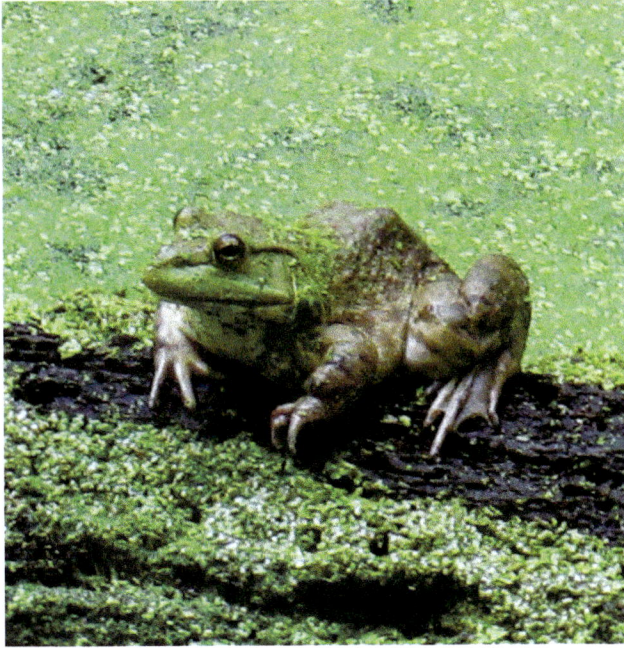

FIGURE 2.1 Frog, Ramapo State Park, Ramapo, New Jersey.

Photo courtesy of John J. Sidtis.

Bass (2014), a distinguished fish scientist, proposed a central pattern generator for fishes and their descendants, sharing an integrated vocal-motor physiological system for processing socially orientated signals. A similar picture is drawn for mammals by Brudzynski (2010), using the term 'ethotransmitter' to designate vocalization as ubiquitous and widespread, comprising 'highly complex coordination and integration of numerous subsystems, including the CNS, autonomic and endocrine systems, and peripheral organs' (p. 3). The encoded calls are both referential and semiotic, providing an 'immensely rich combination of features for encoding signals' (p. 3). These and other animal studies describe properties of the vocal signal that suggest a primordially early complexity in form and function. Brudzynski (2010) proposes a common origin for vocalization processes across biological species, citing the 'homology in transmitters, brain structures and neural regulation' present in animals and humans (p. 5).

The very early presence of sophisticated vocal prowess is now known to occur in humans. The elemental status of voice recognition as biological lifeblood has been underscored by the flood of evidence in the past 40 years for very early competence in humans. Studies have demonstrated recognition of the maternal voice by young infants at 3–4 months (Belin & Grosbras, 2010; Mehler et al., 1978; Purhonen et al., 2004). Using a variety of experimental procedures, beginning with the classic study by DeCasper and Fifer (1980), this ability is now known to be present in newborns (Hepper et al., 1993; Querleu et al., 1984) and in the fetus (Kisilevsky at al., 2003; Voegtline et al., 2013), suggesting an innate propensity to imprint on the unique maternal voice.

2.2 A MORE RECENT BEGINNING: LANGUAGE

Human language is a latecomer in evolutionary history. The exact debut of words, estimated to be between 200,000 and 2 million years ago, is less well established than is the appearance of fish and frog vocalization. Language provides a communication vehicle of sophistication and complexity, but the voice is primordial. Language is a cortically based, structured, abstract system; voice is visceral, arising from 'lower' brain structures, and its rich information packet does not readily tolerate decomposition. The potentially infinite set of ideas that can be transmitted in language has been acknowledged, celebrated, and modelled, but the dense constellation of meaning carried in the voice remains a shy partner in verbal behaviour. Structural properties described for language consist of discretely arranged levels, units, and rules; these may evoke dispute in some of their detail (e.g. Port, 2007; Port & Leary, 2005) but the descriptive model is generally accepted throughout the linguistic sciences. Consider, in stark contrast, the vocal pattern. Its communicative means is not discrete, but graded; multiple signals can occur as faster or lower, louder or softer, higher or lower in pitch along a sliding scale. Efforts to create a descriptive apparatus for individual voice quality patterns have not enjoyed wide application (Laver, 1968). Yet since the beginning, vocal elements have remained the same: fundamental frequency, amplitude, temporal cues, and voice quality, woven into complex patterns by frogs (Chagnaud & Bass, 2014), mammals (Ehret & Kurt, 2010), penguins (Lengagne et al., 2001), and primates (Cheney & Seyfarth, 1999), all variants of vocalizing behaviour in biology.

Although it is acknowledged that the human voice transmits linguistic, semantic, syntactic, emotional, attitudinal, psychiatric, and personal information, any attempted beachhead onto an island of description of this overall capability erodes quite quickly. This is due to the non-transparency inherent in the voice as pattern. Especially in humans, and also in many other species, the repertory of attitudes, moods, and emotions, along with gender, age, and geographical background detectable in the vocal signal is considerable, and the potential auditory-acoustic characteristics cueing these pieces of information, occurring in every combination, proliferate immensely. The vocal signal has been aptly characterized as multilayered and polyphonic (Hermans, 1998; Stiles, 1999), with the qualification that layers and levels are not actually organized or arranged in any veridical sense; instead, the constellation of information is integrated or interwoven into and within the vocal pattern (see Figure 2.2).

The consequences of this condition, whereby the vocal pattern is intricately amalgamated, are noteworthy in a number of ways. Science works best through deconstructing and analysing constituent parts. Serious studies of patterns have been limited and they have dealt with vision (Corcoran, 1971; Poljac et al., 2012; Pomerantz, 1986; Pomerantz et al., 1977; Reed, 1972). While the vocal pattern can be broken down into numerous detailed measures of fundamental frequency, timing cues, amplitude, and voice quality, these parameters each have many configurations and facets, and their subparts combine factorially to constitute an actual vocal pattern (Skuk & Schweinberger, 2014). The information transmitted in the signal, much of it present in the earliest appearances of vocalization, is similarly extensive. Determining how the array of auditory acoustic cues, singly and in combination, succeed in communicating such opulent but disparate detail about the

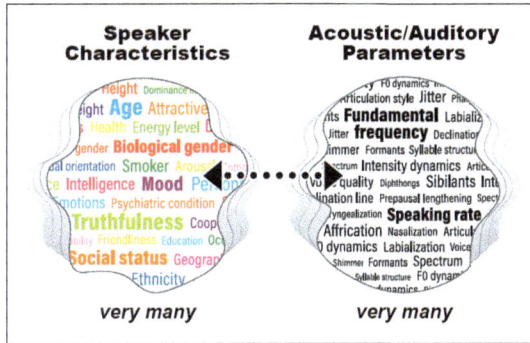

FIGURE 2.2 Schemata depicting the two domains—speaker characteristics and auditory-acoustic parameters.

speaker has proven extremely challenging. Partly because of the longstanding hegemony of the visual modality (as in 'primates are fundamentally visual creatures'; Gould, 2003, p. 136) (see also LeGros Clark, 1959), and partly due to the ephemeral nature of time bound auditory-acoustic material, appreciation of the complexity and sophistication of vocal functionality has emerged only recently.

Properties and functionalities variously described for vocalization evolving in other species remain present in the human vocal signalling system. Social signals, such as aggression and courtship, and personal identity, are the obvious candidates. Signals identifiable as 'emotion' reach a great distance into the biological background, at least to mammals. This very large functionality of vocalization, rudimentarily present from the time of the first larynx and highly elaborated in humans, signals formal linguistic contrasts, the pragmatics of speakers' meanings as revealed in emphasis and theme, emotion, mood, attitude, and personality and psychiatric variables. Every human utterance has the potential of conveying all of this meaning substance, using multifarious, many-to-many mappings of the acoustic-auditory parameters as previously described (see Figure 2.2). Some strands of this rich fabric were present already in the primordial appearance of vocal communication.

The nuances of emotional and attitudinal meanings carried in the human vocal signal border on astronomical in quantity, although for emotion, only happy, angry, surprised, and sad, usually as produced by actors, have been studied (for exceptions see Scherer, 1986). Since the early theories about the physical basis of emotion (James, 1884), some approaches link emotional intonations to physical states (Juslin & Laukka, 2001; Pollermann, 2010). Emotional signals are famously graded (Laukka et al., 2012), similar to signalling systems in non-human animals, and unlike linguistic uses of vocal contrasts, which form discrete units. Attitudes, such as cooperativeness, impatience, willingness, tentativeness—nuances that may be critical in domestic, work, or political contexts—have been studied only a little (Bolinger, 1964a; for review, see Kreiman & Sidtis, 2011). Attitudinal–emotional content pervades verbal expression (Bargh et al., 1992; Geiselman, 1977; Palmeri et al., 1993; Panksepp, 2003; Zajonc, 1980, 1968). How much of this nuance is present in non-human animals remains to be understood. Emotional vocalizations of rats are said to include expressions of pain, separation distress, social joy-play, and laughter (Panksepp, 2010), while those of a non-human primate species convey positive and negative emotions (Zimmerman, 2010). Do non-human animals express anxiety? Contentment? Sarcasm? It is not impossible.

In human speech, sarcasm, distinguishing the insulting 'THAT was a good lecture,' spoken on high, then falling intonation and usually accompanied by distinctive voice quality, from the complimentary, opposite-meaning 'That was a GOOD lecture' is easily identifiable by a native (or non-native) speaker of the language (Audio 2.2). It is a small step from sarcasm to mental states; a few isolated studies of the anxious voice (Laukka et al., 2008) and of the psychopath (Louth et al., 1998) describe vocal signals in association with psychiatric conditions. Mood studies have been essentially limited to depression (Alpert et al., 2001) and non-human animals have been seldom studied. How does the voice reveal attributes of personality, such as confidence, competence, friendliness? Many studies of the vocal cues for personality characteristics have been performed (Revelle & Scherer, 2009), with the results that specifiable features of voice, especially fundamental frequency and rate, produce reliable ratings by listeners. Seldom, or only inconsistently, however, do the ratings match apparent personality parameters in the speakers (Kreiman & Sidtis, 2011, pp. 342–348), indicating the assumption of vocal stereotypes in a given community. In humans, this rich resource—communication via voice—has been elaborated beyond scientists' current abilities to describe it.

2.2.1 Linguistic Uses of Vocal Material

Since the advent of human language as an overlay on the vocal signal, voice, or the prosodic content of a verbal utterance, has contributed importantly to linguistic meanings. The voice is used to signal lexical linguistic contrasts, as in Thai, Chinese, and many African languages (tones) and the word accent contrasts of Swedish and English (Audio 2.3). Grammatical structures, such as those distinguishing statement from question, as well as phrasal types and boundaries, are delineated by vocal cues in many languages. Literal versus idiomatic meanings in ditropic sentences—those with this special kind of ambiguity—are cued by voice alone, as in 'He is at the end of his rope' with a literal meaning versus the figurative one (i.e. having exhausted all escape options) (Van Lancker Sidtis, 2003). The idiomatic–literal contrast cued by voice appears robustly in at least three languages studied—Korean, French, and American English—and each language exploits different auditory-acoustic parameters to cue the contrasts (Abdelli-Beruh et al., 2007; Yang et al., 2015) (Audio 2.4). Speakers' meaning in accent languages is conveyed through sentence focus. For example, 'I gave John the BOOK' contrasts with 'I gave JOHN the book' (Rooth, 1992; Selkirk, 1995; Swerts & Geluykens, 1994) (Audio 2.5). Wearing the cloak of human language, vocalization has assumed a very large burden of communication responsibility, providing linguistic contrasts corresponding to an abstract language system and using discrete categories to reflect speakers' meanings, as well as graded vocal signals. To quote Bolinger (1964b), whose insights about voice in speech spanned several decades, 'An accent language employing relative heights may distinguish old from new or topic from comment, with intonation getting a foothold in the syntax. But the foothold is with one foot; the other one is back there doing its primitive dance' (p. 843). The 'primitive dance' uses graded vocal material to cue emotional/attitudinal/social information arising from physical and personal conditions, and provides signature vocal patterns representing personal identity.

2.3 Brain Processing of the Voice

As suggested by the vocal behaviours of amphibians, vocalization is evolutionarily very old, reaching back as a vehicle of survival among the most rudimentary and primitive of behaviours, utilizing early evolving brain and physical structures, making the most of all manner of functionality including, for example, attracting, repelling, releasing energy, expressing, playing, and enabling individual identity display and recognition. These competences have been accomplished down through the millennia by laryngeal structures, specializing, it is often said, in breathing and airway protection (e.g. Hoh, 2010). In this regard, it is noteworthy that frogs employ the larynx for only a third of their breathing needs, and the process for expelling air for vocalization differs from the respiratory process. The larynx has always been very well fitted to intone, as if, from the beginning, it was anticipated also to produce sound. The human newborn's first lungful of breath is expelled with a cry. The less elaborated brains of fish (employing air bladders) and anurans (utilizing the larynx) sufficed to underwrite a well-elaborated set of behaviours involving voice production and reception of socially orientated calls. It is commonly held, in the spirit of the triune brain (MacLean, 1990), that the vocal expression of emotion originated with the arrival on earth of mammals (e.g. Newman, 2010). However, one might venture to wonder whether 'emotion' of some sort inheres in the advertisement calls of the male frog, whose purpose is to attract the female; or even, going further out on the underwater limb, in the hour-long hums of the midshipman fish. These remarks reflect contemporary intellectual currents in the science of biology that choose to reinterpret the previously strict behaviourist description of animal behaviour, while avoiding the pitfalls of overenthusiastic anthropomorphizing (Hardman, 2014; Panksepp, 1998).

2.3.1 Neural Plasticity

Another change in biologists' perspective can be seen in the view of brain structures responsible for vocal behaviour, departing from previous views of a small set of fixed, hardwired systems. Evidence from frog chorus studies indicates that neural structures in the midbrain, as well as behavioural responses, are shaped by experience in as little as 10 days (Gall & Wilczynski, 2014). Studies reveal dramatic dynamic auditory plasticity in the adult human brainstem (Krishnan et al., 2005). The auditory-acoustic elements are controlled by the central nervous system of the frog, for example, through striatal and limbic audio-vocal integration, and 'social context, learning, and the inner state of the animal (e.g. motivation) can modify the frog's calling' (Walkowiak, 2007, p. 87) in the reception of signals in the auditory midbrain. Male aggressive and advertisement calls, which in some species are graded, show modifications in intensity and duration. Call structures increase in rate, signal-to-noise ratio, frequency, and distribution of spectral energy in association with social conditions, such as the presence of females. Further, timing patterns between males are regulated and shaped (Wells & Schwartz, 2007). The basic foundation of larynx and vocalization has held a conservative line throughout evolution, notwithstanding the overlay of the upstart colossus, human language, which may or may not represent vocalization's material outgrowth— a debate that we need not address here.

2.3.2 Vocalization and Perception

Further, as referred to earlier, the elements of vocalization and the contingencies of audition have formed two sides of a coin from the beginning. Vocalizing and hearing necessarily hinge on each other and they participate in mutually adapting processes. Audio and motor functions converge in the midbrain of the frog (Wilczynski & Endepols, 2007). Coordinated changes in structures for hearing and vocalization have been described for mammals (Porges & Lewis, 2010). The integrative status of audition and vocal production, monitored by temporal lobe structures and stations along the auditory pathway, is seen in humans in adventitious (adult-acquired) hearing impairment, where deleterious changes in the voice occur progressively with ongoing diminished auditory feedback (Leder & Spitzer, 1990).

Early evidence points to elementary and original sensory motor integration for vocalization and its perception, with mutual influences in development and capacity for malleably responding to internal and external environmental contingencies. Given the ancient and conservative nature of vocalization and its perception in evolutionary history, it arguably follows that broadly integrated cerebral levels and systems underlie the ability.

2.4 BRAIN STRUCTURES UNDERLYING VOCALIZATION: UNFAMILIAR AND FAMILIAR VOICES

Here the story requires a few words about the notion of 'familiarity'. Most renditions of this concept attach familiarity as a value to environmental objects, assuming that a face or movie star or a set of keys becomes familiar on an incremental learning curve. Another perspective, one ascribing familiarity to neuropsychology as an independent attribute, arises from observations in neurological disturbance (Van Lancker, 1991). In agnosias, an object or a face or a geographical surrounding can be perceptually described in detail, but the 'feeling' of familiarity is missing. Proposagnosia, familiar face recognition deficit, is a well-known example, and has been associated with right hemisphere specialization (Cutting, 1990; De Renzi, 1986; Gainotti, 2011; Myers, 1998; Neuner & Schweinberger, 2000; Van Lancker, 1997). Alongside vocalization, the familiarity sense is another ancient, well-entrenched attribute, although little studied in its own right. For faces, for example, no upper limit has been found for probes of personally familiar material when recognition is the task (for studies using known faces see Bruck et al., 1991; Bahrick et al., 1975). A condition known as Capgras syndrome, whereby following a right hemisphere stroke, an impaired husband insists adamantly that the woman living in his house, although she looks and acts like his wife and knows all the children, is not his wife, illustrates this notion in a dramatic way (Bourget & Whitehurst, 2004; Ellis & Lewis, 2001; Young et al., 1993).

Some cases ascribed to delusion may well be manifestations of an impairment of the familiarity sense (Silva et al., 1993). Such familiarity agnosias are often associated with damage to the right hemisphere (Cutting, 1990) which, in humans, may specialize in establishing personally relevant phenomena (Van Lancker, 1991); conversely, the disconnected right hemisphere was observed to respond strongly, although non-verbally, to personally relevant material (Sidtis et al., 1981; Sperry et al., 1979). The familiarity trait can inhere in famous or intimately familiar faces and voices, surroundings, landmarks, and handwriting (Heckmann et al., 2001; Herzmann et al., 2004; Landis et al., 1986; Van Lancker & Nicklay, 1992). Our sojourn through the biological emergence and evolution of voice suggests that the familiarity instinct, in an elementary version, was present at the prehistoric beginning. The earlier assertion that 'In the beginning was the familiar voice' (Sidtis & Kreiman, 2011) calls for modification: in the beginning was familiarity, and a favoured vehicle was the voice.

2.4.1 Familiarity has Special Status

There is considerable evidence that familiar and unfamiliar phenomena, manifest most obviously in voices and faces, constitute fundamentally different neuropsychological capacities (Herzmann et al., 2004; Malone et al., 1982; Schweinberger, 2001; Van Lancker & Kreiman, 1987; Van Lancker et al., 1988). While unfamiliar voices potentially carry beneficial social and general personal information (e.g. status, gender, age, size, mood), they may not be given particular attention. It is trivially true that a familiar voice will engage greater arousal and attention systems, and will be imbued with more emotion and cognitive associations, than an unfamiliar voice. An auditory analogue to change blindness was observed from a study using telephone conversation, covertly switching speakers part way through the conversation. The change was not always perceived by the listener (Fenn et al., 2011). Any voice, whether attended to or not, and familiar or not, can and will communicate the array of material reviewed in this chapter. While all voices carry information, the crucial role of the familiar voice in biology—establishing and verifying friend, family, and foe, attracting a mate, repelling the enemy, and distinguishing safety from danger—can hardly be exaggerated.

2.5 WHOLE BRAIN INVOLVEMENT IN VOCAL PRODUCTION AND PERCEPTION

As discussed, a rich palette of vocalization functions, managed by subcortical brain regions, has propagated throughout biological species. In humans, this acquired functionality has been furnished with the vast armamentarium of language and verbal expression. To harness and integrate these prodigious capacities, it is not surprising that, plainly said, it takes a whole brain (Figure 2.3). A whole brain involvement in vocal production and perception holds especially for familiar voices (the most compelling of vocal competence), which pack an assemblage of ingredients for the listener encompassing nuance, history, valence, episodic memory, and knowledge of many kinds. A brief moment of introspection reveals the aura of associations clustered around the mental representation of any personally familiar voice. These are inevitably associated with a broad range of cerebral function. Hearing and producing voice, processes that are believed to be codependent, engage both

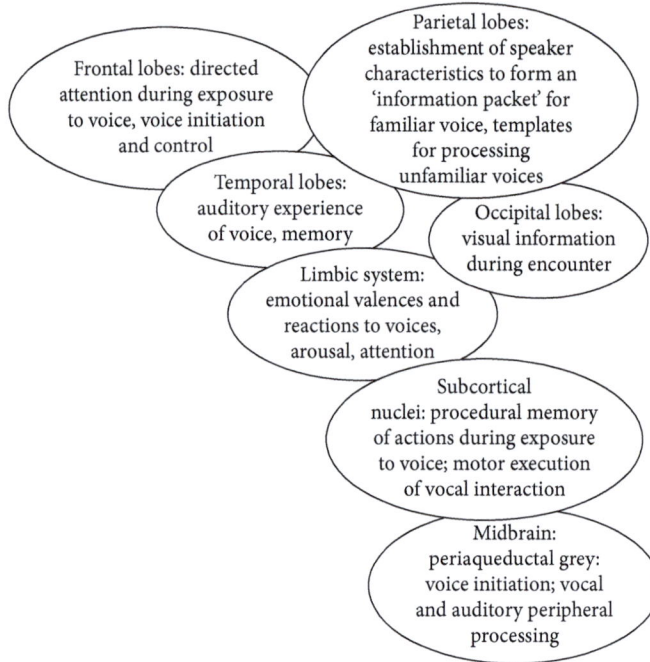

FIGURE 2.3 Schema of brain systems involved in speech production and perception.

cerebral hemispheres, in particular the temporal lobes, site of auditory reception and monitoring of feedback, as well as the parietal lobes, where cross sensory and ideational associations are conducted. The posterior parietal cortex, often neglected in the current approach to structure–function correlations, has been shown from converging studies to allow for cross-modal, multisensory associations of memory (Andersen, 1997; Dobbins et al., 2012; Fair, 1988, 1992; Haramati et al., 2008; Hyvärinen, 1982a,b). Significant connections from the laryngeal motor cortex to parietal cortex have been identified (Simonyan & Horwitz, 2011). In a study using PET functional imaging, merely maintaining stability on the vowel /a/ revealed bilateral, combined increased and decreased blood flow measures, involving sensory, motor, and temporal lobe cortex, caudate and putamen in the basal ganglia, and thalamus (Sidtis, 2015).

There are continuous connections of the frontal lobes, where vocal patterns are organized for production, with nuclei of the basal ganglia (Masterman & Cummings, 1997), sources of motor programmes as well as motivational and emotional contingencies. The basal ganglia sites for vocalization in primates have been known since the early work of Jürgens and his colleagues (1967) and elaborated by later studies (Jürgens, 2002; Simonyan & Jürgens, 2003). Pitch contrasts, the most potent of vocal cues, are produced and processed in numerous sites, including basal ganglia (Sidtis & Van Lancker Sidtis, 2003) and right temporal lobe (Hyde et al., 2008; Sidtis, 1980; Zatorre & Belin, 2001). The limbic system motivates, supplies, and discerns emotional and attitudinal content in the voice (Robinson, 1976; Van Lancker & Cummings, 1999; Vuilleumier, 2005); specific functionality has been identified for the amygdala in processing emotional information in the voice in humans (Frühholz & Grandjean, 2013; Frühholz et al., 2015) and monkeys (Kuraoka & Nakamura, 2010).

A widespread cortico–subcortical network, including auditory cortices, basal ganglia, and frontal regions, was identified underlying human expression of anger (Klaas et al., 2015). Familiarity judgements rely on cortical as well as subcortical nuclei. Depth electrodes implanted in the amygdala, hippocampus, and temporal lobes revealed differential responses to familiar as contrasted to novel faces (Seeck et al., 1993). The cerebellum, key motor area of the brain, manages and configures vocal gestures (Duffy, 2013, pp. 45–7).

The thalamus relays information for sensory and motor impulses to the other vocalizing structures. Vocalization is facilitated and modulated by the periaqueductal grey matter in the midbrain, responsible for respiratory control underlying vocalization (Subramanian et al., 2008), and peripheral structures for vocal and auditory processing emerge from this region. The midbrain periaqueductal grey matter is a particularly ubiquitous structure in the biology of vocalization from the time of fish (Bass, 2014), developing with integrated circuits in limbic and basal ganglia nuclei (Gruber-Dujardin, 2010; Siegel et al., 2010). Its coordinating relationship to breathing further highlights the integrated nature of vocalization: 'it is possible that the periaqueductal grey matter represents an absolutely critical region for the coordination of breathing during involuntary (emotional) and voluntary vocalization' (Davis & Zhang, 1991, p. 65). Damage to this structure in the midbrain in humans has resulted in mutism (Esposito et al., 1999).

2.5.1 Clinical Evidence

Much of our earlier understanding of the brain model underlying voice has come from observing neurological disorders. Some of these findings have been corroborated by evidence from functional imaging methods. Damage to many of the structures outlined here results in abnormal vocalization or voice perception and recognition. Parietal or temporal lobe damage on the right cerebral hemisphere interfered with familiar voice recognition (Assal et al., 1981; Schweinberger, 2001; Sidtis & Kreiman, 2008; Van Lancker & Canter, 1982; Van Lancker et al., 1989) and autobiographical memory (Cimino et al., 1991) in stroke subjects. Functional imaging has identified right-sided cerebral sites for a final common pathway of cortical perception of the human voice (Belin et al., 2000; von Kriegstein & Giraud, 2004).

Cerebellar damage results in a jerky, arrhythmic vocal signal known as scanning or ataxic speech (Duffy, 2013; Sidtis et al., 2011). Basal ganglia dysfunction, as in the well-studied disorder, Parkinson's disease, leads to low volume, distortions of vowel quality (Skodda et al., 2012), monotonic intonation or dysprosody (Skodda et al., 2009), and rate disturbances in speech (Breitenstein et al., 2001; Critchley, 1981; Duffy, 2013; Rusz et al., 2013), all affecting the voice pattern's ability to signal personal identity and other vocally transmitted information (Jaywant & Pell, 2009; Pell & Leonard, 2003). In persons with Parkinson's disease treated with deep brain stimulation (DBS), whereby electrodes are implanted in the subthalamic nucleus of the basal ganglia to reduce tremor, vowel spaces are constricted during the stimulated state compared to healthy speakers, implying a role of the basal ganglia in configuring vowel formants (important cues to vocal identity) in the vocal signal (Sidtis et al., 2016). Lesion and functional imaging studies suggest that frontal lobe damage affects timing features in vocal production, which serve in part to characterize speaker identity, as well as to communicate attitudinal, linguistic, and emotional information (Van Lancker Sidtis et al., 2010).

As indicated by neurological disease, timing in the vocal signal is also impacted by cerebellar and basal ganglia damage. Damage to the brainstem (medulla, pons, and midbrain), site of the periaqueductal grey matter and the emergence of the cranial nerves, affects peripheral processes of audition and vocal production.

2.6 THE VOCAL PATTERN: A SYNOPSIS

These perspectives highlight the challenges in studying the voice. Given its status as a quintessential pattern, deconstruction of a vocal signal into separable components provokes an essential misrepresentation of the stimulus. When studying familiar voices, we are confronted with the fact that each vocal pattern is unique, represented by an exclusive combination of auditory-acoustic elements, which will differ for each personal voice signature. Of the many vocal cues available in a descriptive system, only a few meaningfully characterize a given vocal pattern. Studies using famous voices revealed that different kinds of acoustic alteration, such as changes in rate or backwards presentation, differentially affected listeners' abilities to recognize a voice (Van Lancker et al., 1985). For example, breathy voice, extended syllables, and slow rate may serve to specify one voice; crisp articulation, broad Fo range, and lengthy vowel diphthongization may epitomize another. These observations lead to the notion that there is no additive set of auditory-acoustic characteristics that consistently exist in descending importance as cues to an individual voice pattern.

As for our cerebral studies, the evolutionary depth and breath of vocal behaviours, as well as the assumed broad social and personal functionality at the earliest time, reveal that older as well as later evolving neurological structures contribute importantly to voice production and perception. It is hardly an exaggeration to claim that the whole brain participates in the production and hearing of a vocal signal. Pattern is its essential structural condition. There is a compelling ubiquity of significant auditory-vocal functionality across ontogeny and phylogeny. Human mothers' voices are recognized *in utero*; bat vocal signatures may be genetic; frog vocalizations—possibly the earliest—are themselves sophisticated, giving evidence of being dynamic, malleable, and graded. Midbrain structures, the home of the earliest vocal behaviours, reveal physiological plasticity in response to their own changing sensory-motor behaviours. Key features of vocal expression are its capacity to be graded (louder and longer means more), personally familiar, emotional, socially contextualized, and to express internal states and to instantiate states in others (Kuraoka & Nakamura, 2010; Rendall & Owren, 2010).

Dynamic development of vocal-auditory functionality to accommodate conditions can be seen in frogs, mammals, and primates. For humans, there is compelling literature describing the voice as instantiation of self or personal consciousness (Bertau, 2008; Hermans, 1996; Konopcznski, 2010). The physical signal serves as representative of the being itself, and beings, particularly humans, can be incredibly complex. So are their physical vocal signals. When we identify different dialects or clues to gender, we have merely scratched the surface of a copiously resourceful medium. The voice as preternatural representative of the living being may always have been operative, in one inscrutable way or another, from the time of the frogs to the present manifestation in human life. The voice is the direct ancestor of all vocalized and spoken communication. The evolutionary view reveals the true nature of vocalization—an ancient Ur-faculty of immense variety, astonishing persistence, creative versatility, and high value to biological survival.

ACKNOWLEDGEMENTS

I am grateful to John J. Sidtis for ongoing thoughtful commentary on previous drafts, and to Mona Lindau, Peter Narins, and Binna Lee for reading earlier versions of this paper. Michele Burgevin assisted with editing and graphics. Seung yun Yang, Christina Reuterskiöld, Nassima Abdelli-Baruh, and Silke Mohr generously provided audio samples.

REFERENCES

Abdelli-Beruhs, N., Yang, S., Ahn, J., & Van Lancker Sidtis, D. (2007). *Acoustic cues differentiating idiomatic from literal expressions across languages*. Poster presentation at the Annual Convention of the American Speech-Language-Hearing Association, November, Boston, MA.

Adachi, I., Kuwahata, H., & Fujita, K. (2007). Dogs recall their owner's face upon hearing the owner's voice. *Animal Cognition*, 10, 17–21.

Alpert, M., Pougit, E. T., & Silva, R. R. (2001). Reflections of depression in acoustic measures of the patient's speech. *Journal of Affective Disorders*, 66, 59–69.

Andersen, R. A. (1997). Multimodal integration for the representation of space in the posterior parietal cortex. *Philosophical Transactions of the Royal Society B: Biological Sciences*, 352, 1421–1428.

Arnold, B. D. & Wilkinson, G. S. (2011). Individual specific contact calls of pallid bats (Antrozous pallidus) attract conspecifics at roosting sites. *Behavioral Ecology and Sociobiology*, 65(8), 1581–1593.

Assal, G., Aubert, C., & Buttet, J. (1981). Asymétrie cérébrale et reconnaissance de la voix. *Revue Neurologique* (Paris), 137, 255–268.

Aubin, T., Jouventin, P., & Charrier, I. (2015). Mother vocal recognition in Antarctic fur seal Arctocephalus gazella pups: a two-step process. *PLoS One*. September 2, 2015. doi: 10.1371/journal.pone.0134513

Aubin, T., Jouventin, P., & Hildebrand, C. (2000). Penguins use the two-voice system to recognize each other. *Proceedings of the Royal Society B: Biological Sciences*, 267, 1081–1087.

Bahrick, H., Bahrick, P., & Wittlinger, R. (1975). Fifty years of memory for names and faces: a cross-sectional approach. *Journal of Experimental Psychology: General*, 104, 54–75.

Balcombe, J. P. (1990). Vocal recognition of pups by mother Mexican free-tailed bats, *Tadarida brasiliensis Mexicana. Animal Behaviour*, 39(5), 960–966.

Bargh, J. A., Chaiken, S., Govender, R., & Pratto, F. (1992). The generality of the automatic attitude activation effect. *Journal of Personality and Social Psychology*, 62, 893–912.

Bass, A. H. (2014). Central pattern generator for vocalization: is there a vertebrate morphotype? *Current Opinion in Neurobiology*, 28, 94–100.

Bass, A. H., Chagnaud, B. P., & Feng, N.Y. (2015). Comparative neurobiology of sound production in fishes. In: *Sound Communication in Fishes. Animal Signals and Communication* (vol. 4, pp. 35–75). Vienna: Springer-Verlag. doi: 10.1009/978-3-7091-1846-7

Bee, M. A. (2004). Within-individual variation in bullfrog vocalizations: implications for a vocally mediated social recognition system. *Journal of the Acoustical Society of America*, 116(6), 3770–3781.

Bee, M. A. & Gerhardt, H. C. (2002). Individual voice recognition in a territorial frog (*Rana catesbeiana*). *Proceedings of the Royal Society B: Biological Sciences*, 269, 1443–1448.

Bee, M. A., Kozich, C. E., Blackwell, K. J., & Gerhardt, H. C. (2001). Individual variation in advertisement calls of territorial male green frogs, *Rana clamitans*: implications for individual discrimination. *Ethology*, 107, 65–84.

Belin, P. & Grosbras, M. H. (2010). Before speech: cerebral voice processing in infants. *Neuron*, 65, 733–735.

Belin, P., Zatorre, R. J., Lafaille, P., Ahad, P., & Pike, B. (2000). Voice-selective areas in human auditory cortex. *Nature*, 403, 309–312.

Berg, K. S., Delgado, S., Okawa, R., Beissinger, S. R., & Bradbury, J. W. (2011). Contact calls are used for individual mate recognition in free-ranging green-rumped parrotlets, *Forpus passerines*. *Animal Behaviour*, 81, 241–248.

Bertau, M.-C. (2008). Voice, a pathway to consciousness as 'social contact to oneself'. *Integrative Psychological and Behavioral Science*, 42, 92–113.

Bolinger, D. L. (1964a). Around the edge of language: intonation. *Harvard Educational Review*, 34, 282–296. Reprinted in: D. Bolinger (ed.) *Intonation: Selected Readings* (pp. 19–29). Harmondsworth: Penguin Books.

Bolinger, D. L. (1964b). Intonation as a universal. In: Horace G. Lunt (ed.) *Proceedings of the Ninth International Congress of Linguists* (Cambridge, Mass., 1962) (pp. 833–848). The Hague: Mouton.

Boughman, J. W. & Wilkinson, G. E. (1998). Greater spear-nosed bats discriminate group mates by vocalizations. *Animal Behaviour*, 55(6), 1717–1732.

Bourget, D. & Whitehurst, L. (2004). Capgras syndrome: a review of the neurophysiological correlates and presenting clinical features in cases involving physical violence. *Canadian Journal of Psychiatry*, 49, 719–725.

Breitenstein, C., Van Lancker, D., Daum, I., & Waters, C. (2001). Impaired perception of vocal emotions in Parkinson's disease: influence of speech time processing and executive functioning. *Brain and Cognition*, 45, 277–314. PMID: 11237372.

Bruck, M., Cavanagh, P., & Ceci, S. J. (1991). Fortysomething: recognizing faces at one's 25th reunion. *Memory and Cognition*, 19(3), 221–228.

Brudzynski, S. M. (2010). Vocalization as an ethotransmitter: introduction to the handbook of mammalian vocalization. In: S. M. Brudzynski (ed.) *Handbook of Mammalian Vocalization* (pp. 3–9). London: Elsevier.

Burke, E. J. & Murphy, C. G. (2007). How female barking tree frogs, *Hyla gratiosa*, use multiple call characteristics to select a mate. *Animal Behaviour*, 74, 1463–1472.

Cannatella, D. C. (2007). An integrative phylogeny of Amphibia. In: P. M. Narins, A. L. Feng, R. R. Fay, & A. N. Popper (eds) *Hearing and Sound Communication in Amphibians* (pp. 12–43). New York: Springer.

Chagnaud, P. B. & Bass, A. H. (2014). Vocal behavior and vocal central pattern generator organization diverge among toadfishes. *Brain, Behavior and Evolution*, 84, 51–95.

Charlton, B. D., Reby, D., & McComb, K. (2007). Female perception of size-related formant shifts in red deer, *Cervus elaphus*. *Animal Behaviour*, 74, 707–714.

Charrier, I., Mathevon, N., & Jouventin, P. (2001). Mother's voice recognition by seal pups. *Nature*, 412, 873.

Charrier, I., Mathevon, N., & Jouventin, P. (2003). Individuality in the voice of fur seal females: an analysis study of the pup attraction call in *Arctocephalus tropicalis*. *Marine Mammal Science*, 19, 161–172.

Cheney, D. L. & Seyfarth, R. (1980). Vocal recognition in free-ranging vervet monkeys. *Animal Behaviour*, 28, 362–367.

Cheney, D. L. & Seyfarth, R. M. (1999). Recognition of other individuals' social relationships by female baboons. *Animal Behaviour*, 58, 67–75.

Cimino, C. R., Verfaellie, M., Bowers, D., & Heilman, K. M. (1991). Autobiographical memory: influence of right hemisphere damage on emotionality and specificity. *Brain and Cognition*, 15, 106–118.

Connaughton, M. A., Lunn, M. L., Fine, M. L., & Tayor, M. H. (2002). Characteristics of sounds and their use in two sclaenid species: weakfish and Atlantic croaker. Listening to fish: passive acoustic applications in marine fisheries. Conference Proceedings, 8–10 April. Cambridge: MIT.

Corcoran, D. W. J. (1971). *Pattern Recognition*. Middlesex, England: Penguin Books.

Critchley, E. M. (1981). Speech disorders of Parkinsonism: a review. *Journal of Neurology, Neurosurgery & Psychiatry*, 44(9), 751–758.

Cutting, J. (1990). *The Right Cerebral Hemisphere and Psychiatric Disorders*. Oxford: Oxford University Press.

Davis, P. J. & Zhang, S. P. (1991). What is the role of midbrain periaqueductal grey in respiration and vocalization? In: A. Depaulis & R. Bandler (eds) *The Midbrain Periaqueductal Gray Matter* (pp. 57–67). New York: Plenum Press.

De Casper, A. J. & Fifer, W. P. (1980). Of human bonding: newborns prefer their mothers' voices. *Science*, 208, 1174–1176.

De Renzi, E. (1986). Prosopagnosia in two patients with CT scan evidence of damage confined to the right hemisphere. *Neuropsychologia*, 24, 385–389.

Dobbins, I. G., Jaeger, A., Studet, B., & Simons, J. S. (2012). Use of explicit memory cues following parietal lobe lesions. *Neuropsychologia*, 50, 2992–3003.

Duffy, J. R. (2013). *Motor Speech Disorders: Substrates, Differential Diagnosis, and Management*. Elsevier Health Sciences.

Ehret, G. & Kurt, S. (2010). Selective perception and recognition of vocal signals. In: S. M. Brudzynski (ed.) *Handbook of Mammalian Vocalization* (pp. 125–134). London: Elsevier.

Ellis, H. D. & Lewis, M. B. (2001). Capgras delusion: a window on face recognition. *Trends in Cognitive Sciences*, 5(4), 149–156.

Esposito, A., Demeurisse, G., Alberti, B., & Fabbro, F. (1999). Complete mutism after midbrain periaqueductal gray lesion. *NeuroReport*, 10, 681–685.

Fair, C. M. (1988). *Memory and Central Nervous System Organization*. New York: Paragon House.

Fair, C. M. (1992). *Cortical Memory Functions*. Boston: Birkhäuser.

Feng, A. S., Arch, V. S., Yu, Z., Yu, X.-J., Xu, Z.-M., & Shen, J.-X. (2009). Neighbor-stranger discrimination in concave-eared torrent frogs, *Odorrana tormota*. *Ethology*, 115, 851–856.

Fenn, K. M., Shintel, H., Atkins, A. S., Skipper, J. I., Bond, V. C., & Nusbaum, H. C. (2011). When less is heard than meets the ear: change deafness in a telephone conversation. *Quarterly Journal of Experimental Psychology*, 64, 1442–1456.

Fischer, J. (2004). Emergence of individual recognition in young macaques. *Animal Behaviour*, 67, 655–661.

Frühholz, S. & Grandjean, D. (2013). Amygdala subregions differentially respond and rapidly adapt to threatening voices. *Cortex*, 49, 1395–1403.

Frühholz, S., Hofstetter, C., Cristinzio, C., Saj, A., Seek, M., Builleumier, P., & Grandjean, C. (2015). Asymmetric effects of unilateral or left amygdala damage on auditory cortical processing of vocal emotions. *Proceedings of the National Academy of Sciences of the USA*, 112, 1583–1588.

Fuchs, T., Iacobucci, P., MacKinnon, K. M., & Panksepp, J. (2010). Infant-mother recognition in a social rodent (*Octodon degus*). *Journal of Comparative Psychology*, 124, 166–175.

Gainotti, G. (2011). What the study of voice recognition in normal subjects and brain-damaged patients tells us about models of familiar people recognition. *Neuropsychologia*, 49, 2273–2282.

Gall, M. D. & Wilczynski, W. (2014). Prior experience with conspecific signals enhances auditory midbrain responsiveness to conspecific vocalizations. *Journal of Experimental Biology*, 217, 1977–1982.

Gasser, H., Amézquita, A., & Hödl, W. (2009). Who is calling? Intraspecific call variation in the aromobatid frog *Allobates femoralis*. *Ethology*, 115, 596–607.

Geiselman, R. E. (1977). Incidental retention of a speaker's voice. *Memory and Cognition*, 6, 658–665.

Gerhardt, H. G. & Bee, M. A. (2007). Recognition and localization of acoustic signals. In: P. M., Narins, A. L., Feng, R. R., Fay, & A. N. Popper (eds) *Hearing and Sound Communication in Amphibians* (pp. 113–146). New York: Springer.

Goldman, J. A., Phillips, D. P., & Fentress, J. C. (1995). An acoustic basis for maternal recognition in timber wolves (*Canis lupus*)? *Journal of the Acoustical Society of America*, 97, 1970–1973.

Gould, S. J. (2003). *The Hedgehog, the Fox, and the Magister's Pox: Mending the Gap Between Science and the Humanities*. New York: Harmony.

Gruber-Dujardin, E. (2010). Role of the periaqueductal grey in expressing vocalization. In: S. M. Brudzynski (ed.) *Handbook of Mammalian Vocalization* (pp. 313–327). London: Elsevier.

Guo, X., Luo, B., Liu, Y., Jiang, T.-L., & Feng, J. (2015). Cannot see you but can hear you: vocal identity recognition in bats. *Zoological Research*, 36(5), 257–262.

Hage, S. R. (2010). Neuronal networks involved in the generation of vocalization. In: S. M. Brudzynski (ed.) *Handbook of Mammalian Vocalization* (pp. 339–349). London: Elsevier.

Hansen, E. W. (1976). Selective responding by recently separated juvenile rhesus monkeys to the calls of their mothers. *Developmental Psychobiology*, 9, 83–88.

Haramati, S., Soroker, N., Dudai, Y., & Levy, D. A. (2008). The posterior parietal cortex in recognition memory: a neuropsychological study. *Neuropsychologia*, 46, 1756–1766.

Hardman, S. (2014). Can we use anthropomorphic language in animal behavior research? *Ecologica*, July 14. Online.

Heckmann, J. G., Lang, C. J. G., & Neundörfer, B. (2001). Brief communications: recognition of familiar handwriting in stroke and dementia. *American Academy of Neurology*, 57, 2128–2131.

Hepper, P. G., Scott, D., & Shahidullah, S. (1993). Newborn and fetal response to maternal voice. *Journal of Reproductive and Infant Psychology*, 11, 147–153.

Hermans, H. J. M. (1996). Voicing the self: from information processing to dialogical interchange. *Psychological Bulletin*, 119, 31–50.

Hermans, H. J. M. (1998). The polyphony of the mind: a multivoiced and dialogical self. In: J. Rowan & M. Cooper (eds) *The Plural Self, Polypsychic Perspectives* (pp. 107–131). Thousand Oaks, CA: Sage.

Herzmann, G., Schweinberger, S. R., Jentzsch, I., & Sommer, W. (2004). What's special about personally familiar faces? A multimodal approach. *Psychophysiology*, 41(5), 688–701.

Hoh, J. F. Y. (2010). Laryngeal muscles as highly specialized organs in airway protection, respiration and phonation. In: S. M. Brudzynski (ed.) *Handbook of Mammalian Vocalization* (pp. 13–21). London: Elsevier.

Hyde, K. L., Peretz, I., & Zatorre, R. J. (2008). Evidence for the role of the right auditory cortex in fine pitch resolution. *Neuropsychologia*, 46, 632–639.

Hyvärinen, J. (1982a). Posterior parietal lobe of the primate brain. *Physiological Reviews*, 62(3), 1060–1129.

Hyvärinen, J. (1982b). *The Parietal Cortex of Monkey and Man*. Berlin: Springer-Verlag.

Insley, S. J. (2001). Mother-offspring vocal recognition in northern fur seals is mutual but asymmetrical. *Animal Behaviour*, 61, 129–137.

James, W. (1884). What is an emotion? *Mind*, 9, 188–205.

Jaywant, A. & Pell, M. D. (2009). Listener impressions of speakers with Parkinson's disease. *Journal of the International Neuropsychological Society*, 16, 49–57.

Jouventin, P. & Aubin, T. (2002). Acoustic systems are adapted to breeding ecologies: individual recognition in nesting penguins. *Animal Behaviour*, 64, 747–757.

Jouventin, P., Aubin, T., & Lengagne, T. (1999). Finding a parent in a king penguin colony: the acoustic system of individual recognition. *Animal Behaviour*, 57(6), 1175–1183.

Jürgens, U. (2002). Neural pathways underlying vocal control. *Neuroscience and Biobehavioral Reviews*, 26, 235–258.

Jürgens, U., Maurus, M., Ploog, D., & Winter, P. (1967). Vocalization in the squirrel monkey (*Saimiri sciureus*) elicited by brain stimulation. *Experimental Brain Research*, 4, 114–117.

Juslin, P. N. & Laukka, P. (2001). Impact of intended emotion intensity on cue utilization and decoding accuracy in vocal expression of emotion. *Emotion*, 1, 381–412.

Kisilevsky, B. S., et al. (2003). Effects of experience on fetal voice recognition. *Psychological Science*, 17(3), 200–224.

Klaas, H., Frühholz, S., & Grandjean, D. (2015). Aggressive vocal expressions—an investigation of their underlying neuronal network. *Frontiers in Behavioral Neuroscience*, 9, 1–10.

Kohda, M., et al. (2015). Facial recognition in a group-living cichlid fish. *PloS One*, 10(11), e0142552.

Konopcznski, G. (2010). Les enjeux de la voix. In: M. R. Castarede & G. Konopczynski (eds) *Au Commencement Etait la Voix* (pp. 33–52). Toulouse: Erès.

Kreiman, J. & Sidtis, D. (2011). *Foundations of Voice Studies: Interdisciplinary Approaches to Voice Production and Perception*. Boston: Wiley-Blackwell.

Krishnan, A., Xu, Y., Gandour, J., & Cariani, P. (2005). Encoding of pitch in the human brainstem is sensitive to language experience. *Cognitive Brain Research*, 25, 161–168.

Kuraoka, K. & Nakamura, K. (2010). Vocalization as a specific trigger of emotional responses. In: S. M. Brudzynski (ed.) *Handbook of Mammalian Vocalization* (pp. 167–175). London: Elsevier.

Landis, T., Cummings, J. L., Benson, D. F., & Palmer, E. P. (1986). Loss of topographic familiarity. An environmental agnosia. *Archives of Neurology*, 43(2), 132–136.

Laukka, P., Audibert, N., & Auberge, V. (2012). Exploring the determinants of the graded structure of vocal emotion expressions. *Cognition & Emotion*, 26(4), 710–719.

Laukka, P., Linnman, C., Åhs, F., et al. (2008). In a nervous voice: acoustic analysis and perception of anxiety in social phobics' speech. *Journal of Nonverbal Behavior*, 32, 195–214.

Laver, J. (1968). Voice quality and indexical information. *British Journal of Disorders of Communication*, 3, 43–54.

Le Gros Clark, W. E. (1959). *The Antecedents of Man*. New York: Harper.

Leder, S. B. & Spitzer, J. B. (1990). A perceptual evaluation of the speech of adventitiously deaf adult males. *Ear Hear*, 11(3), 169–75.

Lengagne, T., Lauga, J., & Aubin, T. (2001). Intra-syllabic acoustic signatures used by the king penguin in parent-chick recognition: an experimental approach. *Journal of Experimental Biology*, 204, 663–672.

Louth, S. M., Williamson, S., Alpert, M., Pougeet, E. R., & Hare, R. (1998). Acoustic distinctions in the speech of male psychopaths. *Journal of Psycholinguistic Research*, 27(3), 375–384.

MacLean, P. D. (1990). *The Triune Brain in Evolution*. New York: Plenum.

Malone, D. R., Morris, H. H., Kay, M. C., & Levin, H. S. (1982). Prosopagnosia: a double dissociation between recognition of familiar and unfamiliar faces. *Journal of Neurology, Neurosurgery, and Psychiatry*, 45, 820–822.

Masataka, N. (1985). Development of vocal recognition of mothers in infant Japanese macaques. *Developmental Psychobiology*, 18, 107–114.

Masterman, D. L. & Cummings, J. L. (1997). Frontal-subcortical circuits, the anatomic basis of executive, social, and motivated behaviors. *Journal of Psychopharmacology*, 11, 107–114.

McComb, K., Moss, C., Sayialel, S., & Baker, L. (2002). Unusually extensive networks of vocal recognition in African elephants. *Animal Behaviour*, 59, 1103–1109.

Mehler, J., Bertoncini, J., Barriere, M., & Jassik-Gerschenfeld, D. (1978). Infant recognition of mother's voice. *Perception*, 7, 491–497.

Myers, P. (1998). *Right Hemisphere Damage*. San Diego: Singular Publishing.

Narins, P. M. & Feng, A. L. (2007). Hearing and sound communication in amphibians: prologue and prognostication. In: P. M. Narins, A. L. Feng, R. R. Fay, & A. N. Popper (eds) *Hearing and Sound Communication in Amphibians* (pp. 1–11). New York: Springer.

Neuner, F. & Schweinberger, S. R. (2000). Neuropsychological impairments in the recognition of faces, voices, and personal names. *Brain and Cognition*, 44, 342–366.

Newman, J. D. (2010). Evolution of the communication brain in control of mammalian vocalization. In: S. M. Brudzynski (ed.) *Handbook of Mammalian Vocalization* (pp. 23–28). London: Elsevier.

National Science Foundation (NSF) (2008). Sorry, Charlie, you and Nemo aren't the only fish that talk. Press release with video, July 17, Arlington, VA.

Palmeri, T. J., Goldinger, S. D., & Pisoni, D. B. (1993). Episodic encoding of voice attributes and recognition memory for spoken words. *Journal of Experimental Psychology: Learning, Memory, and Cognition*, 19, 309–328.

Panksepp, J. (1998). *Affective Neuroscience: The Foundations of Human and Animal Emotions*. New York: Oxford University Press.

Panksepp, J. (2003). At the interface of affective, behavioral and cognitive neurosciences: decoding the emotional feelings of the brain. *Brain and Cognition*, 52, 4–14.

Panksepp, J. (2010). Emotional causes and consequences of social-affective vocalization. In: S. M. Brudzynski (ed.) *Handbook of Mammalian Vocalization* (pp. 201–208). London: Elsevier.

Pell, M. D. & Leonard, C. L. (2003). Processing emotional tone from speech in Parkinson's disease: a role for the basal ganglia. *Cognitive, Affective, & Behavioral Neuroscience*, 3(4), 275–288.

Pitcher, B. J., Harcourt, R. G., & Charrier, I. (2010). Rapid onset of maternal vocal recognition in a colonially breeding animal, the Australian sea lion. *PloS One*, 5, e12195.

Poljac, E., de-Wit, L., & Wagemans, J. (2012). Perceptual wholes can reduce the conscious accessibility of their parts. *Cognition*, 123, 308–312.

Pollermann, B. Z. (2010). Qu'exprime la prosodie affective: l'état du corps ou l'état de l'esprit? Proposition d'un modèle de l'émotion et de cognition. In: M. F. Castarede & G. Konopczynski (eds) *Au Commencement Etait la Voix* (pp. 97–104). Toulouse: Erès.

Pomerantz, J. R. (1986). Visual form perception: An overview. In: E. C. Schwab & H. C. Nusbaum (eds) *Pattern Recognition by Humans and Machines* (pp. 1–30). New York: Academic Press.

Pomerantz, J. R., Sager, L. C., & Stoever, R. J. (1977). Perception of wholes and of their component parts: some configural superiority effects. *Journal of Experimental Psychology: Human Perception and Performance*, 3(3), 422–435.

Porges, S. W. & Lewis, G. F. (2010). The polyvagal hypothesis: common mechanisms mediating autonomic regulation, vocalizations, and listening. In: S. M. Brudzynski (ed.) *Handbook of Mammalian Vocalization* (pp. 255–263). London: Elsevier.

Port, R. F. (2007). The graphical basis of phones and phonemes. In: M. Monro & O-S. Bohn (eds) *Second-language Speech Learning: The Role of Language Experienced in Speech Perception and Production* (pp. 349–365). Amsterdam: Benjamins Publishing Co.

Port, R. & Leary, A. (2005). Against formal phonology. *Language*, 81(4), 927–964.

Purhonen, M., Kilpelainen-Lees, R., Valkonen-Korhonen, M., Karhu, J., & Lehtonen, J. (2004). Cerebral processing of mother's voice compared to unfamiliar voice in 4-month-old infants. *International Journal of Psychophysiology*, 52, 257–266.

Querleu, D., Lefebvre, C., Titran, M., Renard, X., Morillion, M., & Crepin, G. (1984). Reactivité du nouveau-né de moins de deux heures de vie à la voix maternelle. *Journal de Gynécologie, Obstétrique et Biologie de la Reproduction*, 13, 125–134.

Reed, S. (1972). Pattern recognition and categorization, *Cognitive Psychology*, 3, 382–407.

Rendall, D. & Owren, M. (2010). Vocalizations as tools for influencing the affect and behavior of others. In: S. M. Brudzynski (ed.) *Handbook of Mammalian Vocalization* (pp. 177–185). London: Elsevier.

Rendall, D., Rodman, P. S., & Edmond, R. E. (1996). Vocal recognition of individuals and kin in free ranging rhesus monkeys. *Animal Behaviour*, 51, 1007–1015.

Revelle, W. & Scherer, K. (2009). Personality and emotion. In: D. Sander & K. Scherer (eds) *Oxford Companion to Emotion and the Affective Sciences* (pp. 304–306). Oxford: Oxford University Press.

Robinson, B.W. (1976). Limbic influences on human speech. *Annals of the New York Academy of Sciences*, 280, 761–771.

Rooth, M. (1992). A theory of focus interpretation. *Natural Language Semantics*, 1, 75–116.

Roundtree, R., Goudey, C., & Hawkins, T. (2002). Listening to fish. Proceedings of the International Workshop on the Applications of Passive Acoustics to Fisheries, MIT Sea Grant, April 8–10 (pp. 4–11). Dedham, MA.

Rusz, J., Cmejla, R., Tykalová, T., & Ruzika, E. (2013). Imprecise vowel articulation as a potential early marker of Parkinson's disease. *Journal of the Acoustical Society of America*, 134(3), 2171–2781.

Ryan, M. J. & Guerra, M. A. (2014). The mechanism of sound production in túngara frogs and its role in sexual selection and speciation. *Current Opinion in Neurobiology*, 28, 54–59.

Scherer, K. R. (1986). Vocal affect expression: a review and a model for future research. *Psychological Bulletin*, 99, 143–165.

Scherrer, J. A. & Wilkinson, G. S. (1993). Evening bat isolation calls provide evidence for herit-able signatures. *Animal Behaviour*, 46, 847–860.

Schweinberger, S. R. (2001). Human brain potential correlates of voice priming and voice rec-ognition. *Neuropsychologia*, 39, 921–936.

Searby, A. & Jouventin, P. (2003). Mother-lamb acoustic recognition in sheep: a frequency coding. *Proceedings of the Royal Society B: Biological Sciences*, 270, 1765–1771.

Searby, A., Jouventin, P., & Aubin, T. (2004). Acoustic recognition in macaroni penguins: an original signature system. *Animal Behaviour*, 67, 615–625.

Sèbe, F., Duboscq, J., Aubin, T., Ligout, S., & Poindron, P. (2010). Early vocal recognition of mother by lambs: contribution of low- and high-frequency vocalizations, *Animal Behaviour*, 79, 1055–1066.

Seeck, M., et al. (1993). Differential neural activity in the human temporal lobe evoked by faces of family members and friends. *Annals of Neurology*, 34(3), 369–372.

Selkirk, E. (1995). Sentence prosody: intonation, stress, and phrasing. In: J. A. Goldsmith (ed.) *The Handbook of Phonological Theory* (pp. 550–569). London: Basil Blackwell.

Sidtis, D. & Kreiman, J. (2008). Let's face it, phonagnosia happens, and voice recognition is fi-nally familiar. In: M. Pachalska & M. Weber (eds) *Neuropsychology and Philosophy of Mind in Process: Essays in Honor of Jason W. Brown* (pp. 298–334). Frankfurt/Lancaster: Ontos Verlag.

Sidtis, D. & Kreiman, J. (2011). In the beginning was the familiar voice: personally familiar voices in the evolutionary and contemporary biology of communication. *Journal of Integrative Psychological and Behavioral Science*, 46(2), 146–159.

Sidtis, J. J. (2015). Functional connectivity associated with acoustic stability during vowel pro-duction: implications for vocal-motor control. *Brain Connectivity*, 5(2), 115–125.

Sidtis, J. J. (1980). On the nature of the cortical function underlying right hemisphere auditory perception. *Neuropsychologia*, 18, 321–330.

Sidtis, J. J., Ahn, J-S., Gomez, C., & Sidtis, D. (2011). Speech characteristics associated with three genotypes of ataxia. *Journal of Communication Disorders*, 44, 478–492.

Sidtis, J. J., Alken, A., Tagliati, M., Alterman, R., & Van Lancker Sidtis, D. (2016). Subthalamic stimulation reduces vowel space at the initiation of sustained production: implications for articulatory motor control in Parkinson's disease. *Journal of Parkinson's Disease*, 6(2), 361–370.

Sidtis, J. J. & Van Lancker-Sidtis, D. (2003). A neurobehavioral approach to dysprosody. *Seminars in Speech and Language*, 24(2), 93–105. PMID: 127098883

Sidtis, J. J., Volpe, B. T., Holtzman, J. D., Wilson, D. H., & Gazzaniga, M. S. (1981). Cognitive interaction after staged callosal section: evidence for transfer of semantic activation. *Science*, 212, 344–346.

Siegel, A., Bhatt, S., Bhatt, R., & Zalcman, S. S. (2010). Limbic, hypothalamic and periaqueductal gray circuitry and mechanisms controlling rage and vocalization in the cat. In: S. M. Brudzynski (ed.) *Handbook of Mammalian Vocalization* (pp. 243–253). London: Elsevier.

Silva, J. A., Leong, G. B., & Wine, D. B. (1993). Misidentification delusions, facial misrecognition, and right brain injury. *Canadian Journal of Psychiatry*, 38, 239–241.

Simmons, A. M. (2004). Call recognition in the bullfrog, *Rana catesbeiana*: generalization along the duration continuum. *Journal of the Acoustical Society of America*, 115, 1345–1355.

Simonyan, K. & Horwitz, B. (2011). Laryngeal motor cortex and control of speech in humans. *The Neuroscientist*, 17(2), 197–208.

Simonyan, K. & Jürgens, U. (2003). Subcortical projections of the laryngeal motor cortex in the rhesus monkey. *Brain Research*, 974, 43–59.

Skodda, S., Grönheit, W., & Schlegel, U. (2012). Impairment of vowel articulation as a possible marker of disease progression in Parkinson's disease. *PLoS One*, 7(2), e32132.

Skodda, S., Rinsche, H., & Schlegel, U. (2009). Progression of dysprosody in Parkinson's disease over time —a longitudinal study. *Movement Disorders*, 24(5), 716–722.

Skuk, V. G. & Schweinberger, S. R. (2014). Influences of fundamental frequency, formant frequencies, aperiodicity and spectral level information on the perception of voice gender. *Journal of Speech, Language, and Hearing Research*, 57(1), 285–296.

Sperry, R. W., Zaidel, E., & Zaidel, D. (1979). Self-recognition and social awareness in the disconnected minor hemisphere. *Neuropsychologia*, 17, 153–166.

Stiles, W. B. (1999). Signs and voices in psychotherapy. *Psychotherapy Research*, 9, 1–21.

Subramanian, H. H., Balnave, R. J., & Holstege, G. (2008). The midbrain periaqueductal gray control of respiration. *Journal of Neuroscience*, 28(47), 12274–12283.

Swerts, M. & Geluykens, R. (1994). Prosody as a marker of information flow in spoken discourse. *Language and Speech*, 37, 21–43.

Terrazas, A., Serafin, N., Hernandez, H., Nowak, R., & Poindron, P. (2003). Early recognition of newborn goat kids by their mother, II. Auditory recognition and evidence of an individual acoustic signature in the neonate. *Developmental Psychobiology*, 43, 311–320.

Than, K. (2008). Humming fish reveal ancient origin of vocalization. *National Geographic News*, July 17.

Torriani, M. V. G., Vannoni, E., & McElligott, A. G. (2006). Mother-young recognition in an ungulate hider species: a unidirectional process. *The American Naturalist*, 168, 412–420.

Van Lancker Sidtis, D. (2003). Auditory recognition of idioms by first and second speakers of English: it takes one to know one. *Applied Psycholinguistics*, 24, 45–57.

Van Lancker Sidtis, D., Kempler, D., Jackson, C., & Metter, E. J. (2010). Prosodic changes in aphasic speech: timing. *Journal of Clinical Linguistics and Phonetics*, 24(2), 155-67. PMID: 20100044

Van Lancker, D. (1991). Personal relevance and the human right hemisphere. *Brain and Cognition*, 17, 64–92.

Van Lancker, D. (1997). Rags to riches: our increasing appreciation of cognitive and communicative abilities of the human right cerebral hemisphere. *Brain and Language*, 57, 1–11.

Van Lancker, D. & Canter, G. J. (1982). Impairment of voice and face recognition in patients with hemispheric damage. *Brain and Cognition*, 1, 185–195.

Van Lancker, D. & Cummings, J. L. (1999). Expletives: neurolinguistic and neurobehavioral inquiries into swearing. *Brain Research Reviews*, 31, 81–104. PMID: 10611497

Van Lancker, D., Cummings, J., Kreiman, J., & Dobkin, B. H. (1988). Phonagnosia: a dissociation between familiar and unfamiliar voices. *Cortex*, 24, 195–209.

Van Lancker, D. & Kreiman, J. (1987). Unfamiliar voice discrimination and familiar voice recognition are independent and unordered abilities. *Neuropsychologia*, 25, 829–834.

Van Lancker, D., Kreiman, J., & Cummings, J. (1989). Voice perception deficits: neuroanatomic correlates of phonagnosia. *Journal of Clinical and Experimental Neuropsychology*, 11, 665–674.

Van Lancker, D., Kreiman, J., & Wickens, T. D. (1985). Familiar voice recognition: patterns and parameters. Part II: recognition of rate-altered voices. *Journal of Phonetics*, 13, 39–52.

Van Lancker, D. & Nicklay, C. (1992). Comprehension of personally relevant (PERL) versus novel language in two globally aphasic patients. *Aphasiology*, 6, 37–61.

Voegtline, K. M., Costigan, K. A., Pater, H. A., & DiPietro, J. A. (2013). Near-term fetal response to maternal spoken voice. *Infant Behavior and Development*, 36, 526–533.

Voigt-Heucke, S. L., Taborsky, M., & Dechmann, D. K. N. (2010). A dual function of echolocation: bats use echolocation calls to identify familiar and unfamiliar individuals. *Animal Behaviour*, 80, 59–67.

von Kriegstein, K. & Giraud, A.-L. (2004). Distinct functional substrates along the right superior temporal sulcus for the processing of voices. *NeuroImage*, 22, 948–955.

Vuilleumier, P. (2005). How brains beware: neural mechanisms of emotional attention. *Trends in Cognitive Sciences*, 9(12), 585–594.

Walkowiak, W. (2007). Call production and neural basis of vocalization. In: P. M. Narins, A. L. Feng, R. R. Fay, & A. N. Popper (eds) *Hearing and Sound Communication in Amphibians* (pp. 87–112). New York: Springer.

Wells, D. K. & Schwartz, J. J. (2007). The behavioral ecology of anuran communication. In: P. M. Narins, A. L. Feng, R. R. Fay, & A. N. Popper (eds) *Hearing and Sound Communication in Amphibians* (pp. 45–86). New York: Springer.

Wilczynski, W. & Endepols, H. (2007). Central auditory pathways in anuran amphibians: the anatomical basis of hearing and sound communication. In: P. M. Narins, A. L. Feng, R. R. Fay, & A. N. Popper (eds) *Hearing and Sound Communication in Amphibians* (pp. 221–249). New York: Springer.

Wolskia, T. R., Houpta, K. A., & Aronson, R. (1980). The role of the senses in mare-foal recognition. *Applied Animal Ethology*, 6, 121–138.

Yang, S.Y., Ahn, J-S., & Van Lancker Sidtis, D. (2015). Listening and acoustic studies of idiomatic-literal contrastive sentences in Korean. *Speech, Language, and Hearing*, 18, 166–178.

Young, A. W., Reid, I., Wright, S., & Hellawell, D. J. (1993). Face-processing impairments and the Capgras delusion. *British Journal of Psychiatry*, 162, 695–698.

Yovel, Y., Melcon, M. L., Franz, M. O., Denziger, A., & Schnitzler, H. U. (2009). The voice of bats: how greater mouse-eared bats recognize individuals based on their echolocation calls. *PLoS Computational Biology*, 5(6), e1000400.

Zajonc, R. B. (1968). Attitudinal effects of mere exposure. *Journal of Personality and Social Psychology Monograph*, 9 (Part 2), 1–28.

Zajonc, R. B. (1980). Feeling and thinking: preferences need no inferences. *American Psychologist*, 35, 151–175.

Zatorre, R. & Belin, P. (2001). Spectral and temporal processing in human auditory cortex. *Cerebral Cortex*, 11, 946–953.

Zimmerman, E. (2010). Vocal expression of emotion in a nocturnal prosimian primate group, mouse lemurs. In: S. M. Brudzynski (ed.) *Handbook of Mammalian Vocalization* (pp. 215–225). London: Elsevier.

CHAPTER 3

··

THE 'VOCAL BRAIN'
Core and Extended Cerebral Networks for Voice Processing

··

PASCAL BELIN

3.1 INTRODUCTION

3.1.1 Speech and Voice

Imagine hearing a woman screaming, a young girl yawning, a man clearing his throat, a boy coughing, a girl laughing, a baby crying (Audio 3.1)—none of these sounds are speech yet we extract much information from them. First, we recognize that these sounds were all produced by the vocal apparatus of a fellow human being: we recognize the sound of a human voice as a conspecific vocalization and that in itself is already precious information. Further, we are able to extract much information on the *person* who produced this vocalization— their gender, approximate age, emotional state, etc.—and this information is highly important for our social interactions (Belin et al., 2004, 2011).

Voice and speech are two different things: voice is the carrier of speech information and it is under this angle that it has been most studied by psychologists and neuroscientists. However, in addition to speech (or even where it carries no speech as in Audio 3.1), the voice is rich in socially-relevant, person-related information, and we have evolved sophisticated cognitive abilities to extract this information robustly and accurately.

First, when hearing a voice we extract information on the *stable physical characteristics* of the speaker. We are really good at identifying the gender of a speaker by combining pitch and timbre cues (Pernet & Belin, 2012), the age (Zaske et al., 2013), an estimate of weight and size, etc. (Kreiman, 1997), allowing us to form a 'vocal signature' of a given person that we can use to later recognize that person from novel utterances (Schweinberger et al., 2014) (see Part V, this volume). We also extract information on *more transient aspects of the speaker's characteristics* such as his/her emotional (Schirmer & Kotz, 2006), motivational, or even hormonal state (see Part IV, this volume). Further, when hearing a voice we extract more subtle cues that we use to form an *impression of the speaker's personality* traits such as dominance, competence, or attractiveness (see Part V, this volume)—an impression that goes a long way in predicting future interactions with that person.

3.1.2 Voices as 'Auditory Faces'

Interestingly, the different types of information that we perceive in the voice, and listed in the previous paragraph, are also perceived in faces—in fact in everyday life we often perceive this information from the voice and face combined—so it is interesting to think of voices as 'auditory faces'. As for faces, we appear to have developed exquisite abilities to rapidly and accurately extract available information from voices, making us genuine voice experts. Indeed, we have been extracting information from many voices every day, since even before birth.

One can regroup, under the general term of '*voice cognition*', the set of auditory cognitive abilities, including speech perception, allowing us to extract information from vocal sounds as a particular sound category. A number of these abilities actually *only* apply to vocal sounds, for example the perception of voice gender. Voice cognition develops early in ontogenesis (see Part II, this volume): long before the child masters the sound and words of her maternal tongue, she is able to identify familiar persons by their voice and recognize affective states. On the day of birth, the newborn baby already shows voice discrimination and recognition abilities; there is even evidence for limited voice discrimination abilities in third-trimester fetuses. So voice cognition actually develops before birth!

Likewise, voice cognition appeared early in phylogenesis (see Part III, this volume): we share abilities to extract information from conspecific vocalizations with many other animal species. So unlike speech perception—for which analogous abilities are hard to identify in the animal kingdom—voice cognition offers a unique comparative window onto the evolution of vocal communication. Indeed, research into the psychological and cerebral bases of voice cognition has direct implications for understanding the evolution of speech: when our ancestors started speaking, a few tens or hundreds of thousand of years ago, they were probably already equipped with sophisticated voice cognition abilities that provided a solid foundation upon which speech-specific mechanisms could evolve.

3.1.3 Are Voices Special?

The similarity in the types of information carried by voices and faces suggests that the underlying neuronal mechanisms could also share some degree of similarity. As such, the vast literature on the psychological and neural mechanisms of face perception offers an invaluable theoretical and methodological guide for voice perception research.

In particular, one of the central tenets of face perception research, confirmed by converging evidence from several experimental sources, is that '*faces are special*'. First, cognitive psychology experiments have evidenced psychological effects such as the 'face inversion effect' (Yin, 1969) (beautifully illustrated in the 'Thatcher illusion' (Thompson, 1980)) indicating that face perception mechanisms require an upright orientation unlike that of other object categories. Second, a syndrome called 'prosopagnosia' has been described, occurring most often after cerebrovascular lesions in right occipito-temporal cortex, in which face identity processing is specifically impaired while the perception of other objects appears spared (Assal, 2001; Bodamer, 1947; Rossion, 2014). Third, electrophysiological and neuroimaging studies have provided accumulating evidence in the brain of macaques and humans for a set of areas showing particular sensitivity to face stimuli (Haxby et al., 2000; Tsao et al., 2003, 2006), including the well-known 'fusiform face area' (FFA) (Kanwisher et al., 1997). Results from these three lines of evidence converge to the notion that faces are processed using perceptual and neural mechanisms that are not engaged by other object categories. Does this apply to voices? Are voices special too?

At all three levels of face perception, recently available evidence indeed suggests the involvement of specific cerebral mechanisms for processing voice information. First, behavioural studies of rapid sound categorization indicate an advantage at categorizing very brief vocal sounds compared to sounds of musical instruments (Suied et al., 2014). The same group recently obtained compelling behavioural evidence for a much more accurate detection of vocal targets in a stream of rapidly presented auditory stimuli (unpublished evidence). Second, at the clinical level, a small number of patients with the syndrome analogous to prosopagnosia, called 'phonagnosia' (Van Lancker et al., 1988), have been described, in whom the inability to recognize familiar persons from their voice is apparently dissociated from a normal recognition of other sounds and normal speech comprehension. Recent cases of 'developmental phonagnosia', that is a behavioural impairment akin to phonagnosia albeit in the absence of any cerebral damage, have been described (Garrido et al., 2009; Roswandowitz et al., 2014; Xu et al., 2015; see Roswandowitz et al., this volume), analogous to developmental prosopagnosia (Duchaine & Nakayama, 2006) and further underscoring the similarity between the two syndromes. Third, neuroimaging provides compelling evidence for voice-sensitive regions in the temporal lobe of humans and macaques, which is reviewed in the next sections.

3.2 A CORE CEREBRAL NETWORK FOR VOICE PROCESSING

3.2.1 Temporal Voice Areas

The first evidence for voice-sensitive cortical areas was provided by a study that Robert Zatorre and I performed at the end of the 1990s. At that time the recent fMRI evidence for face-selective cortical areas in visual cortex and the famous FFA was making quite some noise, and we wondered whether the notion of domain-specific cortical areas could be transposed to auditory perception and auditory cortex. There were indeed some hints in the literature that the extensive cortical response to speech sounds observed with neuroimaging were not only reflecting linguistic processing. A compelling example came from a study by Jeff Binder and colleagues (1999) who observed extensive auditory cortex activation of superior temporal sulcus (STS) areas nearly indistinguishable for English words and their unintelligible time-reversed versions!

We transposed to auditory cortex the 'face localizer' protocol using a 'sparse sampling' (Hall et al., 1999; Petkov, Kayser, et al., 2009) fMRI protocol minimizing the scanner noise artefact thanks to long (10s) repetition times between consecutive fMRI volume acquisitions. We scanned normal volunteers while they were passively listening to 20s-blocks of complex natural sounds belonging to one of two categories—vocal and non-vocal sounds. Vocal sounds consisted of a large number of vocalizations produced by a number of different speakers. They included speech in various languages but also a number of non-speech vocalizations such as coughing, yawning, laughing, etc. (Audio 3.2). Non-vocal sounds were matched in diversity and number of sources per block and included sounds from mechanical, musical, or environmental sources (Audio 3.3) (Belin et al., 2000).

Both vocal and non-vocal sounds produced extensive bilateral activation of auditory cortex in each individual subject when compared to the silent baseline, reflecting their complex acoustical structure and diversity within each block. When compared to one another, however, the two categories were found to elicit statistically significant differences in several discrete areas of secondary auditory cortex in each participant. These areas were all responding significantly more to vocal sounds than to non-vocal sounds—no single area showed the reverse pattern of preferring non-vocal sounds over vocal sounds. Although the location of these areas, termed the 'temporal voice areas' (TVAs), varied from one participant to the other, they were found in most subjects along the upper bank of the middle part of the STS bilaterally, as was the group-averaged maximum of voice sensitivity (Belin et al., 2000) (Figure 3.1).

Follow-up experiments using control sound categories such as bells (to control for within-category homogeneity) and scrambled voices (to disrupt frequency spectrum while preserving temporal envelope) showed that the TVAs are not only sensitive but also quite selective to voices. Whereas the bilateral TVAs responded to all sound categories more to the silent baseline—showing they do not exclusively process vocal sounds—they were significantly more active for the original vocal sounds (Belin et al., 2000).

The comparison of responses between speech and non-speech vocal sounds (e.g. coughs, laughs) reveals an interesting pattern of results: speech sounds are found to drive the activity of all voice-sensitive regions to a high degree, and yield a much greater response than their scrambled version in most parts of auditory cortex (Belin et al., 2002). Part of this response recruits anterior STS regions of the left hemisphere involved in speech comprehension (Davis & Johnsrude, 2003; Obleser et al., 2007; Scott et al., 2000). In contrast, vocal sounds devoid of linguistic content, such as laughs, cries, humming, induce only little activity in left

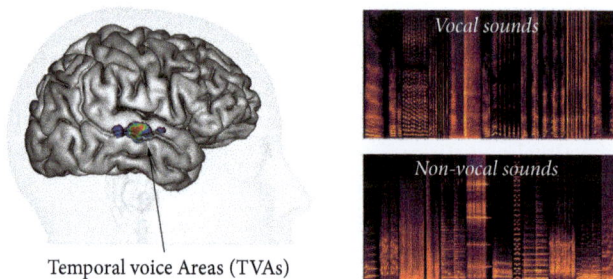

Temporal voice Areas (TVAs)

FIGURE 3.1 Temporal voice areas (TVAs) in the human brain. The comparison of fMRI measures of brain activity obtained in normal adult volunteers during stimulation with vocal vs. non-vocal sounds highlights voice-sensitive TVAs in auditory cortex bilaterally.

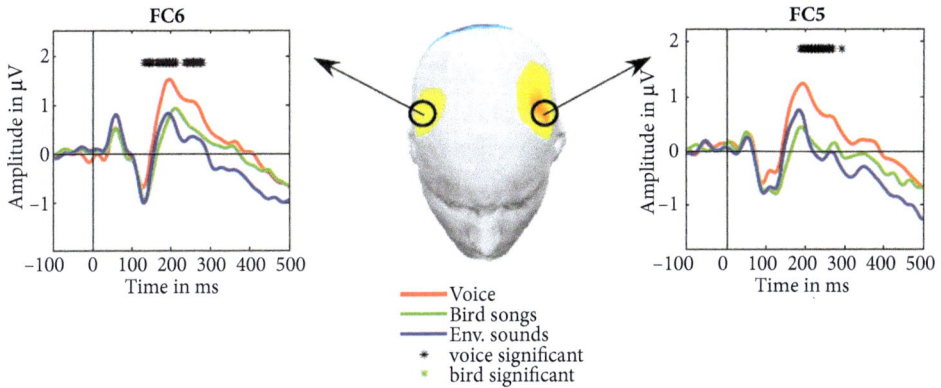

FIGURE 3.2 The fronto-temporal sensitivity to the voice. Auditory evoked potentials recorded during stimulation with brief vocal (red) or non-vocal (green and blue) sound stimuli. The two fronto-temporal electrodes FC5 and FC6 show a strongly significant difference between vocal and non-vocal sounds at a latency of about 200ms after stimulus onset.

Reproduced from Charest I. et al., 'Electrophysiological evidence for an early processing of human voices', *BMC Neuroscience*, Volume 10, Issue 127, doi: 10.1186/1471-2202-10-127, Copyright © 2009 Charest et al., under the terms of the Creative Commons Attribution License (CC by 2.0).

hemisphere auditory cortex regions. It is only in right anterior temporal lobe regions that those non-speech vocal sounds drive neuronal activity more than their scrambled counterpart, suggesting that these regions of the right hemisphere are likely to be involved in processing paralinguistic information in voices (Belin et al., 2002).

The TVAs have been observed by several groups since these initial experiments (e.g. Blank et al., 2011; Ethofer et al., 2007, 2009; Gervais et al., 2004; Grandjean et al., 2005; Linden et al., 2011; Moerel et al., 2013; Von Kriegstein & Giraud, 2004). The sound stimuli necessary for a 'voice localizer' fMRI scan are publicly available (https://neuralbasesofcommunication.eu/download/).

3.2.2 Speed of Voice Processing

How long does the brain take to differentiate vocal from non-vocal sounds? For faces, the earliest electrophysiological component showing reliable differences between face and non-face objects is the 'N170' (Bentin et al., 1996)—a negativity observed on occipito-temporal electrodes 170ms after stimulus onset with greater amplitude for faces (but see Bentin et al., 2007; Thierry et al., 2007). The first estimate of the speed of voice processing also came from Shlomo Bentin's group who found that sung notes produced a positivity at around 320ms after sound onset that was not observed for comparable notes played by instruments (Levy et al., 2001) and with a topography different from that of the attention-related P300. Yet only midline electrodes were observed in that study that provided a surprisingly long duration for voice compared to face detection.

In a later study using high-density EEG we could observe a much earlier voice-sensitive component, termed the 'fronto-temporal sensitivity to voice' (FTPV). Fronto-temporal electrodes showed, in the latency of the P200, a large amplitude difference between vocal sounds and different categories of non-vocal sounds (Charest et al., 2009) (Figure 3.2). A subsequent magnetoencephalography study confirmed this dissociation between neuronal activity at the N100m latency with generators located close to primary auditory cortex (A1) and no amplitude difference between vocal and non-vocal sounds, and the FTPVm close to the P200 latency with strong amplitude differences between vocal and non-vocal sounds and generators located along anterior and posterior superior temporal gyrus bilaterally in cortical locations consistent with the fMRI-localized TVAs (Capilla et al., 2013). Thus, it takes about 200ms for vocal and non-vocal sounds to be differentiated by the brain—a value very comparable to the 170ms required to differentiating face from non-face objects in visual cortex.

3.3 INTER-INDIVIDUAL VARIABILITY OF THE TEMPORAL VOICE AREAS

3.3.1 Three 'Voice Patches'

The TVAs are fairly variable in exact anatomical location across individuals and hemispheres. Yet they are highly reliable within subject as indicated by test–retest reliability analysis (Pernet et al., 2015). A recent 'mega-analysis' of the voice localizer collected in several hundred participants (Pernet et al., 2015) included a cluster analysis of local voice-sensitivity maxima that suggested an organization in three 'voice patches' along the antero-posterior axis of the superior temporal gyrus (STG) and STS bilaterally. The power afforded by the large sample size also showed that the TVAs are but the most salient part of an extended 'vocal brain', a bilateral, distributed network of cortical and subcortical regions showing small but significant voice sensitivity (Figure 3.3). Thus, as for face processing (Haxby et al., 2000), evidence suggests the TVAs constitute a *core network* for voice processing in the temporal lobe connected to an extended network comprised of additional areas in inferior prefrontal cortex bilaterally (Fecteau et al., 2005) as well as the amygdala. The network dynamics of information processing within and between the core and extended voice processing networks is a crucial overarching goal for future research.

3.3.2 Gender Differences

A number of gender differences have been documented at the behavioural level in voice perception (Belin et al., 2008; Schirmer & Kotz, 2006; Schirmer et al., 2002). For instance, female listeners are more accurate than male listeners at recognizing the emotion expressed by non-verbal affect bursts (Belin et al., 2008). We used a large sample of localizer scans collected at the Voice Neurocognition Laboratory in Glasgow to ask whether gender differences could be observed in the distribution of the TVAs (Ahrens et al., 2014). We compared the

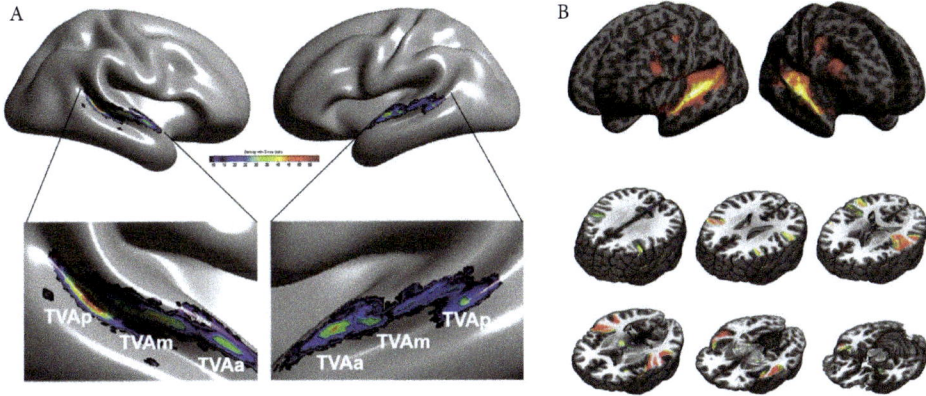

FIGURE 3.3 The core and extended voice networks. **(A)** The core network: three bilateral voice patches in the TVAs as suggested by cluster analysis of individual voice sensitivity maxima. **(B)** The extended network: group analyses with large sample sizes reveal voice sensitivity in a number of extra temporal areas, notably in inferior prefrontal cortex and the amygdala.

Reprinted from *NeuroImage*, Volume 119, Pernet C.R. et al., 'The human voice areas: Spatial organization and inter-individual variability in temporal and extra-temporal cortices', Figures 2 and 4, pp. 164–74, Copyright © Elsevier Ltd., under the terms of the Creative Commons Attribution Licence (CC BY 4.0), http://www.sciencedirect.com/science/article/pii/S1053811915005558.

localizer scans of 149 female and 123 male volunteers. Despite the good statistical power only minute differences emerged in conventional univariate analyses: four voxels in left posterior STG showing greater vocal versus non-vocal difference in female than in male listeners. In contrast, when the same gender comparison was performed on multivariate voice/non-voice classification maps from multi-voxel pattern analysis (MVPA; in which the colour for each voxel corresponds to the classification accuracy in % of a classifier based on fMRI signal from a small sphere centred on that voxel) important differences appeared, all in the same direction. A number of subareas within the TVAs in both hemispheres showed significantly larger voice/non-voice classification accuracy in females—no area showed greater classification accuracy in male listeners (Ahrens et al., 2014). This result suggests that while the TVAs are equally active in male and female listeners, they have a greater informational content in females.

3.3.3 Behavioural Differences

Listeners vary considerably in their voice perception abilities. This has been verified by several studies (Kreiman, 1997; Kreiman & Gerratt, 2010) although often with small sample sizes (but see Roswandowitz et al., 2014) and always using study- and language-specific material. Unfortunately, the lack of a standardized, language-independent battery of voice perception similar to those available for face perception has probably hindered the research into the cerebral correlates of voice processing and its disorders. In an effort to make such a tool available to the scientific community, we have developed the 'Glasgow Voice Memory Test' (GVMT), a brief, standardized test of memory for unfamiliar voices validated in a large sample of more than 1,000 listeners and with minimal linguistic content so as to be usable in different countries (Aglieri et al., 2016). The GVMT is available online at: http://experiments.psy.gla.ac.uk/experiments/assessment.php?id = 127

We examined the link between TVA activation and behaviour by correlating brain activity measured with the TVA localizer scan with performance at the GVMT in a group of thirty-six normal participants (Watson et al., 2009). A highly significant correlation was found between TVA activation in response to sounds—both vocal and non-vocal—and immediate recall performance at the GVMT (Watson et al., 2009). Subjects in whom TVA response to sounds (both vocal and non-vocal) was higher correctly recalled more of the voices they had just heard. Interestingly, memory for bell sounds (the control sound category), although similar in the group to memory for voices, was not predicted by TVA activation. These preliminary findings are strong evidence that neuronal populations in the TVA are specifically involved in the encoding of individual voices, but not other sound categories such as bells, for storage in memory. Further studies investigating the link between voice perception performance and cerebral anatomy, for example using voxel-based morphometry and diffusion tensor imaging, should yield important complementary information.

3.3.4 Temporal Voice Area in Autism Spectrum Disorders

Gervais et al. (2004) examined the TVAs in a group of individuals with autistic spectrum disorders (ASD) and age-matched normal controls using the voice localizer (Belin et al., 2000). Whereas the control group showed typical activation of the TVA when activity elicited by vocal versus non-vocal sound was compared, the autistic group did not show activation of the TVA (Gervais et al., 2004). Interestingly, the response to the non-vocal sounds was similar in the two groups, suggesting normal processing of non-vocal sounds in the autistic group. It is only for the vocal sounds that a difference emerged, the autistic sample failing to show the additional TVA activation that controls showed (Gervais et al., 2004). This suggests a potential link between the communicative disorders associated with autism, particularly for vocal sounds (Klin, 1991; Rutherford et al., 2002) and the abnormal activation of the TVA. This possibility received additional support by behavioural results of the study. When subjects were asked after scanning to recall as many sounds that they had heard as possible, the normal subjects recalled an equal proportion of vocal and non-vocal sounds. In contrast, the autistic subjects recalled an overwhelming (91.5%) proportion of non-vocal sounds, suggesting that the lack of TVA activation was associated at the behavioural level with an attentional bias towards non-vocal sounds. An fMRI study of auditory stimulation in sleeping infants recently provided interesting confirmation of these results by showing a lack of TVA activation in 7-month-old infants with a family history of ASD (Blasi et al., 2015) (see Part II, this volume).

3.4 Functional Role of the Temporal Voice Areas

3.4.1 What are the Temporal Voice Areas Doing?

The existence of TVAs in the cortex of the vast majority of normal listeners has been veri-fied by several groups and can hardly be disputed. What remains less clear is the functional role of the different voice patches. Are these cortical areas even performing computations related to voice perception? The TVA patches do not only respond to voices but also to other complex sounds, although less strongly. One possibility is that these areas are part of a larger set of areas performing general timbre analysis—analogous to cortical areas performing general visual shape analysis of which the FFA and occipital face area (OFA) constitute prominent nodes (Haxby et al., 2001). This potential analogy is reinforced by neuroimaging studies of timbre processing that show that areas of anterior temporal lobe close to the location of the central TVAm cluster respond to the manipulation of different timbre cues in complex sounds (Menon et al., 2002; Warren et al., 2005). Another clue to the TVA's functional role comes from studies of social cognition that indicate a striking involvement of neuronal populations along the STS for processing social signals in gen-eral, that is stimuli from other humans such as mouth, hand, eyes, etc. The observation of voice-sensitive neuronal populations along the STS, particularly in the most posterior voice patch TVAp, constitutes additional evidence for a strong involvement of STS cortex in representing social stimuli.

3.4.2 Causal Link with Voice Perception

Neuroimaging studies consistently report TVA activation during voice stimulation, but is TVA activity *causally* related to voice perception? Neuroimaging indeed only provides cor-relational evidence that can be misleading when trying to infer causal links. For instance, neuroimaging studies of speech perception typically show comparable involvement of audi-tory cortex in the left and right hemispheres, yet left-hemisphere lesions are known to have a much stronger impact on speech comprehension.

In order to examine the potential causal link between TVA activation and voice percep-tion, we conducted a study using repetitive transcranial magnetic stimulation (rTMS) to temporally interfere with the normal function of neuronal populations in the TVAm of the right hemisphere. Eight participants were scanned using the localizer scan to individually localize the anatomical location of their peak of voice sensitivity in the right hemisphere. They were stimulated with rTMS over their right TVAm or at a control site not related to voice perception (right supramarginal gyrus) for 10 minutes at 1Hz. Then they were asked to perform either a voice/non-voice categorization task, or a control auditory task unre-lated to voice perception (loudness change detection). We observed the predicted signifi-cant interaction between the effects of task and stimulation site, with a marked drop in voice categorization, but not loudness detection performance, for TVA compared to control site

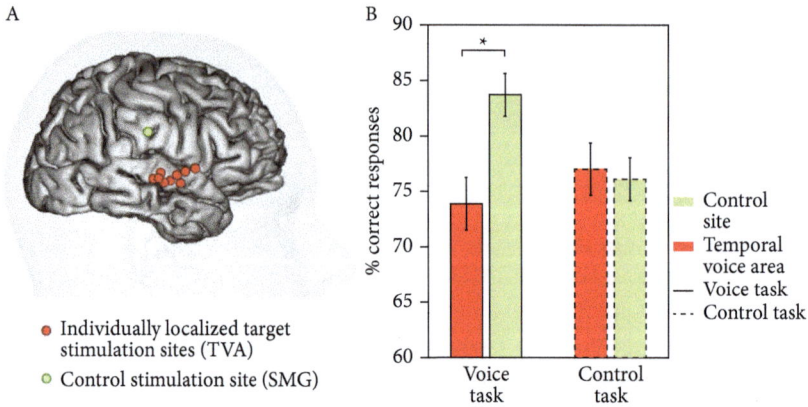

FIGURE 3.4 Right temporal TMS impairs voice detection. (A) Illustration of stimulation sites. Individually localized right temporal voice area (TVA) in red; control site (supramarginal gyrus, SMG) in green. (B) Bar graph illustrates results of both tasks when stimulating the TVA or the control site. Stimulating the TVA caused significantly poorer performance compared with the control site on the voice/non-voice discrimination task. The control task was not affected by rTMS at either stimulation site. Error bars represent standard error of the mean.

stimulation (Bestelmeyer et al., 2011) (Figure 3.4). This result, which calls for replication and extension, constitutes so far the only established causal link between TVA activation and voice perception.

3.4.3 A Voice Detection Gating Stage?

One influential hypothesis on the functional significance of the FFA activations in response to faces is that they reflect a computational stage of face detection (Tsao & Livingstone, 2008). This face detection stage would constitute a mandatory computational stage before processing further facial information according to behavioural goals. Indeed, automatic face processing research suggests it is computationally much more rapid and efficient to first detect face stimuli and then apply specific fine-grained template matching or filter mechanisms only on the detected faces to extract higher-level face information (identity, affect, etc.) than to apply those filters or match internal templates directly on all incoming stimuli, faces as well as non-face objects (Tsao & Livingstone, 2008). Such a mandatory face detection stage before more advanced goal-orientated processing is akin to what Vicky Bruce and Andy Young conceptualize as a face 'structural encoding' stage in their influential model of face processing (Bruce & Young, 1986; Young & Bruce, 2011): a processing stage where a stimulus is recognized as a face and at which its internal structure is encoded for further processing along three main processing routes.

The analogy between face and voice processing suggests that the notion of a mandatory detection stage could also apply for the TVAs. Indeed, we have proposed a model of voice perception directly inspired by Bruce and Young's model (see Section 3.5.1) that includes such a 'voice structural encoding' stage. This first processing stage would correspond to voice detection, that is the recognition that an incoming sound stimulus is a human voice. As for faces, this stage could consist of a mandatory processing stage before higher-level processing of different types of voice information.

This 'structural encoding' stage would not only detect a voice but also at the same time match it to internal voice templates. This notion is consistent with evidence that the TVAs encode novel voices using a norm-based code (Latinus et al., 2013; see Latinus & Zäske, this volume). Voices more acoustically different from an internal voice template (actually two—one male and one female; Audios 3.4 and 3.5) are perceived as more distinctive and elicit greater activity in the TVAs than voices more similar to the prototype (see Kawahara & Skuk; Vinciarelli; this volume). This encoding scheme, strikingly similar to face-encoding schemes (Leopold et al., 2006; Loffler et al., 2005), would constitute a parsimonious way of encoding voice information for further processing in the extended voice network.

3.5 AN EXTENDED CEREBRAL NETWORK FOR VOICE PROCESSING

3.5.1 Modelling Voice Perception

As discussed in Section 3.1, voice cognition consists of a number of different abilities. In parallel, a number of areas beyond the core TVAs show significant voice sensitivity in what seems to constitute an extended network for voice processing. In an effort to establish the functional architecture of this voice information processing network, we once again emphasized the similarities in informational content between face and voice, and observed that the nature of the computational complexity imposed on the brain in processing these signals (categorization, invariance, identification, etc.) has to be similar across the two modalities, at least at higher-level, relatively abstract stages of processing (Belin et al., 2011). Solving these similar problems using a similar neuronal implementation would seem an effective principle of cerebral organization (Ellis, 1989).

We conceptualized the notion of cerebral organization by extending Bruce and Young's (1986) seminal model of cerebral face processing (Bruce & Young, 1986; Young & Bruce, 2011) and proposed a similar functional architecture for voice processing (Belin et al., 2004), as already suggested by other authors (Burton et al., 1990; Ellis, 1989). After low-level analysis in subcortical nuclei and core regions of auditory cortex, voices would be processed in a voice-specific stage of 'structural encoding' probably constituting a mandatory voice detection and encoding stage, before further processing.

After this, the incoming signal would be further processed in three main processing routes or streams, corresponding to processing of the three main types of vocal information (Figure 3.5): (i) a pathway for analysis of speech information, involving anterior and posterior superior temporal sulcus (STS) as well as inferior prefrontal regions and premotor

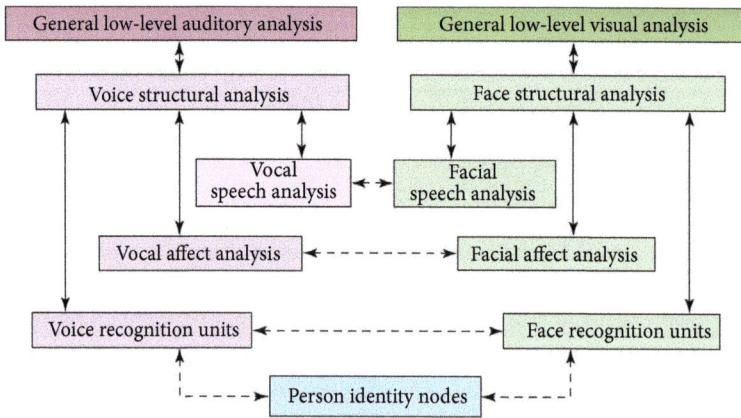

FIGURE 3.5 The 'auditory face' model of voice perception. The right-hand part of the figure is adapted from Bruce and Young's model of face perception (Bruce & Young, 1986). The left-hand part proposes a similar functional organization for voice processing. Dashed arrows indicate multimodal interactions.

Reprinted from *Trends in Cognitive Sciences*, Volume 8, Issue 3, Belin P., Fecteau S., & Bedard C., 'Thinking the voice: neural correlates of voice perception', Figure 1, pp. 129–35, Copyright © 2004 Elsevier Ltd., with permission from Elsevier, http://www.sciencedirect.com/science/article/ pii/S1364661304000257.

cortex predominantly in the left hemisphere; (ii) a pathway for analysis of vocal affective information, involving temporo-medial regions, anterior insula, and amygdala and inferior prefrontal regions predominantly in the right hemisphere; and (iii) a pathway for analysis of vocal identity, involving 'voice recognition units' each activated by one of the voices known to the person, and a putative supra-modal stage of person recognition ('person identity nodes')—although direct anatomical and functional links between face- and voice-selective cortex could be involved in identification of familiar persons (von Kriegstein & Giraud, 2006; von Kriegstein et al., 2005).

As for the face processing streams, these three functional pathways are proposed to interact with each other during normal processing but they can be selectively impaired, resulting in deficits for one type of voice information, while the other voice cognition abilities are spared. This model, which is necessarily wrong like all other models, has the advantage of proposing testable predictions. A number of these predictions have already been verified. The speech perception and identity perception pathways do interact during normal behaviour, as indicated by the better word memory for speech spoken in a familiar voice, or the 'language familiarity effect' (Goggin et al., 1991; Perrachione et al., 2010), by which we are better at discriminating and recognizing speakers of our own language (see Perrachione, this volume). Similarly, the double dissociation between receptive aphasia, in which patients have disrupted speech comprehension but normal voice recognition ability, and phonagnosia, for which patients have impaired speaker recognition but normal speech comprehension, further underscores that the speech and identity processing pathways are dissociable.

3.5.2 Interplay of Core and Extended Networks

Our voice cognition abilities most often involve more than simply detecting a voice, and our behavioural goals often make us focus on one specific type of voice information such as speech content, identity, affective state. Results from neuroimaging studies on the perception of voice gender (Charest et al., 2013), identity (Latinus et al., 2011, 2013), affect (Bestelmeyer, Maurage, et al., 2014), and attractiveness (Bestelmeyer et al., 2012) converge on the notion of an interplay between the core and extended voice processing networks to extract voice information relevant to behavioural goals. These studies all suggest that neuronal activity in the core network is essentially related to extracting voice acoustics, principally driven by acoustical proximity to the voice template in the middle voice patches TVAm, and by acoustical differences with the previously heard voice stimulus in more anterior TVAa. That acoustical information is further processed by the extended network as a function of the task demands, involving subcortical areas such as the amygdala (Bestelmeyer, Belin et al., 2014; Bestelmeyer, Maurage et al., 2014) and several areas of prefrontal cortex bilaterally (Bestelmeyer et al., 2012; Bestelmeyer, Maurage, et al., 2014; Charest et al., 2013; Latinus et al., 2011, 2013). Understanding the functional role and organization of the prefrontal areas of the extended voice network, and their functional connectivity with the core network in the temporal lobe, is an important topic for future research.

3.6 Development of the Vocal Brain

3.6.1 Cerebral Voice Processing in the Newborn

In humans, voice cognition develops faster than speech perception (see Part II, this volume). While phoneme discrimination emerges in babies around 2 months after birth and lexical–semantic processing only around 12 to 14 months after birth (Friederici, 2005), infants aged a few weeks show already well-developed voice perception abilities. Experiments measuring changes in heart rates in neonates during presentation of different voices demonstrate an ability to discriminate voices and to recognize the voices of their parents (Ockleford et al., 1988). This ability is apparently even present in fetuses before birth (Kisilevsky et al., 2003), as the maturing auditory system during the last trimester of pregnancy is daily exposed to voices, in particular the mother's voice.

The earliest evidence for a cerebral signature of voice perception is provided by an EEG study of mother's voice recognition in newborn babies (Beauchemin et al., 2011). On the day of birth, babies underwent a mismatch negativity (MMN) protocol in which they were exposed to a stream of rapid auditory stimulation with a standard voice stimulus interspersed with rare deviant stimuli consisting of the mother's voice or a stranger's voice. The comparison of electrical activity induced by the deviant versus the standard stimuli highlighted a well-formed MMN, indicating that the newborn brain could detect the change in voice identity between the different voice stimuli. Moreover, the MMN in response to the mother's voice was stronger than that to the stranger's voice, demonstrating voice recognition on the first day of life and providing an electrophysiological marker.

3.6.2 Development of the Temporal Voice Areas

However, the first evidence for TVAs in the infant brain occurs at a later age (Figure 3.6). One study used near infrared spectroscopy (NIRS) to contrast measures of blood oxygenation acquired during stimulation with brief vocal or non-vocal stimuli taken from the 'voice localizer' scan routinely used in fMRI studies of adult voice processing (Grossman et al.,

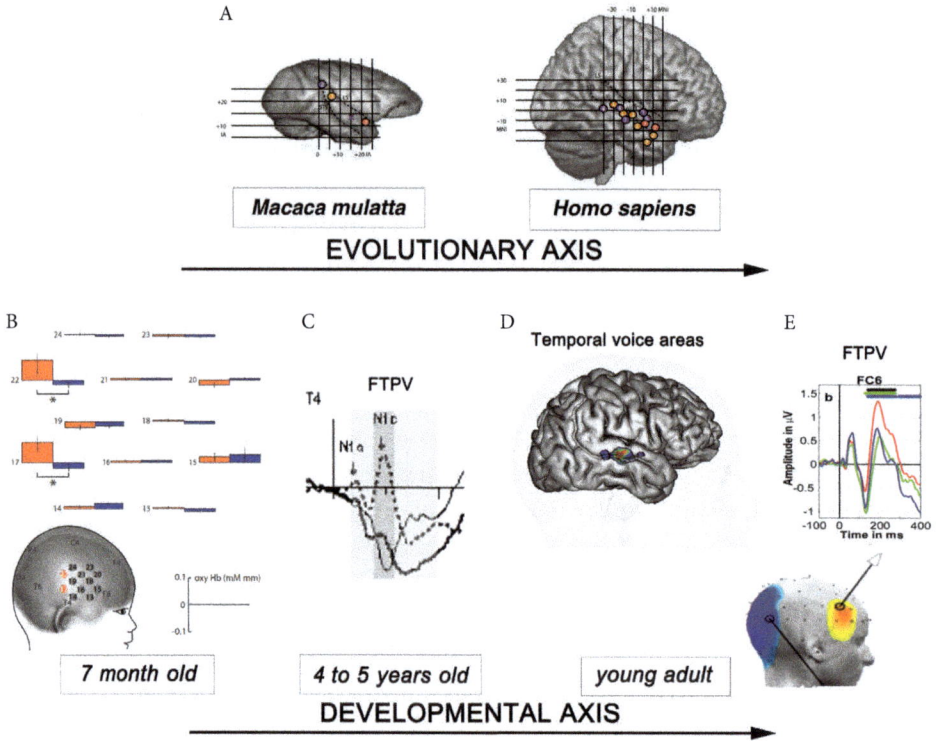

FIGURE 3.6 Phylogeny and ontogeny of cerebral voice processing. (A) Meta-analysis of neuroimaging studies of voice processing in monkeys and humans. Orange and purple circles: voice-selective regions showing greater activity in response to species-specific vocalizations compared to control sounds. Red circles: regions sensitive to speaker identity (Petkov et al., 2009). (B) NIRS study of cerebral response to vocal (orange) and nonvocal (blue) sounds in 7-month-old infants highlights bilateral regions of preferential response to voices in posterior temporal lobe, with greater voice sensitivity in the right hemisphere (Grossman et al., 2010). (C) Auditory evoked potentials in 4- to 5-year-old children comparing vocal (bold line) to non-vocal (dashed line) sounds reveal a 'fronto-temporal sensitivity to voice' (FTPV; light line = vocal–non-vocal) at electrode T4, peaking around 200ms after sound onset, mostly apparent in the right hemisphere (Rogier et al., 2010). (D) TVAs in a young adult subject. (E) The FTPV observed in young adult subjects (Charest et al., 2009).

2010). Seven-month-old infants showed greater oxygenation levels in response to voices versus non-vocal sounds in the posterior part of the temporal lobe bilaterally, with greater voice-sensitive response in the right hemisphere, while no brain region was found exhibiting the opposite pattern. In the 4-month-old infants, however, no such voice-sensitive response was observed (Grossman et al., 2010). Another group used fMRI in sleeping babies (see Paquette et al., this volume) to contrast brain oxygenation levels during exposure to vocal versus non-vocal sounds with a much better spatial resolution than NIRS (Blasi et al., 2011), and observed voice-sensitive responses in the right anterior temporal lobe of 7-month-old infants comparable to evidence obtained in adults. Interestingly, children at risk for autism spectrum disorders did not show this voice-sensitive activity (Blasi et al., 2015), consistent with results in the adult brain (Gervais et al., 2004). Thus these two studies, although they differ on the exact anatomical location of the voice-sensitive activity they observe, converge on the notion that the TVAs emerge and can be detected between 4 and 7 months after birth.

3.7 EVOLUTION OF THE VOCAL BRAIN

3.7.1 Are the Temporal Voice Areas Species-Specific?

Are the TVAs exclusively interested in human voices? Or are they sensitive to the structure of vocal sounds in general, regardless of species? To answer this question we used an event-related design and two categories of animal sounds—a category of mixed animal calls and a homogeneous category of calls from a single species (cats)—to compare the response of the TVAs to human voices versus animal vocalizations (Fecteau et al., 2004). Primary auditory cortices bilaterally showed similar response profiles for the human voices, animal vocalizations, and non-vocal control sounds. At the level of the STS, the TVAs showed greater response to the two human vocal sound categories than to the control sounds, replicating earlier findings. However, their response to the two categories of animal vocalizations was not different from the non-vocal controls, suggesting a high degree of species specificity of the TVAs (Fecteau et al., 2004): the TVAs are not just interested in any type of vocalization—they like *human* voices.

3.7.2 Temporal Voice Areas in the Macaque Brain

Are the TVAs uniquely human? Did the TVAs appear only recently in evolution, perhaps along with the emergence of speech? Or could they also be observed in other animal species, suggesting a longer evolutionary history? In the macaque, electrophysiological and lesion studies have clearly established a sensitivity of auditory (Heffner & Heffner, 1984; Rauschecker et al., 1995) and prefrontal (Cohen et al., 2009; Romanski et al., 2005) cortex to macaque vocalizations. More recently, positron emission tomography and fMRI imaging have provided increasing detail of the functional organization of macaque auditory cortex, initially in anaesthetized then, increasingly, in awake, behaving animals (Gil-da-Costa et al., 2004, 2006; Joly, Pallier, et al., 2012; Joly, Ramus, et al., 2012; Ortiz-Rios et al., 2015; Petkov et al., 2006, 2008; Poremba et al., 2003). These studies show that stimulation with (macaque) voice induces increased activity in a wide network of temporal lobe areas extending to belt and parabelt fields of auditory cortex.

The comparison of activity induced by vocal versus other sound categories, potentially highlighting TVAs, has also yielded mixed results, probably because of the small sample size (typically two or three individuals only). One group found no significant voice-selective activity (Joly, Pallier, et al., 2012), while other groups have shown differences in variable cortical areas (Gil-da-Costa et al., 2004, 2006; Ortiz-Rios et al., 2015; Petkov et al., 2008). Petkov et al. (2008), using fMRI and a design inspired from the human voice localizer (Belin et al., 2000), reported convincing evidence in two awake macaques of several areas showing larger response to voice than other control sounds, including one right anterior temporal area that, as found in humans (Belin & Zatorre, 2003), showed adaptation to speaker repetition (Petkov et al., 2008). The differing anatomical locations of the human and macaque TVAs raise the interesting possibility that the TVAs may have positioned differently with evolution in the two species (Ghazanfar, 2008). However, this finding may also be an artefact related to group averaging in human subjects and to the small macaque sample size studied so far.

That anterior voice area was later found, using electrophysiology, to contain 'voice cells', that is neurons showing significant voice selectivity at the individual level (Perrodin et al., 2011), in an interesting analogy with the 'face cells' of macaque visual cortex (Tsao et al., 2006). Recent experiments using electrical stimulation during fMRI scanning, as a direct way of measuring effective connectivity with the area stimulated, reveal an interesting pattern of effective connectivity between the anterior voice area and inferior prefrontal regions (Petkov et al., 2015; see Perrodin & Petkov, this volume).

3.7.3   Temporal Voice Areas in the Canine Brain

Recently, a group in Budapest developed a brilliant dog fMRI scanning strategy where dogs are trained, using operant conditioning with positive food and social reinforcement, to stay still in the scanner for about 10 minutes (which they learn to do much faster than the macaques!). A group of dogs was scanned during auditory stimulation with sounds of dog vocalizations, human voices, and environmental sounds, allowing the delineation of functionally sensitive auditory cortex and the comparison of selectivity in different cortical areas (Andics et al., 2014). The contrast of images of brain activity measured during stimulation with dog vocalizations versus the other sounds highlighted a small region of middle ectosylvian gyrus that shows significant preference for dog vocalizations—a dog homologue of the voice areas. Furthermore, that area was found to be modulated by the affective content of the vocalizations (Andics et al., 2014), much like the human TVAs (Ethofer et al., 2009, 2012).

3.7.4   An Evolutionary Ancient Vocal Brain

Together, the macaque and dog findings of TVA homologues provide strong evidence for a long evolutionary history of voice processing (see Part III, this volume). The most parsimonious explanation for the fact that voice areas can be found today in these species is that the voice areas were already present in some rudimentary form in the last common ancestor of humans, macaques, and dogs, some 80 million years ago. Thus the neural mechanisms dedicated to analysing conspecific vocalizations have been evolving during these tens of millions of years and it is not surprising that they are highly developed in our brain. This notion implies that we should be able to find voice areas in the brain of many other living animals for whom accurate processing of conspecific vocalizations has some adaptive significance. This also implies that when they started speaking some 0.1–0.2 million years ago, our ancestors were already equipped with sophisticated neural machinery for processing voice information which they could bootstrap to develop a novel mode of vocal communication—speech.

3.8 CONCLUSION

Research into the cerebral mechanisms of the non-linguistic aspects of voice cognition has been lagging compared to speech or face perception research, but it is gaining increasing momentum. Current results suggest, in a strong analogy with known mechanisms of cerebral face processing, a distributed vocal brain with a core network of areas centred on the TVAs and an extended network including extra-temporal areas such as the amygdala and inferior prefrontal cortex. The core network corresponds to a stage of 'voice structural encoding' that performs voice detection and acoustical template matching, while the extended network performs higher-level goal-related computations organized in three interacting processing streams specialized in extracting one particular type of vocal information.

Many open questions remain for a better understanding of the functional architecture of the vocal brain. About the core network in the TVAs: how different is the vocal stimulus representation in the different voice patches? Can homologues of the voice patches be found in macaques and do they show a progression in the voice representation similar to what has been evidenced for the macaque face patches (Freiwald & Tsao, 2010; Freiwald et al., 2009)? Are there precise anatomo-functional correspondences in the human TVAs that could help interpret their large inter-individual variability, and could such correspondences be observed in simplified form in the macaque brain? About the extended network: what is the precise functional topography of prefrontal areas engaged by voices? What is their pattern of anatomical connectivity with the core TVAs and how does this co-vary with inter-individual differences in behavioural performance? How is the pattern of functional connectivity between core and extended networks modulated by task demands and how is it affected in acquired or developmental phonagnosia? There is much exciting work ahead to bring elements of answers to these important questions on the functioning of one of our most ancient and important abilities to extract information from conspecific vocalizations.

ACKNOWLEDGEMENTS

Supported by grant BB/E003958/1 from BBSRC (UK), large grant RES-060-25-0010 by ESRC/MRC (UK), grant AJE201214 by the Fondation pour la Recherche Médicale (France) and by

Labex BLRI (ANR-11-LABX-0036), supported by the French National Agency for Research (ANR) under the programme 'Investissements d'Avenir' (ANR-11-IDEX-0001-02).

REFERENCES

Aglieri, V., Watson, R., Pernet, C., Latinus, M., Garrido, L., & Belin, P. (2016). The Glasgow Voice Memory Test: assessing the ability to memorize and recognize unfamiliar voices. *Behavior Research Methods*, 49(1). doi: 10.3758/s13428-015-0689-6

Ahrens, M. M., Awwad Shiekh Hasan, B., Giordano, B. L., & Belin, P. (2014). Gender differences in the temporal voice areas. *Frontiers in Neuroscience*, 8, 228. doi: 10.3389/fnins.2014.00228

Andics, A., Gacsi, M., Farago, T., Kis, A., & Miklosi, A. (2014). Voice-sensitive regions in the dog and human brain are revealed by comparative fMRI. *Current Biology*, 24(5), 574–578. doi: 10.1016/j.cub.2014.01.058

Assal, G. (2001). Prosopagnosia. *Bulletin De L Academie Nationale De Medecine*, 185(3), 525–536.

Beauchemin, M., Gonzalez-Frankenberger, B., Tremblay, J., Vannasing, P., Martinez-Montes, E., Belin, P., . . . Lassonde, M. (2011). Mother and stranger: an electrophysiological study of voice processing in newborns. *Cerebral Cortex*, 21(8), 1705–1711. doi: 10.1093/cercor/bhq242

Belin, P., Bestelmeyer, P. E., Latinus, M., & Watson, R. (2011). Understanding voice perception. *British Journal of Psychology*, 102(4), 711–725. doi: 10.1111/j.2044-8295.2011.02041.x

Belin, P., Fecteau, S., & Bedard, C. (2004). Thinking the voice: neural correlates of voice perception. *Trends in Cognitive Sciences*, 8, 129–135.

Belin, P., Fillion-Bilodeau, S., & Gosselin, F. (2008). The 'Montreal Affective Voices': a validated set of nonverbal affect bursts for research on auditory affective processing. *Behavioural Brain Research*, 40, 531–539.

Belin, P., & Grosbas, M. H. (2010). Before speech: cerebral voice processing in infants. *Neuron*, 65, 852–858.

Belin, P., & Zatorre, R. J. (2003). Adaptation to speaker's voice in right anterior temporal lobe. *NeuroReport*, 14(16), 2105–2109. doi: 10.1097/01.wnr.0000091689.94870.85

Belin, P., Zatorre, R. J., & Ahad, P. (2002). Human temporal-lobe response to vocal sounds. *Cognitive Brain Research*, 13, 17–26.

Belin, P., Zatorre, R. J., Lafaille, P., Ahad, P., & Pike, B. (2000). Voice-selective areas in human auditory cortex. *Nature*, 403, 309–312.

Bentin, S., Allison, T., Puce, A., Perez, E., & McCarthy, G. (1996). Electrophysiological studies of face perception in humans. *Journal of Cognitive Neuroscience*, 8, 551–565.

Bentin, S., Taylor, M. J., Rousselet, G. A., Itier, R. J., Caldara, R., Schyns, P. G., . . . Rossion, B. (2007). Controlling interstimulus perceptual variance does not abolish N170 face sensitivity. *Nature Neuroscience*, 10, 802–803.

Bestelmeyer, P. E., Belin, P., & Grosbras, M. H. (2011). Right temporal TMS impairs voice detection. *Current Biology*, 21(20), R838–839. doi: 10.1016/j.cub.2011.08.046

Bestelmeyer, P. E., Belin, P., & Ladd, D. R. (2014). A neural marker for social bias toward in-group accents. *Cerebral Cortex*. doi: 10.1093/cercor/bhu282

Bestelmeyer, P. E., Latinus, M., Bruckert, L., Rouger, J., Crabbe, F., & Belin, P. (2012). Implicitly perceived vocal attractiveness modulates prefrontal cortex activity. *Cerebral Cortex*, 22(6), 1263–1270. doi: 10.1093/cercor/bhr204

Bestelmeyer, P. E., Maurage, P., Rouger, J., Latinus, M., & Belin, P. (2014). Adaptation to vocal expressions reveals multistep perception of auditory emotion. *Journal of Neuroscience*, 34(24), 8098–8105. doi: 10.1523/JNEUROSCI.4820-13.2014

Binder, J. R., Frost, J. A., & Bellgowan, P. S. F. (1999). Superior temporal sulcus (STS) responses to speech and nonspeech auditory stimuli. *Journal of Cognitive Neuroscience*, 11(suppl 1), 99.

Blank, H., Anwander, A., & von Kriegstein, K. (2011). Direct structural connections between voice- and face-recognition areas. *Journal of Neuroscience*, 31(36), 12906–12915. doi: 10.1523/JNEUROSCI.2091-11.2011

Blasi, A., Lloyd-Fox, S., Sethna, V., Brammer, M. J., Mercure, E., Murray, L., … Johnson, M. H. (2015). Atypical processing of voice sounds in infants at risk for autism spectrum disorder. *Cortex*, 71, 122–133. doi: 10.1016/j.cortex.2015.06.015

Blasi, A., Mercure, E., Lloyd-Fox, S., Thomson, A., Brammer, M., Sauter, D., … Murphy, D. G. (2011). Early specialization for voice and emotion processing in the infant brain. *Current Biology*, 21(14), 1220–1224. doi: 10.1016/j.cub.2011.06.009

Bodamer, J. (1947). Die prosop-agnosie. *Archiv fur Psychiatrie und Nervenkrankheiten*, 179, 6–53.

Bruce, V. & Young, A. (1986). Understanding face recognition. *British Journal of Psychology*, 77, 305–327.

Burton, A. M., Bruce, V., & Johnston, R. A. (1990). Understanding face recognition with an interactive activation model. *British Journal of Psychology*, 81, 361–380.

Capilla, A., Belin, P., & Gross, J. (2013). The early spatio-temporal correlates and task independence of cerebral voice processing studied with MEG. *Cerebral Cortex*, 23(6), 1388–1395. doi: 10.1093/cercor/bhs119

Charest, I., Pernet, C., Latinus, M., Crabbe, F., & Belin, P. (2013). Cerebral processing of voice gender studied using a continuous carryover FMRI design. *Cerebral Cortex*, 23(4), 958–966. doi: 10.1093/cercor/bhs090

Charest, I., Pernet, C. R., Rousselet, G. A., Quinones, I., Latinus, M., Fillion-Bilodeau, S., … Belin, P. (2009). Electrophysiological evidence for an early processing of human voices. *BMC Neuroscience*, 10, 127. doi: 10.1186/1471-2202-10-127

Cohen, Y. E., Russ, B. E., Davis, S. J., Baker, A. E., Ackelson, A. L., & Nitecki, R. (2009). A functional role for the ventrolateral prefrontal cortex in non-spatial auditory cognition. *Proceedings of the National Academy of Sciences of the United States of America*, 106, 20045–20050.

Davis, M. H. & Johnsrude, I. S. (2003). Hierarchical processing in spoken language comprehension. *Journal of Neuroscience*, 23, 3423–3431.

Duchaine, B. C. & Nakayama, K. (2006). Developmental prosopagnosia: a window to content-specific face processing. *Current Opinion in Neurobiology*, 16, 166–173.

Ellis, A. W. (1989). Neuro-cognitive processing of faces and voices. In: A. W. Young & H. D. Ellis (eds) *Handbook of Research on Face Processing* (pp. 207–215). Elsevier Science Publishers BV.

Ethofer, T., Bretscher, J., Gschwind, M., Kreifelts, B., Wildgruber, D., & Vuilleumier, P. (2012). Emotional voice areas: anatomic location, functional properties, and structural connections revealed by combined fMRI/DTI. *Cerebral Cortex*, 22(1), 191–200. doi: 10.1093/cercor/bhr113

Ethofer, T., Van De Ville, D., Scherer, K., & Vuilleumier, P. (2009). Decoding of emotional information in voice-sensitive cortices. *Current Biology*, 19, 1028–1033.

Ethofer, T., Wiethoff, S., Anders, S., Kreifelts, B., Grodd, W., & Wildgruber, D. (2007). The voices of seduction: cross-gender effects in processing of erotic prosody. *Social, Cognitive, and Affective Neuroscience*, 2, 334–337.

Fecteau, S., Armony, J. L., Joanette, Y., & Belin, P. (2004). Is voice processing species-specific in human auditory cortex? An fMRI study. *NeuroImage*, 23(3), 840–848. doi: 10.1016/j.neuroimage.2004.09.019

Fecteau, S., Armony, J. L., Joanette, Y., & Belin, P. (2005). Sensitivity to voice in human prefrontal cortex. *Journal of Neurophysiology*, 94, 2251–2254.

Freiwald, W. A. & Tsao, D. Y. (2010). Functional compartmentalization and viewpoint generalization within the macaque face-processing system. *Science*, 330(6005), 845–851. doi: 10.1126/science.1194908

Freiwald, W. A., Tsao, D. Y., & Livingstone, M. S. (2009). A face feature space in the macaque temporal lobe. *Nature Neuroscience*, 12, 1187–1196.

Friederici, A. D. (2005). Neurophysiological markers of early language acquisition: from syllables to sentences. *Trends in Cognitive Sciences*, 9, 481–488.

Garrido, L., Eisner, F., McGettigan, C., Stewart, L., Sauter, D., Hanley, J. R., ... Duchaine, B. (2009). Developmental phonagnosia: a selective deficit of vocal identity recognition. *Neuropsychologia*, 47, 123–131.

Gervais, H., Belin, P., Boddaert, N., Leboyer, M., Coez, A., Sfaello, I., ... Zilbovicius, M. (2004). Abnormal cortical voice processing in autism. *Nature Neuroscience*, 7(8), 801–802. doi: 10.1038/nn1291

Ghazanfar, A. A. (2008). Language evolution: neural differences that make a difference. *Nature Neuroscience*, 11, 382–384.

Gil-da-Costa, R., Braun, A., Lopes, M., Hauser, M. D., Carson, R. E., Herscovitch, P., & Martin, A. (2004). Toward an evolutionary perspective on conceptual representation: species-specific calls activate visual and affective processing systems in the macaque. *Proceedings of the National Academy of Sciences of the United States of America*, 101, 17516–17521.

Gil-da-Costa, R., Martin, A., Lopes, M. A., Munoz, M., Fritz, J. B., & Braun, A. R. (2006). Species-specific calls activate homologs of Broca's and Wernicke's areas in the macaque. *Nature Neuroscience*, 9(8), 1064–1070.

Goggin, J. P., Thompson, C. P., Strube, G., & Simental, L. R. (1991). The role of language familiarity in voice identification. *Memory and Cognition*, 19, 448–458.

Grandjean, D., Sander, D., Pourtois, G., Schwartz, S., Seghier, M. L., Scherer, K. R., & Vuilleumier, P. (2005). The voices of wrath: brain responses to angry prosody in meaningless speech. *Nature Neuroscience*, 8, 145–146.

Grossman, T., Oberecker, R., Koch, S. P., & Friederici, A. D. (2010). The developmental origins of voice processing in the human brain. *Neuron*, 65, 852–858.

Hall, D., Haggard, M. P., Akeroyd, M. A., Palmer, A. R., Quentin Summerfield, A., Elliott, M. R., ... Bowtell, R. W. (1999). 'Sparse' temporal sampling in auditory fMRI. *Human Brain Mapping*, 7, 213–223.

Haxby, J. V., Gobbini, M. I., Furey, M. L., Ishai, A., Schouten, J. L., & Pietrini, P. (2001). Distributed and overlapping representations of faces and objects in ventral temporal cortex. *Science*, 293, 2425–2430.

Haxby, J. V., Hoffman, E. A., & Ida Gobbini, M. (2000). The distributed human neural system for face perception. *Trends in Cognitive Sciences*, 4, 223–233.

Heffner, H. E. & Heffner, R. S. (1984). Temporal lobe lesions and perception of species-specific vocalizations by macaques. *Science*, 226, 75–76.

Joly, O., Pallier, C., Ramus, F., Pressnitzer, D., Vanduffel, W., & Orban, G. A. (2012). Processing of vocalizations in humans and monkeys: a comparative fMRI study. *NeuroImage*, 62(3), 1376–1389. doi: 10.1016/j.neuroimage.2012.05.070

Joly, O., Ramus, F., Pressnitzer, D., Vanduffel, W., & Orban, G. A. (2012). Interhemispheric differences in auditory processing revealed by FMRI in awake rhesus monkeys. *Cerebral Cortex*, 22(4), 838–853. doi: 10.1093/cercor/bhr150

Kanwisher, N., McDermott, J., & Chun, M. M. (1997). The fusiform face area: a module in human extrastriate cortex specialized for face perception. *Journal of Neuroscience*, 17(11), 4302–4311.

Kisilevsky, B. S., Hains, S. M., Lee, K., Xie, X., Huang, H., Ye, H. H., ... Wang, Z. (2003). Effects of experience on fetal voice recognition. *Psychological Science*, 14, 220–224.

Klin, A. (1991). Young autistic children's listening preferences in regard to speech: a possible characterization of the symptom of social withdrawal. *Journal of Autism and Developmental Disorders*, 21, 29–42.

Kreiman, J. (1997). Listening to voices: theory and practice in voice perception research. In: K. Johnson & J. Mullenix (eds) *Talker Variability in Speech Research* (pp. 85–108). New York: Academic Press.

Kreiman, J. & Gerratt, B. R. (2010). Perceptual sensitivity to first harmonic amplitude in the voice source. *Journal of the Acoustical Society of America*, 128(4), 2085–2089. doi: 10.1121/1.3478/84

Latinus, M., Crabbe, F., & Belin, P. (2011). Learning-induced changes in the cerebral processing of voice identity. *Cerebral Cortex*, 21, 2820–2828. doi: 10.1093/cercor/bhr077

Latinus, M., McAleer, P., Bestelmeyer, P. E., & Belin, P. (2013). Norm-based coding of voice identity in human auditory cortex. *Current Biology*, 23(12), 1075–1080. doi: 10.1016/j.cub.2013.04.055

Leopold, D. A., Bondar, I. V., & Giese, M. A. (2006). Norm-based face encoding by single neurons in the monkey inferotemporal cortex. *Nature*, 442(7102), 572–575.

Levy, D. A., Granot, R., & Bentin, S. (2001). Processing specificity for human voice stimuli: electrophysiological evidence. *NeuroReport*, 12(12), 2653–2657.

Linden, D. E., Thornton, K., Kuswanto, C. N., Johnston, S. J., Van de Ven, V., & Jackson, M. C. (2011). The brain's voices: comparing nonclinical auditory hallucinations and imagery. *Cerebral Cortex*, 21, 330–337.

Loffler, G., Yourganov, G., Wilkinson, F., & Wilson, H. R. (2005). fMRI evidence for the neural representation of faces. *Nature Neuroscience*, 8, 1386–1390.

Menon, V., Levitin, D. J., Smith, B. K., Lembke, A., Krasnow, B. D., Glazer, D., ... McAdams, S. (2002). Neural correlates of timbre change in harmonic sounds. *NeuroImage*, 17, 1742–1754.

Moerel, M., De Martino, F., Santoro, R., Ugurbil, K., Goebel, R., Yacoub, E., & Formisano, E. (2013). Processing of natural sounds: characterization of multipeak spectral tuning in human auditory cortex. *Journal of Neuroscience*, 33(29), 11888–11898. doi: 10.1523/JNEUROSCI.5306-12.2013

Obleser, J., Zimmermann, J., Van Meter, J., & Rauschecker, J. P. (2007). Multiple stages of auditory speech perception reflected in event-related FMRI. *Cerebral Cortex*, 17, 2251–2257.

Ockleford, E. M., Vince, M. A., Layton, C., & Reader, M. R. (1988). Responses of neonates to parents' and others' voices. *Early Human Development*, 18, 27–36.

Ortiz-Rios, M., Kusmierek, P., DeWitt, I., Archakov, D., Azevedo, F. A., Sams, M., ... Rauschecker, J. P. (2015). Functional MRI of the vocalization-processing network in the macaque brain. *Frontiers in Neuroscience*, 9, 113. doi: 10.3389/fnins.2015.00113

Pernet, C. R., & Belin, P. (2012). The role of pitch and timbre in voice gender categorization. *Frontiers in Psychology*, 3, 23. doi: 10.3389/fpsyg.2012.00023

Pernet, C. R., McAleer, P., Latinus, M., Gorgolewski, K. J., Charest, I., Bestelmeyer, P. E., … Belin, P. (2015). The human voice areas: spatial organization and inter-individual variability in temporal and extra-temporal cortices. *NeuroImage*, 119, 164–174. doi: 10.1016/j.neuroimage.2015.06.050

Perrachione, T. K., Chiao, J. Y., & Wong, P. C. (2010). Asymmetric cultural effects on perceptual expertise underlie an own-race bias for voices. *Cognition*, 114, 42–55.

Perrodin, C., Kayser, C., Logothetis, N. K., & Petkov, C. I. (2011). Voice cells in the primate temporal lobe. *Current Biology*, 21(16). doi:10.1016/ j.cub.2011.07.028

Petkov, C. I., Kayser, C., Augath, M., & Logothetis, N. K. (2006). Functional imaging reveals numerous fields in the monkey auditory cortex. *PLoS Biology*, 4, 1213–1226.

Petkov, C. I., Kayser, C., Augath, M., & Logothetis, N. K. (2009). Optimizing the imaging of the monkey auditory cortex: sparse vs. continuous fMRI. *Journal of Magnetic Resonance Imaging*, 27(8), 1065–1073. doi: 10.1016/j.mri.2009.01.018

Petkov, C. I., Kayser, C., Steudel, T., Whittingstall, K., Augath, M., & Logothetis, N. K. (2008). A voice region in the monkey brain. *Nature Neuroscience*, 11(2), 367–374.

Petkov, C. I., Kikuchi, Y., Milne, A. E., Mishkin, M., Rauschecker, J. P., & Logothetis, N. K. (2015). Different forms of effective connectivity in primate frontotemporal pathways. *Nature Communications*, 6, 6000. doi: 10.1038/ncomms7000

Petkov, C. I., Logothetis, N. K., & Obleser, J. (2009). Where are the human speech and voice regions, and do other animals have anything like them? *Neuroscientist*, 15, 419–429.

Poremba, A., Saunders, R. C., Crane, A. M., Cook, M., Sokoloff, L., & Mishkin, M. (2003). Functional mapping of the primate auditory system. *Science*, 299, 568–572.

Rauschecker, J. P., Tian, B., & Hauser, M. (1995). Processing of complex sounds in the macaque nonprimary auditory cortex. *Science*, 268, 111–114.

Rogier, O., Roux, S., Belin, P., Bonnet-Brilhault, F., & Bruneau, N. (2010). An electrophysiological correlate of voice processing in 4- to 5-year-old children. *International Journal of Psychophysiology*, 75, 44–47.

Romanski, L. M., Averbeck, B. B., & Diltz, M. (2005). Neural representation of vocalizations in the primate ventrolateral prefrontal cortex. *Journal of Neurophysiology*, 93(2), 734–747.

Rossion, B. (2014). Understanding face perception by means of prosopagnosia and neuroimaging. *Frontiers in Bioscience (Elite Edition)*, 6, 258–307.

Roswandowitz, C., Mathias, S. R., Hintz, F., Kreitewolf, J., Schelinski, S., & von Kriegstein, K. (2014). Two cases of selective developmental voice-recognition impairments. *Current Biology*, 24(19), 2348–2353. doi: 10.1016/j.cub.2014.08.048

Rutherford, M. D., Baron-Cohen, S., & Wheelwright, S. (2002). Reading the mind in the voice: a study with normal adults and adults with Asperger syndrome and high functioning autism. *Journal of Autism and Developmental Disorders*, 32, 189–194.

Schirmer, A., & Kotz, S. A. (2006). Beyond the right hemisphere: brain mechanisms mediating vocal emotional processing. *Trends in Cognitive Sciences*, 10, 24–30.

Schirmer, A., Kotz, S. A., & Friederici, A. D. (2002). Sex differentiates the role of emotional prosody during word processing. *Cognitive Brain Research*, 14, 228–233.

Schweinberger, S. R., Kawahara, H., Simpson, A. P., Skuk, V. G., & Zaske, R. (2014). Speaker perception. *Wiley Interdisciplinary Reviews: Cognitive Science*, 5(1), 15–25. doi: 10.1002/wcs.1261

Scott, S. K., Blank, C. C., Rosen, S., & Wise, R. J. (2000). Identification of a pathway for intelligible speech in the left temporal lobe. *Brain*, 123, 2400–2406.

Suied, C., Agus, T. R., Thorpe, S. J., Mesgarani, N., & Pressnitzer, D. (2014). Auditory gist: recognition of very short sounds from timbre cues. *Journal of the Acoustical Society of America*, 135(3), 1380–1391. doi: 10.1121/1.4863659

Thierry, G., Martin, C. D., Downing, P., & Pegna, A. J. (2007). Controlling for interstimulus perceptual variance abolishes N170 face selectivity. *Nature Neuroscience*, 10, 505–511.

Thompson, P. (1980). Margaret Thatcher: a new illusion. *Perception*, 9, 483–484.

Tsao, D. Y., Freiwald, W. A., Knutsen, T. A., Mandeville, J. B., & Tootell, R. B. (2003). Faces and objects in macaque cerebral cortex. *Nature Neuroscience*, 6, 989–995.

Tsao, D. Y., Freiwald, W. A., Tootell, R. B. H., & Livingstone, M. S. (2006). A cortical region consisting entirely of face-selective cells. *Science*, 311, 670–674.

Tsao, D. Y. & Livingstone, M. S. (2008). Mechanisms of face perception. *Annual Review of Neuroscience*, 31, 411–437. doi: 10.1146/annurev.neuro.30.051606.094238

Van Lancker, D. R., Cummings, J. L., Kreiman, J., & Dobkin, B. H. (1988). Phonagnosia: a dissociation between familiar and unfamiliar voices. *Cortex*, 24, 195–209.

von Kriegstein, K. & Giraud, A. L. (2004). Distinct functional substrates along the right superior temporal sulcus for the processing of voices. *NeuroImage*, 22, 948–955.

von Kriegstein, K. & Giraud, A. L. (2006). Implicit multisensory associations influence voice recognition. *PLoS Biology*, 4, e326.

von Kriegstein, K., Kleinschmidt, A., Sterzer, P., & Giraud, A.-L. (2005). Interaction of face and voice areas during speaker recognition. *Journal of Cognitive Neuroscience*, 17, 367–376.

Warren, J. D., Jennings, A. R., & Griffiths, T. D. (2005). Analysis of the spectral envelope of sounds by the human brain. *NeuroImage*, 24, 1052–1057.

Watson, R., Crabbe, F., Quinones, I., Charest, I., Bestelmeyer, P., Latinus, M., & Belin, P. (2009). *Auditory response of the temporal voice areas (TVA) predicts memory performance for voices, but not bells.* Paper presented at the Human Brain Mapping meeting, San Francisco, USA.

Xu, X., Biederman, I., Shilowich, B. E., Herald, S. B., Amir, O., & Allen, N. E. (2015). Developmental phonagnosia: neural correlates and a behavioral marker. *Brain and Language*, 149, 106–117. doi: 10.1016/j.bandl.2015.06.007

Yin, R. K. (1969). Looking at upside-down faces. *Journal of Experimental Psychology*, 81, 141–145.

Young, A. W. & Bruce, V. (2011). Understanding person perception. *British Journal of Psychology*, 102(4), 959–974. doi: 10.1111/j.2044-8295.2011.02045.x

Zaske, R., Skuk, V. G., Kaufmann, J. M., & Schweinberger, S. R. (2013). Perceiving vocal age and gender: an adaptation approach. *Acta Psychologica (Amsterdam)*, 144(3), 583–593. doi: 10.1016/j.actpsy.2013.09.009

CHAPTER 4

ACOUSTIC PATTERNING OF EMOTION VOCALIZATIONS

KLAUS R. SCHERER

4.1 THE EVOLUTIONARY ORIGIN AND COMMUNICATIVE FUNCTION OF VOCAL EMOTION EXPRESSION

THE voice is one of the prime channels for the expression of emotion, a fact that has been commented upon ever since the ancient schools of rhetoric (Aristoteles, Cicero, Quintilian). It can be reasonably argued that the phylogenetic continuity of vocalization as a medium of emotion expression provides important information for the emergence of speech and music in the human species (Scheiner & Fischer, 2011). Both animals and humans produce different kinds of vocal 'affect bursts' under conditions of strong affective arousal, traces of which can be found in the form of interjections in many languages (Scherer, 1994). Early on, Darwin provided some pertinent examples in an argument for the functionality of emotional expression: 'under the feeling of contempt or disgust, there is a tendency, from intelligible causes, to blow out of the mouth or nostrils, and this produces sounds like pooh or pish' (Darwin, 1872/1998, pp. 92–93). Darwin thought that expression followed adaptive actions of the body. For example, in the case of disgust, the avoidance of a bad odour or bad taste is a normal kind of instinctive reaction, and the vocalization that follows is a by-product which takes on a very particular kind of function in the context of social interaction, both within and across species, by informing the observer of the state of the expressor and their respective action or intention to act (Scherer, 1992, 1994). Once a behaviour has acquired this communicative functionality, then this function obviously becomes an object of evolutionary selection, as Darwin showed with many examples. Due to the selective advantage of communicating emotion through motor expression, primitive affect bursts may be the precursors, not only of emotional expression in humans, but also of speech, language, and music (Scherer, 1991, 2013a). This hypothesis is not unreasonable considering how humans use affect vocalizations as a means of communication, for example, when we are unable to produce speech or when we use the same conventionalized vocal emblems across different languages, such as the wailing patterns in mourning rituals.

Affect bursts generally consist of single sounds or repeated sounds. In protohuman and human species, these have evolved into more complex sound sequence patterns, showing the rudiments of syntax, and melody-like intonation patterns (with singing possibly pre-dating speech and a subsequent parallelism in development, at least, with respect to the pragmatic functions such as emotion signalling). Brown (2000) has argued for what he calls a 'musilanguage' model of music evolution, and Mithen (2005) hypothesized that Neanderthals possibly used a form of protomusical language (the 'Hmmmmm communication system'). Specifically, Mithen proposed that the system was (a) holistic, because it relied on whole phrases rather than words, rather like music; (b) manipulative, because it focused on manipulating behaviour of others rather than the transmission of information; (c) multimodal, because it used the body as well as the voice; (d) musical, because it used the variations in pitch, rhythm, and timbre for emotion expression, care of infants, sexual display, and group bonding; and (e) mimetic, because it involved a high degree of mime and mimicry of the natural world.

The evolutionary origin and communicative function of vocal emotion expression are highlighted here as they are essential for the understanding of the mechanisms underlying the acoustic patterning of emotion vocalizations. Due to the important role in communication of vocal emotion expression, both the production of the acoustic emotion signal by the sender and the perception and interpretation by the receiver need to be taken into account. This process can be illustrated by the dynamic Tripartite Emotion Expression and Perception (TEEP) model, based on a modified Brunswikian lens model (Brunswik, 1956; Scherer, 2003, 2013a). The model, shown in Figure 4.1, illustrates how the sender continuously expresses ongoing emotion processes through a multitude of distal cues to the observer, who perceives these as proximal cues and probabilistically attributes the emotion processes unfolding in the sender. The degree to which the proximal cues capture the information content of the distal cues depends on the quality of the transmission channel and the response characteristics of sensory organs. The model is dynamic as it reflects the process nature of the underlying emotion episodes. In contrast to the general assumption in the literature that a stable emotional 'state' is expressed and recognized, the model assumes that the event, the appraisals, and the consequent response patterns continuously change (as do, in consequence, the observer attributions). The model is 'tripartite' as it calls attention to the fact that any sign has three functions (Bühler, 1934/1984; Scherer, 1988):

1. It provides symptoms of an ongoing emotional process in the sender.
2. It signals the emotion and thus appeals to the observer.
3. It symbolizes or represents meaning in the respective species or group (due to the ritualization of the link between symptom and appeal, or the existence of a shared code for encoding and decoding).

It should be noted that the respective elliptic shapes in Figure 4.1 are not active elements of the dynamic model but serve to highlight these three functions.

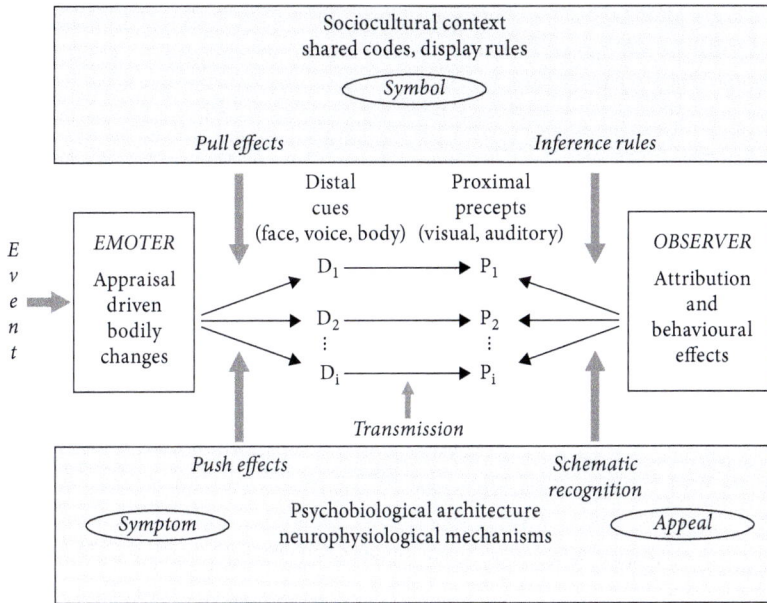

FIGURE 4.1 The tripartite emotion expression and perception (TEEP) model showing the communication of emotion through non-verbal cues. TEEP provides a framework to empirically assess cue validity and observer perception capacity. The left side of the model represents the production; the right side, the perception and inference phase of the communication process.

Adapted from Scherer K.R. (2013) 'Emotion in action, interaction, music, and speech'. In: Arbib A. (ed), *Language, music, and the brain: a mysterious relationship*, pp. 107–139, Cambridge, MA: MIT Press.

The TEEP model highlights the fact that the production of the distal expressive cues and their proximal interpretation are determined both by psychobiological mechanisms and the rules or expectations generated by the sociocultural context. In consequence, the model distinguishes between push and pull effects on the production side, and schematic recognition and inference rules on the perception side (Scherer, 1988). Push effects are motor response patterns due to physiological changes within the individual and to the preparation of motor actions as a consequence of emotion-antecedent appraisal. In contrast, pull effects are expressive configurations that are part of a socially shared communication code serving as socio-communicative signals used to inform or influence other group members. The distal cue characteristics are 'pulled' into the acoustic patterns required by strategic sender intentions or the social context (for further detail, see Scherer, 2013a, pp. 119–120).

In the context of this chapter, it is interesting to discuss the difference between non-verbal vocal expressions and emotional prosody. Both are covered by the TEEP model but one would expect differences in the underlying mechanisms. Thus, unintentional changes in voice quality are most likely produced by pure push effects. In contrast, emotional prosody, for example, emotion-specific intonation contours (see Bänziger & Scherer, 2005), are probably produced by pull effects exerted by language- or culture-specific rules.

However, there are likely to be exceptions. For example, the adoption of a particular voice quality (e.g. dark and hoarse, as found in some female subcultures), even unintentionally, would be driven by push effects.

4.2 VOICE PRODUCTION
AND ACOUSTIC PARAMETERS

Humans produce vocal sounds by pressing a column of air from the lungs through the glottis. The air stream is transformed into an oscillating waveform through the action of opening and closing the vocal folds (the source). This waveform is then 'filtered' through the shape of the upper vocal tract, especially the pharynx, mouth, and nose areas (the filter), producing specific energy distributions in the spectrum of the resulting sound waves. The major characteristics of the complex vocal sound waves are:

1) their fundamental frequency, mostly determined by the rate of vibration of the vocal folds, and heard as pitch;
2) their amplitude or energy, determined in particular by the subglottal air pressure, and heard as loudness;
3) the spectrum of the sound (the energy distribution across the upper frequency components), determined by the vocal tract configuration including phonation and articulation parameters, heard as voice quality and serving phoneme identification in speech contexts.

As voice production is a dynamic phenomenon, all these production processes unfold in the time domain (for further information on voice production, see Kreiman & Sidtis, 2011).

While modern imagery technology now makes it possible to actually observe, and to some extent, measure these processes *in vivo* (Echternach et al., 2012), the royal road to empirically study the process of voice production and the resulting vocal signals has been the extraction of a large number of acoustic parameters in the domains of frequency, amplitude, frequency × amplitude (spectrum), and time. Given the ease of extraction of these parameters with modern digital audio-processing capacity, the number of acoustic variables used in voice research has sky-rocketed, especially in the area of machine learning (e.g. automatic classification of vocally expressed emotions). To provide some guidelines for parameter selection, an interdisciplinary group of voice researchers has drawn up a list of the 'must have' parameters—the Geneva Minimalistic Acoustic Parameter Set (GEMAPS; Eyben et al., 2015). Box 4.1 shows a slightly expanded version of the GEMAPS that will be referred to in this chapter (for more detailed information on vocal acoustic parameters, see Juslin & Scherer, 2005; Kreiman & Sidtis, 2011).

Box 4.1 Expanded listing of the GEMAPS parameter set

Frequency related parameters

Fundamental frequency (Fo; estimation of pitch), logarithmic Fo on a semitone frequency scale, starting at 27.5 Hz (semitone 0)
 Jitter, deviations in individual consecutive Fo period lengths
 Formant 1, 2, and 3 frequency, centre frequency of first, second, and third formant
 Formant 1, bandwidth of first formant

Energy/amplitude related parameters (estimation of loudness)

Formant 1, 2, and 3 relative energy, as well as the ratio of the energy of the spectral harmonic peak at the first, second, third formant's centre frequency to the energy of the spectral peak at Fo
 Shimmer, difference of the peak amplitudes of consecutive Fo periods
 Loudness, estimate of perceived signal intensity from an auditory spectrum
 Harmonics-to-noise ratio (HNR), relation of energy in harmonic components to energy in noise-like components

Spectral parameters (estimation of spectral balance and relative prominence)

Alpha ratio, ratio of the summed energy from 50–1000 Hz and 1–5 kHz
 Hammarberg index, ratio of the strongest energy peak in the 0–2 kHz region to the strongest peak in the 2–5 kHz region
 Spectral slope 0–500 Hz and 500–1500 Hz, linear regression slope of the logarithmic power spectrum within the two given bands
 Harmonic difference H1–H2, ratio of energy of the first Fo harmonic (H1) to the energy of the second Fo harmonic (H2)
 Harmonic difference H1–A3, ratio of energy of the first Fo harmonic (H1) to the energy of the highest harmonic in the third formant range (A3)

Time-related parameters (estimation of duration and tempo)

The **rate of loudness peaks**, i.e. the number of loudness peaks per second
 The **mean length** and the **standard deviation** of continuously **voiced regions** (Fo > 0)
 The **mean length** and the **standard deviation** of **unvoiced regions** (Fo = 0; approximating pauses)
 The **number of continuous voiced regions per second** (pseudo syllable rate)

Source: data from Eyben F. et al., 'The Geneva Minimalistic Acoustic Parameter Set (GeMAPS) for Voice Research and Affective Computing', *IEEE Transactions on Affective Computing*, Copyright © 2016, IEEE, doi: 10.1109/TAFFC.2015.2457417

4.3 THE IMPACT OF EMOTIONS ON VOICE PRODUCTION (ENCODING)

4.3.1 Theory

As shown in the TEEP model in Figure 4.1, appraisal-driven emotional processes will produce bodily changes that impact voice production parameters and consequently result in specific changes in the acoustic patterning of the vocal signal, corresponding to the 'push effects' described in this chapter's introductory section 'The evolutionary origin and communicative function of vocal emotion expression'. Concretely, the assumption is that the efferent response patterns (including physiological changes and facial/vocal expression) accompanying emotion episodes are produced by specific results of *appraisal* processes, that is, the evaluation of the relevance and the consequences of a specific event for the individual, constituting adaptive responses to the need for information processing and action tendencies to cope with the event (Ellsworth & Scherer, 2003; Scherer, 2009). For example, it is well established that autonomic arousal and muscle tension will increase in preparation for action (e.g. fighting). Changes in muscle tension and breathing will strongly affect voice production. In addition, vocal signals, expressing the size and power of an individual, are important elements of dominance fights in both many animals and humans (Fitch, 2000). In consequence, it can be reasonably argued that the specificity in the acoustic patterning of emotions can be predicted on the basis of the cumulative result of the adaptive changes produced by a specific appraisal profile and its efferent consequences (for detailed reviews of this hypothetical patterning mechanism see Scherer, 1986a; Smith & Scott, 1997).

Based on these assumptions, Scherer (1986a, pp. 149–159) has produced an extensive set of predictions concerning the physiological changes, and the ensuing consequences for the voice production mechanism, that can be expected for appraisal results on specific dimensions (based on functional considerations). The complexity of these predictions does not allow for their presentation in detail here. Briefly put, the justification for the predictions rests in using the assumed functional consequence of a particular appraisal result to predict the pattern of peripheral physiological arousal that is likely to result. Then, the effects of the respective physiological pattern on the voice production process are estimated and the acoustic concomitants are inferred. For example, appraising an event as being obstructive to reaching an important goal requires strong action (e.g. fighting), which should lead to high sympathetic arousal with the consequent changes for respiration and muscle tension, and thereby changes in phonation (higher Fo, different glottal pulse shape producing energy changes in the spectrum). Similarly, it is predicted that an appraisal of high coping potential (e.g. power to deal with an obstacle) will lead to orofacial changes evolutionarily linked to biting behaviour. The configuration of the vocal tract produced by this setting will privilege certain filter characteristics of the vocal tract (see Ladefoged, 1975; Laver, 1980; Scherer, 1986a) and will thus affect energy distribution in the spectrum. Given that the bodily changes that affect vocalization are directly caused by the appraisal of the consequences of the eliciting event, it seems reasonable to focus on the differential effects of different appraisal checks in order to understand the underlying mechanisms. Table 4.1 summarizes some of the hypotheses concerning the vocal parameter configurations to be expected for a number of specific appraisal results.

Based on the expected effects of different appraisal checks, specific hypotheses for the acoustic patterning of individual, discrete emotions (like anger, fear, joy, or sadness) can be derived, as there is well-established knowledge about the appraisal outcome configurations that tend to produce the major discrete emotions (Scherer & Meuleman, 2013). Table 4.2 reproduces these early predictions (Scherer, 1986a, Table 6) together with the empirical evidence available today, more than 30 years later, as described in the next section.

Table 4.1 Predicted effects of different appraisal check results on vocalization processes and the resulting acoustic patterning (adapted from Scherer, 1986a)

Check	Production	Type of voice	Acoustic parameters
Pleasant	faucal and pharyngeal expansion, relaxation of tract walls, vocal tract shortened due to AU 25 action	wide	increase in low-frequency energy, F1 falling, slightly broader F1 bandwidth, velopharyngeal nasality, resonances raised
Unpleasant	faucal and pharyngeal constriction, tensing of tract walls, vocal tract shortened due to AU 15 action	narrow	more high-frequency energy, F1 rising, F2 and F3 falling, narrow F1 bandwidth, laryngopharyngeal nasality, resonances raised
Relevant and consistent	overall relaxation of vocal apparatus	relaxed	F0 at lower end of range, low-to-moderate amplitude, balanced resonance with slight decrease in high-frequency energy
Relevant and discrepant	overall tensing of vocal apparatus	tense	F0 and amplitude increase, jitter and shimmer, increase in high-frequency energy, narrow F1 bandwidth, pronounced formant frequency differences
Low control	hypotonus of vocal apparatus	lax	low F0 and restricted F0 range, low amplitude, weak pulses, very low high-frequency energy, spectral noise, format frequencies tending toward neutral setting, broad F1 bandwidth
High control	tensing	tense	see tense voice
High power	chest register phonation	full	low F0, high amplitude, strong energy in entire frequency range
Low power	head register phonation	thin	raised F0, widely spaced harmonics with relatively low energy

Adapted with permission from Scherer, K.R. 'Vocal affect expression: A review and a model for future research', *Pychological Bulletin*, Volume 99, Issue 2, pp. 143–65, Copyright © 1986 American Psychological Association, doi: 10.1037/0033-2909.99.2.143

4.3.2 Empirical Studies

The basis of any functionally valid communication of emotion via vocal expression is that different types of emotion are actually characterized by unique patterns or configurations of acoustic cues. In the context of the TEEP model described at the outset, this means that identifiable emotional states of the sender are in fact externalized by a specific set of objectively measurable distal cues. Without such distinguishable acoustic patterns for different emotions, the nature of the underlying speaker state could not be communicated reliably. A sizeable number of empirical studies (although much inferior to the mass of work in the neighbouring area of facial expression) over the last seven decades have attempted to determine to what extent elicitation of emotional speaker states will produce corresponding acoustic changes.

Table 4.2 Predictions for the direction of acoustic parameter changes for major emotions as based on theoretical considerations (TP) and cumulated empirical findings (EP)

Emotion	Happiness/joy		Disgust/contempt		Sadness/grief		Fear/anxiety		Hot anger		Boredom	
Source	TP	EP	TP	EP	TP	EP	TP	EP	TP	EP	TP	EP
F0 mean	↑=	↑	↑	↓↑	↓↑	↑	↑↑	↑	↓↑	↑	↓	↑
F0 SD	↑	↑	↑	↑	↓	↑	↑↑	↑	↑↑	↑	↑	↑
F0 contour	↑	=			↓=	=	↑	=	=			=
Jitter	↑		↑	=	↑		↑		↑↑	↑		=
Intensity mean	↑=	↑	↑	↑	↓	↑	↓	↑	↑↑	↑	↓	↑
Intensity SD	↑	↑		↑	↑	↑	↑	↑	↑	↑	↑	↑
F1 mean	↓	↑	↑	↓	↑	↑	↑	↑	↑↑	↑		↑
F1 bandwidth	↓↓	↓	↓↓	↑	↓↑		↑↑				↓↑	↑
Formant precision	↑		↑	↑		↑	↑	↑	↑	↑		↑
High-frequency energy	↓↑	=		↑	↓↑	↑	↑	↑	↑↑	↑	↓↑	↑
Speech rate	↑=	↑	↑	↑	↓↑	↑		↑	↑	↑		↑

Note: TP based on Scherer (1986a, Table 6); EP based on Juslin & Scherer (2005, Table 3.2); ˅ decrease, ^ increase, = no change; shaded cells indicate instances of major disagreement between TP and EP

These production-side *encoding* studies can be classified into three major categories— natural vocal expression, induced emotional expression, and simulated emotional expression. Scherer (2003) has extensively documented this literature and the different approaches. Recording during naturally occurring emotional states, such as dangerous flight situations for pilots, journalists reporting emotion-eliciting events, affectively loaded therapy sessions, or talk and game shows on TV, have high ecological validity but often suffer from serious methodological problems (usually only a single or a very small number of speakers, generally very brief durations, low recording quality, difficulty to determine the precise nature of the underlying emotion, potential effects of social control).

Most induction studies have used indirect paradigms that include stress induction via difficult tasks to be completed under time pressure, the presentation of emotion-inducing films or slides, or imagery methods. While this approach, generally favoured by experimental psychologists because of the degree of control it affords, does result in comparable voice samples for all participants, there are a number of serious drawbacks including relatively weak affective arousal and the fact that there is no guarantee that similar emotional states are produced in all individuals (precisely because of the individual differences in event appraisal mentioned in Section 4.3.1 of this chapter). Scherer and his collaborators, in the context of a large-scale study on emotion effects in automatic speaker verification, have attempted to remedy some of these shortcomings by developing a computerized induction battery for a variety of different states (Scherer et al., 2000). Another successful procedure to induce realistic, spontaneous emotions in the laboratory consists of experimentally manipulated computer games (e.g. Johnstone et al., 2005).

The preferred way of obtaining emotional voice samples in this field consists of obtaining simulated (portrayed) or enacted vocal expressions. Professional or lay actors are asked to produce vocal expressions of emotion (often using standard verbal content) as based on emotion labels and/or typical scenarios. This procedure yields much more intense, prototypical expressions than are found for induced states or even natural emotions (especially when highly controlled, as for example in public settings). However, it cannot be excluded that actors overemphasize relatively obvious cues and miss more subtle ones that might appear in natural expression of emotion (Scherer, 1986a, p. 144). It has often been argued that emotion portrayals reflect sociocultural norms or expectations more than the psychophysiological effects on the voice as they occur under natural conditions. However, it can also be argued that all publicly observable expressions are to some extent 'portrayals' (given the social constraints on expression and unconscious tendencies toward self-presentation; see Scherer & Bänziger, 2010). Furthermore, since vocal portrayals are reliably recognized by listener-judges (see Sections 4 and 5) it can be assumed that they reflect, at least in part, 'normal' expression patterns (if the two were to diverge too much, the acted version would lose its credibility). However, there can be little doubt that actors' portrayals are influenced by conventionalized stereotypes of vocal expression (the 'pull' factors mentioned in the description of the TEEP model) and may be prone to overacting. Because of the presumed lack of ecological validity, this approach is regularly criticized in the literature. However, after an extensive discussion of the issues involved, Scherer and Bänziger (2010, p. 166) conclude:

> ... that an analysis of pure push factors, spontaneous unregulated expressions, is unrealistic in practice and probably of little interest, given the scarcity of such pure expressions in social

life. We suggest that one focus of current research should instead be directed toward the explicit study of pull effects, the use of actor portrayals being a highly appropriate methodological choice for this aim, given the possibility of manipulating and standardizing pull effects. The central role of actor portrayals clearly lies in the empirical and experimental study of the shared code of emotional signalling and the examination of cue utilization in emotion perception and inference.

Jürgens and colleagues (2011) collected affect expressions in radio interviews and had them re-enacted by lay and professional actors. The authors report no differences in arousal but variations in voice quality and Fo contour. However, these might also be due to the fact that affective expression in radio interviews is generally based on recalled feelings and subject to display rules imposed by the public setting of a radio interview (see Kappas & Polikova, 2008, on the role of situational context). A recent paper by Juslin et al. (2018) provides important new insights on the issue of real versus enacted emotions. The authors assembled a new database consisting of 1,877 voice clips from 23 datasets, and used it to systematically compare spontaneous and posed expressions across four experiments. Results indicated that (a) spontaneous expressions were generally rated as less emotionally intense, and more positive in valence, than posed expressions; (b) spontaneous expressions were generally rated as more genuinely emotional than were posed expressions even after controlling for differences in emotion intensity; (c) there were significant though small acoustic differences between the stimulus types; and (d) spontaneous expressions with high intensity conveyed discrete emotions to listeners to a similar degree as has been found for posed expressions.

As shown in the preceding paragraphs, all of the methods that have been used to obtain vocal emotion expression samples have both advantages and disadvantages. In the long run, the best strategies seem to look for convergences between all three approaches in the results for the acoustic patterning found for the major emotions. Juslin and Scherer (2005, Table 3.3, p. 91) have reviewed the converging evidence for portrayed and naturally occurring emotions, showing that the observed patterns are extremely similar. In a recent experimental study with participants from three different language groups, the effects of an established psychological mood induction technique (the Velten procedure) with a classic acting/portrayal approach on a set of major acoustic parameters were directly compared. The results showed that the elicitation of positive/happy and negative/sad utterance through both tasks yields essentially the same differences in both tasks for energy, Fo, spectral, and temporal parameters. In comparison, task differences had much less effect (Scherer, 2013b).

4.3.3 The Evidence

Following Williams and Stevens (1972), an ever-growing number of studies have examined the acoustic correlates of vocal emotion expression. Juslin and Laukka (2003, Tables 2 and 7) and Scherer et al. (2003, Table 23.2) reviewed the empirical evidence on the acoustic patterns found for the major discrete emotions (mostly anger, fear, happiness, and sadness; in some studies also boredom, disgust/contempt, love/tenderness, surprise, stress/arousal). Juslin and Scherer (2005, Table 3.2) have synthesized these results and generated a set of empirically based predictions for fifteen voice cues associated with the most commonly investigated discrete emotions, as well as stress/arousal. These *empirically derived* predictions (EP) are shown in Table 4.2 next to the theoretically based predictions (TP) published in Scherer (1986a). The comparison shows that by and large the theoretical predictions are confirmed or compatible with the empirically determined patterns—except in the case of the frequency and bandwidth of formant 1 (F1). Given the relatively large number of studies, performed in different countries and different languages, with widely varying recording conditions and emotion induction or portrayal conditions, this suggests a remarkable stability of the effects of major emotions on the voice and the acoustic patterns that characterize these.

Importantly, the state of the empirical evidence shows that the assumption, often found in the literature, that, contrary to the face, which is capable of communicating qualitative differences between emotions, the voice could only signal levels of physiological arousal (for a detailed discussion see Juslin & Laukka, 2003; Juslin & Scherer, 2005; Scherer, 1986a) is erroneous. Many studies have shown that acoustic properties of speech vary with respect to the emotional quality, intensity, and context (see also Bachorowski & Owren, 1995). Furthermore, studies of emotion encoding in voice from a cross-cultural perspective (comparing tonal and non-tonal languages) found that fundamental frequency and speech rate were used in different ways by speakers of different cultures (Anolli et al., 2008; Ross et al., 1986). This finding confirms that vocal expression does not exclusively signal physiological arousal but also qualitative and culturally sensitive differences between emotions.

There are three limitations to this generally rather satisfactory account:

1) Most studies have focused on only four emotion families—anger, fear, happiness, and sadness. However, in many cases, members of these families may show rather different vocal patterns (e.g. irritation, cold anger vs. hot anger, rage; anxiety vs. panic fear), mostly related to important differences in arousal. In addition, these four families constitute only a small portion of the large number of emotions that seem to be vocally communicated in everyday life.

2) Only a relatively small number of acoustic parameters, mostly related to pitch (Fo), loudness (energy), and tempo (see Table 3.2 in Juslin & Scherer, 2005), have been used consistently in studies in this domain, with the result that the evidence for more advanced parameters (e.g. in the spectral domain) is rather weak. However, a larger set of parameters is required to differentiate a larger number of different emotions, including more subtle ones.

3) There has been little study of the physiological production mechanisms that underlie emotion-induced changes in different acoustic parameters. However, this is an important link if one wants to compare the empirical results on digitally measured acoustic parameters of the waveform to the theoretical predictions about the influence of emotional changes on voice production (see Scherer, 1986a).

There have been some efforts to remedy these shortcomings. As to the focus on only limited emotion families, Banse and Scherer (1996) studied a representative number of fourteen different emotions enacted by German-speaking professional actors, including members of the same emotion family with similar emotion quality and different arousal and intensity levels (hot anger, cold anger, panic fear, anxiety, despair, sadness, elation, happiness, interest, boredom, shame, pride, disgust, and contempt). Using

a factorial design, out of a total of 1,344 recordings, 224 of the best recognized enactments were subjected to the extraction of approximately thirty acoustic parameters in
the time, frequency, energy, and spectral domains. Multivariate discriminant analyses
(MDA) showed that the fourteen emotions could be distinguished at a higher hit rate
than the recognition by human judges (Table 9 in Banse & Scherer, 1996). Extending
this approach, Bänziger and Scherer (2010) recorded the Geneva Multimodal Emotion
Portrayal (GEMEP), consisting of more than 7,000 audio–video emotion portrayals, representing eighteen emotions (including rarely studied subtle emotions), portrayed by ten
French-speaking professional actors who were coached by a professional director (see
also Bänziger et al., 2012).

Goudbeek and Scherer (2010) chose the 120 best recognized enactments of twelve emotions (one per actor), in a factorial design controlling for the dimensions of valence and intensity (and identifying control/power), and again analysed approximately thirty acoustic
parameters representing the major measurement domains. Multivariate analysis of variance (MANOVA) showed highly significant differences between the twelve emotions on
virtually all of these parameters (see Goudbeek & Scherer, 2010, pp. 1326–1329). The authors also compared the pattern of the results for the standardized variables to the earlier
study by Banse and Scherer (1996). Eight parameters (duration, duration of the voiced segments, Fo mean, Fo standard deviation, intensity mean, proportion of energy below 500
Hz, proportion of energy below 1000 Hz, and the Hammarberg index) and nine emotions
(anger, anxiety, despair, fear, interest, irritation, joy, pride, and sadness) that were present
in both corpora could be directly compared. The results showed virtually no significant differences in the patterns and profile correlation parameters (see Goudbeek & Scherer, 2010,
pp. 1328–1330).

In a more recent study, Scherer et al. (2017a) used a larger number of well-recognized
portrayals from the GEMEP corpus (N = 474) to replicate the earlier results and established more stable estimates for the acoustic patterning of this set of twelve major emotions, using a new standard set of acoustic parameters (GEMAPS) (see Eyben et al., 2015).
The results, confirming most of the patterns found earlier, are shown in Table 4.3 and compared to recent results of a cross-cultural study reported by Laukka et al. (2016; see details
below).

These and other studies (e.g. Laukka et al., 2005; Sauter et al., 2010) have remedied the
concern regarding the number and nature of acoustic parameters measured.

As to concern that there has been little study of the physiological production mechanisms that underlie emotion-induced changes in different acoustic parameters, Patel
et al. (2011) have examined voice characteristics in ten actors' productions of a sustained /a/ vowel in five emotions (drawn from the GEMEP corpus already described)
according to physiological variations in phonation (using acoustic parameters derived
from the acoustic signal and the inverse filter estimated voice source waveform). Results
show significant emotion main effects for eleven of twelve parameters. Subsequent principal components analysis revealed three components that explain acoustic variations
due to emotion, including 'tension', 'perturbation', and 'voicing frequency'. Furthermore,
Sundberg et al. (2011) studied the interdependencies among these twelve acoustic parameters and grouped them according to the underlying physiological mechanisms—three
being related to subglottal pressure, five to the transglottal air flow waveform derived
from inverse filtering the audio signal, and four to vocal fold vibration. Each emotion

Table 4.3 Comparison of analysis of variance results for selected acoustic parameters (based on GEMAPS) for vocal expressions for major emotions in two large-scale actor enactment corpora (GEMEP and VENEC) (adapted from Scherer et al., 2017a)

Acoustic cue		Emotion Effect			Trends for the Emotion Effect		
		F	p	Eta	High (↑)	Medium (=)	Low (↓)
Frequency related cues							
F0sem_M	GEMEP	59.90	0.000	0.61	pan, joy, amu, ang, des >	pri	irr > anx, int, rel > ple, sad
	VENEC	38.79	0.001	0.44	Fe, Ha, In, An	Sa	Pr, Re, (Co), Sh, Ne, (Lu)
F0sem_pctlrange13	GEMEP	7.01	0.000	0.15	pri > int > amu, rel >	ang, des, irr, joy >	anx, fea, ple, sad
	VENEC	5.60	0.001	0.10	In, (Lu), (Co)	Pr, Ha, An, Sa, Re, Sh	Fe, Ne
F0sem_M_Rise Slp	GEMEP	3.02	0.001	0.07	Amu, des, irr, sad	ang, anx, fea, int, joy, ple, pri, rel	
	VENEC	3.81	0.001	0.07	Fe, Sa	Ne, Sh, Pr, (Lu), (Co), Re, An	Ha, In
F0sem_M_Fall_Slp	GEMEP	4.35	0.000	0.10	des > amu > irr, sad, joy	ang, fea, int, irr, ple, pri, rel, sad > anx	
	VENEC	1.90	0.043	0.04	(Lu)	Sa, Li, Sh, (Co), Pr, An, Fe, Ha, Ne	Re
FlFreqM	GEMEP	26.54	0.000	0.41	fea > joy > amu, ang, des >	rel > int, ple >	anx, irr, pri, sad
	VENEC	5.74	0.001	0.10	Fe, An	Ha, In, (Lu), Re, Sa, (Co), Sh, Pr	Ne
FlFreqSD	GEMEP	3.25	0.000	0.08	sad > amu, ang, des, int, irr, ple	arx, joy, pri, rel > fea	
	VENEC	3.79	0.001	0.07	An, Ha, Sa	Fe, Pr, (Co), Re, In, (Lu), Sh	Ne
Energy related cues							
Loudness_M	GEMEP	13.23	0.000	0.25	ang >	fea, rel, des, joy > ple, pri	amu, anx, int, irr > sad
	VENEC	60.60	0.001	0.55	An, Ha, Fe	In, (Co), Pr, Re	Sa, Ne, Sh, (Lu)
HNR_M	GEMEP	21.15	0.000	0.35	fea, joy > des > amu > ang	irr > anx, int, pri	ple, rel > sad
	VENEC	16.44	0.001	0.25	In, Fe, Sa	Ha, Sh, Re	Pr, An, Ne, (Co), (Lu)

(continued)

Table 4.3 Continued

Acoustic cue		Emotion Effect			Trends for the Emotion Effect		
		F	p	Eta	High (↑)	Medium (=)	Low (↓)
Spectral balance cues							
F1amp_M	GEMEP	9.71	0.000	0.20		ang > des > joy, pri >	fea > anx > amu, int, irr, ple, sad > rel
	VENEC	19.54	0.001	0.28	Ha, Ne, An, In	Pr, (Co), Fe, Sa	Sh, Re, (Lu)
HammarbergV_M	GEMEP	32.55	0.000	0.46	sad > int > ple > irr	anx, pri, rel > amu	des, joy > ang, fea
	VENEC	25.09	0.001	0.34	Ne, Sa, Sh, In	(Lu), Pr	(Co), Fe, Ha, Re, An
H1A3_M	GEMEP	25.53	0.000	0.46	sad > int > irr	ple, pri > anx > rel >	amu > ang, des, joy > fea
	VENEC	30.15	0.000	0.44	Ne, Sh, Sa	In, (Co), (Lu), Pr, Re	Ha, Fe, An
Temporal cues							
V_SegLengthSec_M	GEMEP	7.22	0.000	0.16		ple, pri > des, joy > ang >	anx, fea, int, irr, rel > amu, sad
	VENEC	3.66	0.001	0.07	Ha	(Co), Pr, An, Fe, In, Sa, (Lu), Ne, Re	Sh
UV_SegLengthSec_M	GEMEP	7.10	0.000	0.15	ple >	sad > anx > int, irr, pri, rel	ang, des, fea, joy > amu
	VENEC	17.70	0.001	0.26	(Lu), Re, Sh	(Co), Pr, Sa, An, Fe	Ha, In, Ne

Note. GEMAPS (Eyben et al., 2015); GEMEP Swiss French corpus, twelve emotions (Scherer et al., 2017a); VENEC English corpus in five cultures, ten emotions (Laukka et al., 2016, values reproduced from Tables 2 and S3). Underlined F-values remained significant p< .05 after Bonferroni adjustment for multiple testing. High (↑) and low (↓) denotes cues with z-values above 0 or below 0, respectively; as indicated by 95% CI not overlapping with 0. Medium (=) denotes cues with z-values around 0, as indicated by 95% CI that includes 0. VENEC: An = anger, Co = contempt; Fe = fear, Ha = happiness, In = interest; (Lu = lust, Ne = neutral), Pr = pride, Re = relief, Sa = sadness, (Sh = shame). GEMEP: pri, pride; joy, joy; amu, amusement; int, interest; ple, pleasure; rel, relief; hot, hot anger; pan, panic fear; des, despair; irr, irritation; anx, anxiety; sad, sadness. For GEMEP, labels indicate homogeneous subsets at extremes according to Tukey's b criterion in post hoc comparisons.

appeared to possess a specific combination of acoustic parameters, reflecting a specific mixture of physiological voice control parameters. Features related to subglottal pressure showed strong within-group and between-group correlations, demonstrating the importance of accounting for vocal loudness in voice analyses. Multiple discriminant analysis revealed that a parameter selection that was based, in a principled fashion, on production processes could yield rather satisfactory discrimination outcomes (87.1% based on twelve parameters and 78% based on three parameters). The results of this study suggest that systems to automatically detect emotions use a hypothesis-driven approach to selecting parameters that directly reflect the physiological parameters underlying voice and speech production.

The literature covered here has been exclusively concerned with the speaking voice. However, it is an issue of great interest to study emotion-induced voice changes in the singing voice, an essential aspect of artistic interpretation in opera and the recital of lieder, given the importance of subtle affect in these domains. Scherer et al. (2015) examined the similarities and differences in the expression of emotion in the singing and the speaking voice. Three internationally renowned opera singers produced 'vocalises' (using a schwa vowel) and short nonsense phrases in different interpretations for ten emotions. Acoustic analyses of emotional expression in the singing samples show significant differences between the emotions. In addition to the obvious effects of loudness and tempo, spectral balance and perturbation make significant contributions (high effect sizes) to this differentiation. A comparison of the emotion-specific patterns produced by the singers in this study with published data for professional actors portraying different emotions in speech generally show a very high degree of similarity. However, singers tend to rely more than actors on the use of voice perturbation, specifically vibrato, in particular in the case of high arousal emotions. The authors suggest that this may be due to the restrictions and constraints imposed by the musical structure (see also Scherer et al., 2017b, on acoustic patterns in singers' vocal expression of emotion).

4.4 TRANSMISSION AND PERCEPTION

The TEEP model already described highlights the need to separately model the transmission of the distal signals from the sender to the receiver/listener before perception and inference become possible. Studies in the area of the vocal communication of emotion have paid little attention to this intermediate stage. However, as the transmission of the relevant cues may be faulty, researchers attempting to model the complete expression/ impression process need to include this stage into their models and measurements. For example, if the transmission process systematically changes the nature of the distal cues, the proximal cues are unlikely to be representative of the characteristics of the distal cues at the source. Thus, limited frequency range of the transmission (e.g. on a telephone) will eliminate much of the higher frequency information in the voice signal. One effect on the listener is to hear the pitch of the voice as lower than it really is—with the well-known ensuing effect of overestimating the age of the speaker at the other end. Scherer et al. (2003) discuss two of the contributing factors in detail—the transmission of sound through space and electronic channels, and the transform functions in perception, as determined by the nature of human hearing mechanisms.

4.4.1 Transmission of Sound

The transmission of vocal sound through physical space is affected by many environmental and atmospheric factors including the distance between sender and receiver (weakening the signal), the presence of other sounds such as background noise (disturbing the signal), or the presence of natural barriers such as walls (filtering the signal). All of these factors will lessen the likelihood that the proximal cues can be a faithful representation of the distal cues with respect to their acoustic characteristics. Importantly, the knowledge about such constraints on the part of the speaker can lead to a modification of the distal cues by way of an effort to modify voice production to offset such transmission effects. For example, a speaker may attempt to produce more intense speech, requiring more vocal effort, and greater articulatory precision, if communicating over large distances. Greater vocal effort in turn, will affect a large number of other acoustic characteristics related to voice production at the larynx. Furthermore, the distance between speaker and listener may have an effect on posture, facial expression, and gestures, all of which are likely to have effects on the intensity and spectral distribution of the acoustic signal (see also Laver, 1991).

Just as distance, physical environment, and atmospheric conditions play a part in the case of immediate voice transmission, the nature of the medium may have potentially strong effects on proximal cues in the case of mediated transmission by intercom, telephone, internet, or other technical means. The band restrictions of the line, as well as the quality of the encoding and decoding components of the system, can systematically affect many aspects of the distal voice cues by disturbing, masking, or filtering, and thus render the proximal cues less representative of the distal cues. While much of this work has been done in the field of engineering, only little has been directly applied to modelling the process of the vocal communication of emotion (but see Baber & Noyes, 1996). In consequence, future research efforts in this area should pay greater attention to this important aspect of the vocal expression/impression chain.

4.4.2 Transform Functions in Perception

Another factor that is well known but generally neglected in research on vocal communication is the transformation of the distal signal through the transfer characteristics of the human hearing system. For example, the perceived loudness of voiced speech signals correlates more strongly with the amplitude of a few harmonics or even a single harmonic than with its overall intensity (Gramming & Sundberg, 1988; Titze, 1992).

Given space limitations, the issue of voice perception which is centrally implicated in the distal–proximal relationship cannot be reviewed here. Recent research paints an increasingly more complex picture of this process which is characterized by a multitude of feedforward and feedback processes between modalities (e.g. visual–vocal), levels of processing (e.g. peripheral–central), and input versus stored schemata. There is, for example, the well-documented phenomenon of the effects of facial expression perception on voice perception (e.g. de Gelder & Vroomen, 2000). Things are further complicated by the fact that the voice generally carries linguistic information with all that this entails with respect to the influence of phonetic-linguistic categories on perception. A particularly intriguing phenomenon is the perception and interpretation of prosodic features which are strongly affected by centrally stored templates. There is currently an upsurge in neuropsychological research activity in this area (e.g. Belin et al., 2011; Frühholz et al., 2014; Grandjean et al., 2005; Wildgruber et al., 2009).

The fact that the role of voice sound transmission and the transform functions specific to the human hearing system have been rarely studied, is not only regrettable for theoretical reasons (preventing one from modelling the communication process in its entirety) but also because one may have missed parameters that are central in the differentiation of the vocal expression of different emotions. Thus, rather than basing all analyses on objective measures of emotional speech, it might be fruitful to employ, in addition, variables that reflect the transformations that distal cues undergo in their representation as proximal cues after passage through the hearing mechanism.

One possibility to assess the proximal representation of the voice quality, as specified by the TEEP model, which serves as an input to inference processes, is to obtain ratings by naïve participants using common language terms that describe the qualities of a voice (e.g. high-pitched, sharp, dark, gravelly). This approach has been occasionally used in the past both for basic and clinical research on the voice (Kreiman & Gerratt, 1998; van Bezooijen, 1986). Recently, a validated rating instrument to measure proximal voice perception has been proposed by Bänziger et al. (2014). In two studies, using two different sets of emotion portrayals by German and French actors, ratings of perceived voice and speech characteristics (loudness, pitch, intonation, sharpness, articulation, roughness, instability, and speech rate) were obtained from non-expert (untrained) listeners. In addition, standard acoustic parameters were extracted from the voice samples. Overall, highly similar patterns of results were found in both studies. Rater agreement (reliability) reached highly satisfactory levels for most features. Multiple discriminant analysis results reveal that both perceived vocal features and acoustic parameters allow a high degree of differentiation of the actor-portrayed emotions. Positive emotions can be classified with a higher hit rate on the basis of perceived vocal features as compared to acoustic parameters, confirming suggestions in the literature that it is difficult to find acoustic valence indicators. The results show that the suggested scales (Geneva Voice Perception Scales) can be reliably used to measure proximal perception of voice quality.

4.5 EMOTION INFERENCE
AND RECOGNITION (DECODING)

As in the field of facial expression recognition, the inference of emotions from the voice is generally studied by presenting vocal emotion portrayals to the participants and asking them to choose the correct label out of a list of emotion terms, allowing to determine the hit rate in the form of proportions or per cent. As vocal expression generally consists of speech or meaningful vocal sounds, research in this area encounters the problem of separating emotion inference from content or meaning versus pure voice quality and dynamic delivery. Researchers have chosen different types of content for their experiments, from standard sentences, to sentence fragments, to strings of nonsense syllables (simulated speech), or simply to sustained vowels. Another possibility is to mask content in the spontaneous speech sample by low-pass filtering of the signal, randomization of signal segments, or backwards presentation (for further details see Scherer et al, 1985).

Scherer et al. (2011) have reviewed the major studies in this area, all of which found better-than-chance accuracy in recognition of vocally expressed emotion. Table 4.4 (column 'Past research', adapted from Table 2 in Scherer et al., 2011) reports the average recognition accuracy (based on some of the major studies) for six emotions from vocal expressions as enacted by Western and non-Western encoders. Vocal emotion expressions are inherently dynamic and generally much less iconic than static facial expression patterns (with the exception of affect vocalizations like laughter or vocal emblems, e.g. 'Yuk'; see Scherer, 1994). It is thus not surprising that the overall recognition accuracy is somewhat lower than for photos of facial expression. However, hit rates are quite comparable for dynamic video presentations of facial expression (for a comparison see Table 2 in Scherer et al., 2011). As expected, higher accuracy scores are found for iconic vocal expressions or vocal affect bursts (Simon-Thomas et al., 2009). Similarly, Hawk and colleagues (2009) found that accuracy scores for non-linguistic affective vocalizations and facial expressions were almost equivalent across nine emotions, and both were generally higher than the accuracy for speech-embedded prosody (with a few emotion-specific exceptions, e.g. surprise). In the data reported in Table 4.4, the best recognized emotions are sadness and anger. This may reflect the importance of the arousal dimension as discussed earlier, with sadness being very low and anger rather high on that dimension.

As for the work on vocal expression encoding, a major drawback of past research is that only a very small number of the major emotions have been studied, again mostly happiness, sadness, fear, and anger (as well as in a few cases, disgust and surprise; but for affect bursts see Simon-Thomas et al., 2009). Apart from the insufficient coverage of the emotion domain, there are two problems with this:

1) The number of negative emotions is larger than that for positive emotions. 2) One consequence of the small number of categories in a recognition study is that guessing becomes easier and raters may resort to strategic classification rather than true recognition (a danger which is exacerbated by problem 1).

It is therefore instructive to examine the recognition data obtained in studies with the full set of the GEMEP corpus (Bänziger & Scherer, 2010) shown in Table 4.4 ('GEMEP' column). These data can be compared (Table 4.4, 'VENEC' column) with accuracy data reported in a recent large-scale study of cross-cultural emotion recognition (Laukka et al., 2016; see Section 7 on cross-cultural differences). In addition, the column 'Past research' in Table 4.4 shows the average accuracy proportions in the literature up to 2011, as reviewed by Scherer et al. (2011). The amount of agreement between the results of the many different relevant studies, involving encoders and decoders from many different cultures, is quite striking.

For a more detailed interpretation, the accuracy hit rates obtained in the different studies need to be seen in the context of the respective confusion patterns in a matrix of target versus judgement. Overall, anger and fear are best recognized, despite the fact that both are negative, high-arousal emotions and thus share the vocal cues for both valence and arousal (a result which cannot be accounted for by two-dimensional valence × arousal

Table 4.4 Mean proportions of recognition accuracy for major emotions across relevant studies

Valence/Arousal	Target	GEMEP		VENEC	Past research	
		Vocal burst /aaa/ (schwa)	Sentence (random phonemes)	Standard sentence	Western encoders	Non-Western encoders
Positive high arousal	pride	0.10	0.24	0.18		
	joy	0.20	0.35	0.56	0.54	0.52
	amusement	0.78	0.57			
Positive low arousal	interest	0.30	0.26	0.43		
	pleasure	0.40	0.31			
	relief	0.73	0.49	0.35		
Negative high arousal	hot anger	0.72	0.67	0.56	0.75	0.66
	panic fear	0.81	0.66	0.55	0.62	0.52
	despair	0.33	0.31			
Negative low arousal	irritation	0.31	0.51			
	anxiety	0.29	0.40			
	sadness	0.23	0.45	0.49	0.69	0.79
Additional emotions	admiration	0.23	0.39			
	shame	0.03	0.11	0.27		
	contempt	0.10	0.25	0.25		
	tenderness	0.22	0.30			
	disgust	0.59	0.12		0.35	
	surprise	0.47	0.33		0.57	

Note: GEMEP corpus as described in Bänziger and Scherer, 2010, adapted from Table 6.1.4; VENEC corpus as described by Laukka et al., 2016, adapted from Table 5; Past research as summarized in the review by Scherer et al., 2011, adapted from Table 2.

emotion theories). For example, the discrepancy in the case of joy is explained by the fact that in the GEMEP study, two additional emotions that are very similar to joy—pleasure and amusement—were studied, which obviously increases the likelihood of within-family confusions. In most studies, the major confusions are easily explained—either they involve members of the same emotion family or a high probability of mixed emotions (e.g. despair/sadness, pride/contempt). These results confirm that emotions can be reliably inferred from vocal expression with better-than-chance accuracy, even within the same quadrants of the valence × arousal space. Also, the extensive study by Juslin et al. (2018) showed that at comparable high intensity of the expression, there is no difference in recognition rate for spontaneous versus posed emotions. However, there are major differences in recognition rates between different emotions and thus one of the challenges for future research will be to better understand the mechanisms underlying vocal emotion communication.

In addition to emotion differences with respect to discriminability, there are major individual differences in the ability to recognize vocally expressed emotions (which is part of the emotional competence to correctly infer the affective state of one's interaction partners in order to respond appropriately). In recent years, a number of instruments have been developed to test this ability (Nowicki & Duke, 1994; Rosenthal et al., 1979; Scherer & Scherer, 2011). Bänziger et al. (2009) developed an instrument that objectively measures this ability on the basis of actor portrayals of dynamic expressions of ten emotions, operationalized as recognition accuracy in four presentation modes combining the visual and auditory sense modalities (audio/video, audio only, video only, still picture). Data from a large validation study showed strong construct validation using related tests (as already mentioned). The results show the utility of a test designed to measure both coarse- and fine-grained emotion differentiation and modality-specific skills. Factor analysis of the data suggested two separate abilities—visual (face) and auditory (voice) recognition—which are largely independent of personality dispositions.

4.6 PATH ANALYSES OF THE EMOTION COMMUNICATION PROCESS

It has been suggested repeatedly (Scherer, 1978, 2003) to use the Brunswikian lens model to study the complete process of expression and impression/inference, including both the sender/encoder and the receiver/decoder side in a combined analysis model (see also Juslin & Laukka, 2001). Unfortunately, until very recently there was a clean split between groups of researchers studying emotion expression and the distal cues produced by the sender, and another, larger group, studying emotion recognition (mostly just in terms of accuracy). This has been true for both facial and vocal expression work.

Spurned by the TEEP model previously described (which is based on the Brunswikian lens model), a first empirical demonstration for the vocal emotion communication process has been published by Bänziger et al. (2015) for two datasets from two different cultures and languages, based on corpora of vocal emotion enactment by professional actors and emotion inference by naïve listeners (the corpora produced by Banse & Scherer, 1996 and Bänziger & Scherer, 2010, previously mentioned). Lens model equations, hierarchical regression, and multivariate path analysis were used to compare the relative contributions of objectively measured acoustic cues in the enacted expressions and subjective voice cues as perceived by listeners (obtained with the Geneva Voice Perception Scales already mentioned) to the variance in emotion inference from vocal expressions for four emotion families (fear, anger, happiness, and sadness). While the results confirm the central role of arousal in vocal emotion communication, the utility of applying an extended path modelling framework is demonstrated by the identification of unique combinations of distal cues and proximal percepts carrying information about specific emotion families, independent of arousal (see illustration of the anger model in Figure 4.2). The statistical models generated show that more sophisticated acoustic parameters need to be developed to explain the distal underpinnings of subjective voice quality percepts that account for much of the variance in emotion inference, in particular voice instability and roughness.

In their large-scale intercultural study on vocal emotion expression and impression, Laukka et al. (2016; see Section 7) also successfully used the Brunswikian lens model to quantify cue validity (the link between specific emotions and specific patterns of distal acoustic

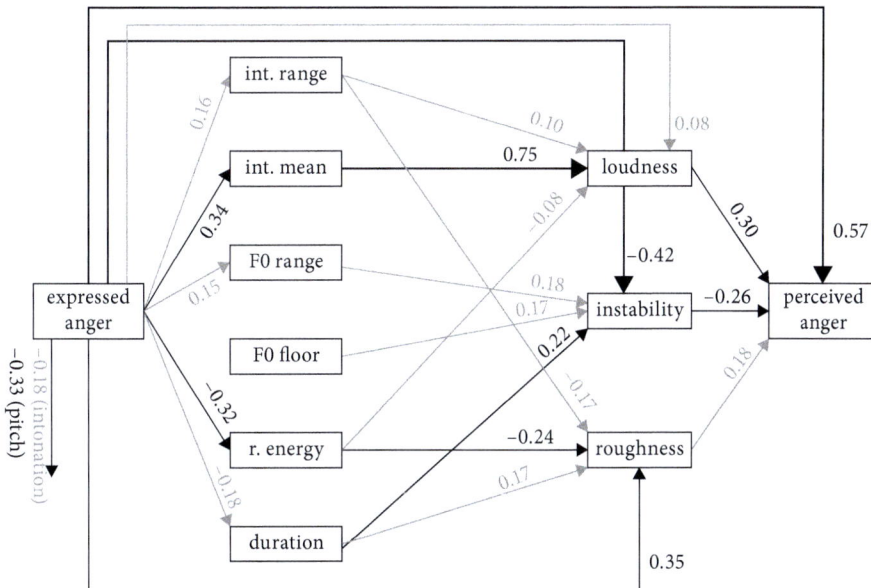

FIGURE 4.2 Standardized path coefficients of the estimated model for the expression and perception of anger (adapted from Bänziger et al., 2015).

Note: Only significant path coefficients are shown (p< 0.02). Significant paths with an absolute value > 0.2 are depicted in black, significant paths with an absolute value < 0.2 are depicted in grey, int. = intensity; r. energy = relative energy.

Adaped from Bänziger T., Hosoya G., & Scherer K.R., 'Path Models of Vocal Emotion Communication', *PLoS One*, Volume 10, Issue 9, e0136675, Copyright © 2015 Bänziger et al., doi: 10.1371/journal.pone.0136675.

parameters) and cue utilization (the use made by listener raters of these acoustic cues) to demonstrate the role of intercultural differences in this process.

4.7 CULTURE AND LANGUAGE DIFFERENCES

The issue of whether emotional expressions are universal across cultures or subject to cultural differences has been hotly debated in the literature. The question is all the more important for the issue of vocal expression, as cultures differ with respect to the languages spoken and one might thus expect differences due to phonemic and suprasegmental (e.g. intonation, rhythm) differences in the respective speech patterns. Ross et al. (1986) performed acoustic analyses of a standard sentence spoken with happy, sad, angry, surprised, and neutral affective prosody by five speakers each of Mandarin, Taiwanese, Thai, and American English. They discovered that for all of the tone languages, the use of Fo variation and Fo slope to express affect was reduced compared to American English. In addition, in the three tone languages the shape of the intonation contours of affective utterances differed less from neutral utterances than was the case for American English. This suggests that the use of a particular acoustic feature (in this case, Fo) in spoken language can constrain its use for the communication of emotion.

In consequence, it seems feasible that the encoding of emotion expression in different cultures may differ, particularly in the case of major differences between the respective language families. If there are such differences, one would expect that the accuracy of decoding, emotion recognition, will be reduced if listeners infer emotions from speech in a foreign language. Scherer et al. (2001) conducted a study in seven countries in Europe, the United States, and Indonesia on vocal emotion portrayals of anger, sadness, fear, joy, and neutral voice as produced by professional German actors. Data showed an overall accuracy of 66% across all emotions and countries. Although accuracy was substantially better than chance, there were sizeable differences ranging from 74% in Germany to 52% in Indonesia. However, patterns of confusion were very similar across all countries, suggesting the existence of similar inference rules from vocal expression across cultures. Generally, accuracy decreased with increasing language dissimilarity from German (in spite of the use of language-free speech samples), confirming the potentially important role of language in the vocal expression of emotion.

In their review of cross-cultural studies, Scherer et al. (2011) indeed found that the few studies in which non-Western decoders were asked to recognize emotions portrayed by Western encoders show reduced accuracy percentages for both facial and vocal expressions. However, the differences were more pronounced in vocal expression recognition —particularly for happiness, fear, and anger. This may be due to the fact that in vocal expression there are no such unequivocal cues as the zygomaticus or frontalis actions found in facial expression. Rather, as fundamental frequency (pitch) of the voice is a reliable cue for arousal, highly aroused emotions are likely to be confused if the perceiver focuses too much on this cue which may be in part determined by language (see Ross et al., 1986). As to encoder differences, comparison of studies using non-Western encoders with Western encoders (in both cases for Western decoders) also shows that accuracy percentages are somewhat lower for non-Western encoders. However, the differences are not very strong (and even in the opposite direction for sadness).

In recent years, an attempt has been made to account for such cultural differences by an integrative theoretical framework—in particular, the dialect theory of emotion expression and recognition (Elfenbein, 2013; Elfenbein & Ambady, 2002), originally developed to help explain the phenomenon of in-group advantage in the recognition of facial expressions (whereby individuals more accurately judge emotional expressions from their own cultural group compared to expressions from foreign groups). In-group advantage has been shown for the recognition of vocal expressions as well (Juslin & Laukka, 2003; Laukka et al., 2014) and it can be argued that, like facial dialects, paralinguistic dialects should involve subtle yet systematic differences across cultures in the style of expressing emotion, in this case via acoustic cues in the voice. In addition, consistent with dialect theory, it can be argued that individuals tend to judge the vocal expressions of other people based on their own cultural style. Although the dialects of a language are still mutually intelligible, some of the meaning may be less well communicated.

Laukka et al. (2016) have conducted a large-scale cross-cultural study to empirically examine these hypotheses. They used the Vocal Expressions of Nineteen Emotions across Cultures (VENEC) database, which consists of scenario-based emotion portrayals (via short standard English sentences) by one hundred professional actors across five countries where English is an official language (Australia, India, Kenya, Singapore, and the USA; Laukka et al., 2010). Three hundred and eighty expressions for ten major affective states (anger, contempt, fear, happiness, interest, sexual lust, pride, relief, sadness, and shame), produced with a moderately high level of emotion intensity and well recognized in a pretest, were selected and analysed with the GEMAPS parameter set (see previous description). These data were analysed for significant differences between the levels of the emotion and culture factors. The results for the emotion factor are compared to the results obtained in a comparable study with French-speaking actors by Scherer et al. (2017a) in Table 4.3. The results for the culture factor show significant culture effects for quite a large number of the acoustic parameters measured (Laukka et al., 2016, Tables 2 and 3), demonstrating the encoding effects predicted by dialect theory. As to decoding, the authors present a confusion matrix (Laukka et al., 2016, Table 4) showing, as expected, that accuracy rates tend to be somewhat higher for the recognition of in-group emotion expressions. However, the differences are relatively small and, as in the study by Scherer et al. (2001), the patterns of confusion are remarkably similar.

In conclusion, the evidence available to date suggests that there are indeed vocal emotion expression dialects, leading to some differential encoding patterns and somewhat different inference rules, but that on the whole emotion communication in the vocal channel functions rather well. Desiderata for further research include, in particular, the study of different language families with well-known differences with respect to phonological structure and suprasegmental dynamics, to better understand the sources of dialectal differences. In other words, to what extent is expression constrained by language features (as in tone languages) and to what extent are non-linguistic features of culture (e.g. traditional display and inference rules) involved?

4.8 APPLIED RESEARCH ON ACOUSTIC PATTERNING OF VOCAL EMOTION EXPRESSION

Much of the literature reviewed so far has been conducted on speech communication and may seem restricted to academic interest in understanding one of the channels of emotion expression and communication. However, there is a long tradition of applied concerns involving the detection of emotion in the voice. The interest in the voice as an indicator of emotion and emotion disturbances has recently gained major impetus through the development of automatic classification techniques in machine learning algorithms (see Schuller et al., 2011). Given space constraints, only a few brief examples can be provided here.

4.8.1 Clinical Diagnostics

For quite some considerable time, psychiatrists have noted, based on their clinical experience, that the voice and speech can provide valuable indicators for emotional disorders such as neurosis, depression, and flat affect in schizophrenia, as well as changes in the course of treatment. In consequence, clinical research has had a pioneering role in fostering the acoustic analysis of the voice in the interest of gaining insights into the severity of symptoms and indicators of therapeutic effects (Alpert et al., 1963; Moses, 1954; Ostwald, 1973). Given the potential of this approach to obtain valuable behavioural indicators for emotional disturbance, research in this domain has been scant. However, a number of studies over the years have investigated acoustic patterns indicative of depression (Alpert et al., 2001; Cannizzaro et al., 2004; Darby et al., 1984; Hill & Holmquist, 1975; Klein, 1996; Levin et al., 1985; Nilsonne et al., 1988) and flat affect in schizophrenic patients (Alpert et al., 1989, 2002; Andreasen et al., 1981; Stassen et al., 1995). In addition, the possibility to trace therapy effects via vocal-acoustic indicators has been successfully demonstrated (Ellgring & Scherer, 1996; Kuny & Stassen, 1993; Mundt et al., 2012; Tolkmitt et al., 1982).

Clinical aspects of voice analysis are also being increasingly investigated in affective computing, using automatic classification via machine-learning techniques (Valstar et al., 2014). Furthermore, attempts to develop automated voice-interactive programs for screening depression via telephone are currently under way (e.g. González & Shriver, 2004; Mundt et al., 2007).

In consequence, the empirical evidence and the technological advances available today (rapid automatic analysis, GEMAPS—as described, and machine classification) suggest the utility of pursuing research efforts to obtain validated acoustic indicators for differential diagnosis, severity of symptoms, and therapy effects.

4.8.2 Stress Detection

There was a flurry of excitement more than thirty years ago when 'voice lie detectors' came on the market. Needless to say, these devices were useless because lies are not emotional states but cognitive operations, and thus cannot be detected on the basis of peripheral physiological signals such as the voice waveform (see overview by Hollien et al., 2014). Stress, however, is a kind of special emotion (see Scherer, 1986b) and should be detectable by vocal analyses (which does not help lie detection as honest people accused of lying are generally much more stressed than inveterate liars).

Despite the obvious potential of continuously monitoring speech for stress symptoms in a variety of contexts and high-risk situations (e.g. pilots, power plant operators) (see Rothkrantz et al., 2004), as well as detecting urgency in emergency calls (Lefter et al., 2011), there has been remarkably little scientific research to explore the voice as a potential stress indicator (but see Murray et al., 1996). One reason might be the extraordinary diversity of different types of stress which are likely to have different effects on voice production and strong individual differences in stress susceptibility. Thus, Tolkmitt and Scherer (1986) found, in an early study, that the Fo floor of high-anxiety and anxiety-denying subjects increased with stress, probably due to physiologically based changes in muscle tension. For anxiety-denying female subjects only, precision of articulation increased under cognitive stress and decreased under emotional stress. This was confirmed by Wallbott and Scherer (1991) who found complex interactions between the type and degree of stress, coping style, and gender of participants, confirming findings on vocal parameters of stress.

Overall, research on the effects of stress on voice and speech has been beset by the problems of an insufficient specification of the type of stress studied and by a neglect of strong individual differences in the susceptibility to experience stress. As a result, there has been little evidence for the existence of a replicable acoustic profile for stressed speech. However, the potential is clearly there. By experimentally separating cognitive stress due to high task load and psychological stress, Scherer et al. (2002) were able to show that cognitive load due to task engagement reliably increases speech rate, energy attack and decay gradients, mean Fo, and the proportion of energy in the higher frequency range. In contrast, only Fo and spectral energy distribution changed in response to the induction of psychological stress.

4.9 CONCLUSION

By necessity, the overview provided in this chapter has had to be somewhat cursory. The reader is referred to the literature covered in many of the cited articles and chapters. It is fair to say that the study of the vocal expression and recognition of emotion has been a poor sibling to the concern with facial expression. However, the ready availability of digital voice analysis programs and the exploding interest in vocal emotion analysis in the areas of affective computing and machine learning has given a much needed impetus to this important research domain. In consequence, it is to be expected that this important part of vocal communication—the expression of emotion and other affective states—will be the subject of a greater number of investigations with more sophisticated experimental designs and methods of assessment.

REFERENCES

Alpert, M., Kurtzberg, R. L., & Friedhoff, A. J. (1963). Transient voice changes associated with emotional stimuli. *Archives of General Psychiatry*, 8(4), 362–365.

Alpert, M., Pouget, E. R., & Silva, R. R. (2001). Reflections of depression in acoustic measures of the patient's speech. *Journal of Affective Disorders*, 66(1), 59–69.

Alpert, M., Rosen, A., Welkowitz, J., Sobin, C. et al. (1989). Vocal acoustic correlates of flat affect in schizophrenia: similarity to Parkinson's disease and right hemisphere disease and contrast with depression. *The British Journal of Psychiatry*, 4. Retrieved from http://psycnet. apa.org/psycinfo/1989-40063-001

Alpert, M., Shaw, R. J., Pouget, E. R., & Lim, K. O. (2002). A comparison of clinical ratings with vocal acoustic measures of flat affect and alogia. *Journal of Psychiatric Research*, 36(5), 347–353.

Andreasen, N. C., Alpert, M., & Martz, M. J. (1981). Acoustic analysis: an objective measure of affective flattening. *Archives of General Psychiatry*, 38(3), 281–285.

Anolli, L., Wang, L., Mantovani, F., & De Toni, A. (2008). The voice of emotion in Chinese and Italian young adults. *Journal of Cross-Cultural Psychology*, 39, 565–598.

Baber, C. & Noyes, J. (1996). Automatic speech recognition in adverse environments. *Human Factors: The Journal of the Human Factors and Ergonomics Society*, 38(1), 142–155.

Bachorowski, J.-A. & Owren, M. J. (1995). Vocal expression of emotion: acoustic properties of speech are associated with emotional intensity and context. *Psychological Science*, 6, 219–224.

Banse, R. & Scherer, K. R. (1996). Acoustic profiles in vocal emotion expression. *Journal of Personality and Social Psychology*, 70(3), 614–636.

Bänziger, T., Grandjean, D., & Scherer, K. R. (2009). Emotion recognition from expressions in face, voice, and body: the multimodal emotion recognition test (MERT). *Emotion*, 9(5), 691–704.

Bänziger, T., Mortillaro, M., & Scherer, K. R. (2012). Introducing the Geneva Multimodal Expression corpus for experimental research on emotion perception. *Emotion*, 12(5), 1161–1179. doi: 10.1037/a0025827

Bänziger, T., Patel, S., & Scherer, K. R. (2014). Perceived voice and speech characteristics in emotional expression. *Journal of Nonverbal Behavior*, 38(1), 31–52.

Bänziger, T., Hosoya, G., & Scherer, K. R. (2015). Path models of vocal emotion communication. *PlosOne*, 10(9): e0136675. doi:10.1371/journal.pone.0136675

Bänziger, T. & Scherer, K. R. (2005). The role of intonation in emotional expressions. *Speech Communication*, 46, 252–267.

Bänziger, T. & Scherer, K. R. (2010). Introducing the Geneva Multimodal Emotion Portrayal (GEMEP) corpus. In: K. R. Scherer, T. Bänziger, & E. B. Roesch (eds) *Blueprint for Affective Computing: A Sourcebook* (pp. 271–294). Oxford: Oxford University Press.

Belin P., Bestelmeyer P. E. G., Latinus M., & Watson, R. (2011). Understanding voice perception. *British Journal of Psychology*, 102, 711–725.

Brown, S. (2000). The 'musilanguage' model of music evolution. In: N. L. Wallin, B. Merker, & S. Brown (eds) *The Origins of Music* (pp. 271–300). Cambridge, MA: MIT Press.

Brunswik, E. (1956). *Perception and the Representative Design of Psychological Experiments*. Berkeley: University of California Press.

Bühler, K. (1934) (new edition 1984). *Sprachtheorie* [Theory of speech]. Jena: Fischer..

Cannizzaro, M., Harel, B., Reilly, N., Chappell, P., & Snyder, P. J. (2004). Voice acoustical measurement of the severity of major depression. *Brain and Cognition*, 56(1), 30–35.

Darby, J. K., Simmons, N., & Berger, P. A. (1984). Speech and voice parameters of depression: a pilot study. *Journal of Communication Disorders*, 17(2), 75–85.

Darwin, C. (1872). *The Expression of Emotions in Man and Animals* (3rd edition, 1998). P. Ekman (ed.). London: HarperCollins.

de Gelder, B. & Vroomen, J. (2000). Bimodal emotion perception: integration across separate modalities, cross-modal perceptual grouping or perception of multimodal events? *Cognition and Emotion*, 14, 321–324.

Echternach, M., Markl, M., & Richter, B. (2012). Dynamic real-time magnetic resonance imaging for the analysis of voice physiology. *Current Opinion in Otolaryngology & Head and Neck Surgery*, 20(6), 450–457.

Elfenbein, H. A. (2013). Nonverbal dialects and accents in facial expressions of emotion. *Emotion Review*, 5, 90–96. doi: 10.1177/1754073912451332

Elfenbein, H. A. & Ambady, N. (2002). On the universality and cultural specificity of emotion recognition: a meta-analysis. *Psychological Bulletin*, 128, 203–235. doi: 10.1037/0033-2909.128.2.203

Ellgring, H. & Scherer, K. R. (1996). Vocal indicators of mood change in depression. *Journal of Nonverbal Behavior*, 20(2), 83–110.

Ellsworth, P. C. & Scherer, K. R. (2003). Appraisal processes in emotion. In: R. J. Davidson, K. R. Scherer, & H. Goldsmith (eds) *Handbook of the Affective Sciences* (pp. 572–595). New York and Oxford: Oxford University Press.

Eyben, F., Scherer, K. R., Schuller, B. W., Sundberg, J., André, E., Busso, C., & Truong, K. P. (2015). The Geneva Minimalistic Acoustic Parameter Set (GeMAPS) for voice research and affective computing. *IEEE Transactions on Affective Computing*, 7(2), 190–202.

Fitch, W. T. (2000). The evolution of speech: a comparative review. *Trends in Cognitive Sciences*, 4(7), 258–267.

Frühholz, S., Trost, W., & Grandjean, D. (2014). The role of the medial temporal limbic system in processing emotions in voice and music. *Progress in Neurobiology*, 123, 1–17.

González, G. M. & Shriver, C. (2004). A bilingual computerized voice-interactive system for screening depression symptoms. *Journal of Technology in Human Services*, 22(4), 1–20.

Goudbeek, M. & Scherer, K. R. (2010). Beyond arousal: valence and potency/control in the vocal expression of emotion. *Journal of the Acoustical Society of America*, 128(3), 1322–1336.

Gramming, P. & Sundberg, J. (1988). Spectrum factors relevant to phonetogram measurement, *Journal of the Acoustical Society of America*, 83, 2352–2360.

Grandjean, D., Sander, D., Pourtois, G., Schwartz, S., Seghier, M. L., Scherer, K. R., & Vuilleumier, P. (2005). The voices of wrath: brain responses to angry prosody in meaningless speech. *Nature Neuroscience*, 8(2), 145–146.

Hawk, S. T., Van Kleef, G. A., Fischer, A. H., & Van Der Schalk, J. (2009). "Worth a thousand words": absolute and relative decoding of nonlinguistic affect vocalizations. *Emotion*, 9(3), 293.

Hill, K. & Holmquist, B. (1975). Voice qualities of depressed patients. *Nordisk Psykiatrisk Tidsskrift*, 29(5), 383–384.

Hollien, H., Bahr, R. H., & Harnsberger, J. D. (2014). Issues in forensic voice. *Journal of Voice*, 28(2), 170–184.

Johnstone, T., van Reekum, C. M., Hird, K., Kirsner, K., & Scherer, K. R. (2005). Affective speech elicited with a computer game. *Emotion*, 5(4), 513–518.

Jürgens, R., Hammerschmidt, K., & Fischer, J. (2011). Authentic and play-acted vocal emotion expressions reveal acoustic differences. *Frontiers in Psychology*, 2, 180.

Juslin, P. N. & Scherer, K. R. (2005). Vocal expression of affect. In: J. A. Harrigan, R. Rosenthal, & K. Scherer (eds) *The New Handbook of Methods in Nonverbal Behavior Research* (pp. 65–135). Oxford: Oxford University Press.

Juslin, P. N. & Laukka, P. (2001). Impact of intended emotion intensity on cue utilization and decoding accuracy in vocal expression of emotion. *Emotion*, 1, 381–412.

Juslin, P. N. & Laukka, P. (2003). Communication of emotions in vocal expression and music performance: different channels, same code? *Psychological Bulletin*, 129, 770–814.

Juslin, P. N., Laukka, P., & Bänziger, T. (2018). The mirror to our soul? Comparisons of spontaneous and posed vocal expression of emotion. *Journal of Nonverbal Behavior*, 42(1), 1–40.

Kappas, A. & Polikova, N. (2008). Judgments of the affective valence of spontaneous vocalizations: the influence of situational context. In: K. Izdebski (ed.) *Emotions in the Human Voice*, Vol. 1 (pp. 109–122). San Diego, CA: Plural Publishing.

Klein, L. B. (1996). Vocal acoustic correlates of geriatric depression. ProQuest Information & Learning, US. Retrieved from http://search.ebscohost.com/login.aspx?direct=true&db=psyh&AN=1996-95017-331&site=ehost-live

Kreiman, J. & Gerratt, B. R. (1998). Validity of rating scale measures of voice quality. *Journal of the Acoustical Society of America*, 104(3), 1598–1608.

Kreiman, J. & Sidtis, D. (2011). *Foundations of Voice Studies: An Interdisciplinary Approach to Voice Production and Perception*. Oxford: John Wiley & Sons.

Kuny, S. & Stassen, H. H. (1993). Speaking behavior and voice sound characteristics in depressive patients during recovery. *Journal of Psychiatric Research*, 27(3), 289–307.

Ladefoged P. (1975). *A Course in Phonetics*. New York: Harcourt Brace Jovanovich.

Laukka, P., Elfenbein, H. A., Chui, W., Thingujam, N. S., Iraki, F. K., Rockstuhl, T., & Althoff, J. (2010). Presenting the VENEC corpus: development of a cross-cultural corpus of vocal emotion expressions and a novel method of annotating emotion appraisals. In: L. Devillers, B. Schuller, R. Cowie, E. Douglas-Cowie, & A. Batliner (eds) *Proceedings of the LREC 2010 Workshop on Corpora for Research on Emotion and Affect* (pp. 53–57). Paris: European Language Resources Association.

Laukka, P., Elfenbein, H. A., Thingujam, N. S., Rockstuhl, T., Iraki, F. K., Chui, W., & Althoff, J. (2016). The expression and recognition of emotions in the voice across five cultures: a lens model analysis based on acoustic features. *Journal of Personality and Social Psychology*, 111, 686–705.

Laukka, P., Juslin, P. N., & Bresin, R. (2005). A dimensional approach to vocal expression of emotion. *Cognition and Emotion*, 19, 633–653.

Laukka, P., Neiberg, D., & Elfenbein, H. A. (2014). Evidence for cultural dialects in vocal emotion expression: acoustic classification within and across five nations. *Emotion*, 14, 445–449. doi: 10.1037/a0036048

Laver J. (1980). *The Phonetic Description of Voice Quality*. Cambridge: Cambridge University Press.

Laver, J. (1991). *The Gift of Speech*. Edinburgh: Edinburgh University Press.

Lefter, I., Rothkrantz, L. J., Van Leeuwen, D. A., & Wiggers, P. (2011). Automatic stress detection in emergency (telephone) calls. *International Journal of Intelligent Defence Support Systems*, 4(2), 148–168.

Levin, S., Hall, J. A., Knight, R. A., & Alpert, M. (1985). Verbal and nonverbal expression of affect in speech of schizophrenic and depressed patients. *Journal of Abnormal Psychology*, 94(4), 487.

Mithen, S. (2005). *The Singing Neanderthals: The Origins of Music, Language, Mind and Body*. London: Weidenfeld and Nicolson.

Moses, P. J. (1954). *The Voice of Neurosis*. New York: Grune & Stratton.

Mundt, J. C., Snyder, P. J., Cannizzaro, M. S., Chappie, K., & Geralts, D. S. (2007). Voice acoustic measures of depression severity and treatment response collected via interactive voice response (IVR) technology. *Journal of Neurolinguistics*, 20(1), 50–64. http://doi.org/10.1016/j.jneuroling.2006.04.001

Mundt, J. C., Vogel, A. P., Feltner, D. E., & Lenderking, W. R. (2012). Vocal acoustic biomarkers of depression severity and treatment response. *Biological Psychiatry*, 72(7), 580–587. http://doi.org/10.1016/j.biopsych.2012.03.015

Murray, I. R., Baber, C., & South, A. (1996). Towards a definition and working model of stress and its effects on speech. *Speech Communication*, 20, 3–12.

Nilsonne, Å., Sundberg, J., Ternström, S., & Askenfelt, A. (1988). Measuring the rate of change of voice fundamental frequency in fluent speech during mental depression. *Journal of the Acoustical Society of America*, 83(2), 716–728.

Nowicki. S. & Duke. M. P. (1994). Individual differences in the nonverbal communication of affect: the diagnostic analysis of nonverbal accuracy. *Journal of Nonverbal Behavior*, 18, 9–35.

Ostwald, P.F. (1973). *The Semiotics of Human Sound*. Mouton: De Gruyter.

Patel, S., Scherer, K. R., Bjorkner, E., & Sundberg, J. (2011). Mapping emotions into acoustic space: the role of voice production. *Biological Psychology*, 87, 93–98.

Rosenthal, R., Hall, J. A., DiMatteo, M. R., Rogers, P. L., & Archer, D. (1979). *Sensitivity to Nonverbal Communication: The PONS Test*. Baltimore: John Hopkins University Press.

Ross, E. D., Edmondson, J. A., & Seibert, G. B. (1986). The effect of affect on various acoustic measures of prosody in tone and non-tone languages: a comparison based on computer analysis of voice. *Journal of Phonetics*, 14, 283–302.

Rothkrantz, L. J., Wiggers, P., van Wees, J.-W. A., & van Vark, R. J. (2004). Voice stress analysis. In: *International Conference on Text, Speech and Dialogue* (pp. 449–456). Springer. Retrieved from http://link.springer.com/chapter/10.1007/978-3-540-30120-2_57

Sauter, D. A., Eisner, F., Calder, A. J., & Scott, S. K. (2010). Perceptual cues in nonverbal vocal expressions of emotion. *The Quarterly Journal of Experimental Psychology*, 63(11), 2251–2272.

Scheiner, E. & Fischer, J. (2011). Emotion expression—the evolutionary heritage in the human voice. In: W. Welsch, W. Singer, & A. Wunder (eds) *Interdisciplinary Anthropology: The Continuing Evolution of Man* (pp. 105–130). Heidelberg: Springer.

Scherer, K. R. (1978). Personality inference from voice quality: the loud voice of extroversion. *European Journal of Social Psychology*, 8, 467–487.

Scherer, K. R. (1986a). Vocal affect expression: a review and a model for future research. *Psychological Bulletin*, 99(2), 143–165.

Scherer, K. R. (1986b). Voice, stress, and emotion. In: M. H. Appley & R. Trumbull (eds) *Dynamics of Stress* (pp. 159–181). New York: Plenum.

Scherer, K. R. (1988). On the symbolic functions of vocal affect expression. *Journal of Language and Social Psychology*, 7, 79–100.

Scherer, K. R. (1991). Emotion expression in speech and music. In: J. Sundberg, L. Nord, & R. Carlson (eds) *Music, Language, Speech, and Brain* (pp. 146–156). Wenner-Gren Center International Symposium Series. London: Macmillan.

Scherer, K. R. (1992). Vocal affect expression as symptom, symbol, and appeal. In: H. Papousek, U. Jürgens, & M. Papousek (eds) *Nonverbal Vocal Communication: Comparative and Developmental Approaches* (pp. 43–60). Cambridge and New York: Cambridge University Press.

Scherer, K. R. (1994). Affect bursts. In: S. van Goozen, N. E. van de Poll, & J. A. Sergeant (eds) *Emotions: Essays on Emotion Theory* (pp. 161–196). Hillsdale, NJ: Erlbaum.

Scherer, K. R. (2003). Vocal communication of emotion: a review of research paradigms. *Speech Communication*, 40, 227–256.

Scherer, K. R. (2009). The dynamic architecture of emotion: evidence for the component process model. *Cognition and Emotion*, 23(7), 1307–1351.

Scherer K. R. (2013a). Emotion in action, interaction, music, and speech. In: M. A. Arbib (ed.) *Language, Music, and the Brain: A Mysterious Relationship* (pp. 107–139). Cambridge, MA: MIT Press.

Scherer, K.R. (2013b). Vocal markers of emotion: comparing induction and acting elicitation. *Computer Speech and Language*, 27(1), 40–58.

Scherer, K. R., Banse, R., & Wallbott, H. G. (2001). Emotion inferences from vocal expression correlate across languages and cultures. *Journal of Cross-Cultural Psychology*, 32(1), 76–92.

Scherer, K. R. & Bänziger, T. (2010). On the use of actor portrayals in research on emotional expression. In: K. R. Scherer, T. Bänziger, & E. B. Roesch (eds) *Blueprint for Affective Computing: A Sourcebook* (pp. 166–178). Oxford: Oxford University Press.

Scherer, K. R., Clark-Polner, E., & Mortillaro, M. (2011). In the eye of the beholder? Universality and cultural specificity in the expression and perception of emotion. *International Journal of Psychology*, 46(6), 401–435.

Scherer, K. R., Feldstein, S., Bond, R.N., & Rosenthal, R. (1985). Vocal cues to deception: a comparative channel approach. *Journal of Psycholinguistic Research*, 14, 409–425.

Scherer, K. R., Johnstone, T., & Klasmeyer, G. (2003). Vocal expression of emotion. In: R. J. Davidson, K. R. Scherer, & H. Goldsmith (eds) *Handbook of the Affective Sciences* (pp. 433–456). New York and Oxford: Oxford University Press.

Scherer, K. R., Johnstone, T., Klasmeyer, G., & Bänziger, T. (2000). Can automatic speaker verification be improved by training the algorithms on emotional speech? Proceedings, Sixth International Conference on Spoken Language Processing (ICSLP 2000), Beijing, China, October 16–20, 2000, vol. 2, pp. 807–810. [ISCA Archive, http://www.isca-speech.org/archive/icslp_2000]

Scherer, K. R. & Meuleman, B. (2013). Human emotion experiences can be predicted on theoretical grounds: evidence from verbal labeling. *PLoS One*, 8(3): e58166. doi:10.1371/journal.pone.0058166

Scherer, K. R. & Scherer, U. (2011). Assessing the ability to recognize facial and vocal expressions of emotion: construction and validation of the emotion recognition index. *Journal of Nonverbal Behavior*, 35, 305–326.

Scherer, K. R., Sundberg, J., Tamarit, L., & Salomão, G. L. (2015). Comparing the expression of emotion in the speaking and the singing voice. *Computer Speech and Language*, 29(1), 218–235.

Scherer, K. R., Trznadel, S., & Eyben, F. (2017a). Differentiating vocally expressed emotions with a standard acoustic parameter set. Manuscript in preparation.

Scherer, K.R., Sundberg, J., Fantini, B., Trznadel, S., & Eyben, F. (2017b). The expression of emotion in the singing voice: acoustic patterns in vocal performance. *Journal of the Acoustical Society of America*, 142, 1805–1815. doi: 10.1121/1.5002886

Scherer, K.R., Grandjean, D., Johnstone, T., Klasmeyer, G., & Bänziger, T. (2002). Acoustic correlates of task load and stress. Proceedings of the International Conference on Spoken

Language Processing, Denver, Colorado, USA, ICSLP-2002, 2017–2020. [ISCA Archive, http://www.isca-speech.org/archive/icslp_2002]

Schuller, B., Batliner, A., Steidl, S., & Seppi, D. (2011). Recognising realistic emotions and affect in speech: state of the art and lessons learnt from the first challenge. *Speech Communication*, 53(9), 1062–1087.

Simon-Thomas, E. R., Keltner, D. J., Sauter, D., Sinicropi-Yao, L., & Abramson, A. (2009). The voice conveys specific emotions: evidence from vocal burst displays. *Emotion*, 9(6), 838–846. http://doi.org/10.1037/a0017810

Smith, C. A. & Scott, H. S. (1997). A componential approach to the meaning of facial expressions. In: J. A. Russell & J. M. Fernández-Dols (eds) *The Psychology of Facial Expression* (pp. 229–254). Cambridge and New York: Cambridge University Press.

Stassen, H. H., Albers, M., Püschel, J., & Scharfetter, C. (1995). Speaking behavior and voice sound characteristics associated with negative schizophrenia. *Journal of Psychiatric Research*, 29(4), 277–296.

Sundberg, J., Patel, S., Björkner, E., & Scherer, K. R. (2011). Interdependencies among voice source parameters in emotional speech. *IEEE Transactions on Affective Computing*, 2(3), 162–174.

Titze, I. (1992). Acoustic interpretation of the voice range profile (phonetogram). *Speech & Hearing Research*, 35, 21–34.

Tolkmitt, F. J. & Scherer, K. R. (1986). Effect of experimentally induced stress on vocal parameters. *Journal of Experimental Psychology: Human Perception and Performance*, 12(3), 302–313.

Tolkmitt, F., Helfrich, H., Standke, R., & Scherer, K. R. (1982). Vocal indicators of psychiatric treatment effects in depressives and schizophrenics. *Journal of Communication Disorders*, 15(3), 209–222.

Valstar, M., Schuller, B., Smith, K., Almaev, T., Eyben, F., Krajewski, J., ... Pantic, M. (2014). AVEC 2014: 3D Dimensional Affect and Depression Recognition Challenge. In: *Proceedings of the 4th International Workshop on Audio/Visual Emotion Challenge* (pp. 3–10). New York, NY, USA: ACM. http://doi.org/10.1145/2661806.2661807

van Bezooijen, R. (1986). Lay ratings of long-term voice-and-speech characteristics. In: F. Beukema & A. Hulk (eds) *Linguistics in the Netherlands 1986* (pp. 1–7). Dordrecht, The Netherlands: Foris Publications.

Wallbott, H. G. & Scherer, K. R. (1991). Stress specificities: differential effects of coping style, gender, and type of stressor on autonomic arousal, facial expression, and subjective feeling. *Journal of Personality and Social Psychology*, 61, 147–156.

Wildgruber, D., Ethofer, T., Grandjean, D., & Kreifelts, B. (2009). A cerebral network model of speech prosody comprehension. *International Journal of Speech-Language Pathology*, 11(4), 277–281.

Williams, C. E. and Stevens, K. N. (1972). Emotions and speech: some acoustical correlates. *Journal of the Acoustical Society of America*, 52, 1238–1250.

CHAPTER 5

ACOUSTIC PROPERTIES OF INFANT-DIRECTED SPEECH

YUANYUAN WANG, DEREK M. HOUSTON,
AND AMANDA SEIDL

5.1 INTRODUCTION

INFANTS take their first steps in language acquisition in the domain of speech perception. During the first year of life, they reach important milestones in language development by showing increased sensitivity to native linguistic categories and decreased sensitivity to non-native ones both at the segmental (Werker & Lalonde, 1988; Werker & Tees, 1984) and suprasegmental levels (Johnson & Seidl, 2008; Jusczyk et al., 1993). This language-specific attunement in infancy seems to predict later language abilities (Cristia et al., 2014; Morgan & Demuth, 1996; Newman et al., 2006). For example, it has been suggested that infants' tuning of their perception to native language categories affords them a strong platform from which to acquire the rest of their native phonological system (Jusczyk, 1993), as well as to bootstrap aspects of their lexical (Curtin, 2009; Curtin et al., 2005) and syntactic structures (Morgan & Demuth, 1996), and ultimately become competent processors of the language spoken around them in just a few years.

Young infants acquire native language skills at an incredible rate and with apparent ease. This points to the possibility that the input to the child during infancy may play a crucial role in language acquisition, either because infants are particularly attentive to it or because the input somehow highlights language-specific properties of the signal. Indeed, a substantial body of research examining the relation between early linguistic input and later development has demonstrated that both the quantity and quality of infant-directed speech (IDS) contribute to infants' speech, language, and cognitive development (Greenwood et al., 2011; Hart & Risley, 1995; Hoff & Naigles, 2002; Kaplan et al., 2002; Weizman & Snow, 2001).

In a landmark longitudinal study, Hart and Risley (1995) recorded natural in-home interactions between parents and infants once each week across two and a half years. They found that the quantity of caregiver talk was a better predictor of children's language outcomes than any other factors in their early language-learning environments. Follow-up studies provided supporting evidence for this conclusion. For example, children who received a larger amount of linguistic input showed faster vocabulary growth and lexical processing than children who received less linguistic input (Hoff & Naigles, 2002; Hurtado et al., 2008). While input quantity is clearly important, mere exposure to speech may not be sufficient. Recent research suggests that speech must be directed to the infant in order to promote language development. Indeed, infants who experience more IDS become more efficient in word recognition and have larger expressive vocabulary by 24 months of age; however, the speech overheard by children does not predict later vocabulary (Weisleder & Fernald, 2013).

Other properties, specifically the quality of IDS, is beneficial over and above the quantity of IDS for language development. Although speech quality can refer to a wide range of linguistic characteristics, in this chapter, we specifically focus on one aspect of the speech directed from the caregivers to the child—namely, the acoustic properties of IDS. Our aim was to conduct a non-exhaustive review of the literature concerning the acoustic characteristics of the input that infants receive and the role this input plays in the process of language development.

When interacting with infants, caregivers, regardless of sex, age, culture, or social status, modify their speech by using a special speech register— IDS (e.g. Ferguson, 1964; Fernald, 1993; Papoušek & Papoušek, 1981; Snow, 1977). This special register has also been alternately labelled 'motherese' or 'parentese'. However, given that it is used by more than just mothers or even parents, we adopt the broader term of IDS and will use this term to refer to the register of speech that is used when addressing infants.

Decades of research on the properties of IDS have revealed that it differs from adult-directed speech (ADS) along both suprasegmental and segmental dimensions, and additionally in the domains of morphology, semantics, and syntax (e.g. Albin & Echols, 1996; Burnham et al., 2002; Cristia, 2010; Dilley et al., 2014; Fernald, 1989; Kuhl et al., 1997; Ratner, 1984; Soderstrom, 2007; Stern et al., 1983; Wang et al., 2015). These modifications present in IDS may be helpful to language learners since typically developing infants, even newborns, prefer listening to speech containing IDS properties over ADS ones (e.g. Cooper & Aslin, 1990; Fernald & Simon, 1984; Fernald et al., 1989; Kitamura et al., 2002; Kuhl et al., 1997; Pegg et al., 1992; Werker & McLeod, 1989), at least during the first six months (Cooper & Aslin, 1990; Fernald, 1985; Werker & McLeod, 1989), although the findings regarding infants' preference for IDS after 9 months is less consistent (Hayashi et al., 2001; McRoberts et al., 2009; Newman & Hussain, 2006; Segal & Newman, 2015). Further, the preference for IDS is very robust as it is present even when speech samples are presented in a foreign language (Werker et al., 1994) or in low-pass filtered speech which contains only prosodic information (Fernald, 1985; Fernald & Kuhl, 1987). Taken together, this body of evidence indicates that infants are perceptually predisposed to attend to IDS over ADS.

In light of these findings, as well as the tremendous progress infants make in speech perception during the first several months of life, a growing number of scholars have hypothesized that some of the properties in IDS, especially its acoustic properties, may play an important role in language development (Fernald & Kuhl, 1987; Schachner & Hannon, 2011; Werker & McLeod, 1989). Thus, an ensuing question in this chapter explores the function and usefulness of IDS in infant speech perception.

Researchers thus far have proposed three major hypotheses regarding the possible roles of IDS. First, IDS may serve to direct and engage attention (Benders, 2013; Fernald & Simon, 1984; Papoušek et al., 1991). For example, acoustically salient properties, particularly pitch range and affect information in the speech, are found to modulate interaction between caregiver and child (Fernald & Kuhl, 1987; Singh et al., 2002), such as to engage and maintain infant attention. Evidence for this function mainly comes from studies showing infants' preferences for IDS over ADS (Cooper & Aslin, 1990; Fernald, 1985; Werker & McLeod, 1989). Second, IDS may serve to communicate caregivers' positive affect (Fernald, 1989; Papoušek et al., 1990; Werker & McLeod, 1989). The melodic contours and exaggerated prosodic features of typical IDS present language-independent sources of information that reflect speakers' positive emotions (Ferguson et al., 1992; Fernald, 1989). In contrast, depressed mothers use less exaggerated and more flat prosody when directing speech to their infants (Kaplan et al., 2002). Additionally, infants are able to discriminate positive and negative emotions in speech, and prefer the speech that contains positive information (Fernald, 1993; Papoušek et al., 1990). Both of these hypotheses suggest that IDS may be used to help maintain an attentional or emotional bond between caregivers and their prelinguistic infants. This increased attention to speech may enhance the processing of speech signal and thus drive language development (Houston & Bergeson, 2014; Vouloumanos & Curtin, 2014).

Finally, the other hypothesis that has been widely discussed is that IDS may be a didactic register. Note that our discussion on this question only focuses on the acoustic distribution of IDS, regardless of the caregiver's intention. Proponents of this hypothesis suggest that IDS serves to facilitate language acquisition by exaggerating language-specific properties of the input signal (Kuhl et al., 1997; Uther et al., 2007). However, this hypothesis is highly controversial. While past studies have suggested that some linguistic categories are exaggerated or clearer in IDS (Kuhl et al., 1997), much recent work has called this finding into question (Cristia & Seidl, 2014; Martin et al., 2015; McMurray et al., 2013; Wang, Lee, & Houston, 2016; Wang et al., 2015). This emerging literature suggests that IDS is not a specifically didactic signal (Cristia & Seidl, 2014; McMurray et al., 2013; Wang et al., 2015), and may even illustrate language-specific properties of speech less clearly than ADS (Lee et al., 2014; Martin et al., 2015). We will discuss these hypotheses and present evidence in favour or against them in more detail.

Crucially, this debate also relates to caregivers' intentions in producing IDS. Some have argued that caregivers modify their speech out of didactic considerations when talking to infants (e.g. Uther et al., 2007). That is, caregivers consciously modify their speech in order to convey clearer linguistic structures to infants. Others have proposed that the modifications to IDS primarily arise from caregivers' intentions to express affect (Benders, 2013).

Unfortunately, the question of caregiver intention has usually been discussed only with regard to the function of IDS, instead of being considered from the speaker's (caregiver's) perspective. For instance, evidence concerning the fact that IDS facilitates language acquisition has been used to support the view that caregivers intentionally provide more salient linguistic categories and structures to their infants. However, it should be noted that the facilitative role of IDS in speech and language development can be independent of the caregivers' intentions when using this speech register. In other words, the changes associated with IDS may be an unintended by-product of other prosodic properties, and do not necessarily derive from a motivation to enhance infants' learning language. Further, there might be individual differences in caregivers' intentions in using IDS which may be taken into consideration such as infants' developmental status, environment, and even the caregiver's mood, etc. As a consequence, the previous discussion on caregivers' intentions in using IDS from acoustic analysis of this speech register may well be uninformative, if not misleading.

This chapter seeks to bring together evidence from experimental work and corpus analyses in the literature on IDS and ADS in order to address the following four major questions: (1) What are the acoustic characteristics of IDS that distinguish it from ADS? (2) What are the functions of this unique speech register in language development? (3) Which aspects of IDS are particularly beneficial to language acquisition? (4) Why do caregivers use this speech register? The examination of this strand of the literature is important because it will serve to inform us about the nature of IDS and the development of language in human infants, and to highlight areas in need of further research.

5.2 ACOUSTIC PROPERTIES OF INFANT-DIRECTED SPEECH

During the past 50 years, a rather extensive body of research has produced an impressive amount of data concerning the acoustic differences between IDS and ADS. Results of this work suggest that despite some cross-cultural and cross-linguistic differences, similar prosodic acoustic properties are found in IDS across world languages (e.g. Fernald et al., 1989; Grieser & Kuhl, 1988; McMurray et al., 2013; Papoušek & Hwang, 1991; Ratner & Luberoff, 1984; Werker et al., 1994). Moreover, a sizeable body of research has further demonstrated that an infant's preference for IDS, as well as the characteristics of IDS, change as the infant develops (e.g. Kitamura et al., 2002; Liu et al., 2009; Stern et al., 1983). In this section, we will examine previous research on the acoustic differences between IDS and ADS, and also report work on the ways in which the acoustic properties of IDS change over the course of infant development.

5.2.1 Prosodic Properties of Infant-Directed Speech

One of the most marked differences between IDS and ADS is the exaggeration of prosodic properties in IDS over ADS (Figure 5.1). Specifically, IDS shows higher pitch, increased pitch range, distinctive pitch contours, slower tempo, and longer pauses than ADS (Bergeson et al., 2006; Bergeson & Trehub, 2002; Fernald, 1992; Fernald & Simon, 1984; Papoušek et al., 1985; Van de Weijer, 1997). In a recent systematic review of this literature, 92% of studies were found to have higher fundamental frequency (typically measured through F0); 67% showed larger pitch variability or pitch range; and 85% reported slower tempo and/or longer vowel duration in IDS as compared to ADS (Cristia, 2013). These prosodic modifications are widely attested across a large variety of Indo-European languages, such as English, French, Italian, and German (Fernald, 1989), and also in languages with different prosodic typologies, including tonal languages such as Mandarin (Grieser & Kuhl, 1988), Cantonese (Rattanasone et al., 2013), Thai (Kitamura et al., 2002), and pitch-accent languages such as Japanese (Fernald, 1989). Samples of IDS and ADS, showing prosodic modifications, can be found in Audios 5.1 and 5.2.

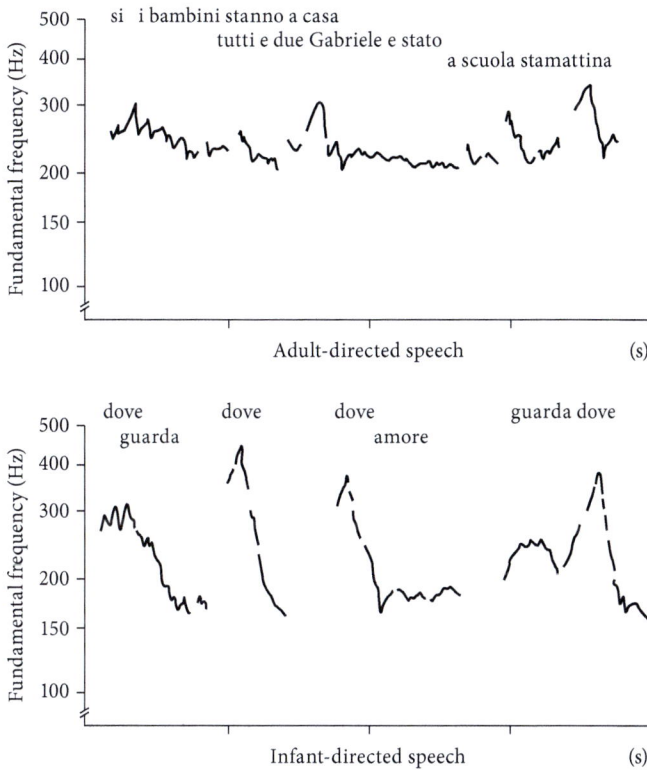

FIGURE 5.1 Fo contours of IDS and ADS in the speech of an Italian mother.

Reproduced from Fernald A. et al., 'A cross-language study of prosodic modifications in mothers' and fathers' speech to preverbal infants', *Journal of Child Language*, Volume 16, Issue 3, Figure 1, pp. 477–501, Copyright © 2014 Cambridge University Press, doi: 10.1017/S0305000900010679, reprinted with permission.

However, there are some differences between languages, at least some of which may be mediated by cultural or social factors. For example, Quiche-speaking mothers may avoid using a high pitch when speaking to their children because high pitch is typically used when addressing people with higher social status in this culture (Ingram, 1995; Ratner & Pye, 1984). In addition, British fathers use higher pitch, but not larger pitch range in IDS (Shute & Wheldall, 1999) as compared with ADS, suggesting that caregivers of different genders may use different combinations of prosodic modifications when talking to infants.

In addition to the general prosodic expansions detailed in the previous paragraphs, IDS also includes a smaller set of prosodic contour types (Fernald & Simon, 1984) and uses specific intonational contours in particular contexts (Fernald & Simon, 1984; Katz et al., 1996; Papoušek et al., 1991; Stern et al., 1982). For instance, mothers use more rising contours in a turn-encouraging context in IDS than in ADS (Papoušek et al., 1991). Moreover, the special characteristics of prosody in IDS also affect smaller linguistic units. For example, mothers consistently place focused words with pitch peaks in utterance-final position, whereas prosodic emphasis in ADS is more variable (Fernald & Mazzie, 1991). Similarly, Kondaurova and Bergeson (2011) compared pitch, pause, and duration cues to large prosodic boundaries in IDS and ADS, and found that most of these cues were enhanced in vowels located in pre-boundary positions (utterance-final) as compared to those in post-boundary positions (utterance-initial).

In sum, evidence suggests that although there are some cross-cultural and cross-linguistic variations, IDS seems to show prosodic exaggeration, as well as to include special contour types, when compared with ADS.

5.2.2 Segmental Properties of Infant-Directed Speech

While there are ample studies on the prosodic properties of IDS as compared with ADS, the number of studies on register differences between phonemes (vowels and consonants), particularly consonants, is relatively small. With respect to vowels, past studies have mainly explored differences in vowel space size, as reflected by the first and second formant frequencies of the corner vowels in IDS and ADS. These studies have yielded mixed results, as the vowel space has been variably reported to be expanded, shifted, reduced, or maintained in IDS. Some studies have demonstrated more extreme formant frequencies in IDS relative to ADS (e.g. Cristia & Seidl, 2014; Kuhl et al., 1997; Liu et al., 2003). For example, Kuhl et al. (1997) examined the vowel spaces for IDS and ADS in mothers who spoke American-English, Swedish, and Russian. They found expanded vowel spaces in IDS across the three languages. Others, however, found smaller vowel space sizes instead (e.g. Benders, 2013; Englund & Behne, 2006) and/or shifted vowel spaces (e.g. Dodane & Al-Tamimi, 2007; Englund & Behne, 2006). These findings may suggest that the vowels produced by caregivers can be overspecified (Figure 5.2), underspecified (Figure 5.3), or maintained in IDS as compared to those in ADS.

It should be kept in mind that the modifications, or lack thereof, in IDS may be conditioned by factors other than the specific nature of IDS. These factors include language typology, culture, infant developmental stage, and even methodologies used to elicit speech or measure the formants. For example, it has been proposed that Cantonese mothers do not hyperarticulate vowels because they pay more attention to, and thus exaggerate, tonal information (Rattanasone et al., 2013). In addition, one obvious difference between most studies reporting expanded vowel space size is that these studies elicited speech to infants with a few objects, whereas most studies reporting no such expansion used many more toys (and hence produced speech in more contexts). One possible explanation for this difference is that when provided with fewer toys or objects, parents may be aware that this small contrastive set is the focus of the experiment and consequently emphasize the relevant cues in the target objects. This points to the need to collect IDS samples in the infant's natural environment so as to examine whether IDS collected with limited objects really allows for generalization to real-life situations.

With respect to consonants, the most well-examined acoustic property is voice onset time (VOT), which has also been variably found to be increased, decreased, or maintained in IDS as compared with that in ADS (Baran et al., 1977; Englund, 2005; Sundberg & Lacerda, 1999). For example, Englund (2005) reported longer VOT in six Norwegian mothers' IDS for the majority of stop consonants examined. On the other hand, Baran et al. (1977) found no overall VOT differences between IDS and ADS. In contrast, when examining speech to Swedish 3-month-olds, Sundberg and Lacerda (1999) found an overall *decrease* of VOT in both voiced and voiceless consonants in IDS. The fact that VOT is also used to cue

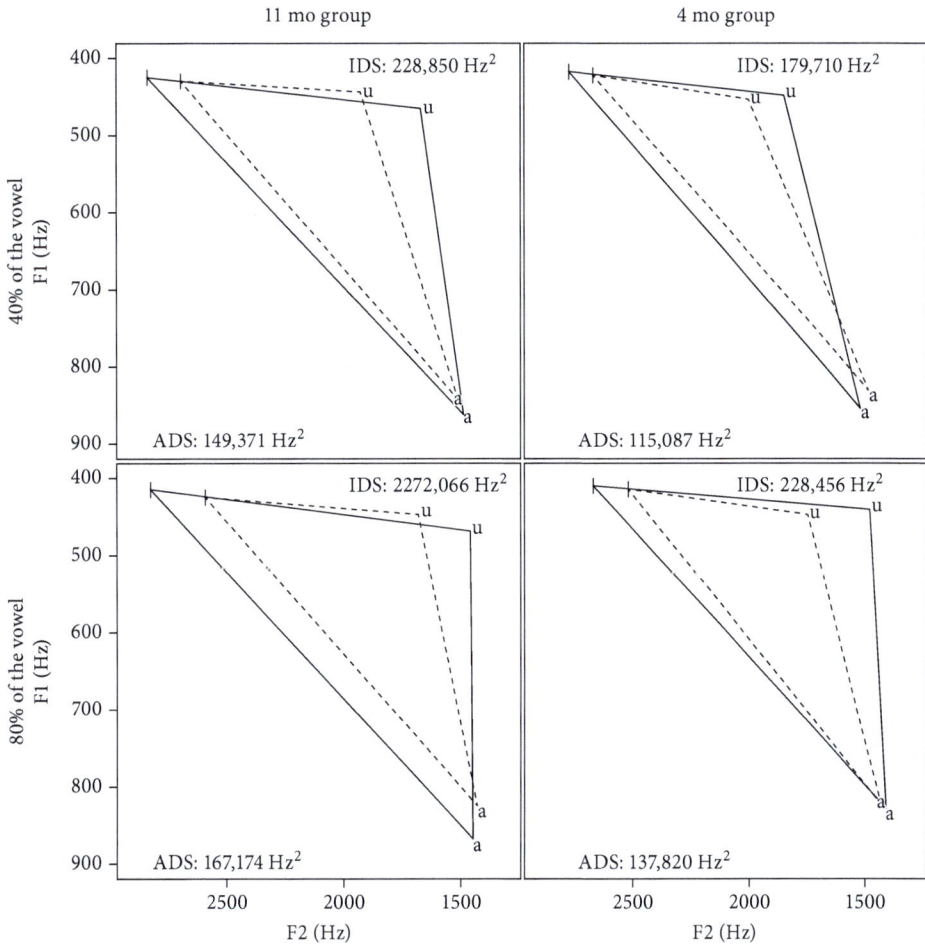

FIGURE 5.2 Vowel space in speech addressed to infants (black, solid) and adults (grey, dashed). The top row shows the averages for the measurement taken 40% into the vowel; the bottom row shows the averages corresponding to 80% measurement. Graphs on the left side correspond to talkers addressing 11-month-olds; on the right, those addressing 4-month-olds.

Reproduced from Cristia A. & Seidl A., 'The hyperarticulation hypothesis of infant-directed speech', *Journal of Child Language*, Volume 41, Issue 4, pp. 913–34, Copyright © 2014 Cambridge University Press, doi: 10.1017/S0305000912000669, reprinted with permission.

phonological voicing contrast for stops in these languages renders the interpretation of these mixed findings even more complex. This is because if VOTs for both voiced and voiceless stops move in the same direction, this can entail larger, similar, or even smaller phonetic distinctions between these two types of stops. In addition, as a temporal variable, VOT is also entangled with the slower-speaking rate present in IDS. In this regard, a recent study by McMurray et al. (2013) offers some new insights. They measured VOT values for both voiced and voiceless stops in IDS and ADS, and found that VOTs increased for both sounds in IDS, as compared to ADS. Most importantly, they further calculated the ratio of VOT to vowel

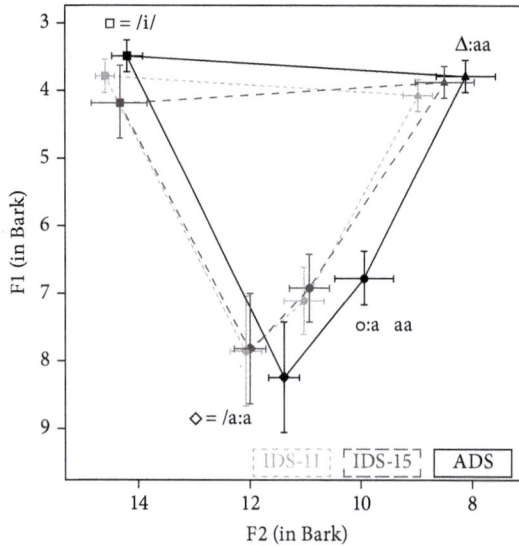

FIGURE 5.3 Vowel space formed by vowels /i/, /aː/, /a/, and /u/, in IDS (dotted lines) and ADS (solid lines) in Dutch.

Reprinted from *Infant Behavior and Development*, Volume 36, Issue 4, Benders T. 'Mommy is only happy! Dutch mothers' realisation of speech sounds in infant directed speech expresses emotion, not didactic intent', Figure 2, pp. 847–62, Copyright © 2013 Elsevier Ltd., with permission from Elsevier, http://www.sciencedirect.com/science/article/pii/S0163638313000908.

length (CV ratio) to create a measure of voicing that accounts for differences in speech rate. The results showed that after controlling for rate differences, no difference was found between IDS and ADS in terms of voicing contrasts. In sum, their study suggests that although absolute measures of VOT are different in IDS and ADS, they do not differ in a way that necessarily provides clearer linguistic information in speech to infants.

Direct evidence supporting the suggestion that consonants may be more clearly articulated in IDS comes from a corpus study by Cristia (2010). Specifically, she examined the location of the centroid in /s/ and /ʃ/ and found that it is higher for /s/ than for /ʃ/ in IDS, thus distinguishing /s/ from its acoustic neighbour /ʃ/. Similarly, Dilley et al. (2014) examined the pronunciation variation of word-final alveolar stops in the environments where regressive assimilation could occur, and found a reliable tendency for canonical or clear variants to occur more often in IDS than in ADS. Despite this work, there is also evidence in other recent work running contrary to the view that IDS provides more discriminable acoustic cues for consonants. Specifically, in a recent comprehensive analysis comparing many types of consonant contrasts in a spontaneous Japanese speech corpus, Martin et al. (2015) found a small but significant advantage for phonetic contrasts in ADS as compared to IDS. Specifically, they calculated the discriminability between each of the onsets and every other onset from using minimal-pair ABX scores (for more discussion of discriminability and ABX scores, see Martin et al., 2015), and found that the phonetic contrasts were reduced in IDS.

To summarize, with respect to the segmental properties of IDS, there are few studies that clearly point to increased clarity of phonetic contrasts in IDS over ADS. In addition, segmental clarity may be impacted by other properties of speech, such as higher-level modification in prosodic contour, and speaking rate. Thus, in a way distinct from the prosodic modifications in IDS, enhanced segmental contrast might not be a universal characteristic of IDS.

5.2.3 Effects of Developmental Status on the Characteristics of Infant-Directed Speech

Before turning to the question of how IDS properties change as a function of infant development, it is necessary to briefly review work on the change of infant preference for IDS, because there might be possible synergies between infant preferences and adult register modifications.

Although young infants in general prefer listening to IDS over ADS (Fernald & Simon, 1984; Fernald et al., 1989; Kitamura et al., 2002; Kuhl et al., 1997; Panneton et al., 2006), evidence has also shown developmental changes in infants' auditory preferences for this speech register. For example, Hayashi et al. (2001) found a U-shaped developmental shift in Japanese-learning infants, with very young infants preferring IDS, 7- to 9-month-olds showing no preferences, and a subsequent recovery in preference for IDS in 10- to 14-month-olds. Similarly, Newman and Hussain (2006) found a similar lack of preference for IDS in 9-month-old English-learning infants, although they did not find a recovery in preference for IDS at 13 months. A recent study, however, has demonstrated that 12- and 16-month-olds continue to prefer listening to speech with the prosodic properties of IDS (Segal & Newman, 2015). Despite the discrepancy among these studies, which could be due to factors such as language typology, culture, or even differences in stimuli, cumulatively these studies suggest that the preference for IDS changes across development.

Recent studies also show a corresponding age-related preference for the prosodic information in IDS (Kitamura & Notley, 2009; McRoberts et al., 2009). For instance, 4-month-olds pay more attention to speech with higher positive affect and a slowed speech rate, whereas 8-month-olds prefer normal-rate speech with a lower level of positive affect (Panneton et al., 2006). McRoberts et al. (2009) suggest that this shift may be related to changes in infants' linguistic development, such that older infants, who have tuned to the linguistic structure of their native language, may be more inclined to attend to signals with clearer structural information.

Taken together, young infants attend to the acoustic properties in the speech signal and their weighting of these cues changes over the first year. If infants' responses to IDS play a role in regulating caregivers' speech, then we would expect that the properties of IDS may also change over time (they would diminish or become more ADS-like). We will now specifically discuss how IDS characteristics change with infant developmental status.

The first aspect we will consider is the age of the infant. Although an infant's linguistic skill and age are clearly not orthogonal dimensions, some studies have focused more on the former, and we will discuss these data here. A few studies have demonstrated age-specific adjustment in the acoustic characteristics of IDS (e.g. Kitamura & Burnham, 2003; Liu et al., 2009; Stern et al., 1983). For example, in a longitudinal study, Stern et al. (1983) compared speech to infants of different ages, and found that IDS addressed to 4-month-olds had a higher pitch than IDS addressed to neonates, and to 1- and 2-year-olds. Similarly, Kitamura and Burnham (2003) reported that Australian mothers adjusted their pitch level and pitch range when addressing infants at a variety of ages from birth to 12 months (0, 3, 6, 9, and 12 months). Particularly, mothers tended to use higher mean F0 to convey positive affect in their phrases addressed to 6- and 12-month-olds, and to use more directive utterances with greater F0 range and lower mean F0 in speech directed to 9-month-olds. The impact of age on IDS–ADS differences is also found in languages from other prosodic typologies, such as tonal languages. For example, Rattanasone et al. (2013) measured tonal triangles (a measure of tone space size as defined by the three tones of 'High Rising', 'High Level', and 'Falling') in ADS and IDS collected from twenty-two native Cantonese-speaking mother–infant dyads at four different ages—3 months, 6 months, 9 months, and 12 months. Comparisons revealed that tonal triangles were larger in IDS than in ADS at 3, 6, and 9 months, but not at 12 months.

In addition to the literature examining how age affects IDS properties, there has been a recent growing body of research examining the acoustic and prosodic features of maternal speech to preverbal infants with paediatric hearing loss, who receive hearing aids or cochlear implants later on. For example, Bergeson et al. (2006) compared the prosodic characteristics of speech directed to three populations—infants who are profoundly deaf with a cochlear implant (CI), normal hearing infants (NH) with matched chronological age, and NH infants with matched hearing experience (younger infant matches). They found that the increase in average and minimum pitch from ADS to IDS in mothers' speech to CI infants was more similar to that in speech to NH infants with matched auditory experience and distinct from NH infants with matched chronological age. In the same vein, Kondaurova and Bergeson (2011) examined the effects of infant age and hearing status on maternal use of prosodic and structural features in IDS. They compared pitch change, pre-boundary vowel lengthening, and pause duration in the speech directed to these three same populations. Results demonstrated that, despite the exaggerated prosodic properties in IDS regardless of infants' hearing status, pre-boundary vowel lengthening was tailored to infants' hearing experience rather than to chronological age. Specifically, they found that the vowel duration difference scores were larger in IDS than ADS in the CI group and the NH group with matched hearing experience, but not in the NH group with matched chronological age.

The findings from Kondaurova and Bergeson (2011) suggest that the degree of exaggeration of IDS changes over infant development and may be impacted by both chronological age and linguistic ability. These findings may imply that caregivers modify their speech, be it consciously or unconsciously, to suit the developmental needs of their infants. For younger infants, who pay more attention to the emotional and affective information in the speech (Kitamura & Burnham, 1998; Singh et al., 2002), IDS may show exaggerated prosodic properties, and thus play an important role in engaging in attention. On the other hand, older infants, who have more mature speech perception abilities, may be actively seeking enhanced perceptual cues and well-specified linguistic information that are beneficial to speech processing (Newman & Hussain, 2006). Therefore IDS directed to this age group may show less prosodic exaggeration, but provide clearer cues to linguistic structure.

5.3 EFFECTS OF INFANT-DIRECTED SPEECH ON LANGUAGE ACQUISITION

In this section, we turn to the question of the functions of IDS on infant language acquisition; we also review work on IDS modification that is conditioned by development. Researchers thus far have proposed three major hypotheses regarding the possible functions of IDS in communication and language acquisition, such as to direct and engage attention (Fernald & Simon, 1984; Papoušek et al., 1991), to communicate affect (Fernald, 1989; Papoušek et al., 1990; Werker & McLeod, 1989), and to facilitate language acquisition (Kaplan et al., 2002; Kuhl et al., 1997; Thiessen et al., 2005). In IDS, engaging attention and expressing affect are mostly implemented by exaggerated prosodic properties of IDS (Fernald & Mazzie, 1991; Fernald & Simon, 1984) and positive affect (Singh et al., 2002). Indeed, infants and adults are better at tracking emotion and communicative intent in IDS than in ADS (Fernald, 1989).

Although there has been substantial discussion of possible properties of IDS that might enhance speech processing, very few studies have systematically investigated the role of IDS in promoting performance on linguistic tasks, that is, comparing learners' capacity to process speech produced in IDS versus ADS. Research along these lines has been primarily *descriptive* in nature (Fernald & Mazzie, 1991; Fernald & Simon, 1984; Gleitman et al., 1989; Peters, 1983; Thiessen et al., 2005) and the investigation of the input infants receive and infant linguistic ability have been studied separately. For example, Fernald and Simon (1984) found that when German-speaking mothers talked to their infants, they spoke with higher pitch, wider pitch range, longer pauses, shorter utterances, and more prosodic repetitions. Likewise, Kuhl et al. (1997) examined vowel spaces cross-linguistically, and found that mothers' vowel spaces were expanded, and thus were *potentially* more discriminable in IDS as compared to ADS. On the basis of these findings, researchers speculated that there may be causal effects between exaggerated prosodic and segmental properties in IDS and infant speech perception.

However, it should be noted that the changes in IDS may enhance language development only if they pattern in a way that could facilitate learning. A second critical question is whether the degree of modifications in IDS is sufficient to promote infant speech processing. These questions have benefited from a few empirical studies that have explored whether there is a direct link between IDS and language acquisition. Some of these studies revealed that IDS may play an important role in speech processing (e.g. Karzon, 1985; Liu et al., 2003; Ma et al., 2011; Singh et al., 2009; Thiessen et al., 2005). For example, infants between 1 and 4 months old discriminate 'malana' from 'marana' only when the syllables are produced in IDS (Karzon, 1985). IDS also appears to facilitate 7.5-month-olds' extraction of statistical regularities in speech (Thiessen et al., 2005). Similarly, 10.5-month-old British-English-learning infants succeeded in a word segmentation task only when they were presented with exaggerated IDS (Floccia et al., 2016). Two recent studies have also demonstrated that IDS promotes word learning. For example, Song et al. (2010) assessed 7- and 8-month-olds' memory for words when the words were produced in IDS and ADS. They found that infants showed successful recognition of the words 24 hours later, but only when the words were produced in IDS. Additionally, Ma et al. (2011) showed that 21-month-old children learn novel words only from IDS, but not from ADS. Nevertheless, the effects of IDS on speech processing seem to attenuate in older children, as 27-month-old children in the same study learned the words under both IDS and ADS conditions (Ma et al., 2011). In addition, recent studies showed that there were no differences in 16-month-olds' ability to segment words from IDS and ADS (Mani & Pätzold, 2016), as well as that 12-month-olds showed reduced sensitivity to trochaic stress pattern from IDS than ADS (Wang et al., 2016).

Despite the limited number of studies on the relation between IDS and speech perception, the aforementioned studies provide some evidence that the unique properties of IDS may have important effects during the course of infants' language development, at least for younger infants. However, it is important to note that we do not know *why* infants in these studies learned better from IDS than from ADS, and we cannot rule out a simple attentional explanation, because increased attention to speech could provide a foundation for language development (Houston & Bergeson, 2014; Vouloumanos & Curtin, 2014; Wang, Shafto, & Houston, 2018).

5.4 WHY DO INFANTS LEARN BETTER FROM INFANT-DIRECTED SPEECH?

In the previous section, we reviewed empirical studies on the direct links between IDS and infant language acquisition. However, in order to have a better understanding of the role of IDS in infant speech processing, it is also very important to consider the question of why young infants might learn better from IDS. In particular, we would like to know which aspects of IDS are most beneficial to learning.

As mentioned earlier, researchers hold different views regarding why IDS facilitates learning. Some have argued that the facilitative role of IDS on language learning is a by-product of learners' enhanced attention to this speech register (e.g. Cristia & Seidl, 2014; Drotar & Sturm, 1988; Trainor et al., 2000). Indeed, a large body of research now exists supporting the view that pitch modulation serves to mediate infants' attention (Cooper & Aslin, 1990; Fernald & Kuhl, 1987; Pegg et al., 1992; Werker & McLeod, 1989). Among all factors (duration, pitch, and intensity), 4-month-olds preferred IDS when the pitch information was maintained (Fernald & Kuhl, 1987). In contrast, when IDS differed from ADS only in amplitude or duration, infants showed no such preference. A follow-up study further demonstrated that infants were especially responsive to the melodic quality of IDS (Fernald, 1989). On the other hand, other researchers have argued that IDS provides better perceptual cues and well-specified linguistic information that are beneficial to speech processing. Indeed, vowel space size in IDS is found to be related to infants' rate of phoneme perception development (Liu et al., 2003) and children's word recognition (Song et al., 2010). However, there are controversies regarding each of these two hypotheses; in addition, these two possibilities are not mutually exclusive.

With regard to the first hypothesis, researchers have raised different ideas about the effectiveness of pitch modulation in attracting infants' attention (Colombo & Horowitz, 1986; Cooper & Aslin, 1994; Kaplan et al., 2002). For example, Colombo and Horowitz (1986) examined 4-month-olds' responses to 1-s, bell-shaped, frequency-modulated tone sweeps stimulating either an IDS pitch range or an ADS range. They found that infants did not prefer IDS over ADS, suggesting that the extent of pitch modulation did not affect infants' attention to other types of auditory stimuli. Likewise, Kitamura and Burnham (1998) and Singh et al.

(2002) suggest that it is the positive affect, instead of purely pitch characteristics of IDS that is the key to infants' general preference for IDS. Specifically, Singh et al. (2002) examined 6-month-olds' listening preferences by manipulating affect and speech register separately (IDS versus ADS). When affect was held constant, they found that infants did not show any preference for listenening to IDS; however, infants preferred ADS stimuli when they were presented with more positive affect than IDS.

Second, with regard to the hypothesis concerning the didactic nature of IDS, there is ample debate regarding whether IDS provides enhanced auditory contrasts and thus clearer examples of native phoneme categories. The expansion of vowel space in IDS is not replicated in all studies (Dodane & Al-Tamimi, 2007; Englund & Behne, 2006; Van de Weijer, 2009). Moreover, an expanded vowel space does not necessarily entail overall clearer speech, as it is found to be not as good a predictor of speech intelligibility as the acoustic distinctiveness of neighbouring vowels (Neel, 2008). In this regard, Cristia and Seidl (2014) gathered acoustic correlates of phonological contrastiveness in terms of the degree of separation between pairs of vowel; they found that /i-ɪ/ actually had greater acoustic overlap in IDS, making discriminability of the two vowels ostensibly more difficult. This finding was replicated in a recent study by McMurray et al. (2013) which showed that IDS may collapse the distinction for some interior vowels.

Another similar line of research comes from studies examining the properties of IDS as a function of prosodic prominence. This line of research makes the assumption that if IDS exaggerates acoustic characteristics only in prosodically salient positions, learners may then be receiving a very different input than would be heard in typical ADS. This is because such selective exaggeration may make linguistic categories more distinct from each other, and thus may potentially facilitate their speech processing. However, if IDS–ADS differences are not modulated by prosodic prominence, then the unique IDS characteristics that we see may instead be more likely to be the by-product of caregivers' expression of affect. In a recent study, Wang et al. (2015) elicited IDS and ADS from mothers of 4- and 11-month-olds. They compared the average duration, average Fo, and vowel peripherality in vowels across the two registers in both stressed and unstressed syllables. The results showed that vowels in both stressed and unstressed syllables exhibited higher Fo and wider vowel peripherality in IDS as compared to those in ADS. However, the IDS–ADS differences were not modulated by lexical stress, suggesting that IDS may not be specifically didactic. In a similar vein, Lee et al. (2014) examined prominence, cued by maximum loudness (Lmax), of vocalic intervals in IDS and ADS in a corpus of utterances from Australian-English mothers. They found that the prominence contrasts were reduced in IDS as compared to in ADS.

Nevertheless, the attentional and the didactic hypotheses may, to a certain degree, not be mutually exclusive, as it is possible that some acoustic properties may be involved in both functions. For example, expanded pitch range, which has been regarded to mainly serve the purpose of attracting infant attention, may also contribute to more intelligible speech. For example, Bradlow et al. (1996) found a tendency for pitch range to be positively correlated with higher speech intelligibility. Similarly, Trainor and Desjardins (2002) demonstrated that large pitch contours in IDS facilitate 6- to 7-month-olds' ability to discriminate vowels. The fact that large pitch contours contribute to better vowel discrimination has a physiological and acoustic basis. Although the Fo and frequencies of vowel harmonics change when there is a pitch contour, the frequencies of formant resonances remain constant (Hillenbrand & Gayvert, 1993). Thus, it is likely that larger pitch changes will enable harmonic sweeps through the frequencies of the formants (Figure 5.4), thereby revealing the locations of the vocal tract resonances of the vowel (Trainor & Desjardins, 2002).

To summarize, it is not clear which acoustic cues of IDS are recruited to maintain infants' attention. Moreover, IDS does not necessarily provide more salient cues for speech processing. Finally, even if IDS does provide clearer cues for processing, there are various

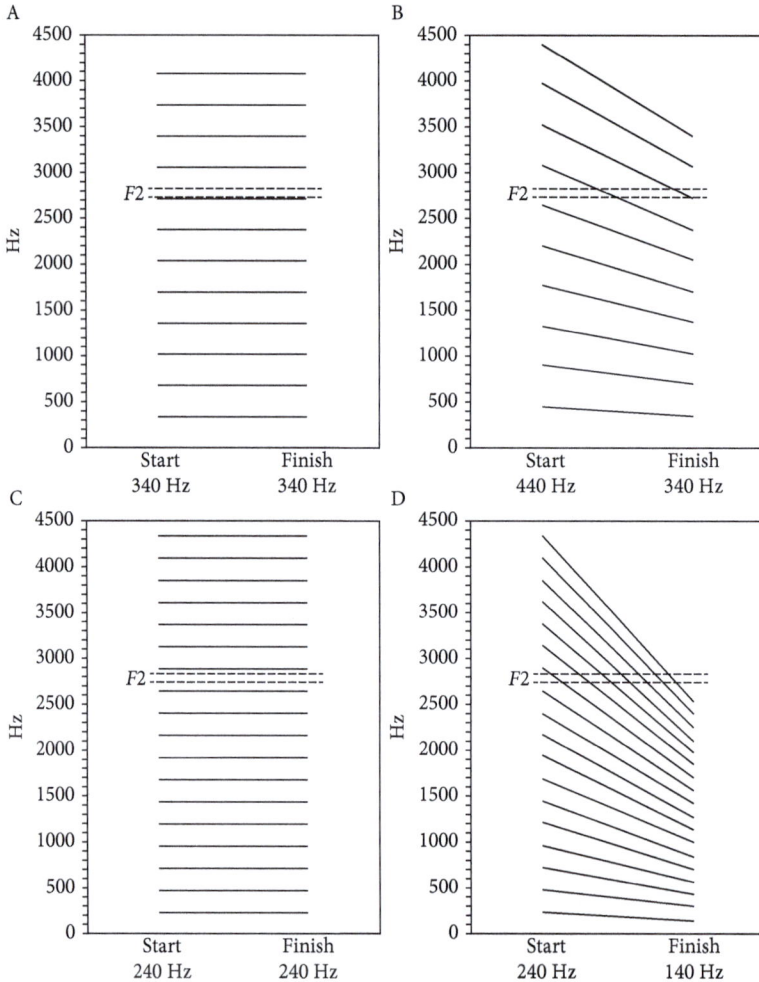

FIGURE 5.4 The harmonic structures for steady-state tokens are shown in panels A and C, and those for contour tokens are shown in panels B and D. Note that for the higher-pitched tokens, shown in panels A and B, the harmonics are more widely spaced than those for the lower-pitched tokens, shown in panels C and D. In the steady-state tokens (panels A and C), the harmonics fall outside the second formant (F2), whereas when pitch contour is added (panels B and D), the harmonics pass through the F2 band.

Reproduced from Trainor J.T. & Renée N.D., 'Pitch characteristics of infant-directed speech affect infants' ability to discriminate vowels', *Psychonomic Bulletin Review*, Volume 9, Issue 2, Figure 1, pp. 335-40, Copyright © 2002 Psychonomic Society, Inc. doi: 10.3758/BF03196290, by permission of Springer.

ways in which the cueing may unfold. One possibility is that different features of IDS are involved in each of these functions. It is also possible that some features may be involved in both processes. Due to these reasons, there is insufficient evidence as to the question of why IDS promotes language acquisition. Perhaps IDS initially serves to express caregivers' emotion, but is conveniently recruited to serve the didactic function. What is clearly known, as we have concluded in the last section, is that IDS plays a crucial role in infants' language development. It seems evident that the more data we gather concerning the previously mentioned problems, the better we will be able to achieve a thorough understanding of this research question. Thus, we encourage future research to disentangle these possibilities under an agnostic lens.

5.5 Why Do Caregivers Use Infant-Directed Speech?

The last question we would like to broach in this chapter concerns why caregivers adopt this unique register. As mentioned, one possibility is that they modify their speech out of a didactic consideration for their language-learning infants. That is, caregivers consciously and explicitly enhance the auditory contrasts between sounds because they intend to convey clear exemplars of categories present in their language. The major supporting evidence for this view comes from the enhanced auditory contrasts between the corner vowels in IDS over ADS (e.g. Bradlow et al., 1996; Burnham et al., 2002), in speech to adult second-language learners (Uther et al., 2007), but not in speech to adult pets (Burnham et al., 2002).

Another option is that the possibly expanded vowel space in IDS, as well as other enhanced sounds or phonological contrasts, might be side effects from other caregiver intentions, such as communicating affect or garnering infant attention, such that the segmental enhancement (when present) or prosodic enhancement may occur only as a consequence of other IDS prosodic propertiesincluding slower speech rate, increased number of syllables and words at the utterance focal positions, and positive affect. This possibility has received some support from Schaeffler (2007) who demonstrated that the caregiver only showed an expanded vowel space for the child for whom she displayed greater emotional availability. In addition, expanded vowel spaces were found in speech to puppies and infants, but not to adult dogs or adult humans (Kim et al., 2006).

Nevertheless, despite all these correlations, it is not clear what the physical or psychological mechanisms are that underlie this connection. Perhaps the best way of testing this hypothesis is to design work that gets at the relation between caregiver intentions and the acoustic properties of IDS, rather than merely focuses on the properties of IDS.

5.6 Conclusions and Future Directions

This chapter has provided a non-exhaustive review of the IDS literature with the aim of addressing four key questions. First, what are the acoustic differences between IDS and ADS?

Second, what are the functions of IDS in linguistic development? Third, why do infants learn better from IDS? Finally, why do caregivers adopt this register? This section summarizes previous findings and concludes by outlining some prospects for future research, some of which are not commonly addressed in the field of IDS/ADS studies. The answers to these questions will not only optimize our understanding of IDS per se, but may also deepen the theoretical and clinical significance of this body of work.

With respect to the first question, the findings discussed in this chapter point to a tendency for IDS and ADS to be clearly distinct registers even across a diverse set of languages. In sum, while IDS and ADS might not diverge from each other in exactly the same way across all languages and cultures there are (a) key differences between IDS and ADS, and (b) some differences that we see across all languages and cultures. Specifically, IDS tends to be prosodically distinct from ADS, for example, being produced at a higher pitch than ADS in most languages and cultures. That said, differences between IDS and ADS at the segmental level seem much less clear and data explored here seems to support the idea that IDS does not specifically exaggerate the segmental properties of the signal.

One possibility that might account for differences in language and culture with regard to IDS is that speakers may enhance dimensions that are more informative over others that are less so in the infant's native language. For example, as we mentioned earlier, Cantonese mothers exaggerate tonal information, but not vowels in IDS, probably because as a tonal language, Cantonese uses tones to distinguish meaning. Thus, lexical tones provide more salient language-specific information over vowels at an early stage of infant development. This hypothesis would greatly benefit from data concerning how exactly this trade-off occurs— whether at the physiological level or at a higher cognitive level. Clearly, this points to the need for more cross-linguistic research as well as more research concerning caregivers' intentions.

To address the second question concerning the function of IDS for the infant, we discussed the effects of IDS on language acquisition. There are three major hypotheses about the possible functions of IDS, such as to maintain infants' attention, to communicate affect, and to be didactic. While there is ample evidence in support of the first two hypotheses showing that infants learn better from happy, affective speech, and from IDS in general, it is less clear that IDS has a purely didactic function. Moreover, efforts thus far along these lines have been focused on only a limited domain, particularly on phoneme perception, word recognition, as well as boundary detection; whereas the degree to which IDS may shape infants' rhythmic processing is less understood. It is possible that the exaggerated prosodic properties of IDS may conflict with the realization of the rhythmic properties of speech, resulting in reduced rhythmic contrasts in IDS (Wang et al., 2016). If this were true, then the role of IDS in speech processing may be task-dependent.

It should be noted that this discussion is based on the assumption that exaggerated acoustic contrasts would promote speech processing. However, direct evidence regarding the correlation between an exaggerated acoustic signal and enhanced speech processing is scarce. It is less clear whether infants are able to take advantage of the more salient acoustic contrasts in IDS, if there are any, in processing speech. This is an important question that warrants future investigation because it not only contributes to the understanding of the effects of IDS in infant acquisition of the structure of their ambient languages, but may also provide a window to look beneath the surface of the acoustic characteristics of IDS and discover what is its fundamental mechanism for promoting language acquisition. Further, the functions of IDS and why parents use it are highly integral and thus should be examined as a cohesive unit, both from a theoretical and practical perspective. However, research endeavours in the past have devoted less attention to this issue. Specifically, most previous research on the effects of IDS on infant learning was conducted in standard laboratory settings, with IDS speech stimuli being recorded from a single, unfamiliar speaker. Results obtained in the laboratory may not allow for generalization to learning in the 'wild'. Therefore, future research to address these questions is highly recommended. In addition to the theoretical significance, the findings from this body of research may also have profound clinical implications because they will indicate what kind of input is most effective for language acquisition, including that for atypically developing populations at risk for language impairment.

Third, we discussed two possibilities as to why infants learn better from IDS over ADS. One possibility is that IDS serves to engage attention and show positive affect, and the facilitative role of IDS on learning is a by-product of infants' increased attention to IDS. Alternatively, the other possibility is that IDS provides better perceptual cues for speech processing. However, we do not yet have a conclusive answer to this question due to mixed results, as well as to the fact that these two possibilities are not mutually exclusive. Another possibility that we need to consider, in light of the discussion on the developmental change of infant preference for IDS, is that the mechanisms underlying the facilitative role of IDS in language acquisition may change as well. Specifically, for young infants, who pay more attention to the intonational and affect information in the speech, the facilitative role of IDS may be through engaging their attention. However, for older infants who seem to prefer speech that provides clearer linguistic structure, IDS may be better at serving a didactic role.

Finally, we briefly discussed mothers' intentions in using IDS, a topic that has received little attention in the literature. This question is far from answerable due to the limited number of empirical studies available and the difficulty in experimentally measuring something as amorphous as intentions. While it seems that caregivers are good at adjusting prosodic properties in IDS, their modification with respect to segmental cues is inconsistent. One further possibility that we may want to consider is that caregivers are attempting to speak more clearly in IDS; however, they are simply unable to exert control over finer segmental cues, such as VOT or vowel formants. Future studies examining both caregiver intentions and IDS properties may disentangle these confounds.

In sum, in this chapter we have reviewed a non-exhaustive list of work on the properties of IDS as compared with ADS. We have also discussed the possible roles of IDS for several aspects of language development (e.g. speech discrimination, word learning). Finally, we have touched upon the ways in which IDS facilitates language acquisition and why caregivers might use IDS when talking to their infants. However, future investigations are encouraged to address the remaining issues in the field of IDS research in order to facilitate our understanding of this unique register, as well as to provide information regarding the theoretical and clinical significance of IDS.

References

Albin, D. D. & Echols, C. H. (1996). Stressed and word-final syllables in infant-directed speech. *Infant Behavior and Development*, 19(4), 401–418.

Baran, J. A., Laufer, M. Z., & Daniloff, R. (1977). Phonological contrastivity in conversation: a comparative study of voice onset time. *Journal of Phonetics*, 5, 339–350.

Benders, T. (2013). Mommy is only happy! Dutch mothers' realisation of speech sounds in infant-directed speech expresses emotion, not didactic intent. *Infant Behavior and Development*, 36(4), 847–862. doi: http://dx.doi.org/10.1016/j.infbeh.2013.09.001

Bergeson, T. R., Miller, R. J., & McCune, K. (2006). Mothers' speech to hearing-impaired infants and children with cochlear implants. *Infancy*, 10(3), 221–240.

Bergeson, T. R. & Trehub, S. E. (2002). Absolute pitch and tempo in mothers' songs to infants. *Psychological Science*, 13(1), 72–75.

Bradlow, A. R., Torretta, G. M., & Pisoni, D. B. (1996). Intelligibility of normal speech I: global and fine-grained acoustic-phonetic talker characteristics. *Speech Communication*, 20(3), 255–272.

Burnham, D., Kitamura, C., & Vollmer-Conna, U. (2002). What's new, pussycat? On talking to babies and animals. *Science*, 296(5572), 1435–1435.

Colombo, J. & Horowitz, F. D. (1986). Infants' attentional responses to frequency modulated sweeps. *Child Development*, 57(2), 287–291.

Cooper, R. P. & Aslin, R. N. (1990). Preference for infant-directed speech in the first month after birth. *Child Development*, 61(5), 1584–1595.

Cooper, R. P. & Aslin, R. N. (1994). Developmental differences in infant attention to the spectral properties of infant-directed speech. *Child Development*, 65(6), 1663–1677.

Cristia, A. (2010). Phonetic enhancement of sibilants in infant-directed speech. *The Journal of the Acoustical Society of America*, 128(1), 424–434.

Cristia, A. (2013). Input to language: the phonetics and perception of infant-directed speech. *Language and Linguistics Compass*, 7(3), 157–170.

Cristia, A. & Seidl, A. (2014). The hyperarticulation hypothesis of infant-directed speech. *Journal of Child Language*, 41(04), 913–934.

Cristia, A., Seidl, A., Junge, C., Soderstrom, M., & Hagoort, P. (2014). Predicting individual variation in language from infant speech perception measures. *Child Development*, 85(4), 1330–1345.

Curtin, S. (2009). Twelve-month-olds learn novel word–object pairings differing only in stress pattern. *Journal of Child Language*, 36(05), 1157–1165.

Curtin, S., Mintz, T. H., & Christiansen, M. H. (2005). Stress changes the representational landscape: evidence from word segmentation. *Cognition*, 96(3), 233–262.

Dilley, L. C., Millett, A. L., Mcauley, J. D., & Bergeson, T. R. (2014). Phonetic variation in consonants in infant-directed and adult-directed speech: the case of regressive place assimilation in word-final alveolar stops. *Journal of Child Language*, 41(01), 155–175.

Dodane, C. & Al-Tamimi, J. (2007). An acoustic comparison of vowel systems in adult-directed speech and child-directed speech: evidence from French, English & Japanese. In: *Proceedings of the 16th International Congress of Phonetic Sciences (ICPhS)* (pp. 1573–1576). Saarbrucken, Germany.

Drotar, D. & Sturm, L. (1988). Prediction of intellectual development in young children with early histories of nonorganic failure-to-thrive. *Journal of Pediatric Psychology*, 13(2), 281–296.

Englund, K. T. (2005). Voice onset time in infant directed speech over the first six months. *First Language*, 25(2), 219–234.

Englund, K. T. & Behne, D. (2006). Changes in infant directed speech in the first six months. *Infant and Child Development*, 15(2), 139–160.

Ferguson, C. A. (1964). Baby talk in six languages. *American Anthropologist*, 66(6), 103–114.

Ferguson, C. A., Menn, L., & Stoel-Gammon, C. (1992). *Phonological Development: Models, Research, Implications*. Timonium, MD: York Press.

Fernald, A. (1985). Four-month-old infants prefer to listen to motherese. *Infant Behavior and Development*, 8(2), 181–195.

Fernald, A. (1989). Intonation and communicative intent in mothers' speech to infants: Is the melody the message? *Child Development*, 60(6), 1497–1510.

Fernald, A. (1992). Meaningful melodies in mothers' speech to infants. In: H. Papoušek, U. Jürgens, & M. Papoušek (eds) *Nonverbal Vocal Communication: Comparative and Developmental Approaches* (pp. 262–282). Cambridge, MA: Cambridge University Press.

Fernald, A. (1993). Approval and disapproval: infant responsiveness to vocal affect in familiar and unfamiliar languages. *Child Development*, 64(3), 657–674.

Fernald, A. & Kuhl, P. (1987). Acoustic determinants of infant preference for motherese speech. *Infant Behavior and Development*, 10(3), 279–293.

Fernald, A. & Mazzie, C. (1991). Prosody and focus in speech to infants and adults. *Developmental Psychology*, 27(2), 209–221.

Fernald, A. & Simon, T. (1984). Expanded intonation contours in mothers' speech to newborns. *Developmental Psychology*, 20(1), 104–113.

Fernald, A., Taeschner, T., Dunn, J., Papousek, M., de Boysson-Bardies, B., & Fukui, I. (1989). A cross-language study of prosodic modifications in mothers' and fathers' speech to preverbal infants. *Journal of Child Language*, 16(03), 477–501.

Floccia, C., Keren-Portnoy, T., DePaolis, R., Duffy, H., Delle Luche, C., Durrant, S., ... Vihman, M. (2016). British english infants segment words only with exaggerated infant-directed speech stimuli. *Cognition*, 148, 1–9.

Gleitman, L. R., Gleitman, H., Landau, B., & Wanner, E. (1989). Where learning begins: initial representations for language learning. In: F. J. Newmeyer (ed.) *Linguistics: The Cambridge Survey. Language: Psychological and Biological Aspects* (Vol. 3, pp. 150–193). Cambridge, MA: Cambridge University Press.

Greenwood, C. R., Thiemann-Bourque, K., Walker, D., Buzhardt, J., & Gilkerson, J. (2011). Assessing children's home language environments using automatic speech recognition technology. *Communication Disorders Quarterly*, 32(2), 83–92.

Grieser, D. L. & Kuhl, P. K. (1988). Maternal speech to infants in a tonal language: support for universal prosodic features in motherese. *Developmental Psychology*, 24(1), 14–20.

Hart, B. & Risley, T. R. (1995). *Meaningful Differences in the Everyday Experience of Young American Children*. Baltimore, MD: Paul H. Brookes Publishing.

Hayashi, A., Tamekawa, Y., & Kiritani, S. (2001). Developmental change in auditory preferences for speech stimuli in Japanese infants. *Journal of Speech, Language, and Hearing Research*, 44(6), 1189–1200.

Hillenbrand, J. & Gayvert, R. T. (1993). Identification of steady-state vowels synthesized from the Peterson and Barney measurements. *The Journal of the Acoustical Society of America*, 94(2), 668–674.

Hoff, E. & Naigles, L. (2002). How children use input to acquire a lexicon. *Child Development*, 73(2), 418–433.

Houston, D. M. & Bergeson, T. R. (2014). Hearing versus listening: attention to speech and its role in language acquisition in deaf infants with cochlear implants. *Lingua*, 139, 10–25.

Hurtado, N., Marchman, V. A., & Fernald, A. (2008). Does input influence uptake? Links between maternal talk, processing speed and vocabulary size in Spanish-learning children. *Developmental Science*, 11(6), F31–F39.

Ingram, D. (1995). The cultural basis of prosodic modifications to infants and children: a response to Fernald's universalist theory. *Journal of Child Language*, 22(01), 223–233.

Johnson, E. K. & Seidl, A. (2008). Clause segmentation by 6-month-old infants: a crosslinguistic perspective. *Infancy*, 13(5), 440–455.

Jusczyk, P. W. (1993). From general to language-specific capacities: the WRAPSA model of how speech perception develops. *Journal of Phonetics*, 21, 3–28.

Jusczyk, P. W., Cutler, A., & Redanz, N. J. (1993). Infants' preference for the predominant stress patterns of English words. *Child Development*, 64(3), 675–687.

Kaplan, P. S., Bachorowski, J.-A., Smoski, M. J., & Hudenko, W. J. (2002). Infants of depressed mothers, although competent learners, fail to learn in response to their own mothers' infant-directed speech. *Psychological Science*, 13(3), 268–271.

Karzon, R. G. (1985). Discrimination of polysyllabic sequences by one- to four-month-old infants. *Journal of Experimental Child Psychology*, 39(2), 326–342.

Katz, G. S., Cohn, J. F., & Moore, C. A. (1996). A combination of vocal fo dynamic and summary features discriminates between three pragmatic categories of infant-directed speech. *Child Development*, 67(1), 205–217.

Kim, H., Diehl, M., Panneton, R., & Moon, C. (2006). Hyperarticulation in mothers' speech to babies and puppies. Paper presented at the annual meeting of the XVth Biennial International Conference on Infant Studies. Kyoto, Japan.

Kitamura, C. & Burnham, D. (1998). The infant's response to maternal vocal affect. *Advances in Infancy Research*, 12, 221–236.

Kitamura, C. & Burnham, D. (2003). Pitch and communicative intent in mother's speech: adjustments for age and sex in the first year. *Infancy*, 4(1), 85–110.

Kitamura, C. & Notley, A. (2009). The shift in infant preferences for vowel duration and pitch contour between 6 and 10 months of age. *Developmental Science*, 12(5), 706–714.

Kitamura, C., Thanavishuth, C., Burnham, D., & Luksaneeyanawin, S. (2002). Universality and specificity in infant-directed speech: pitch modifications as a function of infant age and sex in a tonal and non-tonal language. *Infant Behavior and Development*, 24(4), 372–392.

Kondaurova, M. V. & Bergeson, T. R. (2011). The effects of age and infant hearing status on maternal use of prosodic cues for clause boundaries in speech. *Journal of Speech, Language, and Hearing Research*, 54(3), 740–754.

Kuhl, P. K., Andruski, J. E., Chistovich, I. A., Chistovich, L. A., Kozhevnikova, E. V., Ryskina, V. L., … Lacerda, F. (1997). Cross-language analysis of phonetic units in language addressed to infants. *Science*, 277(5326), 684–686.

Lee, C. S., Kitamura, C., Burnham, D., & Todd, N. P. M. (2014). On the rhythm of infant- versus adult-directed speech in Australian English. *The Journal of the Acoustical Society of America*, 136(1), 357–365.

Liu, H.-M., Kuhl, P. K., & Tsao, F.-M. (2003). An association between mothers' speech clarity and infants' speech discrimination skills. *Developmental Science*, 6(3), F1–F10.

Liu, H.-M., Tsao, F.-M., & Kuhl, P. K. (2009). Age-related changes in acoustic modifications of Mandarin maternal speech to preverbal infants and five-year-old children: a longitudinal study. *Journal of Child Language*, 36(04), 909–922.

Ma, W., Golinkoff, R. M., Houston, D. M., & Hirsh-Pasek, K. (2011). Word learning in infant- and adult-directed speech. *Language Learning and Development*, 7(3), 185–201.

Mani, N. & Pätzold, W. (2016). Sixteen-month-old infants segment words from infant-and adult-directed speech. *Language Learning and Development*, 12(4), 499–508.

Martin, A., Schatz, T., Versteegh, M., Miyazawa, K., Mazuka, R., Dupoux, E., & Cristia, A. (2015). Mothers speak less clearly to infants than to adults: a comprehensive test of the hyperarticulation hypothesis. *Psychological Science*, 26(3), 341–347.

McMurray, B., Kovack-Lesh, K. A., Goodwin, D., & McEchron, W. (2013). Infant directed speech and the development of speech perception: enhancing development or an unintended consequence? *Cognition*, 129(2), 362–378.

McRoberts, G. W., McDonough, C., & Lakusta, L. (2009). The role of verbal repetition in the development of infant speech preferences from 4 to 14 months of age. *Infancy*, 14(2), 162–194.

Morgan, J. L. & Demuth, K. (1996). Signal to syntax: an overview. In: J. L. Morgan & K. Demuth (eds) *Signal to Syntax: Bootstrapping from Speech to Grammar in Early Acquisition* (pp. 1–22). Mahwah, NJ: Lawrence Erlbaum Associates.

Neel, A. T. (2008). Vowel space characteristics and vowel identification accuracy. *Journal of Speech, Language, and Hearing Research*, 51(3), 574–585.

Newman, R. S. & Hussain, I. (2006). Changes in preference for infant-directed speech in low and moderate noise by 4.5- to 13-month-olds. *Infancy*, 10(1), 61–76.

Newman, R. S., Ratner, N. B., Jusczyk, A. M., Jusczyk, P. W., & Dow, K. A. (2006). Infants' early ability to segment the conversational speech signal predicts later language development: a retrospective analysis. *Developmental Psychology*, 42(4), 643–655.

Panneton, R., Kitamura, C., Mattock, K., & Burnham, D. (2006). Slow speech enhances younger but not older infants' perception of vocal emotion. *Research in Human Development*, 3(1), 7–19.

Papoušek, M., Bornstein, M. H., Nuzzo, C., Papoušek, H., & Symmes, D. (1990). Infant responses to prototypical melodic contours in parental speech. *Infant Behavior and Development*, 13(4), 539–545.

Papoušek, M. & Hwang, S.-F. C. (1991). Tone and intonation in Mandarin babytalk to presyllabic infants: comparison with registers of adult conversation and foreign language instruction. *Applied Psycholinguistics*, 12(04), 481–504.

Papoušek, M. & Papoušek, H. (1981). Musical elements in the infant's vocalization: their significance for communication, cognition, and creativity. *Advances in Infancy Research*, 1, 163–224.

Papoušek, M., Papoušek, H., & Bornstein, M. (1985). The naturalistic vocal environment of young infants: on the significance of homogeneity and variability in parental speech. In: T. Field & N. Fox (eds) *Social Perception in Infants* (pp. 269–297). Norwood, NJ: Ablex.

Papoušek, M., Papoušek, H., & Symmes, D. (1991). The meanings of melodies in motherese in tone and stress languages. *Infant Behavior and Development*, 14(4), 415–440.

Pegg, J. E., Werker, J. F., & McLeod, P. J. (1992). Preference for infant-directed over adult-directed speech: evidence from 7-week-old infants. *Infant Behavior and Development*, 15(3), 325–345.

Peters, A. M. (1983). *The Units of Language Acquisition* (Vol. 1 of Cambridge Monographs and Texts in Applied Psycholiguistics). Cambridge University Press Archive.

Ratner, N. B. (1984). Patterns of vowel modification in mother–child speech. *Journal of Child Language*, 11(03), 557–578.

Ratner, N. B. & Luberoff, A. (1984). Cues to post-vocalic voicing in mother–child speech. *Journal of Phonetics*, 12, 285–289.

Ratner, N. B. & Pye, C. (1984). Higher pitch in BT is not universal: acoustic evidence from Quiche Mayan. *Journal of Child Language*, 11(03), 515–522.

Rattanasone, N. X., Burnham, D., & Reilly, R. G. (2013). Tone and vowel enhancement in Cantonese infant-directed speech at 3, 6, 9, and 12 months of age. *Journal of Phonetics*, 41(5), 332–343.

Schachner, A. & Hannon, E. E. (2011). Infant-directed speech drives social preferences in 5-month-old infants. *Developmental Psychology*, 47(1), 19–25.

Schaeffler, S. S. (2007). Are Affective Speakers Effective Speakers? Exploring the Link Between the Vocal Expression of Positive Emotions and Communicative Effectiveness (Doctoral thesis). University of Stirling.

Segal, J. & Newman, R. S. (2015). Infant preferences for structural and prosodic properties of infant-directed speech in the second year of life. *Infancy*, 20(3), 339–351.

Shute, B. & Wheldall, K. (1999). Fundamental frequency and temporal modifications in the speech of British fathers to their children. *Educational Psychology*, 19(2), 221–233.

Singh, L., Morgan, J. L., & Best, C. T. (2002). Infants' listening preferences: baby talk or happy talk? *Infancy*, 3(3), 365–394.

Singh, L., Nestor, S., Parikh, C., & Yull, A. (2009). Influences of infant-directed speech on early word recognition. *Infancy*, 14(6), 654–666.

Snow, C. E. (1977). The development of conversation between mothers and babies. *Journal of Child Language*, 4(01), 1–22.

Soderstrom, M. (2007). Beyond babytalk: re-evaluating the nature and content of speech input to preverbal infants. *Developmental Review*, 27(4), 501–532.

Song, J. Y., Demuth, K., & Morgan, J. (2010). Effects of the acoustic properties of infant-directed speech on infant word recognition. *The Journal of the Acoustical Society of America*, 128(1), 389–400.

Stern, D. N., Spieker, S., Barnett, R., & MacKain, K. (1983). The prosody of maternal speech: infant age and context related changes. *Journal of Child Language*, 10(01), 1–15.

Stern, D. N., Spieker, S., & MacKain, K. (1982). Intonation contours as signals in maternal speech to prelinguistic infants. *Developmental Psychology*, 18(5), 727-735.

Sundberg, U. & Lacerda, F. (1999). Voice onset time in speech to infants and adults. *Phonetica*, 56(3-4), 186–199.

Thiessen, E. D., Hill, E. A., & Saffran, J. R. (2005). Infant-directed speech facilitates word segmentation. *Infancy*, 7(1), 53–71.

Trainor, L. J., Austin, C. M., & Desjardins, R. N. (2000). Is infant-directed speech prosody a result of the vocal expression of emotion? *Psychological Science*, 11(3), 188–195.

Trainor, L. J. & Desjardins, R. N. (2002). Pitch characteristics of infant-directed speech affect infants' ability to discriminate vowels. *Psychonomic Bulletin & Review*, 9(2), 335–340.

Uther, M., Knoll, M. A., & Burnham, D. (2007). Do you speak E-ng-li-sh? a comparison of foreigner- and infant-directed speech. *Speech Communication*, 49(1), 2–7.

Van de Weijer, J. (1997). Language input to a prelingual infant. In: A. Sorace, C. Heycock, & R. Shillcock (eds) *The Gala '97 Conference on Language Acquisition* (pp. 290–293). Edinburgh, United Kingdom: Edinburgh University Press.

Van de Weijer, J. (2009). Vowels in infant- and adult-directed speech. *Working Papers in Linguistics*, 49, 172–175.

Vouloumanos, A. & Curtin, S. (2014). Foundational tuning: how infants' attention to speech predicts language development. *Cognitive Science*, 38(8), 1675–1686.

Wang, Y., Seidl, A., & Cristia, A. (2015). Acoustic-phonetic differences between infant-and adult-directed speech: the role of stress and utterance position. *Journal of Child Language*, 42(4), 821–842.

Wang, Y., Lee, C. S., & Houston, D. M. (2016). Infant-directed speech reduces English-learning infants' preference for trochaic words. *The Journal of the Acoustical Society of America*, 140(6), 4101–4110.

Wang, Y., Shafto, C. L., & Houston, D. M. (2018). Attention to speech and spoken language development in deaf children with cochlear implants: a 10-year longitudinal study. *Developmental Science*, e12677.

Weisleder, A. & Fernald, A. (2013). Talking to children matters: early language experience strengthens processing and builds vocabulary. *Psychological Science*, 24(11), 2143–2152.

Weizman, Z. O. & Snow, C. E. (2001). Lexical output as related to children's vocabulary acquisition: effects of sophisticated exposure and support for meaning. *Developmental Psychology*, 37(2), 265–279.

Werker, J. F. & Lalonde, C. E. (1988). Cross-language speech perception: initial capabilities and developmental change. *Developmental Psychology*, 24(5), 672–683.

Werker, J. F. & McLeod, P. J. (1989). Infant preference for both male and female infant-directed talk: a developmental study of attentional and affective responsiveness. *Canadian Journal of Psychology/Revue Canadienne de Psychologie*, 43(2), 230–246.

Werker, J. F., Pegg, J. E., & McLeod, P. J. (1994). A cross-language investigation of infant preference for infant-directed communication. *Infant Behavior and Development*, 17(3), 323–333.

Werker, J. F. & Tees, R. C. (1984). Cross-language speech perception: evidence for perceptual reorganization during the first year of life. *Infant Behavior and Development*, 7(1), 49–63.

CHAPTER 6

....

THE SINGING VOICE

....

JOHAN SUNDBERG

6.1 INTRODUCTION

THE voice is one of the most common, if not the commonest, and probably also the oldest, of all musical instruments. In all cultures in the world, singing is a regular part of human expression. Singing can be regarded as a derivative—or the origin—of speech; both use the same tool, the voice organ. Yet, in many cultures, the voice characteristics used in singing deviate considerably from those used in speech. In this chapter, some of these characteristics and their underlying physiological correlates will be reviewed.

Basically, the voice organ is an instrument that converts airstream to sound. The production of vocal sounds is illustrated schematically in Figure 6.1. It combines three physiological functions: (1) compressing air by means of the respiratory apparatus; (2) converting exhalatory airstream to a pulsating flow; and (3) filtering the signal thus created by vocal tract resonances (Sundberg, 1987). The contributions of each of these functions will be briefly described in the following.

A raw material is generated when the slit between the vocal folds, the *glottis*, is brought to vibration by the airstream from the respiratory system. The vibration converts this stream to a pulsating airflow, the *voice source*, which is equivalent to sound. This raw material sound propagates through the *vocal tract*, which is constituted by the pharynx and the oral cavity, for nasalized sound complemented by the nasal cavity. Like all other tubes, the vocal tract is a resonator, favouring the transport of sounds at its resonances, which are called *formants*. There are at least five formants of great significance to vocal sounds. The resonance frequencies are determined by the shape of the vocal tract (i.e. by articulation).

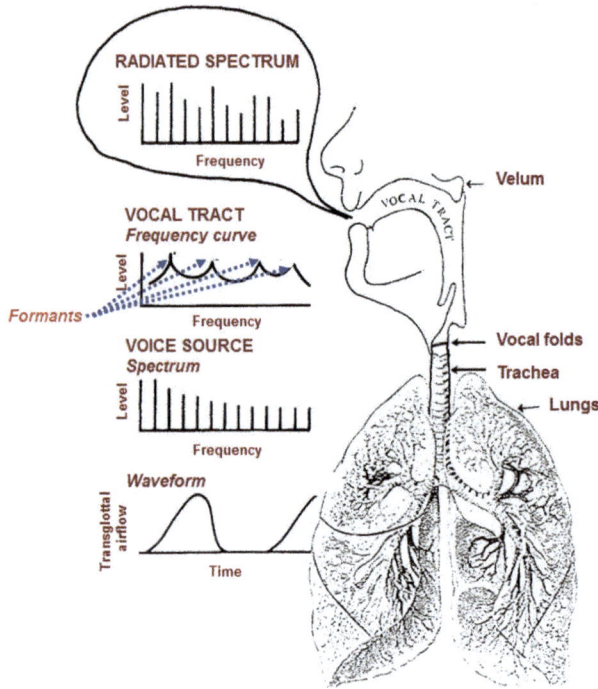

FIGURE 6.1 Schematic illustration of generation of voiced sounds.

Adapted from Sundberg J. (1987) *The Science of the Singing Voice*, DeKalb IL: Northern Illinois University Press.

6.2 PHONATORY BREATHING

Breathing strategy can and does vary between individuals. Why this strategy is relevant to voice timbre may seem unclear. However, voice teachers tend to talk about 'support' when they talk about singers' vocal techniques, and there are good reasons to assume that such support is related to respiratory aspects of phonation.

6.2.1 Subglottal Pressure

To generate an airstream through the glottis it is obviously necessary to create an overpressure of air in the airways, a *subglottal pressure*. This is achieved by reducing the volume of the respiratory organ (i.e. by squeezing the structures surrounding the lungs). There are two major muscle systems that can perform such squeezing. One is the internal intercostal muscles which move the ribs closer to each other and thus reduce the ribcage volume. These muscles are used to increase subglottal pressure. Their antagonist muscles are the inhalatory external intercostal muscles, which lift the ribs, thus widening the ribcage.

The other major respiratory muscle system is the abdominal wall and its antagonist, the diaphragm. The latter is an upward vaulted muscle that constitutes the bottom of the rib-cage. Upon contraction, it flattens and thus expands the ribcage volume, so it is an inhalatory muscle. As the compressibility of the abdominal content is limited, diaphragmatic contraction typically also tends to expand the lower part of the ribcage laterally; if the diaphragm tries to reduce its peripheral length and the abdominal content refuses to move downward correspondingly, the result will be a lifting and expansion of the lateral part of the ribcage. The diaphragm is pushed back into the ribcage by contraction of the muscles in the abdominal wall, so they serve the purpose of exhalation.

Inhalation can result both from lowering the diaphragm and from expanding the ribcage. Breathing patterns vary between singers. Some singers use the diaphragm activation mainly for inhalation, while others use ribcage expansion mainly. Some use both. Some of the singers, who expand the abdominal wall during inhalation, contract it, pushing the diaphragm up into the ribcage, before starting the phrase. Others keep it expanded throughout the phrase and thus rely on ribcage contraction for producing subglottal pressure. Some singers contract both the abdominal wall and ribcage simultaneously.

The respiratory system is elastic and hence possesses recoil force. It is strong and exhalatory at large lung volumes, and strong and inhalatory at low lung volumes. Thus, if after a deep inhalation one relaxes the respiratory muscles and opens the airways, exhalation results. Similarly, inhalation results after relaxing the respiratory muscles after a deep exhalation.

The pressures generated by these recoil forces can be quite high as compared with typical pressures used in conversational speech. In upright position, they can reach 30 cm H_2O after a deep inhalation and -20 cm H_2O after a deep exhalation. Therefore, to control subglottal pressure, respiratory muscles need to be recruited—inspiratory muscles at high lung volumes and exhalatory muscles at low lung volumes. Narrow lung volume ranges are typically used in conversational speech, while in singing, long musical phrases require use of quite wide ranges. This implies that singers have to use their respiratory muscles more than is needed for neutral speech.

As the subglottal pressures generated by the recoil forces are positive at high lung volumes and negative at low lung volumes, they are zero at a particular lung volume. In quiet breathing, inhalations are initiated at this lung volume. It is referred to as the *resting expiratory level* (REL). In neutral speech, as well as in singing, phonation at lung volumes above REL is preferred. Thus, speakers tend to inhale when their lung volumes approach REL and singers tend to inhale deeply enough to sing the entire phrase at lung volumes above REL (Watson & Hixon, 1996).

6.2.2 Subglottal Pressure Control

The main role of the respiratory system in phonation is to control subglottal pressure. This pressure is of crucial importance to phonation. The demands raised on the respiratory system in singing are quite different from those required for speech. While in speech, subglottal pressure is mainly used for varying vocal loudness, in singing it must be varied also with pitch. Thus, high pitches need higher pressures than low pitches. This is illustrated in Figure 6.2, showing the pressures used for singing the exercise shown at the bottom. Note that in both triads not only the pressures are increased with increasing fundamental frequency, but also that the first tone after the bar line, which is only the second highest tone, received the highest pressure. The reason would be that the singer marked the harmony

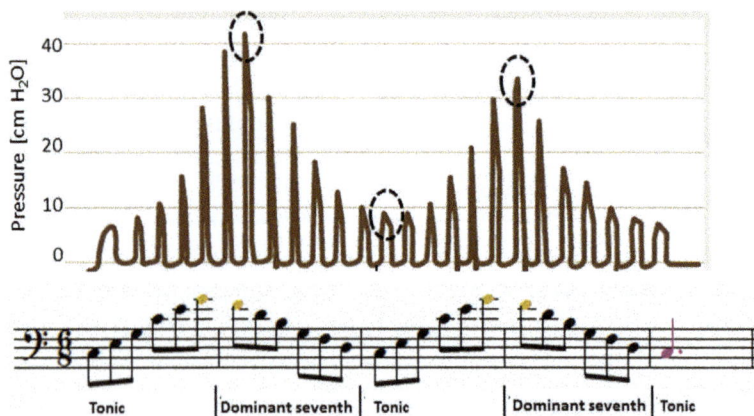

FIGURE 6.2 Subglottal pressures used by a professional, classically trained baritone, singing the exercise shown below the graph. Each peak represents the pressure of the tone shown in the score. Circles mark the first tones appearing after a change of harmonies, which are shown at the bottom.

Reprinted from *Journal of Voice*, Volume 1, Issue 3, Leanderson R., Sundberg J., & von Euler C., 'Breathing muscle activity and subglottal pressure dynamics in singing and speech', pp. 258–61, Copyright © 1987 Elsevier Ltd., with permission from Elsevier, http://www.sciencedirect.com/science/article/pii/S0892199787800097

change at the bar line by means of a crescendo. As pitch and loudness change frequently and according to strict time patterns in music, singers must learn to change subglottal pressure quickly and accurately. The latter is important also for the reason that an increase of subglottal pressure has the side effect to increase pitch. Therefore, the pitch-raising muscles must contract slightly harder when a singer decreases loudness at constant pitch.

The same exercise is often performed first legato, with no pauses between tones, and then staccato, with short pauses between the tones. During these pauses the glottis is open, so subglottal pressure must be reduced to zero to prevent loss of air (McDonnell et al., 2011). Hence, the staccato version would require more skill and accuracy in subglottal pressure control, since the pressure changes between tones are much greater than in the legato version.

6.2.3 Tracheal Pull

The respiratory apparatus is suspended from the skull. Consequently, in upright position it exerts a caudally directed force, the *tracheal pull*. It tends to affect phonation in the sense that it strives to open the glottis. It is stronger at high than at low lung volumes. Thus, at high lung volumes, glottal adduction is generally weaker than at low lung volumes in untrained voices. The significance of this will be described in the following paragraphs.

Watson and Hixon (1985) analysed the breathing patterns of six male, classically trained, professional opera singers in a number of speech and singing conditions. They found two breathing patterns both during inhalation and during singing. For some subjects, the volume contribution of the ribcage was greater than that of the abdomen throughout the phrase. For other subjects, the volume contribution of the abdomen exceeded that of the ribcage in the first part of the phrase, while in the second part, the abdomen and ribcage contributions were similar. In the final part, the ribcage was the dominant contributor.

Thomasson and associates (2001) studied singers' breathing behaviour in an experiment where classically trained, professional singers performed a song together with a professional pianist. Singers were found to be quite consistent in their respiratory behaviour, both for inhalation and during the phrase, but the inter-individual variation was quite substantial. During inhalation, as well as during the phrase, some singers mainly used ribcage expansion while the abdominal wall was kept more or less fixed. Other singers used both the ribcage and abdominal wall.

The term 'support' is commonly used by singers and teachers of singing, but its exact meaning is unclear. The general view seems to be that it refers to breath management or, in other words, to the control of subglottal pressure. Griffin and associates (1995) asked eight classically trained singers to sing the same tasks with and without support. The subjects described supported singing as resonant, clear, and easy to manage. They also reported that it needed 'correct' breath management, but no significant difference was found in their breathing patterns between the two conditions. Furthermore, when singing with support, the singers sang louder and with higher subglottal pressure, and the voice source seemed to be produced with somewhat weaker glottal adduction.

These findings suggest that support is related to both respiratory and phonatory factors. Unlike in speech, subglottal pressure needs to be constantly changed in singing as it needs to be adjusted, taking not only loudness but also pitch into account, as mentioned. If the singer fails to produce the target pressure for a tone, unintended changes of phonation and hence voice quality are likely to happen. It seems possible that support is associated with how successful the singer is in producing the correct subglottal pressure for the tone produced.

6.3 VOICE SOURCE

The waveform of the pulsating airflow through the glottis consists of triangular pulses, created when the glottis is open, surrounded by horizontal segments, produced when the glottis is closed during the vibration period (see Figure 6.3). An example of the sound of the source is presented in Audio 6.1. Normally the voice source is quasi-periodic (i.e. its waveform repeats itself). Because of this, and because the waveform is not a simple sinewave, the signal is complex, constituted by a set of harmonic partials. This means their frequencies are integer multiples of the lowest frequency, the fundamental, which corresponds to the pitch perceived. Thus, when we listen to a sung tone with the pitch A4, the vocal folds are vibrating at 440 Hz.

The partials are harmonic, and so the frequency of the nth partial is

$$f_n = n \times 440 \text{ Hz}$$

and therefore

$$f_1 = 1 \times 440 \text{ Hz} = 440 \text{ Hz}$$
$$f_2 = 2 \times 440 \text{ Hz} = 880 \text{ Hz}$$

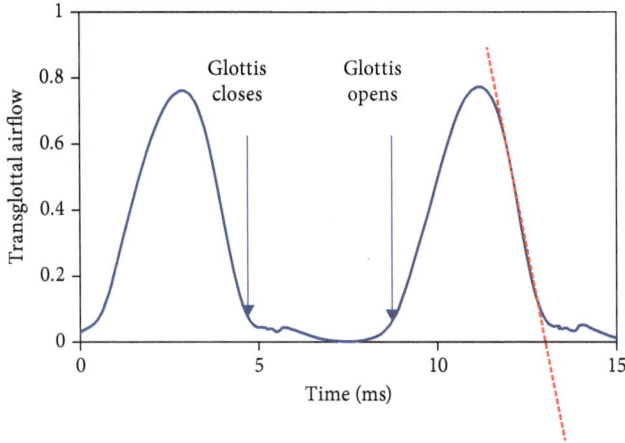

FIGURE 6.3 Typical example of the waveform of the pulsating airflow through the glottis. The steepest slope during the closing phase, marked by the dotted line, represents the strength of the excitation of the vocal tract.

$$f_3 = 3 \times 440 \text{ Hz} = 1320 \text{ Hz}$$
$$f_4 = 4 \times 440 \text{ Hz} = 1760 \text{ Hz}$$

and so on.

The amplitudes of the source spectrum partials tend to decrease with frequency, as illustrated in Figure 6.4. The spectrum slope is mostly described in terms of dB/octave. The steepness varies with vocal loudness—in soft voice approaching −18 dB/octave, and in loud voice −9 dB/octave or even less. As illustrated in Figure 6.4, a 15 dB increase at 600 Hz is accompanied by a 30 dB increase at 3,000 Hz. In other words, increasing subglottal pressure enhances the higher partials more than the lower partials.

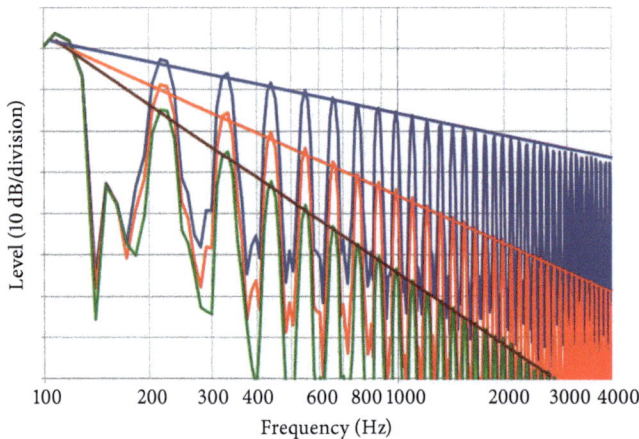

FIGURE 6.4 Schematical illustration of source spectrum for different degrees of vocal loudness. The lines represent the −6, −12, and −18 dB/octave spectrum envelope slope (blue, red, and brown, respectively).

The voice source is controlled by three main physiological parameters—subglottal pressure for vocal loudness, vocal fold length and stiffness for pitch, and glottal adduction for phonation type.

Subglottal pressure has a quite dominant influence on the voice source, as mentioned. With regard to the voice source waveform, a pressure increase results in higher pulse amplitude, quicker termination of the flow pulse, and longer closed phase. Increasing vocal fold length and stiffness, other things being equal, causes the period to shorten and the relative duration of the closed phase to decrease. Increasing glottal adduction causes a reduction of pulse amplitude and lengthening of the closed phase. With regard to the spectrum, increase of subglottal pressure causes a less steep slope, such that the spectrum partials at high frequencies gain more in amplitude than those at low frequencies. Increases of both pitch and glottal adduction are typically accompanied by reduction of the relative amplitude of the fundamental.

For a given vowel, the relation between subglottal pressure and sound level is mostly simple, as illustrated in Figure 6.5; sound levels produced at different pressures typically show a logarithmic relation to subglottal pressure. At 30 cm distance, the sound pressure level produced by 10 cm H_2O generally lies in the neighbourhood of 75 dB, and a doubling of pressure yields about 10 dB increase of sound level.

Also, *glottal adduction* has a strong influence on the voice source. It can exert a quite strong force, as during straining or carrying heavy weights. Weak adduction produces a breathy, hypofunctional type of phonation, while strong adduction results in pressed or hyperfunctional phonation. The type of phonation that results when glottal adduction is reduced to the minimum that still produces glottal closure during the vibration cycle is referred to as *flow phonation*, since it consumes a comparatively large airflow. Acoustically it combines a strong voice source fundamental with strong overtones. Pressed phonation, by contrast, combines strong overtones with a weaker voice source fundamental than flow phonation. Figure 6.6 shows typical flow glottograms for different subglottal pressures and different degrees of glottal adduction.

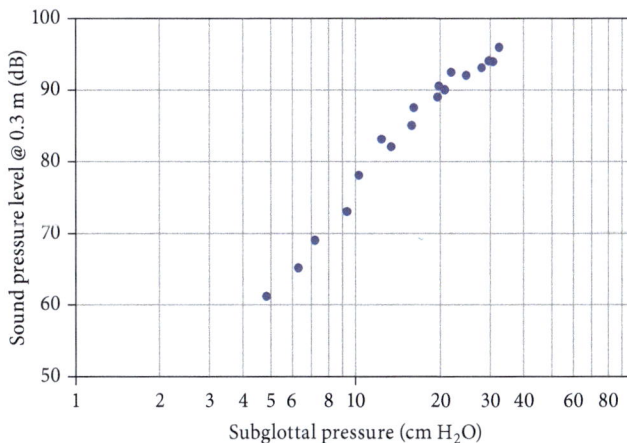

FIGURE 6.5 Typical relationship between sound pressure level and subglottal pressure in a trained voice.

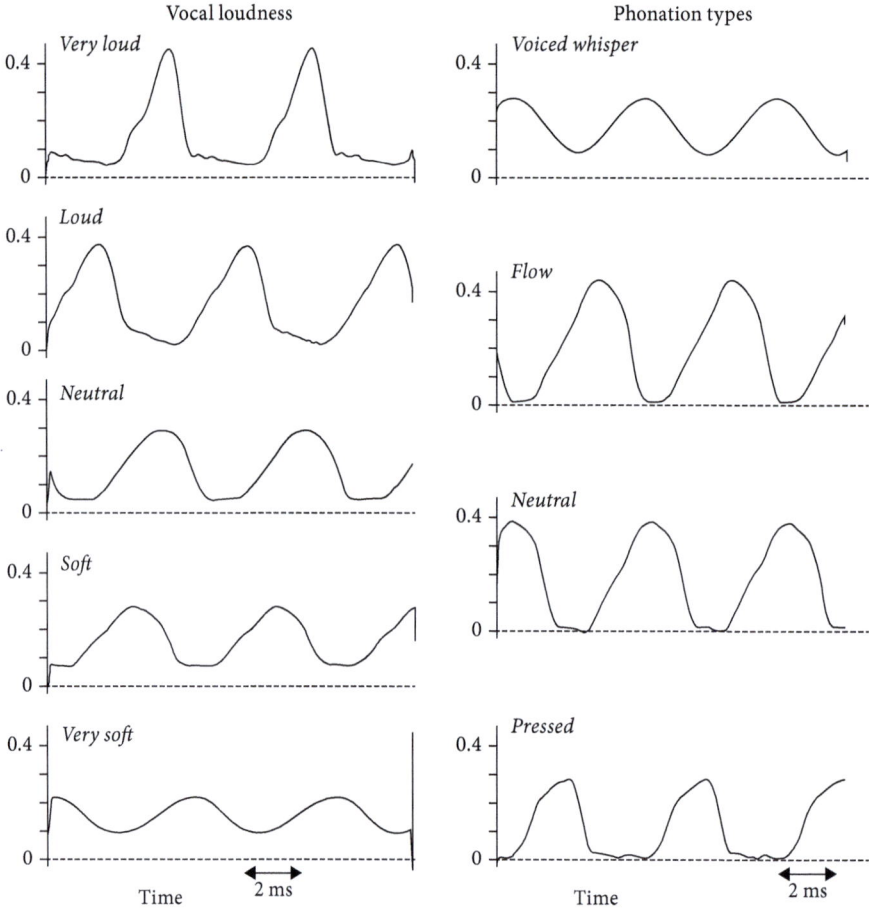

FIGURE 6.6 Typical flow glottograms for different degrees of vocal loudness and different phonation types.

Phonatory pressedness is a clinically relevant aspect of voice. Sundberg and associates (2004) analysed the relationship between expert ratings of phonatory pressedness and flow glottogram parameters in a single singer subject, who voluntarily sang different pitches in breathy, flow, neutral (as in conversational speaking), and pressed phonation and also in different musical styles (Classical, Pop, Jazz, and Blues). The results showed that 88% of the variation in pressedness ratings could be explained by an equation containing subglottal pressure, closed quotient, and the amplitude of the voice source fundamental.

Millgård and associates (2015) analysed the relationship between ratings of phonatory pressedness and voice source parameters and subglottal pressure in eleven subjects (five females and six males), all with healthy voices. They were asked to voluntarily phonate in neutral and pressed phonation, and, if they were able to, also in flow phonation. The stimuli that received the highest and the lowest mean ratings of pressedness are given in Audio 6.2. Also in this study, the ratings were compared with flow glottogram parameters, and also with formant frequencies and spectrum balance, measured in terms of the ratio of summed spectrum energy above and below 1000 Hz. The results showed that about 70% of the variance of the ratings could be explained by voice source parameters. A multiple linear regression analysis suggested that perceived phonatory pressedness was most closely related to subglottal pressure, closed quotient, and the two lowest formants. Thus, unlike in the single-subject study just mentioned, no relationship was found with the amplitude of the voice source fundamental. The reason would be that vocal fold length varies between individuals, so the same subglottal pressure will produce glottal pulses of different amplitudes.

Summarizing, pressed phonation tends to be associated with high subglottal pressure combined with long closed phase, a weak voice source fundamental, and a low amplitude quotient. The relevance of subglottal pressure is logical. A firm glottal adduction must be combined with an elevated subglottal pressure; otherwise there would be no airflow. Likewise, it is easy to imagine that increased glottal adduction will result in lengthening of the closed phase. More interesting, and less expected, is the contribution of weakened voice source fundamental to pressed phonation.

6.3.1 Register

If untrained voices produce ascending or descending glide tones, sudden pitch jumps, so-called register breaks often happen. Audio 6.3 provides an example. Voice register breaks are associated shifts in the vibration mode of the vocal folds.

Generally, voice experts identify three registers—*modal, falsetto*, and *vocal fry*, sometimes referred to as mechanism 1, 2, and 3, respectively. Modal register is used in normal speech, although vocal fry tends to appear at the end of phrases, both in females' and males' relaxed speech. Falsetto is typically used when males mimic female speech, but also female voices have a falsetto register. Classically trained female singers use falsetto register in the upper part of their pitch range, even though many voice experts prefer to call this *mixed register,* thus suggesting it should be regarded as a mixture of modal and falsetto. For the top range they use another register, often referred to as *head register*.

The boundary between modal and falsetto registers appear in a similar pitch range for both female and male adults, somewhere between 300 and 500 Hz (roughly pitches D4 and C5). Vocal fry is aperiodic or has a very low fundamental frequency, well below 100 Hz in both females and males. For this reason it is heard as a sequence of pulses rather than as a continuous tone.

Registers have different acoustic properties and therefore sound quite differently. Falsetto is generally produced with thin vocal folds and incomplete glottal closure. This produces a strong fundamental and weak overtones. Modal voice is produced with thicker vocal folds and often with more or less complete glottal closure. Vocal fry is typically produced with thick folds and complete glottal closure.

In singing, register breaks are used in yodelling, where the voice oscillates in a well-controlled manner between modal and falsetto. In other types of singing, register breaks are avoided. Hence, to iron out timbral differences between registers is an important goal of the training of female singers in the classical tradition.

The so-called *covered* singing mode, which male singers tend to use in the upper part of their pitch range, is regarded as a means to reduce the risk for register breaks. Also, it is regarded as preferable from the point of view of vocal hygiene. Hertegård and associates (1990) asked eleven professionally trained, male singers to sing with and without covering one-octave scales and octave intervals on the vowel /ae/ with the top note near the upper end of their pitch range. Covered voice was found to be associated with increased transglottal airflow and a stronger voice source fundamental, thus showing similarities with flow phonation. Fibreoptic inspection showed that covering was produced with a lowered larynx and a widened pharynx. This lowers the formant frequencies, which leads to a change of vowel quality towards the neutral /shwa/ vowel.

6.3.2 Vibrato

In the classical Western operatic style of singing, *vibrato* is an important characteristic. In Audio 6.4, a synthesized tone is first presented without and then with vibrato. Without vibrato, the vowel sounds almost like a car horn, but then immediately sounds as a singer voice when the vibrato is added.

In the 1930s, vibrato attracted the interest of the music psychologist Carl Seashore, who wrote a number of texts about it (e.g. Seashore, 1938). It typically just develops by itself during a successful education of the singing voice. It corresponds to a quasi-periodic modulation of fundamental frequency with a modulation frequency between 5 and 7 Hz and with peak-to-peak amplitude that is mostly between ±0.5 and ±1 semitone. Audio 6.5 twice presents a synthesized vowel with a vibrato rate of 7, 6, and 5 Hz, first with an extent of ±0.5 semitone and then with an extent of ±1 semitone.

The origin of the vibrato is unclear. One hypothesis is that it is produced by self-oscillation of the pitch control system, which strives to increase frequency when it has drifted downward and to decrease it when it has drifted upward. Titze and associates (1994) found experimental support for this idea. Mostly overlooked are crucial experiments by Hirano and associates (1970) and by Shipp and associates (1990) who measured the electromyography (EMG) signal from the pitch-raising cricothyroid and vocalis muscles. They found contractions in these muscles that were synchronous with the frequency undulations. Thus, it can be concluded that the vibrato is created by a pulsating contraction of the pitch-raising muscles.

A well-defined pitch is perceived of a vibrato tone. It corresponds to the average of the fundamental frequency across one vibrato period (Shonle & Horan, 1980; Sundberg, 1978). However, in rapid tone sequences in florid singing, where the duration of the tone is shorter than one complete vibrato cycle, the final part of the fundamental frequency event seems more influential to the pitch perceived than an average across the tone (d'Alessandro & Castellengo, 1994). The accuracy of the perceived pitch is similar to that of a vibrato-free tone (Sundberg, 1978). In Chinese classical singing, a slower modulation of about 3 Hz is often used. Such slow modulation causes the perceived pitch to undulate.

As the voice source produces a harmonic spectrum with quasi-harmonic partials, the frequency modulation of a vibrato will cause the partials to move toward and away from the formants, thereby varying their amplitudes: amplitude increases as the partial approaches its nearest formant and vice versa. This means that more information on the formant frequency will be generated by the vibrato. At high pitches, where the frequency distance between the partials is great, vowel quality is difficult to perceive, but vibrato could be assumed to help. However, a listening test with synthesized stimuli provided no support for this assumption (Sundberg, 1977).

Vibrato rate is generally quite stable, even though with advancing age it tends to decrease typically by about 0.5 Hz per decade (Sundberg et al., 1998). Thus, elderly singers often sing with a slow vibrato rate. However, Prame (1994) made a surprising observation. He found that the rate typically increased toward the end of long phrase-final notes. The mechanism producing this effect has remained unclear.

6.3.3 Intonation

Pitch control is an important aspect of vocal performance. In general, the fundamental frequencies produced in professional singing are in close agreement with equally tempered tuning. In this tuning system, neighbouring chromatic scale tones are separated by an interval with the frequency ratio

$$1 : \sqrt[12]{2}$$

In other words, if one multiplies the fundamental frequency with this ratio, one obtains the fundamental frequency of a tone that is one equally tempered minor second higher, and the equally tempered tuning divides the octave interval into twelve equally wide minor second intervals.

Listeners' sensitivity to deviations from this tuning system varies considerably, but appears to be around ±10% among trained music listeners (Sundberg, 1978; Sundberg et al., 1996). Yet, tones perceived as perfect in pitch can deviate considerably from this tuning system (Sundberg, 2012). For example, ascending or descending octave intervals obtained by doubling and halving the fundamental frequency respectively are not perceived as acceptable by most musically experienced listeners (Sundberg & Gauffin, 1973). They prefer somewhat wider octaves. Furthermore, the peak tone in phrases with an excited emotional character is often sharpened, sometimes by more than a quartertone. This sharpening can be perceived as intensifying the expressivity of the performance (Sundberg et al., 2013). Because of the vibrato, such deviations do not produce beats with the accompaniment.

6.4 FORMANTS

The sound transfer of the vocal tract resonator is characterized by formant frequencies. Thus, if the vocal tract is excited by a sinewave that sweeps from low to high frequencies with constant amplitude, the response curve recorded at the lip opening rises to peaks at the formant frequencies and these peaks are surrounded by valleys.

As illustrated in Figure 6.7, the frequencies of the two lowest formants determine the vowel quality if we hear, for example, an /i/ or an /a/. The formant combination forms a sail-like pattern, with the vowels /i/, /a/, and /u/ in the corners. These vowels are used in all languages. Figure 6.7 also shows the combinations observed in children and in adult females and males.

The reason why the combinations of the first and second formant frequencies are not identical for children and female and male adults is that formant frequencies are

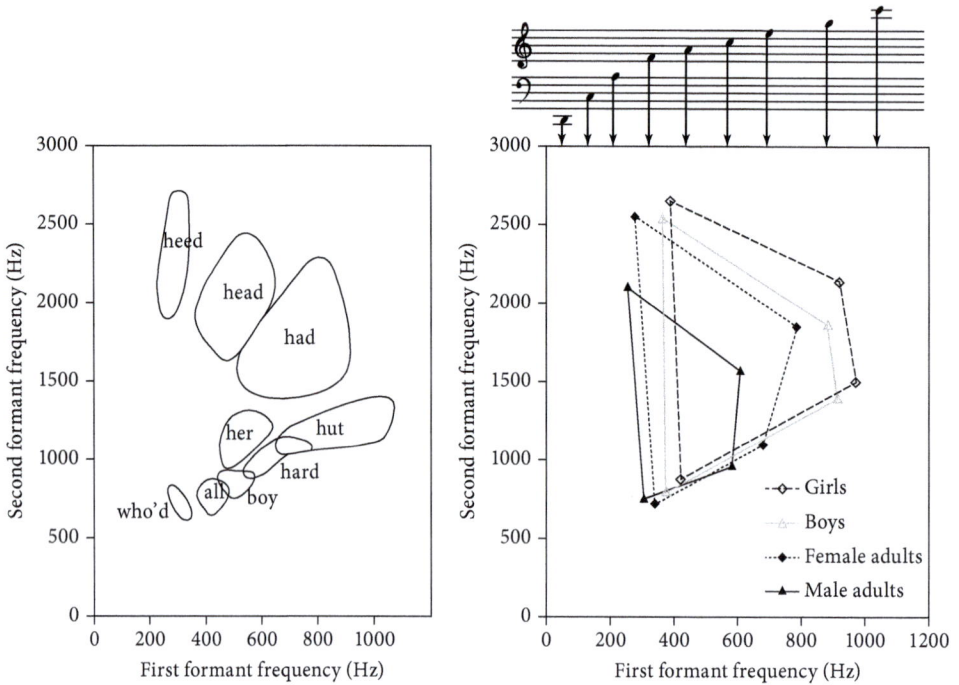

FIGURE 6.7 Left panel: Combinations of the first and the second formats for the vowels in the indicated words. Right panel: Corresponding mean values for the vowels in the words 'who'd', 'hut', 'had', and 'heed' spoken by 10-year-old girls, boys and by female and male adults. The values along the horizontal axis is given in musical notation at the top.

Source: data from White P., 'Formant Frequency Analysis of Children's Spoken and Sung Vowels Using Sweeping Fundamental Frequency Production', *Journal of Voice*, Volume 13, Issue 4, pp. 570–82, Copyright © 1999 Elsevier Inc., http:// www.sciencedirect.com/ science/ article/ pii/ S0892199799800113

determined by the shape of the vocal tract; females have shorter pharynges than males, and children have shorter vocal tracts than females. Typical vocal tract profiles are shown in Figure 6.8. The vowels /i/, /u/, and /a/ are produced with the tongue body in fronted, posterior and caudal position, respectively. Thus, each vowel is produced with a specific shape. It is amazing that children find the correct articulation of the various vowels, even though they cannot produce the combination of first and second formants of their adult environment.

The spectrum of a vowel is heavily influenced by the frequencies of the formants. The general principle is that the amplitudes of the peaks depend on the distance to the other formant peaks. When two formants approach each other in frequency, they both gain in amplitude. For example, halving the frequency separation of two adjacent formants tends to increase the amplitudes of the formant peaks by 6 dB and the valley between them by 12 dB, approximately (Fant, 1960). This implies that the sound level will increase, if the first formant frequency is increased and the other formants are kept constant.

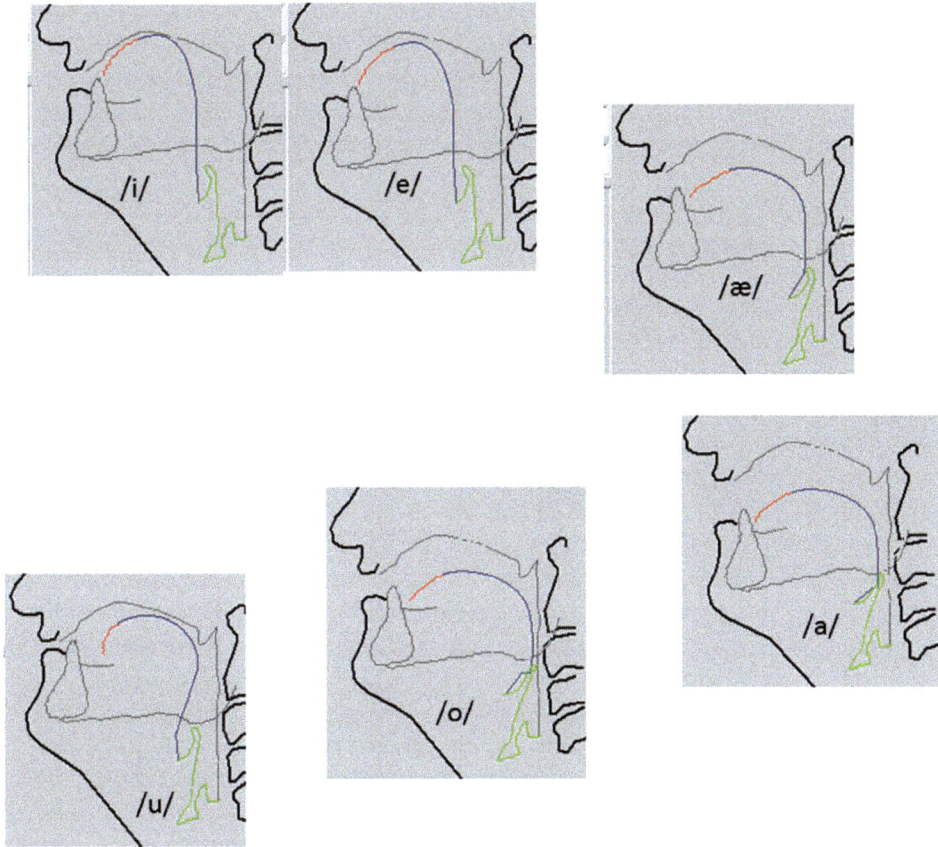

FIGURE 6.8 Schematic illustration of the vocal tract shape for the indicated vowels.

Reproduced with permission from Öhman S.E.G., 'Coarticulation in VCV utterances:
spectrographic measurements', *The Journal of the Acoustical Society of America*, Volume 39, Issue 151,
Copyright © 1966 Acoustical Society of America, doi: 10.1121/1.1909864

6.4.1 Singer's Formant Cluster

Male singers in the classical Western operatic tradition share a spectrum characteristic referred to as the singer's formant cluster, the singer's formant, or the singing formant. It corresponds to a prominent spectrum peak that tends to be present in all voiced sounds. It
can be acoustically explained as a clustering of formants 3, 4, and 5; when formants are
approaching each other in frequency, their amplitudes increase, as mentioned. The timbral
effect of clustering these formants is demonstrated in Audio 6.6. A wide pharynx and a low
larynx seem important for producing it, as this can convert the larynx tube to a separate
resonator with a resonance frequency that falls between the third and fourth formants in
normal spoken vowels. The centre frequency of the cluster tends to vary systematically with
classification, being lower for basses and higher for tenors.

For its generation, the laryngeal ventricle should be important; a large ventricle will produce a lower resonance frequency than a smaller ventricle. Bass singers tend to have longer vocal folds than baritones and tenors, and therefore their laryngeal ventricle should be larger in the anterior-posterior direction. This may be part of the explanation of why basses tend to have a lower centre frequency of the singer's formant cluster than baritones and tenors.

The singer's formant cluster is located in a frequency range where the sound of a competing orchestral accompaniment is rather modest, as illustrated in Figure 6.9. The result is that the singer produces strong partials in a frequency range where the competition with the orchestra is more reasonable than in the low frequency range, where the loudest partials are typically found in normal speech. Considering that the singer's formant cluster is a resonance phenomenon, it is clear that it is an example of vocal economy.

As the singer's formant cluster is created by clustering formants, there must be spectrum partials falling into this cluster in order to produce the spectrum peak. As long as fundamental frequency is low, this condition is always fulfilled since the distance between adjacent partials equals the fundamental frequency. For the same reason, the partials are widely separated in frequency at high pitches. This means that only some of the tones in a scale will contain a partial that falls into the formant cluster and other scale tones will not. As a result, the voice will sound quite different on different scale tones, and this would ruin the timbral similarity between them. This would be the reason why female singers do not have a singer's formant cluster.

Thus, the singer's formant cluster is a typical property of male operatic voices. However, Leino (2008) found a similar but less prominent spectrum peak in voices that he described as 'good'. It appears higher in frequency, between 3,000 and 4,000 Hz. A corresponding peak has been observed also in male pop singer voices (Cleveland et al., 2001). It is possible that it increases the text intelligibility, which is highly dependent on formant patterns in the 2,000 to 4,000 Hz frequency range.

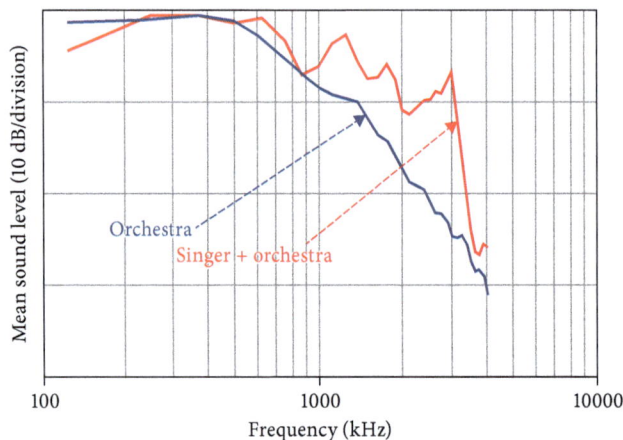

FIGURE 6.9 Long-term average spectra of music played by a symphonic orchestra, with and without a tenor solo singer voice.

6.4.2 Formant Tuning

The range of the first formant frequency in vowels is roughly 250 Hz to 1,000 Hz. Typical top pitches for the various voice classifications are about 350 Hz (F4) for basses, 390 Hz (G4) for baritones, 523 Hz (C5) for tenors, 700 Hz (F5) for altos, and 1,050 Hz (C6) for sopranos. This means that singers often encounter the situation that the fundamental frequency is higher than the normal value of the first formant. They tend to avoid this situation, and for very good reasons—the sound level produced is heavily attenuated, and there is also an increased risk of phonatory instabilities (Titze, 2008; Titze et al., 2008). In such situations, singers have been found to increase the first formant frequency, such that it is somewhat higher than the fundamental frequency. This causes an increase of sound level which may sometimes be as large as 15 dB. As formants are resonance phenomena, this gain in sound level does not cost any effort, so the strategy is an example of vocal economy. The articulatory tools for this are often the jaw and lip openings; female singers are typically seen to widen their lip opening when they sing high pitches. This raises the first formant. Widening the jaw opening also narrows the deeper parts of the pharynx, which has the same effect on the first formant.

The effect on the formant frequencies of a change of the vocal tract shape is dependent on the percentage change of the cross-sectional area. Hence a certain increment of a very narrow constriction has a greater effect than the same increment of an already wide passage. For example, the vowels /i/ and /e/ are produced with an oral constriction, which are important to a low first formant frequency. A simple method to raise the first formant, therefore, is to widen the passage by reducing the bulging of the tongue. At high pitches, however, widening the jaw and lip openings is necessary.

Formant tuning has been observed also under other circumstances than singing at high pitches. Miller and Schutte (1990) and Neumann and associates (2005) have noted that in the upper part of their pitch range, some classically trained male singers tune the first formant to a spectrum partial. On the other hand, Sundberg and associates (2013) found that classically trained baritone and tenor singers tuned their first formant frequency away from the nearest spectrum partials at their top pitches. When the same singers produced the same tones in a vocal style typically used in musical theatre, they mostly tuned their first formant somewhat higher than when they were singing in the operatic style.

As vowel quality is defined in terms of the combination of the formants 1 and 2, the vowels become difficult to identify when sung at high pitches. This is illustrated in Figure 6.10, which shows the highest per cent of correct responses observed in various listening tests with high-pitched vowels. Intelligibility remains good up to about C5 (523 Hz) but decreases sharply with frequency up to F5 (750 Hz). Above this frequency, intelligibility is poor for all vowels, with occasional exceptions for the vowel /a/. It has been reported that an initial consonant can improve intelligibility, but attempts to replicate this finding have failed (Deme, 2014).

Many opera singers have been found to sing the vowels /a/ and /u/ with a small velopharyngeal opening (Birch et al., 2002). The reason for this can be assumed to be that nasalization attenuates the low-frequency part of the spectrum, while leaving the high-frequency parts unaffected. Hence, the high partials become more prominent in the spectrum. This effect can be reached without making the timbre sound nasalized. To reach the same effect without a velopharyngeal opening, the singer would need to increase subglottal pressure (i.e. increase vocal effort); as was mentioned in Section 6.3, 'Voice Source', an increase of subglottal pressure increases the level of

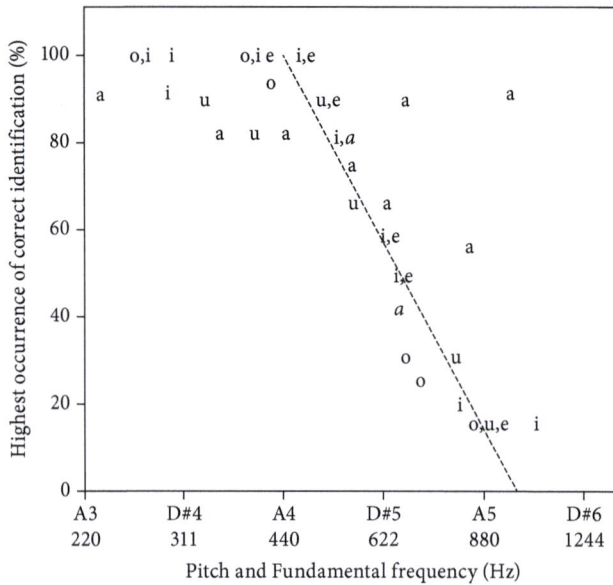

FIGURE 6.10 Highest per cent of correct responses observed in various tests where listeners were asked to identify vowels sung at high pitches.

Adapted from *Journal of Voice*, Volume 8, Issue 2, Sundberg J., 'Perceptual Aspects of Singing', Figure 6, pp. 106–22, Copyright © 1994, with permission from Elsevier, http://www.sciencedirect.com/science/article/pii/S0892199705803030

the higher spectrum partials more than the lower spectrum partials. In this sense, singing with a small velopharyngeal opening seems to be another example of vocal economy. It is interesting that in the singers analysed, no signs of a velopharyngeal opening could be observed for the vowel /i/; for this vowel, the high-frequency part of the spectrum is quite prominent already because of the high second formant.

6.4.3 Formant or Voice Source?

As explained in earlier sections, the fundamental of the radiated spectrum can be strong not only because it is strong in the source spectrum but also because it is close to the first formant. Sundberg and Gauffin (1982) presented synthesized vowels to phonetically experienced listeners who were asked to identify the vowels. In some stimuli, the amplitude of the voice source fundamental was enhanced and, in other stimuli, a similar spectrum was obtained by manipulating the first formant frequency. The results showed that the listeners heard an effect on vowel quality rather than an effect on voice quality.

6.5 TIMING

In so-called syllabic parts of compositions, each syllable in the lyrics is given a new note. In orthography, syllables generally start with a consonant before the vowel and syllables are

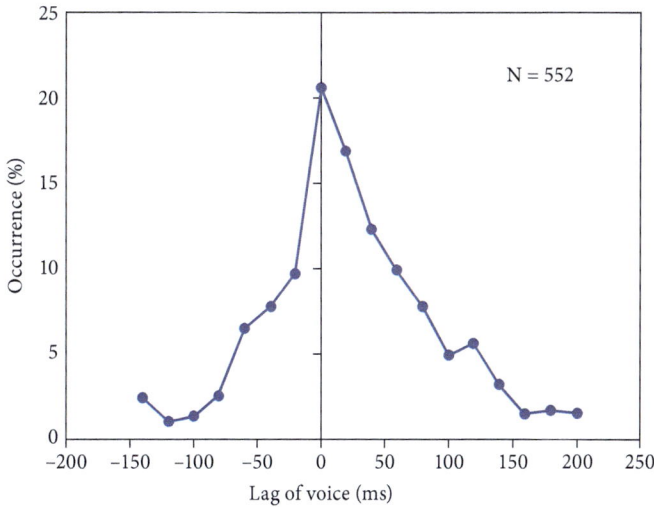

FIGURE 6.11 Histogram of the time lag between vowel onset and the piano chord which, according to the music score, should be synchronous.

Reprinted from *Journal of Voice*, Volume 21, Issue 3, Sundberg J. & Bauer-Huppmann J., 'When Does a Sung Tone Start', pp. 285–93, Copyright © 2007 The Voice Foundation, with permission from Elsevier, http://www.sciencedirect.com/science/article/pii/S0892199706000051

regarded as something like building blocks of words. It is sometimes erroneously assumed that in such cases the tone starts with the consonant. This assumption has been formally tested by measurements (Sundberg & Bauer-Hupmann, 2007). Commercially available phonogram recordings from the lieder repertoire and performed by several singers were analysed with regard to the time difference between the vowel onset and the piano chord, which according to the score should be synchronous with the voice. The time lag between the vowel onset and the piano chord yielded the results shown in Figure 6.11. The distribution has a marked peak at 0 ms. Thus, the vowel onset and the accompaniment chord are mostly in perfect synchrony.

The distribution shown in Figure 6.11 also reveals that both negative and positive time lags occur; sometimes the vowel onset can be more than 100 ms early (i.e. negative lag), and sometimes 200 ms late (i.e. positive lag). Durations of these magnitudes are clearly perceptible, 100 ms being a typical duration of a short note in melodic runs. The high positive and negative lag values tended to occur in different emotional contexts. For example, lead cases were frequently found in excited musical contexts, and lag cases in contexts with a more introvert and contemplative character. Consequently, it seems reasonable to assume that singers use lead and lag of the vowel onset for expressive purposes.

6.6 EMOTIONAL COLOURING

A quite essential aspect of music, as well as that of speech, is the emotional colouring of the message. It is quite likely that the acoustic code used for signalling basic emotions (e.g.

anger, fear, happiness, sadness, love/tenderness) is similar in both these forms of communication. Juslin and Laukka (2003) reviewed and compared the results of 104 studies of vocal expression and forty-one studies of music performance. They found striking similarities concerning both the accuracy with which discrete emotions were communicated to listeners and the emotion-specific patterns of acoustic cues used to communicate each emotion. These similarities concerned speech rate/tempo, intensity variation, spectrum balance between high and low frequencies, pitch contour, tone onset, and microstructural irregularity.

Two major dimensions of emotional communication are excitement (high and low) and valence (positive or negative). Two emotional colours that seem diametrically opposed are angry and sad. Both are obviously of negative valence but typically differing in excitement, the former being high and the latter being low. As can be expected, excitement is signalled by loud voice, fast tempo, quick changes of sound level, and wide vibrato extent. In addition, phonation type is recruited as an expressive means, peaceful ambience being associated with a stronger voice source fundamental than excited ambience (Sundberg, 2000).

Emphasizing important words in the lyrics seems an important property of convincing vocal performances. This can apparently be made by lengthening the note preceding the one that is carrying the important word—the case of 'emphasis by delayed arrival' (Sundberg, 2000).

As was mentioned in Section 6.3.3, 'Intonation', under certain conditions intonation also seems to be available for expressive purposes; in an excited ambience, the highest note of a phrase is often sharpened, and this appears to add to the expressivity (Sundberg et al., 2013).

Siegwart and Scherer (1995) analysed expert listeners' preferences and judgements of emotional expression in five recordings of the cadenza from the 'mad scene' *Ardi gli incensi* from Donizetti's opera *Lucia di Lammermoor*. They expected listeners to disagree about overall preferences and to agree on the emotions expressed, such as tender passion, fear of death, madness, and sadness. However, they found the opposite to be true. Further, based on a factorial-dimensional analysis of acoustic parameters, they constructed a two-component score, which predicted 84% of the variance in the preference ratings. The underlying acoustic parameters were related to the relative level of the fundamental and the strength of the high-frequency components in the spectrum. A voice with a high score on one of the two factors would have a consistently strong fundamental, while a voice with a high score on the other factor would have high energy in frequency near 2,500 Hz, and low energy above this frequency range. A strong fundamental and low high-frequency energy were associated with preference.

Howes et al. (2004) analysed the relevance of vibrato onset, rate, and extent to the findings reported by Siegwart and Scherer. They asked opera-lovers and teachers of singing to rank a number of recordings of the same material. Comparison of the acoustic measurements with preference and emotion judgements suggested that some elements of vibrato may affect listeners' perception of the voice and their preference for a particular singer, and assist the communication of emotion between singer and audience.

6.7 Intensity and Masking

It is commonly assumed that sound pressure level is perceived in terms of vocal loudness. However, the sound level of a vowel sound is almost entirely determined by the sound level of the strongest spectrum partial (Gramming & Sundberg, 1988). Therefore, the sound level can change substantially just by changing the fundamental frequency of the first formant frequency, while the vowel's loudness remains unchanged. Ladefoged and McKenney (1963) asked listeners to rate the loudness of syllables produced at different volumes. Their results revealed that the scatter of the ratings was less if plotted as a function of the subglottal pressure than when plotted as a function of the sound level. Thus, perceived degree of vocal loudness seems more closely related to subglottal pressure than to the acoustical sound level.

Masking implies that a sound becomes impossible to hear in the presence of another sound. In a vowel spectrum, many partials are sounding simultaneously, and some partials then mask other partials. In fact, measurements suggest that many partials in a spectrum are completely masked in the sound reaching a singer's ear while she/he is singing (Gauffin & Sundberg, 1974).

6.8 PLACEMENT

The term 'placement' is quite commonly used in vocal pedagogy to describe an important property of singers' vocal technique. Vurma and Ross (2002) studied its acoustical correlates. They noted that placement can be 'forward,' which is generally considered desirable, and 'backward,' which is considered undesirable. They asked student singers to voluntarily sing triads on different vowels with forward and backward placement. Expert listeners then determined whether the triads were placed forward or backward. Comparing spectral characteristics of triads classified as forward and backward by most expert listeners, they found that the second and third formants tended to be higher in the triads that were classified as placed forward. Also, the singer's formant cluster was much more prominent.

The choice of the term 'forward' and 'backward' is thought-provoking. The fact that it is so commonly used in vocal pedagogy suggests that it is easy to interpret and mostly interpreted in a similar way by different experts. One might speculate that this is related to articulation. The position of the tongue tip has a strong influence on the third formant frequency; retracting the tongue tip tends to lower this formant, while a fronted position raises it. In a similar way, a more fronted position of the tongue body tends to increase the second formant frequency. This seems to support the assumption that forward and backward placement is related to articulation. The increase in level of the singer's formant cluster would be a consequence of the increase of the second and third formants; as mentioned in Section 6.4, 'Formants', a decrease of the frequency separation between two formants automatically increases their levels and the valley between them.

6.9 LARYNX HEIGHT

A change in larynx position affects the vocal tract length and hence the formant frequencies. Sundberg and Nordström (1983) analysed the changes of formants when three trained voices pronounced the same vowels normally and then with a voluntarily raised larynx. Assuming a vocal tract length of 18 cm, an 18-mm rise of the larynx will cause an average 10% increase of the formant frequencies. Such effects are readily perceptible, the difference limen for formant frequency being 1% approximately (Kewley-Port & Watson, 1994).

However, elevation of the larynx is typically accompanied by an increase of glottal adduction and thus a change in phonation type towards a somewhat more hyperfunctional phonation. To explore the perception of an elevation of the larynx, Sundberg and Askenfelt (1983) synthesized ascending scales. The synthesis was modelled to sound like a classically trained baritone. In the top tones of the scale they introduced a gradual increase of the formant frequencies, a weakened voice-source fundamental, and also a decrease of the vibrato extent. The scales were presented to a group of teachers of singing who were asked to decide whether or not the imagined singer was raising his larynx for the top notes of the scale. The results showed that the most salient characteristic of raised larynx was an increase in the formant frequencies. This seems logical as it would be quite difficult to raise the larynx without raising the formant frequencies. However, a reduced amplitude of voice source fundamental also added to the impression of a raised larynx. In addition, a reduced extent of vibrato contributed to this impression, although only if the formant frequencies and the amplitude of the fundamental also suggested a raised larynx.

6.10 SYNTHESIS AND NATURALNESS

Synthesis is an extremely powerful tool for evaluating acoustic descriptions of sound. The strategy is to produce sound with completely defined acoustic properties, corresponding to those found in analysis of the sound considered. If perceptually important properties are missing in the description, synthesis will sound unnatural or synthetic.

During the last half century a great number of attempts have been made to synthesize singing. The seemingly first attempt was made by the Bell Telephone Laboratories in 1961. It efficiently illustrates the difficulties of achieving naturalness. Listening to this synthesis makes it clear that there are several sources of unnaturalness—one is the voice timbre, a second is the intelligibility of the lyrics, a third is the machine-like performance, and a fourth is the limited synchrony between the singer voice and the accompaniment.

Later attempts have been successful in achieving a natural voice timbre. A classic example is the synthesis, by the Institut de Recherche et Coordination Acoustique Musique (IRCAM) in Paris, of the second aria of the *Queen of the Night* from Mozart's opera *Die Zauberflöte*. Examples of baritone synthesis were produced by the Royal Institute of Technology's (KTH) synthesizer 'MUSSE' in 1976 in Stockholm (Sundberg, 2006). In these examples, the text intelligibility is limited; achieving a natural-sounding synthesis of lyrics is much more difficult than synthesizing a realistic voice timbre. The reason would be that consonants are identified by formants that change quickly and precisely in frequency and amplitude, while voice timbre depends on much slower acoustical events. If formant patterns, which cannot be produced by a real singer, occur in synthesis, unnaturalness is likely to happen.

A general and not at all surprising observation is that naturalness increases if the synthesis is complemented by an accompaniment. The sound of the accompaniment is likely to mask details that may decrease naturalness. In addition, it also may distract the listener's attention from the voice quality.

A commonly used technique for synthesizing speech and singing has been to pass a signal corresponding to the voice source through a filter that corresponds to the vocal tract. As long as the frequency response curve of the filter faithfully reflects that of a real vocal tract, the result can sound quite natural. However, to generate natural-sounding synthesis with these means is quite tedious work. The enormous digital storage capacity of today's computers has opened the possibility to store recordings of all consonant–vowel, vowel–consonant, and consonant–consonant combinations that occur in a language and then to splice the appropriate sequences to generate the lyrics. The technique is called concatenation and is presently widely used. An example is the commercially available Vocaloid system, which even allows for transposing a recording of a spoken text to singing. However, the aim has not been to create a natural-sounding synthesis (since real singers are much better at this), as much as to open up new possibilities to music making.

The work with synthesizing singing has demonstrated the relevance of performance: if the synthesis sounds really realistic, listeners are likely to imagine a living singer rather than a machine producing the performance. Under those conditions, demands for musically interesting and convincing performance are likely to appear. This has triggered research on principles underlying musical performance– that is, the gap between a deadpan performance and a real performance (e.g. see Gabrielsson, 1999).

6.11 DIFFERENT STYLES OF SINGING

Voice source and formant characteristics in singing tend to differ more or less widely from conversational speech. A factor of great influence is the demands raised on the acoustic context. For example, in the classical tradition, where no microphone and amplifier system are used, singers are required to produce much louder sound than in conversational speech. In Western operatic singing this has resulted in the singer's formant cluster and in the principle to increase the first formant frequency in cases when otherwise it would become lower than the fundamental. These tricks make the singers' voices easier to hear through a loud orchestral accompaniment, but also create marked deviations from normal speech. Differences between male singers representing the classical Western tradition and musical theatre singers have been analysed with regard to both voice source and formants (Björkner, 2008).

Voice source properties seem to differ between *pop-music styles*. The two panels in Figure 6.12 show an example from a professional vocal artist and pedagogue singing in different pop-music styles—Rock, Soul, Pop, and Dance Band—the latter being a style of singing used by vocalists singing in hotels on weekend evenings (Zangger-Borch & Sundberg, 2012; Audio 6.7). The graphs show subglottal pressure and the mean of a measure of glottal abduction, the so-called normalized amplitude quotient (NAQ) (Alku et al., 2002). Both parameters are plotted as function of fundamental frequency. In the left panel, the chain-dashed curves represent the lowest pressure values which, according to Titze (1992), make the vocal folds vibrate, multiplied by a factor of one, three, six, and nine. Rock is highest in pitch range and uses pressures close to nine times the threshold. Dance Band assumes the opposite extreme, being lowest in pitch and using pressures about three times the threshold. Pop and Soul are higher in pitch range and use pressure values slightly higher than the Dance Band style. The styles also differ markedly in the NAQ parameter, which reflects the degree of glottal abduction. The mean

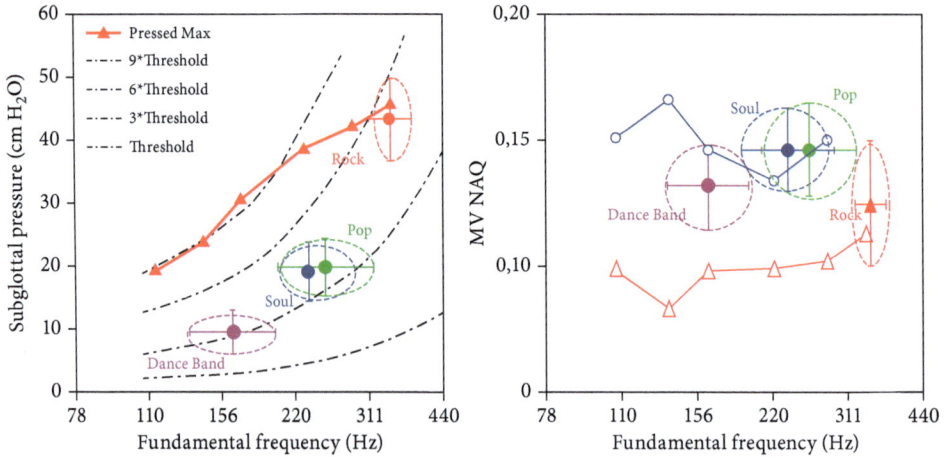

FIGURE 6.12 *Left panel*: Subglottal pressures plotted as functions of the pitch frequency (in logarithmic scale). Chain-dashed curves show one, three, six, and nine times the phonation pressure threshold according to Titze (1992). The red, green, blue, and pink data points show the averages in the indicated styles, and the axes of the ellipses surrounding the points represent the mean plus minus one standard deviation. The red curve represents the singer's highest values when he was singing with deliberately pressed phonation.
Right panel: Corresponding graph showing the mean NAQ values. The blue and red curves refer to the values observed when the singer was singing with neutral and pressed phonation.

Adapted from *Journal of Voice*, Volume 25, Issue 5, Zangger-Borch, D. & Sundberg, J., 'Some Phonatory and Resonatory Characteristics of the Rock, Pop, Soul, and Swedish Dance Band Styles of Singing', Figures 7 and 8, pp. 532–7, Copyright © 2012 The Voice Foundation, with permission from Elsevier, http://www.sciencedirect.com/science/article/pii/S0892199711000137

for Rock is quite close to the value which the subject produced when demonstrating pressed/hyperfunctional phonation (red curve and triangles). Dance Band, Pop, and Soul are much closer to the values that the singer produced when demonstrating neutral phonation (i.e. neither pressed nor breathy).

Twang is a term commonly used and referring to voice timbre. However, some authors use it to describe a special nasal voice quality sometimes used in pop music. Other authors use it to refer to the voice quality that appears when the epilaryngeal tube is narrowed, which would mean that it refers to the sound quality caused by the singer's formant cluster in classically trained male voices. Thus, the term is used with quite different meanings. An attempt has been made to analyse the acoustical correlates of the term when applied to pop-music styles (Sundberg & Thalén, 2010). It was found that subglottal pressure tended to be higher and sound pressure level (SPL) was invariably higher in 'twang' than in non-twang. In 'twang', as compared with neutral, the closed quotient was greater, the pulse amplitude and the voice source fundamental were weaker, and the abduction quotient NAQ tended to be lower. Formants 1 and 2 were higher, whilst formants 3 and 5 were lower. The formant differences, which appeared to be the main cause of the SPL differences, were more important than the source differences for the perception of 'twanginess'. Audio 6.8 demonstrates the timbral effects of successively adding formant and voice source characteristics to a synthesized tone.

Belt is a less ambiguous term referring to a type of voice production commonly used in non-classical genres. It is loud and sounds pressed and expressive, somewhat similar to yelling. It is commonly assumed to require a special type of breathing behaviour. However, an investigation failed to observe a common breathing pattern among six female singers (all professionally performing in the belt styles for many years) neither when they were singing in the belt style nor when they were singing in a more neutral, non-belt style (Sundberg & Thalén, 2015). Subglottal pressures and SPL were quite high in belt, and the abduction parameter NAQ, as well as a weak voice source fundamental, suggested a firmer glottal adduction in belt than in neutral. Also, some of the singers tended to tune the first formant closer to a spectrum harmonic in belt than in neutral.

Summarizing, glottal adduction, and hence also the subglottal pressure range, as well as formant frequencies, differ between different styles of singing. To some extent these differences can be understood as consequences of the acoustical conditions under which the music is being performed. The availability of microphones and sound amplification seems particularly important. In some cases, demands for extreme emotional colours seem relevant. However, as a need to invent new ways to create vocal and musical expressivity seems like an essential factor, the vocal styles change and develop over time.

6.12 OUTLOOK

Not much of the literature reviewed here has explicitly concerned perception of singing. One problem has been the limited possibilities to synthesize singing that sounds perfectly realistic. The perceptual relevance of acoustic properties can be efficiently tested only if varied systematically in synthesized sung tones; as soon as a listener hears that the tone is not sung by a real singer, her/his listening strategy is likely to change.

Perception seems closely related to production. For instance, as demonstrated in Section 6.7, 'Intensity and Masking', ratings of vocal loudness seem more closely related to the subglottal pressure used for producing it than to the sound level. Also thought-provoking is the observation that the terms 'forward placement' and 'backward placement', with regard to the voice, seem related to the placement of the tongue tip. In fact, it seems that the success of a singing teacher's pedagogy would depend on his or her ability to correctly identify the phonatory and articulatory characteristics which the student uses. In this sense, production and perception seem quite closely related; to understand perception, understanding of the production is needed.

REFERENCES

d'Alessandro, C. & Castellengo, M. (1994). The pitch of short-duration vibrato tones. *Journal of the Acoustical Society of America*, 95(3), 1617–1630.

Alku, P., Bäckström, T., & Vilkman, E. (2002). Normalized amplitude quotient for parameterization of the glottal flow. *Journal of the Acoustical Society of America*, 112(2), 701–710.

Birch, P., Gümoes, B., Stavad, H., Prytz, S., Björkner, E., & Sundberg, J. (2002). Velum behavior in professional classic operatic singing. *Journal of Voice*, 16(1), 61–71.

Björkner, E. (2008). Musical theater and opera singing—why so different? A study of subglottal pressure, voice source, and formant frequency characteristics. *Journal of Voice*, 22(5), 533–540.

Cleveland, T., Sundberg, J., & Stone, R. E. (2001). Long-term-average spectrum characteristics of country singers during speaking and singing. *Journal of Voice*, 15(1), 54–60.

Deme, A. (2014). Intelligibility of sung vowels: the effect of consonantal context and the onset of voicing. *Journal of Voice*, 28(4), e19–e25.

Fant, G. (1960). *Acoustic Theory of Speech Production*. The Hague: Mouton.

Gabrielsson, A. (1999). The performance of music. In: D. Deutsch (ed.) *The Psychology of Music*, 2nd edition (pp. 501–579). New York: Academic Press.

Gauffin, J. & Sundberg, J. (1974). Masking effects of one's own voice. *STL-QPSR*, 15(1), 35–41.

Gramming, P. & Sundberg, J. (1988). Spectrum factors relevant to phonetogram measurement. *Journal of the Acoustical Society of America*, 83, 2352–2360.

Griffin, B., Woo, P., Colton, R., Casper, J., & Brewer, D. (1995). Physiological characteristics of the supported singing voice. A preliminary study. *Journal of Voice*, 9(1), 45–56.

Hertegård, S., Gauffin, J., & Sundberg, J. (1990). Open and covered singing as studied by means of fiberoptics, inverse filtering, and spectral analysis. *Journal of Voice*, 4(3), 220–230.

Hirano, M., Vennard, W., & Ohala, J. (1970). Registration of register, pitch and intensity of voice. An electromyographic investigation of intrinsic laryngeal muscles. *Folia Phoniatrica*, 22(1), 1–20.

Howes, P., Callaghan, J., Davis, P., Kenny, D., & Thorpe, W. (2004). The relationship between measured vibrato characteristics and perception in Western operatic singing. *Journal of Voice*, 18(2), 216–230.

Juslin, P. & Laukka, P. (2003). Communication of emotions in vocal expression and music performance: different channels, same code? *Psychological Bulletin*, 129(5), 770–814.

Kewley-Port, D. and Watson, C. S. (1994). Formant-frequency discrimination for isolated English vowels. *Journal of the Acoustical Society of America*, 95(1), 485–496.

Ladefoged, P. and McKenny, N.P. (1963). Loudness, top of form sound pressure, and subglottal pressure in speech. *Journal of the Acoustical Society of America*, 35, 454–460.

Leino, T. (2008). Long-term average spectrum in screening of voice quality in speech. Untrained male university students. *Journal of Voice*, 23(6), 671–676.

McDonnell, M., Sundberg, J., Westerlund, J., Lindestad. P.-Å., & Larsson H. (2011). Vocal fold vibration and phonation start in aspirated, unaspirated, and staccato onset. *Journal of Voice*, 25(5), 526–531.

Miller, D. G. & Schutte, H. K. (1990). Formant tuning in a professional baritone. *Journal of Voice*, 4, 231–237.

Millgård, M., Sundberg, J., & Fors, T. (2015). Flow glottogram characteristics and perceived degree of phonatory pressedness. *Journal of Voice*, 30(3), 287–292.

Neumann, K., Schunda, P., Hoth, S., & Euler, H. A. (2005). The interplay between glottis and vocal tract during the male passaggio. *Folia Phoniatrica Logopedia*, 57, 308–327.

Öhman, S. E. G. (1966). Coarticulation in VCV utterances: spectrographic measurement. *Journal of the Acoustical Society of America*, 39, 151–168.

Prame, E. (1994). Measurements of the vibrato rate of ten singers. *Journal of the Acoustical Society of America*, 96(4), 1979–1984.

Seashore, C. (1938) (reprinted 1967). *Psychology of Music*. New York: McGraw-Hill.

Shipp, T., Doherty, E. T., & Haglund, S. (1990). Physiologic factors in vocal vibrato production. *Journal of Voice* 4(4), 300–304.

Shonle, J. I. & Horan, K. E. (1980). The pitch of vibrato tones. *Journal of the Acoustical Society of America*, 67(1), 246–262.

Siegwart, H. & Scherer, K. R. (1995). Acoustic concomitants of emotional expression in operatic singing: the case of Lucia in 'Ardi gli incense'. *Journal of Voice*, 9(3), 249–260.

Sundberg, J. (1977). Vibrato and vowel identification. *Archives of Acoustics*, 2, 257–266.

Sundberg, J. (1978). Effects of the vibrato and the 'singing formant' on pitch. *Musica Slovaca*, VI, 51–69.

Sundberg, J. (1987). *The Science of the Singing Voice*. DeKalb IL: Northern Illinois University Press.

Sundberg, J. (1994). Perceptual aspects of singing. *Journal of Voice*, 8(2), 106–122.

Sundberg, J. (2000). Emotive transforms. *Phonetica*, 57, 95–112.

Sundberg, J. (2006). The KTH synthesis of singing. *Advances in Cognitive Psychology*, Special Issue on Music Performance, 2(2–3), 131–143.

Sundberg, J. (2012). Some observations on operatic singer's intonation. *Interdisciplinary Studies in Musicology*, 10, 47–59.

Sundberg, J. & Askenfelt, A. (1983). Larynx height and voice source: a relationship? In: J. Abbs & D. Bless (eds) *Voice Physiology* (pp. 307–316). Houston TX: Collegehill.

Sundberg, J. & Bauer-Huppmann, J. (2007). When does a sung tone start? *Journal of Voice*, 21(3), 285–293.

Sundberg, J. & Gauffin, J. (1982). Amplitude of the voice source fundamental and the intelligibility of super pitch vowel. In: R. Carlson & B. Granström (eds) *The Representation of Speech in the Peripheral Auditory System* (pp. 223–228). Amsterdam: Elsevier Biomedical Press.

Sundberg, J. & Gauffin, J. (1973). Musical octaves and pitch. *Journal of the Acoustical Society of America*, 54, 922–929.

Sundberg, J., Lã, F. M. B., & Himonides, E. (2013). Intonation and expressivity: a single case study of classical western singing. *Journal of Voice*, 27(3), e1–e8.

Sundberg, J., Niska-Thörnvik, M., & Söderström, A. M. (1998). Age and voice quality in professional singers. *Logopedics Phoniatrics Vocology*, 23, 169–176.

Sundberg, J. & Nordström, P. E. (1983). Raised and lowered larynx—the effect on vowel formant frequencies. *Journal of Research in Singing*, VI(2), 7–15.

Sundberg, J., Prame, E., & Iwarsson, J. (1996). Replicability and accuracy of pitch patterns in professional singers. In: P. Davis & N. Fletcher (eds) *Vocal Fold Physiology, Controlling Complexity and Chaos* (pp. 291–306). San Diego: Singular Publishing Group.

Sundberg, J. & Thalén, M. (2010). What is 'twang'? *Journal of Voice*, 24(6), 654–660.

Sundberg, J. & Thalén, M. (2015). Respiratory and acoustical differences between belt and neutral style of singing. *Journal of Voice*, 29(4), 418–425.

Sundberg, J., Thalén, M., Alku, P., & Vilkman, E. (2004). Estimating perceived phonatory pressedness in singing from flow glottograms. *Journal of Voice*, 18(1), 56–62.

Thomasson, M. & Sundberg, J. (2001). Consistency of inhalatory breathing patterns in professional operative singers. *Voice*, 15, 373–383. doi: 10.1016/S0892-1997(01)00039-X

Titze, I. R., Riede, T., & Popolo, P. (2008). Nonlinear source–filter coupling in phonation: vocal exercises. *Journal of the Acoustical Society of America*, 123(4), 1902–1915.

Titze, I. R., Solomon, N. P., Luschei, E. S., & Hirano, M. (1994). Interference between normal vibrato and artificial stimulation of laryngeal muscles at near-vibrato rates. *Journal of Voice*, 8(3), 215–223.

Titze, I. R. (2008). Nonlinear source–filter coupling in phonation: theory. *Journal of the Acoustical Society of America*, 123(5), 2733–2749.

Titze, I. R. (1992). Phonation threshold pressure: a missing link in glottal aerodynamics. *Journal of the Acoustical Society of America*, 91(5), 2926–2935.

Vurma, A. & Ross, J. (2002). Where is a singer's voice if it is placed 'forward'? *Journal of Voice*, 16(3), 383–391.

Watson, P. & Hixon, T. (1996). Respiratory behaviour during the learning of a novel aria by a highly trained classical singer. In: P. Davis and N. Fletcher (eds) *Vocal Fold Physiology, Controlling Complexity and Chaos* (pp. 325–343). San Diego: Singular Publishing Group.

Watson, P. & Hixon, T. (1985). Respiratory kinematics in classical (opera) singers. *Journal of Speech, Language, and Hearing Research*, 28(3), 104–122.

White, P. (1999). Formant frequency analysis of children's spoken and sung vowels using sweeping fundamental frequency production. *Journal of Voice*, 13(4), 570–582.

Zangger-Borch, D. & Sundberg, J. (2012). Some phonatory and resonatory characteristics of the Rock, Pop, Soul, and Swedish Dance Band styles of singing. *Journal of Voice*, 25(5), 532–537.

CHAPTER 7

....

SUPRASEGMENTAL SPEECH PROSODY AND THE HUMAN BRAIN

....

MARTIN MEYER, MATTHIAS KELLER, AND NATHALIE GIROUD

7.1 BACKGROUND

....

SPEECH prosody is a key feature of human spoken language. According to Shattuck-Hufnagel and Turk (1996, p. 195) 'a universally acceptable definition of prosody has been elusive' as the understanding and application of the umbrella term 'prosody' is quite inconsistent. However, most authors agree that prosody describes abstract phonological phenomena, such as word stress, sentence accent, sentence mode, and phrasing, which are correlated with the semantic, syntactic, morphological, and segmental organization of speech (Dogil et al., 2002; Frazier et al., 2006). The term prosody is also used to refer to the phonetic attributes used to encode these abstract structures (i.e. pitch, intensity, and duration). As modulations of these parameters are used to transfer linguistically relevant information, the notion of linguistic prosody is often used as a synonym for prosody in general. Listeners can therefore use intonation, duration, and amplitude information to help decode the syntactic mode and focus structure of the sentences they attend to.[1] However tempo, rhythm, and voice can also be conceived as being ensembled under this umbrella term (Cruttenden, 1997). Prosodic aspects of language are superimposed on its segmental, syllabic, and lexical features and are,

---

[1] It should be mentioned that languages differ in their fundamental prosodic structure and patterns. These varieties notwithstanding, modulations of the fundamental frequency (Fo) are considered the main acoustic correlate of prosody and correspond to the perceptual level of intonation. In other words, modulating the slowly and rapidly changing acoustic properties of speech melody may have linguistically relevant implications. Word stress is another example of the linguistic function of prosody. In Indo-European languages, such as English and German, stressed syllables have a higher Fo, are louder, and are longer than unstressed syllables. At the sentence level, modulations of the Fo may mark a semantically neutral spoken utterance as either a question or statement.

hence, regarded as *suprasegmental* (Lehiste, 1970). For most, this information is modulated by the voice of a human individual or by the physical structures of the human vocal tract (larynx, pharynx).[2]

Dellwo et al. (2007) provide a comprehensive overview on the phonetic description of speech and describe how modulations of the human voice relate to suprasegmental and prosodic features.

7.2 EMOTIONAL PROSODY—AN OBSOLETE CONCEPT?

Prosodic modulations may be used to convey not only linguistic but also paralinguistic, emotional information. Some scholars have even formed the notion of *affective prosody* (Berckmoes & Vingerhoets, 2004). The widely held belief in the existence of emotional prosody as a phenomenon that can be acoustically, functionally, and even neurally distinguished from a non-emotional, linguistically driven form of prosody, probably originates from clinical observations more than thirty years ago. By adapting the concept of aphasia as a clinical diagnosis of deficient speech and syntax functions after damage to left perisylvian regions (PR), the notion of aprosodia had been introduced. In patients who suffered from damage to the right perisylvian regions, impairments in expression and perception of prosodic cues, primarily those with an emotional tune, were observed (Ross, 1981; Ross & Monnot, 2008). Since then, prosodic speech with emotional valence has often been conceived as a special case of speech prosody that is organized by distinct neural circuits. According to Ross et al. (2013) injuries of the right frontal operculum and the right superior temporal gyrus (STG) are the best predictors for aprosodic (affective) deficits. However, impairment of affective tune was also observed after damage to the left PR (Ross et al., 1997). A few years later, the task-dependent hypothesis was introduced that attributed emotional prosody to the right PR and linguistically functional prosody to the left PR (Van Lancker, 1980).

Soon, it turned out that this strict division between linguistic and emotional prosody was not corroborated by clinical studies. It rather seemed that damage to either hemisphere may result in any kind of prosodic deficit (Behrens, 1989; Heilman et al., 1984; Pell & Baum, 1997; Ross et al., 2013; Weintraub & Mesulam, 1981; Witteman et al., 2011). An alternative framework proposed that functional lateralization of prosodic cues correlates with distinct acoustic parameters: a left PR dominance for duration and amplitude with the latter encoding loudness at the perception level, and a right PR dominance for the fundamental frequency (Fo) as an acoustic correlate of intonation contour (Van Lancker & Sidtis, 1992). According to this view it is not possible to distinguish between emotional and linguistic prosody until the acoustic modulations underlying prosodic cues have been thoroughly investigated.

---

[2] Beyond conveying a spoken utterance in words and sounds, the speech signal also provides information about the speaker's age, sex, proficiency in a (foreign) language, etc.

However, in a seminal study, Wiethoff et al. (2008) demonstrated, compellingly, that a distinct entity of emotional prosody does not exist because the same acoustic modulations that underlie linguistic functions of prosody—namely mean intensity, mean Fo, variability of Fo, and duration—may also form acoustic patterns that affect the emotional tune of a spoken utterance. Any kind of acoustic cues that carry prosodic information, with or without emotional tune, involve both left and right auditory cortical fields. It remains to be said that we suggest abandoning the notion of *emotional* or *affective prosody* because it is a sole expendable label that lacks a clear definition and distinctiveness. It is primarily of historical origin and has previously been used in the context of clinical neuropsychology. We consider it even misleading as emotional prosody does not automatically mean emotional involvement, which is often accompanied by gestures and facial expression. Notably, humans, like animals, utter affectively-loaded shouts (crying, whining, suspiring, screams of rage, cheers of pleasure) that are completely controlled by subcortical circuits (Ackermann et al., 2014; Hage & Nieder, 2016). On the other hand, everyday spoken language can be deliberately used to feign emotional involvement by imitating acoustic patterns of emotional arousal, even when the speaker only pretends to be emotionally affected. Exactly the same acoustic modulations are used when a speaker wilfully marks a spoken utterance as a question or statement by altering the pitch contour of the final segments of a sentence. Having said this, we again propose an understanding of prosody as a prime organizational structure of spoken utterances that must not be considered a monolithic entity.

7.3 Towards a Parameter-Based Prosody

The last two decades have seen an abundance of studies that sought to identify the neural signature of linguistic domains—namely syntax, semantics, phonology, and prosody (Price, 2012). However, this approach has been challenged in the recent past because there is increasing uncertainty as to whether linguistic domains are of any significance for the human brain and to what extent the realm of neuroscience is compatible with the realm of linguistics (Poeppel, 2012; Poeppel & Embick, 2005). Two main concerns, termed the *maps problem* and the *mapping problem*, are thereby identified. The *maps problem* deals with the question of how informative the insights of domain-based research are in describing the neuronal basis of cognitive functions. While maps of brain function do contribute to a better understanding of which brain regions might (partly) be involved in a task, they are inherently correlational and do not possess any explanatory power regarding the question of how cognitive functions are carried out by the brain.

The second concern, the *mapping problem,* relates to the issue of how to establish formal connections between linguistic (or cognitive theories) and brain function. Based upon the assumption that both language and the brain constitute a set of essential elements of representation and a set of elementary functions, the question arises of how these essentials can be mapped across domains. Representational elements might be morphemes (linguistics) or a cortical column (neuroscience), while concatenation (linguistics) or oscillations (neuroscience) are elementary functions. Thus, in order to achieve an explanatory, mechanistic theory about how the brain does process speech, research has to go beyond a domain-based approach.

How can such an approach be applied to the question of how the brain processes suprasegmental, prosodic information? The first question we may ask is what the representational units and computational functions of prosody are. As it turns out, finding an answer to this question is not trivial and it is difficult to come up with an answer that is not inclusive in nature (Ladd, 2014). We suggest one definition based on phonetic properties, that is, the frequency of temporal modulations of which unfolding acoustic features are made up.

If one looks at speech from an acoustical perspective, it can be described as the superimposition of a multitude of waveforms of varying frequencies, amplitudes, and periodicities. These sound waves are characterized by linguistically relevant categories based on their temporal properties (Rosen, 1992). According to the 'asymmetric sampling in time' (AST) hypothesis (Poeppel, 2003), acoustic information that unfolds in a short timescale (~25 ms) is termed 'temporal fine structure', while modulations that span across several hundreds of milliseconds (~250 ms) are referred to as 'temporal envelope' (see also Meyer, 2008; Rufener et al., 2016; Zatorre & Gandour, 2008). We consider these modulations as the backbone of spoken language as they correspond to linguistic and paralinguistic codes that are indispensable for language comprehension. In particular, the suprasegmental temporal envelope of the speech signal carries pertinent acoustic patterns that transmit prosodic information. You may simply consider the question 'Where do you go?'. Depending on the position of stress, the meaning of the question differs. By putting the stress on the first word ('*Where* do you go?') an emphasis is put on the location (as opposed, for example, to 'when' or 'how'). In contrast, by stressing the personal pronoun ('Where do *you* go?'), the intention of the person addressed, in contrast to any other person, is of interest. The exact meaning of the question can be inferred by evaluating the position of the stress, which is detected by comparing it to its neighbouring segments. From this example we can learn that the relation between segments, that unravel across a time span of tens or hundreds of milliseconds, constitute the prosodic information. This holds true also for other prosodic features, such as accent, tone, and speech rhythm, that typically span across several speech segments. However, it has to be noted that not all of these features can be conceived as suprasegmental (Ladd, 2014).

At least with respect to spoken language, a parameter-based approach is an alternative account. Spoken utterances can be conceived as an acoustic signal which unfolds in time (Meyer, 2008). Thus, speech comprises acoustic information that may be described at the frequency and at the time-scale level. Slow, acoustic modulations that characterize prosodic marking (e.g. intonation contour), occur in a suprasegmental mode that unfolds at a rate of hundreds or even thousands of milliseconds (Phillips & Farmer, 1990).

Taken together, it seems advisable to refrain from viewing prosody as an axiomatic entity to which a corresponding neural correlate can be identified in brain function. Rather, it appears to be more convenient to focus on more general (or elementary) units that are the foundation of prosodic modulations. The issue of how the human brain masters the processing of acoustic information and identifies it as relevant units of spoken language is an impressive example of how the language of the brain works. As opposed to the traditional view proposing that speech and language are an exclusive privilege of the left hemisphere, accumulating research has pointed to an essential role of right temporal areas in speech perception (McGettigan & Scott, 2012; Meyer, 2008; Vigneau et al., 2011), indicating the need of accounting for contributions of both the left and the right peri-auditory fields to speech

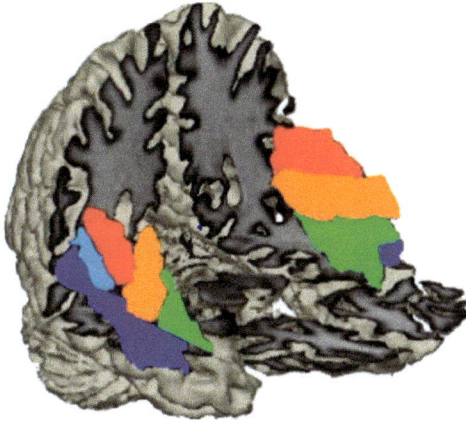

FIGURE 7.1 The distinct bilateral macroanatomical portions of the temporal operculum. Right hemisphere regions are displayed on the left side of the brain. The auditory-related cortex comprises the planum temporale (PT), the posterior superior temporal gyrus (pSTG), Heschl's gyrus/sulcus (HG/HS) and the posterior part of the superior temporal sulcus (STS). Red = PT, turquoise = pSTG, green = planum polare (PP), orange = HG/HS, marine = STG/STS.

processing. In particular, the right posterior auditory association cortex, including the planum temporale, has been attributed to processing speech prosody (Hesling, Clément, et al., 2005; Hesling, Dilharreguy, et al., 2005; Kreitewolf et al., 2014; Kyong et al., 2014; Meyer et al., 2002, 2004; Zhang et al., 2010). However, a meta-analysis suggests that a simple conception of prosody as a right-lateralized brain function per se does not do justice to the complexity of the topic (Belyk & Brown, 2014). It seems appropriate to take a closer look at the brain–prosody relationship to better understand why acoustic cues that underlie prosodic modulations are preferentially governed by the right auditory-related cortex. (See Figure 7.1 for a display of the locations the auditory-related cortex.)

The AST hypothesis provides an explanation for this phenomenon. According to this framework, the left auditory-related cortex is preferentially driven by rapidly changing acoustic cues, while the contralateral auditory fields are specifically amenable to slowly changing suprasegmental information (Poeppel, 2003; Shalom & Poeppel, 2008). Supporting evidence for this view comes from studies that observed right PARC involvement in processing suprasegmental prosodic features other than intonation contour, namely metrical speech rhythm (Geiser et al., 2008), as well as metrical and non-metrical rhymes in spoken utterances (Hurschler et al., 2013, 2015). One study that systematically investigated the effects of parametric degradation of suprasegmental information, following the approach introduced by Saberi and Perrott (1999), also buttresses the AST hypothesis (Liem et al., 2014). In this investigation, acoustic files of spoken sentences were divided into segments of varying duration which were then temporally reversed. Depending on the length of the segments, intelligibility changed. For short segments, intelligibility was almost entirely preserved, while longer segments led to a distortion of temporal envelope information and consequently to a reduced intelligibility. While the primary auditory cortex (Heschl's gyrus) did not show any lateralization effects depending on the segment length, activation in the planum temporale and posterior STG shifted to the right with increasing segment length. The authors concluded that suprasegmental information becomes more strongly weighted with decreasing intelligibility of phonetic information because the brain now only has suprasegmental information at its disposal to achieve an interpretation of the spoken utterance.

Interestingly, Liem et al. (2014) also report a correlation between behavioural and structural measurements in that participants with L > R cortical thickness performed better in an auditory pattern-matching task. This result may imply that individuals with thinner cortex measurements in the right PARC might demonstrate more complementary myelination which might be more suitable for the auditory analysis of suprasegmental acoustic chunks.

Previous neuroanatomical research also provides corroborating evidence for the account that the evolution of spoken language may have shaped the architecture of the human auditory cortex in that it demonstrates structural asymmetry pertaining to the microscopic structure of neuronal microcolumns (Hutsler & Galuske, 2003). Notably, these structural asymmetries are only apparent in the human brain, and not in the brains of apes or monkeys (Buxhoeveden et al., 2001). Hence, the study of Liem and colleagues (2014) confirms one of the most important propositions of the AST hypothesis as it demonstrates a continuum of functional lateralization, with the right PARC becoming more strongly activated, the more suprasegmental information is available for temporal analysis. This view goes against former models that suggested a categorical division of labour between the two hemispheres (Zatorre & Belin, 2001). According to this framework, the right PARC is more strongly devoted to processing spectral information, while the left PARC preferentially subserves the computation of temporal modulations of which acoustic signals are made up.

Even though suggestions have been made on how to reconcile these two accounts (Rufener et al., 2016; Zatorre & Gandour, 2008), we consider the AST model an ideal working hypothesis, as it is more thoroughly built on the temporal dynamics of both spoken language and brain signals. However, while the AST hypothesis, in its original form, addresses the issue of *where* in the brain prosodically relevant information is processed, it does not provide precise information concerning the question of *how* (in a computational sense) prosodic features are decoded during speech perception.

7.3.1 Slow Acoustic Modulations and Slow Neural Oscillations

A complementary framework to address *how* prosodic features are decoded during speech perception, that is grounded on physiologically based assumptions, has been put forward by Anne-Lise Giraud and David Poeppel (2012). Evidently, oscillatory activity in neurons of sensory cortices seems to be a crucial mechanism for sensory integration (Schroeder et al., 2008). This holds true also for speech and its acoustic components. Neuronal oscillations can be found in superficial (II/III) and deep (V/VI) layers of cortical columns. The oscillatory activity in these layers is believed to interact with stimulus-driven spike trains, typically recorded from intermediate layers in column IV. It has been proposed that two populations of pyramidal neurons in layers II and III exist that oscillate in endogenous γ (25–35 Hz) and θ (4–8 Hz) frequencies respectively (Giraud et al., 2007). Auditory input from layer IV modulates the excitatory phases of neurons in superficial layers and leads to a phase reset of oscillations and an alignment between neural oscillations and temporal fluctuations in the input signal. The continuous spike-train signal is hereby transformed into a discontinuous, temporally organized spike-train signal that is then further processed for hierarchically higher computations.

A further proposition is that oscillations exhibit asymmetric properties in terms of the hemispheric contribution. While γ sampling of the input signal mainly dominates the left auditory cortex, θ sampling is more predominant in right auditory fields (Giraud et al., 2007; Giroud et al., 2018; Morillon et al., 2010). Interestingly, the suprasegmental characteristics of temporal fine structure and temporal envelope information is isochronous to the duration of the phases of θ and γ oscillations. The duration of fine-grained acoustic speech events corresponds to the phase duration of a γ oscillation (25 ms). Complementary, temporal envelope cues span about 250 ms, which is the same as the duration of a phase in the θ-frequency range. According to the hypothesis of Giraud and Poeppel (2012), temporal fine structure is sampled through neural γ oscillations, while temporal envelope information is sampled through θ oscillations, which offers a plausible explanation for the aforementioned lateralization effects. Since suprasegmental speech information is related to θ oscillations, preferred computation of this type of information would be expected to be performed in the auditory cortex of the right hemisphere. A further implication of this model is that it also offers a potential explanation for enhanced activity in right auditory cortex during the analysis of spectral information (Belin & Zatorre, 2003; Lattner et al., 2005; Warren et al., 2005) and thus reconciles the models of Poeppel (2003) and Zatorre and Belin (2001).

This framework also provides a link between elementary acoustic units of speech and neural mechanisms, in that the two dimensions have to map onto each other. This mapping has been dubbed *neural entrainment* and has been observed in a variety of studies (for review, see, for example, Peelle & Davis, 2012). However, the exact functional implications of neural entrainment to the temporal envelope of speech are still under debate.

Different hypotheses have been put forward that can be broadly divided into those that view envelope tracking as an analytic mechanism or as a synthesizing mechanism (Ding & Simon, 2014). As part of the initial stage of speech processing, cortical entrainment can be conceived as a way of extracting primitive auditory features from the speech stream (Ding & Simon, 2012b; Howard & Poeppel, 2012). Due to this view, cortical entrainment is seen as a passive mechanism, while other models suggest that cortical entrainment actively serves the integration of features into linguistic units in a top-down manner (Ding & Simon, 2012a; Giraud & Poeppel, 2012; Schroeder et al., 2008). With respect to the latter, attending to a speech stream in a cocktail-party paradigm enhances the neuronal representation of the attended stream in low-level auditory cortex, but the representation of the unattended stream is still preserved (Zion Golumbic et al., 2013). One other study demonstrated enhanced cortical entrainment to temporal envelope of speech when it is intelligible (Peelle et al., 2013).

The confluence of the present evidence at hand implies that neural oscillations are a critical mechanism in the decoding and integration of prosodic features that occur in the time range of ~250 ms. Further, it suggests that at an early stage of speech processing, prosodic information is taken up by neural oscillations irrespective of its linguistic marking or emotional tune (e.g. linguistic vs. emotional prosody).

After the initial (spectrotemporal) analysis of inflowing speech, the preprocessed signal is transferred to processing streams along both right and left dorsal and ventral portions of the perisylvian region executing different language-related computations (Bornkessel-Schlesewsky & Schlesewsky, 2013; Bornkessel-Schlesewsky et al., 2015; Hickok & Poeppel, 2007; Saur et al., 2008).

In a recent study, evidence was found that higher linguistic levels may also be represented by a temporally oscillating code that seems to be driven by linguistic information, namely syllable rate and phrasal peaks, but not acoustic information per se (Ding et al., 2016). Partaking individuals were presented with spoken languages that they were familiar or unfamiliar with. Entrainment to paralinguistic levels occurred only when recipients heard a known language. Thus it seems likely that the neural representation of temporal patterns (either acoustic or linguistic) is essential for language comprehension. This reasoning suggests that in order to understand how prosodic information interacts with the neuronal processing of speech, one has to investigate on which of the various linguistic levels entrainment occurs, how this mapping is temporally encoded, and what linguistic or paralinguistic purpose it subserves. Given the present knowledge, there is consensus that prosodic information supports the prelexical, lexical, syntactic, and discourse structure analysis of speech (Cutler et al., 1997; Frazier et al., 2006).

7.3.2 Prosody as a Structural Device

During prelexical speech perception, concatenated syllables and phrases available in the speech stream, are chunked into segments. Due to this reasoning, low-frequency oscillations entrain to the onset of syllables, which enables the decomposition of the speech stream into syllabic units (Ghitza, 2011). Indeed, it seems like entrainment to the speech envelope is enhanced when rapid changes in the temporal envelope are detectable. A correlation between the sharpness[3] of the envelope with envelope tracking and intelligibility of the stimulus has been observed (Doelling et al., 2014). According to this study, sharper, better-defined fluctuations in the speech signal facilitate tracking and parsing speech input. These sharp temporal fluctuations in the speech envelope can be produced by prosodic manipulations such as syllable stress during production of spoken language (Cutler et al., 1997).

Prosodic cues can also disambiguate information about the syntactic structure of a sentence. Prosodic marking, for instance, can give listeners information about whether a word is a subject or an object. Consider the beginning of a sentence, as follows: 'The mother watched the boy and the girl ...'. Depending on how the sentence continues, *the girl* can be an object ('... eating ice cream') or the subject of a new sentence ('... was eating ice cream'). In this case, the presence or absence of prosodic boundaries help disambiguate the syntactic role of the noun *girl*. Prosodic cues are also involved in the production of discourse structure (i.e. information about the type of sentence, such as a question vs. a declarative sentence) or about stress on specific constituents. The sentence 'Tom writes a letter to Jane' can answer

---

[3] Envelope sharpness is a measure of temporal fluctuations in the speech signal and defined as the mean positive first derivate values of the summed envelope.

questions about *who writes* the letter, about *who receives* the letter, or about *what* is received/ written, depending on after which word the sentence accent is placed.

Even though suprasegmental modulations typically mediate prosodic functions, there are instances where prosodic information unfolds within the scope of a single segment. Prosodic cues that do not span over several segments can be found in the lexical analysis of speech in tonal languages, like Mandarin or Thai. In these languages, syllables have different tone contours and, depending on the contour, the meaning of the word is different. Thus, the distinction between words with different meanings is signalled solely by a different tonal or pitch pattern on the syllable level, and hence are classified as subsegmental. Accordingly, the neural circuits that support lexical, subsegmental prosody in native speakers of tonal languages are preponderantly left lateralized (Gandour et al., 2002a,b, 2003, 2004).

7.4 LANGUAGE EXPERIENCE AND PROSODY

7.4.1 Prosody and the Diversity of Languages

When reasoning about the prosody–brain relationship, one should take into account that languages differ with respect to which role prosody plays for comprehension and production. Furthermore, within languages, prosodic marking may vary between local and regional dialects. Additionally, the meaning of prosody as an important structural device may change across the lifespan, with a particular focus during prelexical infancy and old age.

Internally, humans typically segment speech into smaller units to facilitate processing of complex phrases. Prosody is one acoustic cue that marks linguistic boundaries and therefore segments a speech signal. However, it has also been shown that we internally mark monotonous speech sounds and construct linguistic structures that do not have clear acoustic boundaries (Ding et al., 2016). One open question is whether such implicit prosodic segmentation depends on previous language experience. In other words, do we automatically segment foreign speech based on the experience with our first language (L1) or do we use acoustic cues available in foreign speech? It is well known that languages differ in prosodic information such as speech rhythms and intonation. Does the infant brain use prosodic structures of its L1 and apply these cues to a foreign speech as well?

Hohle et al. (2009) succeeded in demonstrating, with the head-turn preference procedure, that German babies have a preference for stimuli with an accent on the first syllable in a word. Those babies preferred the trochee, which is predominant in German, over the iamb. In an EEG study, Friederici et al. (2007) provided supporting evidence showing that 4-month-old German children only elicited a mismatch negativity response while hearing an unpreferred accent on the second syllable, because in German the initial syllable is usually accented. These results were interpreted by the authors as reflecting a higher perceptual cost for the babies. The studies indicate that humans are biased towards the speech rhythm of L1, while they fail, when transferring this knowledge to unknown languages.

Moreover, it has also been shown that adults too, are sensitive to the rhythmic patterns of an L1. In their event-related potential study, Schmidt-Kassow and Kotz (2009b) demonstrated that German-speaking participants registered subtle deviations in the trochaic speech structure in German sentences, which elicited a P600 response in the neural signal. In another study, the same research team backed up these results by means of event-related potential evidence showing that the rhythmic pattern violations are processed in two succeeding steps— an early left frontal negativity and a late posterior positivity (Schmidt-Kassow & Kotz, 2009a). Comparable results were presented by Magne et al. (2007), where participants also produced an early negativity and a late positivity during the detection of incongruous metrical structures in L1, namely syllable lengthening.

Additionally, some studies have demonstrated, by means of behavioural and neurophysiological data, that violations of words' metric structures hinder lexical access and therefore word comprehension (Magne et al., 2007), and also obscure syntactic processes (Schmidt-Kassow & Kotz, 2009a). In other words, there is evidence that adult listeners use prosodic acoustic features such as stress patterns in their L1 for 'computing the phonetic code that accesses stored lexical entries' (Soto-Faraco et al., 2001, p. 424), which results in facilitated lexical decision responses. So far, it should have become clear that adults and children are sensitive to metric structures in their L1 and that these structures are closely related to semantic and syntactic processes. However, one may wonder to what extent do these patterns in L1 affect speech rhythm decoding in other languages?

The study of Cumming (2011) shows clearly that native speakers of different languages perceive rhythmical patterns in different ways, depending on the features available in the signals of their L1 prosody. Evidently, L1 experience influences the perception of pitch in a way that it enhances the accuracy of pitch representations (Giuliano et al., 2011). There is more conclusive evidence from studies that presented sentences in a foreign language (Colombo et al., 2011; Deguchi et al., 2012; Magne et al., 2007). All three studies used pitch height modifications at the sentence final position. Pitch is closely related to rhythm, having been demonstrated to be a good correlate of lexical stress in different languages (Spitzer et al., 2007). The final word of an utterance had congruous, weakly incongruous, or strongly incongruous pitch patterns. Marques et al. (2007) presented their participants with accordingly modified sentences in the native (French) and in a foreign (Portuguese) language. Processing of weakly and strongly incongruous sentences caused an early negativity and a late positivity in musicians, with both components being more strongly marked in the native language. Other scholars presented similar sentences to native Italian speakers and also constructed French sentences and jabberwocky sentences[4] with legal Italian prosody (Colombo et al., 2011; Deguchi et al., 2012). The congruent conditions revealed an early negativity over temporal sites and a late positivity over parietal sites. The two event-related components occurred earlier and were stronger for the native Italian and jabberwocky sentences compared to the French sentences. From the similar neural responses during listening to the Italian utterances and the jabberwocky utterances, relative to the French sentences, it can be concluded that experience with L1 prototypical pitch patterns facilitates its detection in the L1 but also, to a lesser extent, in foreign languages.

Since those three studies only reported research on pitch deviations at the sentence final position, it would be interesting to study rhythm on a suprasegmental sentence level. Notably, we still do not know much about the learning process during second language

---

[4] Jabberwocky sentences are syntactically correct utterances in which content words are replaced by phonologically legal pseudowords.

acquisition. One study of Schmidt-Kassow et al. (2011) investigated irregular speech rhythm detection at the sentence level of a second language in early second language learners. The participants listened to sentences, which were either correctly accentuated or which had a rhythmic violation (i.e. one word in the sentence had an iambic accent and not the common German trochee). This violation resulted in a P600 component in German native speakers. The same sentences were also presented to French native speakers with a high proficiency level in German. Of note, French natives demonstrate so-called 'stress deafness' because the French speech rhythm is not based on lexical stress (Toro et al., 2009). Accordingly, French participants did not show a P600 component. In a later study, the authors presented the same sentences to Spanish students who were highly proficient in German. The participants also demonstrated an enhanced P600 to metric violations (Schmidt-Kassow et al., 2011), which shows that a rhythm-class problem cannot account for the finding. Both French and Spanish belong to the syllable-timed rhythm class. Hence the result can be explained by the pitch cue insensitivity in the French language. Moreover, further previous research showed that Turkish early L2 learners of German and monolingual German speakers are sensitive to rhythmically irregular German contexts, while late learners of German are not. This suggests that the acquisition of rhythm may be facilitated in younger learners (Roncaglia-Denissen et al., 2015).

In a previous study by our group, we elucidated this issue further. We investigated the processing of rhythmic patterns at the sentence level in an L1-German group, and in an L1-French group and an L1-Italian group of late and low proficiency learners of the German language. We presented jabberwocky sentences with typical German rhythms (trochee) and, for the first time also, rhythms that are unpreferred in the German language (e.g. iamb), to all three groups. French and Italian are languages belonging to the syllable-timed rhythm class and therefore to a different rhythmic category than the German language, which is a stress-timed language. Notably, Italian has similar accent patterns in disyllabic words as German. The two languages differ from French with respect to this feature, because French has a tendency to only accentuate the last syllable in a sentence, which possibly leads to a potential linguistic stress deafness in French individuals. We recorded surface electrical brain activity during auditory sentence processing with and without violations of rhythmic patterns. We calculated P600 effects and predicted its occurrence whenever participants noticed a rhythmical violation due to their L1 rhythmical priming and preference. The words of the jabberwocky sentences were phonotactically legal in German, and the grammatical structure of the sentences was always the same (subject–verb–adjective–object) and was labelled by using real German articles, namely 'der', 'die', and 'das' for the subject and object in the sentences. In relation to the rhythm of the sentences, we created four different conditions: 50% of the sentences were spoken in a trochee style and 50% in an iambic style. The trochee, which is predominant in German, is defined by an accent on the first syllable in a word. The first condition (25% of all sentences) contained, therefore, correctly trochee-stressed sentences (see Figure 7.2 for examples). The second condition (25% of all sentences) had the same structure as the first, but the sentences included a violation of the ongoing trochee stress pattern on the adjective: the accent was reversed, so that the word had an accent on the second syllable and therefore an iambic accent. The third and fourth conditions were both accentuated in an iambic pattern: the sentences of the third condition (25% of all sentences) contained accents on the second or last syllable of the words, without a violation. The fourth condition (25% of all sentences) was constructed with the same pattern as the third, but with a violation of the

Accents	Violation	
	No	Yes
Trochee	Die **Nima bamt** das *weinde* **Koler** 	Der **Schesi friest** das *foste* **Pasteri**
Iamb	Der **Jalulu** razzt **das** *friste* Romi 	Die **Hustel** zippt **die** *lappte* Jafal

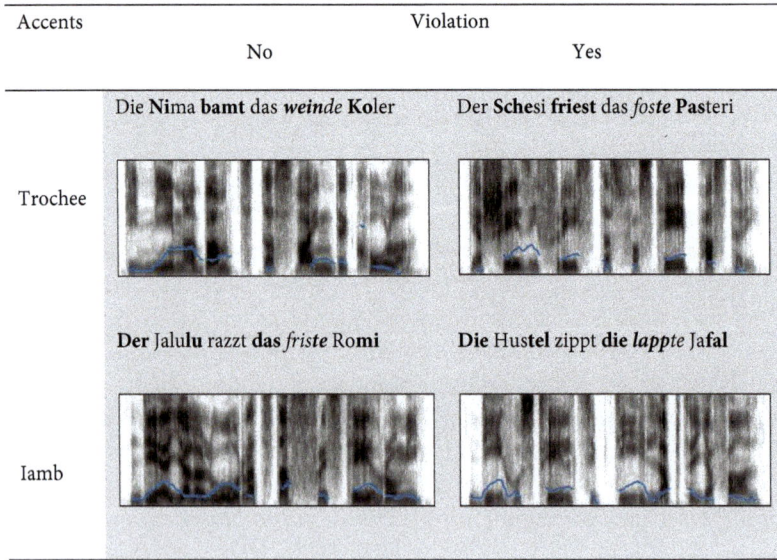

FIGURE 7.2 2×2 design of the study, presenting one example of a sentence for each of the four conditions. The accents are marked with bold letters and the manipulated word is written in italics. The spectrogram and the pitch (in blue), in a range from 75–500 Hz, is also shown for each of the sentences.

rhythmic stress pattern on the adjective: here again the accent was reversed and therefore the first syllable was accentuated, which is conforming to a trochee pattern (see Figure 7.2).

To elucidate the group differences, we compared the mean voltage amplitudes of the P600 between the three experimental groups, as shown in Figure 7.3. In the trochee condition, we demonstrated a significant difference between the L1-French group and the L1-German group: the L1-French participants did not show a significant P600 effect, while the German group showed a late positivity indicating a reanalysis process. The Italian group differed neither from the German group nor from the L1-French sample. Although the event-related potential (ERP) pattern moderately differed in strength from German individuals, the Italian late learners with a low proficiency level processed the same metric mismatches as the German subjects. On the other hand, the L1-French subjects showed a totally different pattern, indicating no processing of rhythmic mismatches in trochaic sentences. As was already shown by Schmidt-Kassow et al. (2011) for Spanish L2 learners of German, the L1-Italian group was sensitive to L2 rhythmic violations in trochee sentences, while L1-French participants were not. This led some researchers to the conclusion that L1-French participants show stress deafness while listening to linguistic rhythmic sentences (Schmidt-Kassow et al., 2011). Apart from that, if we look at the results of the iambic condition, we are the first to demonstrate L1-French learners of the German language to be able to process mismatched rhythmic accents in a foreign language, here in German jabberwocky sentences, depending on their experience with the rhythm.

To conclude, the perceptual processing of pitch incongruity in sentence rhythms seems to be influenced by the familiarity with the rhythmic pattern of a language (Colombo et al., 2011). Our study provides evidence for the hypothesis that L1 experience with a rhythmic

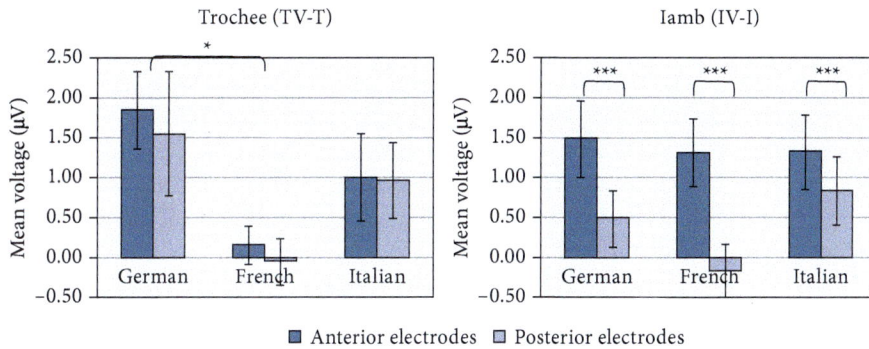

FIGURE 7.3 The mean voltage amplitudes of the neurophysiological P600 responses collected from a pool of anterior and posterior surface electrodes, shown separately for each condition (trochee, iamb) and language (German, French, Italian).

pattern supports the processing of rhythmic information while listening to a foreign language on a qualitatively similar level to native speakers. Neurophysiological evidence implies that processing happens with less intensity, which is reflected by smaller ERP amplitudes. Furthermore, our study supports the assumption that learning the prosody of a foreign language as an adult is characterized and influenced by the rhythmic experiences of the L1 (Roncaglia-Denissen et al., 2015). Overall, the entirety of the above mentioned studies suggest that more focus should be laid on prosody during foreign-language learning (Nickels & Steinhauer, 2016; Nickels et al., 2013), especially when the rhythmic structure of the L1 is different from the foreign language to be learned.

7.4.2 Prosody and Its Role in Natural Language Acquisition

Infants rapidly learn the acoustic and prosodic features of their native language during the very first months of their life. Before infants begin to produce their first speech sounds they have to tune into their first language(s) (Leroy et al., 2011). Apparently, newborn children imitate the stress pattern of their L1 while crying (Mampe et al., 2009). Already at birth, auditory feature analysis is highly developed, but is modified within the first months of life by specific language exposure. Thus, humans have the neurobiological ability to process complex auditory stimuli with high precision, while the specific language acquired is shaped by their environment (Obrig et al., 2010).

During the first year of their life, infants learn a considerable amount of phonology and prosody which are the foundations for linguistic mechanisms including, amongst others, the marking of sentence accents (Friederici, 2005), the categorization of phonemes, and the discrimination of different languages (Dehaene-Lambertz et al., 2008). The structural organization underlying these language-acquiring processes seems to be comparable to adults, although the observed leftwarded lateralization of language-related areas is not yet as strong in infants as it is in adults with more sophisticated language skills.

During the third trimester of gestation and, therefore, at a very early maturation stage, structural brain asymmetries have even been observed to favour the right side in the superior frontal gyrus, the superior temporal gyrus, and Heschl's gyrus (HG) (Dehaene-Lambertz et al., 2008). During further prenatal maturation, the size of the left planum temporale (PT) and the HG is therefore increasing (Kasprian et al., 2011; Steinmetz, 1996). This process has been related to improved computations of fast temporal transitions in regions of the left PARC (Obrig et al., 2010). This view is in line with data, which provides evidence that not only adults, but also newborns and infants, show a functional inter-hemispheric specialization, with a left hemispheric dominance for the processing of segmental information and a right hemispheric dominance for processing of suprasegmental information (Homae et al., 2006; Telkemeyer et al., 2009, 2011; Wartenburger et al., 2007). Additionally, 3-month-old infants recruit areas beyond the temporal lobes, namely the inferior and dorsolateral frontal regions, when engaged in a speech task. The language networks in infants are therefore similar to those in adults (Dehaene-Lambertz et al., 2008).

When infants listen to speech, they are first of all confronted with a continuous auditory stream. However, for the decoding of the meaning of speech, it is indispensable to identify single syllables, words, phrases, or sentences. Since babies have not yet developed lexical representations and acquired the syntactic rules, they have to rely on the acoustic structure of the signal (Obrig et al., 2010). The mechanisms behind this process are generally described as being based on a statistical analysis of the speech input (Leroy et al., 2011). Irrespective of which L1 they are exposed to, infants use auditory regularities in speech, such as repetitive and frequent characteristics, to acquire their native language. Thus, the language acquisition process is bidirectional, because language competence shapes the interpretation of auditory signals. Children recognize regularities in phonological and prosodic features, successively build up a representation of these patterns, and use them as auditory markers to segment the input (Obrig et al., 2010). Evidently, it has been shown that infants are bound to build up such sound representations of their L1 (Friederici, 2005, 2006; Kuhl, 2004, 2010; Kuhl & Rivera-Gaxiola, 2008).

During foreign-language learning in adulthood, we are also initially faced with a continuous auditory stream of foreign language. To decode language and, for example, to attribute meaning to single words, we have to segment this stream into its basic units. Since we have already built up sound representations of our L1, which we have been highly exposed to and are therefore very familiar with, the idea that we probably rely on these familiar patterns during second-language learning has been proposed (Schmidt-Kassow et al., 2011) and shall be further investigated. Since language comprises of segmental but also suprasegmental aspects, it is crucial to investigate language on the sentential level to gain a comprehensive view. Speech rhythm as a prosodic cue that unfolds on a suprasegmental level has been additionally shown to be crucial for the segmentation of an auditory stream (Lee & McAngus Todd, 2004). Interestingly, recent evidence points to a preponderant role of prosodic information not only for infants but also for older adults who partly suffer from age-related brain atrophy and central hearing loss.

7.4.3 The Role of Prosody During Speech Processing in the Elderly

Given the steadily growing proportion of elderly individuals amongst the population, it is of utmost importance to learn more about the specific relationship between brain function and speech processing or hearing in older age. For a long time, a decline of the ability to comprehend spoken language has been conceived as the sole problem of cochlear dysfunction in the inner ear. This age-related impairment has been dubbed *presbycusis* or peripheral hearing loss. In line with this view, the acoustic speech signal that encounters the inner ear is not sufficiently amplified, so that only a fraction of the speech signal reaches the auditory fields in the brain. Thus, this partial interruption of signal transfer leads to a reduction of temporal and spectral cues, typically lacking high-frequency information (> 6 KHz), usually resulting in deficient phonetic perception. Hearing aids that simply amplify the intensity of speech sounds are considered as an optimal intervention tool to treat the problem (Giroud et al., 2017).

However, we know that this reasoning ignores an important part of the problem. Elderly individuals who have been provided with hearing aids often complain that they now hear inflowing sounds louder but still do not understand spoken language properly. Meanwhile, it is assumed that one main reason accounts for this dilemma—namely, a decrease of grey matter in the PARC. Cortical atrophy in auditory fields occurs, in part presumably as a function of peripheral hearing loss due to a significant reduction of auditory information. Lin et al. (2014) investigated this effect in a longitudinal study and demonstrated that peripheral hearing impairment results, sooner or later, in accelerated grey matter atrophy of the PARC. In a seminal position paper, Humes et al. (2012) also emphasized the role of central hearing loss. Its major symptom is the inability to comprehend spoken language properly when it is embedded in acoustic noise or presented in competition to other spoken utterances simultaneously. Surprisingly, older individuals often do not show severe indications of peripheral hearing loss in a pure tone audiogram that measures audibility of sounds. Inevitably, they are hence considered as having 'normal' hearing even though they fail to process spoken sentences under aversive listening conditions (Giroud et al., 2018).

Notably, recent studies have observed stronger rightward brain responses in auditory-related fields even in older adults who were classified as 'normal hearing' (Profant et al., 2015). Complementarily, Giroud and colleagues (2018) noticed that older adults who were classified as 'normal hearing' according to the standards of the World Health Organization, performed significantly worse than normal-hearing young individuals in a speech-in-noise task. Furthermore, this study excavated a relationship between cortical thickness of the right superior temporal sulcus and endogenous θ oscillations, as well as between thickness of other right PARC areas and suprathreshold measurements of hearing.

From these findings it can be concluded that presbycusis can be characterized not only by reduced audibility of inflowing auditory signals but also by deficient processing of temporal sound features and reduced comprehension of spoken language. Despite general age-related cortical atrophy that affects all cortical regions to the same extent, the study by Giroud and colleagues (2018) thus points to a particular role of the right PARC when older individuals are presented with spoken sentences. Evidently, presbycusis has a central component and (at least at the level of the PARC) it should be conceived as a combination of age-related cortical atrophy and altered periphery (Profant et al., 2015).

Eventually, these findings indicate that brain ageing is associated with changes of speech lateralization, in the sense that right auditory-related areas become more dominant in comprehension of spoken language in the older population (Giroud et al., 2018). Based on the reasoning outlined in Section 7.3, right auditory areas preferentially mediate slowly changing acoustic cues. Thus, it comes as no surprise that slow acoustic modulations in spoken language are more relevant for older adults' proficiency in speech comprehension (Wingfield et al., 1992). This view has been underlined by numerous behavioural studies that observed stronger deficits in older individuals when rapidly changing cues available in speech have to be processed. According to the framework of Poeppel (2003) and Zatorre and Gandour (2008), these rapidly changing cues are markers of phonetic information, and their integrity is more severely disrupted by peripheral hearing loss than the audibility of slowly changing cues which characterizes prosody and intonation (Gordon-Salant & Fitzgibbons, 1993; Gordon-Salant et al., 2010; Schneider et al., 2010).

Hence, it seems reasonable to conclude that suprasegmental information plays an important role in spoken language comprehension not only in the earliest but also during the later stages of a lifespan. However, it remains to be investigated as to whether differences in γ and θ oscillations observed in older, contrasted with younger, individuals are a consequence or a trigger for deficient speech comprehension. Another issue that has to be addressed in future research is the presumed intertwining between the integrity of cognitive abilities (inhibitory functions, working memory), general age-related atrophy irrespective of peripheral hearing loss, and the preserved comprehension of spoken utterances (Schneider et al., 2010).

7.5 CONCLUSION

Unlike previous research, we conclude, based on present knowledge, that speech prosody cannot be considered a monolithic, paralinguistic domain. The formerly held proposition of a 'linguistic' prosody, that can be conceived as independent from 'emotional' prosody, is obsolete because various acoustic and vocal modulations form the linguistic marking and emotional tune of spoken utterances. It is rather convenient to consider speech prosody as being made up of a continuum of primarily suprasegmental acoustic features that provide important information which are relevant for a proper interpretation of a spoken utterance.

Brain regions that support receptive aspects of speech prosody reside preferentially in auditory-related fields of the right posterior perisylvian cortex. These regions differ from contralateral areas in macro- and cytoarchitectonics, and appear to be specifically built to process suprasegmental acoustic information. However, there is no compelling evidence for a clear lateralization of prosodic functions to the right hemisphere of the brain, as individual language experience, age-related atrophy, and hearing loss or pertinent experimental tasks may influence the division of labour between the two hemispheres.

Furthermore, we collected evidence for the view that speech prosody plays an eminently important role as the structural device that enables first language acquisition and speech maintenance in many different languages, despite its massive syntactic diversity. Hence, we concur with Kreiner and Eviatar's opinion, who propose that 'the acoustic signal, and in particular prosody, should have a more central role in the study of brain mechanisms of language processing' (Kreiner & Eviatar, 2014, p. 100).

Acknowledgements

This research was supported by the 'Fonds zur Foerderung des akademischen Nachwuchses' (FAN) des 'Zuercher Universitaetsvereins' (ZUNIV) and by the Swiss National Science Foundation (Grant no. 105314-152904). We are indebted to Allison Christen for her helpful comments on this manuscript.

References

Ackermann, H., Hage, S. R., & Ziegler, W. (2014). Brain mechanisms of acoustic communication in humans and nonhuman primates: an evolutionary perspective. *Behavioral & Brain Sciences*, 37, 529–546.

Behrens, S. (1989). Characterizing sentence intonation in a right-hemisphere damaged population. *Brain and Language*, 37, 181–200.

Belin, P. & Zatorre, R. J. (2003). Adaptation to speaker's voice in right anterior temporal lobe. *NeuroReport*, 14, 2105–2109.

Belyk, M. & Brown, S. (2014). Perception of affective and linguistic prosody: an ALE meta-analysis of neuroimaging studies. *Social, Cognitive, and Affective Neuroscience*, 9, 1395–1403.

Berckmoes, C. & Vingerhoets, G. (2004). Neural foundations of emotional speech processing. *Current Directions in Psychological Science*, 13, 182–185.

Bornkessel-Schlesewsky, I. & Schlesewsky, M. (2013). Reconciling time, space and function: a new dorsal-ventral stream model of sentence comprehension. *Brain and Language*, 125, 60–76.

Bornkessel-Schlesewsky, I., Schlesewsky, M., Small, S. L., & Rauschecker, J. P. (2015). Neurobiological roots of language in primate audition: common computational properties. *Trends in Cognitive Science*, 19, 142–150.

Buxhoeveden, D. P., Switala, A. E., Litaker, M., Roy, E., & Casanova, M. F. (2001). Lateralization of minicolums in human planum temporale is absent in nonhuman primate cortex. *Brain, Behavior and Evolution*, 57, 349–358.

Colombo, L., Deguchi, C., Boureux, M., Sarlo, M., & Besson, M. (2011). Detection of pitch violations depends upon the familiarity of intonational contour of sentences. *Cortex*, 47, 557–568.

Cruttenden, A. (1997). *Intonation*. Cambridge: Cambridge University Press.

Cumming, R. E. (2011). The language-specific interdependence of tonal and durational cues in perceived rhythmicality. *Phonetica*, 68, 1–25.

Cutler, A., Dahan, D., & van Donselaar, W. (1997). Prosody in the comprehension of spoken language. A literature review. *Language & Speech*, 40, 141–201.

Deguchi, C., Boureux, M., Sarlo, M., Besson, M., Grassi, M., Schon, D., & Colombo, L. (2012). Sentence pitch change detection in the native and unfamiliar language in musicians and non-musicians: behavioral, electrophysiological and psychoacoustic study. *Brain Research*, 1455, 75–89.

Dehaene-Lambertz, G., Hertz-Pannier, L., Dubois, J., & Dehaene, S. (2008). How does early brain organization promote language acquisition in humans? *European Review*, 16, 399.

Dellwo, V., Fourcin, A., & Abberton, E. (2007). *Rhythmical classification based on voice parameters*. Proceedings of International Congress of Phonetic Sciences, 6–10 August 2007, Saarbruecken, Germany, pp. 1129–1132.

Ding, N., Melloni, L., Zhang, H., Tian, X., & Poeppel, D. (2016). Cortical tracking of hierarchical linguistic structures in connected speech. *Nature Neuroscience*, 19, 158–164.

Ding, N. & Simon, J. Z. (2012a). Emergence of neural encoding of auditory objects while listening to competing speakers. *Proceedings of the National Academy of Science of the United States of America*, 109, 11854–11859.

Ding, N. & Simon, J. Z. (2012b). Neural coding of continuous speech in auditory cortex during monaural and dichotic listening. *Journal of Neurophysiology*, 107, 78–89.

Ding, N. & Simon, J. Z. (2014). Cortical entrainment to continuous speech: functional roles and interpretations. *Frontiers in Human Neuroscience*, 8, 311.

Doelling, K. B., Arnal, L. H., Ghitza, O., & Poeppel, D. (2014). Acoustic landmarks drive delta-theta oscillations to enable speech comprehension by facilitating perceptual parsing. *NeuroImage*, 85, 761–768.

Dogil, G., Ackermann, H., Grodd, W., Haider, H., Kamp, H., Mayer, J., Riecker, A., & Wildgruber, D. (2002). The speaking brain: a tutorial introduction to fMRI experiments in the production of speech, prosody, and syntax. *Journal of Neurolinguistics*, 15, 59–90.

Frazier, L., Carlson, K., & Clifton, C. (2006). Prosodic phrasing is central to language comprehension. *Trends in Cognitive Sciences*, 10, 244–249.

Friederici, A. D. (2005). Neurophysiological markers of early language acquisition: from syllables to sentences. *Trends in Cognitive Sciences*, 9, 481–488.

Friederici, A. D. (2006). The neural basis for language development and its impairment. *Neuron*, 103, 941–952.

Friederici, A. D., Friedrich, M., & Christophe, A. (2007). Brain responses in 4-month-old infants are already language specific. *Current Biology*, 17, 1208–1211.

Gandour, J., Dzemidzic, M., Wong, D., Lowe, M., Tong, Y., Hsieh, L., Satthamnuwong, N., & Lurito, J. (2003). Temporal integration of speech prosody is shaped by language experience: an fMRI study. *Brain and Language*, 84, 318–336.

Gandour, J., Tong, Y., Wong, D., Talavage, T., Dzemidzic, M., Xu, Y., Li, X., & Lowe, M. (2004). Hemispheric roles in the perception of speech prosody. *NeuroImage*, 23, 344–357.

Gandour, J., Wong, D., Lowe, M., Dzemidzic, M., Satthamnuwong, N., Tong, Y., & Li, X. (2002a). A cross-linguistic fMRI study of spectral and temporal cues underlying phonological processing. *Journal of Cognitive Neuroscience*, 14, 1076–1087.

Gandour, J., Wong, D., Lowe, M., Dzemidzic, M., Satthamnuwong, N., Tong, Y., & Lurito, J. (2002b). Neural circuitry underlying perception of duration depends on language experience. *Brain and Language*, 83, 268–290.

Geiser, E., Zaehle, T., Jäncke, L., & Meyer, M. (2008). The neural correlate of speech rhythm as evidenced by metrical speech processing: an fMRI study. *Journal of Cognitive Neuroscience*, 20, 541–552.

Ghitza, O. (2011). Linking speech perception and neurophysiology: speech decoding guided by cascaded oscillators locked to the input rhythm. *Frontiers in Psychology*, 2, 130.

Giraud, A. L., Kleinschmidt, A., Poeppel, D., Lund, T. E., Frackowiak, R. S. J., & Laufs, H. (2007). Endogenous cortical rhythms determine cerebral specialization for speech perception and production. *Neuron*, 56, 1127–1134.

Giraud, A. L. & Poeppel, D. (2012). Cortical oscillations and speech processing: emerging computational principles and operations. *Nature Neuroscience*, 15, 511–517.

Giroud, N., Hirsiger, S., Muri, R., Kegel, A., Dillier, N., & Meyer, M. (2018). Neuroanatomical and resting state EEG power correlates of central hearing loss in older adults. *Brain Structure & Function*, 223(1), 145–163.

Giroud, N., Lemke, U., Reich, P., Matthes, K. L., & Meyer, M. (2017). The impact of hearing aids and age-related hearing loss on auditory plasticity across three months—an electrical neuroimaging study. *Hearing Research*, 353, 162–175.

Giuliano, R. J., Pfordresher, P. Q., Stanley, E. M., Narayana, S., & Wicha, N. Y. Y. (2011). Native experience with a tone language enhances pitch discrimination and the timing of neural responses to pitch change. *Frontiers in Psychology*, 2, 1–12.

Gordon-Salant, S. & Fitzgibbons, P. J. (1993). Temporal factors and speech recognition performance in young and elderly listeners. *Journal of Speech and Hearing Research*, 36, 1276–1285.

Gordon-Salant, S., Frisina, R. D., Popper, A. N., & Fay, R. R. (2010). *Springer Handbook of Auditory Research. The Aging Auditory System*. New York: Springer.

Hage, S. R. & Nieder, A. (2016). Dual neural network model for the evolution of speech and language. *Trends in Neuroscience*, 39, 813–829.

Heilman, K. M., Bowers, D., Speedie, L., & Coslett, H. B. (1984). Comprehension of affective and nonaffective prosody. *Neurology*, 84, 917–921.

Hesling, I., Clément, S., Bordessoules, M., & Allard, M. (2005). Cerebral mechanisms of prosodic integration: evidence from connected speech. *NeuroImage*, 24, 937–947.

Hesling, I., Dilharreguy, B., Clément, S., Bordessoules, M., & Allard, M. (2005). Cerebral mechanisms of prosodic sensory integration using low-frequency bands of connected speech. *Human Brain Mapping*, 26, 157–169.

Hickok, G. & Poeppel, D. (2007). The cortical organization of cortical speech processing. *Nature Reviews Neuroscience*, 8, 393–402.

Hohle, B., Bijeljac-Babic, R., Herold, B., Weissenborn, J., & Nazzi, T. (2009). Language specific prosodic preferences during the first half year of life: evidence from German and French infants. *Infant Behavior & Development*, 32, 262–274.

Homae, F., Watanabe, H., Nakano, T., Asakawa, K., & Taga, G. (2006). The right hemisphere of sleeping infants perceives sentential prosody. *Neuroscience Research*, 54, 276–280.

Howard, M. F. & Poeppel, D. (2012). The neuromagnetic response to spoken sentences: comodulation of theta band amplitude and phase. *NeuroImage*, 60, 2118–2127.

Humes, L. E., Dubno, J. R., Gordon-Salant, S., Lister, J. J., Cacace, A. T., Cruickshanks, K. J., … Wingfield, A. (2012). Central presbycusis: a review and evaluation of the evidence. *Journal of the American Academy of Audiology*, 23, 635–666.

Hurschler, M., Liem, F., Jäncke, L., & Meyer, M. (2013). Right and left perisylvian cortex and left inferior frontal cortex mediate sentence-level rhyme detection in spoken language as revealed by sparse fMRI. *Human Brain Mapping*, 34, 3182–3192.

Hurschler, M. A., Liem, F., Oechslin, M., Stampfli, P., & Meyer, M. (2015). fMRI reveals lateralized pattern of brain activity modulated by the metrics of stimuli during auditory rhyme processing. *Brain and Language*, 147, 41–50.

Hutsler, J. & Galuske, R. A. W. (2003). The specialized structure of human language cortex: pyramidal cell size asymmetries within auditory and language-associated regions of the temporal lobes. *Brain and Language*, 86, 226–242.

Kasprian, G., Langs, G., Brugger, P. C., Bittner, M., Weber, M., Arantes, M., & Prayer, D. (2011). The prenatal origin of hemispheric asymmetry: an in utero neuroimaging study. *Cerebral Cortex*, 21, 1076–1083.

Kreiner, H. & Eviatar, Z. (2014). The missing link in the embodiment of syntax: prosody. *Brain and Language*, 137, 91–102.

Kreitewolf, J., Friederici, A. D., & von Kriegstein, K. (2014). Hemispheric lateralization of linguistic prosody recognition in comparison to speech and speaker recognition. *NeuroImage*, 102, 332–344.

Kuhl, P. & Rivera-Gaxiola, M. (2008). Neural substrates of language acquisition. *Annual Review of Neuroscience*, 31, 511–534.

Kuhl, P. K. (2004). Early language acquisition: cracking the speech code. *Nature Reviews Neuroscience*, 5, 831–843.

Kuhl, P. K. (2010). Brain mechanisms in early language acquisition. *Neuron*, 67, 713–727.

Kyong, J. S., Scott, S. K., Rosen, S., Howe, T. B., Agnew, Z. K., & McGettigan, C. (2014). Exploring the roles of spectral detail and intonation contour in speech intelligibility: an FMRI study. *Journal of Cognitive Neuroscience*, 26, 1748–1763.

Ladd, D. R. (2014). *Simultaneous Structure in Phonology*. Oxford: Oxford University Press.

Lattner, S., Meyer, M., & Friederici, A. (2005). Voice perception: sex, pitch, and the right hemisphere. *Human Brain Mapping*, 24, 11–20.

Lee, C. & McAngus Todd, N. (2004). Towards an auditory account of speech rhythm: application of a model of the auditory 'primal sketch' to two multi-language corpora. *Cognition*, 93, 225–254.

Lehiste, I. (1970). *Suprasegmentals*. Cambridge: MIT Press.

Leroy, F., Glasel, H., Dubois, J., Hertz- Pannier, L., Thirion, B., Mangin, J.-F., & Dehaene-Lambertz, G. (2011). Early maturation of the linguistic dorsal pathway in human infants. *Journal of Neuroscience*, 31, 1500–1506.

Liem, F., Hurschler, M., Jäncke, L., & Meyer, M. (2014). On the planum temporale lateralization in suprasegmental speech perception. Evidence from a study investigating behavior, structure, and function. *Human Brain Mapping*, 35, 1779–1789.

Lin, F. R., Ferrucci, L., An, Y., Goh, J. O., Doshi, J., Metter, E. J., … Resnick, S. M. (2014). Association of hearing impairment with brain volume changes in older adults. *NeuroImage*, 90, 84–92.

Magne, C., Astésano, C., Aramaki, M., Ystad, S., Kronland-Martinet, R., & Besson, M. (2007). Influence of syllabic lengthening on semantic processing in spoken French: behavioral and electrophysiological evidence. *Cerebral Cortex*, 17, 2659–2668.

Mampe, B., Friederici, A. D., Christophe, A., & Wermke, K. (2009). Newborns' cry melody is shaped by their native language. *Current Biology*, 19, 1994–1997.

Marques, C., Moreno, S., Castro, S. L., & Besson, M. (2007). Musicians detect pitch violations in a foreign language better than nonmusicians: behavioral and electrophysiological evidence. *Journal of Cognitive Neuroscience*, 19, 1453–1463.

McGettigan, C. & Scott, S. K. (2012). Cortical asymmetries in speech perception: what's wrong, what's right and what's left? *Trends in Cognitive Sciences*, 16, 269–276.

Meyer, M. (2008). Functions of the left and right posterior temporal lobes during segmental and suprasegmental speech perception. *Zeitschrift für Neuropsychologie*, 19, 93–102.

Meyer, M., Alter, K., Friederici, A. D., Lohmann, G., & von Cramon, D. Y. (2002). Functional MRI reveals brain regions mediating slow prosodic modulations in spoken sentences. *Human Brain Mapping*, 17, 73–88.

Meyer, M., Steinhauer, K., Alter, K., Friederici, A. D., & von Cramon, D. Y. (2004). Brain activity varies with modulation of dynamic pitch variance in sentence melody. *Brain and Language*, 89, 277–289.

Morillon, B., Lehongre, K., Frackowiak, R. J. S., Ducorps, A., Kleinschmidt, A., Poeppel, D., & Giraud, A.-L. (2010). Neurophysiological origin of human brain asymmetry for speech and language. *Proceedings of the National Academy of Sciences of the United States of America*, 107, 18688–18693.

Nickels, S., Opitz, B., & Steinhauer, K. (2013). ERPs show that classroom-instructed late second language learners rely on the same prosodic cues in syntactic parsing as native speakers. *Neuroscience Letters*, 557, 107–111.

Nickels, S. & Steinhauer, K. (2016). Prosody-syntax integration in a second language: contrasting event-related potentials from German and Chinese learners of English using linear mixed effect models. *Second Language Research*, 34(1), 9–37.

Obrig, H., Rossi, S., Telkemeyer, S., & Wartenburger, I. (2010). From acoustic segmentation to language processing: evidence from optical imaging. *Frontiers in Neuroenergetics*, 23(2), pii:13.

Peelle, J. E. & Davis, M. H. (2012). Neural oscillations carry speech rhythm through to comprehension. *Frontiers in Psychology*, 3, 320.

Peelle, J. E., Gross, J., & Davis, M. H. (2013). Phase-locked responses to speech in human auditory cortex are enhanced during comprehension. *Cerebral Cortex*, 23, 1378–1387.

Pell, M. D. & Baum, S. R. (1997). The ability to perceive and comprehend intonation in linguistic and affective contexts by brain-damaged adults. *Brain and Language*, 57, 80–99.

Phillips, D. P. & Farmer, M. E. (1990). Acquired word deafness, and the temporal grain of sound representation in the primary auditory cortex. *Behavioral & Brain Research*, 40, 85–94.

Poeppel, D. (2003). The analysis of speech in different temporal integration windows: cerebral lateralization as 'asymmetric sampling in time'. *Speech Communication*, 41, 245–255.

Poeppel, D. (2012). The maps problem and the mapping problem: two challenges for a cognitive neuroscience of speech and language. *Cognitive Neuropsychology*, 29, 34–55.

Poeppel, D. & Embick, D. (2005). Defining the relation between linguistics and neuroscience. In: A. Cutler (ed.) *Twenty-first Century Psycholinguistics. Four Cornerstones* (pp. 103–118). Mahwah, NJ: Lawrence Erlbaum Associates.

Price, C. J. (2012). A review and synthesis of the first 20 years of PET and fMRI studies of heard speech, spoken language and reading. *NeuroImage*, 62, 816–847.

Profant, O., Tintěra, J., Balogova, Z., Ibrahim, I., Jilek, M., & Syka, J. (2015). Functional changes in the human auditory cortex in ageing. *PloS One*, 10, e0116692.

Roncaglia-Denissen, M. P., Schmidt-Kassow, M., Heine, A., & Kotz, S. (2015). On the impact of L2 speech rhythm on syntactic ambiguity resolution. *Second Language Research*, 31, 157–178.

Rosen, B. R. (1992). Temporal information in speech: acoustic, auditory and linguistic aspects. *Philosophical Transactions of the Royal Society of London B: Biological Sciences*, 33, 367–373.

Ross, E. D. (1981). The aprosodias: functional-anatomic organization of the affective components of language in the right hemisphere. *Archives of Neurology*, 38, 561–569.

Ross, E. D. & Monnot, M. (2008). Neurology of affective prosody and its functional-anatomic organization in right hemisphere. *Brain and Language*, 10, 51–74.

Ross, E. D., Shayya, L., & Rousseau, J. F. (2013). Prosodic stress: acoustic, aphasic and neuroanatomic interactions. *Journal of Neurolinguistics*, 26, 526–551.

Ross, E. D., Thompson, R. D., & Yenkosky, J. (1997). Lateralization of affective prosody in brain and the callosal integration of hemispheric language functions. *Brain and Language*, 56, 27–54.

Rufener, K. S., Oechslin, M. S., Wostmann, M., Dellwo, V., & Meyer, M. (2016). Age-related neural oscillation patterns during the processing of temporally manipulated speech. *Brain Topography*, 29, 440–458.

Saberi, K. & Perrott, D. R. (1999). Cognitive restoration of reversed speech. *Nature*, 398, 760.

Saur, D., Kreher, B. W., Schnell, S., Kümmerer, D., Kellmeyer, P., Vry, M.-S., … Weiller, C. (2008). Ventral and dorsal pathways for language. *Proceedings of the National Academy of Sciences of the United States of America*, 105, 18035–18040.

Schmidt-Kassow, M. & Kotz, S. A. (2009a). Attention and perceptual regularity in speech. *NeuroReport*, 20, 1643–1647.

Schmidt-Kassow, M. & Kotz, S. A. (2009b). Event-related brain potentials suggest a late interaction of meter and syntax in the P600. *Journal of Cognitive Neuroscience*, 21, 1693–1708.

Schmidt-Kassow, M., Roncaglia-Denissen, M. P., & Kotz, S. A. (2011). Why pitch sensitivity matters: event-related potential evidence of metric and syntactic violation detection among Spanish late learners of German. *Frontiers in Psychology*, 2, 131.

Schneider, B. A., Pichora-Fuller, K., & Daneman, M. (2010). Effects of senescent changes in audition and cognition on spoken language comprehension. In: S. Gordon-Salant, R. D. Frisina, A. N. Popper, & R. R. Fay (eds) *The Springer Handbook of Auditory Research. The Aging Auditory System* (pp. 167–210). New York: Springer.

Schroeder, C. E., Lakatos, P., Kajikawa, Y., Partan, S., & Puce, A. (2008). Neuronal oscillations and visual amplification of speech. *Trends in Cognitive Sciences*, 12, 106–113.

Shalom, D. B. & Poeppel, D. (2008). Functional anatomic models of language: assembling the pieces. *Neuroscientist*, 14, 119–127.

Shattuck-Hufnagel, S. & Turk, A. E. (1996). A prosody tutorial for investigators of auditory sentence processing. *Journal of Psycholinguistic Research*, 25, 193–247.

Soto-Faraco, S., Sebastian-Galles, N., & Cutler, A. (2001). Segmental and suprasegmental mismatch in lexical access. *Journal of Memory and Language*, 45, 412–432.

Spitzer, S., Liss, J., & Mattys, S. L. (2007). Acoustic cues to lexical segmentation: a study of resynthesized speech. *Journal of the Acoustical Society of America*, 122, 3678–3687.

Steinmetz, H. (1996). Structure, function and cerebral asymmetry: in vivo-morphometry of the planum temporale. *Neuroscience & Biobehavioral Reviews*, 20, 587–591.

Telkemeyer, S., Rossi, S., Koch, S. P., Nierhaus, T., Steinbrink, J., Poeppel, D., Obrig, H., & Wartenburger, I. (2009). Sensitivity of newborn auditory cortex to the temporal structure of sounds. *Journal of Neuroscience*, 29, 14726–14733.

Telkemeyer, S., Rossi, S., Nierhaus, T., Steinbrink, J., Obrig, H., & Wartenburger, I. (2011). Acoustic processing of temporally modulated sounds in infants: evidence from a combined near-infrared spectroscopy and EEG study. *Frontiers in Psychology*, 1, 62.

Toro, J. M., Sebastian-Galles, N., & Mattys, S. L. (2009). The role of perceptual salience during the segmentation of connected speech. *European Journal of Cognitive Psychology*, 21, 786–800.

Van Lancker, D. (1980). Cerebral lateralization of pitch cues in the linguistic signal. *Papers in Linguistics*, 13, 201–277.

Van Lancker, D. & Sidtis, J. J. (1992). The identification of affective-prosodic stimuli by left- and right-hemisphere-damaged subjects: all errors are not created equal. *Journal of Speech and Hearing Research*, 35, 963–970.

Vigneau, M., Beaucousin, V., Hervé, P. Y., Jobard, G., Petit, L., Crivello, F., … Tzourio-Mazoyer, N. (2011). What is right-hemisphere contribution to phonological, lexico-semantic, and sentence processing? Insights from meta-analysis. *NeuroImage*, 54, 577–593.

Warren, J. D., Jennings, A. R., & Griffiths, T. D. (2005). Analysis of the spectral envelope of sounds by the human brain. *NeuroImage*, 24, 1052–1057.

Wartenburger, I., Steinbrink, J., Telkemeyer, S., Friedrich, M., Friederici, A. D., & Obrig, H. (2007). The processing of prosody: evidence of interhemispheric specialization at the age of four. *NeuroImage*, 34, 416–425.

Weintraub, S. & Mesulam, M.-M. (1981). Disturbances of prosody. A right-hemisphere contribution to language. *Archives of Neurology*, 38, 742–744.

Wiethoff, S., Wildgruber, D., Kreifelts, B., Becker, H., Herbert, C., Grodd, W., & Ethofer, T. (2008). Cerebral processing of emotional prosody–influence of acoustic parameters and arousal. *NeuroImage*, 39, 885–893.

Wingfield, A., Wayland, S. C., & Stine, E. A. (1992). Adult age differences in the use of prosody for syntactic parsing and recall of spoken sentences. *Journal of Gerontology*, 47, 350–356.

Witteman, J., van Ijzendoorn, M. H., van de Velde, D., van Heuven, V. J., & Schiller, N. O. (2011). The nature of hemispheric specialization for linguistic and emotional prosodic perception: a meta-analysis of the lesion literature. *Neuropsychologia*, 49, 3722–3738.

Zatorre, R. J. & Belin, P. (2001). Spectral and temporal processing in human auditory cortex. *Cerebral Cortex*, 11, 946–953.

Zatorre, R. J. & Gandour, J. T. (2008). Neural specializations for speech and pitch: moving beyond the dichotomy. *Proceedings of the Royal Society B: Biological Sciences*, 363, 1087–1104.

Zhang, L., Shu, H., Zhou, F., Wang, X., & Li, P. (2010). Common and distinct neural substrates for the perception of speech rhythm and intonation. *Human Brain Mapping*, 31, 1106–1116.

Zion Golumbic, E. M., Ding, N., Bickel, S., Lakatos, P., Schevon, C. A., McKhann, G. M., ... Schroeder, C. E. (2013). Mechanisms underlying selective neuronal tracking of attended speech at a 'cocktail party'. *Neuron*, 77, 980–991.

CHAPTER 8

RECONSIDERING THE NATURE OF VOICE

JODY KREIMAN AND BRUCE R. GERRATT

8.1 INTRODUCTION

VOICES are everywhere in human experience, to the extent that they inspire hyperbole:

> We constantly inhabit the universe of voices, we are continuously bombarded by voices, we have to make our daily way through a jungle of voices, and we have to use all kinds of machetes and compasses so as not to get lost. There are the voices of other people, the voices of music, the voices of media, our own voice intermingled with the lot. All those voices are shouting, whispering, crying, caressing, threatening, imploring, seducing, commanding, pleading, praying, hypnotizing, confessing, terrorizing, declaring … (Dolar, 2006, p. 13)

These ubiquitous voices carry information about virtually every aspect of existence: the spoken message, of course, but also cues to the speaker's identity, age, gender, physical size, health status, and reproductive fitness (his/her physical self); cues to the speaker's social self, including his/her role in the conversation or social group, attitudes towards other conversational participants or towards the message (attentiveness, truthfulness, superiority, sincerity, curiosity, sarcasm), social status, and dominance; and hints about the speaker's inner self, including clues to personality and emotional state. In some cases, voices actually *are* the information in a message. Consider, for example, the quotes in Box 8.1 from the writing of Raymond Chandler. These quotes reflect the nuanced information about attitudes and emotional states available from voice, as well as the relationships between the speaker and hearer, independent of the lexical meaning of the words uttered.

The many functions subsumed by voice and the many meanings it carries in ordinary, everyday interactions make it notoriously difficult to define or delimit for study. Indeed, Johan Sundberg famously wrote (1987) that everyone knows what voice is until they try to pin it down. Varying research traditions, in disciplines ranging from classics to surgery, have resulted in a wide range of terminological and measurement practices, leading in turn to longstanding and prevalent confusion over how voice should best be characterized, what aspects should be measured, and how this should be accomplished. In this chapter, we will

> **Box 8.1 When the medium is the message: Raymond Chandler on voice quality**
>
> He sounded like a man who had slept well and didn't owe too much money. (*The Big Sleep*, 1939, p. 619)
>
> 'Please don't get up,' she said in a voice like the stuff they use to line summer clouds with. (*The Long Goodbye*, 1953, p. 496)
>
> She slid away from him along the seat but her voice slid away a lot farther than that. (*The Long Goodbye*, 1953, p. 420)
>
> The voice got as cool as a cafeteria dinner. (*Farewell My Lovely*, 1940, p. 843)
>
> Her voice was as dead as the summer before last. (*Nevada Gas*, 1935, p. 166)
>
> And when she spoke her voice had the lucid emptiness of that mechanical voice on the telephone that tells you the time and if you keep on listening, which people don't because they have no reason to, it will keep on telling you the passing seconds forever, without the slightest change of inflection. (*The Long Goodbye*, 1953, pp. 671–672)
>
> All page numbers refer to the 1995 Library of America editions

argue that existing measurement systems for voice are based on an impoverished view of what voice is, and are thus doomed to failure. We will then propose and motivate an alternative view of the nature of voice, and describe a measurement approach that avoids the pitfalls posed by previous protocols.

8.2 CURRENT APPROACHES TO VOICE AND ITS MEASUREMENT

Traditional approaches generally characterize voice as the carrier by which a spoken message is passed from speaker to listener along the 'speech chain' (Denes & Pinson, 1993). Much debate has taken place concerning the precise relationship between language and voice, which appears to be neither part of the message nor wholly separable from it (Butler, 2015). Older traditions insist that voice is not part of language, either in theory or in practice (Butler, in press; Sapir, 1927), while newer approaches focus more on the role of voice in such ostensibly linguistic functions as spoken word recognition (Maibauer et al., 2014; Mullennix et al., 1989), prosodic meanings (for review, see Kreiman & Sidtis, 2011), and so on (for a review of these issues, see Cavarero, 2005).

Regardless of the current state of this debate, the empirical study of voice per se has remained consistently tied to the speech chain model, so that voice production, acoustics, and perception are treated as separate stages that are virtually always studied independently of one another. We begin by reviewing how voice is measured in each of these domains.

8.2.1 Perceptual Evaluation Systems

The term 'quality' is usually defined as a listener's perceptual response to a physical stimulus (ANSI, 1960, p. 45; cf. Helmholtz, 1885), and thus by its nature requires the involvement of someone who hears the signal. The most common approach to the problem of measuring voice quality is simply to create a list of terms to describe listeners' impressions. Listeners then assess quality by indicating which features characterize a given voice—for example, a voice may be deep, brilliant, and attractive, or breathy, high-pitched, and weak, or whining, or sinister, or rough, or harsh, or nasal. This descriptive approach dates back to at least Greco-Roman times, and has the ring of truth that comes with long familiarity. It is also both easy to understand and easy to apply, requiring only vocabulary and imagination (for review, see Butler, 2015; Kreiman & Sidtis, 2011).

As colourful and evocative as such terms for voice quality can be (see Box 8.1), the potential open-endedness of the vocabulary that can be applied to describe phonation ultimately limits the usefulness of such 'protocols' in scientific work. Lists of terms abound in the literature (e.g. Gelfer, 1988; Moore, 1964), but many fundamental issues concerning their construction and use have never been resolved, including which scales to include, how to define the terms selected, and how to eliminate redundancies and ambiguities among terms (for review, see Kreiman & Sidtis, 2011). This approach remains atheoretical and is based on tradition and opinion, rather than evidence.

A number of authors have addressed this problem (at least in cases of vocal pathology) by attempting to constrain and systematize descriptive systems, and by replacing checklists with numerical rating systems to quantify the extent to which a voice possesses each feature. The best-known of these systems is the GRBAS protocol (Isshiki et al., 1966, 1969), so named because it includes the scales Grade (overall severity of disorder), Roughness, Breathiness, Asthenicity (weakness), and Strain. Scales were originally derived using semantic-differential ratings of a small set of hoarse voices on seventeen scales, including eight terms nominally related to voice (e.g. choked, smooth, clear, bad) and nine other terms culled from the general literature on semantic-differential scaling (e.g. dark, sharp, pessimistic, narrow, dry). After factor analysis, factors interpreted as breathy, asthenic, rough, and 'degree' (later re-named 'grade') emerged from these ratings, with the fifth scale for strain subsequently added when the complete GRBAS protocol was adopted by the Japan Society of Logopedics and Phoniatrics (for review, see Hirano, 1981). This protocol, which requires users to rate voices on four-point scales from 'normal' to 'severe', continues to be widely used around the world in both research and clinical applications.

More recently, the Consensus Auditory-Perceptual Evaluation of Voice, or CAPE-V (Kempster et al., 2009), was devised at a consensus conference in 2002 attended by clinicians, voice researchers, and psychometricians (including the authors of this chapter). The goal of this meeting was to create a standardized protocol for both clinical and research application, based on expert recommendations regarding 'best practices' in voice-quality assessment. A certain amount of cynicism accompanied this endeavour: attendees were well aware of the limits of existing protocols for quality assessment, and the paper describing the CAPE-V states, 'The current knowledge base is inadequate for designing a clinical tool that resolves all of the relevant scientific issues' (p. 126). Nevertheless, the hope was that efforts would result in the adoption of a single protocol, which by standardizing practice might 'improve communication and consistency among clinicians' (p. 126) in their clinical assessments.

Loosely following the GRBAS protocol, the CAPE-V includes scales for breathiness, roughness, strain, loudness, and pitch, but uses 100-mm visual analogue scales (with indicators identifying the mild, moderate, and severe ranges) rather than discrete numerical ratings. These particular scales were included because they are in common clinical use, supporting the belief that users find them meaningful. Beyond this, however, the CAPE-V differs significantly from the GRBAS protocol. It specifies the precise tasks used to gather voice samples (spontaneous speech; sustained vowels; and six read sentences including different phonetic contexts believed to elicit behaviours like hard or soft glottal attacks, nasality, and/or voice stoppages) and the recording procedures to be used when collecting voice data. It also includes a standardized form with blank scales for rating additional features, space for the clinician's comments about resonance, and a checklist for features like diplophonia, aphonia, and tremor. The CAPE-V has been reasonably well accepted, particularly in the United States, although clinicians apparently do not adhere consistently to the specified procedures, so it may not promote standardization of clinical practice (Nagle, 2016), and it has proven no more reliable or valid than other subjective protocols for voice assessment (Zraick et al., 2011).

Another 'consensus protocol', the Stockholm Voice Evaluation System (Hammarberg & Gauffin, 1995; Hammarberg, 2000), was developed over a long period of time as colleagues in a single department met to systematically rate voices and discuss and revise their scores and definitions. This protocol is more elaborate than the CAPE-V, including thirteen scales: 'aphonic', 'breathy', 'hyperfunctional/tense', 'hypofunctional/lax', 'vocal fry/creaky', 'rough', 'gratings/high frequency roughness', 'unstable quality/pitch', 'voice breaks', 'diplophonic', 'modal/falsetto register', 'pitch', and 'loudness'—all defined explicitly in terms of how the quality is (hypothetically) produced. For example, 'hyperfunction' is defined as 'voice sounds strained, due to compression/constriction of vocal folds and larynx tube during phonation with insufficient airflow' (Hammarberg, 2000, p. 99). All included qualities are assessed from running speech and scored on continuous visual analogue scales.

One additional quality assessment system—the Vocal Profiles Analysis Scheme (VPAS)—deserves mention here. This system is based on an articulatory model of voice originally developed to describe normal voices (Ball et al., 2000; Laver, 1980, 2000), and subsequently adapted as a clinical voice-evaluation protocol that is used widely in the UK and elsewhere (Laver et al., 1981; Wirz & Mackenzie Beck, 1995). In contrast to the other systems just reviewed, in the VPAS, voice is defined very broadly in terms of the global long-term physiological configuration that (hypothetically) underlies the overall sound of a speaker's voice. That is, it models perception in terms of speech-production processes, without reference to a listener. It includes a large number of parameters for the position of the lips, tongue, and jaw, velopharyngeal opening, larynx position, pitch, loudness, and tremor, in addition to phonation type—all rated on six-point scales. The system is analytic, consistent with phonetic models of speech production, and nearly exhaustive in the physiological domain, and by describing voice quality in detailed terms of the supposed underlying physiological configuration, it indicates where perceptual information about quality *might* be. However, how listeners actually use different features to assess quality, whether (or when, or why) some features might be more important than others, or how dimensions interact perceptually, is not specified.

As already noted, it is not hard to understand the appeal of rating-scale approaches to voice-quality measurement. Ratings from mild to severe are intuitively accessible to everyone, and require no special equipment or technological expertise to gather. Rating systems are also a direct measure of the sound of a voice. In contrast, reported associations of instrumental measures with quality are correlational at best, and can be variable both in strength and in the specific associations proposed (for review, see, for example, Maryn et al., 2009).[1]

Unfortunately, however, both theoretical and practical problems arise from the application of such scales as a measurement system. Theoretically, rating-scale systems require a listener, but cannot accommodate or model differences between listeners or within a single listener across listening contexts. In essence, they treat the listener as a 'black box' that responds in a fixed way as a function of variation in the signal, so that quality ratings reduce to a model of the acoustic signal. This is clearly wrong: many years of behavioural, cognitive, and neuro-psychological research have documented the role listeners play in auditory perception and the extent of variability among listeners in their ratings. For example, a listener's linguistic experience clearly influences the processing of non-linguistic voice quality. The phonemic contrasts present in a listener's native language affect sensitivity to attributes of voice quality, such that listeners who use a contrast to distinguish meanings are able to hear far smaller differences between voices than are other listeners (Kreiman et al., 2010; Krishnan et al., 2009). Ratings of voice quality vary over the short term within listeners as a function of the listening context, such that a voice may sound mildly disordered in isolation, but severely disordered when heard embedded in a set of normal voices (Gerratt et al., 1993; cf. Zäske et al., 2010, for similar findings relating to voice recognition). Differences between listeners also occur: the extent of previous exposure to pathologic voices is reflected in the complexity of perceptual strategies applied when judging vocal similarity (Kreiman et al., 1990, 1992) (for review, see Kreiman & Sidtis, 2011; Schweinberger et al., 2014).

Reliance on scalar quality-assessment protocols is further undermined by studies suggesting that voices are perceived as integral patterns, and not as bundles of perceptually-separable, individually-meaningful features. Many lines of research point to this conclusion. For example, harmonic and inharmonic (noise) components of the voice source interact perceptually due to masking, so that listeners' sensitivity to either acoustic attribute depends on the levels of energy in both (Kreiman & Gerratt, 2012). In priming experiments, responses to 'famous' voices in a famous/not famous task were significantly faster when listeners had previously heard a different exemplar of a famous voice, so that the benefit derived from the complete voice pattern, and not from the specific details of a given sample (Schweinberger et al., 1997). Long-term memory studies indicate that unfamiliar voices are not remembered in terms of their constituent features, but with reference to prototypical patterns (Papcun et al., 1989).

The assumption that listeners are able to separate different features auditorily also appears invalid, given evidence that listeners are unable to isolate individual dimensions of complex patterns (Kreiman & Gerratt, 2000; Kreiman, Gerratt, & Ito, 2007; cf. Poljac et al., 2012, who showed, for the visual system, that perception of a whole renders the parts inaccessible to consciousness). Thus, neither the perceptual meaning of a given quality dimension nor the perceptual significance of an acoustic measure can be assessed without knowledge of the context provided by the complete voice pattern in which the feature or measure functions. In fact, a multidimensional scaling study of expert listeners' judgements of the similarity of 160 voices (eighty female; Kreiman & Gerratt, 1996) produced no evidence of any common dimensions for voice quality, indicating that features like 'breathiness' and 'roughness' may

---

[1] For example, 'rough' voice quality may be correlated with jitter, shimmer, measures of spectral noise, measures of glottal asymmetry or glottal gap, and so on.

simply not exist as part of voice perception, however strongly tradition and belief may argue that they do. Note also that listeners are unable to agree consistently even about which voice samples are or are not breathy or rough, even in cases of severe vocal pathology (Kreiman & Gerratt, 2000).

In practice, rating-scale protocols are plagued with the 'unreliable rater' problem. Studies have repeatedly demonstrated that listeners do not agree in their ratings of voice quality, to the extent that a single voice may be rated as 'normal' or 'mildly disordered' by one rater and as 'severely pathologic' by others (Kreiman & Gerratt, 1998). Many solutions to this problem have been proposed, including training listeners to use scales consistently (Brinca et al., 2015; Chan & Yiu, 2006), providing example stimuli or 'anchors' for each scale value (Awan & Lawson, 2009; Chan & Yiu, 2002), using fewer scale values (Kreiman, Gerratt, & Ito, 2007), averaging ratings to achieve a reliable mean (Shrivastav et al., 2005), or simply giving up and asking patients about their satisfaction with their voice and voice-related quality of life (e.g. Hogikyan & Sethuraman, 1999; Hogikyan et al., 2000; for review, see Franco & Andrus, 2009, who argue that patient surveys may be superior to other methods of evaluating surgical outcomes). Unfortunately, all of these workarounds continue the assumption that quality ratings are straightforward functions of the acoustic characteristics of the voice, and none has provided a satisfactory solution to the problem of listener unreliability, presumably because of their failure to account for listener behaviour.

In summary, feature-based attempts to model voice quality have failed, because such descriptive, dimensional models all require the assumption that a voice pattern is decomposable into features, which is inconsistent with what is known about quality perception. Further, such models do not accommodate the role of the listener in voice perception. We conclude that such models do not measure voice quality in any meaningful way. (We will describe some possible solutions to this unfortunate state of affairs in Section 8.3.)

8.2.2 Acoustic Approaches to Voice-Quality Assessment

Given the operational and theoretical difficulties inherent in measuring voice quality, some authors (particularly those studying pathological voices) have argued that perceptual measures of voice should be replaced with instrumental measures. In contrast to perceptual measures, instrumental measures of acoustic, aerodynamic, or physiological events promise precision, reliability, and replicability. For example, the Acoustic Voice Quality Index (AVQI: Maryn, Corthals, et al., 2010; Maryn, DeBodt, & Roy, 2010; Barsties & Maryn, 2016) comprises a grab bag of acoustic measures (jitter, shimmer, harmonics-to-noise ratio, spectral tilt) generated using Praat software (Boersma & Weenink, 2017) plus variants of the cepstral peak prominence (CPP: Hillenbrand & Houde, 1996). Five expert listeners rated the 'overall voice quality' (analogous to the GRBAS 'Grade' scale) of 251 voices (about twice as many females as males, suffering mostly from mass lesions or functional disorders) on a four-point scale. Stepwise linear regression was then applied to devise a weighted sum of acoustic variables that best predicted the average listener rating:

$$AVQI = (3.295 - 0.111\,CPPs - 0.073\,HNR - 0.213\,\text{percent shimmer}$$
$$+ 2.7893\,\text{shimmer in dB} - 0.032\,\text{slope} + 0.077\,\text{tilt}) \times 2.571$$

where CPPs is the smoothed cepstral peak prominence (Hillenbrand & Houde, 1996), HNR is the harmonics-to-noise ratio, slope is the slope of the long-term average spectrum, and tilt is the tilt of the trend line through the long-term average spectrum. (Subsequent replications produced slightly different predictors and coefficients; e.g. Barsties & Maryn, 2016; Maryn & Weenink, 2015). A correlation of r = 0.78 was obtained between average severity ratings and the acoustic parameter set, but the process of devising this measure was purely empirical. No justification was offered for the choice of parameters included in the analyses, and no explanation was proffered for the particular relationships that emerged.

A similar motivation—the desire for an objective measure that would reliably quantify perceived voice quality—produced the Dysphonia Severity Index (DSI: Wuyts et al., 2000). In this case, the measure represents a function relating five experts' Grade ratings of the voices of 387 adults (sixty-eight normal) to acoustic measures generated by the Multidimensional Voice Program (MDVP: e.g. Al-Nasheri et al., 2017) plus maximum phonation time, vital capacity, phonation quotient; lowest intensity, highest intensity, intensity range; lowest and highest Fo, Fo range, and semitone range. This analysis yielded the following equation:

$$\text{DSI} = 0.13 \text{ maximum phonation time} + 0.0053 \text{ highest F0} - 0.26 \text{ lowest intensity} - 1.18 \text{ percent jitter,}$$

whose result correlated with the Voice Handicap Index (a measure of speakers' satisfaction with their voice; r = −0.79) and correctly predicted the average 'Grade' score 50% of the time.

Another similar measure, the Cepstral Spectral Index of Dysphonia (CSID: Awan et al., 2009, 2010), was derived from ratings of continuous speech rather than steady-state vowels, but again used a set of acoustic measures to predict expert ratings of the severity of vocal disorder. A study of women's voices pre-/post-treatment (Awan et al., 2009) found that mean-rated severity of pathology could be predicted from a weighted sum of the CPP, the mean ratio of low-to-high frequency spectral energy, and the standard deviation associated with that mean:

$$\text{CSID} = 154.59 - 10.39 \text{ CPP} - 3.71 \text{ DFT\_ratio SD} - 1.08 \text{ DFT\_ratio,}$$

where DFT_ratio is the mean ratio of low to high frequency energy in the voice spectrum (R^2 = 0.73). However, a subsequent study, including both male and female voices (Awan et al., 2010), produced somewhat different results[2] (R^2 = 0.65):

$$\text{CSID} = 148.68 - 5.91 \text{ CPP} - 11.17 \text{ CPP sd} - 1.31 \text{ DFT\_ratio} - 3.09 \text{ DFT\_ratio sd}$$

As should be clear by now, these acoustic indices of voice quality do little to solve the issues that plague quality-rating systems, but only kick the can down the road while introducing new concerns of their own. No model of quality underlies or motivates the protocols just

---

[2] DFT ratio is called L/H spectral ratio in their paper.

described, and by focusing solely on severity of vocal pathology, they shed no light on normal voice quality and do little to capture the richness of the sensations alluded to in the 'Introduction' and in Box 8.1. Further, by discarding descriptive terminology in favour of simple ratings of the extent of pathology, they raise major questions regarding their validity as measures of voice quality.

Development of acoustic measures of quality ultimately depends on successfully identifying consistent, motivated correspondences between perceptual measures and the variables included in the measurement protocol. However, no theory exists describing the causational links between physiology, acoustics, and vocal quality, so there is no basis for determining which instrumental measures ought to correspond to perceptually meaningful differences in vocal quality (other than the empirical association, which cannot demonstrate causation), or why such associations should exist. Finally, existing research has produced highly variable results that seem to depend on the particular voices studied and on the acoustic variables chosen for analysis, raising further questions about their validity as measures of voice quality (Maryn et al., 2009). We will discuss another approach to this problem in Section 8.3.

8.2.3 Measuring the Physical Voice

Voice physically originates in the body of the speaker, and another common approach to understanding voice thus focuses on how speakers phonate. At first glance, this seems reasonable enough. After all, bodies are needed to produce voices,[3] and phonation temporally precedes transmission of the acoustic signal and its perception by a listener. By shedding light on the origins of information in voice signals, the details of voice production may provide important clues to the kinds of information listeners have available to them and consequently use. The biological facts of phonation further point to the primacy of production. An acoustic voice signal necessarily encodes the body that produces it, so that characteristics of these signals are partially explainable in terms of the speaker's physical characteristics. This observation applies to many species, including alligators and crocodiles (Chabert, 2015; Reber et al., 2017), frogs (Bee, 2002), birds (Akçay et al., 2016), and most mammals (e.g. Charlton et al., 2012; Frey et al., 2011), adding additional weight to the view that production is the point of entry for understanding voice.

Voice production is enormously complex, and many, many measurement approaches have examined different aspects of phonation. Because the larynx is rather inaccessible in living humans, many of these approaches are necessarily indirect. For example, glottal configurations and patterns of vocal fold vibration can be studied using stroboscopy or high-speed imaging (Echternach et al., 2017; Moore, 1938), or via electroglottography (Fourcin et al., 1995); the air pressure driving phonation can be measured with systems that estimate changes in pressure and airflow as the vocal folds open and close (Rothenberg, 1977); correlations between muscle potentials and movements of the laryngeal cartilages can be measured with electromyography in living humans (Gay et al., 1972) or via direct muscle stimulation in *in vivo* animal models (Chhetri et al., 2012).

---

[3] Putting speech synthesis aside for the present (e.g. Chion, 1999).

Physical models of the vocal folds can be used to evaluate the importance of different details of vocal fold structure (e.g. Z. Zhang et al., 2013), and excised larynx models can provide evidence about anatomy and about the effects of glottal configuration on many aspects of phonation (e.g. Berry et al., 2003; Kakita et al., 1981; Y. Zhang et al., 2017). Even fine details of the motion of air particles through the glottis can be studied with flow-imaging systems or anemometry (Alipour et al., 1994; Bielamowicz et al., 1999) (for an extensive review, see, for example, Baken & Orlikoff, 2000). Finally, computational models (e.g. Ishizaka & Flanagan, 1972; Xue et al., 2014; Z. Zhang, 2016a) have been used extensively to show cause/effect relationships between physiological parameters and patterns of vocal fold vibration.

Unfortunately, most studies of voice production are able to examine only a single facet of the complex production process at a time. This limitation is partly structural: in studies of living humans, both logistical and ethical considerations limit the number of systems that can be studied at once (or studied at all), and associations between systems must always be correlational, because humans cannot control individual muscles, airflow levels, or glottal configurations with any precision. *In vivo* animal models or excised larynx studies allow direct manipulation of some of these factors and permit examination of interactions between parameters (e.g. nerve stimulation levels and glottal configuration); but many studies (e.g. Mau et al., 2012; Regner & Jiang, 2011) have again manipulated parameters one at a time and assessed their individual effects on phonation via correlation. Computational modelling offers great flexibility with respect to covarying parameters, but knowledge of the correct input values for the model (or even of what parameters should be included) is somewhat limited, so it is difficult to know when a system is accurate, or adequately detailed, or too detailed; and, most critically, few models provide acoustic output to demonstrate the importance of the parameters that were studied in the first place.

These issues, while important, mask a more fundamental problem with studies of production as a starting point in voice research. When we begin our exploration of voice from a production point of view, our search for the correct parameters to study is completely unconstrained. Virtually any aspect of the anatomy, physiology, neurophysiology, mechanics, biomechanics, aerodynamics, or aeroacoustics of phonation can be examined, and has been examined; but such studies do not consider how the parameter in question might be involved in creating the message being sent—its perceptual, communicative importance. In the absence of information about a listener's ability to hear changes in a productive parameter, every detail of airflow and tissue movement is potentially interesting. For example, many studies of vortices in the airflow through the glottis have appeared (e.g. Khosla et al., 2008), but none (to our knowledge) considered the perceptibility of changes in vortex location or size. Vortices certainly exist, but they have not been shown to impact the sound of a voice, and thus may be simply epiphenomena. Similarly, dozens of studies addressed the physical origins of jitter and shimmer in phonation, but to no end, given that listeners cannot hear jitter and shimmer separately from overall noise levels in voice (Kreiman & Gerratt, 2005). Studies of glottal asymmetry as evidence of vocal pathology have generally overlooked the fact that voices can sound completely normal despite significant asymmetries (Z. Zhang et al., 2013). Again, such studies provide information about tissue properties and movements, but they are not yet informative about voice production per se, because no body of theory relates them to the sound ultimately produced.

8.2.4 Summary

Most approaches to the study of voice focus on a single aspect of the 'speech chain', largely independently of the others. Researchers study individual pieces of this chain of events, as a result of which no explanation has emerged regarding how to accommodate voice as part of a system for transmitting information from speaker to listener. What we have instead is a plethora of little pieces, so that voice can be defined as the output of vocal fold vibration, or as a system that produces vibration, or as a listener's response to an acoustic signal, or as the acoustic signal itself, with each of these subvoices further divided into more little pieces.

Contemporary research provides no insight into how meaning in voice is constructed and, frankly, current research practice provides no hope of this in the future. The current approach to the study of voice thus appears to us to be a dead end: unless we radically rethink what we mean by voice, and how we approach its study, we are doomed to a situation where voice means something different to everyone who studies it, as bemoaned by Sundberg in 1987 and by everyone who has worked on voice since that time.

8.3 RECONSIDERING VOICE

8.3.1 Its Nature

Having stated that some radical rethinking is required, theoretical perspectives drawn from the critical studies literature may suggest a way out of this most unfortunate state of affairs. We begin by noting that meaning in voice originates in the listener, not in the speaker (Eidsheim, 2014). From the speaker's point of view, phonation exists to convey a message to a listener, and its nature and characteristics depend on what is required to get the desired message across. In the same way that linguistically meaningful (phonemic) contrasts must be phonetically discriminable by listeners for a semantic message to be understood, any part of a voice signal that corresponds to an important speaker attribute must be perceptible by a listener to have any communicative role. The voice necessarily reflects aspects of the speaker's body, as previously discussed, but the way that this happens depends on listeners, because the code relating attributes like size, age, and gender to sound has no meaning or function without a listener who hears and interprets the phonation. Analogous to the tree falling in the forest, without a listener quality does not exist, but only the movement of air particles. Simply put, laryngeal biomechanics and aeroacoustics can be studied as interesting physical problems, but *voice production is impossible to understand out of the context of voice perception*.

At the same time, because voice quality requires a speaker, a listener, and an interaction between them, the concept necessarily implies a social person. Speakers and listeners are both imbedded in a dynamic linguistic, social, and cultural context that shapes both the sound produced and the manner in which it is perceived (for review, see Llamas & Watt, 2010; Podesva, 2007; Podesva & Callier, 2015). For example, Japanese female speakers use Fo values that are higher than those produced by Dutch (van Bezooijen, 1995) or American women (Yuasa, 2008), reflecting different cultural standards for femininity in these countries (see also Starr, 2015). Different kinds of phonation can mark group membership or a regional affiliation; for example, young female speakers of American English (and many men) often use creaky voice (Yuasa, 2010), and a number of studies have shown how voice quality can index social class within a single city (Esling, 1978; for review, see Esling, 2000). As these examples show, phonation expresses not just speakers' physical selves, but also their interior selves in particular social contexts. For this reason, *voice production is impossible to understand in a general way without consideration of the dynamic factors that shape actual utterances.*

Listeners are also affected by the social context in which they perceive a voice. Consider the case of jazz singer Jimmy Scott (1925–2004; Eidsheim, in press; Eidsheim & Kreiman, 2016). Born with Kallman syndrome, which disrupts the growth associated with puberty, Scott's voice sounds unambiguously feminine to most listeners, although his fundamental frequency is consistent with male tenor singing and is considerably lower than the falsetto used by 'high-singing' male vocalists like Smokey Robinson or Marvin Gaye,[4] whose voices sound unambiguously male. In Robinson and Gaye's singing, falsetto in the context of male formant frequencies marks the high-frequency phonation as if with 'timbral scare quotes' that allow it to be heard as masculine despite the very high Fo values. Falsetto is notably absent from Scott's singing; and paradoxically, the lower pitch of his voice and the absence of falsetto contribute to its feminine quality. This example shows how listeners bring a range of culturally and historically contingent conventions (e.g. male formants + falsetto = male voice) to everyday listening that guide how they interpret what they hear, even if acoustic cues (in this case to sex/gender) pull them in different directions.

Finally, in the same way that there is no quality without a listener, there is obviously no quality without a speaker or without the acoustic signal the speaker produces.[5] The complex social and physiological factors already alluded to shape and constrain perceptual processes indirectly by shaping the utterances to be perceived, and directly by influencing listeners' expectations, perceptual biases, and cognitive processing of the stimuli, even at the lowest levels of the auditory system. The perceptual system has co-evolved with the voice-production system, and of course must work with whatever acoustic information speakers send the listeners' way (which depends in part on the speakers' larynges and vocal tract characteristics). At the same time, listeners have learned to interpret these signals in terms of specific, socially- and/or biologically-relevant information, so that the signal to be heard and how it is perceived both depend, in part, on the characteristics of the speaker. We thus conclude that *perception cannot be understood independently from production and acoustics, any more than production can be understood without attention to the listener.*

To conclude the argument thus far, voice quality, voice production, and vocal acoustics have long been treated as essentially independent stages in a sequence of events beginning with phonation and ending with perception. This has led to increasing fragmentation of the literature, such that smaller and smaller pieces of each stage of the sequence have been examined, and less and less attention has been paid to how the pieces go together. We are left with

---

[4] Representative voice samples for all these singers can easily be found on YouTube or iTunes. See, in particular, Jimmy Scott's recording of 'I Wish I Knew' (Warren & Gordon, 1945); Smokey Robinson's lovely 'Ooh Baby Baby' (Robinson & Moore, 1965); and Marvin Gaye's 'Trouble Man' (Gaye, 1972).

[5] We leave aside the problem of so-called 'acousmatic' voices—for example, the disembodied, off-screen narrator in a film—and the problem of auditory hallucinations. (For an extended discussion, see, for example, Chion, 1999.)

the question, 'What is voice?', which in this view appears unanswerable—voice exists in all these domains, so there are many 'voices'. On further consideration, however, we have argued that voice cannot be understood solely as sound, or as descriptive scales like 'breathy' and 'hoarse', or as intraglottal vortices, without taking into consideration the role each 'stage' of the process plays in the others. In a sense, voice is a 'thick object' that exists in all these interacting domains (Eidsheim, 2015), so that voice may be better thought of as a process, rather than a 'thing' or as many things. It is our view that the study of voice faces a choice between characterizing voice as many things, or as one thing, so that production, and acoustics, and quality do not exist independently of each other, but only as a unitary process: no voice quality, no voice production, but only voice, comprising all of these.

8.3.2 Another Approach to the Study of Voice

Such a reconsideration of the nature of voice requires a similar reconsideration of how voice is studied. Quality may be the temporal endpoint of this process, but logically, the process actually begins with the listener, because without the listener, no meaning exists and speakers have no motivation for phonation in the first place. It follows that, because of the interdependence among different aspects of voice, lack of a measurement system for quality undermines our ability to investigate not just the sound of a voice, but biomechanics and acoustics as well, and impedes the study of voice in general. Without knowing what is important to listeners, we cannot identify the important acoustic attributes of a voice signal, and we cannot investigate the sources of those important acoustic attributes in the production system. The listeners' perceptual sensitivities and expectations form a set of constraints on what speakers must do in order to be understood; and both speaker and listener characteristics determine which aspects of the acoustic signal are important. Even studies of why vocal-fold tissue vibrates in the first place imply the question, 'Are these vibrations voice, or simply noise? Would a listener accept them as phonation and as human?' We conclude that, in the final analysis, we must be able to model listeners' responses in order to reach our ultimate goal—*a theoretical understanding sufficient to relate the perceived sound of a voice to the physiology that produced it, and physiology to the resultant percept.* This understanding could then provide a foundation to support further work on the social, cognitive, and evolutionary meaning and uses of voice—of not just what occurs, but of *why* it occurs.

Over the past years, we have developed an approach to the study of quality that we believe begins to address the aforementioned issues raised. We have argued in this chapter that most rating-scale-based protocols for studying voice perception are invalid because listeners are unable to isolate single dimensions in complex auditory patterns. We have further argued that without a model of voice perception, it is impossible to generate meaningful hypotheses about which aspects of production are communicatively important. These two conclusions suggested to us that the way to proceed was to first develop a psychoacoustic model of voice, relating listeners' perceptions of integral voice quality to specific acoustic attributes of voice, and then to address the way that speakers control those parameters (Kreiman et al., 2014). In contrast to previous correlational approaches relating individual vocal attributes to acoustics or production, in our approach, we apply voice synthesis to model voice as a unitary percept—in other words, we model quality, not individual qualities. In the remainder of this chapter, we will briefly describe this model and its development.

To identify candidate acoustic features, we began with the assumption that listeners pay attention to vocal attributes that vary from voice to voice. For example, if every speaker phonated with the same fundamental frequency, vocal pitch would have no value as a cue to identity, age, sex, turn taking in conversation, or anything else. Thus, the first step in developing a psychoacoustic model of voice was to identify the acoustic attributes that best distinguish the individual voices in a large set (Kreiman, Gerratt, & Antoñanzas-Barroso, 2007). Using principal-component analysis to evaluate the source spectra of seventy voices, we arrived at an initial model comprising the source spectral slope above 4 kHz, the slope below 450 Hz, and two parameters modelling the slope between 1.5 kHz and 4 kHz. Parallel analyses of a set of acoustic source parameters produced components associated with the relative difference in the amplitudes of the first two harmonics (H1–H2) and of the second and fourth harmonics (H2-H4), the overall spectral slope, and the amplitude of high-frequency spectral noise.

Model validation then proceeded by using analysis-by-synthesis to demonstrate that all parameters were necessary to model quality (e.g. Garellek et al., 2016; Kreiman & Gerratt, 2010, 2012), and that we had all the parameters we needed (i.e. the model was sufficient) (e.g. Kreiman et al., 2015). The parameter set was modified as a result of these studies; the current set is shown in Table 8.1. Audio 8.1 includes examples of six synthetic voices (three female, three male) created with this model, along with the corresponding original natural voice samples. Because we have demonstrated that this set is sufficient to create copies that are indistinguishable from the vast majority of voice samples, we believe that the model can fairly be held to parametrically quantify the complex pattern that is voice quality.

We emphasize that, by examining cause and effect relationships between acoustic parameters and quality, and by measuring voice as the set of parameter values that allows recreation of the complete perceived pattern, this model differs radically from previous attempts

Table 8.1 Current acoustic parameters in the psychoacoustic model of voice

Model component	Parameters
Harmonic source spectral shape	H1–H2
	H2–H4
	Spectral slope from H4–2 kHz
	Spectral slope from 2 kHz–5 kHz
Inharmonic source spectral shape	Noise spectral amplitude in a band from 0–769 Hz
	Noise spectral amplitude in a band from 769–2115 Hz
	Noise spectral amplitude in a band from 2115–3461 Hz
	Noise spectral amplitude in a band from 3461–5000 Hz
Time-varying source characteristics	F0 mean and standard deviation (or F0 track)
	Amplitude mean and standard deviation (or amplitude track)
Vocal tract transfer function	Formant frequencies and bandwidths
	Spectral zeros and bandwidths

to relate acoustic measures to listeners' perceptions of overall vocal severity or individual qualities like breathiness or roughness. The acoustic model parameters were not arbitrarily chosen, but were selected based on well-motivated hypotheses about the acoustic sources of perceived voice quality; parameters in the model are not redundant with one another; and listeners have demonstrated perceptual sensitivity to all model parameters. This approach thus eliminates objections to acoustic voice profiles and could eventually eliminate the need for subjective quality measures, because the model forms a parametric representation of the complete, integral voice pattern. Thus, parameters can be used validly to evaluate changes in voice quality in the clinic or elsewhere, because they are objective measures whose relationship to quality and to each other is understood theoretically.

8.3.3 The Next Step: A Physiopsychoacoustic Model

The notion that voice is an integral process implies that the ultimate goal of its study must be a model interrelating production, acoustics, and perception, as previously discussed. Such a model would specify causal links from laryngeal physiology, to voice acoustics, to quality, and back. To find such mappings, parameters of the psychoacoustic model can be used as targets for studies of vocal physiology. In this approach, investigators would no longer examine the acoustic effects of changes in vocal-fold stiffness (for example). Instead, they would examine the control of H1–H2 or other model parameters.

This approach has a number of advantages. First, the psychoacoustic model constrains studies of vocal physiology and biomechanics, as already noted, so that there is a basis for understanding which physical or biomechanical attributes are important, and which are epiphenomenal. Secondly, it is likely that there are multiple mechanisms for controlling salient acoustic parameters, in the same way that there are multiple ways to produce important phonemic contrasts in natural languages (for an example, see Kreiman et al., 2012). When research begins with physical processes, such redundancies can only be found by accident; but when the goal of the study is understanding how a specific acoustic parameter is controlled in the context of other parameters, redundancies and interdependencies emerge naturally from modelling efforts.

Research of this sort is in its infancy. For example, in the 'Voice Sim' program, a kind of articulatory synthesizer for voice (Fraj et al., 2012; Lucero et al., 2013), voice synthesis is controlled in terms of laryngeal parameters, with the goal of establishing a direct relationship between physiology and perceived voice quality. Studies to date (Englert et al., 2017) have been limited to modelling roughness, breathiness, and strain, which is accomplished by manipulating frequency perturbation, additive noise, vocal-fold tension, subglottal pressure, and vocal-fold separation. Perceptual evaluation has only assessed the naturalness of the synthesis, which appears to be somewhat limited (over 30% misclassified as synthetic/natural).

Work using computational models of phonation shows somewhat more promise. For example, Z. Zhang (2016a) used a simplified continuum model of phonation to study the roles of vocal-fold stiffness, medial surface thickness, resting glottal opening, and subglottal pressure in regulating source spectral shape (as measured by the parameters in Table 8.1), Fo, and spectral noise levels. He reported a dominant role for the thickness of the medial surface of the vocal folds in regulating spectral shape, while decreasing resting glottal opening served to reduce noise production and increase Fo. (See Z. Zhang, 2016b, for an excellent, thorough review of what is currently known about control of perceptually-important acoustic attributes of voice.)

8.4 Discussion and Conclusions

Both empirical and theoretical arguments have led us to the conclusion that voice must be viewed as a single integral process, and not as a concatenation of separate aspects, subparts, or stages. Voice production, acoustics, aeroacoustics, biomechanics, perception, and all the rest, are conceptually inseparable, and none of these can be understood without knowing how its relationship to the others contributes to its structure and function. Current compartmentalized approaches to studying individual aspects of voice as separate subdisciplines are an inappropriate strategy for unravelling the complex interactions that form the voice process, and impede our progress towards understanding why voice has evolved as it has and how it functions, both physiologically and as a critical aspect of oral communication.

As we have argued, an integral approach to the study of voice would provide a solid grounding for studies of voice in other disciplines, including psychology, sociology, ethology, and even humanistic work in critical theory. Clinical practice in particular could benefit from a reformed approach to voice. The usual clinical goal is to make patients sound like they used to, to restore the voice that sounds like them. A comprehensive understanding of the relationships between the voice-production system and the perceived voice would obviously help target treatment to appropriate functional loci. More than that, however, a broader view of what voice is could help clinicians pinpoint those aspects of patients' voices that are responsible for feelings that this is 'not my voice', with all the complex interwoven cultural, emotional, psychological, and physical meanings implied by such a statement.

In conclusion, we submit that development of such a comprehensive theory of voice should be the primary goal of voice research, both in scientific and humanistic disciplines. Such a theory would form a basis on which to build realistic explanations of how voice functions socially and communicatively, how it has evolved, and how it conveys meanings of all sorts. The benefit of such a labour would be a deeper understanding of what it means to be human and to communicate.

Acknowledgments

This research was supported by grant DC01797 from the National Institute on Deafness and Other Communication Disorders. We thank Zhaoyan Zhang and Nina Eidsheim for many helpful discussions and comments on earlier versions of this chapter. Software for analysis-by-synthesis is available free of charge by request to either author.

References

Akçay, C., Arnold, J. A., Hambury, K. L., & Dickinson, J. L. (2016). Age-based discrimination of rival males in western bluebirds. *Animal Cognition*, 19, 999–1006.

Al-Nasheri, A., Muhammad, G., Alsulaiman, M., Ali, Z., Mesallam, T. A., Farahat, M., Malki, K. H., & Bencherif, M. A. (2017). An investigation of multidimensional voice program parameters in three different databases for voice pathology detection and classification. *Journal of Voice*, 31, 113.e9–113.e18.

Alipour, F., Patel, V. C., & Scherer, R. C. (1994). Measurement of pulsatile flow in excised larynges with hot-wire anemometry. In: F.M. White (ed.) *Individual Papers in Fluids Engineering*, (pp. 1–4). American Society of Mechanical Engineers.

ANSI (1960). *ANSI S1.1-1960: Acoustical Terminology*. New York: American National Standards Institute.

Awan, S. N. & Lawson, L. L. (2009). The effect of anchor modality on the reliability of vocal severity ratings. *Journal of Voice*, 23, 341–352.

Awan, S. N., Roy, N., & Dromey, C. (2009). Estimating dysphonia severity in continuous speech: application of a multi-parameter spectral/cepstral model. *Clinical Linguistics and Phonetics*, 23, 825–841.

Awan, S. N., Roy, N., Jette, M. E., Meltzner, G. S., & Hillman, R. E. (2010). Quantifying dysphonia severity using a spectral/cepstral-based acoustic index: comparisons with auditory-perceptual judgements from the CAPE-V. *Clinical Linguistics and Phonetics*, 24, 742–758.

Ball, M. J., Esling, J., & Dickson, C. (2000). The transcription of voice quality. In: R. D. Kent & M. J. Ball (eds) *Voice Quality Measurement*, (pp. 49–58). San Diego: Singular.

Baken, R. J. & Orlikoff, R. O. (2000). *Clinical Measurement of Speech and Voice* (2nd edn). San Diego: Singular.

Barsties, B. & Maryn, Y. (2016). External validation of the Acoustic Voice Quality Index version 03.01 with extended representativity. *Annals of Otology, Rhinology and Laryngology*, 125, 571–583.

Bee, M. A. (2002). Territorial male bullfrogs (*Rana catesbeiana*) do not assess fighting ability based on size-related variation in acoustic signals. *Behavioral Ecology*, 13, 109–124.

Berry, D. A., Montequin, D. W., Chan, R. W., Titze, I. R., & Hoffman, H. T. (2003). An investigation of cricoarytenoid joint mechanics using simulated muscle forces. *Journal of Voice*, 17, 47–62.

Bielamowicz, S. A., Berke, G. S., Kreiman, J., & Gerratt, B. R. (1999). Exit jet particle velocity in the in vivo canine laryngeal model with variable nerve stimulation. *Journal of Voice*, 13, 153–160.

Boersma, P. & Weenink, D. (2017). Praat: doing phonetics by computer [computer program]. Version 6.0.28, retrieved 23 March 2017 from http://www.praat.org/

Brinca, L., Batista, A. P., Tavares, A. I., Pinto, P. N., & Araújo, L. (2015). The effect of anchors and training on the reliability of voice quality ratings for different types of speech stimuli. *Journal of Voice*, 29, e7–e14.

Butler, S. (2015). *The Ancient Phonograph*. New York: Zone Books.

Butler, S. (in press). What was the voice? In: N. S. Eidsheim & K. L. Meizel (eds) *The Oxford Handbook of Voice Studies*. Oxford: Oxford University Press.

Cavarero, A. (2005). *For More Than One Voice: Toward a Philosophy of Vocal Expression*. Stanford, CA: Stanford University Press.

Chabert, T., Colin, A., Aubin, T., Shacks, V., Bourquin, S. L., Elsey, R. M., Acosta, J. G., & Mathevon, N. (2015). Size does matter: crocodile mothers react more to the voice of smaller offspring. *Scientific Reports*, 5, 15547.

Chan, K. M. K. & Yiu, E. M.-L. (2002). The effect of anchors and training on the reliability of perceptual voice evaluation. *Journal of Speech, Language, and Hearing Research*, 45, 111–126.

Chan, K. M. K. & Yiu, E. M.-L. (2006). A comparison of two perceptual voice evaluation training programs for naive listeners. *Journal of Voice*, 20, 229–241.

Chandler, R. (1995). *Stories and Early Novels*. New York: The Library of America.

Chandler, R. (1995). *Later Novels and Other Writings*. New York: The Library of America.

Charlton, B. D., Reby, D., Ellis, W. A., Brumm, J., & Fitch, W. T. (2012). Estimating the active space of male koala bellows: propagation of cues to size and identity in a eucalyptus forest. *PloS One*, 7, e45420.

Chhetri, D. K., Neubauer, J., & Berry, D. A. (2012). Neuromuscular control of fundamental frequency and glottal posture at phonation onset. *Journal of the Acoustical Society of America*, 131, 1401–1412.

Chion, M. (1999). *The Voice in Cinema*. New York: Columbia University Press.

Denes, P. B. & Pinson, E. N. (1993). *The Speech Chain* (2nd edn). New York: W.H. Freeman.

Dolar, M. (2006). *A Voice and Nothing More*. Cambridge, MA: MIT Press.

Echternach, M., Burk, F., Koberlein, M., Selamtzis, A., Döllinger, M., Burdumy, M., Richter, B., & Herbst, C. T. (2017). Laryngeal evidence for the first and second passaggio in professionally trained sopranos. *PLoS One*, 12, e0175865.

Eidsheim, N. S. (2014). The micropolitics of listening to vocal timbre. *Postmodern Culture*, 24(3).

Eidsheim, N. S. (2015). *Sensing Sound: Singing and Listening as Vibrational Practice*. Durham, NC: Duke University Press.

Eidsheim, N. S. (in press). *Measuring Race: The Micropolitics of Listening to Vocal Timbre and Vocality in African-American Popular Music*. Durham, NC: Duke University Press.

Eidsheim, N. & Kreiman, J. (2016). *Jimmy Scott and the problem of gender in singing*. Invited paper presented at the 170th Meeting of the Acoustical Society of America, May 2016.

Englert, M., Madazio, G., Gielow, I., Lucero, J., & Behlau, M. (2017). Perceptual error analysis of human and synthesized voices. *Journal of Voice*, 31(4), 516.e5–516.e18.

Esling, J. K. (1978). Identification of features of voice quality in social groups. *Journal of the International Phonetic Association*, 8, 18–23.

Esling, J. H. (2000). Crosslinguistic aspects of voice quality. In: R. D. Kent & M. J. Ball (eds) *Voice Quality Measurement*, (pp. 25–36). San Diego: Singular.

Fourcin, A., Abberton, E., Miller, D., & Howells, D. (1995). Laryngograph: speech pattern element tools for therapy, training and assessment. *European Journal of Disorders of Communication*, 30, 101–115.

Fraj, S., Schoentgen, J., & Grenez, F. (2012). Development and perceptual assessment of a synthesizer of disordered voices. *Journal of the Acoustical Society of America*, 132, 2603–2615.

Franco, R. A. & Andrus, J. G. (2009). Aerodynamic and acoustic characteristics of voice before and after adduction arytenopexy and medialization laryngoplasty with GORE-TEX in patients with unilateral vocal fold immobility. *Journal of Voice*, 23, 261–267.

Frey, R., Volodin, I., Volodina, E., Soldatova, N. V., & Juldaschev, E. T. (2011). Descended and mobile larynx, vocal tract elongation and rutting roars in male goitred gazelles (Gazella subgutterosa Guldenstaedt, 1780). *Journal of Anatomy*, 218, 566–585.

Garellek, M., Samlan, R., Gerratt, B. R., & Kreiman, J. (2016). Modeling the voice source in terms of spectral slopes. *Journal of the Acoustical Society of America*, 139, 1404–1410.

Gay, T., Strome, M., Hirose, H., & Sawashima, M. (1972). EMG of the intrinsic laryngeal muscles during phonation. *Annals of Otology, Rhinology and Laryngology*, 81, 401–409.

Gaye, M. (1972). 'Trouble man' on Trouble Man [record]. Los Angeles: Tamla/Motown.

Gelfer, M. P. (1988). Perceptual attributes of voice: development and use of rating scales. *Journal of Voice*, 2, 320–326.

Gerratt, B. R., Kreiman, J., Antoñanzas-Barroso, N., & Berke, G. S. (1993). Comparing internal and external standards in voice quality judgments. *Journal of Speech and Hearing Research*, 36, 14–20.

Hammarberg, B. (2000). Voice research and clinical needs. *Folia Phoniatrica et Logopaedica*, 52, 93–102.

Hammarberg, B. & Gauffin, J. (1995). Perceptual and acoustic characteristics of quality differences in pathological voices as related to physiological aspects. In: O. Fujimura & M. Hirano (eds) *Vocal Fold Physiology: Voice Quality Control* (pp. 283–303). San Diego: Singular.

Helmholtz, H. (1885; reprint 1954). *On the Sensations of Tone*. New York: Dover.

Hillenbrand, J. & Houde, R. A. (1996). Acoustic correlates of breathy vocal quality: dysphonic voices and continuous speech. *Journal of Speech and Hearing Research*, 39, 311–321.

Hirano, M. (1981). *Clinical Examination of Voice*. New York: Springer.

Hogikyan, N. D. & Sethuraman, G. (1999). Validation of an instrument to measure voice-related quality of life (V-RQOL). *Journal of Voice*, 13, 557–569.

Hogikyan, N. D., Wodchis, W. P., Terrell, J. E., Bradford, C. R., & Esclamado, R. M. (2000). Voice-related quality of life (V-RQOL) following type I thyroplasty for unilateral vocal fold paralysis. *Journal of Voice*, 14, 378–386.

Ishizaka, K. & Flanagan, J. L. (1972). Synthesis of voiced sounds from a two-mass model of the vocal cords. *Bell System Technical Journal*, 51, 1233–1268.

Isshiki, N., Okamura, H., Tanabe, M., & Morimoto, M. (1969). Differential diagnosis of hoarseness. *Folia Phoniatrica*, 21, 9–19.

Isshiki, N., Yanagihara, N., & Morimoto, M. (1966). Approach to the objective diagnosis of hoarseness. *Folia Phoniatrica*, 18, 393–400.

Kakita, Y., Hirano, M., & Ohmaru, K. (1981). Physical properties of the vocal fold tissue: measurements on excised larynges. In: K. N. Stevens & M. Hirano (eds) *Vocal Fold Physiology* (pp. 377–396). Tokyo: University of Tokyo Press.

Kempster, G. B., Gerratt, B. R., Verdolini Abbott, K., Barkmeier-Kraemer, J. M., & Hillman, R. E. (2009). Consensus auditory-perceptual evaluation of voice: development of a standardized clinical protocol. *American Journal of Speech-Language Pathology*, 18, 124–132.

Khosla, S., Muruguppan, S., & Gutmark, E. (2008). What can vortices tell us about vocal fold vibration and voice production? *Current Opinion in Otolaryngology Head and Neck Surgery*, 16, 183–187.

Kreiman, J. & Gerratt, B. R. (1996). The perceptual structure of pathologic voice quality. *Journal of the Acoustical Society of America*, 100, 1787–1795.

Kreiman, J. & Gerratt, B. R. (1998). Validity of rating scale measures of voice quality. *Journal of the Acoustical Society of America*, 104, 1598–1608.

Kreiman, J. & Gerratt, B. R. (2000). Sources of listener disagreement in voice quality assessment. *Journal of the Acoustical Society of America*, 108, 1867–1876.

Kreiman, J. & Gerratt, B. R. (2005). Perception of aperiodicity in pathological voice. *Journal of the Acoustical Society of America*, 117, 2201–2211.

Kreiman, J. & Gerratt, B. R. (2010). Perceptual sensitivity to first harmonic amplitude in the voice source. *Journal of the Acoustical Society of America*, 128, 2085–2089.

Kreiman, J. & Gerratt, B. R. (2012). Perceptual interactions of the harmonic source and noise in voice. *Journal of the Acoustical Society of America*, 131, 492–500.

Kreiman, J., Gerratt, B. R., & Antoñanzas-Barroso, N. (2007). Measures of the glottal source spectrum. *Journal of Speech, Language, and Hearing Research*, 50, 595–610.

Kreiman, J., Gerratt, B. R., Garellek, M., Samlan, R., & Zhang, Z. (2014). Toward a unified theory of voice production and perception. *Loquens: Spanish Journal of Speech Science*, 1, e009.

Kreiman, J., Gerratt, B. R., & Ito, M. (2007). When and why listeners disagree in voice quality assessment tasks. *Journal of the Acoustical Society of America*, 122, 2354–2364.

Kreiman, J., Gerratt, B. R., & Khan, S. D. (2010). Effects of native language on perception of voice quality. *Journal of Phonetics*, 38, 588–593.

Kreiman, J., Gerratt, B. R., & Precoda, K. (1990). Listener experience and perception of voice quality. *Journal of Speech and Hearing Research*, 33, 103–115.

Kreiman, J., Gerratt, B. R., Precoda, K., & Berke, G. S. (1992). Individual differences in voice quality perception. *Journal of Speech and Hearing Research*, 35, 512–520.

Kreiman, J., Gerratt, B. R., Signorello, R., & Rastifar, S. (2015). *Sufficiency of a four-parameter spectral model of the voice source*. Paper presented at the 169th Meeting of the Acoustical Society of America, May 2015.

Kreiman, J., Shue, Y-L., Chen, G., Iseli, M., Gerratt, B. R., Neubauer, J., & Alwan, A. (2012). Variability in the relationships among voice quality, harmonic amplitudes, open quotient, and glottal area waveform shape in sustained phonation. *Journal of the Acoustical Society of America*, 132, 2625–2632.

Kreiman, J. & Sidtis, D. (2011). *Foundations of Voice Studies*. Malden, MA: Wiley-Blackwell.

Krishnan, A., Swaminathan, J., & Gandour, J. T. (2009). Experience-dependent enhancement of linguistic pitch representation in the brainstem is not specific to a speech context. *Journal of Cognitive Neuroscience*, 21, 1092–1105.

Laver, J. (1980). *The Phonetic Description of Voice Quality*. Cambridge: Cambridge University Press.

Laver, J. (2000). Phonetic evaluation of voice quality. In: R. D. Kent & M. J. Ball (eds) *Voice Quality Measurement* (pp. 37–48). San Diego: Singular.

Laver, J., Wirz, S., Mackenzie, J., & Hiller, S. M. (1981). A perceptual protocol for the analysis of vocal profiles. *Edinburgh University Department of Linguistics Work in Progress*, 14, 139–155.

Llamas, C. & Watt, D. (eds) (2010). *Language and Identities*. Edinburgh: Edinburgh University Press.

Lucero, J. C., Schoentgen, J., & Behlau, M. (2013). Physics-based synthesis of disordered voices. *Proceedings of Interspeech*, 2013, 587–591.

Maibauer, A. M., Markis, T. A., Newell, J., & McLennan, C. T. (2014). Famous talker effects in spoken word recognition. *Attention, Perception, & Psychophysics*, 76, 11–18.

Maryn, Y., Corthals, P., Van Cauwenberge, P., Roy, N., & De Bodt, M. (2010). Toward improved ecological validity in the acoustic measurement of overall voice quality: combining continuous speech and sustained vowels. *Journal of Voice*, 24, 540–555.

Maryn, Y., De Bodt, M., & Roy, N. (2010). The Acoustic Voice Quality Index: toward improved treatment outcomes assessment in voice disorders. *Journal of Communication Disorders*, 43, 161–174.

Maryn, Y., Roy, N., De Bodt, M., Van Cauwenberge, P., & Corthals, P. (2009). Acoustic measurement of overall voice quality: a meta-analysis. *Journal of the Acoustical Society of America*, 126, 2619–2634.

Maryn, Y. & Weenink, D. (2015). Objective dysphonia measures in the program Praat: smoothed cepstral peak prominence and acoustic voice quality index. *Journal of Voice*, 29, 35–43.

Mau, T., Muhlestein, J., Callahan, S., & Chan, R. W. (2012). Modulating phonation through alteration of vocal fold medial surface contour. *Laryngoscope*, 122, 2005–2014.

Moore, P. (1938). Motion picture studies of the vocal folds and vocal attack. *Journal of Speech and Hearing Disorders*, 1, 235–240.

Moore, P. (1964). *Organic Voice Disorders*. Englewood Cliffs, NJ: Prentice-Hall.

Mullennix, J. W., Pisoni, D. B., & Martin, C. S. (1989). Some effects of talker variability on spoken word recognition. *Journal of the Acoustical Society of America*, 85, 365–378.

Nagle, K. F. (2016). Emerging scientist: challenges to CAPE-V as a standard. *Perspectives of the ASHA Special Interest Groups SIG* 3, Vol. 1(Part 2), 47–53.

Papcun, G., Kreiman, J., & Davis, A. (1989). Long-term memory for unfamiliar voices. *Journal of the Acoustical Society of America*, 85, 913–925.

Podesva, R. J. (2007). Phonation type as a stylistic variable: the use of falsetto in constructing a persona. *Journal of Sociolinguistics*, 11, 478–504.

Podesva, R. J. & Callier, P. (2015). Voice quality and identity. *Annual Review of Applied Linguistics*, 35, 173–194.

Poljac, E., de-Wit, L., & Wagemans, J. (2012). Perceptual wholes can reduce the conscious accessibility of their parts. *Cognition*, 123, 308–312.

Reber, S. A., Janisch, J., Torregrosa, K., Darlington, J., Vliet, K. A., & Fitch, W. T. (2017). Formants provide honest acoustic cues to body size in American alligators. *Scientific Reports* 7, article 1816.

Regner, M. F. & Jiang, J. J. (2011). Phonation threshold power in ex vivo laryngeal models. *Journal of Voice*, 25, 519–525.

Robinson, S. & Moore, P. (1965). 'Ooh, baby baby' [recorded by Smokey Robinson and the Miracles], on Going to a Go Go [record]. Detroit: Tamla/Motown.

Rothenberg, M. (1977). Measurement of airflow in speech. *Journal of Speech and Hearing Research*, 20, 155–176.

Sapir, E. (1927). Speech as a personality trait. *American Journal of Sociology*, 32, 892–905.

Schweinberger, S. R., Herholz, A., & Stief, V. (1997). Auditory long-term memory: repetition priming of voice recognition. *Quarterly Journal of Experimental Psychology: Section A— Human Experimental Psychology*, 50, 498–517.

Schweinberger, S. R., Kawahara, H., Simpson, A. P., Skuk, V. G., & Zäske, R. (2014). Speaker perception. *WIREs Cognitive Science*, 5, 15–25.

Shrivastav, R., Sapienza, C., & Nandur, V. (2005). Application of psychometric theory to the measurement of voice quality using rating scales. *Journal of Speech, Language, and Hearing Research*, 48, 323–335.

Starr, R. L. (2015). Sweet voice: the role of voice quality in a Japanese feminine style. *Language in Society*, 44, 1–34.

Sundberg, J. (1987). *The Science of the Singing Voice*. DeKalb, IL: Northern Illinois University Press.

van Bezooijen, R. (1995). Sociocultural aspects of pitch differences between Japanese and Dutch women. *Language and Speech*, 38, 253–265.

Warren, H. & Gordon, M. (1945). 'I wish I knew' [recorded by Jimmy Scott], on The Source (1969) [record]. Los Angeles: Atlantic.

Wirz, S. & Mackenzie Beck, J. (1995). Assessment of voice quality: the vocal profiles analysis scheme. In: S. Wirz (ed.) *Perceptual Approaches to Communication Disorders* (pp. 39–55). London: Whurr.

Wuyts, F. L., De Bodt, M. S., Molenberghs, G., Remacle, M., Heylen, L., Millet, B., . . . Van de Heyning, P. H. (2000). The dysphonia severity index: an objective measure of vocal quality based on a multiparameter approach. *Journal of Speech, Language, and Hearing Research*, 43, 796–809.

Xue, Q., Zheng, X., Mittal, R., & Bielamowicz, S. (2014). Computational study of effects of tension imbalance on phonation in a three-dimensional tubular larynx model. *Journal of Voice*, 28, 411–419.

Yuasa, I. P. (2008). *Culture and Gender of Voice Pitch*. London: Equinox.

Yuasa, I. P. (2010). Creaky voice: a new feminine voice quality for young urban-oriented upwardly mobile American women? *American Speech*, 85, 315–337.

Zäske, R., Schweinberger, S. R., & Kawahara, H. (2010). Voice aftereffects of adaptation to speaker identity. *Hearing Research*, 268, 38–45.

Zhang, Y., Huang, N., Calawerts, W., Li, L., Maytag, A. L., & Jiang, J. J. (2017). Quantifying the subharmonic mucosal wave in excised larynges via digital kymography. *Journal of Voice*, 31, 123.e7–123.e13.

Zhang, Z. (2016a). Cause-effect relationship between vocal fold physiology and voice production in a three-dimensional phonation model. *Journal of the Acoustical Society of America*, 139, 1493–1507.

Zhang, Z. (2016b). Mechanics of human voice production and control. *Journal of the Acoustical Society of America*, 140, 2614–2635.

Zhang, Z., Kreiman, J., Gerratt, B. R., & Garellek, M. (2013). Acoustic and perceptual effects of changes in body-layer stiffness in symmetric and asymmetric vocal fold models. *Journal of the Acoustical Society of America*, 133, 453–462.

Zraick, R. I., Kempster, G .B., Connor, N. P., Thibeault, S., Klaben, B. K., Bursac, Z., Thrush, C. R., & Glaze, L.E. (2011). Establishing validity of the Consensus Auditory Perceptual Evaluation of Voice (CAPE-V). *American Journal of Speech-Language Pathology*, 20, 14–22.

PART II

ONTOGENETIC
DEVELOPMENT OF
VOICE PERCEPTION

CHAPTER 9

VOICE PERCEPTION IN NEWBORNS AND INFANTS

NATACHA PAQUETTE,
EMMANUELLE DIONNE-DOSTIE,
MARYSE LASSONDE, AND ANNE GALLAGHER

9.1 INTRODUCTION

LIKE a fingerprint, our voice carries important signature information about our identity, gender, approximate age range, and affective state (Belin & Grosbras, 2010). Very early on, children develop the ability to perceive sounds and voices. These abilities are prerequisites for speech and language processing later in life (Belin & Grosbras, 2010). Interestingly, evidence of an evolutionary basis for voice processing has led to the identification of brain regions that show a sensitive response to species-specific vocalization in the macaque brain, located along the superior-temporal plane (Petkov et al., 2008, 2009). Recently, Andics et al. (2014) found evidence of a voice-related area in dogs, responding to both human and dog vocalizations, although stronger for conspecific dog vocalization within the bilateral ventral and left dorsal auditory regions. Similarly, in adult humans, voice perception is associated with activity in specific brain regions: bilaterally along the superior temporal sulcus (STS), with stronger activity in the right hemisphere (Belin et al., 2000, 2004). This region, called the temporal voice area (TVA), has been found to elicit greater neural activity in response to voice—both speech and non-speech—compared to non-vocal environmental sounds or scrambled speech (Belin et al., 2000).

In human infants, however, little is known about how voice perception abilities are developed or which brain regions are recruited in the early voice-processing stages. Nevertheless, recent studies have highlighted the joint influence of the genetic expression underlying structural auditory development and early *in utero* perceptual experience on the development of voice-processing ability in newborns and preverbal infants.

9.2 How Do Newborns and Preverbal Infants Perceive the Human Voice?

9.2.1 The Anatomical Basis of Auditory and Voice Perception

Human auditory development begins very early in fetal life and follows a rapid sequence of events that are crucial for the structural maturation of the cochlea (the organ that receives acoustic information) and the auditory cortex (see Table 9.1). The first trimester of pregnancy extends from the day of conception to the third month of gestation. During this time,

Table 9.1 Fetal auditory development steps

1st trimester (1 to 13 GW)	Days after conception	• Development of the inner ear begins.
	By 7–8 weeks	• All of the auditory centres and pathways within the brainstem are identifiable.
	Around 10–12 weeks	• Auditory synaptogenesis and differentiation of the hair cells begins.
2nd trimester (14 to 26 GW)	At the beginning of the trimester	• Rapid maturation occurs in the cochlea and the cochlear nerve.
	By 20 weeks	• The structural parts of the cochlea in the middle ear are functional.
	After 20 weeks	• Development of the neurosensory parts of the auditory system.
	By 22 weeks	• The process of myelination has begun within the cochlea.
	By 25 weeks	• The auditory system becomes functional.
	By the end of the trimester	• The main components of the brainstem pathways are identifiable.
3rd trimester (27 to 40 GW)	Around 25–27 weeks	• The earliest facial and body movement responses to sounds occur.
	At 27–29 weeks	• Evoked responses to in utero perceived sounds can be recorded (with loud stimuli and slow presentation rates).
	By 28–29 weeks	• Consistent movement responses to sounds.
	Around 28–30 weeks	• The neural connections to the temporal cortical areas are functional.
	At 32 weeks	• Cardiac orienting reflex to the mother's voice can be recorded with ultrasound (using speech stimuli).

GW = gestational weeks
(Graven & Browne, 2008b; Hall, 2000; Kisilevsky & Hains, 2011; Kisilevsky et al., 2000; Pujol & Hilding, 1973; Pujol & Lavigne-Rebillard, 1992)

the initial formation of the organ of Corti occurs, along with the inner and outer hair cells of the cochlea (Moore & Linthicum Jr, 2007). These hair cells convert the physical movements produced by sound vibrations into neural signals, which are transmitted from the cochlea to the auditory cortex via the cochlear nerve (Graven & Browne, 2008a; Hall, 2000; Moore & Linthicum Jr, 2007). The organ of Corti, the cochlea, and the cochlear nerve continue developing during the second trimester of pregnancy (fourth to sixth month). At around 25 to 29 weeks, the main components of the auditory pathways can be identified. By the end of the sixth month, the cochlea has established axonal connections between the inner ear, the brainstem, and the temporal auditory cortex. At this stage, the auditory system becomes functional, and the first evidence of fetal auditory perception can be observed using ultrasound imaging and fetal heart rate monitoring (Graven & Browne, 2008a). During the last trimester, from the seventh month of gestation to birth, the myelination process of the axonal connections initiates, allowing prompt transmission of auditory information, including the voice.

9.2.2 Behavioural Evidence of Fetal Voice Perception

It is thought that fetuses perceive external sounds through bone vibrations and fluids that are conducted from the skull to the inner ear (Sohmer et al., 2001). The earliest evidence of fetal auditory perception can be observed at around 25 to 26 gestational weeks by measuring behavioural changes such as variations in heart rate or body movements in response to loud sounds (Kisilevsky et al., 2000; Morris et al., 2000). Unborn infants are therefore exposed to *in utero* auditory stimulation. Even though the initial development of the basic structures responsible for auditory perception is governed by genetic expression, it is generally accepted that this early exposure allows the fetus to fine-tune the abilities to learn and to respond preferentially to certain auditory stimuli. This is known as an *epigenetic* process, or a process that alters gene activity without changing the DNA sequence, and leads to modifications that can be transmitted to daughter cells (Weinhold, 2006). In this case, the process is the impact of experience and exposure to certain stimuli (such as the mother's voice) on genetic expression and structural development (Graven & Browne, 2008a; Werker & Tees, 1999).

Supporting the epigenetic model, several studies have reported evidence of a voice-sensitive response in fetuses, newborns, and very young infants. The first indications of voice processing in fetuses came from ultrasound imaging studies that investigated heart-rate variations and body-movement patterns. Heart-rate changes, also called the cardiac orienting reflex, have been associated with stimulus-processing ability in fetuses, often elicited by low-intensity stimuli such as the average human voice (Groome et al., 1999, 2000; Lecanuet et al., 1988). However, most of these studies have used speech sounds, thus confounding voice and speech perception in fetuses. For instance, among the first to investigate the fetal response to voice and speech stimuli, Groome et al. (1999) found that from 36 to 40 weeks of gestation, fetal heart rate decelerates in response to speech sounds. More recently, Kisilevsky and Hains (2011) monitored fetal cardiac responses in 143 fetuses in four age groups (29–31, 32–34, 35–37, and more than 37 gestational weeks) while exposed to an audiotape of their mother reading a story segment. They found that the cardiac orienting reflex following the mother's voice onset could be reliably recorded starting at 32 gestation weeks. This heart-rate variability in response to sensory stimuli has been associated with attentional orientation response in infants and fetuses. For instance, Richards and Casey (1991) developed a model of heart-rate variability as an attentional response in infants. According to their model, the influence of attentional mechanisms on heart rate could be observed in distinct phases: 1) initial stimulus detection; 2) heart-rate variability in response to stimulus orientation; 3) sustained attention, characterized by a new, stable heart rate; and 4) declining attention, associated with a return to baseline heart rate.

In order to control for speech perception and to investigate, more specifically, fetus responses to voice, variations in fetal heart rate have also been measured when contrasting the fetal response to the mother's voice to an unfamiliar or the father's voice. For instance, Kisilevsky et al. (2003) measured increased heart rate in term fetuses when their mothers read a story segment. In contrast, when a stranger read the same segment, the fetal heart rate decreased. In a subsequent study, they compared fetal cardiac response to the recorded voices of the mother, the father, and a stranger (Kisilevsky et al., 2009). Results showed a stable fetal heart-rate increase in response to the mother's voice but not the father's or stranger's voice. Instead, fetuses responded at the outset of the father's and stranger's voice with a brief heart-rate increase before returning to baseline. Nevertheless, this suggests that the fetuses heard the voices, although they may not have recognized their father's voice. It was proposed that if fetuses have less exposure to the father's voice, they might need more time to process it compared to the mother's voice. In a replicated study, fetuses were systematically exposed to the father's voice 7 days prior to testing to ensure voice familiarity (Lee & Kisilevsky, 2014). Interestingly, results showed that fetuses responded similarly to both voices (father's and mother's), with a stable heart-rate increase followed by sustained responses throughout the audio recording period. Thus, near-term fetuses can learn and recognize familiar voices to which they are repeatedly exposed.

Overall, findings from studies that have investigated heart-rate variations and behavioural changes in fetuses suggest the presence of basic voice processing recognition such as attentional orientation, learning, and discrimination between familiar and unfamiliar voices.

9.2.3 Birth and Developmental Changes in the First Months of Life

9.2.3.1 *Behavioural Studies*

Most of the pioneering studies of voice perception ability at birth or in the first few months of life have used the high-amplitude-sucking procedure to measure infants' behavioural responses to a variety of auditory stimuli. This method involves presenting the infant with a frequent auditory stimulus while measuring the infant's sucking rate with a specifically designed pacifier (DeCasper & Fifer, 1980). Once the infant demonstrates familiarity, or habituation, with the stimulus by a sucking rate that declines to a preset level, a new set of stimuli is presented. If the infant can discriminate between the two stimuli, a significant change in the sucking rate should be observed (DeCasper & Prescott, 2009; Floccia et al., 2000; Shi et al., 1999). This procedure has allowed researchers to examine the basic cognitive processes as well as the neural networks involved in voice perception. For instance, Floccia et al. (2000) used this procedure with forty newborns while they were presented with a single disyllabic word, spoken by either a single speaker (an unfamiliar male or female) or by the two speakers (male and female) alternately. Their results showed significantly slower sucking rate in newborns presented with the same voice compared to alternated voices.

Interestingly, studies using this procedure have also shown that newborns can use prosodic and rhythmic information to discriminate between languages belonging to separate rhythmic classes, such as English and Japanese (Nazzi et al., 1998), or between two languages they have never heard before, such as French and Russian for American newborns, or English and Italian for French newborns (Mehler et al., 1988). In addition, according to this paradigm, Shi et al. (1999) found that 1- to 3-day-old newborns could use perceptual acoustic cues in voices as well as phonological and rhythmic indices to discriminate between lists of either grammatical or lexical English words. The ability to discriminate between voices and rhythmic information in perceived vocalization very early in life is particularly relevant for the understanding of language acquisition later on. Thus, voice processing is the initial step in learning increasingly complex phonemic and linguistic information in the first months of life.

9.2.3.2 *Neuroimaging and Electroencephalography*

In recent years, the development of neuroimaging techniques such as functional magnetic resonance imaging (fMRI), functional near-infrared spectroscopy (fNIRS), and electrophysiological (EEG) recording have made it possible to assess, non-invasively, brain activity associated with voice and speech processing in infants, without requiring sustained attention or a specific response (see Table 9.2). Accordingly, Beauchemin et al. (2011) used EEG and distributed source analyses to investigate newborns' cortical responses to a voice that was familiar (the mother's), less familiar (the attending nurse's), or unfamiliar. To evoke voice-specific responses, newborns were presented with a short auditory stimulus: the vowel /a/ as in the French word 'allô', spoken by the mother, the nurse, or a female stranger. Results revealed a greater overall discriminative response for the mother's voice than for the two other voices, indicating a significant preferential response to the mother's voice. Figure 9.1 illustrates the source distribution of the activation recorded in response to the mother's and the unfamiliar (the nurse's) voices at four different time points after the stimulus presentation (100 ms, 200 ms, 300 ms, and 525 ms). Interestingly, cerebral source analysis revealed that the newborn's responses to the mother's and the unfamiliar voices were processed in spatially distinct brain areas. Thus, the mother's voice elicited a strong initial activation in the left temporal region, known to be related to language processing later in life. Conversely, unfamiliar voices were preferentially processed in the right temporal region, known to be slightly more lateralized than the left hemisphere in response to voice, at least in adults (Belin et al., 2000, 2002; Pernet et al., 2015). This study was the first to show that newborns process their mother's voice and unfamiliar voices in distinct cortical areas. These results also concur with findings from behavioural studies indicating that infants are better at discriminating phonemes or words spoken by their mothers over an unfamiliar speaker (Barker & Newman, 2004; Liu et al., 2003).

Other recent infant neuroimaging studies have also supported the hypothesis that the speaker's characteristics and voice familiarity could impact speech-processing development in infants. Dehaene-Lambertz et al. (2010) found significant hemispheric asymmetry in 2-month-old infants when listening to speech segments spoken by their mother and a stranger, in favour of the left planum temporale for both conditions. However, when compared to the stranger's voice, the mother's voice elicited stronger activation of the bilateral anterior prefrontal cortex and the left posterior temporal region. Contrary to Beauchemin et al. (2010), the difference between the mother's and the stranger's voice was not significant in the right superior temporal

Table 9.2 Main behavioural, EEG, and brain imaging evidence of voice processing in infants

Age range	Technique	Main findings	Reference
Neonates	Behavioural	• Slower sucking rates when presented with the same voice compared to alternated voices. • Preferential response to words spoken by their mother vs a stranger.	Barker & Newman (2004); Liu et al. (2003)
	EEG	• Spatially distinct and greater overall response for the mother's voice vs the stranger's voice.	Beauchemin et al. (2010)
	EEG	• Happy and fearful syllables elicit higher activation than neutral tone and non-vocal stimuli in the right hemisphere. • Fearful syllables elicit stronger mismatch than happy syllables bilaterally over the frontal regions.	Cheng et al. (2012)
	fNIRS	• Significant haemodynamic concentration increase over the bilateral frontal regions at the beginning of normal-pitched story segment, but not for monotonous flat-pitch segments.	Saito et al. (2007)
3 months	fNIRS	• Greater activation of the right temporo-parietal region in response to unaltered sentences compared to flattened speech.	Homae et al. (2006)
3–7 months	fMRI	• Neutral and emotional vocalizations elicit higher activation than environmental sounds within the right frontal and temporal gyri. • Sad vocalizations elicit activation in regions known to be involved in emotional speech processing (left orbitofrontal and insular cortex).	Blasi et al. (2011)
4–7 months	fNIRS	• The strength of the voice-selective response in the right STS correlates significantly with the infant's age.	Lloyd-Fox et al. (2012)
7 months	EEG	• Stronger reaction to negative (angry voice) than positive or neutral voice stimuli (higher EEG amplitude).	Grossmann et al. (2005)
	fNIRS	• Angry prosody elicits higher activation over the posterior portion of the right temporal area, while happy prosody elicits higher activation over the right inferior frontal region. • The activation recorded in the right temporal cortex is larger in response to angry compared to happy prosody.	Grossmann et al. (2010)
	fNIRS	• An adult-like haemodynamic response is observed in the right anterior temporal region in response to human vocalizations.	Grossmann et al. (2010)
9 months	EEG	• Processing of emotional vocal information is modulated by visual cues on corresponding face stimuli.	Otte et al. (2015)
12 months	Behavioural	• Infants can adjust their emotional behaviours based on emotional vocal stimuli, and can determine other's voice direction without needing visual cues.	Rossano et al. (2012); Vaish & Striano (2004)

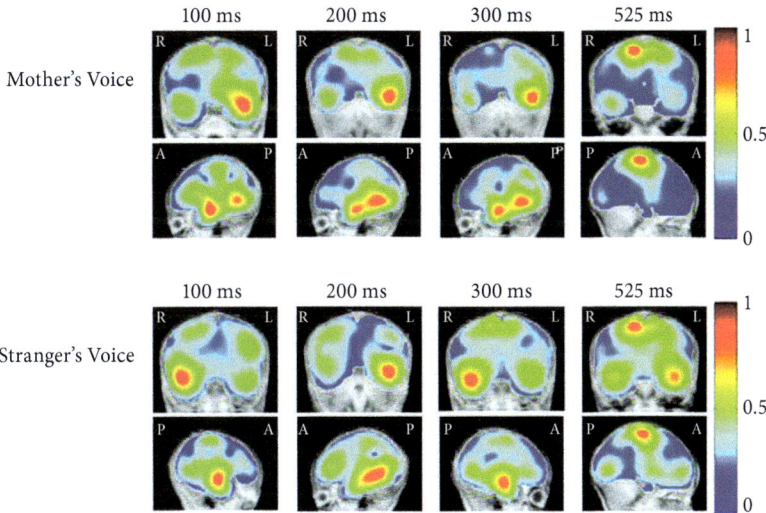

FIGURE 9.1 Coronal and sagittal representations of the sources' distribution of the activation recorded in response to the mother's (top) and the unfamiliar (bottom) voices. The orientation of the sagittal plane (anterior (A)/posterior (P)) varies in order to reflect the lateralization of the activation in the corresponding hemisphere.

Reprinted from Beauchemin M. et al., 'Mother and Stranger: An Electrophysiological Study of Voice Processing in Newborns', *Cerebral Cortex*, Volume 21, Issue 8, Figure 3, pp. 1705–11, Copyright © 2010, doi: 10.1093/cercor/bhq242, by permission of Oxford University Press.

sulcus (STS). These results are most likely due to the processing of full speech segments as opposed to a single vowel. In addition, the two studies used very different neuroimaging techniques (fMRI vs. EEG). Nevertheless, the results suggest that phonetic and speech processing in very young infants is sensitive to the speaker's characteristics as well as voice familiarity.

Grossmann et al. (2010) used fNIRS to determine the emergence of the voice-sensitive area in 4- and 7-month-olds who were presented with vocal (words and non-words) and non-vocal (nature, animal, musical, and environmental) sounds. They found a significantly higher haemodynamic oxyhaemoglobin response in bilateral posterior areas of the temporal cortex in response to the human voice compared to non-vocal sounds. However, this activation pattern was not observed in 4-month-olds, who showed a greater haemodynamic response to non-vocal sounds in the anterior right temporal region. The authors suggested that the voice-sensitive response could still be immature in 4-month-olds, whereas 7-month-olds showed a more adult-like response to voice. It should be noted that the voice stimuli included both speech (words and non-words) and non-speech human vocalizations, whereas the non-voice stimuli included both familiar and unfamiliar sounds. It is possible that the combination of familiar and unfamiliar non-vocal stimuli, as well as using both words and non-words as vocal stimuli, could have generated unspecific activation in the youngest group. To examine this possibility, Lloyd-Fox et al. (2012) also investigated 4- and 7-month-old infants' responses to voice and non-voice stimuli, but using only non-speech voice (e.g. crying, laughing, coughing, yawning) and more familiar non-voice stimuli (naturalistic environmental sounds such as rattling or squeaky toys, running water). Their results revealed that for children of all ages taken together, the posterior portion of the STS showed greater bilateral activation in response to familiar non-voice stimuli, whereas voice stimuli elicited greater activation in the anterior portion of the left STS only. Furthermore, a significant correlation was found between the strength of the voice-selective response in the right STS and the infant's age, suggesting that the cerebral specialization for voice processing becomes more robust in the right hemisphere as the infant's brain develops and the cortical response to different stimulation becomes more specialized.

Similarly, Minagawa-Kawai et al. (2011) analysed native and non-native speech responses in 4-month-olds, along with their responses to three non-speech conditions (emotional human vocalizations, primate vocalizations, and scrambled sounds of all conditions). Results revealed similar patterns of activation within the perisylvian regions for speech and non-speech vocal sounds. However, haemodynamic oxyhaemoglobin responses to the speech (native and non-native) and scramble conditions were lateralized to the left hemisphere, while responses to non-speech vocal condition (human emotional vocalizations) were located within superior temporal regions of the right hemisphere. In contrast, the monkey calls elicited bilateral activations within the temporal regions. Hence, as in adult humans, structural and functional hemispheric asymmetry has often been reported in infant voice perception.

In sum, the debate continues as to whether right cerebral specialization for voice processing is already present in newborns and very young infants. Methodological differences between studies could partially account for the inconsistent results. Differences include familiar and unfamiliar non-vocal sounds as control stimuli, speech and non-speech vocalizations, as well as disparities in the temporal and spatial resolution of the brain-imaging techniques used. That said, the reviewed literature has highlighted the impact of familiarity and emotional information (or prosodic content) on the infant's behavioural and cerebral responses to voice. Infants' perceptions of emotional prosody therefore play a crucial role in social and language development. The next section of this chapter focuses more specifically on how infants process emotional prosody in speech and vocalizations.

9.3 How Do Infants Learn to Extract Social Meaning from Perceived Vocalizations?

Emotional prosody refers to non-verbal cues in vocal expression that communicate information about the speaker's affective state. Prosodic information includes voice intonation (pitch), loudness, pauses, and rhythms (Cutler et al., 1997). The processing of this information has been frequently associated with activation in the right hemisphere in adults, whereas the processing of spectrotemporal changes in pitch and speech sound has been associated with the left hemisphere (Schönwiesner et al., 2007; Zatorre et al., 1992, 2002). Interestingly, neuroimaging studies in adults have shown that the temporal voice area (TVA; Belin et al., 2002) is also associated with the processing of strong-intensity emotional prosody (Beaucousin et al., 2007; Ethofer et al., 2006; Grandjean et al., 2005).

Prosodic processing has been examined in infants using normally spoken speech contrasted with speech with flattened pitch contour, which modifies the sentences' prosodic properties. For instance, in an fNIRS study, full-term newborns were presented with normally pitched and flat-pitched story segments (Saito et al., 2007). Significant increase in the haemodynamic oxyhaemoglobin concentration was observed over the left and right frontal regions at the beginning of the normal pitch condition, but not for the monotonous flat-pitch condition. Moreover, greater activation of the right temporo-parietal regions was also found in quietly sleeping 3-month-olds in response to unaltered sentences compared to flattened speech, suggesting that this region might already be responsive to prosodic processing (Homae et al., 2006). Conversely, in a subsequent study, they found significantly higher activation of the right temporo-parietal and bilateral prefrontal regions in 10-month-olds in response to flattened speech compared to the unaltered speech condition (Homae et al., 2007).

To explain these contrasting results, the authors suggested that the unfamiliarity of the flattened speech induced an additional demand in these cortical regions in older infants. Specifically, speech processing in the infant brain would progress from analysing basic acoustic and pitch information in 3-month-olds to the attentional mechanism modulation involved in comparing and integrating prosodic structures in 10-month-olds. Nevertheless, the cerebral mechanisms responsible for prosodic processing appear to differ or undergo developmental changes between 3 and 10 months of age. Taken together, these studies demonstrated that infants can discriminate prosodic patterns very early in life, and that they respond differentially to pitch variability compared with monotonous speech. However, further investigation is needed to clarify the developmental patterns of speech variability over monotonous flattened speech in the first year of life.

In an EEG experiment, Grossmann et al. (2005) presented words with an angry, happy, or neutral prosody to 7-month-olds to investigate the effect of emotional prosody on voice and speech processing. Results showed that words spoken with an angry voice elicited responses of higher amplitude than words spoken with a happy or neutral tone, suggesting that infants are liable to react more strongly to negative than positive or neutral voice stimuli. The greater response to negative stimuli might be indicative of an evolutionary 'negative bias', as suggested by Vaish et al. (2008). Specifically, as in animals and human adults, infants' propensity to pay attention to and process negative information is fundamental for social and adaptive development. It allows them to learn and to respond quickly to potential danger (Ohman et al., 2001).

In 2010, the same group used fNIRS to further investigate the cerebral network underlying this response in 7-month-olds (Grossmann et al., 2010). They found that happy and angry prosody elicited a significant haemodynamic oxyhaemoglobin increase over the right temporal region, albeit spatially distinct. Whereas angry prosody elicited higher activation over the posterior portion of the right temporal region, happy prosody elicited higher activation over the right inferior frontal region. The activation recorded in the right temporal cortex was larger in response to angry compared to happy prosody. These findings support the notion that the temporal voice area specializes in processing emotional prosody very early in infancy. They also showed that negative and positive prosody differentially impact voice processing within the right hemisphere, supporting the emerging body of evidence for the ontogenetic evolution of a negativity bias in infants (Vaish et al., 2008).

Also supporting this negative bias, Blasi et al. (2011) presented 3- to 7-month-olds with positive, negative, and neutral non-speech vocalizations as well as non-vocal environmental sounds during fMRI recording. Initially they found that, compared to environmental sounds, neutral and emotional vocalizations elicited higher activation in the right frontal and temporal gyri. Sad vocalizations also elicited activation in the left orbitofrontal and insular cortex, known to be involved in emotional processing of speech. In contrast, activation elicited by happy vocalizations did not differ from that elicited by neutral vocalizations. In another recent study, Cheng et al. (2012) measured EEG mismatch responses (corresponding to changes detected in the auditory environment) elicited by the syllables 'dada' spoken with a fearful, happy, or neutral tone and by synthesized non-vocal stimuli in full-term newborns aged 1 to 5 days. In a first experiment, happily uttered syllables elicited a stronger mismatch response than non-vocal sounds, and this response was lateralized to the right hemisphere. In a second experiment, fearful compared to neutral and happy syllables elicited a stronger response in the right hemisphere. Figure 9.2 illustrates the EEG response to emotionally spoken (fearful and happy) and neutral syllables in neonates.

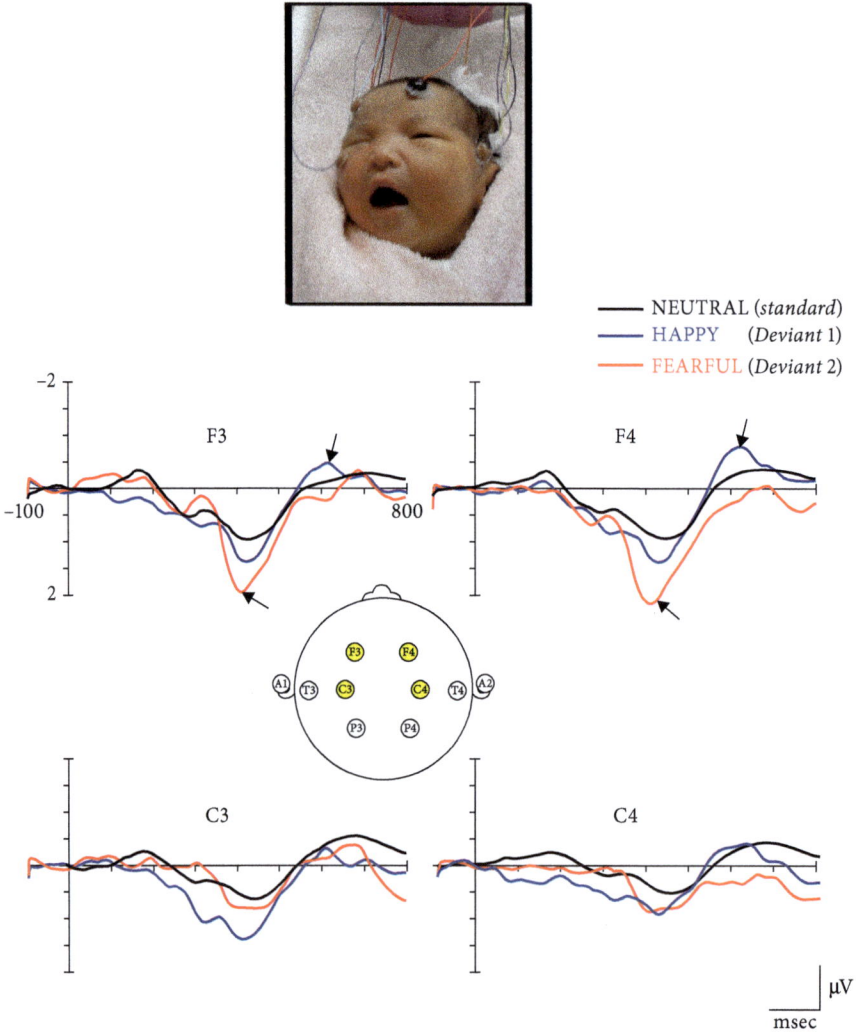

FIGURE 9.2 Average mismatch responses to neutral (black line), happy (blue line), and fearful (red line) syllables in forty-three neonates during an EEG experiment. Negative voltages are plotted up, positive voltages are plotted down. Fearful syllables, compared to neutral, elicited a stronger positive response over the frontal and central regions within the right hemisphere (electrodes F4 and C4). Significant difference between happy and fearful syllables occurred over the right frontal region (electrode F4).

Reproduced from Cheng Y. et al., ' Voice and Emotion Processing in the Human Neonatal Brain', *Journal of Cognitive Neuroscience*, Volume 24, Issue 6, pp. 1411–9, Copyright © 2012 Massachusetts Institute of Technology, doi: 10.1162/jocn_a_00214, reprinted by permission of MIT Press Journals.

Taken together, these findings confirm that even a few days after birth, the infant's brain shows a preference for the human voice and emotional prosody processing. However, although most studies support early specialization for voice and prosody processing in the right hemisphere, the debate continues as to whether or not these abilities are due to early specialization of the neural networks in the infant's brain. Furthermore, little is known to date on how infants use the social and prosodic information transmitted by voice and speech stimuli to learn about their social environment and adjust to it. Nevertheless, developmental studies have clarified the influence of social stimuli and context on learning. For instance, it has been suggested that infants between 9 and 10 months of age can learn and discriminate phonetics in a foreign language as long as the learning sessions are supported by interpersonal interaction, as opposed to exposure to recorded audio tapes only (Kuhl et al., 2003). Additionally, Reeb-Sutherland et al. (2011) recently showed that 1-month-olds who performed an associative learning task showed improved performance when they were exposed to social (a female voice) versus non-social (tone or backward voice) auditory stimuli in a modified eye-blink paradigm. Although more evidence is needed to fully understand how the developing child uses this information in the first few years of life, these results suggest that infants can learn more easily in socially and ecologically meaningful settings.

9.4 FROM VOICE PERCEPTION TO LANGUAGE ACQUISITION: WHAT ARE THE MAJOR DEVELOPMENTAL STEPS?

We have reviewed the literature on the early perception and processing of vocal inputs in fetuses, newborns, and infants. Cognitive and linguistic development is grounded on early sensory experience. The nature of this experience is therefore likely to have long-lasting effects on cognition and language acquisition. Although questions remain as to whether the neural networks underlying these abilities are already specialized in the first few months of life, it is well recognized that these basic auditory skills are a prerequisite for subsequent speech processing and further language development. Specifically, when young infants start learning word forms, they encode not only the word, but also the properties of the speaker's voice, such as the prosody, pitch, and affect that are transmitted (Houston & Jusczyk, 2000). During the first months of life, this process becomes rapidly language-specific as infants start paying attention to phonemes and words that are relevant to their own language. With exposure and experience, they learn that the phonetic information (such as voice onset time and phonemic category boundary) indicates the word's semantic and lexical identity better than the voice characteristics do (Werker & Curtin, 2005). Hence, in this section of the chapter, we briefly describe how infants use these vocal cues to learn language, as well as the major steps in this acquisition process.

9.4.1 Early Phoneme Discrimination and Perceptual Narrowing

From birth, infants have a propensity to attend to vocal and speech sounds over non-speech, and they continue to show this preference over the next several months (Vouloumanos &

Werker, 2004, 2007). During the first months of life, infants can also discriminate speech–sound differences between rhythmically different languages (Werker & Tees, 2002). Furthermore, recent neuroimaging studies indicate that young infants and newborns show a preference for their native language over rhythmically different non-native languages (Minagawa-Kawai et al., 2011; Peña et al., 2010; Sato et al., 2012; Vannasing et al., 2016). This discriminative sensitivity is probably due to the different rhythmic properties of speech, and it is preserved even when phonological cues other than rhythm are removed from the stimuli (Ramus et al., 2000, 2002). Moreover, studies of speech perception in monolingual infants have shown that the ability to differentiate between native and foreign speech sounds improves with exposure and experience (Bosch & Sebastián-Gallés, 2001; Kuhl et al., 2006; Sundara et al., 2006; Tsao et al., 2006).

The infant's ability to distinguish between sounds in a foreign language declines in the second half of the first year (Best & McRoberts, 2003; Kuhl et al., 2006; Kuhl & Rivera-Gaxiola, 2008; Werker & Curtin, 2005). For instance, in a high-amplitude sucking and head-turning paradigm, 4-month-old Japanese babies distinguished between the /r/ and /l/ sounds as reliably as 4-month-olds raised in English-speaking households (Purves et al., 2001). At around ages 10 to 12 months, infants living in English-speaking households, who are consistently exposed to English, become better at detecting the difference between the /r/ and /l/ sounds, which are prevalent in the English language. In contrast, at the same age, Japanese and Hindi babies, with less exposure to these sounds, decline in their ability to detect them (for a review, see Kuhl, 2004; Werker & Tees, 2002).

This dynamic could be explained by the perceptual narrowing that infants show around the end of the first year of life. Throughout this learning process, the sensitivity to vocal cues and phonetic information that are not featured in the child's linguistic and social environment gradually declines. Early experience with different languages therefore has lasting effects on speech perception. For instance, compared to monolingual infants, bilingual-learning infants take longer to establish phonetic categorical boundaries for their native language (Bosch & Sebastián-Gallés, 2001; Kuhl & Rivera-Gaxiola, 2008). Nevertheless, recent studies have also shown that although phonetic discrimination is less mature in bilingual infants aged 6 to 9 months than in same-aged monolingual infants, bilingual infants show increasing ability to discriminate between phonetic units in both languages with increasing age (Garcia-Sierra et al., 2011; Petitto et al., 2012; Rivera-Gaxiola et al., 2005). Infants raised in a multilingual environment therefore appear to benefit from an extended period of sensitivity to learn different languages.

9.5 CONCLUSION

Whereas most previous developmental studies have investigated speech and language processing, very few have focused on the anatomical and functional specificity of voice processing in infants. However, it is now well recognized that language acquisition as well as social development require adequate perceptual skills, and more particularly, voice perception and processing abilities in early infancy. In order to understand how infants learn social cues from perceived vocalization, the initial perceptual abilities that emerge in the late stages of fetal life and early infancy need to be considered, along with the age-related changes associated with speech processing within the first year of life. This chapter was motivated by three critical questions: (1) What are the underlying mechanisms of human voice perception in newborns and young infants? (2) How can infants extract and learn or process socially relevant information from perceived vocalizations? (3) What are the major developmental phases of these learning processes, particularly for language acquisition?

One conclusion that can be drawn from this review is that late prenatal and early postnatal auditory experience helps tune and shape the initial stages of voice perception and speech acquisition. Thus, fetuses and newborns show heightened interest toward social stimuli such as their mother's voice or emotionally charged speech stimuli compared to familiar non-vocal stimuli such as environmental sounds. However, investigations in infants of the cerebral basis for voice perception and the neural networks involved have yielded mixed results, and the developmental mechanisms underlying the functional and structural cerebral specialization for voice processing in infants remain controversial. Although voice-selective specialization may vary considerably across young infants, many researchers have hypothesized that this response becomes more robust by the second half of the first year, especially within the right hemisphere (Lloyd-Fox et al., 2012). Additionally, methodological differences across studies such as stimulus type and familiarity (e.g. speech versus non-speech vocal stimuli), control conditions, paradigms, and imaging techniques, as well as the infant's age, could have produced conflicting results on the lateralization and specialization of a cerebral voice area in infants. Further investigations, particularly with cross-sectional or preferably longitudinal designs, could help clarify the comparative contribution of these factors.

Another significant conclusion that we may draw from this review is that infants show an early preference for social and familiar stimuli. It has been hypothesized that this preference might be the result of an evolutionary process, such that humans are more liable to treat social and familiar stimuli more favourably. Early exposure to human voices and the infant's abilities to process prosodic, phonetic, and familiar information in vocalization help establish the neural basis for language development. Nevertheless, despite recent findings, relatively little is known about the cerebral processing of voice sounds in infancy. Understanding how the infant's brain processes vocal and linguistic information requires an integrative approach that combines evidence from genetic, behavioural, structural, and functional brain imaging areas.

REFERENCES

Andics, A., Gácsi, M., Faragó, T., Kis, A., & Miklósi, A. (2014). Voice-sensitive regions in the dog and human brain are revealed by comparative fMRI. *Current Biology*, 24(5), 574–578. doi: 10.1016/j.cub.2014.01.058

Barker, B. & Newman, R. (2004). Listen to your mother! The role of talker familiarity in infant streaming. *Cognition*, 94(2), B45–B53. http://doi.org/10.1016/j.cognition.2004.06.001

Beauchemin, M., González-Frankenberger, B., Tremblay, J., Vannasing, P., Martínez-Montes, E., Belin, P., … Lassonde, M. (2011). Mother and stranger: an electrophysiological study of voice processing in newborns. *Cerebral Cortex*, 21(8), 1705–1711. http://doi.org/10.1093/cercor/bhq242

Beaucousin, V., Lacheret, A., Turbelin, M.-R., Morel, M., Mazoyer, B., & Tzourio-Mazoyer, N. (2007). FMRI study of emotional speech comprehension. *Cerebral Cortex*, 17(2), 339–352. http://doi.org/10.1093/cercor/bhj151

Belin, P. & Grosbras, M. H. (2010). Before speech: cerebral voice processing in infants. *Neuron*, 65, 733–735. http://doi.org/10.1016/j.neuron.2010.03.018

Belin, P., Zatorre, R. J., & Ahad, P. (2002). Human temporal-lobe response to vocal sounds. *Cognitive Brain Research*, 13(1), 17–26. Retrieved from http://www.ncbi.nlm.nih.gov/pubmed/11867247

Belin, P., Zatorre, R. J., Lafaille, P., Ahad, P., & Pike, B. (2000). Voice-selective areas in human auditory cortex. *Nature*, 403(6767), 309–12. http://doi.org/10.1038/35002078

Best, C. & McRoberts, G. W. (2003). Infant perception of non-native consonant contrasts that adults assimilate in different ways. *Language and Speech*, 46(Pt 2–3), 183–216. http://doi.org/10.1177/00238309030460020701

Blasi, A., Mercure, E., Lloyd-Fox, S., Thomson, A., Brammer, M., Sauter, D., … Murphy, D. G. M. (2011). Early specialization for voice and emotion processing in the infant brain. *Current Biology*, 21(14), 1220–1224. http://doi.org/10.1016/j.cub.2011.06.009

Bosch, L. & Sebastián-Gallés, N. (2001). Evidence of early language discrimination abilities in infants from bilingual environments. *Infancy*, 2(1), 29–49. http://doi.org/10.1207/S15327078IN0201_3

Cheng, Y., Lee, S.-Y., Chen, H.-Y., Wang, P.-Y., & Decety, J. (2012). Voice and emotion processing in the human neonatal brain. *Journal of Cognitive Neuroscience*, 24, 1411–1419. http://doi.org/10.1162/jocn_a_00214

Cutler, A., Dahan, D., & van Donselaar, W. (1997). Prosody in the comprehension of spoken language: a literature review. *Language and Speech*, 40(Pt 2), 141–201. http://doi.org/10.1177/002383099704000203

DeCasper, A. J. & Fifer, W. P. (1980). Of human bonding: newborns prefer their mothers' voices. *Science*, 208(4448), 1174–1176. http://doi.org/10.1126/science.7375928

DeCasper, A. J. & Prescott, P. (2009). Lateralized processes constrain auditory reinforcement in human newborns. *Hearing Research*, 255(1–2), 135–141. http://doi.org/10.1016/j.heares.2009.06.012

Dehaene-Lambertz, G., Montavont, A., Jobert, A., Allirol, L., Dubois, J., Hertz-Pannier, L., & Dehaene, S. (2010). Language or music, mother or Mozart? Structural and environmental influences on infants' language networks. *Brain and Language*, 114(2), 53–65. http://doi.org/10.1016/j.bandl.2009.09.003

Ethofer, T., Anders, S., Wiethoff, S., Erb, M., Herbert, C., Saur, R., … Wildgruber, D. (2006). Effects of prosodic emotional intensity on activation of associative auditory cortex. *NeuroReport*, 17(3), 249–253. http://doi.org/10.1097/01.wnr.0000199466.32036.5d

Floccia, C., Nazzi, T., & Bertoncini, J. (2000). Unfamiliar voice discrimination for short stimuli in newborns. *Developmental Science*, 3(3), 333–343. http://doi.org/10.1111/1467-7687.00128

Garcia-Sierra, A., Rivera-Gaxiola, M., Percaccio, C. R., Conboy, B. T., Romo, H., Klarman, L., … Kuhl, P. K. (2011). Bilingual language learning: an ERP study relating early brain responses to speech, language input, and later word production. *Journal of Phonetics*, 39(4), 546–557. http://doi.org/10.1016/j.wocn.2011.07.002

Grandjean, D., Sander, D., Pourtois, G., Schwartz, S., Seghier, M. L., Scherer, K. R., & Vuilleumier, P. (2005). The voices of wrath: brain responses to angry prosody in meaningless speech. *Nature Neuroscience*, 8(2), 145–146. http://doi.org/10.1038/nn1392

Graven, S. N. & Browne, J. V. (2008a). Auditory development in the fetus and infant. *Newborn and Infant Nursing Reviews*, 8, 187–193. http://doi.org/10.1053/j.nainr.2008.10.010

Graven, S. N. & Browne, J. V. (2008b). Sleep and brain development. *Newborn and Infant Nursing Reviews*, 8(4), 173–179. http://doi.org/10.1053/j.nainr.2008.10.008

Groome, L. J., Mooney, D. M., Holland, S. B., Smith, L. A., Atterbury, J. L., & Dykman, R. A. (1999). Behavioral state affects heart rate response to low-intensity sound in human fetuses. *Early Human Development*, 54(1), 39–54. http://doi.org/10.1016/S0378-3782(98)00083-8

Groome, L. J., Mooney, D. M., Holland, S. B., Smith, Y. D., Atterbury, J. L., & Dykman, R. A. (2000). Temporal pattern and spectral complexity as stimulus parameters for eliciting a cardiac orienting reflex in human fetuses. *Perception & Psychophysics*, 62(2), 313–320. http://doi.org/10.3758/BF03205551

Grossmann, T., Oberecker, R., Koch, S. P., & Friederici, A. D. (2010). The developmental origins of voice processing in the human brain. *Neuron*, 65(6), 852–858. http://doi.org/10.1016/j.neuron.2010.03.001

Grossmann, T., Striano, T., & Friederici, A. D. (2005). Infants' electric brain responses to emotional prosody. *NeuroReport*, 16(16), 1825–1828. http://doi.org/10.1097/01.wnr.0000185964.34336.b1

Hall, J. W. (2000). Development of the ear and hearing. *Journal of Perinatology: Official Journal of the California Perinatal Association*, 20(8 Pt 2), S12–S20. http://doi.org/10.1038/sj.jp.7200439

Homae, F., Watanabe, H., Nakano, T., Asakawa, K., & Taga, G. (2006). The right hemisphere of sleeping infant perceives sentential prosody. *Neuroscience Research*, 54(4), 276–280. http://doi.org/10.1016/j.neures.2005.12.006

Homae, F., Watanabe, H., Nakano, T., & Taga, G. (2007). Prosodic processing in the developing brain. *Neuroscience Research*, 59, 29–39. http://doi.org/10.1016/j.neures.2007.05.005

Houston, D. M. & Jusczyk, P. W. (2000). The role of talker-specific information in word segmentation by infants. *Journal of Experimental Psychology. Human Perception and Performance*, 26(5), 1570–1582. http://doi.org/10.1037/0096-1523.26.5.1570

Kisilevsky, B. S. & Hains, S. M. J. (2011). Onset and maturation of fetal heart rate response to the mother's voice over late gestation. *Developmental Science*, 14(2), 214–223. http://doi.org/10.1111/j.1467-7687.2010.00970.x

Kisilevsky, B. S., Hains, S. M. J., Brown, C. A., Lee, C. T., Cowperthwaite, B., Stutzman, S. S., … Wang, Z. (2009). Fetal sensitivity to properties of maternal speech and language. *Infant Behavior and Development*, 32, 59–71. http://doi.org/10.1016/j.infbeh.2008.10.002

Kisilevsky, B. S., Hains, S. M. J., Lee, K., Xie, X., Huang, H., Ye, H. H., … Wang, Z. (2003). Effects of experience on fetal voice recognition. *Psychological Science*, 14(3), 220–224.

Kisilevsky, B. S., Pang, L., & Hains, S. M. J. (2000). Maturation of human fetal responses to airborne sound in low- and high-risk fetuses. *Early Human Development*, 58, 179–195. http://doi.org/10.1016/S0378-3782(00)00075-X

Kuhl, P. K. (2004). Early language acquisition: cracking the speech code. *Nature Reviews: Neuroscience*, 5(11), 831–43. http://doi.org/10.1038/nrn1533

Kuhl, P. K., Stevens, E., Hayashi, A., Deguchi, T., Kiritani, S., & Iverson, P. (2006). Infants show a facilitation effect for native language phonetic perception between 6 and 12 months. *Developmental Science*, 9(2), F13–F21. http://doi.org/10.1111/j.1467-7687.2006.00468.x

Kuhl, P. K., Tsao, F.-M.-M., & Liu, H.-M.-M. (2003). Foreign-language experience in infancy: effects of short-term exposure and social interaction on phonetic learning. *Proceedings of the National Academy of Sciences of the United States of America*, 100(15), 9096–101. http://doi.org/10.1073/pnas.1532872100

Kuhl, P. & Rivera-Gaxiola, M. (2008). Neural substrates of language acquisition. *Annual Review of Neuroscience*, 31, 511–534. http://doi.org/10.1146/annurev.neuro.30.051606.094321

Lecanuet, J. P., Granier-Deferre, C., & Busnel, M. C. (1988). Fetal cardiac and motor responses to octave-band noises as a function of central frequency, intensity and heart rate variability. *Early Human Development*, 18(2–3), 81–93. http://doi.org/10.1016/0378-3782(88)90045-X

Lee, G. Y. & Kisilevsky, B. S. (2014). Fetuses respond to father's voice but prefer mother's voice after birth. *Developmental Psychobiology*, 56, 1–11. http://doi.org/10.1002/dev.21084

Liu, H. M., Kuhl, P. K., & Tsao, F. M. (2003). An association between mothers' speech clarity and infants' speech discrimination skills. *Developmental Science*, 6(3), 1–10. http://doi.org/10.1111/1467-7687.00275

Lloyd-Fox, S., Blasi, A., Mercure, E., Elwell, C. E., & Johnson, M. H. (2012). The emergence of cerebral specialization for the human voice over the first months of life. *Social Neuroscience*, 7(3), 317–330. http://doi.org/10.1080/17470919.2011.614696

Mehler, J., Jusczyk, P., Lambertz, G., Halsted, N., Bertoncini, J., & Amiel-Tison, C. (1988). A precursor of language acquisition in young infants. *Cognition*, 29(2), 143–178. http://doi.org/10.1016/0010-0277(88)90035-2

Minagawa-Kawai, Y., van der Lely, H., Ramus, F., Sato, Y., Mazuka, R., & Dupoux, E. (2011). Optical brain imaging reveals general auditory and language-specific processing in early infant development. *Cerebral Cortex*, 21(2), 254–261. http://doi.org/10.1093/cercor/bhq082

Moore, J. K. & Linthicum Jr, F. H. (2007). The human auditory system: a timeline of development. *International Journal of Audiology*, 46, 460–478. http://doi.org/10.1080/14992020701383019

Morris, B. H., Philbin, M. K., & Bose, C. (2000). Physiological effects of sound on the newborn. *Journal of Perinatology: Official Journal of the California Perinatal Association*, 20(8 Pt 2), S55–S60. http://doi.org/10.1038/sj.jp.7200451

Nazzi, T., Bertoncini, J., & Mehler, J. (1998). Language discrimination by newborns: toward an understanding of the role of rhythm. *Journal of Experimental Psychology: Human Perception and Performance*, 24(3), 756–766. http://doi.org/10.1037/0096-1523.24.3.756

Ohman, A., Lundqvist, D., & Esteves, F. (2001). The face in the crowd revisited: a threat advantage with schematic stimuli. *Journal of Personality and Social Psychology*, 80, 381–396. http://doi.org/10.1037/0022-3514.80.3.381

Otte, R. A., Donkers, F. C. L., Braeken, M. A. K. A., & Van den Bergh, B. R. H. (2015). Multimodal processing of emotional information in 9-month-old infants. I: emotional faces and voices. *Brain and Cognition*, 95, 99–106. http://doi.org/10.1016/j.bandc.2014.09.007

Peña, M., Pittaluga, E., & Mehler, J. (2010). Language acquisition in premature and full-term infants. *PNAS*, 107(8), 3823–3828. http://doi.org/10.1073/pnas.0914326107

Pernet, C. R., McAleer, P., Latinus, M., Gorgolewski, K. J., Charest, I., Bestelmeyer, P. E. G., ... Belin, P. (2015). The human voice areas: spatial organization and inter-individual variability in temporal and extra-temporal cortices. *NeuroImage*, 119, 164–74. http://doi.org/10.1016/j.neuroimage.2015.06.050

Petitto, L. A., Berens, M. S., Kovelman, I., Dubins, M. H., Jasinska, K., & Shalinsky, M. (2012). The 'Perceptual Wedge Hypothesis' as the basis for bilingual babies' phonetic processing advantage: new insights from fNIRS brain imaging. *Brain and Language*, 121(2), 130–143. http://doi.org/10.1016/j.bandl.2011.05.003

Petkov, C. I., Kayser, C., Steudel, T., Whittingstall, K., Augath, M., & Logothetis, N. K. (2008). A voice region in the monkey brain. *Nature Neuroscience*, 11(3), 367–374. http://doi.org/10.1038/nn2043

Petkov, C. I., Logothetis, N. K., & Obleser, J. (2009). Where are the human speech and voice regions, and do other animals have anything like them? *The Neuroscientist*, 15, 419–429. http://doi.org/10.1177/1073858408326430

Pujol, R. & Hilding, D. (1973). Anatomy and physiology of the onset of auditory function. *Acta Oto-Laryngologica*, 76(1), 1–10.

Pujol, R. & Lavigne-Rebillard, M. (1992). Development of neurosensory structures in the human cochlea. *Acta Oto-Laryngologica*, 112(2), 259–264. Retrieved from http://eutils.ncbi.nlm.nih.gov/entrez/eutils/elink.fcgi?dbfrom=pubmed&id=1604989&retmode=ref&cmd=prlinks\npapers2://publication/uuid/30538E90-3E29-494F-BDD1-61A39472EFDF

Purves, D., Augustine, G. J., Fitzpatrick, D., Katz, L. C., LaMantia, A. S., McNamara, J. O., & Williams, S. M. (eds) (2001). The development of language: a critical period in humans. In: *Neuroscience* (2nd edn). Sunderland, MA: Sinauer Associates.

Ramus, F., Hauser, M. D., Miller, C., Morris, D., & Mehler, J. (2000). Language discrimination by human newborns and by cotton-top tamarin monkeys. *Science*, 288(5464), 349–351. http://doi.org/10.1126/science.288.5464.349

Ramus, F., Pallier, C., Dupoux, E., & Dehaene-, G. (2002). Language discrimination by newborns: teasing apart phonotactic, rhythmic, and intonational cues. *Annual Review of Language Acquisition*, 2, 1–14. http://doi.org/10.1075/arla.2.05ram

Reeb-Sutherland, B. C., Fifer, W. P., Byrd, D. L., Elizabeth, A. D., Levitt, P., & Fox, N. A. (2011). One-month-old human infants learn about the social world while they sleep. *Developmental Science*, 14(5), 1134–1141. http://doi.org/10.1111/j.1467-7687.2011.01062.x

Richards, J. E. & Casey, B. J. (1991). Heart rate variability during attention phases in young infants. *Psychophysiology*, 28(1), 43–53.

Rivera-Gaxiola, M., Silva-Pereyra, J., & Kuhl, P. K. (2005). Brain potentials to native and non-native speech contrasts in 7- and 11-month-old American infants. *Developmental Science*, 8, 162–172. http://doi.org/10.1111/j.1467-7687.2005.00403.x

Rossano, F., Carpenter, M., & Tomasello, M. (2012). One-year-old infants follow others' voice direction. *Psychological Science*, 23(11), 1298–1302. http://doi.org/10.1177/0956797612450032

Saito, Y., Kondo, T., Aoyama, S., Fukumoto, R., Konishi, N., Nakamura, K., … Toshima, T. (2007). The function of the frontal lobe in neonates for response to a prosodic voice. *Early Human Development*, 83, 225–230. http://doi.org/10.1016/j.earlhumdev.2006.05.017

Sato, H., Hirabayashi, Y., Tsubokura, H., Kanai, M., Ashida, T., Konishi, I., … Maki, A. (2012). Cerebral hemodynamics in newborn infants exposed to speech sounds: a whole-head optical topography study. *Human Brain Mapping*, 33, 2092–2103. http://doi.org/10.1002/hbm.21350

Schönwiesner, M., Krumbholz, K., Rübsamen, R., Fink, G. R., & von Cramon, D. Y. (2007). Hemispheric asymmetry for auditory processing in the human auditory brain stem, thalamus, and cortex. *Cerebral Cortex*, 17(2), 492–9. http://doi.org/10.1093/cercor/bhj165

Shi, R., Werker, J. F., & Morgan, J. L. (1999). Newborn infants' sensitivity to perceptual cues to lexical and grammatical words. *Cognition*, 72(2), B11–21. http://doi.org/10.1016/S0010-0277(99)00047-5

Sohmer, H., Perez, R., Sichel, J. Y., Priner, R., & Freeman, S. (2001). The pathway enabling external sounds to reach and excite the fetal inner ear. *Audiology & Neuro-Otology*, 6(3), 109–116. http://doi.org/46817

Sundara, M., Polka, L., & Genesee, F. (2006). Language-experience facilitates discrimination of /d-th/ in monolingual and bilingual acquisition of English. *Cognition*, 100(2), 369–388. http://doi.org/10.1016/j.cognition.2005.04.007

Tsao, F. M., Liu, H. M., & Kuhl, P. K. (2006). Perception of native and non-native fricative-affricate contrasts: cross language tests on adults and infants. *Journal of the Acoustical Society of America*, 120, 2285–2294.

Vaish, A., Grossmann, T., & Woodward, A. (2008). Not all emotions are created equal: the negativity bias in social-emotional development. *Psychological Bulletin*, 134(3), 383–403. http://doi.org/10.1037/0033-2909.134.3.383.

Vaish, A. & Striano, T. (2004). Is visual reference necessary? Contributions of facial versus vocal cues in 12-month-olds' social referencing behavior. *Developmental Science*, 7(3), 261–269. http://doi.org/10.1111/j.1467-7687.2004.00344.x

Vannasing, P., González-Frankenberger, B., Florea, O., Tremblay, J., Paquette, N., Safi, D., … Gallagher, A. (2016). Distinct hemispheric specializations for native and non-native languages in one-day-old newborns identified by fNIRS. *Neuropsychologia*, 84, 63–69.

Vouloumanos, A. & Werker, J. F. (2004). Tuned to the signal: the privileged status of speech for young infants. *Developmental Science*, 7(3), 270–6. http://doi.org/10.1111/j.1467-7687.2004.00345.x

Vouloumanos, A. & Werker, J. F. (2007). Listening to language at birth: evidence for a bias for speech in neonates. *Developmental Science*, 10(2), 159–164. http://doi.org/10.1111/j.1467-7687.2007.00549.x

Weinhold, B. (2006). Epigenetics: the science of change. *Environmental Health Perspectives*, 114(3), 160–167.

Werker, J. & Curtin, S. (2005). PRIMIR: a developmental framework of infant speech processing. *Language Learning and Development*, 1(2), 197–234. http://doi.org/10.1207/s15473341lld0102_4

Werker, J. F. & Tees, R. C. (1999). Influences on infant speech processing: toward a new synthesis. *Annual Review of Psychology*, 50, 509–535. http://doi.org/10.1146/annurev.psych.50.1.509

Werker, J. F., & Tees, R. C. (2002). Cross-language speech perception: evidence for perceptual reorganization during the first year of life. *Infant Behavior and Development*, 25(1), 121–133. http://doi.org/10.1016/S0163-6383(02)00093-0

Zatorre, R. J., Belin, P., & Penhune, V. B. (2002). Structure and function of auditory cortex. *Music and Speech*, 6(1), 37–46.

Zatorre, R. J., Evans, A. C., Meyer, E., & Gjedde, A. (1992). Lateralization of phonetic and pitch discrimination in speech processing. *Science*, 256(5058), 846–849.

CHAPTER 10

ONE STEP BEYOND
Musical Expertise and Word Learning

STEFAN ELMER, EVA DITTINGER,
AND MIREILLE BESSON

10.1 A CORTICAL FRAMEWORK OF SPEECH AND LANGUAGE PROCESSING

10.1.1 The Faculty of Language and its Neural Substrate

Speech and language processing constitute a uniquely human faculty that can be distinguished from other forms of communication in the animal kingdom. In fact, even though it has been proposed that different species possess the faculty of language in a broad sense (i.e. mimic, gesture, olfactory cues, etc.), only human language is characterized by a recursive structure (Fitch, 2010), the latter referring to the ability to produce an infinite number of phrases from a finite number of entities (i.e. phonemes and words). Until now, different evolutionary theories have attempted to explain the possible origin of speech and language processing in human beings, ranging from the expansion of brain size relative to body weight, genetics, brain asymmetries, anatomical characteristics of the larynx, and mirror neurons, to cultural and societal aspects (among others) (Fitch, 2010; Fitch & Reby, 2001; Hauser, 2002). From a linguistic perspective, speech and language processing can be subdivided into different subsystems including phonology, syntax, semantics, morphology, and pragmatics. Phonology refers to knowledge of the sound structure, syntax deals with the rules governing the combination and the order of words in a sentence, semantics addresses the meaning of single words and sentences, morphology is concerned with the structure of words, whereas pragmatics examines language in contexts (e.g. discourse, inference, interaction). Furthermore, depending on intonations and stresses, semantics can be influenced.

In the last decades, both lesion studies and neuroimaging techniques have fundamentally contributed to a better understanding of the cortical organization of speech and language processing. For more than a century, the classical Wernicke-Lichtheim-Geschwind model (Boland, 2014) was considered an accurate representation. This simplistic model was purely based on lesion studies with patients suffering from receptive (i.e. Wernicke's), expressive (i.e. Broca's), or conduction aphasia, and postulated that Broca's area is crucial for language production, whereas Wernicke's area subserves language comprehension functions. In addition, the arcuate fasciculus, a major fibre bundle connecting posterior superior temporal regions (i.e. Brodmann's area 42, Wernicke's area) with Broca's region (i.e. Brodmann's area 44 and 45, pars opercularis and triangularis), was recognized to mediate information exchange between these areas. Even though this historical neurological model enabled the description of a variety of aphasic symptoms, recognizing the contribution of left-sided perisylvian areas to perception and articulation, it is reductive, oversimplified, and relies on brain lesions instead of healthy functioning.

Since that time, several branches of research have fundamentally contributed to improve and ameliorate the cartography of speech and language processing in the human brain. In analogy to the visual system (Milner & Goodale, 2008; Miskin & Ungerleider, 1982), current models conjointly postulate the involvement of two parallel, bidirectional, and hierarchically-organized processing streams stretching from the auditory-related cortex toward the temporal pole (ventral stream) and the frontal lobe (dorsal stream) (Rauschecker & Scott, 2009), and meshing at two points of convergence, namely in the posterior supratemporal plane and in the ventral part of the frontal cortex (see Figure 10.1). However, these models diverge somewhat in the description of the processes supported by the two processing streams, as well as in their linguistic and neurological conceptualization. In turn, we will summarize some of the most popular frameworks of cortical speech and language processing proposed by Hickok and Poeppel (2007), Bornkessel-Schlesewsky and Schlesewsky (2013), Friederici (2009, 2011, 2012), Hagoort (2014), and Rauschecker and Scott (2009). It is important to

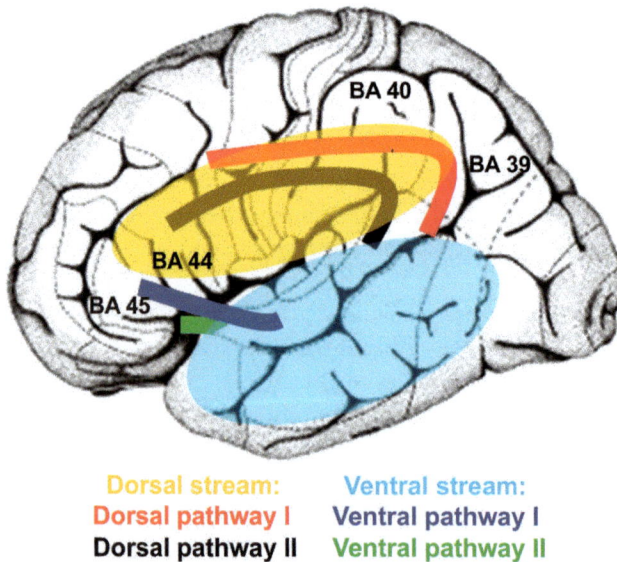

Dorsal stream: Ventral stream:
Dorsal pathway I   Ventral pathway I
Dorsal pathway II   Ventral pathway II

FIGURE 10.1 Ventral and dorsal streams of language processing.

Table 10.1 Summary of current models of cortical speech and language processing proposed by Hickok and Poeppel (2007), Bornkessel–Schlesewsky and Schlesewsky (2013), Friederici (2009, 2011, 2012), Hagoort (2014), and Rauschecker and Scott (2009)

Authors	Type of model	Short description
Hickok and Poeppel	Dual-stream model	The ventral stream is responsible for sound-to-meaning mapping, whereas the dorsal one supports sensory-motor mapping mechanisms and articulation. The ventral stream is bilaterally organized, whereas the dorsal one is lateralized to the left hemisphere.
Bornkessel-Schlesewsky and Schlesewsky	Dual-stream model	The ventral stream operates in a time-independent manner by activating and unifying conceptual schemata necessary for creating units of increased complexity and enabling semantic integration. Otherwise, the dorsal stream subserves general time-dependent processes and is engaged in segmenting the input into prosodic words, combining these elements into a syntactic structure, as well as in assessing them into action-centred representations.
Friederici	Dual-stream model	This model postulates a dorsal and a ventral processing stream that is compatible with the underlying white matter architecture. Within this framework, the dorsal and ventral streams are responsible for more than one isolated function, and based on the underlying white matter architecture, each of them can be segregated into two subpathways (i.e. pathway I & II).
Hagoort	Dynamic and cognitive model	This model acts on the assumption that for central aspects of language processing the neural infrastructure is shared between comprehension and production systems in the form of dynamic networks, and that this neural substrate is not language-specific. Frontal, temporal, and parietal brain regions are differentially recruited based on task-related network characteristics, meaning that the functional role of a specific brain area is influenced by the other regions of the network depending on information type, processing demands, and cognitive control.
Rauschecker and Scott	Dual-stream model	This model is based on physiological and anatomical data from non-human primates, but also integrates findings from speech and music processing in humans, and takes into account similarities between the visual and auditory systems. The model postulates a ventral stream for object identification ('what') and a dorsal one for spatial analyses ('where'), sensorimotor processes, and higher-order linguistic functions.

mention that, besides these models (outlined in Table 10.1), there are a multiplicity of other frameworks that are not discussed in this chapter.

10.1.2 Current Models of Speech and Language Processing

The dual-stream model proposed by Hickok and Poeppel (2007) relies on evidence from both lesion- and task-related neuroimaging studies, and postulates a ventral stream that processes speech signals for comprehension and a dorsal one that maps acoustic speech signals to frontal lobe articulatory networks. When speech signals reach the auditory-related cortex, the model already postulates a division of labour between the two hemispheres (Giraud et al., 2007; Zatorre & Belin, 2001), and highlights a relative specialization of the left hemisphere for the processing of transient and fast-changing acoustic cues (i.e. segmental, time windows of about 25 ms, 40 Hz). By contrast, the right-sided counterpart is more sensitive to slow acoustic modulations and frequency information (i.e. suprasegmental, time windows of about 250 ms, 4 Hz). Even though this relative processing asymmetry is controversial (Overath et al., 2015; Santoro et al., 2014), it has previously been associated with a differential spacing between microcolumns, myelination (Harasty et al., 2003; Seldon, 1981), as well as with asymmetric spontaneous neural oscillations in the theta (right-sided asymmetry) and gamma (left-sided asymmetry) frequency range (Giraud et al., 2007). These specific oscillations have been proposed to play an important role in 'packing' the multitime speech signal (i.e. phonemes, words, etc.) into units of the appropriate temporal granularity (Giraud & Poeppel, 2012) necessary for further processing steps along the ventral and dorsal streams.

In the Hickok and Poeppel (2007) model, the speech signal, after acoustic analysis, spreads along a bilaterally distributed ventral route engaged in meaning extraction (i.e. lexical-semantic processing) through a cascade of hierarchical processes. The posterior supratemporal plane and the posterior part of the superior temporal sulcus (STS) act as an interface between spectrotemporal and phonological processes. At the next hierarchical level, phonological information is mapped onto lexical representations in memory by recruiting posterior, middle, and inferior portions of the temporal lobe. Finally, information converges on a combinatorial network situated in the proximity of the temporal pole and supporting lexical-semantic integration, sentence-level processing, as well as syntactic and semantic nesting. In contrast to the bilateral organization of the ventral route (with a slight left-hemispheric bias), the dorsal stream is strongly left-dominant, maps sensory and phonological representations onto articulatory motor representations in the frontal cortex, and constitutes a bridge between the speech perception and production systems. The dorsal pathway originates from the posterior supratemporal plane, runs through a sensory-motor interface at the parieto-temporal junction, and projects to Broca's area as well as to the dorsal part of the premotor cortex. The model proposed by Hickok and Poeppel is anatomically well-defined. However, it only focuses on speech and not generally on language processing, and lacks a certain linguistic depth, especially regarding syntactic and lexical-semantic processes.

Recently, Bornkessel-Schlesewsky and Schlesewsky (2013) presented an alternative dual-stream model that attempts to unify neurobiological assumptions and linguistic sentence comprehension. Similar to Hickok and Poeppel, the authors postulate the engagement of bidirectional ventral and dorsal processing streams, however with important computational differences regarding time dependence. The ventral stream projects from auditory core areas along the superior temporal plane toward the anterior temporal cortex and ventral frontal cortex, whereas the dorsal stream runs, via a relay station situated in the inferior parietal lobe, to the inferior frontal cortex. In their framework, the authors abstain from a conceptual dichotomy between comprehension and articulation and instead propose time-dependent processes along the dorsal stream and time-independent ones along the ventral stream. Thereby, it is assumed that the ventral stream operates in a time-independent manner by activating and unifying conceptual schemata necessary for creating units of increased complexity and enabling semantic integration. Furthermore, the model postulates that the ventral stream enables word-level semantic information, as well as phrase-structure comprehension, by the activation and unification of actor-event schemata (e.g. who and what) that are actor-centred (i.e. focus on persons or objects responsible for a certain events) and category neutral (i.e. nouns or verbs). Unification occurs by integrating one schema (e.g. who) into another one (e.g. what). According to the same model, the dorsal stream does not specifically subserve articulation and repetition but, rather, general time-dependent processes. Therefore, this stream supports both speech production and comprehension and is engaged in segmenting the input into prosodic words, combining these elements into a syntactic structure, as well as in assessing them in action-centred representations (i.e. who is responsible for a certain event).

Finally, it is important to mention that even though the two processing streams converge in the ventral part of the frontal cortex, this brain region is not assumed to support specific linguistic functions but, rather, accommodates action planning and general executive functions such as verbal and non-verbal memory, inhibitory control, switching, and updating. This framework fundamentally contributes to a better understanding of the cortical implementation of linguistic processes (especially phonology, semantics, and syntax). Otherwise, the model is anatomically vaguely defined and does not explicitly address processing asymmetries along the ventral and dorsal streams.

An alternative dual-stream model is the one proposed by Friederici (2009, 2011, 2012). This model is based on sentence processing, is anatomically as well as linguistically well-defined, and reconciles precise cortical cartography with the underlying white matter pathways. Within this framework, the dorsal and ventral streams are responsible for more than one isolated function, and based on the underlying white matter architecture, each of them can be segregated into two subpathways. The dorsal stream constitutes one fibre bundle connecting the superior temporal cortex to the premotor cortex (via the superior longitudinal fasciculus, dorsal pathway I) as well as by a second pathway linking the temporal cortex to pars opercularis (via the arcuate fasciculus, dorsal pathway II). By contrast, the ventral stream relies on the fibre bundle running from the anterior temporal cortex to pars triangularis (via the extreme capsule, ventral pathway I) as well as on the connection between the anterior supratemporal regions and the frontal operculum (via the uncinate fasciculus, ventral pathway II) (see Figure 10.1).

Initial acoustic and phonological analyses involve the primary and secondary auditory cortex, from where activity spreads along the ventral stream to anterior and posterior supratemporal regions. In successive processing steps, initial phrase structure building is conjointly analysed by the left anterior temporal cortex and the frontal operculum (i.e. ventral pathway II). Successively, semantic, grammatical, and thematic relations are processed in a parallel manner. Semantic analyses are supported by middle-posterior areas of the superior and middle temporal gyrus, as well as by pars triangularis and orbitalis (i.e. ventral pathway I). Otherwise, syntactically complex sentences are dependent upon pars opercularis and the posterior temporal cortex (i.e. dorsal pathway II). Furthermore, within this framework, the anterior part of the temporal lobe supports both semantic and syntactic processing and subserves combinatorial processes. Finally, the connection between the posterior supratemporal plane and the premotor cortex (i.e. dorsal pathway I) promotes auditory-to-motor mapping mechanisms, whereas the fibre bundle bridging the posterior temporal cortex and pars opercularis (i.e. dorsal pathway I) supports syntactic processes (especially when sentences are complex). Prosodic information is assumed to be predominantly processed in the right hemisphere and integrated with left-hemispheric syntactic information through the posterior part of the corpus callosum (i.e. isthmus).

The model proposed by Hagoort (2014) overlaps with the models described above in that it posits the engagement of temporal, parietal, and frontal brain regions as the constitutional entities of speech and language processing. However, this model acts on the assumption that for central aspects of language processing, the neural infrastructure is shared between comprehension and production systems in the form of dynamic networks, and that this neural substrate is not language-specific (see also Friederici & Singer, 2015). Within this framework, brain regions situated along the ventral and dorsal streams are differentially recruited based on task-related network characteristics, meaning that the functional role of a specific brain area is influenced by the other regions of the network depending on information type (i.e. phonological, syntactic, and semantic), processing demands, and cognitive control mechanisms.

This perspective has been implemented in a 'Memory, Unification, and Control' (MUC) model that postulates that regions situated in distributed networks in the temporal and inferior parietal cortex generally subserve mnemonic representations (i.e. phonological word forms, morphological information, and the syntactic templates associated with nouns, verbs, and adjectives). Otherwise, frontal regions (including Broca's area) are crucially involved in unification operations by generating larger structures (i.e. phonologic, semantic, and syntactic) from the templates retrieved from memory. Finally, the model also posits that 'memory' and 'unification' mechanisms are hierarchically subordinated to higher executive control mechanisms that are executed by the dorsolateral prefrontal cortex, the anterior cingulate cortex, as well as by the parietal attention system. This model is compatible with studies on non-human primates militating that diverse perceptual and cognitive functions are based on similar neural mechanisms, leading to suggestions of a general rather than a language-specific intrinsic organization of the human brain (Rauschecker & Scott, 2009; Friederici & Singer, 2015).

Last but not least, it is noteworthy to mention the hierarchical dual-stream model of Rauschecker and Scott (Rauschecker & Scott, 2009) that emphasizes how our understanding of speech processing has profited from findings in non-human primates. According to the visual system, this model postulates an antero-ventral processing stream supporting auditory object recognition (i.e. 'what stream', including communication sounds), whereas a postero-dorsal stream facilitates spatial and motion perception (i.e. 'where stream'), sensorimotor functions as well as higher-order linguistic processing. Furthermore, the model implies that connections between temporal, frontal, and parietal areas link speech perception and production systems, and extends beyond speech processing by generally integrating both vision and audition.

10.2 Perceptual and Cognitive Demands on Speech- and Language-Learning Mechanisms

The investigation of speech- and language-learning mechanisms in infants provides an empirically-based framework for better comprehending the perceptual and cognitive processing underlying this uniquely human faculty. Currently, it is known that the auditory cortex starts functioning at about 24 weeks of gestation and that shortly after birth, infants are characterized by some left-hemispheric language specialization (Dehaene-Lambertz & Spelke, 2015; Perani et al., 2011). These functional-anatomical constraints, in association with neural commitment (Kuhl, 2004), facilitate language-learning mechanisms in infants, including the perception and discrimination of vowels, consonants, phonetic contrasts, and stress patterns in words. Nowadays, it is also recognized that a part of the dorsal stream (i.e. dorsal pathway I) linking the auditory cortex with the premotor cortex is observable shortly after birth, whereas a second pathway connecting the auditory cortex with Broca's area (i.e. dorsal pathway II) matures only later during development (Brauer et al., 2013).

Speech constitutes a concatenated acoustic signal whose parameters (e.g. pitch and envelope) not only vary in time but also depend on the talker (e.g. gender), speech rate, as well as on the context (e.g. loudness of the environment). Consequently, before acquiring single words, infants have to learn to decrypt the 'speech code' by figuring out the composition of the phonetic categories of a specific language. This mechanism, called 'categorical perception', is (at least partially) mediated by the 'magnet effect', a phenomenon where prototypical phonetic representations stored in memory attract surrounding deviant sounds (Kuhl, 2004). A commonplace example of this effect can be observed in English infants who learn that /r/ and /l/ pertain to different phonetic categories, whereas Japanese children treat these two phonemes as equivalent because they are not lexically contrastive in Japanese.

Aside from categorical perception, a further important phenomenon is speech segmentation (i.e. the ability to extract meaningful sounds from continuous speech). The recognition of words' boundaries is at least partly based on 'statistical learning'—an implicit faculty that enables infants to analyse statistical distributions and relationships between speech sounds (Kuhl, 2004; Saffran, 2003). For example, within the German language it is more probable (i.e. there is a higher transitional probability) that the consonant /r/ follows the consonants /t/ and /p/ than /z/. Importantly, infants also strongly rely on prosodic cues (e.g. linguistic stress on the first syllable in German) for the segmentation of a continuous speech signal into different subunits and to identify potential word candidates.

Certainly, speech- and language-learning mechanisms are also strongly influenced by social factors that enable infants to be attracted to infant-directed speech (e.g. motherese) by providing enriched referential information through action-based forms (Kuhl, 2007). In this context, there is evidence showing that language-learning mechanisms rely on the functional contribution of phylogenetically older subcortical reward systems (Péron et al., 2016) possibly involved in reinforcing human motivation to learn a language (Ripollés et al., 2014).

One of the most distinctive differences between infants' and adults' speech and language acquisition is that, in the latter, several of the processes described above are established and the brain has already committed to the mother tongue. In fact, in adults, the neural circuits underlying speech processing are fully developed and prefrontal brain regions supporting higher cognitive functions (i.e. attention, memory, planning, inhibition, etc.) and explicit learning strategies have reached a maturational ceiling (Gogtay et al., 2004). On the other hand, a common experience, such as being exposed to a new language in a foreign country, brings to light several analogies between speech and language acquisition in infants and adults. Similar to infants, adults have to learn to recognize the phonetic repertoire of a foreign language as well as to segregate continuous speech into subunits in order to recognize words' boundaries and to identify single words. Depending on the phonetic overlap between native and foreign language (e.g. Indo-European, Asian, or neo-Latin), the acquisition process can be either facilitated or hindered. A further point is that not only the phonetic properties of a language but also its spectrotemporal attributes, as well as its syntactic complexity, have an influence on the learning process. This is, for example, the case for tonal (e.g. Mandarin or Cantonese Chinese) and quantitative languages (e.g. Finnish) where phonemes vary in pitch (i.e. rising or falling), temporal extension of the vowel (i.e. short or long), or even by a combination of such spectral and temporal attributes that contribute to differences in word meaning (e.g. Thai).

Currently, there is a significant amount of literature addressing differential aspects of speech- and language-learning mechanisms in both adults and children, ranging from the articulation of foreign speech sounds, categorical perception, speech segmentation, and word learning, to the implicit or explicit acquisition of syntactic knowledge. Even though all these studies cannot be discussed in detail here, it is important to emphasize that the neural circuits underlying different aspects of language-learning mechanisms are the same as those described in Section 10.1, 'A Cortical Framework of Speech and Language Processing'. Therefore, we will only provide a few examples of some of these studies.

Recently, López-Barroso and colleagues (2013) measured a sample of adult participants who performed an artificial language-learning task consisting of segmenting and learning single pseudo-words presented in the form of concatenated speech. Results demonstrated that word-learning ability was related to increased functional and structural connectivity between the left auditory cortex and Broca's region (dorsal pathway). In other studies, Golestani and colleagues reported that French participants who more accurately learnt to discriminate (Golestani & Zatorre, 2004) or pronounce (Golestani & Pallier, 2007) non-native phonetic contrasts were characterized by increased brain activity in left perisylvian areas as well as by enhanced grey-matter density in brain regions supporting speech articulation, respectively. Finally, previous electrophysiological studies on vocabulary learning were able to demonstrate lexical-semantic facilitation effects (i.e. as reflected by increased N400 amplitudes) after only a few hours of training (McLaughlin et al., 2004; Perfetti et al., 2005).

In the next section, we will introduce professional musicians, as well as children undergoing short- or long-term music training, as a vehicle for better understanding the mutual interdependence between perception and cognition during different aspects of speech and language learning. Thereby, we will draw a bridge between functional and structural training-related brain changes, perceptual and cognitive benefits, and several aspects of language learning.

10.3   MUSIC TO SPEECH TRANSFER EFFECTS

Compared to language research, the neuroscience of music is a relatively new field that has also led to fascinating discoveries. This is at least partly based on the fact that, while all normally-developing children end up being language experts, not all human beings are professional musicians. In fact, much has been learned about the anatomo-functional organization of the brain and about brain plasticity by studying the musician's brain and the impact of long-term music training on different perceptual and cognitive functions (Elbert et al., 1995; Jäncke, 2012; Münte et al., 2002; Schlaug et al., 1995; Schneider et al., 2002; Sluming et al., 2002).

Here, we focus on transfer effects, defined as the influence of training in one domain on the level of performance in another domain. Specifically, we address transfer effects from music training to several aspects of language processing (in a broad sense that includes speech processing), to cross-modal integration, and to executive functions (see Asaridou & McQueen, 2013, for the influence of linguistic experience on music processing). The results described in this section were obtained using different methodologies: behavioural measurements, electrophysiological recordings at the level of the brainstem and at the cortical level (event-related potentials—ERPs), and functional magnetic resonance imaging (fMRI). First, we review the growing evidence for transfer effects; then, we consider two main interpretations of such transfers; and finally, we address the questions of the influence of music training or of genetic predispositions for music, and whether music and language processing rely on shared or distinct neural substrates.

10.3.1   Growing Evidence for Transfer Effects

Results of many experiments have demonstrated the positive influence of music training on speech perception (Besson et al., 2011; Kraus & Chandrasekaran, 2010). For instance, there is clear evidence that music training influences the segmental processing of speech sounds (consonants, vowels, and syllables) (see Appendix 10.1 and Audio 10.1 for examples of consonant-vowel syllables) at multiple levels of the auditory system from the brainstem (Bidelman & Krishnan, 2010; Musacchia et al., 2007; Wong et al., 2007) to cortical regions (Bidelman & Alain, 2015; Bidelman et al., 2011; Chobert et al., 2014; Elmer et al., 2012; Meyer et al., 2012; Ott, 2011). Music training also positively influences pitch processing in tonal languages such as Mandarin Chinese and Thai, in which pitch variations in vowels change the meaning of words (Alexander et al., 2005; Bidleman et al., 2011; Bidelman et al., 2013; Lee & Hung, 2008; Wong et al., 2007). At the suprasegmental level (couple of syllables, words, and sentences), results have shown that musicians are typically more sensitive than nonmusicians to linguistic and emotional prosody (i.e. speech melody and rhythm) (Cason & Schön, 2012; Lima & Castro, 2011; Ma & Thompson, 2015; Magne et al., 2006; Marques et al., 2007; Moreno et al., 2009; Schön et al., 2004; Thompson et al., 2004, 2012; and for contrastive results, Trimmer & Cuddy, 2008), as well as to the timbre of human voices (Chartrand & Belin, 2006).

As reviewed in Section 10.2, categorical perception and speech segmentation are the cornerstones of speech perception. In this context, Bidelman and collaborators (2013) demonstrated an influence of music training on the categorical perception of speech sounds (/u/ to /a/ continuum) at the cortical level: the P2 component of the ERPs was sensitive to between-categories' phonetic boundaries defined by psychometric functions. By contrast, this effect was not significant at the brainstem level. Results of subsequent experiments also showed that younger (Bidelman et al., 2014) and older musicians (Bidelman & Alain, 2015) were faster and showed steeper boundaries between phonetic categories in a vowel categorization task than non-musicians. Increased auditory sensitivity may thus be one of the driving forces behind enhanced categorical perception and enhanced speech processing in musicians.

Speech segmentation is also fundamental to speech comprehension. This is clearly exemplified when learning a foreign language that is perceived as a continuous stream of nonsense words. François and colleagues (2013) used a longitudinal approach in children, over a period of two school years, during which the children were trained in music or in painting (45 minutes, twice a week in the first year and once a week in the second year). Children first listened to 5 minutes of an artificial, continuous, sung language in which syllables varied in their transitional probability (as previously described) and was higher within three syllabic items (hence considered as familiar) than between two consecutive items (hence considered as unfamiliar). Children were then asked which of two items was most familiar. At the behavioural level, implicit recognition of familiar and unfamiliar items steadily increased over the course of the two years of music training—but not of painting training. At the cortical level, and similarly to adults (François & Schön, 2011), only the music-trained children were characterized by a fronto-central negative component that was larger to unfamiliar than to familiar items. Thus, this longitudinal study demonstrated that music training improved speech segmentation.

Certainly, transfer from music to language is by no means limited to low-level speech processing, such as categorical perception or speech segmentation, but has also been shown to extend to higher-level language processing. For example, based on the idea that both music and language are structured sequences of events that unfold in time, several studies have investigated the influence of music training on syntactic processing in adults (Fitzroy & Sanders, 2012) and in children (Janus et al., 2016; Jentschke & Koelsch, 2009). Jentschke and Koelsch (2009) compared the ERPs to violations of linguistic and musical syntax in musically trained and untrained 10–11-year-old children. The electrophysiological markers of both types of violations were larger in the former group. Not surprisingly, musically trained children were more sensitive to harmonic structure than children without such training. What was more surprising is that they also showed more comprehensive knowledge of the syntactic structure of sentences, possibly through faster implicit syntactic processing and/or a more efficient use of the prosodic and rhythmic cues that constrain syntactic constructions (Roncaglia-Denissen et al., 2013; Schmidt-Kassow & Kotz, 2009).

A hotly debated issue in the literature is whether the influence of music training on different abilities is causally linked to music training or rather results from genetic predispositions for music. Cross-sectional studies comparing (professional) musicians and non-musicians, children or adults, do not allow for this issue to be addressed since, as pointed out by Schellenberg (2004), correlation is not causality. To our knowledge, the only way to test causality in humans is to use a test–training–retest longitudinal approach that compares two groups of non-musicians (children or adults)—one group trained with music and the other group trained with an equally interesting activity, such as painting or cooking. Participants are pseudo-randomly assigned to one of the two groups, thereby ensuring that no between-group differences on the different tests of interest are found before training. If musically trained participants outperformed painting-/cooking-trained participants in the retest session, this is evidence that the type of training strongly influenced the results. This approach has been successfully used to demonstrate the influence of music training on the perception of pitch variations in sentence context (Moreno et al., 2009) and on the preattentive processing of the temporal aspects of speech (Chobert et al., 2014) and on speech segmentation (Francois et al., 2013), as previously mentioned.

10.3.2   Interpretations of Transfer Effects

Having summarized some of the evidence for music to language transfer effects, we now turn to the most important question: *How can we explain music to speech processing transfer effects?* Two main interpretations, that we refer to as the cascade and multidimensional hypotheses, have been proposed in the literature.

Following the cascade hypothesis, transfer effects arise because speech and music are auditory signals relying on the same acoustic parameters (i.e. duration, frequency, intensity, and timbre). As musicians are highly trained in perceiving the acoustic structure of sounds, sound encoding is facilitated not only in music but also in speech. Thus, enhanced perceptual encoding and categorization of speech sounds in musicians facilitates higher levels of speech processing. Let us take the example of novel word learning, that will be considered in detail later. If a learner is able to differentiate the subtle acoustic features of different phonemes, he/she may form a more precise phonological representation of the new word. Consequently, it will be easier to associate such a phonological representation with the corresponding word meaning than a less distinct one. This bottom-up interpretation may explain why musicians are more sensitive to the spectro-temporal aspects of speech processing at the segmental and suprasegmental levels, as already reviewed, as well as to other aspects of speech perception (e.g. speech in noise perception, speech segmentation, sentence syntactic structure).

The multidimensional hypothesis is based on the fact that music training is multidimensional. Playing a musical instrument involves auditory and visual perception (the notes on the score), visuo-auditory-motor integration (transforming visual notes into sounds through movements), selective and divided attention (focusing attention on one's own instrument and dividing attention between the different instruments of the orchestra), and motor control (adapting posture and fine distal movements). Playing a musical piece also requires memory (most musicians play by heart), executive functions (switching between visual and auditory codes), inhibitory control (withholding a movement to play at the right moment and updating information), and emotion (as translated into the interpretation of the musical piece). Since professional musicians are at their advantage in these different functions, they may outperform non-musicians when these functions are necessary for the task at hand.

Evidence for this multidimensional hypothesis is accumulating from several results showing transfer from music training to cross-modal integration (Chen et al., 2008; Lee & Noppeney, 2011; Pantev et al., 2009) and to executive functions. Executive functions are defined as top-down processes that control behaviour, and typically include selective attention, working memory (WM), short- and long-term memory, and cognitive control (inhibitory control, cognitive flexibility, updating), although this is still a matter of controversy

(Diamond, 2013). In this respect, musicians have been shown to be more efficient at audio-motor learning than non-musicians (Barrett et al., 2013; Lahav et al., 2007; Mathias et al., 2015), possibly because they use different integration strategies, with musicians relying more on auditory and non-musicians more on visual information (Paraskevopoulos et al., 2012, 2014, 2015). In addition, there is evidence that adult musicians outperform non-musicians in WM tasks based on musical stimuli (George & Coch, 2011; Pallesen et al., 2010; Schulze & Koelsch, 2012; Schulze, Mueller, et al., 2011; Schulze, Zysset, et al., 2011; Schulze et al., 2012; Williamson et al., 2010), even though the influence of music training on verbal memory is more controversial (Brandler & Rammsayer, 2003; Chan et al., 1998; Williamson et al., 2010). Importantly, WM, short-term memory, and long-term memory are tightly intertwined, and more work is clearly needed to disentangle the different components of executive functions (Franklin et al., 2008; Jakobson et al., 2008). Research in children also demonstrated that music training can have an influence on executive functions (cognitive flexibility, processing speed, inhibitory control, non-verbal intelligence) as well as on short-term and long-term memory (Bergman Nutley et al., 2014; Janus et al., 2016; Moreno et al., 2011; Roden et al., 2012; Zuk et al., 2014).

In summary, results of a number of studies suggest that music training in adults and in children positively influences several aspects of language processing, executive functions, WM, as well as short-term and long-term memory. Importantly, differences between adult musicians or children with music training and controls are generally larger for the most demanding tasks, when most resources are needed to perform the task at hand (Besson et al., 2011; Diamond, 2013). However, in line with a dynamic and interactive view of human cognition, results also showed that these different functions are intrinsically linked. For instance, Diamond (2013) reported that the training of task-switching abilities transferred to verbal and non-verbal WM, inhibition (Stroop interference), and reasoning tasks. Better understanding of these intricate relationships is an exciting aim of future research, keeping in mind that we need to use well-controlled experimental designs, standardized tests when they are available (e.g. forward digit span for short-term memory, backward digit span for WM), and data-analysis methods that allow controlling for the effects of the many different factors that can also influence the results.

10.3.3 Transfer Effects and Shared Neural Networks

Finally, one current hotly debated topic is whether the music to language and cognition transfer effects already reviewed are supported by *shared neural networks*. In fact, the question of whether brain networks involved in music and language processing are similar or different is a long-standing question that recently received new answers.

Let us take the example of syntactic processing and Broca's area. Using fMRI, early results demonstrated that Broca's area, considered as specifically involved in the processing of linguistic syntactic structures for over a century (Berwick et al., 2013; Friederici et al., 2006), was also activated when processing musical structures (Koelsch et al., 2002; Levitin & Menon, 2003; Maess et al., 2001; Tillmann et al., 2003; Vuust et al., 2006). These results provided evidence that processing syntax in music and language relied on shared neural substrates. This conclusion was further supported by recent results of Abrams et al. (2011) and Rogalsky et al. (2011) showing that similar activations of frontal and temporal regions in both hemispheres are activated by temporal violations in linguistic sentences

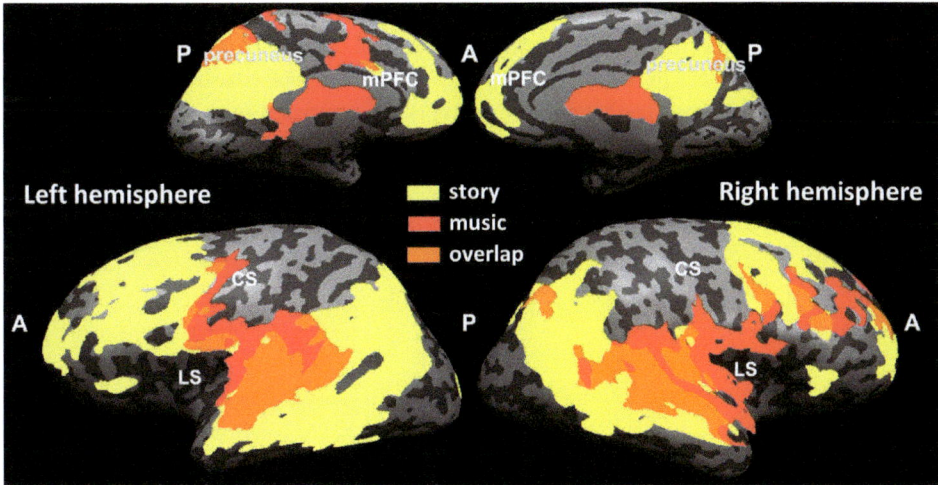

FIGURE 10.2 Maps of brain activation whilst attentively listening to an intact story (yellow) or an intact musical excerpt (red) are shown for experienced pianists. Story listening evoked reliable responses in the temporo-parietal junction, angular gyrus, inferior frontal gyrus, lateral and medial prefrontal areas, and orbitofrontal cortex. Reliable responses to music were found in the lateral sulcus, pre-central gyrus, and middle frontal gyrus. Overlapping regions of reliable responses to both stimuli (orange) were evident in early auditory areas along the superior temporal gyrus (STG). mPFC = middle pre-frontal cortex, A = anterior, P = posterior, CS = central sulcus, LS = lateral sulcus.

and melodies. However, results based on a more fine-grained approach—multivariate pattern analysis—showed that the two types of stimuli elicited spatially distinct activity. Thus, based on these results, the authors concluded that temporal structure is encoded differently within the two domains and that distinct cortical networks are activated. Interestingly, brain structures in these networks involved the voice-selective areas identified by Belin and collaborators (2000) and the speech-selective component that emerged from the hypothesis-free voxel decomposition method recently used by Norman-Haignere and colleagues (2015).

In summary, through the example of Broca's and temporal areas, the most studied brain structures in the neuroscience of language, we have seen evidence both for shared and for distinct networks involved in processing syntax and temporal structures in music and language. Importantly, evidence is tightly linked to the specific aspects of music and language that are compared and to the methods chosen for analysis. Depending upon the temporo-spatial resolution of the method, upon the characteristics of the stimuli, and upon the task at hand, results may show overlap of brain regions involved in music and language processing or distinct local networks involved in specific aspects of language and music processing (see Figure 10.2). There is no doubt that tremendous progress in our understanding of the language–music relationship will be made in the years to come by using finer-grained analyses of the spatio-temporal dynamics of brain networks in well-controlled experiments. Moreover, language and music are complex human functions that are not processed independently of other cognitive and emotional functions. As a consequence, we consider the cascade and the multidimensional interpretations of transfer effects as strongly complementary. Finally, as we will see in the following section, the ERPs method, that allows us to continuously record on-line changes in brain activity associated to the stimuli and task at hand, has also provided interesting results regarding the spatio-temporal dynamics of music to language transfer effects.

10.4 MUSIC TRAINING AND WORD LEARNING

In previous parts of this chapter, we considered word learning as an example of a multi-dimensional task relying on both perceptual and cognitive functions. Therefore, in this section, we specifically examine meaning acquisition of novel words, and we illustrate why word learning constitutes a wonderful opportunity to study the influence of music training on semantic processing, one of the key features of language.

When it comes to learning the meaning of novel words, the learner has to focus attention to the stimuli in order to discriminate spectral and temporal phonetic contrasts, build new phonological representations, and associate these representations with meaning by re-cruiting working-, short-term-, episodic-, and semantic-memory processes. Finally, initial word representations have to be consolidated to build longer-lasting and more robust forms of these representations.

Based on its high temporal resolution, the ERPs method has been frequently used to capture the dynamics of word learning. Thereby, the building up of initial word representations has been shown to be reflected by the rapid emergence of a frontally distributed N400, a negative-going ERP component that develops between 300 and 600 ms after stimulus presentation. For instance, McLaughlin and colleagues (2004) were able to show increased N400 amplitudes in native English speakers after 14 hours of training with French words. Perfetti and colleagues (2005) revealed similar results after only 45 minutes of learning the meaning of low-frequency words.

Finally, in the case of learning a novel word's meaning from highly constraining meaningful contexts, Batterink and Neville (2011) showed the integration of such novel meanings into semantic networks after ten repetitions, Mestres-Missé and colleagues (2007) demonstrated the rapid development of an N400 after only three exposures to such words, and Borovsky and collaborators (2010) even after a single exposure to the words. In conclusion, while learning the meaning of novel words may seem to be slow and laborious, initial word representations can be built up within short training sessions and after only a few repetitions depending on the context in which novel words are presented.

In Section 10.3, we provided evidence for transfer from music to a variety of levels of language processing, including the perception of acoustic-phonetic parameters, segmentation, phonology, and syntax. To go one step beyond, we examined whether professional music training also facilitates semantic processing. We tested the hypothesis that professional music training facilitates word learning, designing an ecologically valid series of experiments aimed at tracking the electrophysiological dynamics of phonological categorization, semantic acquisition, as well as semantic retrieval (Dittinger et al., 2016) (see Figure 10.3). Specifically, two groups of adult French speakers, comprising fifteen professional musicians and fifteen non-musicians, performed first a phonological categorization task, consisting of

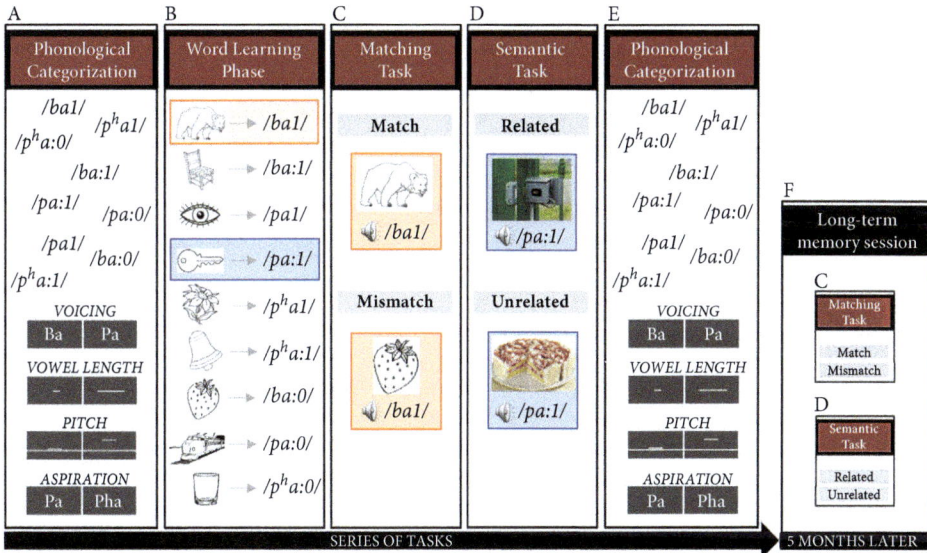

FIGURE 10.3 Participants performed a series of tasks. First, in the phonological categorization task (**A**), nine natural Thai monosyllabic words had to be categorized based on voicing, vowel length, pitch, or aspiration contrasts. Second, in the word-learning phase (**B**), each word was paired with its respective picture. Third, in the matching task (**C**), the words were presented with one of the pictures, either matching or mismatching the previously learned associations. Fourth, in the semantic task (**D**), the words were presented with novel pictures that were either semantically related or unrelated to the novel words. Fifth, participants again completed the four subtasks of the phonological categorization task (**E**). Finally, participants came back 5 months after the main session to perform again the matching and semantic tasks (**F**).

identifying nine natural Thai monosyllabic words containing either a simple voicing contrast, a tonal, a vowel length, or an aspiration contrast. Importantly, two (/ba/ and /pa/) out of these nine words were part of the French phonemic repertoire and therefore simple to categorize. By contrast, the other seven words contained contrasts which are linguistically irrelevant for French speakers, but relevant for quantitative or tonal languages (i.e. vowel length, pitch, and aspiration contrasts that are lexically relevant in Thai), resulting in more difficult categorization tasks (Dittinger et al., 2018). Following the categorization task, participants learned the meaning of these nine words through picture–word associations during a word-learning phase of about 6 minutes. Then, participants were tested for training success by asking them if a presented picture–word pair matched or mismatched the previously learned association (i.e. matching task). Moreover, to determine whether word learning was restricted to the picture–word pairs learned during the training phase or whether the meaning of the newly learned words was already integrated into semantic networks so that priming effects generalized to new pictures, participants performed a semantic task during which novel pictures that had not been seen in the former task were presented in combination with the previously learned words. They were asked to decide whether the picture and the word were semantically related or unrelated. Finally, participants were behaviourally retested 5 months after the main experimental session, to assess first, how long rapidly installed word representations can last, and second, whether professional music training influences long-term memory—two aspects that had not been investigated before.

The originality of this series of experiments is that EEG was simultaneously recorded in all these tasks (except in the long-term-memory session). This allowed us to follow the temporal dynamics of word learning from the early stages of word categorization and initial word encoding to subsequent stages of word-meaning retrieval once the novel words had been integrated into pre-existing semantic networks. Thus, we aimed at studying different processes underlying word learning that have previously only been explored in isolation in single experiments, to gain a more complete and integrated view of word learning. Since, as already noted, several studies have evidenced a positive influence of music not only on auditory perception, but also on attention, audiovisual integration abilities, as well as memory functions, we expected that professional musicians would be at an advantage to learn these novel words compared to non-musicians.

In line with this hypothesis, results showed that professional musicians learned the meaning of novel words more efficiently than controls, and this result was supported by both behavioural and electrophysiological data. Behaviourally, musicians outperformed non-musicians in word categorization and, as expected, group differences were particularly large for the tonal and aspiration contrasts (Dittinger et al., 2016). While these contrasts are not part of the French phonetic repertoire, the ability to discriminate them is inevitable for the acquisition of several foreign languages. For meaning acquisition, musicians performed similarly to non-musicians in the matching task, but outperformed non-musicians in the semantic task. These results were taken as evidence that musicians had already better integrated the novel words' meanings into semantic networks (i.e. enabling them to generalize the knowledge to novel pictures). Importantly, these behavioural results were supported by group differences in electrophysiological markers. In line with the development of a frontal N400 during novel-word encoding (Batterink & Neville, 2011; Borovsky et al., 2010, 2012; McLaughlin et al., 2004; Mestres-Misse et al., 2007; Perfetti et al., 2005), all participants showed enhanced N400s over frontal scalp sites after the first half (i.e. only 3 minutes) of the word-learning phase. However, only musicians showed additional N400 increases over left centro-parietal scalp regions after the second half of the word-learning phase, suggesting that musicians were faster in encoding word meaning and integrating novel words into existing semantic networks.

During the test phase (i.e. matching and semantic tasks), musicians were characterized by a typical centro-parietal N400 effect (Kutas & Federmeier, 2011) resulting from larger N400 amplitudes for unexpected (i.e. mismatching or unrelated) than for expected (i.e. matching or related) conditions (see Figure 10.4). By contrast, the N400 was still frontally distributed in non-musicians. In summary, while both groups showed the typical electrophysiological marker of word learning (i.e. the frontal N400) during the learning phase, only musicians showed semantic priming effects during the test phase that were similar to those typically found for known words. In line with this conclusion, a correlation between musical aptitudes and the amplitude of the semantic N400 effect was found for musicians, but not for non-musicians, thereby clearly pointing to a relationship between musicality and word learning. Finally, in the behavioural retest 5 months after the main session, musicians remembered more words compared to non-musicians, thereby showing evidence for long-lasting word representations and an influence of music training on verbal long-term memory.

In a second step, data from this word-learning experiment was reanalysed by means of functional connectivity (Dittinger et al., 2017). Functional connectivity is defined as the statistical association or dependency among two or more anatomically distinct functional time series (Friston et al., 1996). Functional connectivity is a useful method for studying

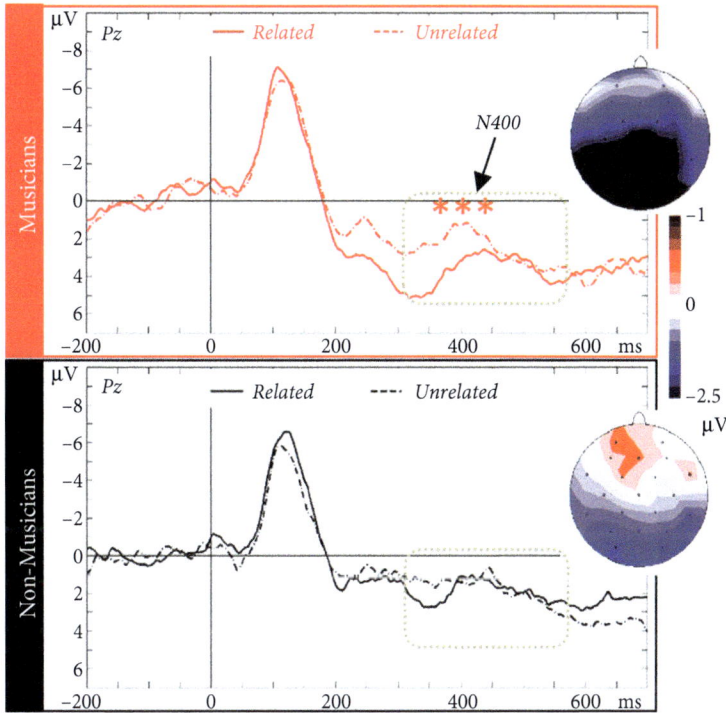

FIGURE 10.4 Semantic task. ERPs recorded at parietal sites (Pz) are overlapped for semantically related (solid lines) and unrelated (dotted lines) words, separately for musicians (red) and non-musicians (black). Time in milliseconds is in abscissa, the amplitude of the effects in microvolts is in ordinate, time zero corresponds to word onset, and negativity is plotted upwards. The grey dotted rectangles represent the typical N400 latency window, and the level of significance of the related vs unrelated difference in the two groups is represented by asterisks (with ***p < 0.001). Topographic voltage distribution maps of the unrelated minus related differences in musicians and non-musicians are illustrated for the N400 component and voltage values are scaled from −2.5 to +1.0 μV.

functional relationships between regions as a function of expertise. In the first part of this chapter, we reviewed some of the current models of speech processing that converge on the view that two main processing streams, the ventral (i.e. sound-to-meaning mapping) and the dorsal (i.e. sound-to-articulation mapping) pathways, are involved in speech processing (Friederici, 2009). Specifically, the dorsal pathway relies on a fibre tract corresponding to the superior longitudinal fasciculus (SLF)/arcuate fasciculus (AF) complex, sprawling from inferior parietal and superior-posterior temporal brain regions towards Broca's area and promoting auditory-to-motor mapping mechanisms. Recently, Lopez-Barroso and colleagues (2013) showed that word learning was correlated with the strength of functional and structural connectivity between Broca's and Wernicke's territory. Moreover, there is evidence that the functional-structural architecture of the left dorsal processing stream is influenced by professional musical training (Halwani et al., 2011; Klein et al., 2016; Oechslin et al., 2009).

Based on these results, we investigated functional connectivity between angular/supramarginal gyrus (AG/SMG) (region of interest (ROI) 1, Brodmann area (BA) 39/40) and Broca's area (ROI 2, BA 44/45) in the three tasks related to word learning previously described (i.e. word learning phase, matching tasks, and semantic tasks) and compared patterns of connectivity between musicians and the non-musician controls. Specifically, we evaluated non-linear functional connectivity by using lagged coherence, that is, a measure of the variability of time differences between two signals (e.g. coming from ROI 1 and from ROI 2) in a specific frequency band (Lehmann et al., 2006; Thatcher, 2012). We focused on theta (4–7 Hz) oscillations based on previous literature evidencing that theta reflects neuronal communications over long-range circuits and is a reliable frequency band to examine mnemonic processes (Ward, 2003).

As expected, results revealed increased left-hemispheric functional connectivity in musicians compared to controls, but only in the semantic task. In addition, this increased connectivity was correlated with the cumulative number of training years. Results were interpreted as showing facilitated feed-forward and feed-backward exchanges between AG/SMG and Broca's area in musicians, thereby facilitating the rehearsal and learning of novel words in musicians. These results are in line with previous results (Klein et al., 2016; López-Barroso et al., 2013) and with the group differences in ERPs and behaviour described previously. Furthermore, the data indicates a relationship between the musicians' superiority in word learning and the temporal alignment of neural oscillations in the theta frequency band in the left dorsal stream.

Taken together, ERPs and functional connectivity revealed two main findings. First, word learning was reflected in the spatio-temporal dynamics of the N400 component: while initial word learning was reflected by frontally increasing N400s, centro-parietal N400s only developed once the novel words started being integrated into the pool of well-known words. This difference in scalp distribution may reflect different cognitive processes and clearly points to distinct neural generators. For instance, frontal N400s to novel words are compatible with results showing that prefrontal and temporal brain regions are associated with the maintenance of novel information in working or short-term memory (Hagoort, 2014) and with the initial building up of episodic memory traces (Rodriguez-Fornells et al., 2009). By contrast, centro-parietally distributed N400s are in line with results showing that semantic representations are possibly stored in the left inferior parietal cortex (Catani & Ffytche, 2005) and/or in the left temporal lobe (Geranmayeh et al., 2015). Furthermore, our experimental design allowed us to track the fast spatio-temporal dynamics of word learning that were characterized by a shift in N400 distribution from frontal to parietal networks after only 3–6 minutes of training. These results open new perspectives for further research on brain plasticity and word learning. In addition, we provide the first behavioural evidence for the longevity of these rapidly established word representations, highlighting that even rapid brain plasticity can have long-lasting consequences.

Second, our results revealed that word learning was facilitated by professional music training. How can we account for such a transfer and what could be the implications of these results? As already mentioned in Section 10.3.2, two main interpretations have been proposed to explain why musicians learn novel words more efficiently than non-musicians. The first one, in terms of cascading effects, claims that enhanced auditory perception facilitates word learning in musicians. Such an interpretation would be in line with bottom–up accounts of transfer effects. Support for this interpretation was provided by Wong and Perrachione (2007) and by Cooper and Wang (2012) who showed that both tone pitch identification and musical aptitudes were significantly correlated with word-learning success in adult English speakers. To directly test for the causality of these effects, Cooper and

Wang (2013) trained English non-musicians on the perception of Cantonese tones, and results demonstrated that enhanced perception at the tone level significantly improved word learning. By contrast, the multidimensional interpretation acknowledges potential top–down influences on word learning, as well as interactions between the acoustic properties of sounds, task demands, and expertise of the listener.

While our experimental design does not allow for the disentangling of the cascade and multidimensional accounts, the present results clearly reveal that music training influences the semantic level of language processing, thereby going one step beyond previous studies on transfer effects. Certainly, further studies are needed to replicate these results, possibly with children and older adults, and to disentangle the respective contribution of perceptive and cognitive functions to word learning, thereby possibly lifting the exciting secret of why musicians seem to be better at learning novel words.

10.5 Conclusion

The issue of music to speech transfer effects has generated great interest in the scientific community, as well as in the lay public, probably because music and speech are fascinating domains. The multidimensional aspects of music and speech—how they both rely on perceptual, cognitive, emotional, and motor processes through multiple interactions—are important new avenues for future research. Similarly, much more needs to be done to fully understand how these two abilities are implemented in the brain and whether they rely on shared or distinct neural resources. Based on the current state of knowledge, it is clear that results are tightly linked to the tasks and stimuli that are presented and to the methods that are used for data analysis. Also clear is that music exerts a profound influence on the brain's structural and functional organization, thanks to brain plasticity. It is worth noting in this respect that recent results demonstrated changes in brain electric activity in less than 3 minutes in a novel word-learning task (Dittinger et al., 2017). Taken together, these results open exciting new perspectives for the rehabilitation of patients (children, young adults, and older adults) with various neurological or psychiatric deficits. In this respect, music training may have a strong societal impact.

Acknowledgements

We are grateful for the help provided by the Labex BLRI (ANR-11-LABX-0036), supported by the French National Agency for Research (ANR), under the programme 'Investissements d'Avenir' (ANR-11-IDEX-0001-02). ED is supported by a doctoral fellowship from the BLRI. The authors declare no competing financial interests.

References

Abrams, D. A. et al. (2011). Decoding temporal structure in music and speech relies on shared brain resources but elicits different fine-scale spatial patterns. *Cerebral Cortex*, 21, 1507–1518.

Alexander, J. A., Wong, P. C., & Bradlow, A. R. (2005). *Lexical tone perception in musicians and non-musicians.* Paper presented at 9th European Conference on Speech Communication and Technology, Lisbon, Portugal (pp. 397–400).

Asaridou, S. S. & McQueen, J. M. (2013). Speech and music shape the listening brain: evidence for shared domain-general mechanisms. *Frontiers in Psychology*, 4, article 321.

Barrett, K. C., Ashley, R., Strait, D. L., & Kraus, N. (2013). Art and science: how musical training shapes the brain. *Frontiers in Psychology*, 4, article 713.

Batterink, L. & Neville, H. (2011). Implicit and explicit mechanisms of word learning in a narrative context: an event-related potential study. *Journal of Cognitive Neuroscience*, 23, 3181–3196.

Belin, P., Zatorre, R. J., Lafaille, P., Ahad, P., & Pike, B. (2000). Voice-selective areas in human auditory cortex. *Nature*, 403, 309–312.

Bergman Nutley, S., Darki, F., & Klingberg, T. (2014). Music practice is associated with development of working memory during childhood and adolescence. *Frontiers in Human Neuroscience*, 7, 926.

Berwick, R. C., Friederici, A. D., Chomsky, N., & Bolhuis, J. J. (2013). Evolution, brain, and the nature of language. *Trends in Cognitive Sciences*, 17, 89–98.

Besson, M., Chobert, J., & Marie, C. (2011). Transfer of training between music and speech: common processing, attention, and memory. *Frontiers in Psychology*, 2, article 94.

Bidelman, G. M. & Alain, C. (2015). Musical training orchestrates coordinated neuroplasticity in auditory brainstem and cortex to counteract age-related declines in categorical vowel perception. *Journal of Neuroscience*, 35, 1240–1249.

Bidelman, G. M. & Krishnan, A. (2010). Effects of reverberation on brainstem representation of speech in musicians and non-musicians. *Brain Research*, 1355, 112–125.

Bidelman, G. M., Gandour, J. T., & Krishnan, A. (2011). Musicians and tone-language speakers share enhanced brainstem encoding but not perceptual benefits for musical pitch. *Brain and Cognition*, 77, 1–10.

Bidelman, G. M., Moreno, S., & Alain, C. (2013). Tracing the emergence of categorical speech perception in the human auditory system. *NeuroImage*, 79, 201–212.

Bidelman, G. M., Weiss, M. W., Moreno, S., & Alain, C. (2014). Coordinated plasticity in brainstem and auditory cortex contributes to enhanced categorical speech perception in musicians. *European Journal of Neuroscience*, 40, 2662–2673.

Boland, J. E. (2014). A history of psycholinguistics: the pre-Chomskyan era. *Historiographia Linguistica*, 41(1), 168–175.

Bornkessel-Schlesewsky, I. & Schlesewsky, M. (2013). Reconciling time, space and function: a new dorsal-ventral stream model of sentence comprehension. *Brain and Language*, 125, 60–76.

Borovsky, A., Elman, J. L., & Kutas, M. (2012). Once is enough: N400 indexes semantic integration of novel word meanings from a single exposure in context. *Language Learning and Development*, 8, 278–302.

Borovsky, A., Kutas, M., & Elman, J. (2010). Learning to use words: event-related potentials index single-shot contextual word learning. *Cognition*, 116, 289–296.

Brandler, S. & Rammsayer, T. H. (2003). Differences in mental abilities between musicians and non-musicians. *Psychology of Music*, 31, 123–138.

Brauer, J., Anwander, A., Perani, D., & Friederici, A. D. (2013). Dorsal and ventral pathways in language development. *Brain and Language*, 127, 289–295.

Cason, N. & Schön, D. (2012). Rhythmic priming enhances the phonological processing of speech. *Neuropsychologia*, 50, 2652–2658.

Catani, M. & Ffytche, D. H. (2005). The rises and falls of disconnection syndromes. *Journal of Brain and Neurology*, 128, 2224–2239.

Chan, A. S., Ho, Y. C., & Cheung, M. C. (1998). Music training improves verbal memory. *Nature*, 396, 128.

Chartrand, J.-P. & Belin, P. (2006). Superior voice timbre processing in musicians. *Neuroscience Letters*, 405, 164–167.

Chen, J. L., Penhune, V. B., & Zatorre, R. J. (2008). Moving on time: brain network for auditory-motor synchronization is modulated by rhythm complexity and musical training. *Journal of Cognitive Neuroscience*, 20, 226–239.

Chobert, J., Francois, C., Velay, J.-L., & Besson, M. (2014). Twelve months of active musical training in 8- to 10-year-old children enhances the preattentive processing of syllabic duration and voice onset time. *Cerebral Cortex*, 24, 956–967.

Cooper, A. & Wang, Y. (2013). Effects of tone training on Cantonese tone-word learning. *Journal of the Acoustical Society of America*, 134, EL133–EL139.

Cooper, A. & Wang, Y. (2012). The influence of linguistic and musical experience on Cantonese word learning. *Journal of the Acoustical Society of America*, 131, 4756–4769.

Dehaene-Lambertz, G. & Spelke, E. S. (2015). The infancy of the human brain. *Neuron*, 88, 93–109.

Diamond, A. (2013). Executive functions. *Annual Review of Psychology*, 64, 135–168.

Dittinger, E. et al. (2016). Professional music training and novel word learning: from faster semantic encoding to longer-lasting word representations. *Journal of Cognitive Neuroscience*, 28(10), 1584–1602.

Dittinger, E., Valizadeh, S. A., Jäncke, L., Besson, M., & Elmer, S. (2017). Increased functional connectivity in the ventral and dorsal streams during retrieval of novel words in professional musicians. *Human Brain Mapping*, 39, 722–734.

Dittinger, E., D'império, M., & Besson, M. (2018). Enhanced neural and behavioral processing of a non-native phonemic contrast in professional musicians. *European Journal of Neuroscience*, 1–13. doi: 10.1111/ejn.13939

Elbert, T., Pantev, C., Wienbruch, C., Rockstroh, B., & Taub, E. (1995). Increased cortical representation of the fingers of the left hand in string players. *Science*, 270, 305–307.

Elmer, S., Meyer, M., & Jancke, L. (2012). Neurofunctional and behavioral correlates of phonetic and temporal categorization in musically trained and untrained subjects. *Cerebral Cortex*, 22, 650–658.

Farbood, M. M., Heeger, D. J., Marcus, G., Hasson, U., & Lerner, Y. (2015). The neural processing of hierarchical structure in music and speech at different timescales. *Frontiers in Neuroscience*, 9, 157.

Fitch, W. T. (2010). *The Evolution of Language*. Cambridge University Press.

Fitch, W. T. & Reby, D. (2001). The descended larynx is not uniquely human. *Proceedings of the Royal Society B: Biological Sciences*, 268, 1669–1675.

Fitzroy, A. B. & Sanders, L. D. (2012). Musical expertise modulates early processing of syntactic violations in language. *Frontiers in Psychology*, 3, 603.

Francois, C., Chobert, J., Besson, M., & Schon, D. (2013). Music training for the development of speech segmentation. *Cerebral Cortex*, 23, 2038–2043.

Francois, C. & Schön, D. (2011). Musical expertise boosts implicit learning of both musical and linguistic structures. *Cerebral Cortex*, 21, 2357–2365.

Franklin, M. S. et al. (2008). The effects of musical training on verbal memory. *Psychology of Music*, 36, 353–365.

Friederici, A. D. (2009). Pathways to language: fiber tracts in the human brain. *Trends in Cognitive Sciences*, 13, 175–181.

Friederici, A. D. (2011). The brain basis of language processing: from structure to function. *Physiology Review*, 91, 1357–1392.

Friederici, A. D. (2012). The cortical language circuit: from auditory perception to sentence comprehension. *Trends in Cognitive Sciences*, 16, 262–268.

Friederici, A. D., Bahlmann, J., Heim, S., Schubotz, R. I., & Anwander, A. (2006). The brain differentiates human and non-human grammars: functional localization and structural connectivity. *Proceedings of the National Academy of Sciences of the United States of America*, 103, 2458–2463.

Friederici, A. D. & Singer, W. (2015). Grounding language processing on basic neurophysiological principles. *Trends in Cognitive Sciences*, 19, 329–338.

Friston, K. J., Frith, C. D., Fletcher, P., Liddle, P. F., & Frackowiak, R. S. (1996). Functional topography: multidimensional scaling and functional connectivity in the brain. *Cerebral Cortex*, 6, 156–164.

George, E. M. & Coch, D. (2011). Music training and working memory: an ERP study. *Neuropsychologia*, 49, 1083–1094.

Geranmayeh, F., Leech, R., & Wise, R. J. S. (2015). Semantic retrieval during overt picture description: left anterior temporal or the parietal lobe? *Neuropsychologia*, 76, 125–135.

Giraud, A.-L. & Poeppel, D. (2012). Cortical oscillations and speech processing: emerging computational principles and operations. *Nature Neuroscience*, 15, 511–517.

Giraud, A.-L. et al. (2007). Endogenous cortical rhythms determine cerebral specialization for speech perception and production. *Neuron*, 56, 1127–1134.

Gogtay, N. et al. (2004). Dynamic mapping of human cortical development during childhood through early adulthood. *Proceedings of the National Academy of Sciences of the United States of America*, 101, 8174–8179.

Golestani, N. & Pallier, C. (2007). Anatomical correlates of foreign speech sound production. *Cerebral Cortex*, 17, 929–934.

Golestani, N. & Zatorre, R. J. (2004). Learning new sounds of speech: reallocation of neural substrates. *NeuroImage*, 21, 494–506.

Hagoort, P. (2014). Nodes and networks in the neural architecture for language: Broca's region and beyond. *Current Opinion in Neurobiology*, 28, 136–141.

Halwani, G. F., Loui, P., Rüber, T., & Schlaug, G. (2011). Effects of practice and experience on the arcuate fasciculus: comparing singers, instrumentalists, and non-musicians. *Frontiers in Psychology*, 2, 156.

Harasty, J., Seldon, H. L., Chan, P., Halliday, G., & Harding, A. (2003). The left human speech-processing cortex is thinner but longer than the right. *Laterality*, 8, 247–260.

Hauser, M. D. (2002). The faculty of language: what is it, who has it, and how did it evolve? *Science*, 298, 1569–1579.

Hickok, G. & Poeppel, D. (2007). The cortical organization of speech processing. *Nature Reviews Neuroscience*, 8, 393–402.

Jakobson, L. S., Lewycky, S. T., Kilgour, A. R., & Stoesz, B. M. (2008). Memory for verbal and visual material in highly trained musicians. *Music Perception: An Interdisciplinary Journal*, 26, 41–55.

Jäncke, L. (2012). The relationship between music and language. *Frontiers in Psychology*, 3, article 123.

Janus, M., Lee, Y., Moreno, S., & Bialystok, E. (2016). Effects of short-term music and second-language training on executive control. *Journal of Experimental Child Psychology*, 144, 84–97.

Jentschke, S. & Koelsch, S. (2009). Musical training modulates the development of syntax processing in children. *NeuroImage*, 47, 735–744.

Klein, C., Liem, F., Hänggi, J., Elmer, S., & Jäncke, L. (2016). The 'silent' imprint of musical training. *Human Brain Mapping*, 37, 536–546.

Koelsch, S. et al. (2002). Bach speaks: a cortical 'language-network' serves the processing of music. *NeuroImage*, 17, 956–966.

Kraus, N. & Chandrasekaran, B. (2010). Music training for the development of auditory skills. *Nature Reviews Neuroscience*, 11, 599–605.

Kuhl, P. K. (2004). Early language acquisition: cracking the speech code. *Nature Reviews Neuroscience*, 5, 831–843.

Kuhl, P. K. (2007). Is speech learning 'gated' by the social brain? *Developmental Science*, 10, 110–20.

Kutas, M. & Federmeier, K. D. (2011). Thirty years and counting: finding meaning in the N400 component of the event-related brain potential (ERP). *Annual Review of Psychology*, 62, 621–647.

Lahav, A., Saltzman, E., & Schlaug, G. (2007). Action representation of sound: audiomotor recognition network while listening to newly acquired actions. *Journal of Neuroscience*, 27, 308–314.

Lee, C.-Y. & Hung, T.-H. (2008). Identification of Mandarin tones by English-speaking musicians and nonmusicians. *Journal of the Acoustical Society of America*, 124, 3235–3248.

Lee, H. & Noppeney, U. (2011). Long-term music training tunes how the brain temporally binds signals from multiple senses. *Proceedings of the National Academy of Sciences of the United States of America*, 108, E1441–1450.

Lehmann, D., Faber, P. L., Gianotti, L. R. R., Kochi, K., & Pascual-Marqui, R. D. (2006). Coherence and phase locking in the scalp EEG and between LORETA model sources, and microstates as putative mechanisms of brain temporo-spatial functional organization. *Journal of Physiology (Paris)*, 99, 29–36.

Levitin, D. J. & Menon, V. (2003). Musical structure is processed in 'language' areas of the brain: a possible role for Brodmann Area 47 in temporal coherence. *NeuroImage*, 20, 2142–2152.

Lima, C. F. & Castro, S. L. (2011). Speaking to the trained ear: musical expertise enhances the recognition of emotions in speech prosody. *Emotion (Washington DC)*, 11, 1021–1031.

López-Barroso, D. et al. (2013). Word learning is mediated by the left arcuate fasciculus. *Proceedings of the National Academy of Sciences of the United States of America*, 110, 13168–13173.

Ma, W. & Thompson, W. F. (2015). Human emotions track changes in the acoustic environment. *Proceedings of the National Academy of Sciences of the United States of America*, 112, 14563–14568.

Maess, B., Koelsch, S., Gunter, T. C., & Friederici, A. D. (2001). Musical syntax is processed in Broca's area: an MEG study. *Nature Neuroscience*, 4, 540–545.

Magne, C., Schön, D., & Besson, M. (2006). Musician children detect pitch violations in both music and language better than nonmusician children: behavioral and electrophysiological approaches. *Journal of Cognitive Neuroscience*, 18, 199–211.

Marques, C., Moreno, S., Castro, S. L., & Besson, M. (2007). Musicians detect pitch violation in a foreign language better than nonmusicians: behavioral and electrophysiological evidence. *Journal of Cognitive Neuroscience*, 19, 1453–1463.

Mathias, B., Palmer, C., Perrin, F., & Tillmann, B. (2015). Sensorimotor learning enhances expectations during auditory perception. *Cerebral Cortex*, 25, 2238–2254.

McLaughlin, J., Osterhout, L., & Kim, A. (2004). Neural correlates of second-language word learning: minimal instruction produces rapid change. *Nature Neuroscience*, 7, 703–704.

Mestres- Misse, A., Rodriguez-Fornells, A., & Munte, T. F. (2007). Watching the brain during meaning acquisition. *Cerebral Cortex*, 17, 1858–1866.

Meyer, M., Elmer, S., & Jäncke, L. (2012). Musical expertise induces neuroplasticity of the planum temporale. *Annals of the New York Academy of Sciences*, 1252, 116–123.

Milner, A. D. & Goodale, M. A. (2008). Two visual systems re-viewed. *Neuropsychologia*, 46, 774–785.

Mishkin, M. & Ungerleider, L. G. (1982). Contribution of striate inputs to the visuospatial functions of parieto-preoccipital cortex in monkeys. *Behavioural Brain Research*, 6, 57–77.

Moreno, S. et al. (2009). Musical training influences linguistic abilities in 8-year-old children: more evidence for brain plasticity. *Cerebral Cortex*, 19, 712–723.

Moreno, S. et al. (2011). Short-term music training enhances verbal intelligence and executive function. *Psychological Science*, 22, 1425–1433.

Münte, T. F., Altenmüller, E., & Jäncke, L. (2002). The musician's brain as a model of neuroplasticity. *Nature Reviews Neuroscience*, 3, 473–478.

Musacchia, G., Sams, M., Skoe, E., & Kraus, N. (2007). Musicians have enhanced subcortical auditory and audiovisual processing of speech and music. *Proceedings of the National Academy of Sciences of the United States of America*, 104, 15894–15898.

Norman-Haignere, S., Kanwisher, N. G., & McDermott, J. H. (2015). Distinct cortical pathways for music and speech revealed by hypothesis-free voxel decomposition. *Neuron*, 88, 1281–1296.

Oechslin, M. S., Imfeld, A., Loenneker, T., Meyer, M., & Jäncke, L. (2009). The plasticity of the superior longitudinal fasciculus as a function of musical expertise: a diffusion tensor imaging study. *Frontiers in Human Neuroscience*, 3, 76.

Ott, C. (2011). Processing of voiced and unvoiced acoustic stimuli in musicians. *Frontiers in Psychology*, 2, article 195.

Overath, T., McDermott, J. H., Zarate, J. M., & Poeppel, D. (2015). The cortical analysis of speech- specific temporal structure revealed by responses to sound quilts. *Nature Neuroscience*, 18, 903–911.

Pallesen, K. J. et al. (2010). Cognitive control in auditory working memory is enhanced in musicians. *PLoS One*, 5, e11120.

Pantev, C., Lappe, C., Herholz, S. C., & Trainor, L. (2009). Auditory-somatosensory integration and cortical plasticity in musical training. *Annals of the New York Academy of Sciences*, 1169, 143–150.

Paraskevopoulos, E., Kraneburg, A., Herholz, S. C., Bamidis, P. D., & Pantev, C. (2015). Musical expertise is related to altered functional connectivity during audiovisual integration. *Proceedings of the National Academy of Sciences of the United States of America*, 112, 12522–12527.

Paraskevopoulos, E., Kuchenbuch, A., Herholz, S. C., & Pantev, C. (2012). Musical expertise induces audiovisual integration of abstract congruency rules. *Journal of Neuroscience*, 32, 18196–18203.

Paraskevopoulos, E., Kuchenbuch, A., Herholz, S. C., & Pantev, C. (2014). Multisensory integration during short-term music reading training enhances both uni- and multisensory cortical processing. *Journal of Cognitive Neuroscience*, 26, 2224–2238.

Perani, D. et al. (2011). Neural language networks at birth. *Proceedings of the National Academy of Sciences of the United States of America*, 108, 16056–16061.

Perfetti, C. A., Wlotko, E. W., & Hart, L. A. (2005). Word learning and individual differences in word learning reflected in event-related potentials. *Journal of Experimental Psychology: Learning, Memory and Cognition*, 31, 1281–1292.

Péron, J., Frühholz, S., Ceravolo, L., & Grandjean, D. (2016). Structural and functional connectivity of the subthalamic nucleus during vocal emotion decoding. *Social, Cognitive, and Affective Neuroscience*, 11, 349–356.

Rauschecker, J. P. & Scott, S. K. (2009). Maps and streams in the auditory cortex: nonhuman primates illuminate human speech processing. *Nature Neuroscience*, 12, 718–724.

Ripollés, P. et al. (2014). The role of reward in word learning and its implications for language acquisition. *Current Biology*, 24, 2606–2611.

Roden, I., Kreutz, G., & Bongard, S. (2012). Effects of a school-based instrumental music program on verbal and visual memory in primary school children: a longitudinal study. *Frontiers in Psychology*, 3, article 572.

Rodríguez-Fornells, A., Cunillera, T., Mestres-Missé, A., & de Diego-Balaguer, R. (2009). Neurophysiological mechanisms involved in language learning in adults. *Philosophical Transactions of the Royal Society B: Biological Sciences*, 364, 3711–3735.

Rogalsky, C., Rong, F., Saberi, K., & Hickok, G. (2011). Functional anatomy of language and music perception: temporal and structural factors investigated using functional magnetic resonance imaging. *Journal of Neuroscience*, 31, 3843–3852.

Roncaglia-Denissen, M. P., Schmidt-Kassow, M., & Kotz, S. A. (2013). Speech rhythm facilitates syntactic ambiguity resolution: ERP evidence. *PLoS One*, 8, e56000.

Saffran, J. R. (2003). Statistical language learning mechanisms and constraints. *Current Directions in Psychological Science*, 12, 110–114.

Santoro, R. et al. (2014). Encoding of natural sounds at multiple spectral and temporal resolutions in the human auditory cortex. *PLoS Computational Biology*, 10, e1003412.

Schellenberg, E. G. (2004). Music lessons enhance IQ. *Psychological Science*, 15, 511–514.

Schlaug, G., Jancke, L., Huang, Y., & Steinmetz, H. (1995). In vivo evidence of structural brain asymmetry in musicians. *Science*, 267, 699–701.

Schmidt-Kassow, M. & Kotz, S. A. (2009). Event-related brain potentials suggest a late interaction of meter and syntax in the P600. *Journal of Cognitive Neuroscience*, 21, 1693–1708.

Schneider, P. et al. (2002). Morphology of Heschl's gyrus reflects enhanced activation in the auditory cortex of musicians. *Nature Neuroscience*, 5, 688–694.

Schön, D., Magne, C., & Besson, M. (2004). The music of speech: music training facilitates pitch processing in both music and language. *Psychophysiology*, 41, 341–349.

Schulze, K., Dowling, W. J., & Tillmann, B. (2012). Working memory for tonal and atonal sequences during a forward and a backward recognition task. *Music Perception: An Interdisciplinary Journal*, 29, 255–267.

Schulze, K. & Koelsch, S. (2012). Working memory for speech and music. *Annals of the New York Academy of Sciences*, 1252, 229–236.

Schulze, K., Mueller, K., & Koelsch, S. (2011). Neural correlates of strategy use during auditory working memory in musicians and non-musicians. *European Journal of Neuroscience*, 33, 189–196.

Schulze, K., Zysset, S., Mueller, K., Friederici, A. D., & Koelsch, S. (2011). Neuroarchitecture of verbal and tonal working memory in nonmusicians and musicians. *Human Brain Mapping*, 32, 771–783.

Seldon, H. L. (1981). Structure of human auditory cortex. I. Cytoarchitectonics and dendritic distributions. *Brain Research*, 229, 277–294.

Sluming, V. et al. (2002). Voxel-based morphometry reveals increased gray matter density in Broca's area in male symphony orchestra musicians. *NeuroImage*, 17, 1613–1622.

Thatcher, R. W. (2012). Coherence, phase differences, phase shift, and phase lock in EEG/ERP analyses. *Developmental Neuropsychology*, 37, 476–496.

Thompson, W. F., Marin, M. M., & Stewart, L. (2012). Reduced sensitivity to emotional prosody in congenital amusia rekindles the musical protolanguage hypothesis. *Proceedings of the National Academy of Sciences of the United States of America*, 109, 19027–19032.

Thompson, W. F., Schellenberg, E. G., & Husain, G. (2004). Decoding speech prosody: do music lessons help? *Emotion (Washington DC)*, 4, 46–64.

Tillmann, B., Janata, P., & Bharucha, J. J. (2003). Activation of the inferior frontal cortex in musical priming. *Annals of the New York Academy of Sciences*, 999, 209–211.

Trimmer, C. G. & Cuddy, L. L. (2008). Emotional intelligence, not music training, predicts recognition of emotional speech prosody. *Emotion (Washington DC)*, 8, 838–849.

Vuust, P., Roepstorff, A., Wallentin, M., Mouridsen, K., & Østergaard, L. (2006). It don't mean a thing... Keeping the rhythm during polyrhythmic tension activates language areas (BA47). *NeuroImage*, 31, 832–841.

Ward, L. M. (2003). Synchronous neural oscillations and cognitive processes. *Trends in Cognitive Sciences*, 7, 553–559.

Williamson, V. J., Baddeley, A. D., & Hitch, G. J. (2010). Musicians' and nonmusicians' short-term memory for verbal and musical sequences: comparing phonological similarity and pitch proximity. *Memory and Cognition*, 38, 163–175.

Wong, P. C. M. & Perrachione, T. K. (2007). Learning pitch patterns in lexical identification by native English-speaking adults. *Applied Psycholinguistics*, 28(4), 565–585.

Wong, P. C. M., Skoe, E., Russo, N. M., Dees, T., & Kraus, N. (2007). Musical experience shapes human brainstem encoding of linguistic pitch patterns. *Nature Neuroscience*, 10, 420–422.

Zatorre, R. J. & Belin, P. (2001). Spectral and temporal processing in human auditory cortex. *Cerebral Cortex*, 11, 946–953.

Zuk, J., Benjamin, C., Kenyon, A., & Gaab, N. (2014). Behavioral and neural correlates of executive functioning in musicians and non-musicians. *PLoS One*, 9, e99868.

APPENDIX 10.1

AUDITORY STIMULI

The four consonant-vowel (CV) syllables (two natural German consonant-vowel syllables and two reduced-spectrum analogues; see Audio 10.1) were used in three previous publications in order to assess putative advantages of musicians in processing fast-changing phonetic cues. These stimuli consisted of the German CV syllables /ka/ (voiceless initial consonant) and /da/ (voiced initial consonant) as well as of its reduced-spectrum analogues. The duration of the syllables was about 350 ms, and the voice-onset time (VOT) of /da/ and /ka/ was approximately 13 ms and 53 ms, respectively. For the reduced-spectrum analogues, spectral information was removed from the CV syllables by replacing the frequency-specific information in a broad frequency region with band-limited white noise (band 1: 500–1500 Hz, band 2: 2500–3500 Hz). Amplitude and temporal cues were preserved in each spectral band, resulting in double-band-pass filtered noise with temporal CV-amplitude dynamics. A detailed description of the stimuli can be found here:

Elmer, S., Meyer, M., & Jäncke, L. (2012). Neurofunctional and behavioral correlates of phonetic and temporal categorization in musically trained and untrained subjects. *Cerebral Cortex*, 22, 650–658.

Elmer, S., Hänggi, J., Meyer, M., & Jäncke, L. (2013). Increased cortical surface area of the left planum temporale in musicians facilitates the categorization of phonetic and temporal speech sounds. *Cortex*, 49, 2812–2821.

Elmer, S., Hänggi, J., & Jäncke, L. (2016). Interhemispheric transcallosal connectivity between the left and right planum temporale predicts musicianship, performance in temporal speech processing, and functional specialization. *Brain Structure and Function*, 221, 331–344.

CHAPTER 11

....

SOCIAL PERCEPTION IN INFANCY

An Integrative Perspective on the Development of Voice and Face Perception

....

EVELYNE MERCURE AND LAURA KISCHKEL

11.1 INTRODUCTION

HUMAN neonates are born social beings, and seek out human interaction and communication. The ability to perceive, judge, and evaluate social cues in a vast array of situations requires considerable amounts of expertise, which is developed over the course of life. Despite their complexity, babies and children learn these abilities in a seemingly effortless manner from a very early age onwards.

From the first days of life, babies appear to be naturally attracted to human faces and voices, and have a bias to preferentially attend these social stimuli over competing stimuli. Indeed, it has been shown that neonates prefer to look at schemas representing the natural configuration of a human face than to abstract patterns (Johnson et al., 1991). They also preferentially attend to pictures displaying a face that directly looks at them over a face with an averted gaze (Farroni et al., 2002), which further suggests a preference for potential communication. These attentional biases in the visual modality are observed without extensive experience of human faces since neonates are only exposed to human faces after birth.

In the auditory modality, human neonates also show a preference for social stimuli. They preferentially listen to speech, compared to complex non-speech analogues (Vouloumanos & Werker, 2007). However, unlike in the visual modality, this preference may result from prenatal experience and learning. Indeed, since human infants can hear from the twenty-fourth week of gestation (Birnholz & Benacerraf, 1983), they are born with experience of human voices, particularly their mother's. The sounds and vibrations of their mother's voice are perceived prenatally and used to learn about human vocalizations, speech, and language. Newborns also prefer to listen to their own mother's voice in contrast with the voice of another woman, and prefer their mother tongue to an unfamiliar language (DeCasper & Fifer 1980; Moon et al., 1993), which suggests that infants benefit from a head start in learning about voices when compared to faces.

These newborn biases to preferentially attend to facial and vocal cues put babies on a trajectory that maximize exposure to social signals from the first days of life. This strengthens their expertise in collecting and analysing information from other human beings to gain information about the world around them and to develop their own means of social communication. In parallel to this perceptual and cognitive development, the brain also develops specialized networks to process faces and voices.

In this chapter, we will address the earliest steps in the human development of voice processing, as well as its integration with face processing during infancy. We will start by discussing recent neuroimaging findings relating to brain processing of human vocalizations in infancy, before presenting behavioural and neurocognitive evidence of audiovisual integration in social perception.

11.2 Voice Processing in the Infant Brain

Human voices play a fundamental role in social communication since they communicate information through speech, as well as cues about a person's gender, age, emotional state, and well-being (Latinus & Belin, 2011). As discussed in Part IV of this handbook, the human voice and the emotional information conveyed by human vocalizations have been found to modulate the activity of a number of areas of the adult brain, including the superior temporal sulcus (STS), inferior prefrontal cortex, premotor cortical regions, amygdala, and insula (Fecteau et al., 2005, 2007; Morris et al., 1999; Sander & Scheich, 2001; Warren et al., 2006). A few recent neuroimaging studies suggest that specialized brain networks for processing human voices develop very early in infancy.

11.2.1 Voice-Sensitive Activation

Preferential activation for human voices has been repeatedly observed along the STS in adulthood (Belin et al., 2000), but the developmental trajectory of this cortical specialization is less clear. To address this question, Blasi et al. (2011) examined activation patterns to vocal and non-vocal stimuli in 3- to 7-month-old infants using functional magnetic resonance imaging (fMRI). Infants were presented with three types of adult vocalizations (emotionally neutral, emotionally positive, and emotionally negative) and a mixture of non-vocal environmental sounds likely to be familiar to infants of that age. All vocal stimuli were non-speech natural vocalizations that preverbal infants produce themselves from a very early age (sneezing, coughing, crying, laughing). When comparing emotionally neutral vocalizations with non-vocal sounds, a strong voice-sensitive activation was found in the temporal cortex of 3- to 7-month-old infants (see Figure 11.1A). The strongest activation was found in the right middle temporal gyrus close to the temporal pole, in a location similar to the anterior portion of the voice-sensitive area reported in adults (Belin et al., 2000). These results suggest that the functional specialization of the superior temporal cortex for human voices develops within the first few months of life. Interestingly, a significant cluster in the left superior temporal gyrus (Brodmann area 22) showed a positive correlation with age in the vocal versus non-vocal activation pattern. This suggests that the sensitivity for human voices further increases in the temporal cortex between 3 and 7 months.

For methodological reasons, infants in this fMRI study were scanned during their natural sleep. It is unclear how brain activation was influenced by the infants' sleeping state. Studies using functional near infrared spectroscopy (fNIRS) could clarify this question, since this method can be reliably used with awake and attending infants. Using fNIRS, Grossmann et al. (2010) investigated cortical activation in two groups of infants (4- and 7-month-olds) in response to vocal sounds (a mixture of speech and non-speech vocalizations) and non-vocal sounds (sounds from nature, animals, cars, telephones, airplanes, and musical instruments). Increased activation for vocal versus non-vocal stimuli was found in the superior temporal cortex. Interestingly, this pattern was observed in 7-month-olds but not 4-month-olds, which suggests a rapid development of voice sensitivity within the temporal cortex between 4 and 7 months.

Convergent evidence stems from another fNIRS study by Lloyd-Fox et al. (2011) in which 4- to 7-month-old infants were presented with vocal and non-vocal sounds (see Appendix 11.1 for stimuli used). In this study, both types of sounds resulted in activation of temporal lobe areas. Vocal sounds were associated with stronger activation than non-vocal sounds in the anterior portion of the STS area, an area which showed striking similarity with the one found by Blasi et al. (2011) with a subset of the same infants (see Figure 11.1B). This activation was only significant in the left hemisphere, with a non-significant trend being observed in two channels of the right hemisphere. This voice-sensitive activation further increased with

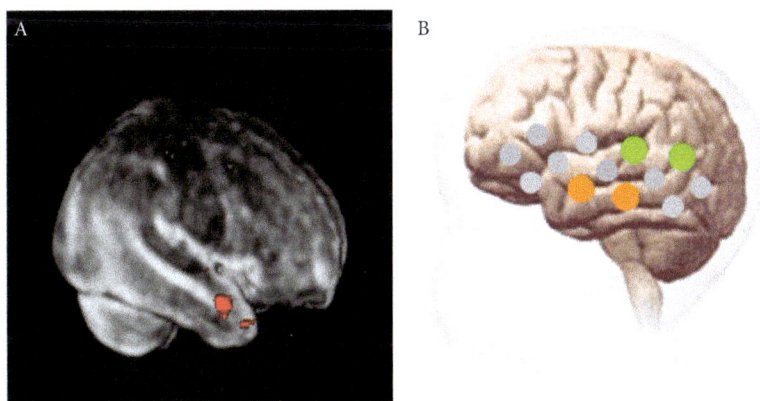

FIGURE 11.1 (A) Three-dimensional rendering of fMRI significant voice > non-voice contrast in 3–7-month-old infants. (B) Schematic of infant head with fNIRS channels that revealed a significantly greater response (p < 0.05; either HbO2 or HHb) for voice > non-voice (in orange) and for non-voice > voice (in green) in 4–7-month-old infants.

age, and activity in the right hemisphere was more strongly observed for vocal stimuli in older infants.

Blasi et al. (2011) and Grossman et al. (2010) both found right lateralized voice-sensitive activation in the temporal cortex, which is congruent with adult findings (Belin & Grosbras, 2010; Fecteau et al., 2004). Also congruent with adult findings, Minagawa-Kawai et al. (2010) found right lateralized temporal activation to emotional non-speech vocalizations in 3–4-month-old infants, while speech activated preferentially the left hemisphere. The right anterior STS has been specifically related to the analysis of non-verbal features of speech in adults, showing more activation when focusing on the speaker's voice than when focusing on the semantic content of spoken sentences (von Kriegstein et al., 2003).

The results of these studies suggest that a right-hemisphere bias for processing human vocalizations may emerge early in development. However, in Lloyd-Fox et al.'s (2011) fNIRS study, voice-sensitive activation was found to be significant only in the left hemisphere. Despite these findings at the group level, a non-significant trend for voice-sensitive activation was also observed in the homologous region of the right hemisphere, which suggests bilateral activation. It is unclear why lateralization differs in group analyses between these different infant studies. Given relatively small sample sizes in these studies, it is possible that group analyses were influenced by the vast amount of inter-individual differences in this lateralization pattern.

11.2.2 Emotion-Modulated Activation

In adulthood, the emotional information conveyed by human vocalizations modulates the activity of many brain areas, including the temporal voice-sensitive area, inferior prefrontal cortex, premotor cortical regions, amygdala, and insula (Fecteau et al., 2005, 2007; Morris et al., 1999; Sander & Scheich, 2001; Warren et al., 2006).

In order to clarify the early development of emotion processing in the brain, a few recent studies examined the effects of emotional valence on vocal activation in the infant brain. Blasi et al. (2011) compared vocalizations of happy, sad, and neutral emotions, using emotional signals that preverbal infants produce themselves from a very early age (cries and laughter) and that are thought to reflect innate behaviours to communicate emotional states (Barr et al., 2000). Infants did not show any significant difference in their activation to happy versus neutral vocalizations. However, sad vocalizations elicited increased responses in the insula and orbitofrontal cortex as opposed to neutral vocalizations.

These results are congruent with findings of increased activation in the insula when adults listen to emotionally salient non-speech vocalizations (especially sad and fearful vocalizations) (Morris et al., 1999; Sander & Scheich, 2001). The orbitofrontal cortex has also been involved in the processing of affective stimuli in adulthood (Kringelbach, 2005), such as recognizing emotions from facial expressions (Leppänen & Nelson, 2009). Blasi et al.'s (2011) results suggest that the role of the orbitofrontal cortex for processing emotions extends to emotions presented in the auditory modality and emerges early in human development.

Another way of studying emotion processing in infancy is by looking at brain activation to emotional prosody in speech. Using fNIRS, Grossman et al. (2011) found that words spoken with a clear emotional prosody (happy or angry) were associated with increased activity in the voice-sensitive area of the right temporal cortex. Interestingly, this effect was found in

7-month-olds, but not 4-month-olds, which suggests a rapid development of emotional processing of speech prosody. In the same age group, event-related potentials (ERPs) revealed a positive slow wave over temporal electrodes when words were spoken with a happy or angry prosody, but not with a neutral prosody (Grossmann et al., 2005). Contrary to these findings, no difference in activation was found between happy and neutral emotional vocalizations in sleeping infants using fMRI (Blasi et al., 2011). The sleeping state of the infants may have reduced the potential differences in activation between emotional conditions. This could explain the discrepancy between the results for happy vocalization obtained in sleeping infants using fMRI and awake infants using fNIRS and ERPs.

One point that remains to be clarified from these results is the potential influence of acoustic properties on these patterns of brain activation. Indeed, the difference in brain response between stimulus categories could reflect low-level differences in acoustic properties of these stimuli. Unfortunately, the number of stimulus categories that can be successfully presented in an infant study is considerably limited by the short attention span of awake infants in fNIRS and ERP studies, and the short duration of their nap in fMRI studies. For this reason, none of the studies discussed in the previous paragraph included acoustically matched stimuli to assess the potential influence of acoustic properties of the stimuli on brain activation. Moreover, another unexplored factor is the potential influence of stimulus familiarity on these patterns of brain activation. Indeed, the finding that activation was evident for sad versus neutral, but not happy versus neutral vocalizations in Blasi et al.'s (2011) study could reflect the likely unfamiliarity of young infants with adult expression of sadness (cries). The same increased activation for sad vocalizations may not be observed when studying the response to the sound of a child crying in a group of infants who have older siblings or who attend childcare settings from an early age.

Studying the infants of depressed mothers may also be a way of assessing the role of early experience, because these infants may be exposed to an atypical balance of neutral, happy, sad, and angry vocalizations. Research examining infants of depressed mothers found that those infants habituated to sad faces more quickly than infants of non-depressed mothers and showed a novelty effect when watching videos of happy emotional expression (Field et al., 2009). This most likely reflects the emotional expression the infants were frequently exposed to. It would be interesting to see if these effects of experience also influence brain activation to emotional vocalization and facial expression.

11.2.3 Voice-Sensitive Activation in Atypical Development

Recent neuroimaging findings indicate a development towards a more specialized voice-sensitive network within the infant brain. The picture is complicated by the vast amount of variability that accompanies child development. It becomes even more opaque when considering children that diverge from typical developmental trajectories. For example, in autism spectrum disorder (ASD), there are well-studied behavioural atypicalities in language development, which can be observed at different ages (Frith & Happe, 1994). ASD is diagnosed based on behavioural markers observed from 18 months at the earliest (Baron-Cohen et al., 1992). These behavioural markers could be associated with atypical neural development, which can potentially be observed at an earlier stage. For example, in the domain of face processing, Elsabbagh et al. (2012) showed that ERP components evoked in response to dynamic eye-gaze shifts differed in a group of infants at high-risk of ASD compared to infants at lower risk of ASD. More interestingly, a longitudinal study of these infants revealed that characteristics of these ERP components were associated with ASD diagnosed at 36 months. These findings suggest that the study of brain signals associated with social stimuli may lead to earlier identification of infants at highest risk for developing later impairments such as ASD.

In the same line of thought, Blasi et al. (2015) and Lloyd-Fox et al. (2013) studied young infants at high risk of developing ASD in that they had an older sibling who had previously been diagnosed with ASD. These children were presented with vocal and non-vocal stimuli, and compared to a group of infants of the same age who were at lower risk of developing ASD since they had no family history of ASD. In their fNIRS study, Lloyd-Fox et al. (2013) found voice-sensitive activation in the temporal cortex of low-risk but not high-risk infants. Similarly, more extensive activation was found for *visual* social stimuli (videos of female actors who either moved their eyes left or right, or performed hand games such as 'peek-a-boo' and 'incy-wincy spider') (see Appendix 11.1 for examples of stimuli) in the low-risk than the high-risk group. In an fMRI study with a subgroup of the same infants, Blasi et al. (2015) found voice-sensitive activation in low-risk infants in the right temporal and medial frontal regions, while this effect was not observed in high-risk infants. Moreover, low-risk infants showed stronger sensitivity than high-risk infants to sad vocalizations in the right fusiform gyrus and left hippocampus. Despite the fact that at the time of the study it was not yet known whether or not the high-risk infants were going to be diagnosed with ASD, it is striking to see the reduction in brain selectivity for social cues in this group.

These infant results are congruent with adult neuroimaging suggesting that adults diagnosed with ASD show reduced voice sensitivity in similar cortical areas (Gervais et al., 2004). More recently, Schelinski et al. (2016) have observed a typical voice-sensitive response in a group of high-functioning adults with ASD when passively listening to vocal and non-vocal sounds. However, a dysfunction of this voice sensitivity of the right posterior superior temporal sulcus/gyrus (STS/STG) was observed when the same group of high-functioning adults with ASD was performing a voice-identity recognition task, but not a speech recognition task. Moreover, functional activation of the right STS/STG correlated with voice-identity recognition performance in typical adults, but not in adults with ASD, suggesting that adults with ASD performed voice-identity recognition tasks in a functionally different manner that may not involve the right STS/STG to the same degree as in typical adults.

Taken together, these results suggest that the brain of infants at high risk of developing ASD can show markers of autism in its functional processing of social stimuli even though ASD can only be diagnosed years later. This is both relevant in clarifying the development of the social brain and as hope for further development of early diagnosis of atypical development.

11.2.4 Cross-Cultural Development of Voice-Sensitive Activation

Some evidence has been presented showing that the development of voice sensitivity is a stable phenomenon that can be observed cross-culturally. Lloyd-Fox et al. (2014) conducted an fNIRS study in the Gambia, a rural area of Africa, assessing vocal processing of

4- to 8-month-olds growing up in a vastly different cultural environment (see Appendix 11.1 for stimuli). As in British infants, they found that vocal stimuli produced greater activation than non-vocal stimuli in the STS region and the inferior frontal cortex. The pattern of voice-sensitive activation observed in infants growing up in the Gambia was broadly similar to the results observed in infants growing up in Europe (Blasi et al., 2011; Grossman et al., 2010; Lloyd-Fox et al., 2012), but was generally more widespread and extended to the inferior frontal cortex. More variation within the sample could explain these results, as the age range of Gambian infants was slightly broader than in European infants. Also, the development of children in the Gambia is even more varied than that of British children, due to less stable environmental factors. Nevertheless, this study has shown that neural activation patterns are similar cross-culturally and despite substantial differences in socioeconomic, cultural, and geographic environments.

11.3 VOICE AND FACE INTEGRATION IN INFANCY

The exposure to voices begins *in utero*, but after birth, voices are most frequently encountered in combination with faces. Making sense of social cues is crucial as infants learn how to interact with the world around them. By being able to perceive input from various modalities, infants can get much richer information about subtle social cues. Therefore it is of interest to examine how infants integrate both auditory and visual social cues in order to extract meaningful information about their social communication partner. Combining the input from both modalities allows inference about information on a broad range of characteristics, including the identity of the speaker, the emotion displayed, as well as the content of messages conveyed by speech. In this section, we will discuss the behavioural and brain evidence of the development of audiovisual integration in infants' social perception.

11.3.1 Audiovisual Identity Integration

Being able to match the appropriate voice with a corresponding face seems trivial to adults, but is a complex process that enables infants to interact with their social environment. In the first few months of life, infants' ability to integrate faces and voices into unified person perception progresses rapidly. Indeed, 4- and 6-month-olds, but not 2-month-olds, can detect changes in face–voice pairings of unfamiliar adults, suggesting that by 4 months, they can perceive, learn, and remember an unfamiliar pairing in face and voice (Bahrick et al., 2005). When listening to an adult's voice, 4- and 7-month-olds also look longer at the face of an adult, and longer at the face of a child when listening to a child's voice of the same gender, suggesting that they are able to extract age cues from both faces and voices and are able to integrate these (Bahrick et al., 1998). Furthermore, 6-month-olds look longer at a video of a speaking face when a voice of the same gender is played, suggesting that they can also extract and integrate gender information from faces and voices (Walker-Andrews & Lennon, 1991). Infants of 9 and 12 months are also able to match gender of a voice that they have heard with a still picture of a face, but in both age groups, this effect was driven by an ability to match gender in female and not male faces and voices. This likely reflects the increased experience of most infants with adults of the female gender. It was also observed that 12-month-olds were more reliable in gender matching than 9-month-olds, suggesting that these skills are still under development in the last few months of an infant's first year (Poulin-Dubois et al., 1994).

11.3.2 Audiovisual Emotion Integration

By adulthood, integration of visual and auditory cues has become so ingrained that it is hard to inhibit. Affective cues from faces and voices are integrated by adults even when instructed to ignore the vocal emotions (de Gelder & Vroomen., 2000) and in the absence of conscious perception (de Gelder et al., 2002). ERPs reveal that auditory and visual displays of emotions are integrated at very early latencies often believed to reflect unimodal processing and involve an interactive network of brain areas such as the amygdala, fusiform face area, and superior and middle temporal region (Campanella & Belin, 2007).

Infants appear to be especially sensitive to the integration of emotional cues from human faces and voices. Indeed, infants as young as 5 and 7 months look longer at a video of a face expressing an emotion congruent with a vocal emotion simultaneously presented than the video of a face expressing a different emotion (Walker, 1981). Even when the temporal synchrony of the voice and face is disrupted, infants looked longer to the face displaying congruent emotion, suggesting that this response is not driven by audiovisual temporal synchrony. When the lower third of each face is obscured, 7-month-olds, but not 5-month-olds, increase their fixation to a filmed facial expression that is emotionally congruent with vocalizations (Walker-Andrews, 1986). This suggests that older infants have more refined analyses of the emotional information present in the eye region, while younger infants may rely mainly on information provided in the mouth region, such as the presence of a smile. However, preferential looking at a congruent emotion is disrupted by face inversion in both 5- and 7-month-olds, suggesting a global analysis of emotional faces (Walker, 1981). In line with this, Vaillant-Molina et al. (2013) presented 3.5- and 5-month-old infants with an auditory stimulus of either positive or negative emotional valence. Concurrently, infants were presented two faces with either a happy or a sad expression. Looking time was analysed in order to see if infants looked at the matching faces more often than could be expected by chance. Indeed, they found that infants directed their gaze more often to the matching picture, this finding being more stable in the group of 5-month-olds.

Even younger infants can integrate vocal and facial emotions when displayed by a familiar individual. Indeed, 3.5-month-olds were presented with two filmed facial expressions (happy and sad), accompanied by a vocal expression. When their own mother modelled the emotional expression, infants looked longer at the facial expression congruent with emotional vocalizations, but infants who were presented videos of an unfamiliar woman did not (Kahana-Kalman & Walker-Andrews, 2001).

Further evidence that 7-month-old infants can integrate emotional prosody with pictures of happy and angry facial expression was provided by ERPs (Grossmann et al., 2006). When the emotional content was incongruent between the face and voice, infants demonstrated a larger negative component (400–600 ms latency interval) than when emotional prosody was congruent with the facial emotion. Conversely, the amplitude of a subsequent positive component (600–1,000 ms latency interval) was larger to emotionally congruent than to incongruent faces and voices.

Like unisensory perception of faces and voices, the ability to integrate auditory and visual aspects of faces and voices gradually narrows down to *human* faces and voices in the first year of life. When presented with human faces, infants show equal amounts of activation no matter if the face is upright or inverted, indicating no fixed preference at 6 months of age. Rather, this preference seems to develop gradually, and adults show a much greater occipital response to faces that are upright and in line with our visual expertise. Interestingly, this effect does not generalize to monkey faces, which have been associated with equal amounts of cortical activation no matter if presented upright or inverted (de Haan et al., 2002). With regard to integrating visual and auditory cues, when presented with pairs of monkey faces producing two different vocal expressions, 4- and 6-month-olds correctly matched the face with the vocalization, while 8- and 10-month-olds did not exhibit this audiovisual matching skill with non-human faces and voices (Lewkowicz & Ghazanfar, 2006).

11.3.3 Audiovisual Speech Integration

Adults automatically integrate the audio and visual aspects of spoken language to the extent that the visual perception of speech can influence its auditory perception. A well-documented example of audiovisual integration is the McGurk effect, in which an individual is exposed to non-matching auditory and visual speech stimuli (McGurk & MacDonald, 1976). Classically, participants are exposed to stimuli with the verbal presentation of one consonant overlaid with the auditory presentation of another (e.g. visual /g/ sound, auditory /b/ sound). In adults, this creates a combined percept of a third sound, which is neither the auditory nor the visual stimulus. In the aforementioned example, the result is the perception of a /d/ sound in the majority of adults. However, not all combinations of consonants lend themselves to the McGurk effect. Whereas a combination of a visual /g/ and an auditory /b/ leads to a fusion of a percept of /d/, the reverse stimulus is more difficult to reconcile. A visual /b/ and an auditory /g/ do not regularly lead to fusion, but to combination. The resulting percept is more analogous to a /bg/ sound. This combination is more difficult to integrate to speakers of English and many other languages, and therefore leads to a different process than the fusion stimulus where the mismatch leads to unnoticed integration.

The McGurk effect has also been studied in infants. Kushnerenko et al. (2008) utilized ERPs in order to assess whether infants integrate the audiovisual aspect of speech. Mismatch negativity is a negative ERP component that reflects the violation of an expectation that the child might hold, such as an interruption of a uniform stream of stimuli by a non-matching stimulus. When studying 5-month-old infants, Kushnerenko et al. (2008) presented the infants with incongruent stimulus pairs, such as the visual /g/ and an auditory /b/, which was expected to lead to fusion, as well as a combination of a visual /b/ and a verbal /g/, which was more likely to be unfamiliar to the infant. They found that mismatch negativity did not occur when presenting stimuli that easily fuse into one in adults (see Figure 11.2). In the case of stimuli that rather lead to an unfamiliar combined percept, the mismatch response was higher in the ERPs measured in infants. This is suggesting that young infants can experience the McGurk effect, and the findings can be taken as an indication for very early integration of cross-modal stimuli.

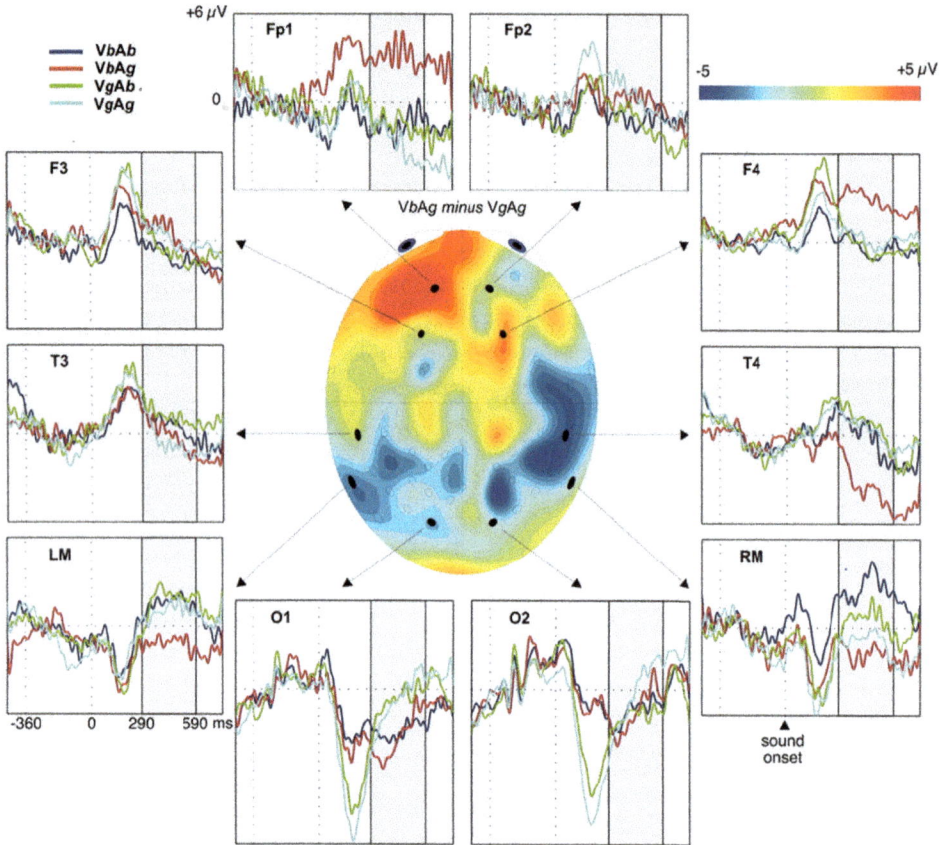

FIGURE 11.2 Grand-averaged responses to the audiovisual pairs Visual /b/– Auditory /b/ (VbAb - dark blue), Visual /b/– Auditory /g/ (VbAg - red), Visual /g/– Auditory /b/ (VgAb - green), and Visual /g/–Auditory /g/ (VgAg - light blue), time-locked to the sound onset at 0 ms. Selected channels are shown according to 10–20 system (LM and RM refer to the left and right mastoid, respectively). The highlighted area corresponds to a time window within which the ERP to the VbAg stimulus significantly deviated from the others. The topographic map in the middle represents the voltage difference between responses to VbAg and VgAg pairs within the highlighted window.

Evidence of audiovisual speech integration can also be observed in even younger infants. Infants as young as 2 months looked longer at a face articulating a phoneme when it was congruent with the phoneme that they were hearing at the same time (Kuhl & Meltzoff, 1984; Patterson & Werker, 1999, 2002, 2003).

Not only are babies able to integrate the audio and visual aspects of speech, but they can also use visual cues of speech articulation to enhance phoneme discrimination (Teinonen et al., 2008). Indeed, 6-month-old infants were exposed to speech sounds from a continuum between /ba/ and /da/. One group of infants saw a visual articulation of a canonical /ba/ or /da/, congruent with the auditory token, while the other group was always presented with the same visual articulation (/ba/ or /da/) with all auditory tokens. A stimulus-alternation preference procedure revealed that infants in the congruent articulation group discriminated the /ba/–/da/ contrast, while infants in the second group did not.

At the brain level, the combination of infant-directed speech *and* direct gaze was observed to enhance infant brain activation (Lloyd-Fox et al., 2015). Participants were presented with actors who naturalistically interacted with them while brain responses were recorded using fNIRS imaging. Activation was observed in response to this interaction, with the strongest response resulting from a combination of infant-directed speech and infant-directed gaze. This activation could be localized in inferior frontal and temporal regions of the brain, regions known to be involved in processing auditory and visual aspects of social communication.

11.4 Conclusions

From the first days of life, infants are naturally attracted to human faces and voices. These early biases maximize their social interaction and experience of social stimuli. This leads to impressively early and sophisticated processing of human faces and voices in infancy. Recent advances in neuroimaging methods have allowed the study of the earliest steps in the development of the social brain. These studies suggest that the infant's temporal cortex shows patterns of voice sensitivity that resemble the ones observed later in adulthood, although the functional lateralization of this network appears to be more variable across different infants and different infant studies than in the adult literature. Moreover, available data suggests a rapid increase of voice sensitivity along the infant STS in the first few months of life. This voice-sensitive activation is observed cross-culturally, but is reduced in infants at risk of developing autism spectrum disorder. The activation of the infant brain is also modulated by the emotional content of human vocalizations in regions involved in emotion processing in adulthood, such as the temporal voice-sensitive area, amygdala, and orbitofrontal cortex.

Very young infants also appear to be sensitive to the integration of facial and vocal cues. Indeed, they show very early and increasing skills in integrating gender, age, identity, and emotional cues of faces and voices. They can also integrate visual articulation with auditory spoken language, an ability that appears to be used in phoneme discrimination. All these skills are present from the first months of life and are increasingly more sophisticated as infants get closer to their first birthday.

The brain network involved in the integration of facial and vocal cues is still unknown. Moreover, the respective influence of anatomical maturation and experience on the development of the social brain still remains to be clarified. Behavioural data suggests that the integration of facial and vocal cues is influenced by familiarity, in that infants often show more advanced processing and integration skills when presented with their mother's face and voice. These results suggest that this development is experience-dependent and not merely a product of maturation. A better understanding of the development of social perception in the infant brain could be gained by studying infants with a different social experience from that of the majority—for example, hearing infants with deaf parents, sighted infants with blind parents, bilingual infants, and infants of clinically depressed mothers.

REFERENCES

Bahrick, L. E., Hernandez-Reif, M., & Flom, R. (2005). The development of infant learning about specific face-voice relations. *Developmental Psychology,* 41(3), 541.

Bahrick, L. E., Netto, D., & Hernandez-Keif, M. (1998). Intermodal perception of adult and child faces and voices by infants. *Child Development,* 69(5), 1263–1275.

Baron-Cohen, S., Allen, J., & Gillberg, C. (1992). Can autism be detected at 18 months? The needle, the haystack, and the CHAT. *The British Journal of Psychiatry,* 161, 839–843.

Barr, R. G., Hopkins, B., & Green, J. A. (2000). *Crying as a Sign, a Symptom, and a Signal: Clinical, Emotional and Developmental Aspects of Infant and Toddler Crying.* Cambridge, UK: Cambridge University Press.

Belin, P., Fillion-Bilodeau, S., & Gosselin, F. (2008). The Montreal Affective Voices: a validated set of nonverbal affect bursts for research on auditory affective processing. *Behavior Research Methods,* 40(2), 531–539.

Belin, P. & Grosbras, M. (2010). Before speech: cerebral voice processing in infants. *Neuron,* 65(6), 733–735.

Belin, P., Zatorre, R. J., Lafaille, P., Ahad, P., & Pike, B. (2000). Voice-selective areas in human auditory cortex. *Nature,* 403(6767), 309–312.

Birnholz, J. C. & Benacerraf, B. R. (1983). The development of human fetal hearing. *Science,* 222(4623), 516–518.

Blasi, A., Lloyd-Fox, S., Sethna, V., Brammer, M. J., Mercure, E., Murray, L., ... Johnson, M. H. (2015). Atypical processing of voice sounds in infants at risk for autism spectrum disorder. *Cortex,* 71, 122–133.

Blasi, A., Mercure, E., Lloyd-Fox, S., Thomson, A., Brammer, M., Sauter, D., ... Deoni, S. (2011). Early specialization for voice and emotion processing in the infant brain. *Current Biology,* 21(14), 1220–1224.

Campanella, S. & Belin, P. (2007). Integrating face and voice in person perception. *Trends in Cognitive Sciences,* 11(12), 535–543.

De Gelder, B. & Vroomen, J. (2000). The perception of emotions by ear and by eye. *Cognition & Emotion,* 14(3), 289–311.

de Gelder, B., Pourtois, G., & Weiskrantz, L. (2002). Fear recognition in the voice is modulated by unconsciously recognized facial expressions but not by unconsciously recognized affective pictures. *Proceedings of the National Academy of Sciences of the United States of America,* 99(6), 4121–4126. doi:10.1073/pnas.062018499

de Haan, M., Pascalis, O., & Johnson, M. (2002). Specialization of neural mechanisms underlying face recognition in human infants. *Journal of Cognitive Neuroscience,* 14(2), 199–209.

DeCasper, A. J. & Fifer, W. P. (1980). Of human bonding: newborns prefer their mothers' voices. *Science,* 208(4448), 1174–1176.

Elsabbagh, M., Divan, G., Koh, Y., Kim, Y. S., Kauchali, S., Marcín, C., ... Wang, C. (2012). Global prevalence of autism and other pervasive developmental disorders. *Autism Research,* 5(3), 160–179.

Farroni, T., Csibra, G., Simion, F., & Johnson, M. H. (2002). Eye contact detection in humans from birth. *Proceedings of the National Academy of Sciences of the United States of America,* 99(14), 9602–9605. doi:10.1073/pnas.152159999

Fecteau, S., Armony, J. L., Joanette, Y., & Belin, P. (2004). Is voice processing species-specific in human auditory cortex? An fMRI study. *NeuroImage,* 23(3), 840–848.

Fecteau, S., Armony, J. L., Joanette, Y., & Belin, P. (2005). Sensitivity to voice in human prefrontal cortex. *Journal of Neurophysiology*, 94(3), 2251–2254. doi:00329.2005 [pii]

Fecteau, S., Belin, P., Joanette, Y., & Armony, J. L. (2007). Amygdala responses to nonlinguistic emotional vocalizations. *NeuroImage*, 36(2), 480–487.

Field, T., Diego, M., & Hernandez-Reif, M. (2009). Depressed mothers' infants are less responsive to faces and voices. *Infant Behavior and Development*, 32(3), 239–244.

Frith, U. & Happe, F. (1994). Language and communication in autistic disorders. *Philosophical Transactions of the Royal Society of London. Series B, Biological Sciences*, 346(1315), 97–104. doi:10.1098/rstb.1994.0133

Gervais, H., Belin, P., Boddaert, N., Leboyer, M., Coez, A., Sfaello, I., ... Zilbovicius, M. (2004). Abnormal cortical voice processing in autism. *Nature Neuroscience*, 7(8), 801–802.

Grossmann, T., Johnson, M. H., Vaish, A., Hughes, D. A., Quinque, D., Stoneking, M., & Friederici, A. D. (2011). Genetic and neural dissociation of individual responses to emotional expressions in human infants. *Developmental Cognitive Neuroscience*, 1(1), 57–66.

Grossmann, T., Oberecker, R., Koch, S. P., & Friederici, A. D. (2010). The developmental origins of voice processing in the human brain. *Neuron*, 65(6), 852–858.

Grossmann, T., Striano, T., & Friederici, A. D. (2005). Infants' electric brain responses to emotional prosody. *NeuroReport*, 16(16), 1825–1828.

Grossmann, T., Striano, T., & Friederici, A. D. (2006). Crossmodal integration of emotional information from face and voice in the infant brain. *Developmental Science*, 9(3), 309–315.

Johnson, M. H., Dziurawiec, S., Ellis, H., & Morton, J. (1991). Newborns' preferential tracking of face-like stimuli and its subsequent decline. *Cognition*, 40(1–2), 1–19.

Kahana-Kalman, R. & Walker-Andrews, A. S. (2001). The role of person familiarity in young infants' perception of emotional expressions. *Child Development*, 72(2), 352–369.

Kringelbach, M. L. (2005). The human orbitofrontal cortex: linking reward to hedonic experience. *Nature Reviews Neuroscience*, 6(9), 691–702.

Kuhl, P. K. & Meltzoff, A. N. (1984). The intermodal representation of speech in infants. *Infant Behavior and Development*, 7(3), 361–381.

Kushnerenko, E., Teinonen, T., Volein, A., & Csibra, G. (2008). Electrophysiological evidence of illusory audiovisual speech percept in human infants. *Proceedings of the National Academy of Sciences of the United States of America*, 105(32), 11442–11445. doi:10.1073/pnas.0804275105

Latinus, M. & Belin, P. (2011). Human voice perception. *Current Biology*, 21(4), R143–R145.

Leppänen, J. M. & Nelson, C. A. (2009). Tuning the developing brain to social signals of emotions. *Nature Reviews Neuroscience*, 10(1), 37–47.

Lewkowicz, D. J. & Ghazanfar, A. A. (2006). The decline of cross-species intersensory perception in human infants. *Proceedings of the National Academy of Sciences of the United States of America*, 103(17), 6771–6774. doi:0602027103 [pii]

Lloyd-Fox, S., Blasi, A., Everdell, N., Elwell, C. E., & Johnson, M. H. (2011). Selective cortical mapping of biological motion processing in young infants. *Journal of Cognitive Neuroscience*, 23(9), 2521–2532.

Lloyd-Fox, S., Blasi, A., Elwell, C. E., Charman, T., Murphy, D., & Johnson, M. H. (2013). Reduced neural sensitivity to social stimuli in infants at risk for autism. *Proceedings of the Royal Society B: Biological Sciences*, 280(1758), 20123026. doi:10.1098/rspb.2012.3026

Lloyd-Fox, S., Blasi, A., Mercure, E., Elwell, C. E., & Johnson, M. H. (2012). The emergence of cerebral specialization for the human voice over the first months of life. *Social Neuroscience*, 7(3), 317–330.

Lloyd-Fox, S., Papademetriou, M., Darboe, M. K., Everdell, N. L., Wegmuller, R., Prentice, A. M., ... Elwell, C. E. (2014). Functional near infrared spectroscopy (fNIRS) to assess cognitive function in infants in rural Africa. *Scientific Reports*, 4, 4740.

Lloyd-Fox, S., Széplaki-Köllőd, B., Yin, J., & Csibra, G. (2015). Are you talking to me? Neural activations in 6-month-old infants in response to being addressed during natural interactions. *Cortex*, 70, 35–48.

McGurk, H. & MacDonald, J. (1976). Hearing lips and seeing voices. *Nature*, 264, 746–748.

Minagawa-Kawai, Y., Van Der Lely, H., Ramus, F., Sato, Y., Mazuka, R., & Dupoux, E. (2010). Optical brain imaging reveals general auditory and language-specific processing in early infant development. *Cerebral Cortex*, 21(2), 254–261.

Moon, C., Cooper, R. P., & Fifer, W. P. (1993). Two-day-olds prefer their native language. *Infant Behavior and Development*, 16(4), 495–500.

Morris, J. S., Scott, S. K., & Dolan, R. J. (1999). Saying it with feeling: neural responses to emotional vocalizations. *Neuropsychologia*, 37(10), 1155–1163.

Patterson, M. L. & Werker, J. F. (1999). Matching phonetic information in lips and voice is robust in 4.5-month-old infants. *Infant Behavior and Development*, 22(2), 237–247.

Patterson, M. L. & Werker, J. F. (2002). Infants' ability to match dynamic phonetic and gender information in the face and voice. *Journal of Experimental Child Psychology*, 81(1), 93–115.

Patterson, M. L. & Werker, J. F. (2003). Two-month-old infants match phonetic information in lips and voice. *Developmental Science*, 6(2), 191–196.

Poulin-Dubois, D., Serbin, L. A., Kenyon, B., & Derbyshire, A. (1994). Infants' intermodal knowledge about gender. *Developmental Psychology*, 30(3), 436.

Sander, K. & Scheich, H. (2001). Auditory perception of laughing and crying activates human amygdala regardless of attentional state. *Cognitive Brain Research*, 12(2), 181–198.

Schelinski, S., Borowiak, K., & von Kriegstein, K. (2016). Temporal voice areas exist in autism spectrum disorder but are dysfunctional for voice identity recognition. *Social Cognitive and Affective Neuroscience*, 11(11), 1812–1822.

Teinonen, T., Aslin, R. N., Alku, P., & Csibra, G. (2008). Visual speech contributes to phonetic learning in 6-month-old infants. *Cognition*, 108(3), 850–855.

Vaillant-Molina, M., Bahrick, L. E., & Flom, R. (2013). Young infants match facial and vocal emotional expressions of other infants. *Infancy*, 18(s1), E97–E111.

von Kriegstein, K., Eger, E., Kleinschmidt, A., & Giraud, A. L. (2003). Modulation of neural responses to speech by directing attention to voices or verbal content. *Cognitive Brain Research*, 17(1), 48–55.

Vouloumanos, A. & Werker, J. F. (2007). Listening to language at birth: evidence for a bias for speech in neonates. *Developmental Science*, 10(2), 159–164.

Walker, E. (1981). Emotion recognition in disturbed and normal children: a research note. *Journal of Child Psychology and Psychiatry*, 22(3), 263–268.

Walker-Andrews, A. S. (1986). Intermodal perception of expressive behaviors: relation of eye and voice? *Developmental Psychology*, 22(3), 373.

Walker-Andrews, A. S. & Lennon, E. (1991). Infants' discrimination of vocal expressions: contributions of auditory and visual information. *Infant Behavior and Development*, 14(2), 131–142.

Warren, J. E., Sauter, D. A., Eisner, F., Wiland, J., Dresner, M. A., Wise, R. J., ... Scott, S. K. (2006). Positive emotions preferentially engage an auditory-motor 'mirror' system. *The Journal of Neuroscience*, 26(50), 13067–13075. doi:26/50/13067 [pii]

VISUAL AND AUDITORY SOCIAL/NON-SOCIAL STIMULI USED IN LLOYD-FOX ET AL. (2011, 2012, AND 2013)

Auditory Stimuli

The *voice* condition represented non-speech adult vocalizations, including coughing, yawning, throat clearing, laughing, and crying, produced by a range of male and female speakers. The *non-voice* condition represented naturalistic environmental sounds (that were not human or animal produced, but were likely to be familiar to infants of that age, including water running and toys such as rattles, squeaky toys, spinning balls). Voice and non-voice stimuli were chosen from the Montreal Affective Voices (for more detail, see Belin et al., 2008), the stimuli of the voice functional localizer (http://vnl.psy.gla.ac.uk/resources_main.php), or were recorded by the author EM (toy sounds). Each stimulus sequence lasted 8 s and consisted of four different sounds (of voice or non-voice stimuli) presented for 0.37–2.92 s each, interleaved with short periods of silence (0.16–0.24 s). The stimulus categories were equivalent in terms of average sound intensity and duration ($p > .65$). Each of the four sounds within a stimulus sequence (trial) differed (e.g. laughing, crying, yawning, coughing) but over the course of the session, these sounds were presented repeatedly, as they were taken from a range of sixteen different voice/non-voice stimuli.

Visual Stimuli

Social stimuli consisted of full-colour, life-size (head and shoulders only) videos of female actors who either moved their eyes left or right, or performed hand games ('peek-a-boo' and 'incy wincy spider'). Two visual social videos were presented per trial, lasting 9–12 s. Six different visual social videos (two actors; three types of social videos) were presented over the course of the study. Baseline *non-social stimuli* represented full-colour, still images of different types of transport (e.g. cars and helicopters) presented randomly for a pseudo-random duration (1–3 s) for 9–12 s.

CHAPTER 12

NEURAL RESPONSES TO INFANT VOCALIZATIONS IN ADULT LISTENERS

KATHERINE S. YOUNG, CHRISTINE E. PARSONS,
ALAN STEIN, PETER VUUST, MICHELLE G. CRASKE,
AND MORTEN L. KRINGELBACH

12.1 INTRODUCTION

THE evolving parent–infant relationship relies on bidirectional communication between adult and offspring. This communication forms a base for the development of a complex social and affective relationship between the pair. Given the extent and complexity of human infant needs, parental sensitivity to infant cues promotes infant survival, and ultimately helps to ensure survival of the species (Darwin, 1872; Konner, 2010). The two primary modes of communication available to an infant are vocalizations and facial expressions. These signals provide parents with vital information about their infants' needs which, in combination with other contextual factors, help to determine the selection of caregiving behaviour. Vocalizations form an essential part of this multimodal communication. Infant distress cries, in particular, are salient signals serving both to alert a caregiver from a distance and to provide acoustic information about the infant's physiological and affective state.

In this chapter, we first describe characteristics of infant vocalizations and provide some theoretical considerations regarding adults' responses to these cues. We then describe a neural network, termed the 'parental brain', implicated in responding to infant cries based on fMRI studies. Next, we discuss evidence from studies investigating the temporal dynamics of activity within this network, followed by findings assessing experience-dependent plasticity in the parental brain. We end with a description of strategies for future directions in this developing field of research.

12.2 ACOUSTICS OF INFANT VOCALIZATIONS

From immediately postpartum, human infants cry. An infant's cry is characterized by its high and dynamic pitch (ranging between 250–700 Hz; Golub & Corwin, 1985). A single-cry burst has a duration of one to three seconds and generally has a 'falling' or 'rising–falling' melody (see Figure 12.1; Audio 12.1a; cf. Audio 12.1b; Wasz-Höckert et al., 1985). In early life, crying is considered to be largely reflexive (Bell & Ainsworth, 1972), occurring in response

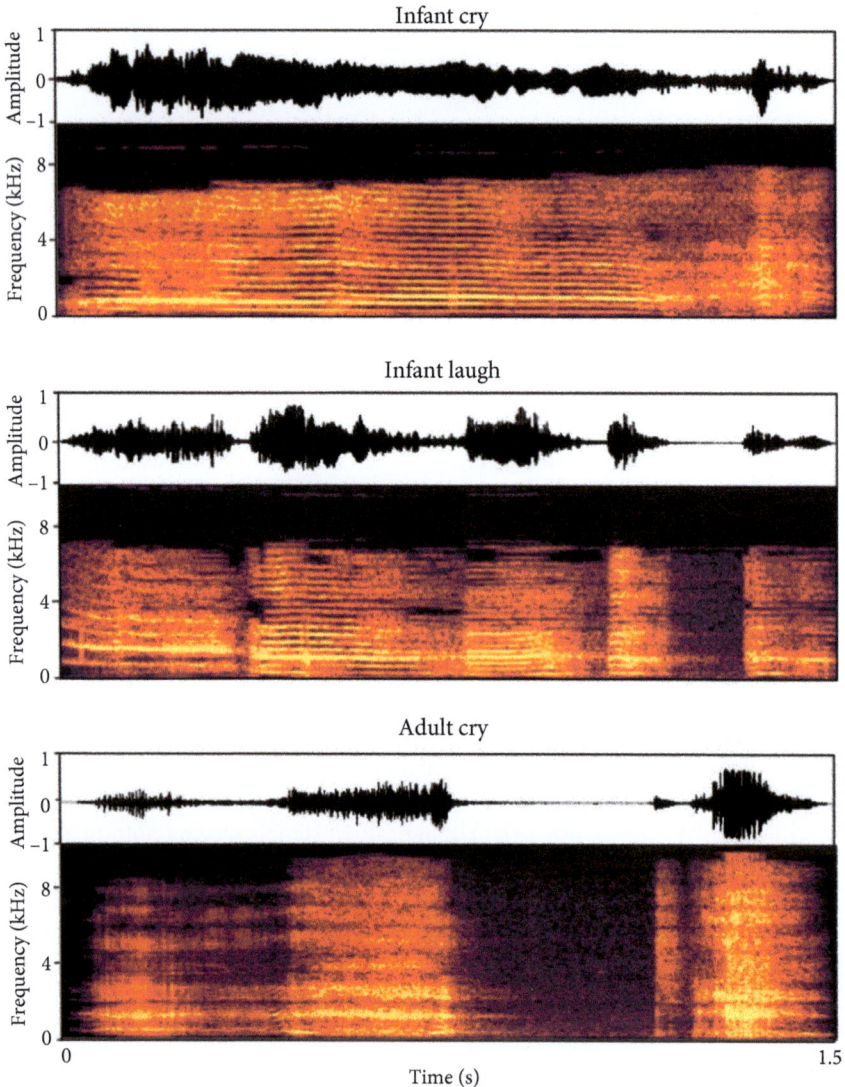

FIGURE 12.1 Waveforms and spectrograms demonstrating acoustic features of infant cry, infant laugh, and adult (female) cry sounds. While all types of vocalizations presented here have similar frequency ranges, the fundamental frequency (F0) of the infant cry (522 Hz) and infant laugh (562 Hz) are higher than that of the adult female cry (403 Hz). Patterns of burst duration also vary across sound type (Audio 12.1a; cf. Audio 12.1b.).

to pain, hunger, or separation from a caregiver. After two to three months postpartum, there is a clear change in infant vocalizations. Cries become more differentiated, reflecting greater motor control of the vocal tract (Ostwald & Murray, 1985; Soltis, 2004). At around four months of age, infants begin to produce a wider range of vocalizations, including positive emotional cues, such as laughter (Audio 12.1c) and preverbal vocalizations referred to as 'babbling' (Kuhl, 2004; Nwokah et al., 1994; Oller & Eilers, 1988).

A number of studies have investigated whether infant cries could be categorized into distinct 'types' (e.g. a pain cry, a hunger cry) (see Gustafson et al., 2000 for a review). While gaining initial empirical support (e.g. Wasz-Höckert et al., 1964), more recent studies have demonstrated low accuracy rates in the identification of cry 'cause' (Muller et al., 1974). In a different conceptualization, an infant's cry is referred to as a 'graded signal', with varying acoustical properties reflecting different levels of distress (Izard, 1971). This is a characteristic readily recognized by adult listeners, with studies showing that higher-pitched cries are perceived as sounding more distressed (Parsons, Young, Jegindó, et al., 2014; Porter et al., 1986; Young et al., 2012; Zeskind & Marshall, 1988).

12.3 SENSITIVITY TO INFANT VOCALIZATIONS

The ability to respond promptly and appropriately to an infant's communicative cues is a parenting capacity key to survival of the species (Ainsworth et al., 1974). There is a general scientific consensus that the quality of early parenting has a profound effect on child development (Bornstein et al., 2011; Feldman, 2015; Parsons, Stark, et al., 2013; Parsons et al., 2010). In particular, the sensitivity with which parents respond to their infant's communicative cues has been shown to impact cognitive and socio-emotional outcomes (Murray et al., 1999; Stein et al., 2013).

Early theoretical descriptions of adult responsiveness to infant cries suggested various motivations for caregiving behaviour including: i) a desire to terminate an aversive stimulus; ii) an empathic response to reduce distress in another; or iii) an evolutionary desire to ensure the well-being of offspring (for overview, see Murray, 1979). Murray alternatively proposed a 'motivational entity' model of infant cries, suggesting that there are two separable stages to responding to an infant cry (Murray, 1979). First, the specific acoustic structure of an infant cry acts as the 'motivational entity', rapidly alerting the listener. Second, other factors such as caregiving context and cognitive appraisal of the sound influence the selection of specific behavioural responses (Murray, 1985). The concept of a motivational entity is comparable to the often described 'Kindchenschema' (Lorenz, 1943) in which the particular configuration of infant facial features is thought to act as an 'innate releaser' of caregiving behaviour. More generally, this can be likened to a framework of emotional experience that considers initial reactions to situations as 'core-affect', which can be modulated by attentional states and contextual factors (Barrett et al., 2007).

Understanding the neural mechanisms that facilitate parental behaviour can likewise be considered as a two-stage process. First, there is rapid initiation of a non-specific motivational state. Second is slower, detailed appraisal to facilitate the selection of appropriate behavioural responses. This is consistent with general models of 'dual-stream' emotional processing, with a broad evidence base supporting the notion of quick, imprecise processing, followed by slower, more detailed analysis (Barrett & Bar, 2009; LeDoux, 2000; Rolls, 2000).

In the context of caregiving behaviour, the rapid initiation of a motivational state might be considered largely reflexive. We consider findings of this type that are *common* across a number of studies to be evidence of a generalized 'caregiving instinct'. We use the term 'instinct' here as shorthand to describe phenomena that do not appear to depend on extensive experience, occurring across different groups of individuals (e.g. males and females, parents and non-parents). We do not mean to imply that such responses are 'hard-wired' or unchangeable by experience. Selection of 'appropriate' responses is influenced by a range of factors and is adaptable through learning and experience-dependent brain plasticity. We consider findings that are *specific* to certain groups of individuals as evidence of experience-dependent plasticity in the parental brain. Notably, these effects might include 'sensitization' or 'optimization' of previously described 'instincts'.

12.4 NEURAL REACTIVITY TO INFANT CRIES: NETWORKS OF THE 'PARENTAL BRAIN'

The sound of an infant cry has a range of effects on the listener. Infant cries are generally perceived as distressing, piercing, or aversive, and promote a desire in adults to provide care (e.g. Del Vecchio et al., 2009; Dessureau et al., 1998; Frodi et al., 1978). Physiologically, hearing infant cries can impact the listener's heart rate, respiration, and hand-grip strength (although the direction of these effects varies across studies; Bakermans-Kranenburg et al., 2012; Bleichfeld & Moely, 1984; Del Vecchio et al., 2009; Furedy et al., 1989; Joosen et al., 2012; Wiesenfeld et al., 1981). In addition, when presented as a background sound, infant cries can interfere with performance on simple cognitive tasks, suggesting a strong capacity to capture attention (Chang & Thompson, 2011; Neuhoff et al., 2014).

Research into the neural architecture supporting caregiving behaviour has primarily used functional magnetic resonance imaging (fMRI) to study regions of the brain reactive to infant cues (both vocalizations and facial expressions). To date, at least seven of these studies have focused on regions reactive to the sound of infant cries, compared to 'control sounds' (white noise or scrambled sounds). Two regions most consistently reported, across groups of mothers, fathers, and childless women investigated in this way, are the superior temporal gyrus (STG) and basal ganglia (see Table 12.1). Other regions reported in multiple studies include temporal lobe regions (middle temporal gyrus, MTG), frontal regions (orbitofrontal cortex, OFC; inferior frontal gyrus, IFG; prefrontal cortex, PFC; cingulate cortex), premotor regions (premotor cortex and supplementary motor area, SMA) and the cerebellum. Together, these studies highlight cortical neural circuitry for the perception (temporal), appraisal (frontal), and preparation of motor responses (premotor and basal ganglia) to infant cries (see Figure 12.2).

 Considering the dual-stream model of emotional processing, subcortical regions are thought to support rapid responses while cortical regions allow more detailed appraisal (Adolphs, 2002). The OFC is considered a critical hub in this system, providing an interface between the two routes (Barrett & Bar, 2009). Cortical areas highlighted here in the 'parental brain' are similar to models of the 'social brain', a network of neural areas

Table 12.1 Functional MRI studies reporting greater activity to infant cries versus control sounds across different populations

Study Control stimulus	Temporal lobe regions	Frontal lobe regions	Subcortical regions	Motor regions	Other regions
Mothers					
Kim et al., 2010 *Unknown cry > intensity-matched white noise*	MTG STG	IFG insula PCC PFC		Motor cortex Premotor/SMA	Visual cortex
Lorberbaum et al., 2002 *Unknown cry > intensity-matched white noise*	ITG MTG STG	d/ACC IFG PCC PFC	Basal ganglia[a] Hypothalamus Thalamus		
Laurent et al., 2012a *Unknown cry > frequency-matched pure tone*		Insula PCC PFC OFC	Basal ganglia[a,b,c] PAG/VTA		Angular gyrus Supramarginal gyrus Cerebellum
Own infant cry > unknown infant cry		dACC insula			Visual cortex
Fathers					
Mascaro et al., 2014 *Unknown cry > frequency- and intensity-matched pure tone*	STG STS	IFG insula MFG OFC	Basal ganglia[d]		

(continued)

Table 12.1 Continued

Study Control stimulus	Temporal lobe regions	Frontal lobe regions	Subcortical regions	Motor regions	Other regions
Childless women					
Bos et al., 2010 *Unknown infant cry > intensity- matched scrambled infant cry*	STG				
Riem et al., 2011 *Unknown infant cry > intensity- and frequency-matched scrambled infant cry*	MTG STG		Amygdala		
Montoya et al., 2012 *Unknown infant cry > pink noise*	MTG STG		Basal ganglia[c]	Premotor/SMA	Cerebellum

(Regions listed— (d)ACC: (dorsal) anterior cingulate cortex; IFG: inferior frontal gyrus; ITG: inferior temporal gyrus; MTG: middle temporal gyrus; OFC: orbitofrontal cortex; PAG: periaqueductal grey; PCC: posterior cingulate cortex; PFC: prefrontal cortex; SMA: supplementary motor area; STG/S: superior temporal gyrus/sulcus; VTA: ventral tegmental area. Superscript letters denote basal ganglia nuclei as follows: [a]substantia nigra; [b]caudate, nucleus accumbens; [c]putamen; [d]globus pallidus.)

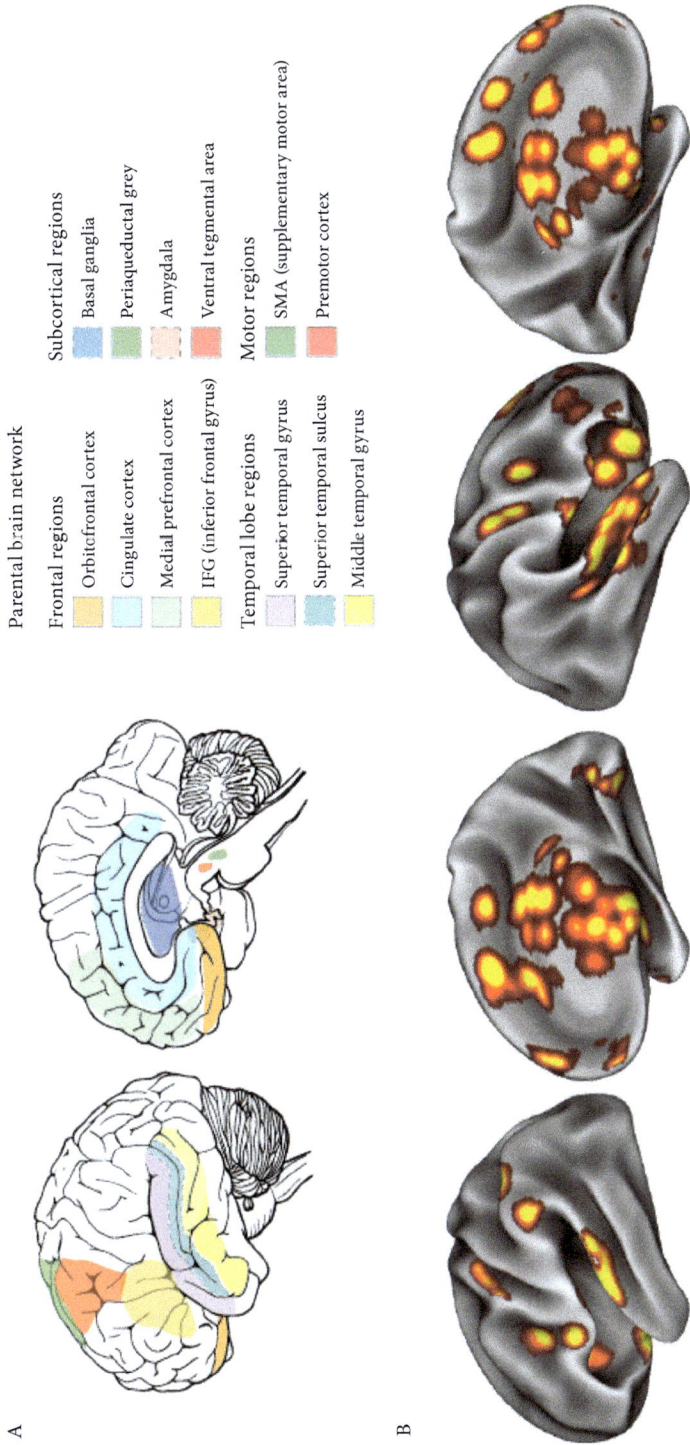

Parental brain network

Frontal regions
- ☐ Orbitfrontal cortex
- ☐ Cingulate cortex
- ☐ Medial prefrontal cortex
- ☐ IFG (inferior frontal gyrus)

Temporal lobe regions
- ☐ Superior temporal gyrus
- ☐ Superior temporal sulcus
- ☐ Middle temporal gyrus

Subcortical regions
- ☐ Basal ganglia
- ☐ Periaqueductal grey
- ☐ Amygdala
- ☐ Ventral tegmental area

Motor regions
- ☐ SMA (supplementary motor area)
- ☐ Premotor cortex

FIGURE 12.2 (A) Schematic diagram of 'parental brain' — networks of regions recruited in responding to the sound of an infant cry. (B) Findings from fMRI studies demonstrating regions of differential reactivity to infant cries, compared to control sounds (collated using GingerALe, Eickhoff et al., 2009).

sensitive to emotional social cues (for reviews, see Amodio & Frith, 2006; Adolphs, 2003; Frith, 2007; Frith & Frith, 2010). Early processing of the affective content of voices is known to recruit both cortical (STS/STG, MTG) and subcortical (amygdala) regions of the temporal lobe (Belin et al., 2004; Ethofer et al., 2006; Frühholz et al., 2014; Yovel & Belin, 2013). Activity in these regions is then thought to project to frontal regions, such as the OFC and IFG, for appraisal and higher-order processing (Frühholz & Grandjean, 2013; Frühholz et al., 2015; Schirmer & Kotz, 2006).

One key difference between models of the social brain and the proposed parental brain is the greater involvement of 'survival circuitry' in the parental brain, namely subcortical and brainstem regions that enable more reflexive-like responses. While not activated consistently in this set of fMRI studies, robust evidence from animal studies implicates a number of subcortical regions, including the amygdala, periaqueductal grey (PAG), and ventral tegmental area (VTA) in rapid responding to infant vocalizations (Rilling & Young, 2014). The amygdala has been proposed to play a 'vigilance' role in the parental brain, supporting preferential attending towards the infant (Feldman, 2015), while the PAG and VTA have been highlighted in the animal literature for the selection and initiation of care-giving behaviour (Lonstein et al., 2015; Rilling & Young, 2014). These studies typically employ techniques that disrupt the functioning of specific brain regions (e.g. through surgical lesioning or chemical infusion) and subsequent behavioural changes. Compared to the correlational nature of human neuroimaging, these methods allow stronger inferences to be made regarding the role of specific neural regions in behaviours of interest. As these regions are phylogenetically older than the neocortex and are conserved across evolution, it is likely that they perform similar functions in both animal and human brains (Corter & Fleming, 1990).

Investigation of the specific roles of nodes within the parental brain network is under way, using three key strategies. First, temporally sensitive neuroimaging techniques are being used to better understand the timing of activity in these regions, specifically in response to infant cries. Secondly, comparisons of groups of individuals varying in levels of caregiving experience are being conducted to assess experience-dependent brain plasticity. Thirdly, studies are beginning to incorporate behaviourally-relevant measures to assess correlations with activity across different regions. The following sections will elaborate on each of these research areas in turn.

12.5 INVESTIGATING THE TEMPORAL DYNAMICS OF THE 'PARENTAL BRAIN'

Data from neuroimaging techniques with high temporal resolution can complement the high-spatial sensitivity of data from fMRI studies. Specifically, investigation of the time windows in which specific regions are differentially sensitive to stimuli can inform theories of functioning for nodes within a network (see Figure 12.3 for a summary). In the following section, we describe three studies using magnetoencephalography (MEG) and one study using local field potential (LFP) recordings that have begun to inform the temporal dynamics within the parental brain.

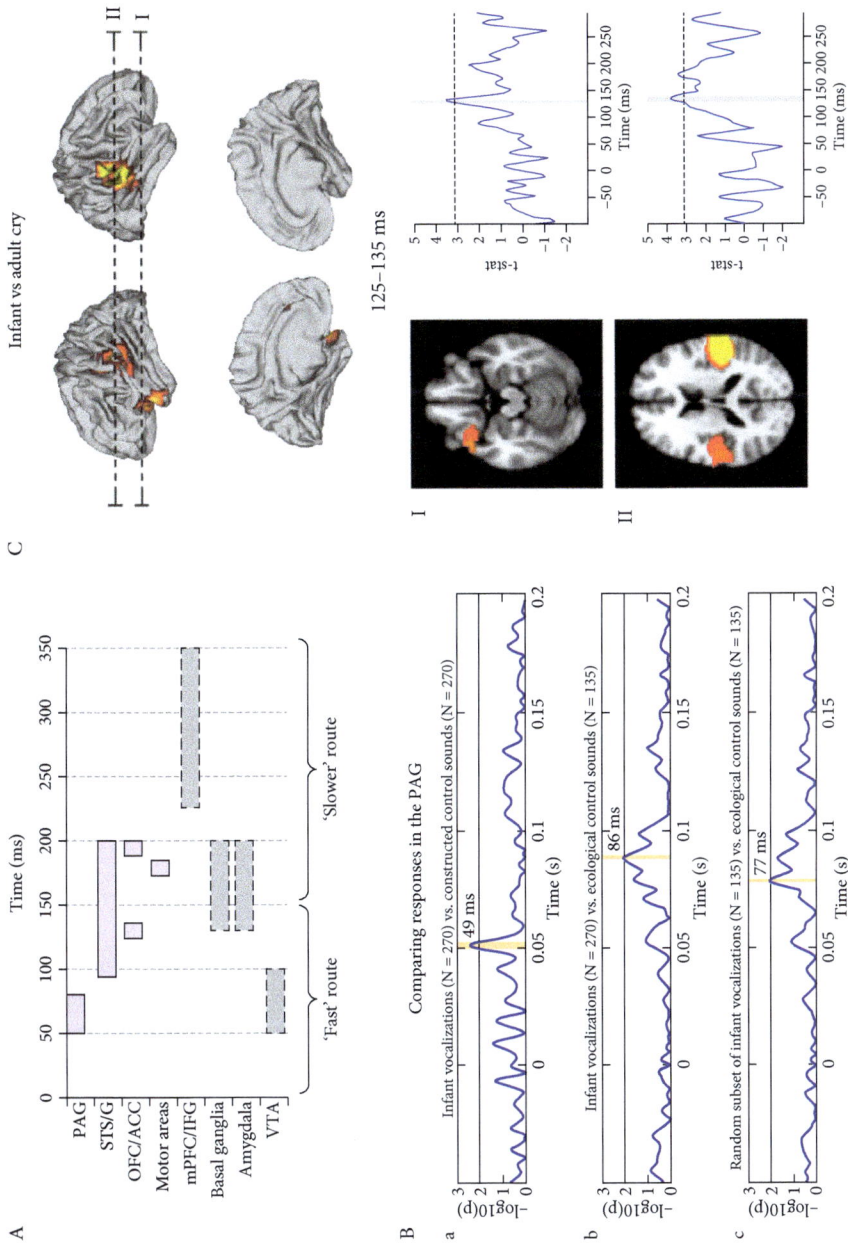

FIGURE 12.3 Temporal dynamics of neural responses to infant cries. (A) Proposed timing of recruitment of brain regions to infant cries within the 'fast' and 'slower' routes of emotional processing. Purple bars represent data from LFP and MEG studies, grey dashed bars represent suggested timings for other regions. (B) LFP evidence for rapid sensitivity to infant cry vocalizations in the PAG of the brainstem. (C) MEG evidence for early differential activity between infant and adult cry vocalizations in the (I) OFC and (II) STG.

12.5.1 Role of the Orbitofrontal Cortex in Rapid Orientating Responses: Evidence from MEG Studies

The OFC is a region of particular interest in the investigation of responsive caregiving be-haviour. It has established roles in both reward processing and social cognition (Berridge & Kringelbach, 2015; Kringelbach, 2005; Parsons, Stark, et al., 2013; Rudebeck & Murray, 2014). It is uniquely placed as an interface of the 'dual-stream' routes of emotional processing (Adolphs, 2002; LeDoux, 2000), receiving input from both cortical and subcortical path-ways (Kringelbach, 2005; Zald & Pardo, 2002). The 'affective prediction hypothesis' sug-gests that the OFC plays a crucial role in the coordination of both fast and slow responses to emotional stimuli (Bar, 2007; Barrett & Bar, 2009). Early in time, the OFC coordinates the 'tagging' of salient stimuli, influencing ongoing sensory processing and priming rapid motor reactions (Bar et al., 2006; Chaumon et al., 2013; D'Hondt et al., 2013). Later in time, activity in the OFC represents the reward value of stimuli, based on more refined identifica-tion, which may influence higher-order processing (Kringelbach & Rolls, 2003). Both these processes are plausibly implicated in parenting, with swift identification supporting rapid orientating responses and sustained representation of reward influencing selection of care-giving behaviour (Parsons, Stark, et al., 2013).

We recently examined the temporal dynamics of neural responses to infant cries com-pared to adult cries in a novel MEG paradigm (Young, Parsons, Elmholdt, et al., 2015). As both stimuli were hypothesized to elicit activity in vocal-processing regions of the social brain, differences observed reflected neural processing sensitive to 'infancy'. Results of beam-forming source-localization analyses demonstrated two types of response: sustained differential activity, localized to temporal lobe regions (95–200 ms); and transient responses in the OFC, anterior cingulate cortex (ACC) (125–135 ms; 190–200 ms; see Figure 12.3C), and cortical motor regions (175–185 ms). This activity is consistent with the affective prediction hypothesis: early activity in the OFC may rapidly 'tag' infant vocalizations as salient stimuli and affect ongoing sensory processing as well as priming motor responses. Of note, these findings implicate the OFC in differential processing earlier in time (125–200 ms) than gen-eral theories of auditory processing (at around 300 ms; Schirmer & Kotz, 2006).

These findings are similar to previous work in the visual domain, which demonstrated rapid differential activity in the OFC (130 ms) in response to images of infant and adult faces (Kringelbach et al., 2008). This OFC response to 'infancy' was diminished by the presence of a structural abnormality in the infant face (cleft lip; Parsons, Young, Mohseni, et al., 2013). This supports the notion that early OFC reactivity is based on rapid stereotyped responses, such that when there is a deviation from the expected template (as in the case of a structural abnormality), rapid detection may be attenuated. Behavioural studies have demonstrated reduced motivation to view infant faces with cleft lip in non-parent adults (Parsons et al., 2011) as well as less sensitive maternal behaviour when an infant has a cleft lip (Murray et al., 2008). Disruption to rapid, reflexive neural responses to infant cues might be one mech-anism through which this reduction in motivation and maternal sensitivity occurs.

The timing of these responses—in the range of 100–300 ms post-stimulus—is most likely 'preconscious' in nature. In seminal work, Libet demonstrated a typical delay of around 500 ms between the onset of neural activity and the emergence of mental awareness (Libet, 2002, 2006). Similarly, work by Dehaene and colleagues has demonstrated that awareness of stimuli can modulate ERP components from 250–300 ms onwards, while components occurring earlier in time were unaffected by whether stimuli were subsequently consciously perceived or not (Gaillard et al., 2009; Sergent et al., 2005). In combination, MEG studies of responses to infant vocalizations and facial expressions suggest a modality-independent function of the OFC in the detection of infant cues at a speed faster than conscious processing. Importantly, these effects were observed in adults who were not parents, suggesting that this early OFC reactivity may be relatively universal in nature. As such, we propose this reactivity may constitute part of a so-called 'caregiving instinct', not dependent on extensive exposure or training. Further investigation of this proposal, comparing parents with non-parents would be of much interest.

12.5.2 Early Detection in the Subcortical Pathway: Evidence from Local Field Potentials

Rodent studies have highlighted the role of subcortical regions in maternal responsiveness. In particular, it has been demonstrated that lesioning of the PAG results in impaired maternal caregiving behaviour (Lonstein & Stern, 1997; Miranda-Paiva et al., 2007; Sukikara et al., 2010). Located in the midbrain, the PAG has an extensive network of anatomical connections including the nearby inferior colliculus (Dujardin & Jürgens, 2005) and frontal lobe regions, including the OFC (Cavada et al., 2000). Some fMRI studies have demonstrated activity in the PAG in response to infant cries (Laurent & Ablow, 2012a) and infant faces (Bartels & Zeki, 2004; Noriuchi et al., 2008). However, activity in the PAG can be difficult to detect with fMRI due to its small size and motion artefacts caused by pulsatile blood flow in the brainstem (Zhang et al., 2006). Intracranial recordings from electrodes implanted for deep brain stimulation (DBS) provide rare opportunities for direct recording of activity from such regions.

Our laboratory conducted a study investigating PAG responsiveness to infant cries using recordings from DBS electrodes implanted in this region (Parsons, Young, Joensson, et al., 2014). We demonstrated significant differences in local field potential (LFP) recordings from the PAG in response to infant cries compared to constructed control sounds as early as 49 ms after stimulus onset (see Figure 12.3B). Compared to natural control sounds (adult cries and animal distress sounds), significant differences were observed at 86 ms. It should be noted that while electrodes were implanted in the PAG, it is possible that activity recorded at this site was influenced by reactivity in neighbouring subcortical regions, such as the inferior colliculus. These findings support the proposal that the human brain subcortical regions, such as the PAG, might aid selection of caregiving behaviour, perhaps through rapid discrimination of infant vocalizations.

In summary, the use of temporally-sensitive neuroimaging techniques suggests that early reactivity in the OFC is sensitive to 'infancy', with evidence of specialized recruitment of this region of the social brain. This reactivity might be supported by rapid differentiation of these cues in the PAG, a phylogenetically older 'survival' region. Further investigation of this network, particularly of how regions might act in concert with one another and their impact on behaviour, would be essential for investigating this proposal. Previous reviews have suggested that this 'bottom–up' activation of the parental brain (i.e. activation by sensory stimuli) may facilitate the initiation of caregiving behaviour in non-parents ('alloparental care'; Feldman, 2015). We propose that early detection of salient infant cues supports rapid orientating responses towards infants, a crucial first step in the initiation of caregiving behaviour, alloparental or otherwise.

12.6 EXPERIENCE-DEPENDENT PLASTICITY IN THE 'PARENTAL BRAIN'

The demands of parenting change considerably as the infant develops. Beyond initial orientating of attention towards the infant, parents rapidly learn to identify their own infant by sound, smell, or touch alone (see Figure 12.4; Parsons et al., 2010). As the infant's perceptual and communicative skills develop, parents automatically adapt their own interactive style, a phenomenon aptly termed 'intuitive parenting' (Papoušek, 2007). Throughout early infancy, parents demonstrate 'primary parental preoccupation', in which a high degree of focus and attention is directed towards the infant (Leckman et al., 2004; Winnicott, 1956). These parenting behaviours support behavioural, social, and cognitive development in the infant. Around 6 months of age, infants begin to show a strong preference for primary caregiver(s) over other individuals, a developmental landmark called 'attachment' (Bowlby, 1982). Beyond this stage, infants' social competencies develop further, with the capacity to consider the subjective state of others ('intersubjectivity'/theory of mind) and the foundations of empathy and self-awareness (Ruddy & Bornstein, 1982; Trevarthen et al., 1981).

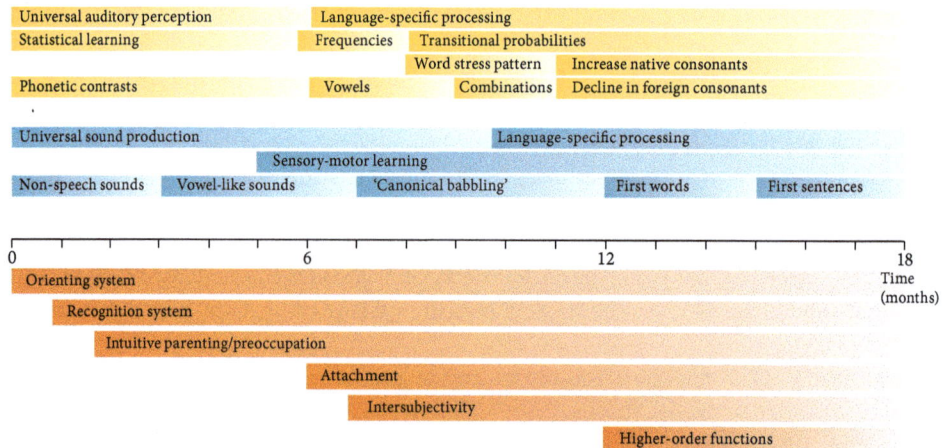

FIGURE 12.4 A behavioural framework of parenting (red) alongside a timeline of infant auditory/vocal developmental milestones.

Reprinted with permission from *Progress in Neurobiology*, Volume 91, Issue 3, Parsons C.E., Young K.S., Murray L., Stein A., & Kringelbachab M.L., 'The functional neuroanatomy of the evolving parent–infant relationship', Copyright © 2010 Elsevier Ltd., with permission from Elsevier, http://www.sciencedirect.com/science/article/pii/S0301008210000651

12.6.1 Individual Differences in Responses to Infant Cries: Effects of Gender and Parental Status

It is generally assumed that males differ from females, and parents differ from non-parents in their reactions to infant crying. However, research to date has demonstrated mixed evidence on the nature of such differences. Studies of physiological reactivity to the sound of infant cries has shown differential heart-rate reactivity between males and females, yet the direction of these effects varies across studies (Furedy et al., 1989; Out et al., 2010; Wiesenfeld et al., 1981). Similar studies comparing parents to childless adults support between-group differences, yet the direction of effects is also unclear (Hall & Morsbach, 1989; Out et al., 2010). Studies of adults' perceptions of infant cries have shown that both men and women perceive distress in infant cries and report a desire to respond (Donate-Bartfield & Passman, 1985; Leger et al., 1996). Some studies suggest that parents rate infant cries as less distressed and less aversive compared to non-parents (Irwin, 2003; Zeskind & Lester, 1978), while other work suggests no differences between these groups (Lin & McFatter, 2012).

One effect that is apparent across this body of work is that parents rapidly acquire specific sensitivity to cries from their own infants (Cismaresco & Montagner, 1990; Parsons et al., 2010). While early studies of this effect suggested a female advantage in this process, with mothers acquiring selective sensitivity to own-infant cues more rapidly than fathers (Wiesenfeld et al., 1981), recent work has challenged this view. When the amount of time spent in caregiving was taken into account, mothers and fathers did not differ in their ability to recognize their own infant's cry (Gustafsson et al., 2013). This would suggest that sensitivity is more related to experience-dependent plasticity than innate gender differences.

Two fMRI studies investigating gender differences in response to infant cries showed greater 'deactivation' in the cingulate cortex in females compared to males, independent of parental status (De Pisapia et al., 2013; Seifritz et al., 2003). One of these studies additionally demonstrated stronger amygdala responses to infant cries than infant laughter in parents compared to non-parents, independent of gender (Seifritz et al., 2003). Inclusion of a measure of the amount of time spent in close proximity with infants in studies such as these would allow investigation of 'innate' versus experience-dependent differences in the brain. One such study using multimodal infant cues demonstrated an association of time spent in childcare with amygdala–STS connectivity in fathers (Abraham et al., 2014). Further support for this type of mechanism, however, requires replication. Longitudinal studies, comparing the same individuals over time as they gain parenting experience would be particularly informative in this regard.

12.6.2 Individual Differences: Correlating Neural Activity with Behavioural Responses

Studies have begun to investigate relationships between neural responses to infant cries and behavioural measures of parenting. Overall, these studies point to an association between more adaptive caregiving responses with reduced subcortical and greater prefrontal reactivity to infant cries. Focusing first on subcortical regions, reduced amygdala reactivity to infant cries was observed in mothers with higher-quality relationships with their infants (Laurent & Ablow, 2012b), as well as among adults with better-quality relationships with other adults (Riem et al., 2012). Both these studies used measures of attachment, a measure of the emotional bond between two individuals (Bowlby, 1982). While not implicated directly in the parental brain circuitry, decreased activity in the hippocampus in response to infant cries was also associated with greater attachment security and retrospective reports of good maternal care during participants' own childhoods (Kim et al., 2010; Laurent & Ablow, 2012b). The hippocampus is classically implicated in memory processes, supporting claims of experience-dependent differences in neural responses (Eichenbaum, 2000).

For frontal regions, findings generally suggest that greater reactivity to infant cries is associated with more sensitive parenting behaviour. Greater OFC and right ventrolateral PFC activity was associated with better quality of attachment between mothers and their infants (Laurent & Ablow, 2012b). A similar pattern was observed for the IFG, with greater reactivity in this region associated with more sensitive maternal behaviour (Musser et al., 2012) and with less 'restrictive paternal attitudes' (a measure of fathers' controlling approach to caregiving; Mascaro et al., 2014). In addition, more middle frontal gyrus activity was associated with better perceived maternal care in childhood (Kim et al., 2010).

This pattern of increased prefrontal activity, paired with decreased subcortical activity, has been highlighted in work investigating emotion regulation capacities—the ability of individuals to control their affective responses to experiences (Ochsner et al., 2012). Prefrontal regions are proposed to help regulate activity among subcortical limbic regions (primarily the amygdala), promoting changes in emotional reactions. Of note, dysregulation of this system is the dominant neural model of anxiety disorders, whereby hyper-reactivity of the amygdala to potentially threatening cues, paired with failure to regulate using prefrontal regions, is thought to impair the capacity to regulate emotional experiences (Jazaieri et al., 2015). By this model, greater frontal reactivity to infant cries might be considered as a measure of engagement of regulation capacities. Those individuals with more adaptive parenting behaviours might engage frontal regions more effectively, perhaps promoting selection of appropriate caregiving responses.

Plasticity in the parental brain also involves changes in other cortical regions. Greater activity in auditory cortex was associated with better reported maternal care in mothers (Kim et al., 2010) and more positive parenting thoughts in fathers (Kim et al., 2015). These findings are indicative of experience-dependent changes in sensory cortices, perhaps promoting more sensitive analysis of infant cues. In addition, the insula has been implicated in different processes in different studies, linked to less 'restrictive paternal attitude' in fathers (Montoya et al., 2012) or poorer attachment quality and more 'intrusive' behaviour in mothers (Laurent & Ablow, 2012b; Musser et al., 2012). One study also implicated plasticity in subregions of the basal ganglia, with reports of maternal anxiety linked to substantia nigra activity and paternal positivity linked to caudate activity (Kim et al., 2015).

One recent study investigated neural responses to infant cries in young mothers (aged 19–22 years) from low socioeconomic settings, and demonstrated a different pattern of effects (Hipwell et al., 2015). Maternal sensitivity in this study was correlated with increased reactivity across cortical and subcortical regions (thalamus, hippocampus, putamen, and insula). The measure of maternal behaviour used was 'maternal mental state talk' (MMST). MMST is thought to be an adaptive behaviour in which the parent treats the infant as an intentional agent, and also includes the parent's understanding that the child has representations of the world (also known as 'mind-mindedness'; Meins et al., 2003). In contrast to work previously discussed, this study suggests more adaptive maternal behaviour is linked to greater activity across both subcortical and cortical regions. Further research directly comparing groups of mothers of different ages and from different backgrounds would allow investigation of whether neural reactivity might differ according to these demographic variables.

As an emerging field, the study of experience-dependent plasticity in the parental brain would benefit from standardization and replication of effects to inform current models more effectively. As exemplified here, 'parenting' can be operationalized in vastly different ways, from observation of specific caregiving behaviours to recollection of perceived parenting attitudes. The use of a common framework to define key components of parenting behaviour, taking into account the varying demands of childcare as infants develop, is crucial. Careful measurement of parenting sensitivity and participant demographics, combined with high-quality, large imaging studies will enable more sensitive analysis of individual differences.

12.6.3 Neural Correlates of Disrupted Parent–Infant Interactions

Conditions in which parental behaviour is disrupted can also inform theories of the parental brain. Three such studies investigated different aspects of disrupted behaviour—postnatal depression and substance abuse in mothers, and autism spectrum disorder (ASD) in infants. Postnatal depression (PND) affects 13–19% of mothers (O'Hara & McCabe, 2013) and is associated with difficulties in parent–infant interactions, including reduced responsiveness to infant cues (Field, 1995; Murray et al., 1996; Stein et al., 1991). Depression has been shown to negatively impact emotional appraisal and recognition accuracy of infant facial expressions (Arteche et al., 2011; Stein et al., 2010), as well as discrimination of distress and psychomotor reactivity to infant cries (Young et al., 2012; Young, Parsons, Stein, et al., 2015). The behavioural impact of substance abuse in mothers varies according to substance and severity. Broadly speaking, substance-abusing mothers tend to use more harsh discipline (Mayes & Sean, 2002) and spend less time interacting with their infants (Gottwald & Thurman, 1994) compared to healthy mothers. In late infancy, ASD is associated with disrupted mother–infant interactions (from 12 months of age; Rozga et al., 2011). Prior to this age, there is evidence suggesting that infants at risk of ASD have atypical cry acoustics (abnormally high and variable pitch; Sheinkopf et al., 2012).

Neuroimaging findings have demonstrated that, compared to healthy mothers, mothers with depression had reduced reactivity to infant cries in frontal (OFC, PFC, ACC) and reward regions (nucleus accumbens; Laurent & Ablow, 2012a). Mothers with substance abuse had more widespread effects, with reduced reactivity across sensory (STG), frontal (IFG, PFC, ACC, insula), motor, and subcortical (thalamus and amygdala) regions (Landi et al., 2011). In healthy adults, neural reactivity to cries of infants at risk for ASD, compared to typically developing infants, was greater in auditory and frontal regions (STG, IFG, and OFC; Venuti et al., 2012). Together, these preliminary findings confirm suggestions that the reward value of infant cries is supported by activity in frontal and reward circuitry (as in depression); that global dampening of responsiveness might impair the motivation to interact with an infant (as in substance abuse); and that atypical infant cues can disrupt sensory and appraisal processing (as in ASD). Collectively, these studies elucidate the importance of considering disruptions to both interactive partners, altered parental behaviour, and abnormal infant signalling. Further investigation of these and other disorders can additionally inform understanding of disrupted interactions.

12.6.4 The Influence of Hormonal Levels on the Parental Brain

Pregnancy, childbirth, and caregiving are all associated with changes in neuroendocrinal states (Lonstein et al., 2015). Oxytocin (OT) in particular has been ascribed a central role in maternal and social behaviour in animals (Carter, 1998; Insel & Young, 2001). Its role in human behaviour however is somewhat less clear, partly due to inconsistencies in methodological approaches (Bakermans-Kranenburg & Van Ijzendoorn, 2013; Nave et al., 2015). One fMRI study investigating the effects of oxytocin (compared to placebo) administration on brain responses to infant cries found greater reactivity in the insula and IFG, along with reduced amygdala activity in childless women (Riem et al., 2011). A similar study, administering testosterone, also demonstrated increased insula activity, along with greater reactivity in the thalamus and posterior cingulate cortex (Bos et al., 2010). Testosterone may serve to 'sensitize' neural circuitry involved in responsive caregiving, while OT may additionally 'dampen' amygdala responses, potentially serving an anxiolytic effect.

Three studies have investigated natural fluctuations in hormonal levels in motherhood by comparing: i) mothers who had vaginal deliveries (VD) with those who had Caesarean section deliveries (CSD); ii) breastfeeding versus formula-feeding mothers; and iii) natural variation in cortisol responses. Compared to CSD mothers, VD mothers had stronger reactivity to their own infant cries (compared to cries of other infants) in auditory (STG/MTG), frontal (superior frontal gyrus), and subcortical (thalamus/hypothalamus, amygdala) regions (Swain et al., 2008). Compared to formula-feeding mothers, breastfeeding mothers also had stronger reactivity in frontal (SFG, insula) and subcortical (striatum, amygdala) regions—activity which was associated with greater maternal sensitivity in observed mother–infant interactions (Kim et al., 2011). Cortisol reactivity, on the other hand, was associated with reduced levels of activity in the PAG and frontal brain regions (OFC, ACC, mPFC, and insula; Laurent et al., 2011). Together, these studies suggest that higher levels of sex hormones (through administration studies or behavioural differences) might promote more sensitive caregiving behaviour through generally enhancing activity across regions of the parental brain. Higher levels of cortisol (conceptualized as the 'stress' hormone), however, may impair appraisal of and responding to infant cries. Inclusion of the independent measurement of hormonal levels in future studies would allow a more nuanced understanding of the differing effects of hormones in a natural context.

12.7 FUTURE DIRECTIONS

As an emerging research field, there are many possible future avenues for improving our understanding of the parental brain. A principal concern is to combine multiple levels of analysis in the same individuals in order to build a more complete picture of the range of effects that parenting confers on the individual (e.g. physiological, neural, behavioural). Neuroimaging studies with careful assessment of behavioural responses, both inside and outside the scanner, combined with measurements of physiological reactivity and hormonal levels, hold much potential in this regard. Standardization of terminology, measurement tools, and theoretical frameworks would also enable easy comparison of novel findings with current trends and permit assessment of the reproducibility of effects observed.

Research to date has focused on responses to negative vocal affect (i.e. infant cries). Parenting behaviour is likely to be motivated as much by approach behaviour towards positive infant cues (e.g. infant laughter) as it is by avoidance or reduction of exposure to negative cues. Processing of positive infant cues is likely to recruit reward circuitry in the brain (such as the nucleus accumbens, VTA, and OFC), providing a better understanding of other aspects of caregiving behaviour. The majority of studies described here are passive listening paradigms in socially isolated contexts. Such studies are rightly criticized for a lack of ecological validity, attempting to measure aspects of social behaviour in the absence of interaction with another individual (Schilbach, 2010). One opportunity to overcome this limitation is the use of 'hyperscanning'—simultaneous measurement of neural activity from two individuals (Konvalinka & Roepstorff, 2012). This would be of particular interest in investigating the formation of emotional bonds between parent and infant.

Another essential future strategy is the use of longitudinal designs to map changes in the parental brain. In particular, following individuals from before pregnancy through to parenthood would provide novel insight into the experience-dependent neural plasticity supporting parenting. Studies investigating clinically assessed impairments in parent–infant relationships also hold hope for a better understanding of critical neural functioning. Similarly, investigation of naturally occurring disruptions to infant vocalizations, such as the high-pitched cries of infants with cri-du-chat syndrome, allow novel insight into the neural underpinnings of 'instinctive' neural responses. Assessment of impaired responsiveness, alongside treatment studies investigating the impact of interventions for parenting behaviour, may help develop a mechanistic description of neural processes facilitating caregiving.

12.8 Conclusion

In this chapter, we present current evidence for the neural circuitry supporting detection and responding to infant cry vocalizations. Regions identified, labelled the 'parental brain', largely overlap with the 'social brain', with the addition of a number of survival-related subcortical regions. We propose that the 'social brain' is preferentially recruited during parent–infant interactions. Rapid identification and orientating responses to infant vocalizations might be facilitated by discriminative activity in this system, with the PAG and OFC as proposed subcortical and cortical hubs supporting this. Studies investigating differential neural responses to infant cries in parenthood suggest that there is experience-dependent plasticity in the parental brain which may support the ever-changing demands of parenthood through infant development. Emerging results highlight the potential importance of 'emotion regulation' neural processes, potentially mediating perception of and reaction to infant cries. Future work should aim to combine levels of analysis and standardize measures used in a common framework to enable a more holistic view of the parental brain. In addition, more research is needed to examine whether a detailed understanding of these parental neural processes could guide more precise clinical interventions. Longitudinal studies focusing on different stages of parenthood, as well as conditions in which parenting is disrupted, will be particularly important for understanding at a more mechanistic level.

REFERENCES

Abraham, E., Hendler, T., Shapira-Lichter, I., Kanat-Maymon, Y., Zagoory-Sharon, O., & Feldman, R. (2014). Father's brain is sensitive to childcare experiences. *Proceedings of the National Academy of Sciences,* 111, 9792–9797.

Adolphs, R. (2002). Neural systems for recognizing emotion. *Current Opinion in Neurobiology,* 12, 169–177.

Adolphs, R. (2003). Cognitive neuroscience of human social behaviour. *Nature Reviews Neuroscience,* 4, 165–178.

Ainsworth, M. D., Bell, S. M., & Stayton, D. J. (eds) (1974). *Infant–mother Attachment and Social Development: Socialization as a Product of Reciprocal Responsiveness to Signals.* London: Cambridge University Press.

Amodio, D. M. & Frith, C. D. (2006). Meeting of minds: the medial frontal cortex and social cognition. *Nature Reviews Neuroscience,* 7, 268–277.

Arteche, A., Joormann, J., Harvey, A., Craske, M., Gotlib, I. H., Lehtonen, A., Counsell, N., & Stein, A. (2011). The effects of postnatal maternal depression and anxiety on the processing of infant faces. *Journal of Affective Disorders,* 133, 197–203.

Bakermans-Kranenburg, M. J. & Van Ijzendoorn, M. (2013). Sniffing around oxytocin: review and meta-analyses of trials in healthy and clinical groups with implications for pharmaco-therapy. *Translational Psychiatry,* 3, e258.

Bakermans-Kranenburg, M. J., Van Ijzendoorn, M. H., Riem, M. M. E., Tops, M., & Alink, L. R. A. (2012). Oxytocin decreases handgrip force in reaction to infant crying in females without harsh parenting experiences. *Social Cognitive and Affective Neuroscience,* 7, 951–957.

Bar, M. (2007). The proactive brain: using analogies and associations to generate predictions. *Trends in Cognitive Sciences,* 11, 280–289.

Bar, M., Kassam, K. S., Ghuman, A. S., Boshyan, J., Schmid, A. M., Dale, A. M., ... Rosen, B. R. (2006). Top-down facilitation of visual recognition. *Proceedings of the National Academy of Sciences of the United States of America,* 103, 449–454.

Barrett, L. F. & Bar, M. (2009). See it with feeling: affective predictions during object perception. *Philosophical Transactions of the Royal Society B: Biological Sciences,* 364, 1325–1334.

Barrett, L. F., Mesquita, B., Ochsner, K. N., & Gross, J. J. (2007). The experience of emotion. *Annual Review of Psychology,* 58, 373.

Bartels, A. & Zeki, S. (2004). The neural correlates of maternal and romantic love. *NeuroImage,* 21, 1155–1166.

Belin, P., Fecteau, S., & Bedard, C. (2004). Thinking the voice: neural correlates of voice perception. *Trends in Cognitive Sciences,* 8, 129–135.

Bell, S. M. & Ainsworth, M. D. (1972). Infant crying and maternal responsiveness. *Child Development,* 43, 1171–1190.

Berridge, K. C. & Kringelbach, M. L. (2015). Pleasure systems in the brain. *Neuron,* 86, 646–664.

Bleichfeld, B. & Moely, B. E. (1984). Psychophysiological responses to an infant cry: comparison of groups of women in different phases of the maternal cycle. *Developmental Psychology*, 20, 1082–1091.

Bornstein, M. H., Hahn, C.-S., & Haynes, O. M. (2011). Maternal personality, parenting cognitions, and parenting practices. *Developmental Psychology*, 47, 658.

Bos, P. A., Hermans, E. J., Montoya, E. R., Ramsey, N. F., & Van Honk, J. (2010). Testosterone administration modulates neural responses to crying infants in young females. *Psychoneuroendocrinology*, 35, 114–121.

Bowlby, J. (1982). Attachment and loss: retrospect and prospect. *American Journal of Orthopsychiatry*, 52, 664–678.

Carter, C. S. (1998). Neuroendocrine perspectives on social attachment and love. *Psychoneuroendocrinology*, 23, 779–818.

Cavada, C., Compañy, T., Tejedor, J., Cruz-Rizzolo, R. J., & Reinoso-Suárez, F. (2000). The anatomical connections of the macaque monkey orbitofrontal cortex. A review. *Cerebral Cortex*, 10, 220–242.

Chang, R. S. & Thompson, N. S. (2011). Whines, cries, and motherese: their relative power to distract. *Journal of Social, Evolutionary, and Cultural Psychology*, 5, 131–141.

Chaumon, M., Kveraga, K., Barrett, L., & Bar, M. (2013). Visual predictions in the orbitofrontal cortex rely on associative content. *Cerebral Cortex*, 24(11), 2899–2907.

Cismaresco, A. & Montagner, H. (1990). Mothers' discrimination of their neonates' cry in relation to cry acoustics: the first week of life. *Early Child Development and Care*, 65, 3–11.

Corter, C. M. & Fleming, A. S. (1990). Maternal responsiveness in humans: emotional, cognitive and biological factors. *Advances in the Study of Behavior*, 19, 83–136.

D'hondt, F., Lassonde, M., Collignon, O., Lepore, F., Honoré, J., & Sequeira, H. (2013). 'Emotions guide us': behavioral and MEG correlates. *Cortex*, 49, 2473–2483.

Darwin, C. (1872). *The Expression of the Emotions in Man and Animals*. London: John Murray.

De Pisapia, N., Bornstein, M. H., Rigo, P., Esposito, G., De Falco, S., & Venuti, P. (2013). Gender differences in directional brain responses to infant hunger cries. *NeuroReport*, 24, 142.

Del Vecchio, T., Walter, A., & O'Leary, S. G. (2009). Affective and physiological factors predicting maternal response to infant crying. *Infant Behavior and Development*, 32, 117–122.

Dessureau, B. K., Kurowski, C. O., & Thompson, N. S. (1998). A reassessment of the role of pitch and duration in adults' responses to infant crying. *Infant Behavior and Development*, 21, 367–371.

Donate-Bartfield, E. & Passman, R. H. (1985). Attentiveness of mothers and fathers to their baby's cries. *Infant Behavior and Development*, 8, 385–393.

Dujardin, E. & Jürgens, U. (2005). Afferents of vocalization-controlling periaqueductal regions in the squirrel monkey. *Brain Research*, 1034, 114–131.

Eichenbaum, H. (2000). A cortical–hippocampal system for declarative memory. *Nature Reviews Neuroscience*, 1, 41–50.

Eickhoff, S. B., Laird, A. R., Grefkes, C., Wang, L. E., Zilles, K., & Fox, P. T. (2009). Coordinate-based activation likelihood estimation meta-analysis of neuroimaging data: a random-effects approach based on empirical estimates of spatial uncertainty. *Human Brain Mapping*, 30, 2907–2926.

Ethofer, T., Anders, S., Wiethoff, S., Erb, M., Herbert, C., Saur, R., Grodd, W., & Wildgruber, D. (2006). Effects of prosodic emotional intensity on activation of associative auditory cortex. *NeuroReport*, 17, 249–253.

Feldman, R. (2015). The adaptive human parental brain: implications for children's social development. *Trends in Neurosciences*, 38(6), 387–399.

Field, T. (1995). Infants of depressed mothers. *Infant Behavior and Development*, 18, 1–13.

Frith, C. D. (2007). The social brain? *Philosophical Transactions of the Royal Society B: Biological Sciences*, 362, 671–678.

Frith, U. & Frith, C. (2010). The social brain: allowing humans to boldly go where no other species has been. *Philosophical Transactions of the Royal Society B: Biological Sciences*, 365, 165–175.

Frodi, A. M., Lamb, M. E., Leavitt, L. A., & Donovan, W. L. (1978). Fathers' and mothers' responses to infant smiles and cries. *Infant Behavior and Development*, 1, 187–198.

Frühholz, S. & Grandjean, D. (2013). Processing of emotional vocalizations in bilateral inferior frontal cortex. *Neuroscience & Biobehavioral Reviews*, 37, 2847–2855.

Frühholz, S., Gschwind, M., & Grandjean, D. (2015). Bilateral dorsal and ventral fiber pathways for the processing of affective prosody identified by probabilistic fiber tracking. *NeuroImage*, 109, 27–34.

Frühholz, S., Trost, W., & Grandjean, D. (2014). The role of the medial temporal limbic system in processing emotions in voice and music. *Progress in Neurobiology*, 123, 1–17.

Furedy, J. J., Fleming, A. S., Ruble, D., Scher, H., Daly, J., Day, D., & Loewen, R. (1989). Sex differences in small-magnitude heart-rate responses to sexual and infant-related stimuli: a psychophysiological approach. *Physiology and Behavior*, 46, 903–905.

Gaillard, R., Dehaene, S., Adam, C., Clémenceau, S., Hasboun, D., Baulac, M., Cohen, L., & Naccache, L. (2009). Converging intracranial markers of conscious access. *PLoS Biology*, 7, e1000061.

Golub, H. L. & Corwin, M. J. (1985). A physioacoustic model of the infant cry. In: B. M. Lester & C. F. Boukydis (eds) *Infant Crying: Theoretical and Research Perspectives*. New York: Plenum Press.

Gottwald, S. R. & Thurman, S. K. (1994). The effects of prenatal cocaine exposure on mother–infant interaction and infant arousal in the newborn period. *Topics in Early Childhood Special Education*, 14, 217–231.

Gustafson, G. E., Wood, R. M., & Green, J. A. (2000). Can we hear the causes of infants' crying? In: R. G. Barr, B. Hopkins, & J. A. Green (eds) *Crying as a Sign, a Symptom, and a Signal*. Cambridge: Cambridge University Press.

Gustafsson, E., Levréro, F., Reby, D., & Mathevon, N. (2013). Fathers are just as good as mothers at recognizing the cries of their baby. *Nature Communications*, 4, 1698.

Hall, A. & Morsbach, G. (1989). Differential stress responses in mothers and non-mothers to infant crying. In: F. J. Mcguigan, W. E. Sime, & J. M. Wallace (eds) *Stress and Tension Control 3*. Boston, MA: Springer.

Hipwell, A., Guo, C., Phillips, M., Swain, J., & Moses-Kolko, E. (2015). Right frontoinsular cortex and subcortical activity to infant cry is associated with maternal mental state talk. *Journal of Neuroscience*, 35, 12725–12732.

Insel, T. R. & Young, L. J. (2001). The neurobiology of attachment. *Nature Reviews Neuroscience*, 2, 129–136.

Irwin, J. R. (2003). Parent and nonparent perception of the multimodal infant cry. *Infancy*, 4, 503–516.

Izard, C. E. (1971). *The Face of Emotion*. New York: Appleton-Century-Crofts.

Jazaieri, H., Morrison, A. S., Goldin, P. R., & Gross, J. J. (2015). The role of emotion and emotion regulation in social anxiety disorder. *Current Psychiatry Reports*, 17, 1–9.

Joosen, K. J., Mesman, J., Bakermans-Kranenburg, M. J., Pieper, S., Zeskind, P. S., & Van Ijzendoorn, M. H. (2012). Physiological reactivity to infant crying and observed maternal sensitivity. *Infancy*, 18(3), 414–431.

Kim, P., Feldman, R., Mayes, L. C., Eicher, V., Thompson, N., Leckman, J. F., & Swain, J. E. (2011). Breastfeeding, brain activation to own infant cry, and maternal sensitivity. *Journal of Child Psychology and Psychiatry and Allied Disciplines*, 52, 907–915.

Kim, P., Leckman, J. F., Mayes, L. C., Newman, M. A., Feldman, R., & Swain, J. E. (2010). Perceived quality of maternal care in childhood and structure and function of mothers' brain. *Developmental Science*, 13, 662–673.

Kim, P., Rigo, P., Leckman, J. F., Mayes, L. C., Cole, P. M., Feldman, R., & Swain, J. E.(2015). A prospective longitudinal study of perceived infant outcomes at 18–24 months: neural and psychological correlates of parental thoughts and actions assessed during the first month postpartum. *Frontiers in Psychology*, 6, 1772.

Konner, M. (2010). *The Evolution of Childhood: Relationships, Emotion, Mind.* Harvard University Press.

Konvalinka, I. & Roepstorff, A. (2012). The two-brain approach: how can mutually interacting brains teach us something about social interaction? *Frontiers in Human Neuroscience*, 6, 215.

Kringelbach, M. L. (2005). The human orbitofrontal cortex: linking reward to hedonic experience. *Nature Reviews Neuroscience*, 6, 691–702.

Kringelbach, M. L., Lehtonen, A., Squire, S., Harvey, A. G., Craske, M. G., Holliday, I. E., … Cornelissen, P. L. (2008). A specific and rapid neural signature for parental instinct. *PLoS One*, 3, e1664.

Kringelbach, M. L. & Rolls, E. T. (2003). Neural correlates of rapid reversal learning in a simple model of human social interaction. *NeuroImage*, 20, 1371–1383.

Kuhl, P. K. (2004). Early language acquisition: cracking the speech code. *Nature Reviews Neuroscience*, 5, 831–843.

Landi, N., Montoya, J., Kober, H., Rutherford, H. J., Mencl, W. E., Worhunsky, P. D., Potenza, M. N. & Mayes, L. C. (2011). Maternal neural responses to infant cries and faces: relationships with substance use. *Frontiers in Psychiatry*, 2, 32.

Laurent, H. K. & Ablow, J. C. (2012a). A cry in the dark: depressed mothers show reduced neural activation to their own infant's cry. *Social Cognitive and Affective Neuroscience*, 7, 125–134.

Laurent, H. K. & Ablow, J. C. (2012b). The missing link: mothers' neural response to infant cry related to infant attachment behaviors. *Infant Behavior and Development*, 35, 761–772.

Laurent, H. K., Stevens, A., & Ablow, J. C. (2011). Neural correlates of hypothalamic-pituitary-adrenal regulation of mothers with their infants. *Biological Psychiatry*, 70, 826–832.

Leckman, J., Feldman, R., Swain, J., Eicher, V., Thompson, N., & Mayes, L. (2004). Primary parental preoccupation: circuits, genes, and the crucial role of the environment. *Journal of Neural Transmission*, 111, 753–771.

Ledoux, J. E. (2000). Emotion circuits in the brain. *Annual Review of Neuroscience*, 23, 155–184.

Leger, D. W., Thompson, R. A., Merritt, J. A., & Benz, J. J. (1996). Adult perception of emotion intensity in human infant cries: effects of infant age and cry acoustics. *Child Development*, 67, 3238–3249.

Libet, B. (2002). The timing of mental events: Libet's experimental findings and their implications. *Consciousness and Cognition*, 11, 291–299.

Libet, B. (2006). Reflections on the interaction of the mind and brain. *Progress in Neurobiology*, 78, 322–326.

Lin, H.-C. & Mcfatter, R. (2012). Empathy and distress: two distinct but related emotions in response to infant crying. *Infant Behavior and Development*, 35, 887–897.

Lonstein, J. S., Lévy, F., & Fleming, A. S. (2015). Common and divergent psychobiological mechanisms underlying maternal behaviors in non-human and human mammals. *Hormones and Behavior*, 73, 156–185.

Lonstein, J. S. & Stern, J. M. (1997). Role of the midbrain periaqueductal gray in maternal nurturance and aggression: C-fos and electrolytic lesion studies in lactating rats. *Journal of Neuroscience*, 17, 3364–3378.

Lorberbaum, J. P. et al. (2002). A potential role for thalamocingulate circuitry in human maternal behavior. *Biological Psychiatry*, 51, 431–445.

Lorenz, K. (1943). Die angeborenen formen möglicher erfahrung. [Innate forms of potential experience]. *Zeitschrift für Tierpsychologie*, 5, 235–519.

Mascaro, J. S., Hackett, P. D., Gouzoules, H., Lori, A., & Rilling, J. K. (2014). Behavioral and genetic correlates of the neural response to infant crying among human fathers. *Social, Cognitive and Affective Neuroscience*, 9, 1704–1712.

Mayes, L. C. & Sean, T. D. (2002). Substance abuse and parenting. In: M. H. Bornstein (ed.) *Handbook of Parenting* (2nd edn). Mahwah, NJ: Lawrence Erlbaum Associates Publishers.

Meins, E., Fernyhough, C., Wainwright, R., Clark-Carter, D., Das Gupta, M., Fradley, E., & Tuckey, M. (2003). Pathways to understanding mind: construct validity and predictive validity of maternal mind-mindedness. *Child Development*, 74, 1194–1211.

Miranda-Paiva, C. M., Canteras, N. S., Sukikara, M. H., Nasello, A. G., Mackowiak, I., & Felicio, L. F. (2007). Periaqueductal gray cholecystokinin infusions block morphine-induced disruption of maternal behavior. *Peptides*, 28, 657–662.

Montoya, J. L., Landi, N., Kober, H., Worhunsky, P. D., Rutherford, H. J. V., Mencl, W. E., Mayes, L. C., & Potenza, M. N. (2012). Regional brain responses in nulliparous women to emotional infant stimuli. *PLoS One*, 7(5), e36270.

Muller, E., Hollien, H., & Murry, T. (1974). Perceptual responses to infant crying: identification of cry types. *Journal of Child Language*, 1, 89–95.

Murray, A. D. (1979). Infant crying as an elicitor of parental behavior: an examination of two models. *Psychological Bulletin*, 86, 191.

Murray, A. D. (1985). Aversiveness is in the mind of the beholder: perception of infant crying by adults. In: B. M. Lester & C. F. Boukydis (eds) *Infant Crying: Theoretical and Research Perspectives*. New York: Plenum Press.

Murray, L., Fiori-Cowley, A., Hooper, R., & Cooper, P. (1996). The impact of postnatal depression and associated adversity on early mother–infant interactions and later infant outcome. *Child Development*, 67, 2512–2526.

Murray, L., Hentges, F., Hill, J., Karpf, J., Mistry, B., Kreutz, M., … Goodacre, T. (2008). The effect of cleft lip and palate, and the timing of lip repair on mother–infant interactions and infant development. *Journal of Child Psychology and Psychiatry*, 49, 115–123.

Murray, L., Sinclair, D., Cooper, P., Ducournau, P., Turner, P., & Stein, A. (1999). The socioemotional development of 5-year-old children of postnatally depressed mothers. *Journal of Child Psychology and Psychiatry and Allied Disciplines*, 40, 1259–1271.

Musser, E. D., Kaiser-Laurent, H., & Ablow, J. C. (2012). The neural correlates of maternal sensitivity: an fMRI study. *Developmental Cognitive Neuroscience*, 2, 428–436.

Nave, G., Camerer, C., & Mccullough, M. (2015). Does oxytocin increase trust in humans? A critical review of research. *Perspectives on Psychological Science*, 10, 772–789.

Neuhoff, J. G., Hamilton, G. R., Gittleson, A. L., & Mejia, A. (2014). Babies in traffic: infant vocalizations and listener sex modulate auditory motion perception. *Journal of Experimental Psychology: Human Perception and Performance*, 40, 775.

Noriuchi, M., Kikuchi, Y., & Senoo, A. (2008). The functional neuroanatomy of maternal love: mother's response to infant's attachment behaviors. *Biological Psychiatry*, 63, 415–423.

Nwokah, E. E., Hsu, H. C., Dobrowolska, O., & Fogel, A. (1994). The development of laughter in mother–infant communication: timing parameters and temporal sequences. *Infant Behavior and Development*, 17, 23–35.

O'hara, M. W. & Mccabe, J. E. (2013). Postpartum depression: current status and future directions. *Annual Review of Clinical Psychology*, 9, 379–407.

Ochsner, K. N., Silvers, J. A., & Buhle, J. T. (2012). Functional imaging studies of emotion regulation: a synthetic review and evolving model of the cognitive control of emotion. *Annals of the New York Academy of Sciences*, 1251, E1–E24.

Oller, D. K. & Eilers, R. E. (1988). The role of audition in infant babbling. *Child Development*, 59, 441–449.

Ostwald, P. F. & Murray, T. (1985). The communicative and diagnostic significance of infant sounds. In: B. M. Lester & C. F. Boukydis (eds) *Infant Crying: Theoretical and Research Perspectives*. New York: Plenum Press.

Out, D., Pieper, S., Bakermans-Kranenburg, M. J., & Van Ijzendoorn, M. H. (2010). Physiological reactivity to infant crying: a behavioral genetic study. *Genes, Brain and Behavior*, 9, 868–876.

Papoušek, M. (2007). Communication in early infancy: an arena of intersubjective learning. *Infant Behavior and Development*, 30, 258–266.

Parsons, C. E., Stark, E. A., Young, K. S., Stein, A., & Kringelbach, M. L. (2013). Understanding the human parental brain: a critical role of the orbitofrontal cortex. *Social Neuroscience*, 8, 525–543.

Parsons, C. E., Young, K. S., Jegindø, E.-M. E., Vuust, P., Stein, A., & Kringelbach, M. L. (2014). Music training and empathy positively impact adults' sensitivity to infant distress. *Frontiers in Psychology*, 5, 1440.

Parsons, C. E., Young, K. S., Joensson, M., Brattico, E., Hyam, J. A., Stein, A., ... Kringelbach, M. L. (2014). Ready for action: a role for the human midbrain in responding to infant vocalizations. *Social Cognitive and Affective Neuroscience*, 9, 977–984.

Parsons, C. E., Young, K. S., Mohseni, H., Woolrich, M. W., Thomsen, K. R., Joensson, M., ... Kringelbach, M. L. (2013). Minor structural abnormalities in the infant face disrupt neural processing: a unique window into early caregiving responses. *Social Neuroscience*, 8, 268–274.

Parsons, C. E., Young, K. S., Murray, L., Stein, A., & Kringelbach, M. L. (2010). The functional neuroanatomy of the evolving parent–infant relationship. *Progress in Neurobiology*, 91, 220–241.

Parsons, C. E., Young, K. S., Parsons, E., Dean, A., Murray, L., Goodacre, T., & Kringelbach, M. L. (2011). The effect of cleft lip on adults' responses to faces: cross-species findings. *PLoS One*, 6, e25897.

Porter, F. L., Miller, R. H., & Marshall, R. E. (1986). Neonatal pain cries: effect of circumcision on acoustic features and perceived urgency. *Child Development*, 57, 790–802.

Riem, M. M. E., Bakermans-Kranenburg, M. J., Pieper, S., Tops, M., Boksem, M. A., Vermeiren, R. R., Van Ijzendoorn, M. H., & Rombouts, S. A. (2011). Oxytocin modulates amygdala, insula, and inferior frontal gyrus responses to infant crying: a randomized controlled trial. *Biological Psychiatry*, 70, 291–297.

Riem, M. M. E., Bakermans-Kranenburg, M. J., Van Ijzendoorn, M. H., Out, D., & Rombouts, S. A. R. B. (2012). Attachment in the brain: adult attachment representations predict amygdala and behavioral responses to infant crying. *Attachment and Human Development*, 14, 533–551.

Rilling, J. K. & Young, L. J. (2014). The biology of mammalian parenting and its effect on off-spring social development. *Science, 345,* 771–776.

Rolls, E. T. (2000). Précis of the brain and emotion. *Behavioral and Brain Sciences, 23,* 177–191.

Rozga, A., Hutman, T., Young, G. S., Rogers, S. J., Ozonoff, S., Dapretto, M., & Sigman, M. (2011). Behavioral profiles of affected and unaffected siblings of children with autism: contribution of measures of mother–infant interaction and nonverbal communication. *Journal of Autism and Developmental Disorders, 41,* 287–301.

Ruddy, M. G. & Bornstein, M. H. (1982). Cognitive correlates of infant attention and maternal stimulation over the first year of life. *Child Development, 53,* 183–188.

Rudebeck, P. H., & Murray, E. A. (2014). The orbitofrontal oracle: cortical mechanisms for the prediction and evaluation of specific behavioral outcomes. *Neuron, 84,* 1143–1156.

Schilbach, L. (2010). A second-person approach to other minds. *Nature Reviews Neuroscience, 11,* 449–449.

Schirmer, A. & Kotz, S. A. (2006). Beyond the right hemisphere: brain mechanisms mediating vocal emotional processing. *Trends in Cognitive Sciences, 10,* 24–30.

Seifritz, E., Esposito, F., Neuhoff, J. G., Lüthi, A., Mustovic, H., Dammann, G., ... Tedeschi, G. (2003). Differential sex-independent amygdala response to infant crying and laughing in parents versus nonparents. *Biological Psychiatry, 54,* 1367–1375.

Sergent, C., Baillet, S., & Dehaene, S. (2005). Timing of the brain events underlying access to consciousness during the attentional blink. *Nature Reviews Neuroscience, 8,* 1391–1400.

Sheinkopf, S. J., Iverson, J. M., Rinaldi, M. L., & Lester, B. M. (2012). Atypical cry acoustics in 6-month-old infants at risk for autism spectrum disorder. *Autism Research, 5,* 331–339.

Soltis, J. (2004). The signal functions of early infant crying. *Behavioral and Brain Sciences, 27,* 443–458.

Stein, A., Arteche, A., Lehtonen, A., Craske, M., Harvey, A., Counsell, N., & Murray, L. (2010). Interpretation of infant facial expression in the context of maternal postnatal depression. *Infant Behavior and Development, 33,* 273–278.

Stein, A., Gath, D. H., Bucher, J., Bond, A., Day, A., & Cooper, P. J. (1991). The relationship between post-natal depression and mother–child interaction. *British Journal of Psychiatry, 158,* 46–52.

Stein, A., Malmberg, L. E., Leach, P., Barnes, J., Sylva, K., & Team, F. (2013). The influence of different forms of early childcare on children's emotional and behavioural development at school entry. *Child: Care, Health and Development, 39,* 676–687.

Sukikara, M. H., Mota-Ortiz, S. R., Baldo, M. V., Felicio, L. F., & Canteras, N. S. (2010). The periaqueductal gray and its potential role in maternal behavior inhibition in response to predatory threats. *Behavioural Brain Research, 209,* 226–233.

Swain, J. E., Tasgin, E., Mayes, L. C., Feldman, R., Todd Constable, R., & Leckman, J. F. (2008). Maternal brain response to own baby-cry is affected by Cesarean section delivery. *Journal of Child Psychology and Psychiatry, 49,* 1042–1052.

Trevarthen, C., Murray, L., & Hubley, P. (1981). Psychology of infants. In: J. A. Davis & J. Dobbing (eds) *Scientific Foundations of Clinical Paediatrics* (pp. 211–274). London: William Heinemann Medical Books Ltd.

Venuti, P., Caria, A., Esposito, G., De Pisapia, N., Bornstein, M. H., & De Falco, S. (2012). Differential brain responses to cries of infants with autistic disorder and typical development: an fMRI study. *Research in Developmental Disabilities, 33,* 2255–2264.

Wasz-Höckert, O., Michelsson, K., & Lind, J. (1985). Twenty-five years of Scandinavian cry research. In: B. M. Lester & C. F. Boukydis (eds) *Infant Crying: Theoretical and Research Perspectives.* New York: Plenum Press.

Wasz-Höckert, O., Partanen, T. J., Vuorenkoski, V., Michelsson, K., & Valanne, E. (1964). The identification of some specific meanings in infant vocalization. *Experientia, 20*, 154.

Wiesenfeld, A. R., Malatesta, C. Z., & Deloach, L. L. (1981). Differential parental response to familial and unfamiliar infant distress signals. *Infant Behavior and Development, 4*, 281–295.

Winnicott, D. (1956). *Primary Maternal Preoccupation.* London: Tavistock.

Young, K. S., Parsons, C. E., Elmholdt, E.-M. J., Woolrich, M. W., Van Hartevelt, T. J., Stevner, A. B., Stein, A., & Kringelbach, M. L. (2015). Evidence for a caregiving instinct: rapid differentiation of infant from adult vocalizations using magnetoencephalography. *Cerebral Cortex, 26*(3), 1309–1321.

Young, K. S., Parsons, C. E., Stein, A., & Kringelbach, M. L. (2012). Interpreting infant vocal distress: the ameliorative effect of musical training in depression. *Emotion, 12*, 1200.

Young, K. S., Parsons, C. E., Stein, A., & Kringelbach, M. L. (2015). Motion and emotion: depression reduces psychomotor performance and alters affective movements in caregiving interactions. *Frontiers in Behavioral Neuroscience, 9*, 26.

Yovel, G. & Belin, P. (2013). A unified coding strategy for processing faces and voices. *Trends in Cognitive Sciences, 17*, 263–271.

Zald, D. H. & Pardo, J. V. (2002). The neural correlates of aversive auditory stimulation. *NeuroImage, 16*, 746–753.

Zeskind, P. S. & Lester, B. M. (1978). Acoustic features and auditory perceptions of the cries of newborns with prenatal and perinatal complications. *Child Development*, 580–589.

Zeskind, P. S. & Marshall, T. R. (1988). The relation between variations in pitch and maternal perceptions of infant crying. *Child Development, 59*, 193–196.

Zhang, W. T., Mainero, C., Kumar, A., Wiggins, C. J., Benner, T., Purdon, P. L., ... Sorensen, A. G. (2006). Strategies for improving the detection of fMRI activation in trigeminal pathways with cardiac gating. *NeuroImage, 31*, 1506–1512.

PART III

EVOLUTION AND
COMPARATIVE
PERSPECTIVE

CHAPTER 13

COMPARATIVE PERSPECTIVES ON COMMUNICATION IN HUMAN AND NON-HUMAN PRIMATES

Grounding Meaning in Broadly Conserved Processes of Voice Production, Perception, Affect, and Cognition

ALAN K.S. NIELSEN AND DREW RENDALL

13.1 INTRODUCTION

COMPARATIVE perspectives on primate and human communication have varied historically and been marked by two equally untenable extremes, one being that language is special, the other that it is not. The former, conventional stance, assumes language is special, unique, and without significant evolutionary precedent. It has struggled, therefore, to explain the origins and evolution of a complex faculty from scratch (Chomsky, 1968; Pinker, 1994). The latter stance reflects more recent comparative research on systems of communication in non-human primates which, in general, has been extremely productive (Fitch, 2010). At times, however, research on systems of primate communication has been focused quite narrowly on high-level linguistic constructs, like *meaning, information,* and *syntax*, and in an effort to demonstrate continuity to language has often appropriated and applied these constructs to primates in relatively loose and metaphorical ways that can distort their linguistic significance (Owren et al., 2010; Rendall & Owren, 2010; Rendall et al., 2009). In the process, such approaches risk trivializing the distinctive properties of language and overstating continuity with primate communication, thereby leaving little to explain about the *evolution* of language.

Here, we try to strike a balance and identify fertile common ground between human and primate communication by focusing on what is indisputably shared, namely the basic units of sound that are the building blocks of vocal communication in each. We then consider how these basic building blocks combine with additional commonalities in fundamental processes of voice perception, affect, and cognition to yield functional outcomes for communication in each group. Critically, this approach points to some novel possibilities for how some of the more complex semantic dimensions of language, not shared with primates, might nevertheless be grounded in and bootstrapped from basic dimensions of voice production and perception that *are* shared. The hope is that this approach will also promote further productive integration in research on both groups and develop some common terms and modes of analysis to facilitate that.

We begin by focusing on language and with a discussion of the pressures for human languages to be both learnable and expressible (Kirby et al., 2006). We outline the outcomes of those pressures in producing languages that take advantage of perceptuo-cognitive processes of human language learning operating on fundamental elements of voice production and perception.

To outline the arguments in brief, we suggest that humans have a suite of perceptual biases that make certain associations between words and meanings more salient than they would be otherwise. For example, 'moo' is a good word for the sound that a cow makes because it is imitative of the sound of that event (i.e. onomatopoeic), and thus potentially more memorable for a naïve language learner. Beyond these simple types of imitative word-meaning mappings, natural languages also take advantage of associations between perception and emotion. Thus, for example, we use curse words like 'fuck' that contain higher proportions of fricative and plosive consonants and also prosodic cues that highlight their affective weight, allowing them to highjack the perceptual machinery of their perceiver to increase their salience. The ability of words like 'fuck' to induce affective or behavioural changes in the listener (or utterer) demonstrates a third pressure that shapes the structure of languages—functional deployability. This fundamental pressure has, heretofore, been largely overlooked because human language is typically characterized as a system for the transfer of propositional content (i.e. information) that is largely free of the influence of affective systems and low-level perceptual and motivational biases of the sort that impel many other sorts of behaviour. Here, we highlight this pressure as especially interesting because it is evidenced widely in animal communication systems and may represent an important, underappreciated link between the two.

In addition to the pressures for learnability and functional deployability in determining the structure of human languages based on an interaction with perceptuo-cognitive processes, constraints in domain-general processes like memory also have important impacts on language structure (Kirby et al., 2006). In terms of iterated learning, languages need to be compressible. That is, languages are easier to learn when they are structured in such a way that storing the rules and representations of the language takes up minimal space. Thus, regular tense marking aids language learning because it is generalizable and compressible.

At the same time, the pressure for expressivity is at odds with both learnability and compressibility: a perfectly compressed language would have only a single word, and thus would be perfectly learnable, but it would fail outright to be expressive. Thus, human languages need to balance these pressures, optimizing learnability, deployability, and expressivity relative to one another.

In Section 13.2, we outline the evidence from human languages that demonstrates the outcomes of these pressures, considering primarily the mechanistic basis for the perceptual and cognitive biases that shape language and their influence on how language is learned. Much of this evidence is relatively new, based on a resurgence of interest in what we call *motivated* associations between words and meanings, but also on configurations of the language that are *systematic* (Nielsen, 2016).

Subsequent to our discussion of human languages, in Section 13.3 we focus on an exploration of whether analogues of the same types of associations can be found in animal communication systems. In English, for example, we see that curse words like 'fuck' often take advantage of associations between acoustic harshness and emotional valence. This type of motivated association between signals and meanings can also be seen in animal communication systems, where harsh, spectrally chaotic calls are often given in aggressive contexts and softer more mellifluous ones in affiliative contexts.

In Section 13.4, we attempt to bridge the gap between discussions of human language and animal communication systems, suggesting that, if considered carefully, the exploration of one can inform us about the other. We suggest, first, that many discussions of human language and its evolutionary origins have ignored the pressure for functional deployability and thus one of the potentially most crucial evolutionary links between humans and other animals. To this end, we propose a biosemantic framework, where meaning at the level of the phoneme (rooted in its underlying acoustic structural features) might represent an important contribution to the evolution of the human-language faculty and communication systems more generally.

From this, we suggest that, to the degree that animal communication systems can be thought of as conveying propositional content, we should look for the fingerprints of functional deployability in establishing this type of reference. We have suggested elsewhere that animal communication systems become more functional by leveraging motivated signal-meaning mappings, but extend this suggestion here to propose that motivated signal-meaning mapping might also make animal signals more learnable. Finally, we suggest that animal-signalling systems might also bear the hallmarks of systematicity.

Ultimately, of course, while we will emphasize the foundational role of a set of systematic, non-arbitrary processes and relationships in the structure, function, and deployment of language and communication systems more generally, we also fully acknowledge that the structures of human languages are, in fact, largely arbitrary. Hence, our emphasis on the potential non-arbitrary elements of them recognizes that these will likely represent only a small component of the realized design of languages. Nevertheless, the relationships we emphasize critically allow for an examination of non-arbitrariness that can explain features of both animal and human communication systems and some productive possible links between them which have been a long-time, but heretofore largely unfulfilled, goal of comparative, evolutionarily orientated research.

13.2 HUMAN LANGUAGE

How do words get their meanings? This question dates back to at least Plato's 'Cratylus' dialogue, which is recognized as the first exploration of the issue. Linguistic tradition has been built around the idea that connections between words and meanings are arbitrary and established only by linguistic convention (de Saussure, 1983; Hockett, 1960; but cf. Joseph, 2015). There is, for example, nothing about the word 'dog' that makes it particularly good for describing a species of domesticated canine, nor any cosmic irony for why, in English, 'god' is just 'dog' backwards—it's arbitrary. The arbitrariness of relationships between words and meanings became one of the central dogmas of linguistics for the majority of the twentieth century, being codified by Hockett (1960) as a design feature of human language. Recently, however, the proposal that languages are entirely arbitrary and conventional (Newman, 1933; Newmeyer, 1993) has come under closer scrutiny. The relationship between words and the objects or events that they describe can be non-arbitrary in two ways, and researchers have increasingly recognized that human languages, far from being entirely arbitrary and conventional, contain many non-arbitrary words. Further, researchers have increasingly suggested that these associations are probably important (Nielsen & Rendall, 2012): they might make words more learnable (Nygaard et al., 2009), expressive (Yardy, 2010), or both (Nielsen, 2011).

The relationship between words and meanings can be non-arbitrary in terms of both their motivatedness and their systematicity (Dingemanse et al., 2015; Nielsen, 2016). Motivatedness refers to non-arbitrary associations between words and meanings where a feature of an individual word is mapped onto some feature of its meaning (Figure 13.1). This type of association is mediated by the perceptual and cognitive organization of the language users such that a dimension of meaning can be mapped onto a dimension of the signal. In some cases, this type of association is imitative or iconic—'oink', for example, is imitative of its meaning (the sound that a pig makes). In other cases, the association can be based on an affective or perceptual feature of meaning. As previously discussed, a swear word like 'fuck' (or, for example, 'tabarnac' in French) has acoustic features that make it particularly evocative for its purpose.

Second, associations between words and meanings can be non-arbitrary by virtue of being systematic (Monaghan et al., 2011). Systematic relationships between words and meanings refer to a configuration where a shared feature of a set of words is mapped onto a shared

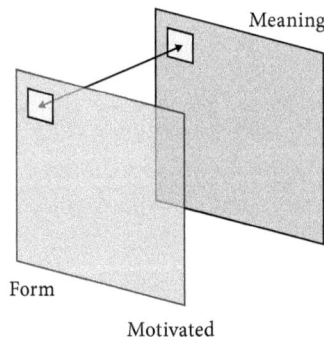

FIGURE 13.1 A diagrammatic representation of a motivated relationship between a word's form and its meaning.

Data from Gasser M., 'The Origins of Arbitrariness in Language', *Proceedings of the Annual Meeting of the Cognitive Science Society*, Volume 26, Issue 26, pp. 434–9, 2004, https://escholarship.org/uc/item/34g8355v

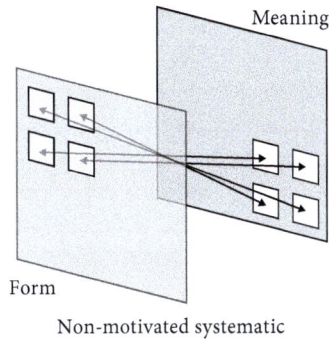

Non-motivated systematic

FIGURE 13.2 A diagrammatic representation of a systematic association between word forms and meanings. Here, word forms that are similar to each other are mapped onto meanings that are similar to one another, but the specific mapping between the form space and the meaning space is arbitrary.

feature of a set of meanings (Figure 13.2). For example, the 'gl-' phonaestheme cluster contains a number of words that share the same initial segment ('glimmer', 'glitter', 'glisten', 'glint', etc.) that all have meanings related to vision or light. In the case of the 'gl-' cluster, there is nothing that motivates the specific form that the systematic association takes, and the use of 'gl-' as a marker for words connoting light is likely a feature of the contingent history of the English language (Cuskley, 2013). However, it bears noting that associations between words and meanings can be both motivated and systematic: the 'sn-' phonaestheme cluster, for example, contains a number of words ('snot', 'sniffle', 'snout', etc.) that have to do with the nose. The fact that this cluster of words contains a heavily nasal consonant segment ('sn-') suggests that, in this case, the specific form of the systematic association is likely also motivated (Figure 13.3), and thus it is not surprising that this association has been observed across a number of other languages (Blasi et al., 2014).

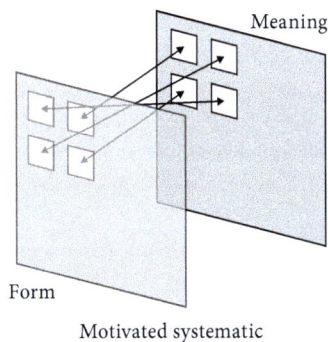

Motivated systematic

FIGURE 13.3 A diagrammatic representation of the association between word forms and meanings that is both motivated and systematic. In this case, the motivated connection between the form of a set of words and the form of its related set of meanings is based not on individual motivated associations but a motivated mapping of the set of word forms to the set of meanings.

13.2.1 Motivatedness

The acknowledgement that cognitive and perceptual biases have downstream effects on human language has proven to be a rich source of explanatory power. Human-language learners share the same basic perceptual and cognitive structures, and thus human languages, despite being different, share some features that reflect the strengths and constraints of human perception and cognition. Languages have a pressure to be learnable (Hockett, 1960; Kirby et al., 2006), and by taking advantage of motivated associations, languages can become easier for their users to learn, which may account for the ability of humans to learn language easily despite a purportedly impoverished stimulus (Chomsky, 1965).

The motivatedness of associations between words and meanings can vary based on both their modality and transparency. In terms of modality, associations can be unimodal and iconic, or crossmodal and mediated by associations between sensory or affective characteristics that seem otherwise unrelated to one another. The types of associations that are leveraged by languages also vary as a function of their transparency. Some are straightforward and iconic, while others are embedded in language systems such that the motivatedness of the association is contingent on knowledge about the rest of the language.

13.2.1.1 *Modality*

Unimodal associations between words and meanings are the most straightforwardly understood and thus perhaps the least surprising type of motivated association in language. Onomatopoeia is the most easily recognized example of a unimodal association between words and meanings. In onomatopoeia, the sound of a word is imitative of the sound of the event that it describes, so 'crash' for example is imitative of the sound of a collision, while 'buzz' is imitative of the sound that a bee makes. Unimodal associations are not however limited to imitating the sound of events. In some cases, such as in Japanese mimetics (Kanera et al., 2014), reduplication can be leveraged to convey the temporal patterning of events. Thus, 'goron' is the word for a large object rolling, while 'gorogoro' is the word for a large object rolling repeatedly (Asano et al., 2015). In this case, the repetition of syllables is imitative of the repeated nature of the event that it describes. Similarly, prosodic cues can leverage unimodal associations, even in words that are already onomatopoeic (Dingemanse et al., 2016). When saying the word 'tweet', for example, one might up-modulate their pitch to make the imitative nature of the token more salient. This type of prosodic enhancement is common in both normative speech patterns and in exaggerated forms, such as motherese (Grieser & Kuhl, 1988).

Although unimodal associations are generally straightforward, they are inherently limited in the types of associations that they can leverage. Onomatopoeia has been observed in the majority of languages that have been analysed for its presence (Cuskley, 2013), but reduplicative mimetics are only found in a smaller (but still substantial) portion of the world's languages (Asano et al., 2015), and there is little, if any, data examining the use of prosodic cues for establishing unimodal associations (Perniss & Vigliocco, 2014). Even if all of these types of unimodal associations were leveraged heavily by all languages, they would still however be limited in their ability to convey meanings beyond a constrained set of possibilities. Many features of meaning do not have unimodal analogues in either the sounds used in languages or the way they are combined to form identifiable words.

Perceptual biases that lead to associations across modalities open up the possibility of expressing a broader range of meanings. A number of studies, for example, have shown that humans demonstrate a persistent bias to associate small objects with higher vocal frequencies, and this is manifest not only linguistically (e.g. Sapir, 1929), but also in expectations about the relationship between speaker body size and voice pitch and resonances or formants (Pisanski & Rendall, 2011). Linguistically, this association can be observed in the frequency with which words connoting small objects contain high front vowels (with a relatively high second formant frequency), while words connoting large objects contain low back vowels (with a relatively low second formant frequency), and this association has been observed cross-linguistically (e.g. English (Johnson, 1967), but also Chinese, Thai (Huang, 1969), Korean (Kim, 1977), and several other languages (Gebels, 1969; Malmberg, 1964; cf Newman, 1933; Newmeyer, 1993))).

In the last decade, the empirical investigation of these types of crossmodal biases has experienced a veritable explosion, centred around the classic *bouba-kiki* or *takete-maluma* effect (Kohler, 1947; Pexman & Sidhu, 2014; Ramachandran & Hubbard, 2001), where novel, visually jagged object forms are reliably associated with novel, nonsense words containing strident consonants (e.g. /k/, /p/, and /t/), while curvier object forms are associated with nonsense words containing more mellifluous, sonorant consonants (e.g. /m/, /n/, /l/). The bouba-kiki effect has been demonstrated in both children (e.g. Ozturk et al., 2013) and adults, as well as with speakers of multiple languages (Davis, 1961; Bremner et al., 2013). (See Figure 13.4 for samples of original object forms used by Kohler in 1947, and Appendix 13.1 for audio samples of speech tokens used in more recent experiments.)

The number of reliable crossmodal relationships using nonsense words that have been observed in the psychological literature is staggering, although the degree to which the relationships involved are manifest in the structure of real words is only now emerging as a field of study (Nielsen, 2016). Certainly, the capacity for crossmodal biases functionally related to a broad range of perceptual features has been described (see Figure 13.5) both among people in the so-called 'normal' population and also among synaesthetes who have exaggerated crossmodal perceptual biases that have been proposed to be simply an exaggeration of biases in the normal population (Bankieris & Simner, 2015).

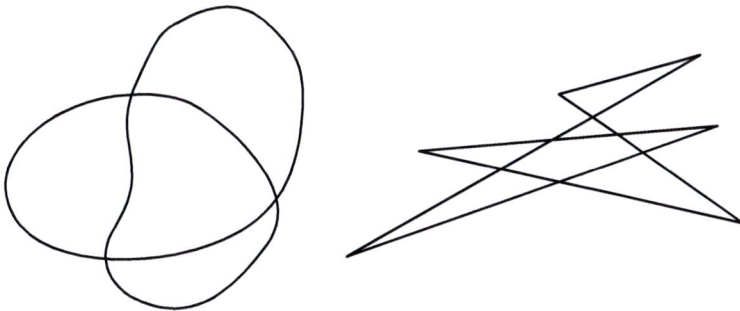

FIGURE 13.4 The original 'maluma' (left) and 'takete' (right) shapes.

Reproduced from Köhler, W. *Gestalt Psychology*, *2e* Copyright © 1947 W. W. Norton & Company, Inc.

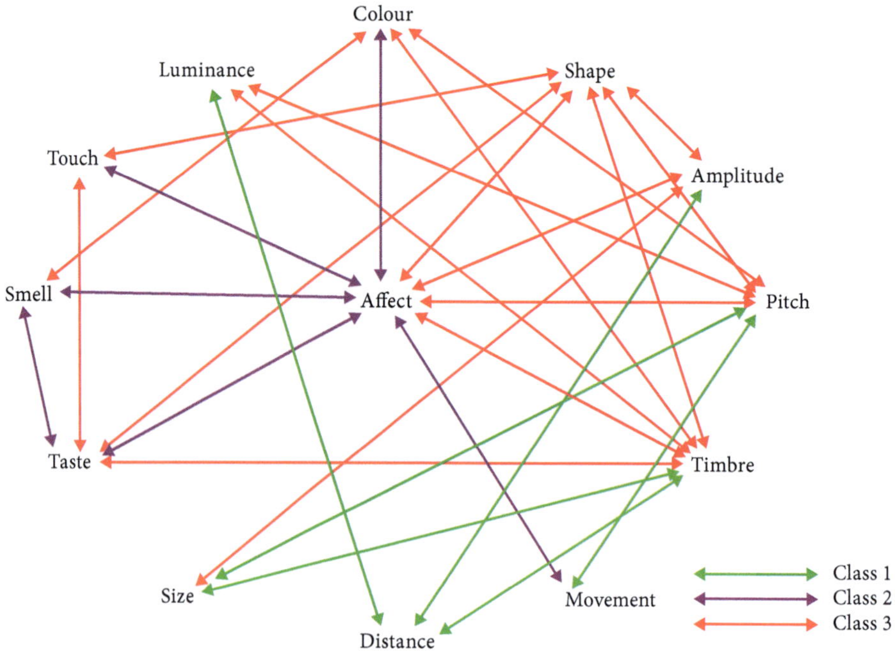

FIGURE 13.5 Web diagram of crossmodal connections, labelled according to their pervasiveness. Class 1 connections are those which seem mandatory given the laws of physics (such as light fading over distance). Class 2 connections are those which do not seem mandatory, but which otherwise seem aberrant (e.g. the association between taste and smell). Class 3 connections are those which are typically labelled as aberrant and attributed to synaesthesia (e.g. between shape and pitch), but have also been observed in non-synaesthetes to some extent.

13.2.1.2 *Transparency*

Both unimodal and crossmodal associations can vary in terms of their transparency, that is, how obvious they would be to a naïve language user. The word 'moo' is more similar to the sound that a cow makes than the word 'cock-a-doodle-doo' is to the sound of a rooster, and thus might be more easily recognized. One of the limitations of motivated associations for expressing certain meanings is thus that some words are more amenable to transmission over certain types of channels. Because English is a spoken language and the call of a rooster is relatively complex, even our onomatopoeic imitation of that sound is constrained. First, human language is unable to perfectly mimic the sounds of some acoustic events because words are composed of strings of speech sounds (i.e. vowels and consonants) that are themselves constrained by the human vocal apparatus. Second, even if phonemes could perfectly mimic environmental sounds, all languages have a constrained set of available phonemes (Assaneo et al., 2011), so some languages would be more apt than others at imitating environmental sounds. Because of the interaction of these features, the onomatopoeic words for a rooster crowing are quite different across languages—German uses 'kikiriki', where French uses 'cocorico'. As an English speaker, I might suggest that 'cock-a-doodle-doo' is more straightforwardly iconic than the other two, but nevertheless all three are quite different from the actual sound made by a rooster (Perniss et al., 2010).

The constrained ability of languages to transparently represent certain types of meanings can also be seen in sign languages, where the communication channel is gestural rather than acoustic. The use of sign affords the possibility of representing a different suite of meanings iconically (Taub, 2001). Thus, sign languages often iconically represent movement and spatial features in ways that spoken languages simply cannot (Thompson et al., 2012). This is especially true early in the development of those signed languages, before signals became smaller, more discrete, and conventionalized (Berent & Goldin-Meadow, 2015). Conversely, because signed languages are non-verbal, they cannot include the acoustic onomatopoeia pervasive in many spoken languages.

Crossmodal associations can also vary in their transparency or saliency. Size-sound symbolism has been observed in a number of the world's languages (though experimental evidence is not very strong; cf. Cuskley, 2013), whereas reduplication is not as common, and arguably exhibits secondary iconicity (Ahlner & Zlatev, 2010), where the reduplication of syllables serving to highlight the repetition of an action is only apparent after exposure to an example.

In addition to varying in transparency based on the ability of the language channel to express a given meaning, associations can be motivated only based on their relationship to other words in a language. Dingemanse (2011) outlines one such example in Siwu, where a group of words that varies in terms of their vowel quality ('pɔmbɔlɔɔ', 'pumbuluu', and 'pimbilii') maps to meanings about the protrusion of the belly, with /ɔ/ being mapped to the largest protrusion and /i/ to the smallest. Considered alone, the motivatedness of these associations might not be salient enough to be recognized by a naïve language user, but considered together, the crossmodal association between vowel roundedness and roundness (protrusion of the belly) becomes more obvious.

13.2.1.3 *Mechanism*

There is converging evidence that the types of motivated biases described in previous paragraphs are underpinned by gross structural and anatomical features of the brain. First, in the normal population, the perceptual biases underlying associations like the bouba-kiki effect have been demonstrated to be underpinned by differential neural activation (Kanera et al., 2014; Lockwood & Dingemanse, 2015). Second, the study of synaesthesia, a condition that results in exaggerated connections between unrelated sensory modalities (Ramachandran & Hubbard, 2001), has demonstrated an increased density of connections between the cortical areas responsible for processing crossmodally associated percepts (Rouw & Scholte, 2007), and that synaesthesia appears to be a heritable condition (Asher et al., 2009). Although some have suggested that synaesthesia relies on cortical wiring that is not present in the normal population (e.g. Brang et al., 2010), others have provided evidence that at least some forms of synaesthesia make use of crossmodal connections that are common in the normal population (e.g. Revill et al., 2014; Ward et al., 2006). Further support for the proposal that synaesthetes and the normal population share the same mechanistic underpinnings is provided by the finding that many, but not all, crossmodal associations observed in synaesthetes have also been demonstrated in the normal population, with synaesthetes showing exaggerated versions of those associations (Bankieris & Simner, 2015).

Taken together, the study of sound-symbolism and crossmodality in the normal population, and the study of synaesthesia, thus illuminate a plausible mechanistic account that appears to be a common organizational feature of the nervous system (Rouw & Scholte, 2007). This further suggests a potentially important role for motivated word-meaning associations in language acquisition, transmission, and use. Determining the specific nature of these associations, and whether they reflect a fundamental feature of neural organization (direct connectivity) or are mediated by a central structural circuit is thus critical for an explanation of their importance or evolutionary trajectory.

As we saw in Figure 13.5, associations between affect and certain perceptual features are amongst the most common of those reported in the literature, which might suggest that some crossmodal perceptual biases are mediated by affect (Nielsen, 2011). For example, there are well-established associations between colour and affect (Valdez & Mehrabian, 1994), and also between pitch and affect (Krumhansl, 2002), which raises the possibility that any one of those three dimensions mediates the connection between the remaining two. For example, if high pitch is associated with bright colours, bright colours with positive affect, and high pitch with positive affect, it is possible that the presence of one of those associations can be explained by one of the others. In this case, we might suggest that high pitch is associated with positive affect, and bright colours are associated with positive affect, and that this creates a third association between high pitch and bright colours.

The possible centrality of affect to motivated associations between words and meanings is further supported by the recognition that language, in addition to being about the transfer of information between conspecifics, is often about influencing the behaviour of others by modulating their affect. Poets and musicians have recognized the importance of sounds and rhythm in inducing affect in their audiences seemingly far longer than the idea has been considered scientifically (Paquette et al., 2013; Trost et al., 2015). The central proposal of affective semantics (Rendall & Owren, 2010) recognizes this type of language use as important in its own right, but also important to the evolutionary history of language, as the modulation of affect has clear homologues in animal communication systems and does not require advanced cognition or the transfer of any propositional content (Rendall et al., 2009).

Swearing serves as a paradigm example of emotionally valenced language illustrating the principle of affective semantics. Lancker and Cummings (1999; also Yardy, 2010), for example, have shown that swear words contain an unusually high number of fricative and plosive consonants. Whether one considers swear words an honest reflection of the underlying emotional or motivational state of utterers (such as when signalling pain), or as being exceptionally effective at grabbing and modulating listener attention and affect (when directed at others), they are undoubtedly effective. By using consonants that are relatively harsh and broadband in their acoustical structure, and also by introducing prosodic cues that accentuate that harshness or amplitude, the use of swear words can hijack the perceptual apparatus of perceivers to produce a desired response.

Gross acoustical characteristics are of course far from the only way in which human language can be modulated. Temporal patterning, pitch, and other aspects of speech prosody are all important for both conveying meaning or emotion and influencing emotions in others. For example, rising or falling pitch can be used to demarcate certain phrase types (e.g. questions from statements; Hirst & Di Cristo, 1998) and also to signal the relative confidence of the speaker (with confident speakers using low or falling pitch and unconfident ones using high or rising pitch; Bolinger, 1980), as well as to modulate the attention and affect of the listener as classically illustrated in the phenomenon of infant-directed speech or 'motherese' (Fernald & Morikawa, 1993).

13.2.2 Systematicity

Where motivatedness refers to associations that operate directly between words and their meanings, the second non-arbitrary dimension along which language can be structured (i.e. systematicity) operates by mapping features of sets of words to features of sets of meanings. Language is uncontroversially systematic at the level of morphosyntax, and it has been suggested that this type of systematicity has important implications for learning (Chater & Vityani, 2003; Tamariz & Kirby, 2015). The use of regular suffixes to mark tense, for example, makes a language more compressible and thus easier to learn than if every morpheme was entirely idiosyncratic.

At the level of the lexicon, however, there has been little work exploring the degree to which languages are systematic. Small systematic pockets of language, like the 'gl-' phonaestheme cluster, exist in a number of languages but are typically treated as marginal. However, Monaghan et al. (2014) conducted a broad corpus analysis of a number of languages and found that the lexica of those languages was more systematic than would be expected by chance. That is, words that were similar to one another based on their phonology were more likely to have meanings that were also similar to one another. The level of systematicity of the analysed languages was overall rather modest and statistical in nature, which might explain why the previous assumption had been that such systematic associations were rare or unimportant. However, even previously recognized systematic mappings, like phonaestheme clusters, are not absolute in their mapping. Although words like 'glimmer', 'glitter', and 'glisten' share both the same initial segment and have similar meanings, many words exist that use that same initial segment but have meanings unrelated to light or vision (e.g. 'glaive', 'glove', 'glum'): systematicity in natural languages operates at a statistical level, rather than an absolute one (Reilly et al., 2012).

Crucially, associations between words and meanings can be both systematic and motivated at the same time. Consider, for example, the 'sn-' phonaestheme cluster ('sneeze', 'snore', 'sniff', etc.) mentioned previously. In this phonaestheme cluster, the use of a word initial segment that is heavily nasalized is unlikely to be explained by historical accident, and thus a word like 'sniffle' has the property of being both systematic and motivated at the same time. In fact, we have suggested elsewhere (Nielsen, 2016) that the leveraging of motivated associations between word forms and meanings can lead towards the establishment of systematic associations between sets of words and sets of meanings, producing what we have called 'incidental systematicity'.

Consider again the structure and meaning of swear words, which, to rehearse, include an abnormal proportion of fricative and plosive consonants (in addition to being marked prosodically). In a language with only a single curse word, say 'shit', for example, the association between 'shit' and its meaning would be motivated, but not systematic. However, in English and most other languages, there is a large repertoire of curse words, and insofar as each of those words leverages the spectral harshness and affective salience of the same set of phonemes, the structure of the set of curse words and the structure of the set of their

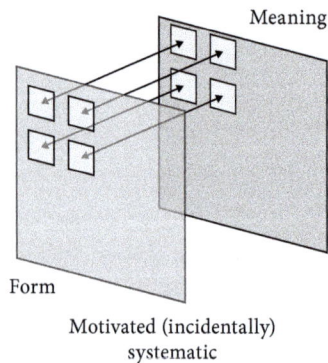

FIGURE 13.6 A diagrammatic representation of the formation of an incidentally systematic mapping between words and meanings. In this case, individual word forms are mapped to meanings based on a motivated association between the two. Because multiple similar word forms are mapped to multiple similar meanings, the resulting configuration of the language can be recognized as being systematic.

meanings could become aligned and gain the property of being systematic, in addition to being motivated (Figure 13.6).

In the remainder of this chapter, we will focus on non-arbitrariness at the level of the lexicon, because it has the clearest analogues in animal communication systems: that is, it is difficult to look for non-arbitrary morphosyntax in animal communication systems that are not generally considered to have either morphology or syntax to begin with (cf. Engesser et al., 2015; Suzuki et al., 2016).

13.2.3 Learnability and Expressivity

The cross-generational transmission of languages is recognized to be subject to a selection process analogous to natural selection, with words or structures that are easier for learners to acquire or retain being passed on more faithfully than other, less suitable variants (Kirby et al., 2015). Crucially, this process does not require intelligent design or deliberate selection by language learners since the constraints on memory, production, saliency, and fidelity of transmission that are imposed by language learners mean that some language variants will win out over others and be retained, while others will be outcompeted and thus eliminated. Because the process of language transmission is operating at all times and across many learners simultaneously, languages can adapt to the constraints of their learners much faster than biological evolution can produce adaptations that shape the cognition and perception of learners to the structure of languages (Thompson et al., 2016).

In addition to being learnable, languages also need to be expressive. A language with only a single word denoting a single meaning would be perfectly learnable, but would not be sufficiently expressive to facilitate communication. As we have discussed, exclusive reliance on motivated associations between words and meanings would lead to a language that could only express a relatively small set of meanings. Words like 'lullaby' and 'shit' can be straightforwardly mapped onto the underlying affective dimensions of their meanings, but motivated signal forms for many other words are hard to fathom and quite unlikely.

Nevertheless, the pressure for languages to be learnable should favour both motivatedness and systematicity (Dingemanse et al., 2014). Motivated associations between words and meanings are easier for language learners to acquire because the association between a word and its meaning is, in some sense, natural. In support of this suggestion, researchers have explored the learnability of motivated words, both experimentally and by analysing the corpora of natural languages. Experimentally, researchers have demonstrated, using both artificial (Aveyard, 2012; Monaghan et al., 2012; Nielsen & Rendall, 2012) and natural languages (Nygaard et al., 2009; Yoshida, 2012), that sound-symbolic, or otherwise motivated, associations between words and meanings facilitate learning not only in children (Kantarzis et al., 2011) but also in adults (Asano et al., 2015). For example, Imai et al. (2008) showed that English-speaking children can learn the meaning of putatively sound-symbolic ideophones in Japanese more easily than non-sound-symbolic synonyms in English. This finding aligns with data from corpus analyses, where researchers have discovered that the degree of motivatedness of word-meaning associations can be predicted by their age of acquisition (Monaghan et al., 2014): children learn sound-symbolic and other motivated words early before progressing to learn the remainder of the lexicon that is predominantly arbitrary.

Systematicity at the level of the lexicon has been less thoroughly explored than has motivatedness, but preliminary results broadly suggest that systematic mappings between sets of words and sets of meanings facilitate learning, at least in some contexts (Monaghan et al., 2011; Nielsen, 2016). Primarily, researchers have suggested that systematicity facilitates the processes of categorization and generalization. Imagine, for example, a language where all words for food ended with the segment '-um'. In this language chicken might be called 'chum', pork called 'pum', bread called 'brum', etc. Because the association between '-um' and edibility is not, necessarily, a motivated one, each of these word-meaning pairs might have to be learned individually, but given sufficient exposure to the language, a learner would find their ability to divine the meaning of unfamiliar labels enhanced by the systematic structure of the language. If, for example, they were told to grab the 'bacum' from the table, they would immediately know that they were being asked to procure some type of edible substance, even if they were not sure which particular substance was being referenced. By learning the rule of their language by which the segment '-um' was mapped systematically to edible objects, a user of this language would gain the ability to generalize to novel tokens, much in the way that learners rely on generalization to guess the correct tense marker for unfamiliar verbs in English (e.g. Rumelhart & McClelland, 1986). In addition to aiding generalization, systematicity can also aid categorization. When presented with a novel type of berry along with its name, the learner of this artificial language could immediately determine its suitability for consumption based on the presence or absence of the '-um' segment—'strums' are edible, whereas 'belladonums' are not.

The structure of human languages is fundamentally determined by the interaction of the pressures for learnability and expressivity with the perceptual, cognitive, and production machinery of its users, which serve to create a selective bottleneck through which language is filtered and undergoes change (Kirby et al., 2015). However, despite the implication that both motivatedness and systematicity enhance learnability at the level of the lexicon, languages are curiously largely arbitrary. Why is this the case? First, as we have discussed earlier in the chapter, motivated associations between words and meanings can only convey a limited number and type of meanings, suggesting that the contribution of motivatedness to the structure of a complete language should be fairly minimal overall (Lockwood & Dingemanse, 2015; Nielsen, 2016). Second, the same features of systematicity that enhance categorization and generalization can negatively influence the learnability of individual words, especially as the number of words to be learned increases (Gasser, 2004; Monaghan et al., 2011). In the example we gave earlier, consider the suggestion that an ideal 'sandum' is made with two slices of 'brum', a smear of 'mustum', a few slices of 'hum', two slices of creamy 'havartum', and a healthy dollop of 'mayonum'. Even with the added contextual information, this set of directions for constructing a sandwich might be confusing, especially when you take into account the imperfect fidelity of both production and reception. Did your partner ask you to pick up 'milum' at the store, or was it 'malum'? Systematic associations, when applied absolutely, constrain the overall flexibility and, thus, the memorability of their language (Gasser, 2004; Nielsen, 2016).

The potential negative influence of systematicity is compounded by the fact that there are so many systematic dimensions along which a language can be divided, and many of those dimensions overlap (e.g. kale is green, it is a vegetable, it is edible (arguably), etc.). The inability of languages to express a sufficient number of meanings while remaining entirely systematic is best exemplified by Wilkins' (1668) attempt to create a 'perfect' language that was entirely systematic. First, Wilkins' perfect language resulted in classifications that were unnatural. The English word 'salmon', for example, was translated as 'zana' and meant 'a scaled river fish with ruddy meat'. Because Wilkins' language was so constrained, it was also easy to confuse similar words. Thus, even Wilkins, who created the language, confused 'gade' (barley) with the similar meaning 'gape' (tulip). These two outcomes explain the dominance of arbitrary word-meaning mappings in the lexicon, while leaving open the possibility that, at lower levels of saturation, systematic associations can be leveraged without introducing any concomitant learning penalty based on confusability or unnaturalness (Gasser, 2004).

The importance of the pressures for learnability and expressivity, and their influence on the structure of language, are well established and accepted, but both pressures are based on the notion that the purpose of language is for the transmission of information between conspecifics. However, as we have suggested here, and elsewhere (Nielsen, 2011; Owren et al., 2010), human language involves more than the exchange of information. Specifically, much of language and communication is about influencing the behaviour of others. In a Machiavellian sense, the behaviour of others can be influenced by sharing or withholding information, but thanks to perceptual biases it is also possible to induce desired affective responses in others separately from the propositional content of a given utterance. Using an affectively valenced word like 'fuck' is effective for grabbing attention not only because of its agreed-upon and conventional naughtiness, but also because of its acoustic characteristics (the former stemming in part from the latter). Thus, in addition to pressures for learnability and expressivity to shape the structure of language, here we suggest that an additional pressure for functional deployability based on affect induction, rather than information transmission, can have important effects on the structure of language.

When it comes to fully-fledged human languages, we suggest that the strength of this pressure will be rather modest, but the relative weakness of the pressure does not preclude it from having an important influence. Specifically, we suggest that because the types of perceptual biases underpinning motivated associations between sensory and perceptual modalities are broadly conserved across a number of species (see Section 13.3; Morton, 1977,

1994), the continuity of those associations might inform our understanding of the evolution of the human-language faculty.

13.3 ANIMAL COMMUNICATION

We suggested earlier that the informational model does not capture the entirety of human communication and thus fails to recognize that the structure of language can be shaped by pressures that do not influence the transmission of propositional content. This applies doubly for animal communication, which displays little evidence of morphology or meaningful syntax (Suzuki et al., 2016; cf. Ouattara et al., 2009). Animals do use discrete signals that some have considered analogous to the (monomorphemic) words of human languages (Seyfarth et al., 1980; Zuberbühler, 2000), but these signals are almost exclusively indexical (Queiroz & Ribeiro, 2002) and the degree to which their production is intentional is highly controversial (Penn & Povinelli, 2007; Tomasello, 2008).

In the following section, we propose that the structure of animal signals is determined by the same pressure for languages to be functionally deployable, namely by being filtered through the perceptuo-cognitive apparatus of the animal.

13.3.1 Motivatedness

Just as associations between words and meanings in human languages can be motivated by links between perception, production, and cognition, so too can animal signals be similarly motivated. Although some early studies in primate communication focused on the possibility that primate vocalizations might be arbitrarily structured, in the main, research on primates (and other animals) has adopted the stance that the particular form that a signal takes is likely to be closely tied to the function it serves. In this, work on animal signalling obeys a broader axiom of evolutionary biology which is that form and function are intimately connected for most (possibly all) organismal traits. To wit, Morton (1977) was among the first to lay out some common principles of the form–function fit for animal signals, with what he termed 'motivation–structural' (MS) rules. MS rules captured some very common associations between the form of broad classes of vocal signal and the context in which they are typically produced, and, in particular, the motivational state underlying signal production. For example, he observed that harsh, spectrally broadband calls tend to be given in agonistic contexts, while more mellifluous calls are used in prosocial affiliative contexts (Morton, 1977, 1994). Sometime later, Owren & Rendall (1997, 2001) elaborated this framework noting that while such structural features may reliably reflect the underlying affect or emotion of signallers, they likewise can have potential effects on the affect and responses of listeners. Indeed, they argued that the latter effects on listeners might ultimately represent the more salient pressure, motivating many of the signal structure patterns first noted by Morton.

For example, across many species, alarm calls produced by animals in the context of encountering dangerous predators are often structured quite similarly and are typically short, high-amplitude calls with very abrupt onsets and harsh spectral structures (see Appendix 13.1 for sample audio files). Not coincidentally, these call features are also exactly those that best elicit a well-documented auditory reflex, termed the 'acoustic startle reflex' (Eaton, 1984). This involuntary response involves immediate attentional shifts and the interruption of ongoing activity, and it induces a host of other basic nervous-system responses, including stimulating reticular formation nuclei in the brainstem that help to regulate overall brain activation—all preparing the listening organism for immediate, dramatic action, highly functional in the context of encountering predators and other dangers. The phenomenon is thought to occur in every hearing species (Eaton, 1984) and clearly demonstrates the way in which sounds can have direct access to low-level nervous-system mechanisms that guide functional behaviours in listening animals. In fact, so direct are the effects that they can be quite difficult, or even impossible, to resist or habituate to. Starlings, for example, are unable to habituate to the sound of their species-typical distress call, which will always elicit a startle reaction regardless of the number of previous presentations (Johnson et al., 1985).

Other examples of sounds with direct effects on listener behaviour are common. For example, both humans and animals are sensitive to signals that incorporate repeated pulses and dramatic frequency sweeps. Frequency up-sweeps are especially effective for capturing receiver attention and increasing arousal or motor activity, and this has been observed both in animals and in humans, through both music (Schneider, 1963) and in infant-directed speech (Fernald & Morikawa, 1993; Kaplan & Owren, 1994; Papousek et al., 1991). Both animal and human infants are also known to take advantage of these motivated signal-meaning associations, producing affiliative cooing and babbling or aversive shrieking and wailing to modulate the behaviour of their caregivers to their own ends (Rendall et al., 2009).

Beyond modulating the behaviour of conspecifics, the ability to functionally leverage motivated signal-meaning associations can be observed where calls are directed from one species to another. For instance, handlers and herders of various domesticated animals have long capitalized on the impact of sounds like whistles, tongue clicks, and lip smacks to manage their charges (McConnell, 1991). Similarly, many prey species, when captured by a predator, produce 'death screams' which are often described as sudden, powerful, and piercing and have been suggested as an attempt to startle the predator and allow the caller a chance to escape (Driver & Humphries, 1969) (cf. Arnal et al., 2015; Belin & Zatorre, 2015 for analysis of the special status of screams for human communication).

In general then, the signals of primates and other animals are fundamentally motivated and the associations between signals and 'meanings' or, more appropriately, 'outcomes', are typically indexical and appear to be mediated often by an association between general arousal or affect, and, for example, gross acoustic features like the spectral density of a signal. This might suggest that animals are able to learn connections between signals and meanings only when those connections are motivated, but we know that this is not the case entirely. For example, the extended history of attempts to teach artificial languages to some species of great ape clearly show that they are capable, when tutored, of learning unmotivated (arbitrary) signal–object associations (Segerdahl et al., 2005). Instead, we suggest that just as in human languages, the presence of motivated signal-meaning mappings over arbitrary ones might be accounted for by the pressure for those signal-meaning pairs to be learnable and functionally deployable. In the following section, we discuss the constraints of animal signalling systems that either further bias them towards motivatedness or limit their expressivity.

13.3.1.1 *Modality*

Animals, much like humans, seem to share associations between sensory modalities that are not limited to those connecting acoustic and affective dimensions, although to date there is no evidence that those crossmodal biases (Hanganu-Opatz et al., 2015) are functionally leveraged in their communication systems. For example, chimpanzees have been shown to share the human bias of associating high-pitched sounds with perceptually bright objects (Ludwig et al., 2011), but do not have calls that denote the presence of bright objects in their environment.

Similarly, animal signals do not make use of unimodal associations in the same way that human languages do. Even in animal species that are vocal mimics, mimicked signals are either used blindly, as when they are incorporated into mating displays (Higgins et al., 1990), or used truly imitatively to attract prey (Calleia et al., 2009) or produce a response from conspecifics or another species that is in some way beneficial to the mimic (Flower, 2014). In no case that we know of are mimicked calls used to refer to the presence of the animal, or event, being imitated.

13.3.1.2 *Transparency*

Whether animal signals can be meaningfully described as either transparent or opaque is difficult to determine, because transparency is so closely tied to the idea of meaning. If, even without any prior learning, an animal responds 'correctly' to an alarm call by becoming startled and surveying their surroundings, for example, should we suggest that the 'meaning' of the alarm call is transparent to them? If their startle response is mediated by an unavoidable association between sound and arousal, and that association leads to appropriate behaviour, by what method can we establish that the animal understands anything about the meaning of the call?

In cases of so-called functionally referential vocalizations, such as the classic example of alarm calls given by vervet monkeys (Seyfarth et al., 1980), evaluating transparency is no easier. The alarm calls the vervets produce for different classes of predator certainly share many broad characteristics that are appropriate for eliciting a startle response (Owren & Rendall, 2001), but the fact that each call elicits a somewhat different response from listeners suggests that either: a) there is something about the call for one type of predator, say 'leopard', that makes it more appropriate for leopards than for other types of predators such as snakes or hawks; or b) the general structure of each alarm call is motivated by the same sound-affect bias, and specific responses are not transparent but are established (learned) by experience (i.e. following or emulating the responses of others). The fact that different populations of Campbell's monkeys are reported to make use of local 'dialects' (Schlenker et al., 2014) suggests that the second possibility is more likely.

13.3.1.3 *Production Constraints*

One potential explanation for the lack of signals that leverage non-affective perceptual biases to more effectively convey meaning in animals is that the anatomy and operation of the vocal apparatus may be more constrained in the range of sounds produced compared to humans (Fitch, 2000). However, even prodigious vocal mimics among birds, who are capable of producing a far broader range of sounds than humans, do not take advantage of these perceptual biases, which may point to a general cognitive deficit in the ability to map signals to specific meanings, even when they have the benefit of being motivated.

13.3.1.4 *Mechanism-Affective Semantics*

Natural forms of crossmodal association have not been systematically studied in animals. However, the evidence from some of the best-documented cases where they are most likely to be found (e.g. the alarm-call system of vervets) points to a mechanism of 'affective semantics'. As reviewed previously, the alarm calls of vervets, and those of many other species, are similar in possessing a common suite of acoustic structural features well suited to stimulating a host of reflexive autonomic, affective responses that immediately prepare listeners for a 'flight-or-fight' type of response, which is obviously functional in the context of confronting predators or other dangers. An interesting element of this phenomenon, as documented in vervet monkeys, is that it takes predator-naïve infants some time to develop adult-like, differentiated escape responses to the alarm calls elicited by different predators (Seyfarth & Cheney, 1986). At first, the different alarm calls simply produce a generalized startle response in infants as a result of the common affect-inducing acoustic features of each call. Over time, infants' responses begin to differentiate into the more adult-like repertoire of different escape options.

Although the details of this process remain undocumented, it is well established that the upregulation of brain activation, glucose metabolism, and stress hormones that accompanies emotion-inducing experiences facilitates learning and memory (McGaugh, 2003). Therefore, the powerful effects that the alarm calls have from the very start on attentional and affective systems likely serve to tag the significance of these events for naïve infants and promote additional learning about the different predators involved and the specific behavioural responses that follow and are appropriate to them. As a result, although predator avoidance is rooted developmentally in the inherent affect-inducing properties the alarm calls have (i.e. inherent sound-affect associations), later, as mature responders, vervets may well develop some sort of representation of the different types of predator they encounter as a result of their accumulated history of experiencing them in association with the alarm calls themselves. Hence, the calls may develop some rudimentary semantic value that is rooted in the original functional perceptual and affective biases that kicked things off.

13.3.2 Systematicity

The question of whether animal signals can be considered systematic, in the sense outlined here, is an interesting and novel one. For species reported to use signals even semi-referentially in ways suggestive of signal-meaning mappings, the repertoire of such signals is typically quite small, on the order of one to three call types. This necessarily makes it challenging to evaluate the potential systematicity of the relationships between the sets of signals and the sets of 'meanings' involved. We might suggest that the small suite of alarm calls produced by vervet monkeys has the property of being incidentally systematic, in having a small number of similarly structured calls pointing out a small set of different predators or classes of danger. However, the meaningfulness of this type of systematicity to the animals themselves is entirely unknown. Given experience with their own set of different alarm calls, would vervets be able to generalize to a novel signal and recognize it as an alarm call for a new predator in their environment?

13.3.3 Learnability and Expressivity

Animal signalling systems are generally characterized by relatively small overall repertoires, at least compared to the lexicons of languages. They are unlikely then to be significantly constrained by a pressure for expressivity. However, the fact that animal calls are typically indexical and often leverage sound-affect associations suggests either that the pressure for those signals to be learnable has influenced their structure, or that the perceptual biases mediating the sound-affect associations actively constrain the possible signals that an animal can produce for a given 'meaning'.

The broadly conserved structure of alarm calls across many species seems to be shaped by the pressure for functional deployability, but is the specific detailed form that individual signals take constrained by some need also to be learnable? Put differently, in the absence of a pressure for functional deployability, would a vervet be able to learn that a quite different and mellifluous 'coo-ing' sound is a signal for a specific kind of predator, or is the normal, affectively-mediated perceptual bias to harsh calls required as a substrate upon which to establish an element of reference?

13.4 SHARED EVOLUTIONARY HISTORY OF COMMUNICATION: FILLING IN THE BLANKS

Both animal and human communication are at least partially structured based on the interaction of a pressure for functional deployability with the perceptuo-cognitive architecture of their users. In a sense, this functional deployability pressure is extra-linguistic, as it deals with the modulation of the behaviour of conspecifics by exploiting associations between perceptual features delivered via the vocal channel and affective and attentional processes. In animal communication systems, the leveraging of affective biases for functional purposes seems to be the only way that signal structures are influenced, but in human language those same affective biases are supplemented by others to influence the learnability and expressivity of the language.

The shared evolutionary history of the perceptual and cognitive apparatus of humans and other animals leads naturally to the suggestion that the pressure for functional deployability might have served as an initial seed from which more complex associations could be leveraged to convey a growing set of meanings. Animal signals, like the alarm calls of vervet monkeys, that are at least putatively referential seem to suggest exactly this possibility. In the following sections, we suggest a number of ways that these areas can inform one another, as well as surveying a number of open questions about the evolution of communication systems and how they might be approached.

13.4.1 Biosemantics

The morphemes of human languages are composed of phonemes, the basic building blocks of language that, by themselves, are conventionally held to carry no meaning. As we have seen, however, that is not necessarily true. Phonemes are processed both as discrete, potentially meaningless units, but also as sounds whose acoustic features can leverage meaning. Thus, phonemes have meaning that is separate from their embeddedness and typical conventionalized use in a language. The ability of sound to carry 'meaning' by virtue of affective or perceptual associations is shared with a number of non-human species, but the possibility that the richer semantics of more robust communication systems can be scaffolded on these simple sound-meaning associations is rarely considered.

For example, infants of all species first learn sound-meaning associations that have clear functional biological relevance. For example, they learn to establish the age, sex, body size, and disposition of caregivers and others in their world based on vocal cues. These distinctions are signalled by differences in basic acoustic features like voice pitch, formants, and prosodic variation that vary predictably and systematically with consequences of clear biological relevance and affective salience such as provision of food, comfort, and care, or danger and threat (Fitch & Giedd, 1999; Rendall et al., 2005; Titze, 1989). Thus, the first sound-meaning associations that infants acquire are not propositional in nature, but are nonetheless highly functional, predicting not only social distinctions but also their concomitant affective and behavioural consequences. Many animals learn similar types of sound-meaning associations early in their development, yet fail to establish the rich semantics of human language. Why is this the case? Also, how much of the 'meaning' of animal signals is given directly by the leveraging of perceptual bias, or facilitated and scaffolded by those associations?

This is what we refer to as biosemantics, which could be characterized, a bit awkwardly, as 'biologically constrained phonological semantics'.

The suggestion is that species' typical biological organization acts as a substrate by which phonological or acoustic features of utterances have 'meaning', or at the very least proto-semantic meaning. Thus, certain phonetic forms might be biologically motivated, grounded in the broader evolutionary history of the structure and use of similar signal forms in animal signalling systems where they mark distinctions of clear functional, biological relevance (e.g. harsh spectral structures and dangers; low pitch or resonance and large size and social potency). Parsimony suggests that the broadly conserved perceptual and cognitive biases that support this long evolutionary history of functionality in animals need not abruptly end or somehow be abandoned uniquely in the human line. Rather, it would be expected to continue and offer communicative possibilities in language as well. By this route, some phonetic forms in language (as reviewed earlier) might thus inherit natural meaning potential based on their specific acoustic structural forms and the conserved history those may have had in signalling functional distinctions with clear biological relevance in animal communication systems.

The novelty in this approach is in seeking continuity between human and animal communication systems, not in the potentially more rarefied features of full-blown language (e.g. intentionality, high-level semantics, syntax) but rather at much more fundamental levels (e.g. the level of individual sound units) that are indisputably shared, and then seeing the evolutionarily conserved pressure for functional deployability at these levels as a potential seed for the evolution of language. The value of this approach may be manifold. First, it may prompt a productive reorientation of analysis in language, where traditionally the assumption has been that linguistic forms are largely arbitrary and constructed from meaningless phonemes. It might also prompt an equally productive reorientation of research in animal communication systems, particularly those of closely related non-human primates, away from attempts to find continuity in the more rarefied features of language, where results to date, even on a favourable reading, have been thin. Finally, it might thus allow better integration and comparability between the two programmes based on adoption of common constructs and methods of analysis.

To this point, a central problem in research on sound-symbolic phenomena in human language and animal communication is that the features of signals from the two systems are described using non-overlapping jargon, or according to measures that cannot easily be translated between the two. Human perceptual bias, for example, is generally explained in terms of phonology (i.e. aspirated voiceless stop consonants are associated with jagged visual images) or by invoking psychological intuitions about sounds (e.g. that 'kiki' is a 'harsher' word than 'bouba'). In contrast, animal signals are typically described based on detailed acoustic measures such as amplitude envelope, harmonics-to-noise ratio, or spectral density, that make the differences between signals more explicit and objectively quantifiable.

Because these metrics are not directly comparable, the degree to which human and animal perceptual and affective biases are similar remains unanswered, with few authors (e.g. Owren & Rendall, 1997, 2001) recognizing that the biases are likely to be conserved and underpinned by the same general mechanisms. To explore this possibility, it is first necessary that researchers should explore human affective and perceptual biases, like the bouba-kiki effect, using stimuli that are characterized based on metrics that can be compared directly to animal signals. That is, biosemantic biases should be described based on their acoustic, rather than their phonological, features.

If human and animal affective and perceptual biases are indeed similar to one another, and those biases are leveraged by the requirement in human language for learnability (and thus have downstream effects on the structure of language), then it stands to reason that animal communication systems might similarly be structured around such biases, or that the leveraging of biases might allow animals to learn motivated signal-meaning mappings with increased ease in the same way that humans do. The exploration of this possibility can serve to bridge the gap between human and animal communication based on both structure and function. It might also generate many further testable predictions that address the importance of biosemantic associations for human language and also highlight the pieces missing in animals that hamper transitioning from a functional leveraging of perceptual and affective biases to a truly semantic leveraging of those same biases.

13.4.2 Human Affective Semantics

An account of the origins of human language that returns to functional pressures and affective biases as a driving pressure raises important questions concerning both the possible centrality of affect to perceptual biases that are leveraged semantically and also the degree to which the use of language in modern humans is still mediated by those same functional pressures.

In the modern era of human communication, the suggestion that language is primarily about the transfer of information seems unimpeachable. We daily consume massive amounts of information and generally take in a large proportion of this information in written form, which is not likely to be as appropriate a channel for leveraging perceptual and affective associations. Historically, however, this was not the case, and only half of the world's extant languages have a formal writing system (Lewis et al., 2016). The informational account of human language also stumbles on questions about its evolutionary trajectory. A fully formed language system is, without a doubt, valuable for transmitting information and doing uniquely human things, but where does that leave the connection between animal and human communication? The recognition that human verbal communication continues to leverage core affective systems and widely conserved perceptual biases embraces the possibility that the arbitrary and conventional semantic components of language, central to its modern functioning in carrying and conveying information, are likely built on a common framework of affective and perceptual biases shared widely among primates, certainly, and possibly other animal groups.

13.4.3 Systematicity in Animal Communication

The degree to which animal communication systems are systematically structured, or that systematic signal-meaning associations might positively influence learnability in animals as they do in humans, are open empirical questions. Nielsen (2016) has suggested that learning systematic associations between words and meanings might enhance the learnability of later-acquired conventional associations by bootstrapping the acquisition of concepts and categories in human-language learners. Might animal signalling systems be less complex than human language partially because they do not take advantage of conceptual bootstrapping? Or are the 'deficiencies' of animal communication systems entirely explained by additional cognitive abilities in humans specifically associated with the elaboration of language?

13.5 CONCLUSIONS

The relatively recent recognition that the structure of languages is shaped by the pressures to be both learnable and expressible, when filtered through the perceptual and cognitive apparatus of users, has been immensely productive for modern linguistic research. Similarly, research into animal communication has recognized the importance of perceptual, productive, and cognitive processes for shaping the behavioural and signalling repertoires of various species. Here, we have proposed that these two streams of research can be productively combined and can inform each other, to develop not only a better understanding of natural languages but also the evolutionary trajectory of language and communication systems more broadly.

Specifically, we have suggested that in addition to pressures for learnability and expressivity, both human and animal communication systems are sculpted by a pressure for their signals to be functionally deployable. This pressure for functional deployability is not merely a filter through which communication signals must pass but, rather, is intimately and directly tied to core perceptual and cognitive biases that thus underpin and determine signal effectiveness. Fully embracing and integrating these points into future work promises a host of additional potential insights into the structural and functional organization of communication systems in humans and animals alike, and, importantly, the potential productive links between them.

REFERENCES

Ahlner, F. & Zlatev, J. (2010). Cross-modal iconicity: a cognitive semiotic approach to sound symbolism. *Sign System Studies,* 38, 294–348.

Arnal, L. H., Flinker, A., Kleinschmidt, A., Giraud, A-L., & Poeppel, D. (2015). Human screams occupy a privileged niche in the communication soundscape. *Current Biology,* 25, 2051–2056.

Asano, M., Imai, M., Kita, S., Katajo, K., Okada, H., & Thierry, G. (2015). Sound symbolism scaffolds language development in preverbal infants. *Cortex,* 63, 196–205

Asher, J. E., Lamb, J. A., Brocklebank, D., Cazier, J. B., Maestrini, E., Addis, L., ... Monaco, A. P. (2009). A whole-genome scan and fine-mapping linkage study of auditory-visual synesthesia reveals evidence of linkage to chromosomes 2q24, 5q33, 6p12, and 12p12. *The American Journal of Human Genetics,* 84(2), 1–7.

Assaneo, M. F., Nichols, J. I., & Trevisan, M. A. (2011). The anatomy of onomatopoeia. *PLoS One,* 6(12), e28317.

Aveyard, M. E. (2012). Some consonants sound curvy: effects of sound symbolism on object recognition. *Memory and Cognition,* 40, 83–92.

Bankieris, K. and Simner, J. (2015). What is the link between synaesthesia and sound symbolism? *Cognition,* 136, 186–195.

Belin, P. & Zatorre, R. J. (2015). Neurobiology: sounding the alarm. *Current Biology,* 25, R793–810.

Berent, I. & Goldin-Meadow, S. (2015). Language by mouth and by hand. *Frontiers in Psychology,* 6, 78. doi:10.3389/fpsyg.2015.00078

Blasi, D., Christiansen, M. H., Wichmann, S., Hammarstrom, H., & Stadler, P. (2014). Sound symbolism and the origins of language. In: E. A. Cartmill, S. Roberts, H. Lyn, & H. Cornish (eds) *The Evolution of Language: Proceedings of the 10th International Conference* (EVOLANG10). Singapore: World Scientific.

Bolinger, D. (1980). *Language: The Loaded Weapon. The Use and Abuse of Language Today.* New York: Longman.

Brang, D., Hubbard, E. M., Coulson, S., Huang, M., & Ramachandran, V. S. (2010). Magnetoencephalography reveals early activation of V4 in grapheme-color synesthesia. *NeuroImage,* 53, 268–274.

Bremner, A. J., Caparos, S., Davidoff, J., de Fockert, J., Linnell, K. J., & Spence, C. (2013). 'Bouba' and 'Kiki' in Namibia? A remote culture makes similar shape-sound matches, but different shape-taste matches to Westerners. *Cognition,* 126, 165–172.

Chater, N. & Vitanyi, P. (2003). Simplicity: a unifying principle in cognitive science. *Trends in Cognitive Sciences,* 7, 19–22

Chomsky, N. (1965). *Aspects of the Theory of Syntax.* Cambridge, MA: MIT Press.

Chomsky, N. (1968). *Language and Mind.* New York: Harcourt Brace Jovanovich.

Cuskley, C. (2013). *Shared Cross-modal Associations and the Emergence of the Lexicon.* University of Edinburgh Doctoral Thesis, Edinburgh, UK.

Davis, R. (1961). The fitness of names to drawings. A cross-cultural study in Tanganyika. *British Journal of Psychology,* 52, 259–268.

de Oliveira Calleia, F., Rohe, F., & Gordo, M. (2009). Hunting strategy of the margay (*Leopardus wiedii*) to attract the wild pied tamarin (*Saguinus bicolor*). *Neotropical Primates,* 16, 32–34.

De Saussure, F. (1983). *Course in General Linguistics.* C. Bally & A. Sechehaye (eds) Translated by R. Harris. La Salle, Illinois: Open Court.

Dingemanse, M. (2011). Ideophones and the aesthetics of everyday language in a West-African society. *Senses and Society,* 6(1), 77–85.

Dingemanse, M., Blasi, D. E., Lupyan, G., Christiansen, M. H., & Monaghan, P. (2015). Arbitrariness, iconicity, and systematicity in language. *Trends in Cognitive Sciences,* 19, 603–615.

Dingemanse, M., Schuerman, W., Reinisch, E., Tufvesson, S., & Mitterer, H. (2016). What sound symbolism can and cannot do: testing the iconicity of ideophones from five languages. *Language,* 92, 117–133.

Dingemanse, M. Verhoeft, T., & Roberts, S. G. (2014). The role of iconicity in the cultural evolution of communicative skills. In: B. De Boer & T. Verhoef (eds) *Proceedings of Evolang X: Workshop on Signals, Speech, and Signs* (pp. 11–15).

Driver, P. M. & Humphries, D. A. (1969). The significance of the high-intensity alarm call in captured passerines. *Ibis,* 111, 243–244.

Eaton, R. C. (1984). *Neural Mechanisms of Startle Behaviour.* New York, NY: Plenum.

Engesser, S., Crane, J. M. S., Savage, J. L., Russell, A. F., & Townsend, S. W. (2015). Experimental evidence for phonemic contrasts in a nonhuman vocal system. *PLoS Biology,* 13(6), e1002171.

Fernald, A. & Morikawa, H. (1993). Common themes and cultural variations in Japanese and American mothers' speech to infants. *Child Development,* 64, 637–656.

Fitch, W. T. (2010). *The Evolution of Language.* Cambridge: Cambridge University Press.

Fitch, W. T. (2000). The evolution of speech: a comparative review. *Trends in Cognitive Sciences,* 4, 258–267.

Fitch, W. T. & Giedd, J. (1999). Morphology and development of the human vocal tract: a study using MRI. *Journal of the Acoustical Society of America,* 106, 1511–1522.

Flower, T. P. (2014). Deception by flexible alarm mimicry in an African bird. *Science,* 344, 513–516.

Gasser, M. (2004). The origins of arbitrariness of language. In: *Proceedings of the 26th Annual Conference of the Cognitive Science Society* (pp. 434–439). Mahwah, NJ: Lawrence Erlbaum Associates.

Gebels, G. (1969). An investigation of phonetic symbolism in different cultures. *Journal of Verbal Learning and Verbal Behavior,* 8, 310–312.

Grieser, D. L. & Kuhl, P. K. (1988). Maternal speech to infants in a tonal language: support for universal prosodic features in motherese. *Developmental Psychology,* 24, 14–20.

Hanganu-Optaz, I. L., Rowland, B. A., Bieler, M., & Sieben, K. (2015). Unraveling cross-modal development in animals: neural substrate, functional coding, and behavioral readout. *Multisensory Research,* 28, 33–69.

Higgins, P. J., Peter, J. M. & Steele, W. K. (1990). Superb lyrebird. In: S. Marchant & P. J. Higgins (eds) *Handbook of Australian, New Zealand and Antarctic Birds* (pp. 142–173). Melbourne: Oxford University Press.

Hirst, D. & Di Cristo, A. (1998). *Intonation Systems: A Survey of Twenty Languages.* Cambridge, UK: Cambridge University Press.

Hockett, C. F. (1960). The origin of speech. *Scientific American,* 203, 88–96.

Huang, Y. H. (1969). Universal magnitude symbolism. *Journal of Verbal Learning and Verbal Behavior,* 8, 155–156.

Imai, M., Kita, S., Nagumo, M., & Okada, H. (2008). Sound symbolism facilitates early verb learning. *Cognition,* 109, 54–65.

Johnson, R. C. (1967). Magnitude symbolism of English words. *Journal of Verbal Learning and Verbal Behavior,* 6, 508–511.

Johnson, R., Cole, P., & Stroup, W. (1985). Starling response to three auditory stimuli. *Journal of Wildlife Management,* 49, 620–625.

Joseph, J. E. (2015). Iconicity in Saussure's linguistic work and why it does not contradict the arbitrariness of the sign. *Historiographia Linguistica,* 32, 85–105.

Kanera, J., Imai, M., Okuda, J., Okada, H., & Matsuda, T. (2014). How sound symbolism is processed in the brain: a study on Japanese mimetic words. *PLoS One,* 9(5), e97905.

Kantarzis, K., Kita, S., & Imai, M. (2011). Japanese sound symbolism facilitates word learning in English speaking children. *Cognitive Science,* 35, 575–586.

Kaplan, P. & Owren, M. (1994). Dishabituation of infant visual attention in 4-month-olds by infant-directed frequency-modulated sweeps. *Infant Behavior and Development,* 17, 347–358.

Kim, K.-O. (1977). Sound symbolism in Korean. *Journal of Linguistics,* 13, 67–75.

Kirby, S., Cornish, H., & Smith, K. (2006). Cumulative cultural evolution in the laboratory: an experimental approach to the origins of structure in human language. *Proceedings of the National Academy of Sciences,* 105, 10681–10686.

Kirby, S., Tamariz, M., Cornish, H., & Smith, K. (2015). Compression and communication in the cultural evolution of linguistic structure. *Cognition,* 141, 87–102.

Köhler, W. (1947). *Gestalt Psychology* (2nd edn). New York, NY: Liveright.

Krumhansl, C. L. (2002). Music: a link between cognition and emotion. *Current Directions in Psychological Science,* 11, 45–50.

Lancker, D. V. & Cummings, J. L. (1999). Expletives: neurolinguistics and neurobehavioral perspectives on swearing. *Brain Research Reviews,* 31, 83–104.

Lewis, M. P., Simons, G. F., & Fennig, C. D. (eds) (2016). *Ethnologue: Languages of the World,* (19th edn). Dallas, Texas: SIL International.

Lockwood, G. & Dingemanse, M. (2015). Iconicity in the lab: a review of behavioural, developmental, and neuroimaging research into sound symbolism. *Frontiers in Psychology,* 6, 1264.

Ludwig, V. U., Adachi, I., & Matsuzawa, T. (2011). Visuoauditory mappings between high luminance and high pitch are shared by chimpanzees (*Pan troglodytes*) and humans. *Proceedings of the National Academy of Sciences,* 108, 20661–20665.

Malmberg, B. (1964). Couches primitives de structure phonologique. *Phonetica,* 1, 221–227.

McConnell, P. B. (1991). Lessons from animal trainers: the effect of acoustic structure on an animal's response. In: P. Bateson & P. Klopfer (eds) *Perspectives in Ethology. Vol. 9: Human Understanding and Animal Awareness* (pp. 165–187). New York: Plenum Press.

McGaugh, J. L. (2003). *Memory and Emotion: The Making of Lasting Memory.* Weidenfeld & Nicolson.

Monaghan, P., Christiansen, M. H., & Fitneva, S. A. (2011). The arbitrariness of the sign: learning advantages from the structure of the vocabulary. *Journal of Experimental Psychology: General,* 140, 325–347.

Monaghan, P., Mattock, K., & Walker, P. (2012). The role of sound symbolism in language learning. *Journal of Experimental Psychology: Learning, Memory, and Cognition,* 38, 1152–1164.

Monaghan, P., Shillcock, R. C., Christiansen, M. H., & Kirby, S. (2014). How arbitrary is language? *Philosophical Transactions of the Royal Society B: Biological Sciences,* 369, 20130299.

Morton, E. S. (1977). On the occurrence and significance of motivation-structural rules in some birds and mammal sounds. *American Naturalist,* 111, 855–869.

Morton, E. S. (1994). Sound symbolism and its role in non-human vertebrate communication. In: L. Hinton, J. Nichols, & J. Ohala (eds) *Sound Symbolism*. Cambridge: Cambridge University Press.

Newman, S. S. (1933). Further experiments in phonetic symbolism. *American Journal of Psychology,* 45, 53–75.

Newmeyer, F. J. (1993). Iconicity and generative grammar. *Language,* 68, 756–796.

Nielsen, A. K. S. (2011). *Sound Symbolism and the Bouba-Kiki Effect: Uniting Function and Mechanism in the Search for Language Universals*. Master's Thesis, University of Lethbridge, Lethbridge, Alberta.

Nielsen, A. K. S. (2016). *Systematicity, Motivatedness, and the Structure of the Lexicon*. Doctoral Thesis, University of Edinburgh, Edinburgh, UK.

Nielsen, A. & Rendall, D. (2011). The sound of round: evaluating the role of consonants in the classic Takete-Maluma phenomenon. *Canadian Journal of Experimental Psychology,* 65, 115–124.

Nielsen, A. & Rendall, D. (2012). The source and magnitude of sound-symbolic biases in processing artificial word material and their implications for language learning and transmission. *Language and Cognition,* 4, 115–125.

Nygaard, L. C., Cook, A. E., & Namy, L. L. (2009). Sound to meaning correspondences facilitate word learning. *Cognition,* 112, 181–186.

Ouattara, K., Lemasson, A., & Zuberbuhler, K. (2009). Campbell's monkeys concatenate vocalisations into context-specific call sequences. *Proceedings of the National Academy of Sciences,* 106, 22026–22031.

Owren, M. J. & Rendall, D. (1997). An affect-conditioning model of nonhuman primate vocalizations. In: D. W. Owings, M. D. Beecher, & N. S. Thompson (eds) *Perspectives in Ethology. Vol. 12: Communication* (pp. 299–346). New York, NY: Plenum Press.

Owren, M. J. & Rendall, D. (2001). Sound on the rebound: returning form and function to the forefront in understanding nonhuman primate vocal signaling. *Evolutionary Anthropology,* 10(2), 58–71.

Owren, M. J., Rendall, D., & Ryan, M. J. (2010). Redefining animal signaling: influence versus information in communication. *Biology & Philosophy,* 25, 755–780.

Ozturk, O., Krehm, M., & Vouloumanos, A. (2013). Sound symbolism in infancy: evidence for sound-shape cross-modal correspondences in 4-month olds. *Journal of Experimental Child Psychology,* 114, 173–186.

Papousek, M., Papousek, H., & Symmes, D. (1991). The meanings of melodies in motherese in tone and stress languages. *Infant Behavior and Development,* 14, 415–440.

Paquette, S., Peretz, I., & Belin, P. (2013). The musical emotional bursts: a validated set of musical affect bursts to investigate auditory affective processing. *Frontiers in Psychology,* 4, 509.

Penn, D. C. & Povinelli, D. J. (2007). On the lack of evidence that non-human animals possess anything remotely resembling a 'theory of mind'. *Philosophical Transactions of the Royal Society B: Biological Sciences,* 362, 731–744.

Perniss, P., Thompson, R., & Vigliocco, G. (2010). Iconicity as a general property of language: evidence from spoken and signed languages. *Frontiers in Psychology*, 1, 1–15.

Perniss, P. & Vigliocco, G.(2014). The bridge of iconicity: from a world of experience to the experience of language. *Philosophical Transactions of the Royal Society B: Biological Sciences*, 369, 20130300.

Pexman, P. & Sidhu, D. M. (2014). Beyond the bouba/kiki effect: the bob/kirk effect. *Canadian Journal of Experimental Psychology*, 68, 253–254.

Pinker, S. (1994). *The Language Instinct*. New York, NY: Harper Perennial Modern Classics.

Pisanski, K. & Rendall, D. (2011). The prioritization of voice fundamental frequency or formants in listeners' assessments of speaker size, masculinity, and attractiveness. *Journal of the Acoustical Society of America*, 129, 2201–2212.

Queiroz, J. & Ribeiro, S. (2002). The biological substrate of icons, indexes, and symbols in animal communication: a neurosemiotic analysis of Vervet monkey alarm calls. In: M. Shapiro (ed.) *The Peirce Seminar Papers: Essays in Semiotic Analysis*, 5 (pp. 69–78). New York: Berghahn Books.

Ramachandran, V. S. & Hubbard, E. M. (2001). Synaesthesia—a window into perception, thought and language. *Journal of Consciousness Studies*, 8, 3–34.

Reilly, J.,Westbury, C., Kean, J., & Peele, J. E. (2012). Arbitrary symbolism in natural language revisited: when forms carry meaning. *PLoS One*, 7(8), 1–15.

Rendall, D., Kollias, S, Ney, C., & Lloyd, P. (2005). Pitch (Fo) and formant profiles of human vowels and vowel-like baboon grunts: the role of vocalizer body size and voice-acoustic allometry. *Journal of the Acoustical Society of America*, 117, 944–955.

Rendall, D., Notman, H., & Owren, M. J. (2009). Asymmetries in the individual distinctiveness and maternal recognition of infant contact calls and distress screams in baboons. *Journal of the Acoustical Society of America*, 125, 1792–1805.

Rendall, D. & Owren, M. J. (2010). Vocalizations as tools for influencing the affect and behavior of others. In: S. Brudzynski (ed.) *Handbook of Mammalian Vocalizations* (pp. 177–186). Oxford: Academic Press.

Rendall, D., Owren, M. J., & Ryan, M. J. (2009). What do animal signals mean? *Animal Behaviour*, 78, 233–240.

Revill, K. P., Namy, L. L., DeFife, L. C., & Nygaard, L. C. (2014). Cross-linguistic sound symbolism and crossmodal correspondence: evidence from fMRI and DTI. *Brain and Language*, 128, 18–24.

Rouw, R. & Scholte, H. S. (2007). Increased structural connectivity in grapheme–color synesthesia. *Nature Neuroscience*, 10, 792–797.

Rumelhart, D. E. & McClelland, J. L.(1986). On learning the past tense of English verbs. In: J. McClelland & D. Rumelhart (eds) *Parallel Distributed Processing: Explorations in the Microstructure of Cognition (Vol. 2)*. Cambridge, MA: MIT Press.

Sapir, E. (1929). A study in phonetic symbolism. *Journal of Experimental Psychology*, 12, 225–239.

Schlenker, P., Chemla, E., Arnold, K., Lemasson, A., Ouattara, K., Keenan, S., … Zuberbuhler, K. (2014). Monkey semantics: two 'dialects' of Campbell's monkey alarm calls. *Linguistics and Philosophy*, 37, 439–501.

Schneider, E. H. (ed.) (1963). *Music Therapy*. Lawrence, KS: Allen Press.

Segerdahl, P., Fields, W. M., & Savage-Rumbaugh, E. S. (2005). *Kanzi's Primal Language: The Cultural Initiation of Apes into Language*. London: Palgrave/Macmillan.

Seyfarth, R. M. & Cheney, D. L. (1986). Vocal development in vervet monkeys. *Animal Behaviour*, 34, 1640–1658.

Seyfarth, R. M., Cheney, D. L., & Marler, P. (1980). Monkey responses to three different alarm calls: evidence of predator classification and semantic communication. *Science,* 210, 801–803.

Suzuki, T. N., Wheatcroft, D., & Griesser, M. (2016). Experimental evidence for compositional syntax in bird calls. *Nature Communications,* 7, 10986.

Tamariz, M. & Kirby, S. (2015). Culture: copying, compression, and conventionality. *Cognitive Science,* 39, 171–183.

Taub, S. F. (2001). *Language from the Body: Iconicity and Metaphor in American Sign Language.* Cambridge: Cambridge University Press.

Thompson, R. L., Vinson, D. P., Woll, B., & Vigliocco, G. (2012). The road to language learning is iconic: evidence from British sign language. *Psychological Science,* 23, 1443–1448.

Thompson, B., Kirby, S., & Smith, K. (2016). Culture shapes the evolution of cognition. *Proceedings of the National Academy of Sciences,* 113(16), 4530–4535.

Titze, I. R. (1989). Physiologic and acoustic differences between male and female voices. *Journal of the Acoustical Society of America,* 85, 1699–1707.

Tomasello, M. (2008). *Origins of Human Communication.* MIT Press.

Trost, W., Frühholz, S., Cochrane, T., Cojan, Y., & Vuilleumier, P. (2015). Temporal dynamics of musical emotions examined through intersubject synchrony of brain activity. *Social Cognition: Affect Neuroscience,* 10, 1705–1721.

Valdez, P. & Mehrabian, A. (1994). Effects of color on emotions. *Journal of Experimental Psychology: General,* 123, 394–409.

Ward, J., Huckstep, B., & Tsakanikos, E. (2006). Sound-colour synaesthesia: to what extent does it use cross-modal mechanisms common to us all? *Cortex,* 42, 264–280.

Wilkins, J. (1668). *An Essay Towards a Real Character, and a Philosophical Language.* London: Royal Society Printer.

Yardy, B. J. (2010). *Sound Symbolism, Sonority, and Swearing: An Affect Induction Perspective.* Master's Thesis, University of Lethbridge, Lethbridge, Alberta.

Yoshida, H. (2012). A cross-linguistic study of sound symbolism in children's verb learning. *Journal of Cognitive Development,* 13, 232–265.

Zuberbühler, K. (2000). Referential labeling in wild Diana monkeys. *Animal Behaviour,* 59, 917–927.

APPENDIX 13.1

SAMPLES OF HUMAN AND PRIMATE SOUNDS

Human Speech

Audio 13.1 provides examples of synthetic speech stimuli used in experiments testing the classic *bouba-kiki* effect, wherein nonsense words containing spectrally harsh or strident consonants (such as /k/ or /t/) tend to be matched to unfamiliar objects or images that are *jagged* or *fractured* in appearance, while nonsense words containing more sonorant consonants (such as /b/ but more especially /l/ or /m/) tend to be matched to unfamiliar objects or images that are *smooth* or *rounded* in appearance. The functional argument is that, although formal linguistic theory typically regards these basic differences in spectral structure between strident and sonorant consonants to be meaningless, it is possible that the differences, in fact, carry some natural semantic potential (i.e. some ability to convey rudimentary semantic contrasts of the sort just noted). Further, the different consonant forms may inherit their semantic potential from the wider use of sounds typifying these same basic distinctions in other species, such as closely related non-human primates.

Primate Vocalizations

Audio 13.2 provides examples of typical primate vocalizations given in one of two different contexts. The first context is characterized by high arousal and excitement and is typified by encounters with dangerous predators, or with social agonism involving hostility, aggression, or fighting with companions. Typically associated vocalizations are loud, strident *barks* and *screams* which are high-amplitude, abrupt, and spectrally harsh, noisy, or chaotic sounds. The second context contrasts sharply with the first and is typified either by relaxed group movement through the landscape or relatively calm, affiliative social interactions with companions involving friendly contact and grooming. In such situations, typically associated vocalizations are sonorant *grunts* and *coos* which are comparatively low-amplitude, with smooth signal onsets and tonal or harmonic spectral structures.

....

CHAPTER 14

LINKING VOCAL LEARNING TO SOCIAL REWARD IN THE BRAIN
Proposed Neural Mechanisms of Socially Guided Song Learning

....

SAMANTHA CAROUSO-PECK
AND MICHAEL H. GOLDSTEIN

14.1 INTRODUCTION

VOCAL learning—the ability to modify or learn new vocalizations—is a rare phenomenon. Although the evolutionary lineage leading to humans diverged from that leading to songbirds 300 million years ago, the process by which birds learn to sing and humans learn to speak shares parallels at multiple levels. Humans and songbirds must both achieve the complex task of learning to produce sounds which are functional for communicating with conspecifics. Song and language both require learning during a critical developmental period, and practice through immature vocalizations for both birds (subsong and plastic song) and babies (babbling).

An additional, and understudied, parallel is the powerful role of social feedback in the development of mature vocal forms. Evidence is rapidly accumulating that vocal learning in humans and songbirds is motivated by social factors and is intrinsically rewarding at the neural level. Functional and neural links between social-motivational brain regions and vocal learning circuitry continue to emerge from new investigations. Without social exposure, both humans and songbirds fail to develop normal vocalizations. Immature vocalizations play an essential role, not only in learning to use the vocal apparatus, but also in eliciting feedback from social partners to guide immature vocalizations into more mature forms. Our chapter will assess mechanisms of vocal learning with respect to the ecological contexts of young learners. A crucially important context, especially in altricial species, is the social environment.

Early work on vocal development across species found that, for both birdsong and human language, learning primarily requires exposure to species-typical sounds during a sensitive period. Experimental manipulations found the amount of input necessary to be small, and effective regardless of the inclusion of social factors, provided that the learning organism had extensive time to practise (Lenneberg, 1967; Marler, 1970). While this paradigm led to increased understanding of the neurological control of vocal production, researchers investigating the ontogeny of communication began to note that it could not explain all that they observed. Social stimulation, or lack thereof, can extend or delay the sensitive period for song learning in birds, or even allow vocalizations to be modified throughout life (Baptista & Gaunt, 1997; Payne & Payne, 1997). Different vocalizations may be utilized in different social contexts, and vocal learning does not merely involve learning to produce sounds, but also when and how to use them appropriately. If raised in an inadequate social environment, cowbirds may develop potent songs but not know how to use them (West et al., 1990), vervet monkeys may learn alarm calls but use them in response to non-threatening stimuli (Seyfarth & Cheney, 1986), and marmosets may learn vocalizations but fail to learn to take turns when communicating with conspecifics (Takahashi et al., 2016). While parrots may learn to mimic human speech through mere exposure, they can only learn to use language referentially and functionally when taught using socially interactive techniques (Pepperberg, 1993). Social partners may influence vocal development through a variety of mechanisms, providing learners with reinforcement, an attentional focus, general stimulation, or selective feedback.

Not all vocally learning species are equally socially influenced, necessitating a comparative, cross-species approach to understand what traits grant a given species the greatest capacity for vocal flexibility during ontogeny. Species with the most unpredictable environments, such as the zebra finches of central Australia, and the greatest mobility, such as migratory birds and mammals, tend to have the greatest capacity for learning new vocalizations and being influenced by social factors. This may be due to selective evolutionary pressures placed on species which would be most likely to encounter unfamiliar conspecifics with different vocal dialects. Species which live in stable, consistent social groups year-round would gain less advantage from vocal plasticity, and are often less flexible vocal learners (Snowdon & Hausberger, 1997). The developmental mechanisms underlying the incorporation of social information into learned vocalizations also vary depending on a given species' ontogeny, sensitive periods, life history, social structure, access to vocal tutors early in life, and, crucially, usage of vocalizations. Bird species which use song primarily for defending territories from competitors, and therefore benefit most by learning songs directly from dominant males, should be expected to learn song very differently from those who use song only for attracting a mate, and may benefit most from paying attention to which songs are most arousing to the opposite sex.

In the study of birdsong development, two primary models of learning processes have been proposed—instructive and selective (Changeux et al., 1984; Jerne, 1967). Instructive models propose that stimulation from the environment adds information not already present in the behavioural repertoire. These models typically consist of young birds listening to a tutor's song, memorizing it, and subsequently practising until they can reproduce the song (e.g. sensorimotor learning; Konishi, 1965). Selective models propose that learning consists of experience leading to the selection and attrition of behaviours from a relatively vast pre-existing repertoire. The best-known example of selective learning is 'action-based learning' (Marler, 1991), also called 'selective attrition' (Marler & Peters, 1982). Primarily studied in territorial sparrows, action-based learning refers to the selection of songs from a large, over-produced repertoire sung during the plastic stage of song learning. When territorial male sparrows engage in counter-singing, they exchange similar song types. During these social interactions, matching songs may be reinforced, while non-matching types are discarded (Marler & Nelson, 1993). Young song sparrows are more likely to select matching songs from tutors they can overhear interacting with other birds than from those with which they can directly interact, and do not learn preferentially from more aggressive or higher-quality adults (Akçay et al., 2014; Beecher, 2016).

While both instructive and selective models explain numerous aspects of song learning, especially the eavesdropping-based (Beecher et al., 2007) song-learning strategy in territorial sparrows, both models rely heavily on imitation. Neither explains invention and improvization of new song types which vary from that of the tutor, or the learning process of any species which utilizes non-vocal feedback or otherwise develops without exposure to an auditory model.

The socially guided learning (SGL) model instead proposes that social partners may selectively reinforce components of immature vocalizations. Much like action-based learning, SGL relies on behavioural shaping, allowing an animal to retain those behaviours most often associated with a positive social response, but rather than relying on selective attrition of non-functional songs, SGL allows young learners to construct mature vocalizations from component sounds. When attempting to write an essay, we find it far easier to be given a blank page and construct the essay using our vocabulary rather than being given a list of all possible combinations of all possible words and whittling it down to only those words we wish to include. In the same way, it is easier for a developing organism to construct an adaptive vocalization from basic parts than by being born already able to produce all possible vocalizations and removing those elements which are non-functional. While action-based learning incorporates aspects of SGL, it only allows for social shaping through selective attrition, not the constructive mechanisms we propose.

14.2 SOCIALLY GUIDED LEARNING IN BIRDSONG FUNCTION AND DEVELOPMENT

There exist over 4,000 species of songbird (oscine), and no two are precisely alike in ecological niche, life-history strategy, or song-learning trajectory. The degree of social interaction necessary and sufficient for normal vocal development varies across species. Song serves two primary functions in birds—to declare a territory from which other birds are aggressively excluded, and to attract members of the opposite sex for mating (Catchpole & Slater, 1995; Kroodsma & Miller, 1996), though some species employ only one of these song functions. In many species of songbird, only males sing, though there are numerous species in which females also produce song (Odom et al., 2014). There is extreme diversity in the types of songs birds produce, and each individual species has a characteristic acoustic structure. The simplest unit of the song is referred to as an 'element' or 'note'. A series of elements that regularly occur together form a song 'syllable', while a sequence of multiple syllables that repeatedly occurs in a song is described as a 'motif' (Brenowitz et al., 1997) (see Figure 14.1). Most juvenile songbirds fail to develop normal song if they do not hear the song of a conspecific adult tutor, or if they cannot hear themselves sing.

Songbirds may be divided into 'open-ended' and 'close-ended' or 'age-limited' learners (Nottebohm, 1993). Open-ended learners, including canaries (*Serinus canaria*), red-winged blackbirds (*Agelaius phoeniceus*), and European starlings (*Sturnus vulgaris*), can continue to learn new songs or song elements for many years or throughout life (Adret-Hausberger et al., 1990; Yasukawa et al., 1980). For close-ended learners, song acquisition is restricted to a short sensitive phase, usually early in development.

Research on vocal learning in birds has been guided by the sensorimotor model, based on studies of song learning in the white-crowned sparrow (*Zonotrichia leucophrys*), a close-ended learner (Konishi, 1965). This model incorporates two developmental stages—the sensory period, during which the song is acquired and memorized, and the sensorimotor period, during which the bird practises the song and uses auditory feedback to compare its own song to its stored memory. The beginning of the sensorimotor phase is accompanied by the production of *subsong*, the first song-like vocalizations, but which is unstructured, varies from moment to moment, and bears little resemblance to adult song (Audio 14.1). Its variability invites comparison with the early stages of babbling in human infants. Subsong and baby babbling both serve to train the vocal apparatus and improve vocal control, as well as to elicit social feedback to facilitate development of more mature sounds (Goldstein et al., 2003). Subsong gradually develops into *plastic song* that incorporates recognizable syllables from the song model (Audio 14.2), but remains variable and requires

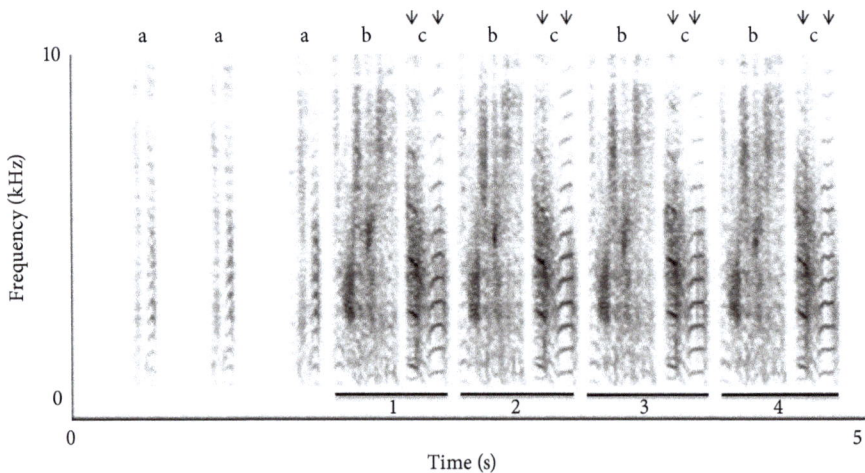

FIGURE 14.1 Spectrogram of adult zebra finch song with labelled structural components. The song begins with repeated introductory notes ('a') followed by a motif which is repeated several times (bars 1–4). Motifs consist of a number of syllables (identified by letters above the spectrogram). Syllables may contain one or more elements or notes. For example, syllable 'c', which is repeated four times, consists of two notes (denoted by arrows).

additional practice before it will mature into the final, *crystallized* adult song (DeWolfe et al., 1989) (Audio 14.3).

Syllable structure tends to reach an adult form prior to the onset of crystallized syntax, such that even after learning to produce mature and stereotyped song elements, young birds will still rearrange the sequence of these elements between song bouts. The crystallization process is rapid compared to the prolonged learning period preceding it (Todt & Geberzahn, 2003). The duration of the sensitive period is not fixed, but may vary depending on social experience. For many species, raising birds in isolation extends the sensitive period, such that adults may still learn song elements when a tutor is finally presented (Slater et al., 1988). For some species, birds exposed only to the song of a different species during development will continue to learn songs from conspecifics at a time when normally raised birds can no longer learn new song (Slater et al., 1988). Insufficient social experience or exposure to the tutor leaves the brain open to learning for longer than normal.

The subject of sensitive periods in the development of song has led to some debate on the differing effects of tutoring birds using live, interactive social partners versus pre-recorded tapes of birdsong. There are a few oscine species in which naïve individuals may produce near-perfect copies of tape-recorded song, including chaffinches (Thorpe, 1958) and white-crowned sparrows (Marler, 1970), which were among the first and most commonly studied model species. Under natural conditions, these species learn via eavesdropping on neighbouring adult males while establishing territories (Beecher et al., 1994; Nice, 1943). It is important to note, however, that social influences can dramatically change song learning, and white-crowned sparrows still learn more readily from a live tutor than a recording (Baptista & Petrinovich, 1984). Early tape-tutoring isolate studies concluded that white-crowned sparrows uniformly reject heterospecific song (Marler, 1970), but when the tutor is a live bird, they will learn from another species (Baptista & Petrinovich, 1984). Furthermore, while conspecific tape-tutored songs are deemed 'normal' to the ears of researchers, they are often functionally useless. A study of tape-tutored wood thrushes (*Hylocichla mustelina*) concluded that they developed normal wild-type song, but when the song was played back to wild wood thrushes it failed to elicit any response (Lanyon, 1979). Many other species fail to learn normal song entirely when solely exposed to tape recordings (Baptista & Petrinovich, 1986; Derégnaucourt et al., 2013; Thielcke, 1970).

Facultative social learners can use recordings to form a song model memory in isolation, but their learning is greatly improved with exposure to a live tutor. Indigo buntings (*Passerina cyanea*), domestic canaries, and European starlings can all learn a few syllables from a recording, but learn far more when exposed to the same song produced by a live tutor (Chaiken et al., 1993; Rice & Thompson, 1968; Waser & Marler, 1977). Obligate social learners, such as Eurasian tree-creepers (*Certhia familiaris*) and North American sedge wrens (*Cistothorus platensis*)[1], do not learn from tape recordings, but will readily learn from one another when naïve individuals are housed together (Kroodsma & Verner, 1978; Thielcke, 1984). Human infants seem to be subject to similar learning constraints, as studies of children raised in isolation found that they fail to develop speech normally (Fromkin et al., 1974; Lane, 1976). It is important to remember, however, that when

---

[1] When housed in acoustic isolation or exposed to passive playback, sedge wrens will improvize song elements, resulting in an approximation of species-typical song.

a social organism such as a human or songbird is raised in isolation, it is deprived not only of normal exposure to vocalizations but also of all typical social exposure. As in the case of isolate-reared monkeys developing severe behavioural abnormalities (Harlow & Harlow, 1962), early social deprivation likely has dramatic developmental impacts beyond vocal learning.

The impact of social factors also seems to shift over the course of development. For example, white-crowned sparrows will readily learn from a tape recording until 50 days of age, but will only accept live tutors as song models past that point (Baptista & Petrinovich, 1986). Conversely, starlings learn better from live tutors than tapes at 4 months of age, but tape tutoring becomes more effective by 12 months (Chaiken et al., 1993). A possible reason for this variation may be the difference in the repertoire sizes of these two species. White-crowned sparrows rarely sing more than one song as adults (Baptista, 1975), while starlings can sing dozens of different song types (Van Hout et al., 2012). This may impose different constraints on learning, such that it becomes too restrictive for a species with a large repertoire to limit learning to only one familiar tutor.

14.3 Socially Guided Vocal Learning in the Zebra Finch

Each oscine species has its own learning requirements and capabilities, and no single species can serve as a model of vocal learning for all oscines. However, the species which has been most thoroughly studied and whose learning mechanisms have been most often compared to those of humans is the zebra finch. For this species, live social interaction of the correct form and timing is vital for normal song learning. Zebra finches (*Taeniopygia guttata*) are highly gregarious, non-territorial, and socially monogamous, using their song solely for the purpose of mate attraction and pair maintenance. Only males sing, and preferentially use the song of their own father as a learning model. Zebra finches raised in isolation develop a song with abnormal properties, including unusual note structure and decreased stereotypy (Price, 1979; Williams et al., 1993). Isolated males often fail to develop a canonical motif, and will only rarely repeat a given sequence of notes. Untutored songs also often include repeated notes, resembling the structure of the trills of canaries (Williams, 2004). While these abnormalities may arise due to the absence of a song model normally provided by a tutor, some features of untutored song appear to arise due to the absence of behavioural feedback from conspecifics.

The zebra finch sensory period lasts from approximately 20–65 days of age, while the sensorimotor period lasts from days 35–90 (Brainard & Doupe, 2000), though young finches deprived of social interaction during the sensitive period will continue to be able to learn for at least several weeks beyond the normal close of the sensitive period (Clayton, 1987; Eales, 1985). Zebra finches require minimal exposure to the tutor song, and can learn to sing well with less than a minute of interactive tutoring per day (Tchernichovski et al., 1999). Sensory responses to songs are traditionally thought to be fixed and immutable, but are increasingly understood to be modulated by prior experience (Gilbert et al., 2009; Thompson & Gentner, 2010). Neural responses to songs are strongly modulated by whether or not they are reinforced by food or social feedback, and differences in acquired salience predict learning rate (Bell et al., 2015).

Throughout song development, zebra finches are naturally exposed to a highly social environment, which favours a function for listeners in song learning. In the gregarious brown-headed cowbird (*Molothrus ater*), female cowbirds selectively respond to immature male vocalizations with a non-vocal signal, in the form of a rapid lateral wing movement called a 'wing stroke'. Juvenile males attend to these cues, which are believed to be indicators of female arousal, and repeat elements which elicited a wing stroke, allowing female listeners to direct the course of song learning (West & King, 1988). Similar mechanisms may influence learning in zebra finches which, like cowbirds, are highly gregarious and experience a high degree of overlap in the sensory and sensorimotor phases of song learning (Roper & Zann, 2006; Slater et al., 1988), allowing the opportunity for social feedback to influence learning.

As with buntings, canaries, and starlings, for zebra finches interaction with a live tutor leads to more effective song learning than passive exposure to a tape-recorded song (Chen et al., 2016; Derégnaucourt et al., 2013; Eales, 1989). The salience of adult-tutor song is based on physical proximity of the tutor (Mann & Slater, 1995), aggression directed towards the fledglings (Clayton, 1987; Jones & Slater, 1996), the tutor's mating status and partner quality (Eales, 1987; Mann & Slater, 1994), visual cues such as colour morph (Mann et al., 1991; Mann & Slater, 1995), and auditory information such as song similarity between the father and subsequent song tutors (Clayton, 1987).

Juvenile males preferentially learn to sing from their fathers, even when other potential tutors are available, although they will learn from alternative tutors depending on the level of parental care they receive (Williams, 1990). Zebra finches cross-fostered under Bengalese finches (*Lonchura striata*) will produce a good copy of their foster-parent's song, even if a zebra finch model is available in a neighbouring cage (Bohner, 1983; Immelmann, 1969). Price (1979) hand-reared zebra finches such that they imprinted on him, and then tutored them each time he fed them by playing an adult song from a tape-recorder hung around his neck. The finches learned only a few syllables from the recording. However, if a finch can control the delivery of a recorded song by pressing a key, causing presentation of the model to be contingent on its own actions, it can learn to produce a good imitation (Adret, 1993). Control over the stimulus, much like interaction with a live tutor, may increase the young bird's attention to the song, leading to better learning. Simply pairing a stimulus with the sound of the model might sufficiently enhance motivation or arousal to improve learning, as in the case of common nightingales (*Luscinia megarhynchos*) which will only learn a taped song when they can observe the researcher operating the loudspeaker (Todt et al., 1979). Furthermore, male siblings have an effect on song learning, as multiple male zebra finches raised together by the same father will develop a highly variable song compared to that learned by a male without siblings (Tchernichovski & Nottebohm, 1998).

As in the brown-headed cowbird, non-singing female listeners are also known to affect song learning in the zebra finch (Jones & Slater, 1993). Males raised with deaf adult females sing more frequently and develop more atypical songs than those raised with hearing females (Williams, 2004), and blindfolded males raised with a tutor develop more accurate song when also raised with a female sibling than without one (Adret, 2004). These cases of enhanced learning in the presence of conspecifics may be the result of heightened arousal or attention in social contexts (ten Cate, 1991), or the result of attendance to song-elicited conspecific behaviours (Vyas et al., 2009).

A recent discovery shows that zebra finch females may guide juvenile male song learning in a manner very similar to that seen in cowbirds, by selectively responding to more mature, complex, or arousing elements with a wing stroke (Menyhart, Carouso-Peck et al., in preparation). These movements are extremely rapid, lasting less than 0.3 seconds, and imperceptible to the human eye, being only visible when video-recorded and then played back at 30% speed. This may explain the failure of earlier efforts to determine what cues may be responsible for differing trajectories of juvenile song learning in the presence of females; past studies observed live zebra finches at real speed, such that their rapid cues could not be detected (e.g. Houx & ten Cate, 1998).

This bias towards using human perceptual capacities to observe avian interactions has led to many interesting behaviours being overlooked in the past. Among the manakins, a South American group of birds known for their spectacular courtship displays, the black manakin (*Xenopipo atronitens*) was thought to have a simple and lacklustre display, with a courtship routine consisting only of repetitive hopping (Kirwan & Green, 2012). However, when the display of the black manakin was captured on high-speed video and slowed down, it was discovered that every 'hop' was a very rapid (360 milliseconds) and technically complex backwards somersault (see Lindsay et al., 2015). But if these movements are too rapid for humans to perceive, might they also be too quick for birds to perceive, much less use as a social cue to alter their own behaviour? The golden-collared manakin (*Manacus vitellinus*) also has a very fast courtship display, which consists of mechanical sounds and rapid lateral leaps between sapling trunks. High-speed video revealed that prior to each leap, the male quickly flares his neck feathers into a 'beard', an action that takes an average of 53 milliseconds (Fusani et al., 2007). The timing of this beard-up motion has the highest rate of inter-individual variability of any aspect of the complex display, and is also the primary basis upon which females decide whether or not to copulate with a given male (Lainy Day, personal communication). At least in some avian species, individuals are able to both perceive and make behavioural alterations based on extremely rapid movements of conspecifics—far too fast for a human researcher to perceive unaided, as human visual-system critical flicker-fusion rate is about half that of a small bird (Healy et al., 2013).

14.4 SONG CONTROL CIRCUITRY IN A SOCIAL BRAIN

Until recently, social behaviour in the brain was thought to be divided into distinct nodes, each of which was the centre for a particular category of social behaviour, such as parental care, territoriality, or pair bonding. An alternative model proposed by Sarah Newman (1999) instead suggested a social system network—a tightly interconnected system of limbic areas across which social behaviour and motivation are distributed. Social behaviours are not localized to a particular area, but rather neural activity distributed in a certain way across the network generates a given behaviour. Exactly what stimulus is necessary to elicit a behaviour and how it manifests in the brain varies by species, sex, age, and life-history traits such as gregariousness and territoriality. This social circuit overlaps significantly with the circuitry governing motivation and reward, in particular the amygdala, which mediates motivational arousal. The connection between the amygdala and ventral tegmental area (VTA) makes up much of the mesolimbic dopamine pathway modulating the behavioural response to rewarding or motivating stimuli (Syal & Finlay, 2011).

Before delving into the neurobiology underlying song learning and production, it is helpful to conceptualize the tasks the brain must accomplish in order to drive vocal learning. First, it must generate motor commands to the vocal organ (the syrinx). It must also modify these commands in response to auditory feedback (i.e. the bird detecting that its own song is not a match to its memorized model) or social feedback (i.e. behaviour from a conspecific updating the bird's mental model of ideal song). This requires the brain to use feedback to evaluate song performance, then alter motor output to minimize the difference between the song and the ideal model (Mooney, 2009). Finally, the brain must motivate the bird both to sing and to adjust its song based on feedback, requiring some form of reward resulting from singing behaviour and accurate matching responses to auditory and social feedback. How the brain accomplishes the comparison between song output and the mental model of ideal song is still being investigated, but the neural mechanisms for song production and variability are better understood. Exploration of the neural circuitry underlying song behaviour, plasticity, and variability may shed light on how this machinery incorporates social feedback into song learning.

Song behaviour and learning is regulated by an interconnected network of discrete brain nuclei referred to as the song system, which distinguishes the songbird brain from that of birds which do not learn to vocalize (Kroodsma & Konishi, 1991; Wild, 2004). During song learning, these nuclei undergo anatomical and neurochemical changes (Alvarez-Buylla & Kirn, 1997). This network is composed of two pathways—the song motor pathway (SMP) and the anterior forebrain pathway (AFP)—which together affect vocalizations through the muscles of the respiratory system and the syrinx (Figure 14.2). The SMP is a posterior motor pathway connecting nucleus RA (robust nucleus of the arcopallium), HVC (proper name, not an abbreviation; previously 'high vocal centre'), and nXIIts (tracheosyringeal portion of the twelfth cranial nerve). Each of the precise individual functions of these regions is a matter of some debate, as discussed in the following paragraphs, but together these connected regions control song production and some aspects of song learning.

Lesions in the SMP will disrupt or entirely abolish singing (Simpson & Vicario, 1990). In contrast, the AFP is involved in evaluation of the bird's song via auditory feedback and adaptive modification of the song, and is essential to both song learning and recognition (Brainard & Doupe, 2000). Lesions to this pathway will not immediately degrade crystallized song, but will prevent accurate vocal learning by reducing song variability and plasticity (Bottjer et al, 1984; Olveczky et al., 2005). The AFP is an anterior cortical–basal ganglia–thalamic loop originating in HVC, which then projects to Area X of the para-olfactory lobe and lateral magnocellular nucleus of the anterior neostriatum (LMAN), ultimately connecting back to the motor pathway at RA (Doupe et al., 2005). Nuclei in the AFP, as well as its connections to the SMP, regress substantially by the time the sensitive period closes (Hermann & Arnold, 1991; Iyengar et al., 1999).

The linkage between these two pathways, as well as the fact that both contain neurons which respond both to song production (Leonardo & Fee, 2005; McCasland, 1987) and auditory or social stimulation (Margoliash, 1983; Vicario & Yohay, 1993; Yanagihara & Hessler, 2006), suggests a mechanism by which social feedback in response to a juvenile's song may influence vocal output.

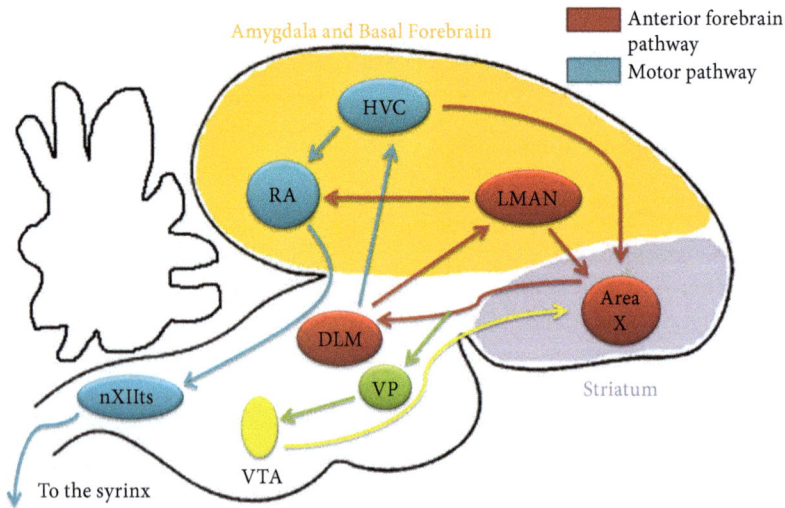

FIGURE 14.2 New thinking on the neural basis for birdsong. The song-production pathway (motor pathway) consists of projections from DLM → HVC → RA → nXIIts (indicated with blue arrows). The song-learning pathway (anterior forebrain pathway) consists of connections between HVC, LMAN, Area X, DLM, and RA (indicated with red arrows). Area X receives dopaminergic projections from VTA (yellow arrow). Area X indirectly projects song-related information back to VTA via the ventral pallidum (VP, green arrows). Based on Syal and Finlay's (2011) concept that brain areas generally believed to be homologous to mammalian pallium (neocortex) more closely resemble amygdala and basal forebrain (in orange) and areas considered homologous to basal ganglia more closely resemble striatum (in purple). This is based on the observation that bird vocal nuclei are located in tissue derived from lateral and ventral pallida, which gives rise to motivational/social circuitry in mammals.

HVC; RA, robust nucleus of the arcopallium; LMAN, lateral magnocellular nucleus of the anterior neostriatum; DLM, medial nucleus of the dorsolateral thalamus; VTA, ventral tegmental area; nXIIts, tracheosyringeal portion of the nucleus hypoglossus.

14.5 THE SONG MOTOR PATHWAY: THE VOCAL GENERATOR

A shared characteristic of human speech and birdsong, but not the majority of other animal vocalizations, is that they are controlled by the telencephalon. In birds, the anatomical basis of this control is the SMP. The nucleus HVC is a target for auditory and motor pathways, and is, conspicuously, a shared component of the SMP and AFP. The size of HVC is also altered by social factors. For example, birds placed in a complex social environment develop a larger HVC than those housed with a single conspecific (Lipkind et al., 2002). This differential growth occurs despite the fact that birds in the simple social context sing far more than those in the complex context, indicating that it is caused not by vocal output levels but instead by the task of processing a rich auditory environment (Adar et al., 2008). HVC's position as a nexus connecting various circuits in the sensorimotor system makes it a good place to begin investigating song circuitry in the social context.

HVC seems to function as a neural clock, firing in time with the elements of the song and generating its tempo. Singing-related activity in the SMP propagates through the system, arising in HVC prior to RA (McCasland, 1987). HVC-firing activity is time-locked to individual syllables, but given that stimulation of HVC disrupts song (Ashmore et al., 2005) and that HVC activity is present even in deaf birds (McCasland & Konishi, 1981), it seems to serve a strictly motor rather than auditory function. HVC neurons projecting to RA rarely fire an action potential unless the bird sings, and even then the firing is very brief (about a 10-millisecond burst at a single point during a 1-second motif) (Hahnloser et al., 2002). Ablation of HVC neurons projecting to RA, but not those projecting to Area X, will severely degrade the structure of the song (Scharff et al., 2000). This indicates that motor commands from HVC proceed directly to RA without passing through the AFP. Different neurons fire at different time points in the motif, suggesting that these neurons function to specify the production timing of different song elements. Given that some of the neurons also fire during intervening gaps of silence, they may also specify the timing of inter-note temporal spacing.

In line with the idea that HVC controls song tempo, when HVC is cooled down, the tempo of all aspects of the song, from individual notes to the entire motif, slow down by about 3% per degree Celsius of cooling (Long & Fee, 2008). Surprisingly, cooling has little effect on any other aspects of the song, such as amplitude or pitch. Cooling RA has little discernible effect on any aspect of song. It is possible that RA simply serves to turn HVC's timing signal into a motor signal, specifying the acoustic features of the song (like the structure of syllables) which should be produced according to the timing HVC specifies.

14.6 The Anterior Forebrain Pathway: Learning and Variation

As previously mentioned, the effect on song of lesioning components of the AFP is dependent on the developmental time at which it occurs. After song has crystallized, AFP lesions seem to have little immediate effect on song in most contexts. Lesions during song learning, however, prevent normal adult song from being fully learned, instead resulting in song with abnormally high stereotypy which never progresses beyond that point, as if premature crystallization has occurred (Scharff & Nottebohm, 1991).

Neural activity in the AFP during singing is strongly modulated by the presence of a conspecific listener. The magnitude and variability of activity in LMAN and Area X are lower and more consistent during singing directed to a female than undirected singing produced when the male is not orientated toward another conspecific (Hessler & Doupe, 1999a). LMAN seems to be the song's 'jitter injector', inserting variability into song during sensorimotor learning, thereby ensuring that the juvenile bird explores its acoustic range (Kao & Brainard, 2006). Stimulation of LMAN during singing will cause perturbation of the song, while LMAN inactivation reduces the bout-to-bout variability of plastic song (Olveczky et al., 2005), resulting in a repetitive and stereotyped song. The firing rate of LMAN neurons changes over developmental time, with their highest rate occurring during sensorimotor learning, suggesting that developmental change in song variability is a direct result of changes in LMAN activity. Supporting this idea, stimulating LMAN alters song structure almost immediately (as early as 30 milliseconds after stimulation) (Kao et al., 2005). LMAN was once thought to mediate song plasticity based on auditory feedback of the bird's own song as it attempted to match the song 'template'—the mental representation of the precise form of the memorized song of the tutor—yet LMAN neurons are entirely unresponsive to manipulated auditory feedback, suggesting that in LMAN, the bird's own song is not used for error detection (Leonardo, 2004).

Much like RA, LMAN serves a motor function, as neural activity in LMAN increases during song production (Hessler & Doupe, 1999b) and persists in deafened birds. Localized cooling of LMAN, much like HVC, slows down the timescale of subsong (Aronov et al., 2011). The timing signal from HVC, coupled with the 'noise' added to the signal from LMAN, may work in concert to deliver a precise motor pattern to the vocal muscles via RA.

It remains unclear whether LMAN is simply acting permissively to allow vocal plasticity, or if it is truly providing an instructive signal by injecting noise. Despite the differing level and timing of activity in LMAN between directed and undirected singing, the average pattern of firing for an individual neuron is similar across these social contexts (Kao et al., 2008). Furthermore, stimulating a single locus of LMAN will consistently change a targeted syllable in the same way—for example, always increasing its pitch—rather than inserting variability at random (Kao et al., 2005). Rather than simply driving variation, LMAN may be systematically biasing acoustic output, instructively driving vocalizations toward a particular goal. When a finch is negatively reinforced by a burst of white noise in response to a particular syllable exceeding a certain pitch threshold, the bird will shift the syllable's pitch downwards (Sober & Brainard, 2009; Tumer & Brainard, 2007). Inactivation of LMAN will cause the syllable to instantly revert to its original pitch (Andalman & Fee, 2009). LMAN thus appears to be actively biasing song away from vocal errors.

Although the influence of the AFP on song is more obvious during song learning, it continues to regulate song variability in adults. After song crystallization, AFP activity and acoustic variability are higher during undirected song than directed song (Jarvis et al., 1998; Sossinka & Bohner, 1980), with more variable spike timing during undirected song (Kao et al., 2008). Lesioning LMAN will abolish this social-context-dependent variability (Kao & Brainard, 2006), but does not prevent a male bird from performing other courtship-related behaviours normally produced only in the presence of a female, such as dancing and beak wiping. Because males seem to be able to interpret female social cues in the absence of LMAN, their capacity to detect and respond to social context must lie elsewhere in the brain and selectively activate LMAN when a female is not present.

The role of Area X in song learning remains as mysterious as its cryptic name implies, with conflicting findings thus far. Neurons in Area X exhibit highly variable patterns of firing during singing, leading some investigators to suggest that they may drive variability downstream in LMAN (Goldberg et al., 2010). Conversely, and in contrast to lesions of LMAN, juveniles with Area X lesions exhibit normal vocal variability (Goldberg & Fee, 2011; Sohrabji et al., 1990). However, eliminating Area X leads to protracted variability in adult song, with abnormal acoustic structure and little resemblance to the song of the tutor (Scharff & Nottebohm, 1991).

It has also been proposed that Area X is the site where the song template is stored and compared to the bird's own song output. This 'AFP comparison hypothesis' posits that auditory information about the bird's own song is transmitted to Area X, where it is evaluated against the template (Mooney, 2004; Sakata & Brainard, 2008). If this is the case, Area X neurons should respond to vocal errors while birds are singing, but distorted auditory feedback does not elicit such responses (Kozhevnikov & Fee, 2007; Leonardo, 2004). Furthermore, singing-related activity in Area X is not altered by deafening the bird (Hessler & Doupe, 1999a), contrary to what one would expect if the region was sensitive to perceived auditory error.

The AFP comparison hypothesis is motivated largely by observations of AFP activation in response to auditory stimuli in birds while not singing, anaesthetized, or asleep (Dave & Margoliash, 2000; Doupe, 1997; Prather et al., 2008). However, response to auditory input is ubiquitous throughout both the AFP and SMP in non-singing birds, even in syringeal motor neurons, and is not a special property of Area X (Fee & Goldberg, 2011; Williams & Nottebohm, 1985). These observations led Fee and Goldberg (2011) to hypothesize that Area X does not store the song template, evaluate match to tutor, process auditory feedback, or receive an error evaluation signal from elsewhere in the AFP. Rather, Area X may receive an evaluation signal conveying the quality of song as it is produced via neuromodulatory inputs. Particularly well suited to carry such a global, rapid (<100 milliseconds), and time-dependent signal indicating good or bad vocal performance is the dopaminergic system, as discussed in the following paragraphs.

14.6 REWARD VALUE OF SONG: PLUGGING INTO SOCIAL CIRCUITRY

A great deal of effort has been made to map out which neural circuits are involved in various social behaviours such as sexual behaviour, aggression, and parental behaviour. Studies of these regions have often led to the unexpected conclusion that there is considerable overlap in the circuitry required for these behaviours, prompting exploration of the possibility that they form an integrated social-behaviour network, much like the song-learning network.

Newman (1999) proposed a system in mammals consisting of six limbic areas, each identified as regulating multiple social behaviours, and each reciprocally connected to each of the others (Figure 14.3). Rather than a single region regulating a single social behaviour, each region responds to a number of stimuli. Social context leads to a distinct pattern of activation across regions, and this determines behavioural response. Evidence increasingly suggests that this network exists in all vertebrates, and some of the most relevant findings come from birds (see Goodson, 2005), with network responses to social stimuli differently patterned in species of songbird with different levels of sociality (Goodson et al., 2005).

The social-behaviour network is also reciprocally connected to the mesolimbic reward system, enabling social decision-making, which requires evaluation of the salience of a given stimulus before a behavioural response is executed (O'Connell & Hofmann, 2011). In order to determine the neural mechanisms by which social feedback may be affecting the trajectory of song learning, we must establish: (a) that singing is rewarding, activating the mesolimbic reward system; (b) that social context modulates this reward value; and (c) that the social-motivation system is connected to the song system and modulates its activity.

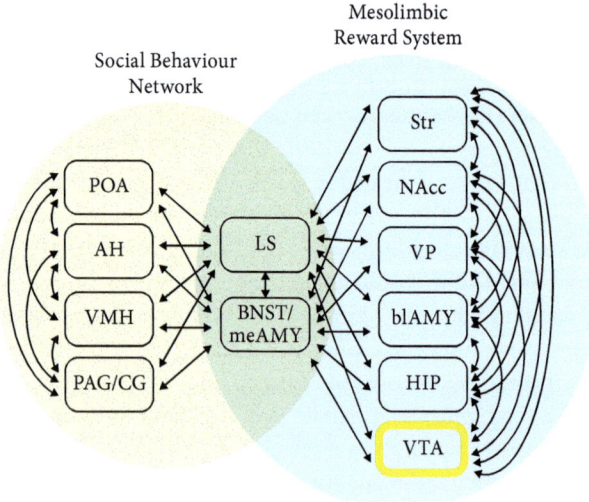

FIGURE 14.3 Interactive nodes of the networks regulating social decision-making, from O'Connell and Hoffmann (2011). Brain regions in the social behaviour network (left) and mesolimbic reward centre (right), as well as those involved in both systems (centre), are shown. VTA has been highlighted yellow to indicate the region by which social/motivational centres project to the song-learning system (as seen in Figure 14.2). Arrows indicate anatomical connections between systems in mammals.

AH, anterior hypothalamus; blAMY, basolateral amygdala; BNST/meAMY, bed nucleus of the stria terminalis/medial amygdala; HIP, hippocampus; LS, lateral septum; NAcc, nucleus accumbens; PAG/CG, periaqueductal grey/central grey; POA, preoptic area; Str, striatum; VMH; ventromedial hypothalamus; VP, ventral pallidum; VTA, ventral tegmental area.

Reproduced with permission from O'Connell L.A. & Hofmann H.A., 'The Vertebrate mesolimbic reward system and social behavior network: A comparative synthesis', *The Journal of Comparative Neurology*, Volume 519, Issue 18, pp. 3599–639, Copyright © 2011 Wiley-Liss, Inc, doi: 10.1002/cne.22735

We know that song learning and singing behaviour are controlled by the neural song system, and that both are affected by social factors. However, we know little about how social reward and song circuitry are linked. Reward associated with certain behaviours can act as a powerful incentive to perform those behaviours, and can influence food intake, copulation, and social interaction (Agmo & Berenfeld, 1990; Berridge & Kringelbach, 2008). For a socially gregarious species like the zebra finch, motivation to seek social affiliation is important for survival, attention to social feedback during development is necessary for learning a reproductively successful song, and attention to social context in adult males is vital for attracting a mate. Given that songbirds are motivated to produce song at high rates in multiple social contexts, it is likely that singing is linked to reward. In humans, adults exhibit robust fMRI activation in the ventral striatum—a region involved in reward processing—when successfully learning new words, suggesting that language learning is intrinsically rewarding (Ripolles et al., 2014).

The idea that vocalization is intrinsically rewarding has also been investigated in a non-oscine bird, the ring dove (*Streptopelia risoria*), in which male courtship involves cooing to a female. Oestrogen then acts on the midbrain song nucleus (mICo) of the female, inducing her to coo in response (Cohen & Cheng, 1981). The female's coo, not the male's, causes an endocrine cascade in the female which results in egg laying (Cheng, 2003).

In order to investigate whether song is intrinsically rewarding in songbirds, Riters and Stevenson (2012) used a conditioned place preference paradigm to assess the reward value of directed singing (at a social partner) versus undirected song. When placed in an apparatus with two distinctive sides, male zebra finches preferred to spend time on the side where they had previously produced undirected song, suggesting that singing is coupled with reward state. They displayed no preference for the side of the apparatus in which they had previously sung directed song. This indicates that the role of reward in song production differs depending on social context, with directed and undirected song relying on different mechanisms of reward. Directed song is likely externally reinforced by conspecifics, with the associated reward value resulting from successful social feedback elicitation, mate attraction, or copulation. In line with this hypothesis, males that produced directed song but failed to attract a female developed an aversion to the side of the apparatus where they had sung. Riters and Stevenson suggest that production of undirected song, without immediate social reinforcement, may instead rely on an intrinsic reward system and the act of producing undirected song could activate neural reward systems. However, in light of work suggesting that undirected song also serves a communicative purpose for more distal recipients, this hypothesis may need to be revisited (Dunn & Zann, 1996). What mechanisms might underlie the reward value of song, and how is it modulated in different social contexts?

A leading candidate for the cause of context-dependent neuronal activity in the AFP is dopamine, a catecholamine neurotransmitter and an important contributor to the neural mechanisms allowing animals to pursue reward (Koob, 1996). Goal-directed, socially motivated vocal behaviours, such as ultrasonic vocalizations in rats anticipating a social reward, can be stimulated by dopamine (Wintink & Brudzynski, 2001). In songbirds, dopamine plays a primary role in sexually motivated song directed towards females (Heimovics et al., 2009), and peripheral injections of dopamine agonists stimulate song produced in response to the introduction of a female, whereas antagonists inhibit song (Rauceo et al., 2007; Schroeder & Riters, 2006). Song produced in a social context appears to be highly rewarding, as elevated dopamine levels in the striatum of birds during directed singing resemble those after drug administration in mammals (Sasaki et al., 2006). The neural song system is strongly innervated by catecholaminergic neurons (Appeltants et al., 2001; Liao et al., 2013), which is not seen in comparable forebrain areas in bird species which do not sing (Moons et al., 1994). Catecholaminergic innervation of the song system is also much stronger in male zebra finches than in non-singing females (Bottjer, 1992).

Dopamine also contributes to behavioural reinforcement that mediates appetitive learning (Panksepp & Moskal, 2008). Dopaminergic neurons in the VTA (a mesolimbic region) of monkeys trained on an operant task encode discrepancies between the expected reward normally delivered to them following a conditioned stimulus, and whether or not the reward is actually delivered (Schultz et al., 1993). Intense social interactions also result in increased glutamate activity in VTA (Huang & Hessler, 2008). In the zebra finch, EGR-1 expression in catecholaminergic neurons in VTA is significantly higher in birds which have been tutored socially than in untutored and passively tutored birds, suggesting that it is social interaction, not merely hearing song, that leads to activity in VTA (Chen et al., 2016). In songbirds, VTA is a primary source of dopaminergic input to both LMAN and Area X (Gale & Perkel, 2006; Lewis et al., 1981), where it also regulates synaptic plasticity (Ding & Perkel, 2004) and may encode prediction errors in song production. VTA neurons are known to exhibit singing-related activity, and projections from VTA to the song system modulate early gene activity related to social context (Hara et al., 2007).

Dopamine levels in Area X are elevated more during directed song than undirected song (Sasaki et al., 2006), and infusion of dopamine antagonist near Area X (though possibly also affecting LMAN) increases variability during directed song (Leblois et al., 2010), hinting that dopamine may function as a regulator of AFP activity. Given that more than 95% of Area-X-projecting VTA neurons are dopaminergic (Person et al., 2008), changes in VTA activity likely affect the release of dopamine in the AFP, leading to changes in song output and variability. When perceived song quality is distorted with auditory feedback, VTA neuron activity is repressed, encoding this performance error (Gadagkar et al., 2016). Therefore, when a bird makes a vocal 'mistake' which does not match the memorized tutor song, or fails to elicit a wing stroke or other positive feedback from a conspecific, VTA neurons may detect this error and modulate song away from it. This idea is supported by the finding that lesions of dopaminergic inputs to Area X greatly impair vocal learning in the Bengalese finch, while having no detectable effect on vocal performance (Hoffmann et al., 2016).

Particularly among neuroscientists, song learning and the reward value driving it is considered strictly internally computed, the sole result of the young bird comparing its vocal output to its memorized template. However, just as monkeys can detect errors and learn to correct them for an external reward of juice, songbird vocal learning can be guided by external factors. A recent study found that spiking activity in Area X neurons was modulated by food rewards and reward signals in an operant task. However, the authors concluded that the role of Area X in general learning is 'limited and vestigial' (Seki et al., 2014). In contrast, we believe that the contribution of Area X to song learning is vital, and it may be the region that allows external social stimuli to affect song. Area X is highly sensitive to social context, and exhibits a marked, consistent, and rapid-onset response in electrophysiological activity when a female is introduced (Hessler & Doupe, 1999a). Several studies also suggest that Area X is primarily driving song learning rather than production, as the influence of the AFP on motor output is reduced in adults singing stable songs compared to juveniles singing plastic songs (Bottjer et al., 1984; Scharff & Nottebohm, 1991; Sohrabji et al., 1990).

Such differing levels of activation in different social contexts may reflect a varying level of arousal, or could be specifically related to the communicative function of singing to another bird. In cowbirds, juveniles actively monitor conspecific listeners (West & King, 1988), and it seems probable that zebra finches are doing the same. Area X, via dopaminergic input from VTA neurons, may be responsible for altering the song in response to social feedback. It may also send song-related information back to VTA via the ventral pallidum, creating a two-way path between socially modulated song learning and reward value. Females have been shown to greatly prefer the song of their mate over the song of other conspecifics (Woolley & Doupe, 2008), suggesting that females are most aroused by song elements similar to those of their mate, resulting in maternal wing strokes that may drive song learning towards paternal song.

In order for rapid social signals to precisely affect the song-learning trajectory by targeting specific syllables, Area X would need to receive information on both the precise time in the song at which feedback was received, and the current variability and structure of the song. Area X receives input from HVC in timed bursts which are brief and precisely locked to one time point in the song with precision on a submillisecond scale (Kozhevnikov & Fee, 2007).

This demonstrates that Area X receives a sparse and precise representation of the current time in the song (Fee & Goldberg, 2011), which could be used for Area X to generate a signal to drive variability in LMAN at a specific moment in the song sequence. LMAN also projects indirectly to Area X via axon collaterals in RA, which enables every neuron in LMAN driving vocal variability to be directly 'observed' by Area X (Bottjer & Sengelaub, 1989; Vates et al., 1997). Together, this would allow Area X to receive a social-reward signal via VTA neurons in response to external feedback, identify the precise time in the song at which the feedback was received, accordingly alter the level of song-structure variability at that time point, and then send this information back to social-reward and motivation centres. This hypothesis has never been directly tested, as the role and form of social feedback in zebra finches is only just being discovered, and no mechanisms of socially guided vocal learning have been investigated at the neural level in this species.

14.7 Conclusions: Social-Motivational Learning in Context

Behavioural similarities between birdsong and human speech are matched by parallels in the neural system (Bolhuis et al., 2010; Doupe & Kuhl, 1999). Both share a neural dissociation between brain regions involved in the production and learning of vocalizations on the one hand, and in auditory memory and perception on the other (Bolhuis et al., 2012; Gobes & Bolhuis, 2007). Speech and language in humans involves Broca's area and associated regions in the frontal lobe, while perception and memory involve Wernicke's area and temporal lobe areas (Bolhuis et al., 2010). Human language is thought to be dependent on the cortex. However, language often develops even in cases of severe cortical damage or complete loss of either the left or right cortical hemisphere (Bates et al., 2001). While catastrophic damage to cortical and sensory systems may leave language unscathed, any alteration to motivational systems proves extremely detrimental (Syal & Finlay, 2011). Until recently, the avian song nuclei were thought to be homologous to mammalian cortical domains (Jarvis et al., 2005), but more recent embryological evidence suggests avian vocal areas are limbic (Medina, 2007). As previously discussed, in mammals, limbic areas such as the amygdala and basal forebrain give rise to circuitry involved in social motivation. Placing song-learning circuitry regions in areas associated with social reward (see Figure 14.2) opens the possibility that vocal learning is directly coupled with social motivation, and that similar processes may underlie human language learning (Syal & Finlay, 2011).

Virtually all behavioural systems that incorporate learning of any sort are driven by a motivational context. The motivation and social circuits of the brain are inextricably connected, predisposing gregarious organisms to attach reward value to social partners. All that is required for socially guided vocal learning to occur is for evolution to lead to the connection of the social-motivation system to the vocal-learning system. If song circuitry is indeed homologous to the basal forebrain and amygdala—regions intimately connected to social-motivational circuitry—rather than the neocortex as traditionally presumed, we must use this new perspective to seek homology to songbirds in other vocally learning organisms. Another commonly studied socially guided vocal learner, and potentially as equally excellent a model organism for birds as birds are for them, is the human infant. Just as zebra finches can learn from a taped song only when playing is contingent on their own key pressing (Adret, 1993) and grey parrots fail to learn from non-interactive vocal models (Pepperberg, 1999), human infants are dependent on response contingency to develop mature vocalizations (Goldstein & Schwade, 2008). Infants are sensitive to social contingencies from a young age, and demonstrate varying levels of sensitivity to contingency depending on the general responsiveness of their caregivers (Bigelow & Rochat, 2006).

In species that have evolved socially guided vocal learning, a unique link has been forged between social circuitry and vocal learning systems, such that learning is driven by social motivation. The 'social gating hypothesis' was first advanced in work on human infant language acquisition, proposing that language is gated by the motivating properties of social interaction such as attention and arousal (Kuhl, 2007). It has long been known that human parents alter their behaviour when interacting with infants, most noticeably changing the prosody of their speech to generate *infant-directed speech*. Compared to adult-directed speech, infant-directed speech is higher in pitch and contains longer pauses, more repetition, and shorter utterances (Fernald et al., 1989), and more effectively attracts and sustains infant attention (Kuhl et al., 2005; Locke, 1993).

It was recently found that adult zebra finches alter the structure of their vocalizations when interacting with juveniles in a manner strikingly similar to human infant-directed speech. When singing to a juvenile, adults lengthen the intervals between motifs, increase goodness of pitch, and repeat more introductory notes before song. Juveniles were also significantly more attentive to this 'pupil-directed' song than to undirected song, and those which received a greater proportion of pupil-directed song during development learned better matches to tutor song (Chen et al., 2016). This presents the intriguing possibility that adult finches could be actively facilitating successful song learning in juveniles, and that, as in human parents and infants, shared attention between tutor and pupil drives vocal learning. Young zebra finches quickly shift the pitch of their song to match that of a movie of an adult tutor facing towards them, but not one facing away from them (Ljubičić et al., 2016).

As with zebra finches learning song, human infants learn from caregiver responses which are contingent on their own vocalizations, be they vocal (a tutor song or a spoken word) or non-vocal (a wing stroke or a smile) (Goldstein et al, 2003; Goldstein & Schwade, 2008). Infants also fail to learn the phonemic contrasts of a foreign language unless they are presented by a live, interactive tutor (Kuhl et al., 2003). Learning in both infants and songbirds may be gated by shared attention and social motivation, a process potentially enabled by similar neural circuitry linking vocal learning and social reward.

An ecologically valid and more complete understanding of vocal learning requires the incorporation of social factors. Social context and motivation affect the vocal-learning system at virtually every level, both behaviourally and neurally. In humans and zebra finches, normal learning fails to occur without social exposure, and moment-to-moment social feedback to immature vocalizations shapes and guides vocal learning. In the songbird brain, social exposure during development leads to growth of HVC, while social context affects activity levels in Area X, which receives dopaminergic input from regions involved in social reward and motivation. Future research efforts should focus on the effects of manipulation of social-motivational circuitry on social behaviour, including sensitivity to social cues, and the resulting effects on song-learning outcomes.

References

Adar, E., Lotem, A., & Barnea, A. (2008). The effect of social environment on singing behavior in the zebra finch (*Taeniopygia guttata*) and its implication for neuronal recruitment. *Behavioural Brain Research*, 187, 178–184.

Adret, P. (1993). Operant conditioning, song learning and imprinting to taped song in the zebra finch. *Animal Behaviour*, 46, 149–159.

Adret, P. (2004). Vocal imitation in blindfolded zebra finches (*Taeniopygia guttata*) is facilitated in the presence of a non-singing conspecific female. *Journal of Ethology*, 22, 29–35.

Adret-Hausberger, M., Guttinger, H. R., & Merkel, F. W. (1990). Individual life history and song repertoire changes in a colony of starlings (*Sturnus vulgaris*). *Ethology*, 84, 265–280.

Agmo, A. & Berenfeld, R. (1990). Reinforcing properties of ejaculation in the male rat: role of opioids and dopamine. *Behavioral Neuroscience*, 104, 177–182.

Akçay, C., Campbell, S. E., Reed, V. A., & Beecher, M. D. (2014). Song sparrows do not learn more song from aggressive tutors. *Animal Behaviour*, 94, 151–159.

Alvarez-Buylla, A. & Kirn, J. R. (1997). Birth, migration, incorporation, and death of vocal control neurons in adult songbirds. *Journal of Neurobiology*, 33, 585–601.

Andalman, A. S. & Fee, M. S. (2009). A basal ganglia–forebrain circuit in the songbird biases motor output to avoid vocal errors. *PNAS*, 106, 12518–12523.

Appeltants D., Ball G. F., & Balthazart J. (2001). The distribution of tyrosine hydroxylase in the canary brain: demonstration of a specific and sexually dimorphic catecholaminergic innervation of the telencephalic song control nulcei. *Cell and Tissue Research*, 304, 237–59.

Aronov D., Veit L., Goldberg J. H., & Fee M. S. (2011). Two distinct modes of forebrain circuit dynamics underlie temporal patterning in the vocalizations of young songbirds. *Journal of Neuroscience*, 31, 3009–3011.

Ashmore, R. C., Wild, J. M., & Schmidt, M. F. (2005). Brainstem and forebrain contributions to the generation of learned motor behaviors for song. *Journal of Neuroscience*, 25, 8543–8554.

Baptista, L. F. (1975). Song dialects and demes in sedentary populations of the white-crowned sparrow (*Zonotrichia leucophrys nuttali*). *University of California Publications in Zoology*, 105, 1–52.

Baptista, L. F. & Gaunt, S. L. L. (1997). Social interaction and vocal development in birds. In: C. T. Snowdon & M. Hausberger (eds) *Social Interaction Influences on Vocal Development* (pp. 23–42). Cambridge: Cambridge University Press.

Baptista, L. F. & Petrinovich, L. (1984). Social interaction, sensitive phases and the song template hypothesis in the white-crowned sparrow. *Animal Behaviour*, 32, 172–181.

Baptista, L. F. & Petrinovich, L. (1986). Song development in the white-crowned sparrow: social factors and sex differences. *Animal Behaviour*, 34, 1359–1371.

Bates, E., Reilly, J., Wulfeck, B., Dronkers, N., Opie, M., Fenson, J., … Herbst, K. (2001). Differential effects of unilateral lesions on language production in children and adults. *Brain and Language*, 79, 223–265.

Beecher, M. D. (2016). Birdsong learning as a social process. *Animal Behaviour*, http://dx.doi.org/10.1016/j.anbehav.2016.09.001

Beecher, M. D., Burt, J. M., O'Loghlen, A. L., Templeton, C. N., & Campbell, S. E. (2007). Bird song learning in an eavesdropping context. *Animal Behaviour*, 73, 929–935.

Beecher, M. D., Campbell, S. F., & Stoddard, P. K. (1994). Correlation of song learning and territory establishment strategies in the song sparrow. *PNAS*, 91, 1450–1454.

Bell, B. A., Phan, M. L., & Vicario, D. S. (2015). Neural responses in songbird forebrain reflect learning rates, acquired salience, and stimulus novelty after auditory discrimination training. *Journal of Neurophysiology*, 113, 1480–1492.

Berridge, K. C. & Kringelbach, M. L. (2008). Affective neuroscience of pleasure: reward in humans and animals. *Psychopharmacology (Berl)*, 199, 457–480.

Bigelow, A. E. & Rochat, P. (2006). Two-month-old infants' sensitivity to social contingency in mother–infant and stranger–infant interaction. *Infancy*, 9, 313–325.

Bohner, J. (1983). Song learning in the zebra finch (*Taeniopygia guttata*): selectivity in choice of a tutor and accuracy of song copies. *Animal Behaviour*, 31, 231–237.

Bolhuis, J. J., Gobes, S. M. H., Terpsta, N. J., den Boer-Visser, A. M., & Zandberger, M. A. (2012). Learning-related neuronal activation in the zebra finch song system nucleus HVC in response to bird's own song. *PLoS One*, 7, e41556.

Bolhuis J. J., Okanoya K., & Scharff C. (2010). Twitter evolution: converging mechanisms in birdsong and human speech. *Nature Reviews Neuroscience*, 11, 747–759.

Bottjer, S. W. (1992). The distribution of tyrosine hydroxylase immunoreactivity in the brains of male and female zebra finches. *Journal of Neurobiology*, 24, 51–69.

Bottjer S. W. & Sengelaub D. R. (1989). Cell death during development of a forebrain nucleus involved with vocal learning in zebra finches. *Journal of Neurobiology*, 20, 609–618.

Bottjer, S. W., Miesner, E. A., & Arnold, A. P. (1984). Forebrain lesions disrupt development but not maintenance of song in passerine birds. *Science*, 224, 901–903.

Brainard, M. S. & Doupe, A. J. (2000). Auditory feedback in learning and maintenance of vocal behaviour. *Nature Reviews Neuroscience*, 1, 31–40.

Brenowitz, E. A., Margoliash, D., & Nordeen, K. W. (1997). An introduction to birdsong and the avian song system. *Journal of Neurobiology*, 33, 485–500.

Catchpole, C. K. & Slater, P. J. B. (1995). *Bird Song: Biological Themes and Variations*. Cambridge: Cambridge University Press.

Chaiken, M., Bohner, J., & Marler, P. (1993). Song acquisition in European starlings (*Sturnus vulgaris*): a comparison of the song of live-tutored, untutored, and wild caught males. *Animal Behaviour*, 46, 1079–1090.

Changeux, J. P., Heidman, T., & Patte, P. (1984). Learning by selection. In: P. Marler & H. S. Terrace (eds) *The Biology of Learning* (pp. 115–133). Berlin: Springer-Verlag.

Chen, Y., Matheson, L. E., & Sakata, J. T. (2016). Mechanisms underlying the social enhancement of vocal learning in songbirds. *PNAS*, 113, 6641–6646.

Cheng, M. F. (2003). Vocal self-stimulation: from the ring dove story to emotion-based vocal communication. *Advances in the Study of Behavior*, 33, 309–353.

Clayton, N. S. (1987). Song tutor choice in Zebra finches. *Animal Behaviour*, 35, 714–721.

Cohen, J. & Cheng, M. F. (1981). The role of the midbrain in courtship behavior of the female ring dove (*Streptopelia risoria*): evidence from radiofrequency lesion and hormone implant studies. *Brain Research*, 207, 279–301.

Dave A. S. & Margoliash D. (2000). Song replay during sleep and computational rules for sensorimotor vocal learning. *Science*, 290, 812–816.

Derégnaucourt, S., Poirier, C., Kant, A. V., Linden, A. V., & Gahr, M. (2013). Comparisons of different methods to train a young zebra finch (*Taeniopygia guttata*) to learn a song. *Journal of Physiology—Paris*, 107, 210–218.

DeWolfe, B. B., Baptista, L. F., & Petrinovich, L. (1989). Song development and territory establishment in Nuttal's white-crowned sparrows. *Condor*, 97, 376–389.

Ding L. & Perkel D. J. (2004). Long-term potentiation in an avian basal ganglia nucleus essential for vocal learning. *Journal of Neuroscience*, 24, 488–494.

Doupe A. J. (1997). Song- and order-selective neurons in the songbird anterior forebrain and their emergence during vocal development. *Journal of Neuroscience,* 17, 1147–1167.

Doupe A. J. & Kuhl P. K. (1999). Birdsong and human speech: common themes and mechanisms. *Annual Review of Neuroscience,* 22, 567–631.

Doupe, A. J., Perkel, D. J., Reiner, A., & Stern, E. A. (2005). Birdbrains could teach basal ganglia research a new song. *Trends in Neuroscience,* 28, 353–363.

Dunn, A. M. & Zann, R. A. (1996). Undirected song in wild zebra finch flocks: contexts and effects of mate removal. *Ethology,* 10, 529–539.

Eales, L. A. (1985). Song learning in zebra finches: some effects of song model availability on what is learnt and when. *Animal Behaviour,* 33, 1293–1300.

Eales, L. A. (1987). Song learning in female-raised zebra finches: another look at the sensitive phase. *Animal Behaviour,* 35, 1356–1365.

Eales, L. A. (1989). The influences of visual and vocal interaction on song learning in zebra finches. *Animal Behaviour,* 37, 507–508.

Fee, M. S. & Goldberg, J. H. (2011). A hypothesis for basal ganglia-dependent reinforcement learning in the songbird. *Neuroscience,* 198, 152–170.

Fernald, A., Taeschner, T., Dun, J., Papousek, M., de Boysson Bardies, B., & Fukui, I. (1989). A cross-language study of prosodic modifications in mothers' and fathers' speech to preverbal infants. *Journal of Child Language,* 16, 477–501.

Fromkin, V., Krashen, S., Curtis, S., Rigler, D., & Rigler, M. (1974). The development of language in Genie: a case of language acquisition beyond the 'critical period'. *Brain and Language,* 1, 81–107.

Fusani, L., Giordano, M., Day, L. B., & Schlinger, B. A. (2007). High-speed video analysis reveals individual variability in the courtship displays of male golden-collared manakins. *Ethology,* 113, 964–972.

Gadagkar, V., Puzerey, P. A., Chen, R., Baird-Daniel, E., Farhand, A. R., & Goldberg, J. H. (2016). Dopamine neurons encode performance error in singing birds. *Science,* 354, 1278–1282.

Gale, S. D. & Perkel D. J. (2006). Physiological properties of zebra finch ventral tegmental area and substantia nigra pars compacta neurons. *Journal of Neurophysiology,* 96, 2295–2306.

Gilbert, C.D., Li, W., & Piesch, V. (2009). Perceptual learning and adult cortical plasticity. *Journal of Physiology,* 587, 2743–2751.

Gobes, S. M. H. & Bolhuis, J. J. (2007). Bird song memory: a neural dissociation between song recognition and production. *Current Biology,* 17, 789–793.

Goldberg, J. H., Adler, A., Bergman, H., & Fee, M. S. (2010). Singing-related neural activity distinguishes two putative pallidal cell types in the songbird basal ganglia: comparison to the primate internal and external pallidal segments. *Journal of Neuroscience,* 30, 7088–7098.

Goldberg, J. H. & Fee, M. S. (2011). Vocal babbling in songbirds requires the basal ganglia-recipient motor thalamus but not the basal ganglia. *Journal of Neurophysiology,* 105, 2729–2739.

Goldstein, M. H., King, A. P., & West, M. J. (2003). Social interaction shapes babbling: testing parallels between birdsong and speech. *PNAS,* 100, 8030–8035.

Goldstein, M. H. & Schwade, J. A. (2008). Social feedback to infants' babbling facilitates rapid phonological learning. *Psychological Science,* 19, 515–523.

Goodson, J. L. (2005). The vertebrate social behavior network: evolutionary themes and variations. *Hormones and Behavior,* 48, 11–22.

Goodson, J. L., Evans, A. K., Lindberg, L., & Allen, C. D. (2005). Neuro-evolutionary patterning of sociality. *Proceedings of the Royal Society B,* 272, 227–235.

Hahnloser, R. H., Kozhevnikov, A. A., & Fee, M. S. (2002). An ultra-sparse code underlies the generation of neural sequences in a songbird. *Nature*, 419, 65–70.

Hara, E., Kubikova, L., Hessler, N. A., & Jarvis, E. D. (2007). Role of the midbrain dopaminergic system in modulation of vocal brain activation by social context. *European Journal of Neuroscience*, 25, 3406–3416.

Harlow, H. F. & Harlow, M. K. (1962). Social deprivation in monkeys. *Scientific American*, 207, 136–146.

Healy, K., McNally, L., Ruxton, G. D., Cooper, N., & Jackson, A. L. (2013). Metabolic rate and body size are linked with perception of temporal information. *Animal Behaviour*, 86, 685–696.

Heimovics, S. A., Cornil, C. A., Ball, G. F., & Riters, L. V. (2009). D1-like dopamine receptor density in nuclei involved in social behavior correlates with song in a context-dependent fashion in male European starlings. *Neuroscience*, 159, 962–73.

Hermann, K. & Arnold, A. P. (1991). The development of afferent projections to the robust archistriatal nucleus in male zebra finches: a quantitative electron microscopic study. *Journal of Neuroscience*, 11, 2063–2074.

Hessler, N. A. & Doupe, A. J. (1999a). Social context modulates singing-related neural activity in the songbird forebrain. *Nature Neuroscience*, 2, 209–211.

Hessler, N. A. & Doupe, A. J. (1999b). Singing-related neural activity in a dorsal forebrain-basal ganglia circuit of adult zebra finches. *Journal of Neuroscience*, 19, 10461–10481.

Hoffmann, L. A., Saravanan, V., Wood, A. N., He, L., & Sober, S. J. (2016). Dopaminergic contribution to vocal learning. *Journal of Neuroscience*, 36, 2176–2189.

Houx, B. B. & ten Cate, C. (1998). Do contingencies with tutor behavior influence song learning in zebra finches? *Behaviour*, 5, 599–614.

Huang, Y. C. & Hessler, N. A. (2008). Social modulation during songbird courtship potentiates midbrain dopaminergic neurons. *PLoS One*, 3, e3281.

Immelmann, K. (1969). Song development in the zebra finch and other estrildid finches. In: R. A. Hinde (ed.) *Bird Vocalizations* (pp. 61–81). Cambridge: Cambridge University Press.

Iyengar, S., Viswanathan, S. S., & Bottjer, S. W. (1999). Development of topography within song control circuitry of zebra finches during the sensitive period for song learning. *Journal of Neuroscience*, 19, 6037–6057.

Jarvis, E. D., Scharff, C., Grossman, M. R., Ramos, J. A., & Nottebohm, F. (1998). For whom the bird sings: context-dependent gene expression. *Neuron*, 21, 775–788.

Jarvis, E. D., Gunturkun, O., Bruce, L., Csillag, A., Karten, H., Kuenzel, W., … Butler, A. B. (2005). Avian brains and a new understanding of vertebrate brain evolution. *Nature Reviews Neuroscience*, 6, 151–159.

Jerne, N. (1967). Antibodies and learning: selection versus instruction. In: G. C. Quarton, T. Melnechuk, & F. O. Schmitt (eds) *The Neurosciences, a Study Program* (pp. 200–205). New York: Rockefeller University Press.

Jones, A. & Slater, P. (1993). Do young male zebra finches prefer to learn songs that are familiar to females with which they are housed? *Animal Behaviour*, 46, 616–617.

Jones, A. & Slater, P. (1996). The role of aggression in song tutor choice in the zebra finch: cause or effect? *Behaviour*, 133, 103–115.

Kao, M. H. & Brainard, M. S. (2006). Lesions of an avian basal ganglia circuit prevent context-dependent changes to song variability. *Journal of Neurophysiology*, 96, 1441–1455.

Kao, M. H., Doupe, A. J., & Brainard, M. S. (2005). Contributions of an avian basal ganglia-forebrain circuit to real-time modulation of song. *Nature*, 433, 638–643

Kao, M. H., Wright, B. D., & Doupe, A. J. (2008). Neurons in a forebrain nucleus required for vocal plasticity rapidly switch between precise firing and variable bursting depending on social context. *Journal of Neuroscience*, 28, 13232–13247.

Kirwan, G. M. & Green, G. (2012). *Cotingas and Manakins*. Princeton, NJ: Princeton University Press.

Konishi, M. (1965). The role of auditory feedback in the control of vocalization in the white-crowned sparrow. *Zeitschrift fur Tierpsychologie*, 22, 770–783.

Koob, G. F. (1996). Hedonic valence, dopamine and motivation. *Molecular Psychiatry*, 1, 186–189.

Kozhevnikov, A. A. & Fee, M. S. (2007). Singing-related activity of identified HVC neurons in the zebra finch. *Journal of Neurophysiology*, 97, 4271–4283.

Kroodsma, D. & Konishi, M. (1991). A suboscine bird (eastern phoebe, *Sayornis phoebe*) develops normal song without auditory feedback. *Animal Behaviour*, 42, 477–484.

Kroodsma, D. E. & Miller, E. H. (1996). *Ecology and Evolution of Acoustic Communication in Birds*. Ithaca, NY: Comstock.

Kroodsma, D. E. & Verner, J. (1978). Complex singing behaviors among *Cistothorus* wrens. *Auk*, 95, 703–716.

Kuhl, P. K. (2007). Is speech learning 'gated' by the social brain? *Developmental Science*, 10, 110–120.

Kuhl, P. K., Coffey-Corina, S., Padden, D., & Dawson, G. (2005). Links between social and linguistic processing of speech in preschool children with autism: behavioral and electrophysiological evidence. *Developmental Science*, 8, F1–F12.

Kuhl, P. K., Tsao, F. M., & Liu, H. M. (2003). Foreign-language experience in infancy: effects of short-term exposure and social interaction on phonetic learning. *PNAS*, 100, 9096–9101.

Lane, H. L. (1976). *The Wild Boy of Aveyron*. Cambridge, MA: Harvard University Press.

Lanyon, W. E. (1979). Development of song in the wood thrush (*Hylocichla mustelina*) with notes on a technique for hand-rearing passerines from the egg. *American Museum Novitates*, 2666, 1–27.

Leblois, A., Wendel, B. J., & Perkel, D. J. (2010). Striatal dopamine modulates basal ganglia output and regulates social context-dependent behavioral variability through D1 receptors. *Journal of Neuroscience*, 30, 5730–5743.

Lenneberg, E. H. (1967). *Biological Foundations of Language*. New York: Wiley.

Leonardo, A. (2004). Experimental test of the birdsong error-correction model. *PNAS*, 101, 16935–16940.

Leonardo, A. & Fee, M. S. (2005). Ensemble coding of vocal control in birdsong. *Journal of Neuroscience*, 25, 652–661.

Lewis, J. W., Ryan, S. M., Arnold, A. P., & Butcher, L. L. (1981). Evidence for a catecholaminergic projection to area X in the zebra finch. *Journal of Comparative Neurology*, 196, 347–354.

Liao, C., Wang, S., Pan, X., Hou, G., & Li, D. (2013). Dopamine modulates the excitability of projection neurons in the robust nucleus of the arcopallium in adult zebra finches. *PLoS One*, 8, e82497.

Lindsay, W. R., Houck, J. T., Giuliano, C. E., & Day, L. B. (2015). Acrobatic courtship display coevolves with brain size in manakins (*Pipridae*). *Brain, Behavior, and Evolution*, 85, 29–36.

Lipkind, D., Nottebohm, F., Rado, R., & Barnea, A. (2002). Social change affects the survival of new neurons in the forebrain of adult songbirds. *Behavioral Brain Research*, 133, 31–43.

Ljubičić, I., Bruno, J. H., & Tchernichovski, O. (2016). Social influences on song learning. *Current Opinion in Behavioral Sciences*, 7, 101–107.

Locke, J. (1993). *The Path to Spoken Language*. Cambridge, MA: Harvard University Press.

Long, M. A. & Fee, M. S. (2008). Using temperature to analyze temporal dynamics in the song-bird motor pathway. *Nature*, 456, 189–194.

Mann, N. I. & Slater, P. J. B. (1994). What causes young male zebra finches, *Taeniopygia guttata*, to choose their father as song tutor? *Animal Behaviour*, 47, 671–677.

Mann, N. I. & Slater, P. J. B. (1995). Song tutor choice by zebra finches in aviaries. *Animal Behaviour*, 49, 811–820.

Mann, N. I., Slater, P. J. B., Eales, L. A., & Richards, C. (1991). The influence of visual stimuli on song tutor choice in the Zebra finch, *Taeniopygia guttata*. *Animal Behaviour*, 42, 285–293.

Margoliash, D. (1983). Acoustic parameters underlying the responses of song-specific neurons in the white-crowned sparrow. *Journal of Neuroscience*, 3, 1039–1057.

Marler, P. (1970). A comparative approach to vocal learning: song development in white-crowned sparrows. *Journal of Comparative and Physiological Psychology*, 71, 1–25.

Marler, P. (1991). Song-learning behavior: the interface with neuroethology. *Trends in Neuroscience*, 14, 199–206.

Marler, P. & Nelson, D. A. (1993). Action-based learning: a new form of developmental plasticity in bird song. *Netherlands Journal of Zoology*, 43, 91–103.

Marler, P. & Peters, S. (1982). Developmental overproduction and selective attrition: new processes in the epigenesis of birdsong. *Developmental Psychobiology*, 15, 369–378.

McCasland, J. S. (1987). Neuronal control of birdsong production. *Journal of Neuroscience*, 7, 23–39.

McCasland, J. S. & Konishi, M. (1981). Interaction between auditory and motor activities in an avian song control nucleus. *PNAS*, 78, 7815–7819.

Medina, L. (2007). Do birds and reptiles possess homologues of mammalian visual, somato-sensory and motor cortices? In: J. H. Kaas (ed.) *Evolution of Nervous Systems* (Vol. 2) (pp. 163–194). New York: Academic Press.

Menyhart, O., Carouso-Peck, S., Chou, R., DeVoogd, T. J., & Goldstein, M.H. (in prep). Socially guided song learning in the zebra finch (*Taeniopygia guttata*): effects at multiple time scales.

Mooney, R. (2004). Synaptic mechanisms for auditory-vocal integration and the correction of vocal errors. *Annals of the New York Academy of Sciences*, 1016, 476–494.

Mooney, R. (2009). Neural mechanisms for learned birdsong. *Learning and Memory*, 16, 655–669.

Moons, L., Van Gils, J., Ghijsels, E., & Vandesande, F. (1994). Immunocytochemical localization of L-DOPA and dopamine in the brain of the chicken (*Gallus domesticus*). *Journal of Comparative Neurology*, 346, 97–118.

Morris, D. (1954). The reproductive behaviour of the zebra finch (*Poephila guttata*), with special reference to pseudofemale behaviour and displacement activities. *Behaviour*, 6, 271–322.

Newman, S. W. (1999). The medial extended amygdala in male reproductive behavior: a node in the mammalian social behavior network. *Annals of the New York Academy of Sciences*, 877, 242–257.

Nice, M. M. (1943). Studies in the life history of the song sparrow II. The behavior of the song sparrow and other passerines. *Transactions of the Linnaean Society*, 6, 1–238.

Nottebohm, F. (1993). The search for neural mechanisms that define the sensitive period for song learning in birds. *Netherlands Journal of Zoology*, 43, 193–234.

O'Connell, L. A. & Hofmann, H. A. (2011). The vertebrate mesolimbic reward system and social behavior network: a comparative synthesis. *Journal of Comparative Neurology*, 519, 3599–3639.

Odom, K. J., Hall, M. L., Riebel, K., Omland, K. E., & Langmore, N. E. (2014). Female song is widespread and ancestral in songbirds. *Nature Communications*, 5, 3379.

Olveczky, B. P., Andalman, A. S., & Fee, M. S. (2005). Vocal experimentation in the juvenile songbird requires a basal ganglia circuit. *PLoS Biology*, 3, e153

Panksepp, J. & Moskal, J. (2008). Dopamine and seeking: subcortical reward systems and appetitive urges. In: A. J. Elliot (ed.) *Handbook of Approach and Avoidance Motivation* (pp. 67–88). New York: Taylor and Francis.

Payne, R. B. & Payne, L. L. (1997). Field observations, experimental design, and the time and place of learning bird song. In: C. T. Snowdon & M. Hausberger (eds) *Social Influences on Vocal Development* (pp. 57–84). Cambridge: Cambridge University Press.

Pepperberg, I. M. (1993). A review of the effects of social interaction on vocal learning in African grey parrots (*Psittacus erithacus*). *Netherlands Journal of Zoology*, 43, 104–124.

Pepperberg, I. M. (1999). *The Alex studies: Cognitive and Communicative Abilities of Grey Parrots.* Cambridge, MA: Harvard University Press.

Person, A. L., Gale, S. D., Farries, M. A., & Perkel, D. J. (2008). Organization of the songbird basal ganglia, including area X. *Journal of Comparative Neurology*, 508, 840–866.

Prather, J. F., Peters, S., Nowicki, S., & Mooney, R. (2008). Precise auditory-vocal mirroring in neurons for learned vocal communication. *Nature*, 451, 305–310.

Price, P. (1979). Developmental determinants of structure in zebra finch song. *Journal of Comparative and Physiological Psychology*, 93, 260–277.

Rauceo, S., Harding, C. F., Maldonado, A., Gaysinkaya, L., Tulloch, I., & Rodriguez, E. (2007). Dopaminergic modulation of reproductive behavior and activity in male zebra finches. *Behavioural Brain Research*, 187, 133–139.

Rice, J. O. & Thompson, W. L. (1968). Song development in the indigo bunting. *Animal Behaviour*, 16, 462–469.

Ripollés, P., Marco-Pallarés, J., Hielscher, U., Mestres-Missé, A., Tempelmann, C., Heinze, H., ... Noesselt, T. (2014). The role of reward in word learning and its implications for language acquisition. *Current Biology*, 24, 1–6.

Riters, L. V. & Stevenson, S. A. (2012). Reward and vocal production: song-associated place preference in songbirds. *Physiology & Behavior*, 106, 87–94.

Roper, A. & Zann, R. (2006). The onset of song learning and song tutor selection in fledgling zebra finches. *Ethology*, 112, 458–470.

Sakata, J. T. & Brainard, M. S. (2008). Online contributions of auditory feedback to neural activity in avian song control circuitry. *Journal of Neuroscience*, 28, 11378–11390.

Sasaki, A., Sotnikova, T. D., Gainetdinov, R. R., & Jarvis, E. D. (2006). Social context-dependent singing-regulated dopamine. *Journal of Neuroscience*, 26, 9010–9014.

Scharff, C., Kirn, J. R., Grossman, M., Macklis, J. D., & Nottebohm, F. (2000). Targeted neuronal death affects neuronal replacement and vocal behavior in adult songbirds. *Neuron*, 25, 481–492.

Scharff, C. & Nottebohm, F. (1991). A comparative study of the behavioral deficits following lesions of various parts of the zebra finch song system: implications for vocal learning. *Journal of Neuroscience*, 11, 2896–2913.

Schroeder, M. B. & Riters, L. V. (2006). Pharmacological manipulations of dopamine and opioids have differential effects on sexually motivated song in male European starlings. *Physiology & Behavior*, 88, 575–584.

Schultz, W., Apicella, P., & Ljungberg, T. (1993). Responses of monkey dopamine neurons to reward and conditioned stimuli during successive steps of learning a delayed response task. *Journal of Neuroscience*, 13, 900–913.

Seki, Y., Hessler, N. A., Xie, K., & Okanoya, K. (2014). Food rewards modulate the activity of song neurons in Bengalese finches. *European Journal of Neuroscience*, 39, 975–983.

Seyfarth, R. M. & Cheney, D. L. (1986). Vocal development in vervet monkeys. *Animal Behaviour*, 34, 1640–1658.

Simpson, H. B. & Vicario, D. S. (1990). Brain pathways for learned and unlearned vocalizations differ in zebra finches. *Journal of Neuroscience*, 10, 1541–1556.

Slater, P. J. B., Eales, L. A., & Clayton, N. S. (1988). Song learning in zebra finches (*Taeniopygia guttata*): progress and prospects. *Advances in the Study of Behavior*, 18, 1–34.

Snowdon, C. T. & Hausberger, M. (1997). Introduction. In: C. T. Snowdon & M. Hausberger (eds) *Social Influences on Vocal Development* (pp. 1–6). Cambridge: Cambridge University Press.

Sober, S. J. & Brainard, M. S. (2009). Adult birdsong is actively maintained by error correction. *Nature Neuroscience*, 12, 927–931.

Sohrabji, F., Nordeen, E. J., & Nordeen, K. W. (1990). Selective impairment of song learning following lesions of a forebrain nucleus in the juvenile zebra finch. *Behavioral and Neural Biology*, 53, 51–63.

Sossinka, R. & Bohner, J. (1980). Song types in the zebra finch *Poephila guttata castanotis*. *Zeitschrift für Tierpsychologie*, 53, 123–132.

Syal, S. & Finlay, B. F. (2011). Thinking outside the cortex: social motivation in the evolution and development of language. *Developmental Science*, 14, 417–430.

Takahashi, D. Y., Fenley, A. R., & Ghazanfar, A. A. (2016). Early development of turn-taking with parents shapes vocal acoustics in infant marmoset monkeys. *Philosophical Transactions of the Royal Society B*, 371, 20150370.

Tchernichovski, O., Lints, T., Mitra, P. P., & Nottebohm, F. (1999). Vocal imitation in zebra finches is inversely related to model abundance. *PNAS*, 96, 12901–12904.

Tchernichovski, O. & Nottebohm, F. (1998). Social inhibition of song imitation among sibling male zebra finches. *PNAS*, 95, 8951–8956.

ten Cate, C. (1991). Behaviour-contingent exposure to taped song and zebra finch song learning. *Animal Behaviour*, 42, 857–859.

Thielcke, G. (1970). Learning of song as a possible pacemaker of evolution. *Zeitschrift fuer Zoologische Systematik und Evolutionsforschung*, 8, 309–320.

Thielcke, G. (1984). Gesangslernen beim Gartenbaumlaufer (*Certhia brachydactyla*). *Die Vogelwarte*, 32, 282–297.

Thompson, J. V. & Gentner, T. Q. (2010). Song recognition learning and stimulus-specific weakening of neural responses in the avian auditory forebrain. *Journal of Neurophysiology*, 103, 1785–1797.

Thorpe, W. H. (1958). The learning of song patterns by birds, with especial reference to the song of the chaffinch *Fringilla coelebs*. *Ibis*, 100, 535–570.

Todt, D. & Geberzahn, N. (2003). Age dependent effects of song exposure: song crystalization sets a boundary between fast and delayed vocal imitation. *Animal Behaviour*, 65, 971–979.

Todt, D., Hultsch, H., & Heike, D. (1979). Conditons affecting song acquisition in nightingales (*Luscinia megarhynchos* L.). *Zeitschrift fur Tierpsychologie*, 51, 23–35.

Tumer, E. C. & Brainard, M. S. (2007). Performance variability enables adaptive plasticity of 'crystallized' adult birdsong. *Nature*, 450, 1240–1244.

Van Hout, A. J. M., Pinxten, R., Darras, V. M., & Eens, M. (2012). Testosterone increases repertoire size in an open-ended learner. *Hormones and Behavior*, 62, 563–568.

Vates, G. E., Vicario, D. S., & Nottebohm, F. (1997). Reafferent thalamo-'cortical' loops in the song system of oscine songbirds. *Journal of Comparative Neurology*, 380, 275–290.

Vicario, D. S. & Yohay, K. H. (1993). Song-selective auditory input to a forebrain vocal control nucleus in the zebra finch. *Journal of Neurobiology*, 24, 488–505.

Vyas, A., Harding, C., Borg, L., & Bogdan, D. (2009). Acoustic characteristics, early experience, and endocrine status interact to modulate female zebra finches' behavioral responses to songs. *Hormones and Behavior*, 55, 50–59.

Waser, M. S. & Marler, P. (1977). Song learning in canaries. *Journal of Comparative and Physiological Psychology*, 91, 1–7.

West, M. J. & King, A. P. (1988). Female visual displays affect the development of male song in the cowbird. *Nature*, 334, 244–246.

West, M. J., King, A. P., & Duff, M. A. (1990). Communicating about communicating: when innate is not enough. *Developmental Psychobiology*, 23, 585–598.

Wild, J. M. (2004). Functional neuroanatomy of the sensorimotor control of singing. *Annals of the New York Academy of Sciences*, 1016, 438–462.

Williams, H. (1990). Models for song learning in the zebra finch: fathers or others? *Animal Behaviour*, 39, 745–757.

Williams, H. (2004). Birdsong and singing behavior. *Annals of the New York Academy of Sciences*, 1016, 1–30.

Williams, H., Kilander, K., & Sotanski, M. L. (1993). Untutored song, reproductive success and song learning. *Animal Behaviour*, 45, 695–705.

Williams, H. & Nottebohm, F. (1985). Auditory responses in avian vocal motor neurons: a motor theory for song perception in birds. *Science*, 229, 279–282.

Wintink, A. J. & Brudzynski, S. M. (2001). The related roles of dopamine and glutamate in the initiation of 50-kHz ultrasonic calls in adult rats. *Pharmacology, Biochemistry, and Behavior*, 70, 317–323.

Woolley, S. C. & Doupe, A. J. (2008). Social context-induced song variation affects female behavior and gene expression. *PLoS Biology*, 6, e62.

Yanagihara, S. & Hessler, N. A. (2006). Modulation of singing-related activity in the songbird ventral tegmental area by social context. *European Journal of Neuroscience*, 24, 3619–3627.

Yasukawa, K., Blank, J. L., & Patterson, C. B. (1980). Song repertoires and sexual selection in the red-winged blackbird. *Behavioral Endocrinology and Sociobiology*, 7, 233–238.

CHAPTER 15

....

VOICE-SENSITIVE REGIONS, NEURONS, AND MULTISENSORY PATHWAYS IN THE PRIMATE BRAIN

....

CATHERINE PERRODIN AND CHRISTOPHER I. PETKOV

There is very little difference in people, but that little difference makes a big difference.

(Rags-to-riches businessman and philanthropist,
W. Clement Stone)

15.1 INTRODUCTION

....

IMAGINE a future world where androids, created for the service of humanity, are mass produced and look and speak identically. Socially it would be a vapid world, and because of this would quickly get replaced with one where there are more natural interactions between humans and machines, where every android is an individual, and, at the very least, has a distinct face and voice. Evolutionary pressures have ensured that individual animals can be readily identified by face, voice, or other physical attributes. So nature's playground is full of dashing variability within and between species, because identifying individuals not only makes life more interesting but is important for social interactions and survival.

This handbook considers the intriguing variability in vocal and facial signals that we and other animals use to communicate with each other, and the neurocognitive operations that work on these signals. Our chapter begins with a cursory background, simply to set the stage, into what is a rich history of scientific pursuit more thoroughly discussed elsewhere in this book and the literature (e.g. Blank et al., 2014; Campanella & Belin, 2007; Young & Bruce, 2011). Our contribution to this narrative focuses on the neurobiological correspondences between neural signals and pathways processing voice and face communication signals in the brains of human and non-human primates. How the artificial neural networks of intelligent machines recognize individuals will remain beyond the scope of this chapter, although it will be enthralling in the future to compare machine recognition with the way that living brains solve the problem of recognizing communication signals and individuals.

15.2 Voice-Sensitive Brain Regions

Studies in the visual sensory modality yielded the earliest insights into how the brain processes identity-related information. Face-sensitive neurons were identified in the monkey inferior temporal cortex, as neurons responding more strongly to faces compared to other non-face objects (Bruce et al., 1981; Perrett et al., 1982). Subsequently, neuroimaging studies revealed face-category preferring regions in the human fusiform gyrus as well as in occipital and other brain areas (Haxby et al., 2001; Kanwisher et al., 1997; Sergent et al., 1992). Monkey neuroimaging studies showed homologous visual face-category sensitivity in the fundus and inferior bank of the superior temporal sulcus (STS) in the temporal lobe (Freiwald & Tsao, 2010; Ku et al., 2011; Logothetis et al., 1999; Tsao & Livingstone, 2008; Tsao et al., 2006).

Scientists have also intensified efforts to investigate the processing of auditory voice-related content in communication sounds. Many neuroimaging studies of human acoustic communication focus on understanding the neural substrates for speech and language (Berwick et al., 2013; Binder et al., 2009; Bornkessel-Schlesewsky et al., 2015; Friederici, 2011; Hickok & Poeppel, 2007). Parallel work in non-human animals has been identifying the neurobiological representations of referential signals (i.e. 'what' was vocalized) as an evolutionarily related process to human communication of meaning via speech (Ghazanfar & Takahashi, 2014; Romanski, 2012). Another strand of work, inspired in part by visual studies of face processing, where neural responses to face versus non-face categories of stimuli are used to identify face-sensitive regions in the brain, led to analogous experiments in the auditory domain. Belin and colleagues used functional magnetic resonance imaging (fMRI) to discover voice-sensitive regions in the human brain that respond stronger to voice versus non-voice categories of sounds (Figure 15.1A; Belin et al., 2000, 2004).

However, human voice regions also respond strongly to speech (Fecteau et al., 2004), and speech and voice content engage overlapping neural processes in the human temporal lobe (Formisano et al., 2008; for more recent evidence, see Mesgarani & Chang, 2012). These observations left open the possibility that voice and speech processes in humans are functionally intertwined, such that human voice regions may have functionally specialized in ways that differ from how voice content is processed in the brains of non-human animals.

In support of the notion that the function of voice regions is evolutionarily conserved in primates, Petkov and colleagues obtained fMRI evidence that rhesus macaques (an Old World monkey species) have, as do humans, temporal lobe voice-sensitive regions that respond more strongly to voice than to non-voice categories of sounds (Petkov et al., 2008). A recent fMRI study in marmosets identified temporal lobe regions that respond more strongly to conspecific vocalizations than other categories of sounds (Sadagopan et al., 2015). The neuroimaging study in marmosets sets the stage for interrogating the sensitivity of these regions to voice content in a New World monkey and provides additional insights into voice regions in the primate order. Separately, temporal lobe voice-sensitive regions have also been identified in domestic dogs (Andics et al., 2014). Thus, the neuroimaging evidence to date

A. Human voice-sensitive sites   B. Monkey voice-sensitive sites

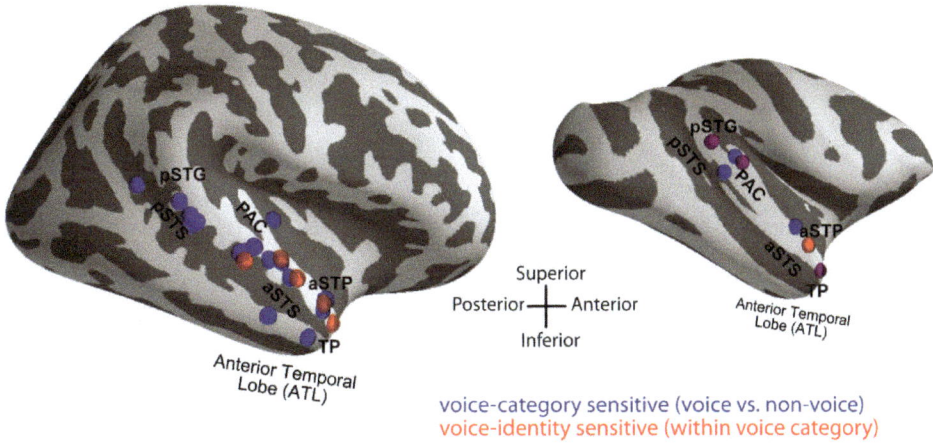

voice-category sensitive (voice vs. non-voice)
voice-identity sensitive (within voice category)

FIGURE 15.1 Imaging voice-sensitive fMRI clusters in the primate temporal lobe. (A) Voice-category sensitive sites (voice vs. non-voice sounds; blue) in the human temporal lobe and those that are voice-identity sensitive (within category; red). The identified sites are projected onto the surface using pySurfer software (https://pysurfer.github.io/) and correspond to the identified peak of activity clusters reported in Andics et al., 2010; Belin & Zatorre, 2003; Belin et al., 2000; Chandrasekaran et al., 2011; Latinus et al., 2013; von Kriegstein et al., 2003; Watson et al., 2014. These representations focus only on the temporal lobe and the right hemisphere, although, as the original reports show, the left hemisphere and other brain areas have voice-sensitive regions that respond selectively to the categorical differences between voice vs non-voice sounds. For a probability map of the location of voice-category sensitive regions in humans see Pernet et al., 2015. (B) Summary of voice-category and voice-identity sensitive sites in the macaque temporal lobe, obtained from peak activity clusters reported in Petkov et al., 2008. Also shown in purple are vocalization-sensitive peak responsive sites as reported in macaque neuroimaging studies using monkey vocalizations for stimuli (Gil-da-Costa et al., 2006; Joly et al., 2011; Poremba et al., 2004).

Abbreviations: a, anterior; p, posterior; PAC, primary auditory cortex; TP, temporal pole; STS, superior temporal sulcus; STG, superior temporal gyrus; STP, superior temporal plane.

Reprinted from *Trends in Cognitive Sciences*, Volume 19, Issue 12, Perrodin C., Kayser, C., Abel T J., Logothetis N.K., & Petkov, C. I., 'Who is That? Brain Networks and Mechanisms for Identifying Individuals', pp. 783-96, Copyright © 2015 Elsevier Inc., under the terms of the Creative Commons Attribution Licence (CC by 4.0), http://www.sciencedirect.com/science/article/pii/S1364661315002260

in humans, monkeys, and dogs supports the notion of broadly conserved voice-sensitive neural clustering of operations and functions. Nonetheless, additional studies in other animals and species are needed to unravel the broader evolutionary picture.

In neuroimaging studies, voice-sensitive regions are typically identified as areas of the brain that show a stronger response preference to a collection of voices in comparison to categories of other types of complex natural sounds. An additional functional property of some of these voice regions is a/their/the selectivity for particular voices within the voice category of vocalization sounds. Namely, several acoustical features, including those resulting from filtering of the sound produced by the vocal source in the mammalian larynx, provide indexical cues that animals use to identify individuals (Fitch & Fritz, 2006;

Ghazanfar et al., 2007; Rendall et al., 1998; Smith et al., 2005). Harnessing this natural variability in the category of vocalizations produced by different individuals (while ensuring that the vocal expression or meaning of the vocalizations produced by these individuals is the same; see Videos 15.1 and 15.2[1]) can be an effective strategy for identifying neural processes sensitive to the acoustical cues that animals use to identify other individuals.

In certain voice-sensitive regions, strong categorical responses to the set of voices could reflect a neural process coding for the species-specific voice characteristics of the sounds (a human voice, a monkey voice, etc.). In the same or other fMRI-identified voice clusters, neural responses may be particularly sensitive to specific individual voices within the voice category of sounds, which is important for identifying individuals. In this regard, anterior temporal lobe regions in the human brain show a sensitivity to the variability in voice identity within the category of human voices producing the same type of vocalization (Figure 15.1A; Andics et al., 2010; Belin & Zatorre, 2003; McLaren et al., 2009; von Kriegstein et al., 2003). A corresponding sensitivity has also been seen in macaque monkeys (Petkov et al., 2008), as follows: of several fMRI clusters identified in the monkey supra-temporal plane, the most anterior one is particularly sensitive to 'who' vocalized rather than 'what' was vocalized, showing more variable responses to different individuals producing the same type of vocalization than to different call types produced by the same individual (Figure 15.1B).

Thus, although the evidence from non-human animal neuroimaging studies on voice-content sensitivity remains relatively sparse, the results from monkey fMRI emulate two of the functional characteristics identified for anterior voice-identity sensitive fMRI clusters in humans. Namely, human and monkey voice-identity sensitive regions show a sensitivity to the category of voice versus non-voice sounds, with more anterior temporal lobe regions also showing a sensitivity to different individual voices within the voice category (Figure 15.1). Other brain regions, such as frontal cortex, can also show voice-category sensitivity (Campanella & Belin, 2007), responding to certain aspects of voice content in communication sounds. How neurons support these intriguing types of regional responses, however, cannot be answered with fMRI, because this neuroimaging approach indirectly measures neuronal ensemble activity by way of the blood oxygen level dependent response. Direct recordings from neurons in the fMRI identified regions in animal models are required to understand the response characteristics of neurons in voice-sensitive brain areas.

15.3 Voice-Sensitive Neurons and their Response Characteristics

In the 1980s, neuronal recordings in non-human primates obtained the first evidence of neurons with robust responses to faces (face cells). In the 1990s, face-sensitive regions were

---

[1] Videos such as these can be used to stimulate neurons and to assess multisensory influences. For instance, the video alone can be played to determine if the neuron is visually driven, the soundtrack alone can be played to see if the neuron is acoustically driven, and the combined audiovisual signal can be presented to determine if the response differs from that produced by the neuron in response to the visual or auditory stimulus alone. Using videos from different individuals producing the same types of vocalizations is also useful for studying identity-sensitive neurons (see text).

discovered in humans using brain neuroimaging, which was followed at the turn of the millennium by comparative fMRI evidence for face-sensitive regions in the brains of macaque monkeys (reviewed in Campanella & Belin, 2007; Tsao & Freiwald, 2006). With the discovery of voice-identity sensitive regions in humans (Belin et al., 2000) and that these regions in the human temporal lobe appear to have evolutionary counterparts in the brains of non-human primates (Petkov et al., 2008; Sadagopan et al., 2015), the stage was set to ask whether voice regions contain 'voice cells', and, if so, whether their response characteristics would closely emulate those that have been described for face cells. Arguably, the auditory system tends to show less tangible and obvious organizational properties than the visual and somatosensory systems (Griffiths et al., 2004; King & Nelken, 2009; Nelken et al., 2003). Namely, acoustical features tend to be processed by large populations of neurons (distributed code), which does not require strong selectivity for particular features to be evident in individual neurons (Bizley et al., 2009; Mizrahi et al., 2014; Rothschild et al., 2010).

15.3.1 Location of the Anterior Voice-Sensitive Cluster and Position within the Auditory Processing Hierarchy

The fMRI-based localization of the anterior voice-identity sensitive cluster in the macaque monkey shows that its position straddles anatomically delineated regions Ts1/Ts2 (Galaburda & Pandya, 1983; or area RTp in the terminology of Saleem & Logothetis, 2007) on the anterior supra-temporal plane. This area is rostral to the primary and immediately adjacent non-primary auditory cortical areas (Figure 15.2B; Kaas & Hackett, 2000; Petkov et al., 2008). The anterior temporal lobe voice-sensitive cluster falls between the fourth and fifth processing stage in the auditory cortical hierarchy, downstream from the tonotopically organized core (1°), belt (2°), and parabelt (3°) fields (Kaas & Hackett, 2000; Kikuchi et al., 2010; Perrodin et al., 2011; Petkov et al., 2006; Petkov et al., 2008; Rauschecker et al., 1995). Thus the anatomical localization of the anterior voice area places it at an intermediate level in the ventral auditory 'object' processing stream, whose feedforward connectivity successively links auditory cortical fields with association areas in the superior temporal sulcus (STS), superior temporal gyrus (STG), and ventral prefrontal cortex (Plakke & Romanski, 2014; Romanski et al., 1999; Scott et al., 2015).

15.3.2 Do Voice Cells Exist, and if so, are their Response Characteristics Comparable to those Known for Face Cells?

In an initial study of neuronal responses from the voice cluster located in the anterior supra-temporal plane, fMRI maps identifying this anterior voice-sensitive cluster were obtained in each of the macaque monkeys and used to guide neurophysiological recordings (Figure 15.2A; Perrodin et al., 2011). Three categories of sounds from the voice-localizer paradigm in the original monkey fMRI study were used to acoustically stimulate neurons (Petkov et al., 2008). The sounds used for stimulation included conspecific macaque vocalizations produced by many individuals (many voices). Neuronal responses to this category of sounds were compared with those to two other categories of sounds—animal vocalizations from other species (again, many voices but not from conspecific individuals) and familiar natural sounds that were recorded from the animal's home environment (e.g. rain, running water). The sounds in each of the three categories were subsampled from a larger stimulus set so that the resulting categories of sounds used in the experiments were as acoustically comparable as possible. This meant that at least two low-level features were matched across the three categories of sounds, the frequency content, and fluctuations in sound energy.

Comparing neuronal response amplitudes to each of the three sound categories showed a rather modest proportion of neurons within the voice-sensitive brain area that could be characterized as 'voice cells' (~25% of the neuronal sample). Voice cells are defined as neurons that respond two-fold stronger to the collection of conspecific voice stimuli than to the stimuli in the other two categories of sounds (Figure 15.2C; Perrodin et al., 2011). Auditory studies in animal models have shown that neuronal responses typically become increasingly more selective for complex sound features along the auditory processing hierarchy (Bizley et al., 2013; Chechik & Nelken, 2012; Kajikawa et al., 2015; Rauschecker et al., 1995; Romanski et al., 2005;). This occurs in particular as one ascends the ventral processing stream in auditory cortex (Kaas & Hackett, 1999; Rauschecker, 1998; Rauschecker & Tian, 2000; Rauschecker et al., 1997; Romanski et al., 1999; Tian et al., 2001), the processing pathway that is more sensitive to object features ('what' stream), in relation to the dorsal stream that by comparison is more sensitive to spatial features ('where' stream).

The response selectivity for species-specific vocalizations seems to increase in the auditory processing hierarchy outside of primary auditory cortex (Fukushima et al., 2014; Kikuchi et al., 2010; Poremba et al., 2004; Rauschecker et al., 1995; Recanzone, 2008; Tian et al., 2001). By comparison, in the initial processing stages of the auditory cortex, the neuronal responses to conspecific vocalizations are often not different to responses given to control sounds containing at least similar spectral content (Rauschecker et al., 1995; Recanzone, 2008; Wang, 2000; Wollberg & Newman, 1972). The results obtained from voice-sensitive neurons in the anterior supra-temporal plane, a few stages of processing further down the ventral processing pathway downstream from primary auditory cortex, show considerable selectivity for voice and other vocalization features (Perrodin et al., 2011, 2014).

How do these impressions about voice cells in the auditory modality compare to those that have been obtained for face cells in the visual modality? Comparing the results from voice-sensitive neurons in the auditory modality to observations in the visual 'face' processing system already shows some discordance between voice and face cells response characteristics, indicating that voice cells do not appear to be direct analogues of visual face cells.

The relatively small proportion of voice cells is in stark contrast to the results of several studies of face cells, which report high clustering of face-selective cells ranging from 60% to 90% (or higher) across different face clusters throughout the macaque monkey inferior temporal cortex (Aparicio et al., 2016; Freiwald & Tsao, 2010; McMahon et al., 2015; Tsao et al., 2006). In addition, comparing voice-cell responses to individual voices showed that voice cells in the anterior temporal cluster are also remarkably stimulus-selective, only responding to a select few voices within the conspecific voice-sound category (Figure 15.2D; Perrodin et al., 2011). Given the anatomical location of the anterior voice region within the auditory ventral processing pathway, the stimulus selectivity of voice cells is expectedly higher than the selectivity for vocalizations reported at several stages of the auditory processing hierarchy, such as the core and belt auditory cortex (Recanzone, 2008; Tian et al., 2001). The stimulus selectivity of neurons in the anterior voice cluster is also higher than those from an auditory region in the insula (Remedios et al., 2009) and lateral portions of auditory cortex on the superior temporal gyrus (Russ et al., 2008). By comparison, the high stimulus selectivity of the voice cells in the anterior temporal lobe is on a par with that measured for neurons responding to conspecific vocalizations in the ventrolateral prefrontal cortex (Gifford et al., 2005; Romanski, 2012; Romanski et al., 2005).

The high neuronal selectivity noted for voice cells also appears to diverge from the response characteristics that have been reported for face cells, which, by comparison, typically respond more broadly to the majority of faces presented within the face-stimulus category (Figure 15.2E; Hasselmo et al., 1989; Tsao et al., 2006). Thereby, comparisons of the proportion and general characteristics of voice-sensitive neurons are in concordance with other data from the auditory ventral processing stream. These comparisons provide complementary information on voice sensitivity that can be related to human voice-sensitive regions by way of the links that can be made to the corresponding monkey fMRI observations. However, when voice-cell response characteristics are compared to those that are known for face cells, the results so far raise the possibility that voice cells are not direct auditory analogues of face cells.

It is possible that the auditory and visual pathways may have specialized in different ways for processing the indexical cues about individual identity (Perrodin et al., 2011). However, methodological differences need to be excluded. For instance, given that sounds are by their nature dynamic and many prior studies of face-sensitive neurons have assessed responses to static images, it is possible that these apparent discrepancies in voice- and face-cell response characteristics may become less apparent when face cells' responses are assessed with dynamic faces. It would also be useful to reassess comparisons between voice- and face-cell characteristics once more data is available from neuronal recordings in other voice clusters in the temporal lobe (such as those closer to the auditory core and belt; Petkov et al., 2008).

15.3.3 Auditory-Feature Sensitivity of Voice-Region Neurons in Relation to Neurons in Adjacent Temporal Lobe Regions

The sensitivity of voice-area neurons to a number of auditory stimulus features was investigated by quantifying neuronal responses to a set of voices from different human and monkey individuals, organized in a multifactorial design. Neuronal spiking rates in the voice-sensitive cluster were differentially modulated by changes in a number of auditory features in the voice stimuli, such as call type ('what' was vocalized), caller identity ('who' vocalized; Figure 15.2F), and caller species (Perrodin et al., 2014). In particular, the results revealed a distinct subpopulation of voice-preferring neurons, which accounts for much of the observed sensitivity to caller-identity features. Thus, the neuronal recordings show that the responses of neurons in voice-sensitive clusters can be both sensitive to the category of voices (responding stronger to it than to non-voice stimulus categories) *and* selective for individual voices within the voice category of stimuli. The dual neuronal sensitivity to these two features of

A. Approach to the aSTP

Superior
Posterior—+—Anterior

STS

Voice
cluster
multi-
sensory
face cluster

C. Voice sensitive cell

Response (spks/s)

MVocs
AVocs
NSnds

20

10

0

-10

Stimulus

0　　200　　400
Time after sound onset (ms)

E. Voice and face cell
response selectivity

Proportion of stimuli >
half-maximum response

60

40

20

0

Voice cells　Face cells

Baylis et al., 1985

Hasselmo et al., 1989

B. Anterior voice cluster fMRI

Monkey # 1

35
30
25
20
15
10
5
0
-5
-10
-15

A1

MVocs preference

0.01　　　　0.0001
p-value

0　5　10　15　20　25　30　35
ML (mm)

D. Sparse coding by
voice cells

Cell number

5

10

15

20

Voice　1　2　3　4　5　6　7　8　9　10 11 12
call　Grunt　Bark　Scream　Coo
type　　　　Harmonic
　　　　arch
　　　MVoc stimulus

Core
(1° aud. Ctx.)　Belt　Parabelt　Higher
auditory
areas

F. Sensitivity to caller
identity

caller M1
caller M2

200

150

100

50

0

**

0　　500　　1000
Time after sound onset (ms)

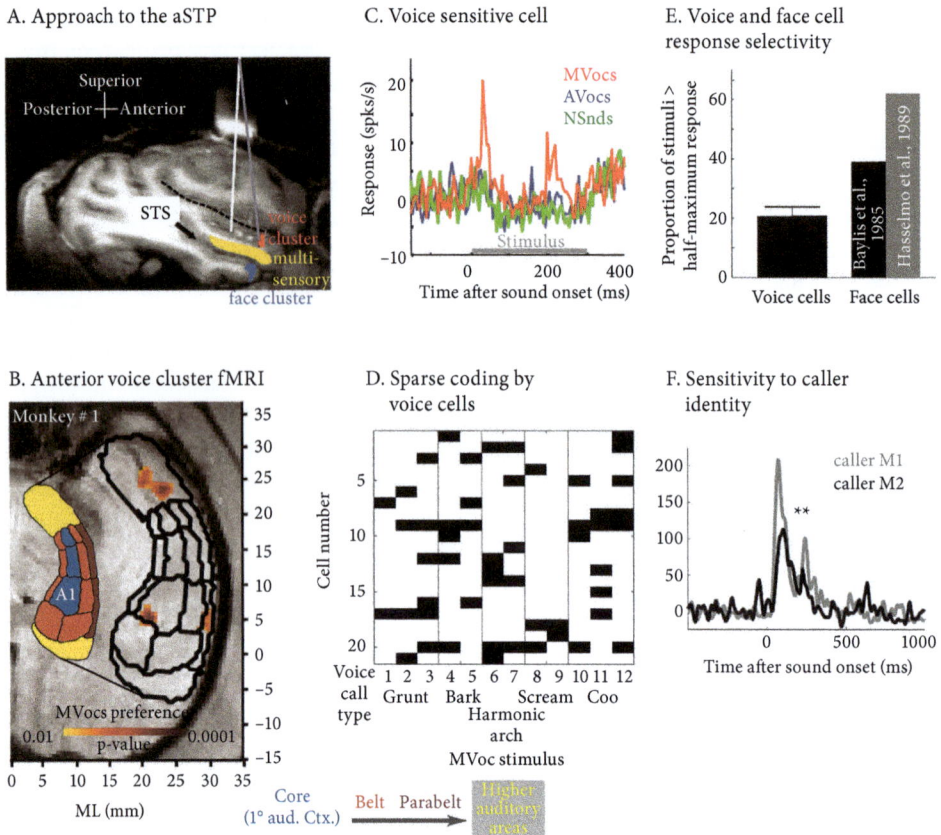

FIGURE 15.2 Probing voice cells and their auditory response characteristics. (A) Targeting approach for recording neurons from the anterior voice-identity sensitive fMRI cluster in the aSTP (anterior superior temporal plane; red), using stereotaxic coordinates and a neurosurgical targeting system to guide electrode placement (purple line). Classical multisensory (association) cortex in the upper bank of the superior temporal sulcus (STS) is illustrated in yellow. The fundus and lower bank of the STS can contain face-sensitive clusters (blue). (B) Individual fMRI map of the voice-sensitive cluster (red heat map) in relation to other parts of auditory cortex in one of the macaques in Perrodin and colleagues' studies (ibid 2011, 2014, 2015). The axial MRI slice is aligned in plane with the STP (dotted black line) from (A). Also shown are the outlines of the separately localized auditory fields (black outlines), such as tonotopically organized core and belt auditory cortex (Petkov et al., 2006, 2008). (AP: antero-posterior; ML: medio-lateral coordinates). (C) Exemplary spiking response of a voice-sensitive cell displaying a two-fold stronger response to the MVocs category (monkey vocalizations from many individual voices) than to the other two sound categories (AVocs: animal vocalizations; NSnds: natural environmental sounds). (D) Voice-sensitive cells ($n = 21$) respond selectively to a small subset of the stimuli presented within the MVocs category. The black squares indicate that the particular MVoc stimulus elicited a response larger than the half maximum response for a particular voice cell. (E) Voice-sensitive cells appear to be more stimulus-selective (i.e. respond well to smaller percentages of the presented voices) (Perrodin et al., 2011), than face cells which, by comparison, tend to respond to ~55% of the faces within the category of face stimuli (Baylis et al., 1985; Hasselmo et al., 1989; Tsao et al., 2006). Shown is mean ± SEM. (F) Neurons

voice processing is paralleled at a very different spatiotemporal scale by the fMRI results in macaques and humans, showing that anterior voice-sensitive clusters are sensitive to both the categorical distinction between voice versus non-voice stimuli *and* to specific conspecific voices within the category of voices (Belin & Zatorre, 2003; Chandrasekaran et al., 2011; Petkov et al., 2008; von Kriegstein et al., 2003).

Converging evidence from the visual and auditory modalities points to anterior subregions of the temporal lobe being more sensitive to identity-related features than posterior temporal lobe sites. In the visual domain, face regions in the anterior inferior temporal (aIT) lobe (see Figure 15.5) are seen to be more sensitive to individual identity-related content than more posterior temporal lobe regions in both humans (Kriegeskorte et al., 2007; Tsao & Livingstone, 2008) and monkeys (Freiwald & Tsao, 2010; Morin et al., 2014). Likewise in the auditory modality, more anterior temporal lobe areas are particularly sensitive to identity-related content in communication sounds in humans (Andics et al., 2010; Belin & Zatorre, 2003; Chandrasekaran et al., 2011; von Kriegstein et al., 2003) and monkeys (Petkov et al., 2008).

A number of theoretical models also highlight the anterior temporal lobe as a region containing sites sensitive to aspects of voice/face identity-related content (Belin et al., 2011; Bruce & Young, 1986; Campanella & Belin, 2007; Perrodin, Kayser, Abel, et al., 2015). However, since anterior temporal lobe sites are nodes in a broader network processing voice and face content (Fecteau et al., 2005; Tsao et al., 2008), more posterior voice- or face-sensitive sites in the temporal lobe network undoubtedly play a complementary role in identity processing, especially when features of facial or vocal expressions can identify individuals (Aparicio et al., 2016; Freiwald & Tsao, 2010; Meyers et al., 2015; Morin et al., 2014). More posterior superior temporal lobe regions can also be sensitive to person-related voice or face content, regardless of the sensory modality (Chan et al., 2011; Deen et al., 2015; Watson et al., 2014).

How auditory are the neurons in the anterior voice-sensitive cluster in relation to adjacent sites in the anterior temporal lobe? To answer this question, the neuronal sensitivity to auditory vocal features in the voice-sensitive cluster in the anterior supratemporal plane (aSTP) was compared to that of a neighbouring population of neurons in the upper bank of the anterior STS (see Figures 15.2A and 15.5). The aSTS is strongly interconnected with adjacent sites including the anterior voice-sensitive cluster and has long been thought of as an association area involved in multisensory object representations (Chandrasekaran & Ghazanfar, 2009; Ghazanfar et al., 2005; Plakke & Romanski, 2014; Romanski, 2012; Saleem et al., 2008), in part because it contains auditory, visual, and bimodal neurons (Beauchamp et al., 2004; Dahl et al., 2009). Neuronal recordings in the aSTS region, using the same collection

---

sensitive to voice (caller) identity tend to show invariant responses to different vocalizations (here, the responses to 'coo' and 'grunt' calls are averaged) but differential responses to different callers (caller M1 vs. M2; Perrodin et al., 2014).

of vocalizations from different callers as used to study aSTP neuronal responses, showed little sensitivity to the auditory features tested, such as call type and caller identity. This comparison indicates that neurons in the aSTP are more auditory-feature sensitive than those in the aSTS (Perrodin et al., 2014). Such a loss of auditory-feature sensitivity by regions such as the aSTS that are downstream from the aSTP is interesting but does not seem to impact upon auditory-responsive neurons in the prefrontal cortex (PFC), which are sensitive to vocalization type (Gifford et al., 2005) and caller identity (Plakke et al., 2013). The auditory-responsive neurons in the ventrolateral PFC must receive their auditory sensitivity from other sources than the aSTS, as we will consider in the next section.

Altogether, these results suggest more similarity in auditory-feature representations at voice-sensitive clusters and auditory-responsive neurons in the ventral PFC than in an association cortical region such as the aSTS (Stein & Stanford, 2008). These impressions substantiate the idea that the neurons in the voice-sensitive cortex in the aSTP reflect the properties of a region that is functionally well integrated in the ventral auditory processing pathway, downstream to tonotopically organized auditory core and belt fields.

15.4 Multisensory Influences and Pathways of Convergence for Voice and Face Information

How is the voice-sensitive cluster within the anterior temporal lobe functionally interconnected with other brain areas in the temporal or frontal lobes, including PFC? Previous neuroanatomical studies using neuronal tractography have identified pathways for sensory input from the temporal lobe into the frontal lobe, including dense projections from the second key stage of auditory cortical processing, the auditory belt, into PFC (Plakke & Romanski, 2014; Romanski et al., 1999). In addition, projections to frontal cortex from association cortex in the anterior superior temporal gyrus are considerable (Petrides & Pandya, 1988; Seltzer & Pandya, 1989). Yet whether neurons in the aSTP voice cluster would project to certain regions of frontal cortex, as strongly as either the upstream auditory belt cortex or downstream STS areas, was unclear.

Insights into the effective connectivity between some of these regions were recently obtained using combined electrical microstimulation and fMRI in monkeys. Electrically stimulating a brain region and using fMRI to assess which regions respond can reveal the synaptic targets of the stimulated site, a presumption supported by the fact that target regions activated by stimulation are often consistent with those identified using neuronal anterograde tractography (e.g. Matsui et al., 2011; Petkov et al., 2015). This approach allows for the charting of the functional effective connectivity of neural pathways. Namely, first a target region is electrically microstimulated and fMRI used to identify the regions activated by stimulating this site. Then a target of the region, identified by its fMRI activity response, is subsequently stimulated to identify with fMRI which additional areas are activated that were not evident when the first site was stimulated.

A. Microstimulating voice sensitive cortex elicits fMRI activity in adjacent ATL regions

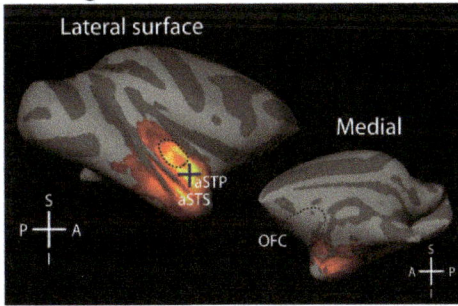

B. Microstimulating the aSTS elicits fMRI activity also in frontal cortex (OFC)

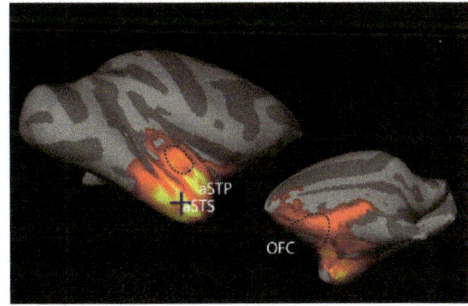

FIGURE 15.3 Imaging voice-sensitive effective connectivity projection patterns. (A) A study of effective functional connectivity using combined microstimulation and brain imaging with fMRI shows that electrically stimulating voice-sensitive cortex (blue cross) results in fMRI activity in adjacent anterior temporal lobe (ATL) regions (Petkov et al., 2015). (B) By comparison, the anterior STS, a multisensory region that appears to be a functional recipient of voice-sensitive cortex and is thought to integrate auditory and visual information (Beauchamp et al., 2004; Chandrasekaran & Ghazanfar, 2009; Dahl et al., 2009; Ghazanfar et al., 2005; Plakke & Romanski, 2014; Romanski, 2012; Saleem et al., 2008), when electrically stimulated also elicits an fMRI-activity response in frontal cortex, in particular the orbitofrontal cortex (OFC).

A: anterior, P: posterior, S: superior, I: inferior.

Interestingly, microstimulating voice-identity sensitive cortex in the aSTP does not strongly activate PFC, unlike stimulation of a downstream multisensory area in the STS or stimulation of upstream auditory cortical areas in the lateral belt (Petkov et al., 2015). Thus, the voice-sensitive cortex in the primate aSTP seems to functionally interact primarily with a local multisensory network in the temporal lobe, which includes the upper bank of the aSTS and regions around the temporal pole (Figure 15.3A). By contrast, stimulating the aSTS resulted in significantly stronger frontal fMRI activation, particularly in orbital frontal cortex (Figure 15.3B). These observations suggest that multisensory voice/face processes can influence each other within a network of anterior temporal lobe regions, only parts of which have a strong functional impact on frontal cortex.

These effective connectivity results complement insights on the inter-regional connectivity of auditory and association cortex areas in the anterior temporal lobe obtained in studies of either neuronal tractography (Frey et al., 2004; Plakke & Romanski, 2014; Saleem et al., 2008; Scott et al., 2015) or neural function (Kikuchi et al., 2010; Perrodin et al., 2014; Poremba et al., 2004). They also link to information obtained from structural and functional connectivity studies in humans showing connections between voice- and face-sensitive regions (Blank et al., 2011; Ethofer et al., 2013).

15.4.1 Multisensory Interactions in Voice-Sensitive Cortex: How Multisensory is the Anterior 'Voice'-Sensitive Region?

The initial neuroimaging and electrophysiological studies in monkeys had perhaps too hastily referred to the anterior temporal fMRI-identified cluster as a 'voice'-sensitive area. These initial results, obtained studying responses exclusively to auditory stimulation, cannot rule out that this region is potentially highly multisensory and may not be an auditory voice region after all.

Human fMRI studies have shown both functional crosstalk (Schall et al., 2013; von Kriegstein et al., 2005; von Kriegstein & Giraud, 2006) and direct structural connections (Blank et al., 2011) between voice- and face-sensitive regions, suggesting that visual face information is available in voice-sensitive regions. Other potential sources of visual input into the auditory STP include cortico-cortical projections from visual areas (Bizley et al., 2007; Blank et al., 2011), feedback projections from association areas, including those in voice-/face-sensitive ventrolateral PFC (Romanski, Bates, et al., 1999; Romanski, Tian, et al., 1999) and the multisensory STS (Cappe & Barone, 2005; Pandya et al., 1969). Multisensory projections with subcortical origins, such as the suprageniculate nucleus of the thalamus or the superior colliculus, could also directly or indirectly support crossmodal influences.

A number of electrophysiological studies have directly evaluated the multisensory influences of face input on voice processing in non-human primates, in a number of cortical sites, including posterior fields closer to the primary auditory cortex (Ghazanfar et al., 2005; Kayser et al., 2008) and classical association cortex such as the STS (Chandrasekaran & Ghazanfar, 2009; Dahl et al., 2009; Ghazanfar et al., 2008) or ventrolateral PFC (Sugihara et al., 2006; Romanski, 2007). In addition, whether the anterior STP would qualify as auditory or association cortex had thus far been ambiguous, the assumption having been based solely on neuroanatomical observations (Galaburda & Pandya, 1983; Kaas & Hackett, 1998). Thus, it was unclear whether multisensory interactions in this region would be qualitatively comparable to those in hierarchically earlier auditory cortical fields, or alternatively, relate better to those seen in a multisensory association area in the temporal lobe such as the aSTS.

15.4.2 How Multisensory are Neurons in the Anterior Voice-Identity Sensitive fMRI Cluster Compared to Neurons at Other Sites in the Temporal Lobe?

To answer whether and how auditory responses to voices are affected by simultaneously presented visual facial information, neuronal recordings were performed from the aSTP voice cluster in macaque monkeys conducting a visual-fixation task during auditory, visual, or audiovisual presentation of dynamic face and voice stimuli. As expected of an auditory cortical area, neurons in voice-sensitive cortex mainly respond to auditory stimuli, while silent visual stimuli are mostly ineffective in eliciting neuronal firing (for example responses, see Figure 15.4; Perrodin et al., 2014). However, comparing the magnitude of spiking rates to unimodal versus bimodal stimulation revealed that auditory firing rates were influenced by the visual modality, mainly via non-linear (subadditive or superadditive) neuronal response modulation (Figure 15.4A). This observation provided the first evidence for robust visual modulation of auditory neuronal responses at

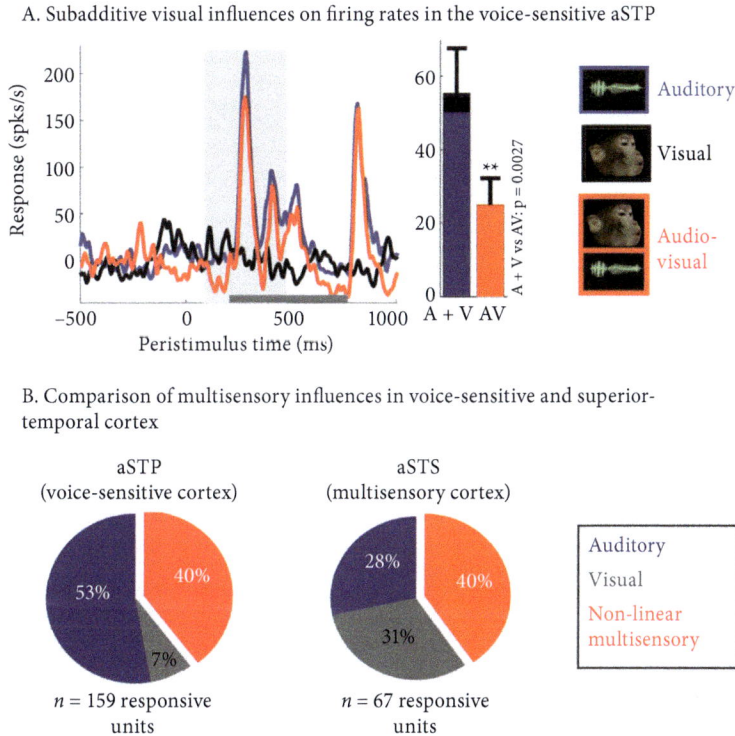

A. Subadditive visual influences on firing rates in the voice-sensitive aSTP

B. Comparison of multisensory influences in voice-sensitive and superior-temporal cortex

aSTP
(voice-sensitive cortex)
n = 159 responsive units

aSTS
(multisensory cortex)
n = 67 responsive units

Auditory
Visual
Non-linear multisensory

FIGURE 15.4 Visual face influences on the responses of neurons in the voice-sensitive aSTP. (A) Example spiking response of a unit in the anterior voice-sensitive fMRI cluster, in the supra-temporal plane, showing non-linear (subadditive) visual modulation of auditory activity. Firing rates in response to combined audiovisual stimulation (AV: voice and face) significantly differ from the sum of the responses to the unimodal stimuli (A: auditory and V: visual; A vs (A+V), z-test, **: p<0.01). The horizontal grey line indicates the duration of the auditory stimulus, and the light grey box represents the 400-ms peak-centred response window. Bar plots indicate the response amplitudes in the 400-ms response window (shown is mean ± SEM). (B) Neuronal multisensory influences are prominent in voice-sensitive cortex (anterior supra-temporal plane; aSTP) but are qualitatively different from those in the anterior superior temporal sulcus (aSTS). For example, aSTS neurons more often display bimodal responses.

a voice-sensitive fMRI cluster in the aSTP (Perrodin et al., 2014). The direction of non-linear visual modulation of neuronal responses was further shown to be predicted by the relative timing between the natural voice and face stimuli onsets, via resetting of the phase of low-frequency oscillations in neuronal ensemble (local field potential) responses (Perrodin, Kayser, Logothetis, et al., 2015). Similar types, proportions, and mechanisms of visual influences have been found to modulate auditory-responsive neurons in the posterior core/belt auditory cortex (Bizley et al., 2007; Ghazanfar et al., 2005; Kayser et al., 2008; Lakatos et al., 2007), suggesting qualitatively comparable neuronal-level multisensory interactions in the voice-sensitive aSTP as seen in other auditory cortical processing sites.

Extracellular recordings of neuronal activity from association cortex in the anterior upper bank of the STS revealed a comparable proportion of non-linear audiovisual interactions as seen in the aSTP neurons using the same set of stimuli and conditions (Figure 15.4B). However, in agreement with previous electrophysiological studies (Benevento et al., 1977; Bruce et al., 1981; Dahl et al., 2009), direct crossmodal convergence was more prevalent in the STS, where neurons showed a balance of both auditory and visual responses (Figure 15.4B). These observations are consistent with those in studies highlighting the STS as an association cortical region that is a prominent target for both auditory and visual afferents (Beauchamp et al., 2004; Seltzer & Pandya, 1994).

Beyond characterizing the proportions and types of multisensory interactions, crossmodal influences on neural responses can also differ in their specificity to behaviourally-relevant multisensory associations (Werner & Noppeney, 2010). To look into this facet of neuronal responses in aSTP and aSTS neurons, the sensitivity of visual influences to speaker congruency was investigated using a set of incongruent audiovisual control stimuli. For instance, a voice could be paired with a mismatched visual (face) context, such as a monkey face being paired with a human voice. Direct electrophysiological recordings showed that multisensory influences on aSTP units were relatively insensitive to speaker congruency and were not strongly affected by mismatched audiovisual stimulus pairs (Perrodin et al., 2014). The relative lack of specificity for visual influences in the aSTP is consistent with this area showing more general crossmodal influences, which at least qualitatively match those seen in and around primary auditory cortex (Ghazanfar & Schroeder, 2006; Kayser & Logothetis, 2007; Schroeder et al., 2003; Werner & Noppeney, 2010). These general comparisons suggest that such auditory regions, perhaps because they are primarily engaged in sensory analysis in the dominant modality, have less obvious cross-sensory specificity. This might avoid disruption of vocal or facial analysis during incongruent cross-sensory situations (such as looking at an individual that is not the one vocalizing).

The presentation of incongruent audiovisual stimuli revealed that, in contrast to the somewhat generic visual influences in aSTP neurons, those modulating the auditory responses of aSTS neurons showed greater specificity. Namely, multisensory interactions in the aSTS were sensitive to the congruency of the presented voice–face pairing, and visual influences on aSTS neuron visual responses occurred more frequently in response to matching than mismatching audiovisual stimuli. As a result, non-linear multisensory responses in aSTS neurons were more likely to be disrupted by incongruent stimulation. Altogether, these observations are consistent with the evidence for integrative multisensory processes in the human and monkey STS (Beauchamp et al., 2004; Dahl et al., 2009), potentially at the cost of decreased specificity for unisensory representations (Werner & Noppeney, 2010).

However, it is also worth noting that incongruent stimuli have so far only rarely been used to probe neurons in auditory cortex. For instance, Ghazanfar and colleagues (2005) noted a sensitivity to the congruency of pairing a voice with an artificial visual mouth movement in caudal auditory cortex. So, additional comparisons of neuronal responses to different voice and face multisensory conditions are warranted and depend on obtaining additional empirical data.

The observations that can currently be made on the forms of audiovisual interactions seen in aSTP neurons complement the impressions obtained by the functional characterization of voice-sensitive neuronal representations in the auditory domain. The results reveal clear visual influences on many auditory neurons in the anterior voice-sensitive cluster. However, visual influences on voice-sensitive neurons are seen to be qualitatively more similar to those reported in early auditory cortical fields, underscoring the predominantly auditory role of the aSTP and the anterior voice-sensitive cortical neurons. In contrast, neurons in an association cortex such as the STS display more specific audiovisual interactions than neurons in the aSTP voice-sensitive cluster. These results can be interpreted as reversed gradients of functional specificity in the unisensory and multisensory processing of communication signals, along their respective processing pathways. The general comparisons of anterior voice-cluster neuron characteristics in relation to processes in early auditory fields and the STS (for reviews see, for example, Campanella & Belin, 2007; Ghazanfar & Schroeder, 2006; Stein & Stanford, 2008) implicate an intermediate functional role for the anterior voice cluster, in terms of both its auditory and audiovisual processing roles within the respective processing hierarchies.

The findings we have overviewed inform our understanding of where and how in the sensory-processing hierarchy, voice and face content is likely to be integrated into a unified multisensory representation. However, these snapshots of the neuronal encoding properties at different processing stages can only hint at the intriguing transformations of sensory representations that are likely to occur from one level to another. It also remains unclear how the specificity in neuronal multisensory influences might causally impact on perception, which can only be gleaned by studying neural responses during active behaviour (Fetsch et al., 2013; Yau et al., 2015) as the animals encode voice/face predictions or prediction errors (Bastos et al., 2012).

15.5 A PRIMATE MODEL FOR STAGES IN VOICE- AND FACE-IDENTITY PROCESSING

The combination of direct extracellular recordings and non-invasive imaging methods considered in this chapter reveal initial insights into voice-sensitive neuronal representations and how they compare qualitatively to relevant data across multiple levels of the ventral sensory processing stream in the primate brain. This information motivates a heuristic

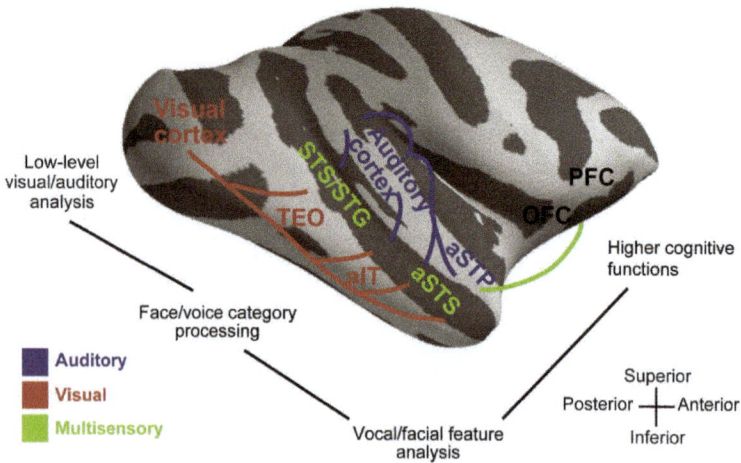

A. Auditory and visual processing pathways in the monkey brain

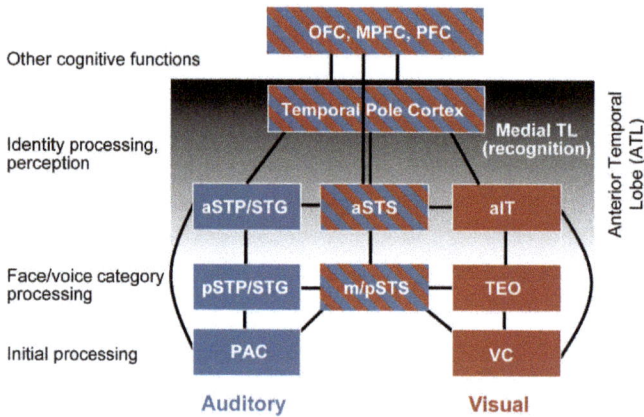

B. A primate model for voice/face processing

FIGURE 15.5 A model for auditory voice and visual face processing pathways in the primate brain. (**A**) A framework focused on the sensory cortical streams for processing auditory voice and visual face information. The model is illustrated on the right hemisphere of a rendered macaque brain. It features early sensory cortices, processing stages extracting face content in visual areas of the inferior temporal lobe TEO and aIT, and auditory regions of the anterior superior temporal plane/gyrus (aSTP/STG) extracting voice-related content. Multisensory interactions are possible between voice- and face-processing regions including by way of association areas along the superior temporal sulcus (STS) and frontal cortex (PFC: prefrontal cortex, OFC: orbitofrontal cortex). The cortical regions are interconnected via bidirectional pathways of inter-regional projections (solid lines—auditory: blue, visual: red, audiovisual: green), and these regions have feedforward and feedback projections to the auditory and visual processing streams (not illustrated). (M: medial, p: posterior, a: anterior.) (**B**) The model focuses on the auditory pathway involved in extracting voice-identity content in communication signals and the analogous visual pathway. Similar principles would apply to other sensory input streams, although the interacting regions involved may differ. The key

model of identity processing in the primate brain and we consider the ways in which it may generalize to humans.

Non-invasive neuroimaging studies in humans initially revealed face- and voice-sensitive areas (Blank et al., 2011; Chan et al., 2011; Deen et al., 2015; Schall et al., 2013; von Kriegstein & Giraud, 2006; von Kriegstein et al., 2005; Watson et al., 2014). These observations were compared with and informed by work in non-human primates, which provide detailed information on neuronal responses at some of the corresponding regions of interest. However, it is currently unclear how voice and face cells in the human temporal lobe would respond to different stimulus features and how voice/face regions are functionally interconnected with multisensory regions in the STS and in frontal cortex. Since this knowledge is already available in monkeys, the extracellular electrophysiological studies in non-human animals can be used to generate hypotheses that can be tested in humans using, for example, intracranial recordings in patients being monitored for surgical resection (Griffiths et al., 2010; Mesgarani & Chang, 2012).

Thus, while direct recordings from the human brain can only be serendipitously obtained in patients from brain regions that are clinically important to monitor for surgery, the available neuroimaging studies and data from non-human primates generate predictions on neuronal processes that may at some point be studied in humans and seen to correspond to the information available from non-human primates. This would also provide another basis upon which to translate insights in animal models obtained using approaches that still cannot be used in humans, e.g. systematic neuronal recordings and pharmacological, optogenetic, or electrical perturbation of the system in animal models. Such reciprocal cross-exchange of insights from human and animal models is crucial for increasing knowledge about the neurobiological substrates of voice and face processing across neural spatiotemporal scales.

Based on the available insights from non-human primates on the auditory and audiovisual voice-sensitive neuronal processes in the anterior temporal lobe described in this chapter, we propose a model of identity-related processing in primates (Figure 15.5; Perrodin, Kayser, Abel et al., 2015). In this model, two independent but interacting auditory and visual ventral processing streams extract voice/face features. Anterior regions of the temporal lobe are more sensitive to identity features, with other, more posterior, areas evaluating other aspects of voice/face content, such as category membership and voice/face expression or location in space. The STS is a key conduit between voice- and face-processing streams, with the aSTS

---

features of the model are the initial sensory and category-sensitive processing stages (m/pSTS; visual area TEO and auditory regions in posterior STP/STG). Multisensory influences are present throughout the visual and auditory pathway, but are thought to be qualitatively different in the STS, in relation to, for example, aSTP regions where the auditory modality is dominant (Chandrasekaran & Ghazanfar, 2009; Perrodin et al., 2014). Identity-related processes would primarily involve ATL regions (anterior STP/STG; aSTS; aIT). (Note: not illustrated are interactions with MTL structures such as the entorhinal cortex and hippocampus that could support the recognition of familiar individuals.)

Reprinted from *Trends in Cognitive Sciences*, Volume 19 Issue 12, Perrodin C., Kayser, C., Abel T J., Logothetis N.K., & Petkov, C. I., 'Who is That? Brain Networks and Mechanisms for Identifying Individuals', pp. 783-96, Copyright © 2015 Elsevier Inc., under the terms of the Creative Commons Attribution Licence (CC by 4.0), http://www.sciencedirect.com/science/article/pii/S1364661315002260

serving as a convergence site that allows multisensory representations to more strongly influence frontal cortex. Neurons in anterior temporal lobe (ATL) subregions such as the aSTS and the temporal pole integrate highly specific information about unique entities, such as individuals. Because of extensive multisensory interactions in the anterior temporal pole, such representations may not be tied to any sensory modality and the neural mechanisms underlying multisensory computations at different ATL sites need to be determined (for discussion, see Perrodin, Kayser, Abel, et al., 2015).

Possibly, the ATL provides crucial feedback to unisensory processing streams to route specific forms of sensory input that might assist in forming multisensory associations crucial for recognizing identity. Anatomical connectivity between the primate ATL regions funnels into the temporopolar cortex (Fan et al., 2014; Pascual et al., 2015), but less is known about this region's functional role in primates, particularly for processing identity. Identity recognition is also likely to involve memory-related structures in the medial temporal lobe (MTL). However, whether auditory pathways to the MTL in primates are less direct than those in humans is currently an open question (Fritz et al., 2005; Munoz-Lopez et al., 2010). Answers to this and other questions will depend upon direct cross-species comparisons of functional and structural connectivity using similar neurobiological approaches in the different species (e.g. Oya et al., 2017; Petkov et al., 2015).

This primate model at a regional level is generally in agreement with human models on face and voice processing contributing towards perception, whereby distinct sensory processing streams have prominent multisensory interactions between face and voice areas (Blank et al., 2014; Belin et al., 2011; Gainotti, 2013). One issue that needs addressing is whether human voice regions in the STG/STS are intrinsically more multisensory than the voice region in the primate aSTP. It is possible that human auditory voice regions in the STG are difficult to distinguish from neighbouring multisensory regions in the STS in group neuroimaging data (Pernet et al., 2015). Thus, the anterior upper bank of the STS may be a key site of multisensory convergence for identity processing in both humans and monkeys. The model highlights ATL areas such as the aSTS and the temporopolar cortex as important sites for identity-related multisensory convergence.

15.6 SUMMARY, CONCLUSIONS, AND LOOK AHEAD

Guided by imaging evidence of voice-sensitive regions in humans, comparative neuroimaging studies located what appear to be functionally homologous voice areas in monkeys. Macaque monkeys have become a prominent animal-model system that is providing neuronal-level insights on the processing of voices at finer neurobiological scales than have been possible in humans. Single-unit electrophysiological recordings in non-human primates from the anterior temporal lobe fMRI voice cluster revealed the existence of a modest proportion of voice-sensitive cells, whose encoding properties and neuronal-response characteristics appear to differ from those reported for face cells in the visual system. Auditory neuronal responses within the anterior voice cluster are influenced by visual face input, but in a mainly modulatory way that is seen to be similar to reported multisensory influences on neuronal responses in regions within and around primary auditory cortex. These types of multisensory responses, however, contrast with those obtained from neurons in association cortical regions of the STS. Close functional interconnectivity and interactions are seen between these regions in the anterior temporal lobe, providing the basis for multisensory face/voice interactions and for certain regions to act as functional conduits, transmitting processes to prefrontal cortex and receiving feedback influences.

Although the gaps in our understanding of voice processes in humans and animal models have begun to close, the next set of empirical questions is in better focus. The following aspects require further study for a better understanding of the neuronal substrates of vocal- and caller-identity processing: a) the transformations of neural representations that occur along the processing hierarchies; b) the causal roles that certain sites might have in influencing perception; and c) the neural dynamics that influence representations, including the form and functional characteristics of feedback inputs. Elucidating these neural operations and the roles of particular sites in the neural network will require studying behaving animals while manipulating neuronal activity with electrical, pharmacological, or molecular-genetic tools. Such research is likely to bring new insights into the neural codes, brain systems, and pathways enabling social communication, one benefit of which would be to provide awareness of how to design better and more flexible recognition of unique entities in artificial systems.

ACKNOWLEDGEMENTS

We thank Christoph Kayser and Nikos Logothetis for useful discussion, support, and encouragement. This work was supported by the Max Planck Society, the Wellcome Trust (CIP, Investigator Award WT092606AIA; CP, Sir Henry Wellcome Fellowship WT110238/Z/15/Z), the European Research Council (CIP, MECHIDENT), the Swiss National Science Foundation (P2SKP3-158691 to CP), and the Biotechnology and Biological Sciences Research Council (BB/J009849/1 to CIP, joint with Q. Vuong).

REFERENCES

Andics, A., Gácsi, M., Faragó, T., Kis, A., & Miklósi, Á. (2014). Voice-sensitive regions in the dog and human brain are revealed by comparative fMRI. *Current Biology*, 24(5), 574–578.

Andics, A., McQueen, J. M., Petersson, K. M., Gal, V., Rudas, G., & Vidnyanszky, Z. (2010). Neural mechanisms for voice recognition. *NeuroImage*, 52(4), 1528–1540.

Aparicio, P. L., Issa, E. B., & DiCarlo, J. J. (2016). Neurophysiological organization of the middle face patch in macaque inferior temporal cortex. *Journal of Neuroscience*, 36(50), 12729–12745.

Bastos, A. M., Usrey, W. M., Adams, R. A., Mangun, G. R., Fries, P., & Friston, K. J. (2012). Canonical microcircuits for predictive coding. *Neuron*, 76(4), 695–711.

Baylis, G. C., Rolls, E. T., & Leonard, C. M. (1985). Selectivity between faces in the responses of a population of neurons in the cortex in the superior temporal sulcus of the monkey. *Brain Research*, 342(1), 91–102.

Beauchamp, M. S., Argall, B. D., Bodurka, J., Duyn, J. H., & Martin, A. (2004). Unraveling multisensory integration: patchy organization within human STS multisensory cortex. *Nature Neuroscience*, 7(11), 1190–1192.

Belin, P., Bestelmeyer, P. E. G., Latinus, M., & Watson, R. (2011). Understanding voice perception. *British Journal of Psychology*, 102(4), 711–725.

Belin, P., Fecteau, S., & Bedard, C. (2004). Thinking the voice: neural correlates of voice perception. *Trends in Cognitive Sciences*, 8(3), 129–135.

Belin, P. & Zatorre, R. J. (2003). Adaptation to speaker's voice in right anterior temporal lobe. *Neuroreport*, 14(16), 2105–2109.

Belin, P., Zatorre, R. J., Lafaille, P., Ahad, P., & Pike, B. (2000). Voice-selective areas in human auditory cortex. *Nature*, 403(6767), 309–312.

Benevento, L. A., Fallon, J., Davis, B. J., & Rezak, M. (1977). Auditory–visual interaction in single cells in the cortex of the superior temporal sulcus and the orbital frontal cortex of the macaque monkey. *Experimental Neurology*, 57(3), 849–872.

Berwick, R. C., Friederici, A. D., Chomsky, N., & Bolhuis, J. J. (2013). Evolution, brain, and the nature of language. *Trends in Cognitive Sciences*, 17(2), 89–98.

Binder, J. R., Desai, R. H., Graves, W. W., & Conant, L. L. (2009). Where is the semantic system? A critical review and meta-analysis of 120 functional neuroimaging studies. *Cerebral Cortex*, 19(12), 2767–2796.

Bizley, J. K., Nodal, F. R., Bajo, V. M., Nelken, I., & King, A. J. (2007). Physiological and anatomical evidence for multisensory interactions in auditory cortex. *Cerebral Cortex*, 17(9), 2172–2189.

Bizley, J. K., Walker, K. M. M., Silverman, B. W., King, A. J., & Schnupp, J. W. H. (2009). Interdependent encoding of pitch, timbre, and spatial location in auditory cortex. *Journal of Neuroscience*, 29(7), 2064–2075.

Bizley, J. K., Walker, K. M., Nodal, F. R., King, A. J., & Schnupp, J. W. (2013). Auditory cortex represents both pitch judgments and the corresponding acoustic cues. *Current Biology*, 23(7), 620–625.

Blank, H., Anwander, A., & von Kriegstein, K. (2011). Direct structural connections between voice- and face-recognition areas. *Journal of Neuroscience*, 31(36), 12906–12915.

Blank, H., Wieland, N., & von Kriegstein, K. (2014). Person recognition and the brain: merging evidence from patients and healthy individuals. *Neuroscience and Biobehavioral Reviews*, 47, 717–734.

Bornkessel-Schlesewsky, I., Schlesewsky, M., Small, S. L., & Rauschecker, J. P. (2015). Neurobiological roots of language in primate audition: common computational properties. *Trends in Cognitive Sciences*, 19(3), 142–150.

Bruce, C., Desimone, R., & Gross, C. G. (1981). Visual properties of neurons in a polysensory area in superior temporal sulcus of the macaque. *Journal of Neurophysiology*, 46(2), 369–384.

Bruce, V. & Young, A. (1986). Understanding face recognition. *British Journal of Psychology*, 77, 305–327.

Campanella, S. & Belin, P. (2007). Integrating face and voice in person perception. *Trends in Cognitive Sciences*, 11(12), 535–543.

Cappe, C. & Barone, P. (2005). Heteromodal connections supporting multisensory integration at low levels of cortical processing in the monkey. *European Journal of Neuroscience*, 22(11), 2886–2902.

Chan, A. M., Baker, J. M., Eskandar, E., Schomer, D., Ulbert, I., Marinkovic, K., Cash, S. S., & Halgren, E. (2011). First-pass selectivity for semantic categories in human anteroventral temporal lobe. *Journal of Neuroscience*, 31(49), 18119–18129.

Chandrasekaran, B., Chan, A. H., & Wong, P. C. (2011). Neural processing of what and who information in speech. *Journal of Cognitive Neuroscience*, 23(10), 2690–2700.

Chandrasekaran, C. & Ghazanfar, A. A. (2009). Different neural frequency bands integrate faces and voices differently in the superior temporal sulcus. *Journal of Neurophysiology*, 101(2), 773–788.

Chechik, G. & Nelken, I. (2012). Auditory abstraction from spectro-temporal features to coding auditory entities. *Proceedings of the National Academy of Sciences of the United States of America*, 109(46), 18968–18973.

Dahl, C. D., Logothetis, N. K., & Kayser, C. (2009). Spatial organization of multisensory responses in temporal association cortex. *Journal of Neuroscience*, 29(38), 11924–11932.

Deen, B., Koldewyn, K., Kanwisher, N., & Saxe, R. (2015). Functional organization of social perception and cognition in the superior temporal sulcus. *Cerebral Cortex*, 25(11), 4596–4609.

Ethofer, T., Bretscher, J., Wiethoff, S., Bisch, J., Schlipf, S., Wildgruber, D., & Kreifelts, B. (2013). Functional responses and structural connections of cortical areas for processing faces and voices in the superior temporal sulcus. *NeuroImage*, 76, 45–56.

Fan, L., Wang, J., Zhang, Y., Han, W., Yu, C., & Jiang, T. (2014). Connectivity-based parcellation of the human temporal pole using diffusion tensor imaging. *Cerebral Cortex*, 24(12), 3365–3378.

Fecteau, S., Armony, J. L., Joanette, Y., & Belin, P. (2004). Is voice processing species- specific in human auditory cortex? An fMRI study. *NeuroImage*, 23(3), 840–848.

Fecteau, S., Armony, J. L., Joanette, Y., & Belin, P. (2005). Sensitivity to voice in human prefrontal cortex. *Journal of Neurophysiology*, 94(3), 2251–2254.

Fetsch, C. R., DeAngelis, G. C., & Angelaki, D. E. (2013). Bridging the gap between theories of sensory cue integration and the physiology of multisensory neurons. *Nature Reviews Neuroscience*, 14(6), 429–442.

Fitch, W. T. & Fritz, J. B. (2006). Rhesus macaques spontaneously perceive formants in conspecific vocalizations. *Journal of the Acoustical Society of America*, 120(4), 2132–2141.

Formisano, E., De Martino, F., Bonte, M., & Goebel, R. (2008). 'Who' is saying 'what'? Brain-based decoding of human voice and speech. *Science*, 322(5903), 970–973.

Freiwald, W. A. & Tsao, D. Y. (2010). Functional compartmentalization and viewpoint generalization within the macaque face-processing system. *Science*, 330(6005), 845–851.

Frey, S., Kostopoulos, P., & Petrides, M. (2004). Orbitofrontal contribution to auditory encoding. *NeuroImage*, 22(3), 1384–1389.

Friederici, A. D. (2011). The brain basis of language processing: from structure to function. *Physiology Reviews*, 91(4), 1357–1392.

Fritz, J., Mishkin, M., & Saunders, R. C. (2005). In search of an auditory engram. *Proceedings of the National Academy of Sciences of the United States of America*, 102(26), 9359–9364.

Fukushima, M., Saunders, R. C., Leopold, D. A., Mishkin, M., & Averbeck, B. B. (2014). Differential coding of conspecific vocalizations in the ventral auditory cortical stream. *Journal of Neuroscience*, 34(13), 4665–4676.

Gainotti, G. (2013). Is the right anterior temporal variant of prosopagnosia a form of 'associative prosopagnosia' or a form of 'multimodal person recognition disorder'? *Neuropsychology Review*, 23(2), 99–110.

Galaburda, A. M. & Pandya, D. N. (1983). The intrinsic architectonic and connectional organization of the superior temporal region of the rhesus monkey. *Journal of Computational Neurology*, 221(2), 169–184.

Ghazanfar, A. A., Chandrasekaran, C., & Logothetis, N. K. (2008). Interactions between the superior temporal sulcus and auditory cortex mediate dynamic face/voice integration in rhesus monkeys. *Journal of Neuroscience*, 28(17), 4457–4469.

Ghazanfar, A. A., Maier, J. X., Hoffman, K. L., & Logothetis, N. K. (2005). Multisensory integration of dynamic faces and voices in rhesus monkey auditory cortex. *Journal of Neuroscience*, 25(20), 5004–5012.

Ghazanfar, A. A. & Schroeder, C. E. (2006). Is neocortex essentially multisensory? *Trends in Cognitive Sciences*, 10(6), 278–285.

Ghazanfar, A. A. & Takahashi, D. Y. (2014). The evolution of speech: vision, rhythm, cooperation. *Trends in Cognitive Sciences*, 18(10), 543–553.

Ghazanfar, A. A., Turesson, H. K., Maier, J. X., van Dinther, R., Patterson, R. D., & Logothetis, N. K. (2007). Vocal-tract resonances as indexical cues in rhesus monkeys. *Current Biology*, 17(5), 425–430.

Gifford III, G. W., MacLean, K. A., Hauser, M. D., & Cohen, Y. E. (2005). The neurophysiology of functionally meaningful categories: macaque ventrolateral prefrontal cortex plays a critical role in spontaneous categorization of species-specific vocalizations. *Journal of Cognitive Neuroscience*, 17(9), 1471–1482.

Gil-da-Costa, R., Martin, A., Lopes, M. A., Munoz, M., Fritz, J. B., & Braun, A. R. (2006). Species-specific calls activate homologs of Broca's and Wernicke's areas in the macaque. *Nature Neuroscience*, 9(8), 1064–1070.

Griffiths, T. D., Kumar, S., Sedley, W., Nourski, K. V., Kawasaki, H., Oya, H., … Howard, M. A. (2010). Direct recordings of pitch responses from human auditory cortex. *Current Biology*, 20(12), 1128–1132.

Griffiths, T. D., Warren, J. D., Scott, S. K., Nelken, I., & King, A. J. (2004). Cortical processing of complex sound: a way forward? *Trends in Neuroscience*, 27(4), 181–185.

Hasselmo, M. E., Rolls, E. T., & Baylis, G. C. (1989). The role of expression and identity in the face-selective responses of neurons in the temporal visual cortex of the monkey. *Behavioral and Brain Research*, 32(3), 203–218.

Haxby, J. V., Gobbini, M. I., Furey, M. L., Ishai, A., Schouten, J. L., & Pietrini, P. (2001). Distributed and overlapping representations of faces and objects in ventral temporal cortex. *Science*, 293(5539), 2425–2430.

Hickok, G. & Poeppel, D. (2007). The cortical organization of speech processing. *Nature Reviews Neuroscience*, 8(5), 393–402.

Joly, O., Ramus, F., Pressnitzer, D., Vanduffel, W., & Orban, G. A. (2011). Interhemispheric differences in auditory processing revealed by fMRI in awake rhesus monkeys. *Cerebral Cortex*, 22(4), 838–853.

Kaas, J. H. & Hackett, T. A. (1998). Subdivisions of auditory cortex and levels of processing in primates. *Audiology and Neurotology*, 3(2–3), 73–85.

Kaas, J. H. & Hackett, T. A. (1999). 'What' and 'where' processing in auditory cortex. *Nature Neuroscience*, 2(12), 1045–1047.

Kaas, J. H. & Hackett, T. A. (2000). Subdivisions of auditory cortex and processing streams in primates. *Proceedings of the National Academy of Sciences of the United States of America*, 97(22), 11793–11799.

Kajikawa, Y., Frey, S., Ross, D., Falchier, A., Hackett, T. A., & Schroeder, C. E. (2015). Auditory properties in the parabelt regions of the superior temporal gyrus in the awake macaque monkey: an initial survey. *Journal of Neuroscience*, 35(10), 4140–4150.

Kanwisher, N., McDermott, J., & Chun, M. M. (1997). The fusiform face area: a module in human extrastriate cortex specialized for face perception. *Journal of Neuroscience*, 17(11), 4302–4311.

Kayser, C. & Logothetis, N. K. (2007). Do early sensory cortices integrate cross-modal information? *Brain Structure and Function*, 212(2), 121–132.

Kayser, C., Petkov, C. I., & Logothetis, N. K. (2008). Visual modulation of neurons in auditory cortex. *Cerebral Cortex*, 18(7), 1560–1574.

Kikuchi, Y., Horwitz, B., & Mishkin, M. (2010). Hierarchical auditory processing directed rostrally along the monkey's supratemporal plane. *Journal of Neuroscience*, 30(39), 13021–13030.

King, A. J. & Nelken, I. (2009). Unraveling the principles of auditory cortical processing: can we learn from the visual system? *Nature Neuroscience*, 12(6), 698–701.

Kriegeskorte, N., Formisano, E., Sorger, B., & Goebel, R. (2007). Individual faces elicit distinct response patterns in human anterior temporal cortex. *Proceedings of the National Academy of Sciences of the United States of America*, 104(51), 20600–20605.

Ku, S. P., Tolias, A. S., Logothetis, N. K., & Goense, J. (2011). fMRI of the face-processing network in the ventral temporal lobe of awake and anesthetized macaques. *Neuron*, 70(2), 352–362.

Lakatos, P., Chen, C. M., O'Connell, M. N., Mills, A., & Schroeder, C. E. (2007). Neuronal oscillations and multisensory interaction in primary auditory cortex. *Neuron*, 53(2), 279–292.

Latinus, M., McAleer, P., Bestelmeyer, P. E., & Belin, P. (2013). Norm-based coding of voice identity in human auditory cortex. *Current Biology*, 23(12), 1075–1080.

Logothetis, N. K., Guggenberger, H., Peled, S., & Pauls, J. (1999). Functional imaging of the monkey brain. *Nature Neuroscience*, 2(6), 555–562.

Matsui, T., Tamura, K., Koyano, K. W., Takeuchi, D., Adachi, Y., Osada, T., & Miyashita, Y. (2011). Direct comparison of spontaneous functional connectivity and effective connectivity measured by intracortical microstimulation: an fMRI study in macaque monkeys. *Cerebral Cortex*, 21(10), 2348–2356.

McLaren, D. G., Kosmatka, K. J., Oakes, T. R., Kroenke, C. D., Kohama, S. G., Matochik, J. A., Ingram, D. K., & Johnson, S. C. (2009). A population-average MRI-based atlas collection of the rhesus macaque. *NeuroImage*, 45(1), 52–59.

McMahon, D. B. T., Russ, B. E., Elnaiem, H. D., Kurnikova, A. I., & Leopold, D. A. (2015). Single-unit activity during natural vision: diversity, consistency, and spatial sensitivity among AF face patch neurons. *Journal of Neuroscience*, 35(14), 5537–5548.

Mesgarani, N. & Chang, E. F. (2012). Selective cortical representation of attended speaker in multi-talker speech perception. *Nature*, 485(7397), 233–236.

Meyers, E. M., Borzello, M., Freiwald, W. A., & Tsao, D. (2015). Intelligent information loss: the coding of facial identity, head pose, and non-face information in the macaque face patch system. *Journal of Neuroscience*, 35(18), 7069–7081.

Mizrahi, A., Shalev, A., & Nelken, I. (2014). Single neuron and population coding of natural sounds in auditory cortex. *Current Opinion in Neurobiology*, 24, 103–110.

Morin, E. L., Hadj-Bouziane, F., Stokes, M., Ungerleider, L. G., & Bell, A. H. (2014). Hierarchical encoding of social cues in primate inferior temporal cortex. *Cerebral Cortex*, 25(9), 3036–3045.

Munoz- Lopez, M. M., Mohedano-Moriano, A., & Insausti, R. (2010). Anatomical pathways for auditory memory in primates. *Frontiers in Neuroanatomy*, 4, 129.

Nelken, I., Fishbach, A., Las, L., Ulanovsky, N., & Farkas, D. (2003). Primary auditory cortex of cats: feature detection or something else? *Biological Cybernetics*, 89(5), 397–406.

Oya, H., Howard, M. A., Magnotta, V. A., Kruger, A., Griffiths, T. D., Lemieux, L., ... Kovach, C. K. (2017). Mapping effective connectivity in the human brain with concurrent intracranial electrical stimulation and BOLD-fMRI. *Journal of Neuroscientific Methods*, 277, 101–112.

Pandya, D. N., Hallett, M., & Mukherjee, S. K. (1969). Intra- and interhemispheric connections of the neocortical auditory system in the rhesus monkey. *Brain Research*, 14(1), 49–65.

Pascual, B., Masdeu, J. C., Hollenbeck, M., Makris, N., Insausti, R., Ding, S. L., & Dickerson, B. C. (2015). Large-scale brain networks of the human left temporal pole: a functional connectivity MRI study. *Cerebral Cortex*, 25(3), 680–702.

Pernet, C. R., McAleer, P., Latinus, M., Gorgolewski, K. J., Charest, I., Bestelmeyer, P. E., ... Belin, P. (2015). The human voice areas: spatial organization and inter-individual variability in temporal and extra-temporal cortices. *NeuroImage*, 119, 164–174.

Perrett, D. I., Rolls, E. T., & Caan, W. (1982). Visual neurones responsive to faces in the monkey temporal cortex. *Experimental Brain Research*, 47(3), 329–342.

Perrodin, C., Kayser, C., Abel, T. J., Logothetis, N. K., & Petkov, C. I. (2015). Who is that? Brain networks and mechanisms for identifying individuals. *Trends in Cognitive Sciences*, 19(12), 783–796.

Perrodin, C., Kayser, C., Logothetis, N. K., & Petkov, C. I. (2011). Voice cells in the primate temporal lobe. *Current Biology*, 21(16), 1408–1415.

Perrodin, C., Kayser, C., Logothetis, N. K., & Petkov, C. I. (2014). Auditory and visual modulation of temporal lobe neurons in voice-sensitive and association cortices. *Journal of Neuroscience*, 34(7), 2524–2537.

Perrodin, C., Kayser, C., Logothetis, N. K., & Petkov, C. I. (2015). Natural asynchronies in audiovisual communication signals regulate neuronal multisensory interactions in voice-sensitive cortex. *Proceedings of the National Academy of Sciences of the United States of America*, 112(1), 273–278.

Petkov, C. I., Kayser, C., Augath, M., & Logothetis, N. K. (2006). Functional imaging reveals numerous fields in the monkey auditory cortex. *PLoS Biology*, 4(7), e215.

Petkov, C. I., Kayser, C., Steudel, T., Whittingstall, K., Augath, M., & Logothetis, N. K. (2008). A voice region in the monkey brain. *Nature Neuroscience*, 11(3), 367–374.

Petkov, C. I., Kikuchi, Y., Milne, A. E., Mishkin, M., Rauschecker, J. P., & Logothetis, N. K. (2015). Different forms of effective connectivity in primate frontotemporal pathways. *Nature Communications*, 6, 10.1038/ncomms7000.

Petrides, M. & Pandya, D. N. (1988). Association fiber pathways to the frontal cortex from the superior temporal region in the rhesus monkey. *Journal of Computational Neurology*, 273(1), 52–66.

Plakke, B., Diltz, M. D., & Romanski, L. M. (2013). Coding of vocalizations by single neurons in ventrolateral prefrontal cortex. *Hearing Research*, 305, 135–143.

Plakke, B. & Romanski, L. M. (2014). Auditory connections and functions of prefrontal cortex. *Frontiers in Neuroscience*, 8, 199.

Poremba, A., Malloy, M., Saunders, R. C., Carson, R. E., Herscovitch, P., & Mishkin, M. (2004). Species-specific calls evoke asymmetric activity in the monkey's temporal poles. *Nature*, 427(6973), 448–451.

Rauschecker, J. P. (1998). Parallel processing in the auditory cortex of primates. *Audiology and Neurotology*, 3(2–3), 86–103.

Rauschecker, J. P. & Tian, B. (2000). Mechanisms and streams for processing of 'what' and 'where' in auditory cortex. *Proceedings of the National Academy of Sciences of the United States of America*, 97(22), 11800–11806.

Rauschecker, J. P., Tian, B., & Hauser, M. (1995). Processing of complex sounds in the macaque nonprimary auditory cortex. *Science*, 268(5207), 111–114.

Rauschecker, J. P., Tian, B., Pons, T., & Mishkin, M. (1997). Serial and parallel processing in rhesus monkey auditory cortex. *Journal of Computational Neurology*, 382(1), 89–103.

Recanzone, G. H. (2008). Representation of con-specific vocalizations in the core and belt areas of the auditory cortex in the alert macaque monkey. *Journal of Neuroscience*, 28(49), 13184–13193.

Remedios, R., Logothetis, N. K., & Kayser, C. (2009). An auditory region in the primate insular cortex responding preferentially to vocal communication sounds. *Journal of Neuroscience*, 29(4), 1034–1045.

Rendall, D., Owren, M. J., & Rodman, P. S. (1998). The role of vocal tract filtering in identity cueing in rhesus monkey (*Macaca mulatta*) vocalizations. *Journal of the Acoustical Society of America*, 103(1), 602–614.

Romanski, L. M. (2007). Representation and integration of auditory and visual stimuli in the primate ventral lateral prefrontal cortex. *Cerebral Cortex*, 17(Suppl 1), i61–69.

Romanski, L. M. (2012). Integration of faces and vocalizations in ventral prefrontal cortex: implications for the evolution of audiovisual speech. *Proceedings of the National Academy of Sciences of the United States of America*, 109(Suppl 1), 10717–10724.

Romanski, L. M., Averbeck, B. B., & Diltz, M. (2005). Neural representation of vocalizations in the primate ventrolateral prefrontal cortex. *Journal of Neurophysiology*, 93(2), 734–747.

Romanski, L. M., Bates, J. F., & Goldman-Rakic, P. S. (1999). Auditory belt and parabelt projections to the prefrontal cortex in the rhesus monkey. *Journal of Computational Neurology*, 403(2), 141–157.

Romanski, L. M., Tian, B., Fritz, J., Mishkin, M., Goldman-Rakic, P. S., & Rauschecker, J. P. (1999). Dual streams of auditory afferents target multiple domains in the primate prefrontal cortex. *Nature Neuroscience*, 2(12), 1131–1136.

Rothschild, G., Nelken, I., & Mizrahi, A. (2010). Functional organization and population dynamics in the mouse primary auditory cortex. *Nature Neuroscience*, 13(3), 353–360.

Russ, B. E., Ackelson, A. L., Baker, A. E., & Cohen, Y. E. (2008). Coding of auditory-stimulus identity in the auditory non-spatial processing stream. *Journal of Neurophysiology*, 99(1), 87–95.

Sadagopan, S., Temiz-Karayol, N. Z., & Voss, H. U. (2015). High-field functional magnetic resonance imaging of vocalization processing in marmosets. *Science Report*, 5, 10950.

Saleem, K. S. & Logothetis, N. K. (2007). *A Combined MRI and Histology Atlas of the Rhesus Monkey Brain in Stereotaxic Coordinates*. London: Academic Press.

Saleem, K. S., Kondo, H., & Price, J. L. (2008). Complementary circuits connecting the orbital and medial prefrontal networks with the temporal, insular, and opercular cortex in the macaque monkey. *Journal of Computational Neurology*, 506(4), 659–693.

Schall, S., Kiebel, S. J., Maess, B., & von Kriegstein, K. (2013). Early auditory sensory processing of voices is facilitated by visual mechanisms. *NeuroImage*, 77, 237–245.

Schroeder, C. E., Smiley, J., Fu, K. G., McGinnis, T., O'Connell, M. N., & Hackett, T. A. (2003). Anatomical mechanisms and functional implications of multisensory convergence in early cortical processing. *International Journal of Psychophysiology*, 50(1–2), 5–17.

Scott, B. H., Leccese, P. A., Saleem, K. S., Kikuchi, Y., Mullarkey, M. P., Fukushima, M., Mishkin, M., & Saunders, R. C. (2015). Intrinsic connections of the core auditory cortical regions and rostral supratemporal plane. *Cerebral Cortex*, 27(1), 809–840.

Seltzer, B. & Pandya, D. N. (1989). Frontal lobe connections of the superior temporal sulcus in the rhesus monkey. *Journal of Computational Neurology*, 281(1), 97–113.

Seltzer, B. & Pandya, D. N. (1994). Parietal, temporal, and occipital projections to cortex of the superior temporal sulcus in the rhesus monkey: a retrograde tracer study. *Journal of Computational Neurology*, 343(3), 445–463.

Sergent, J., Ohta, S., & MacDonald, B. (1992). Functional neuroanatomy of face and object processing. A positron emission tomography study. *Brain*, 115 Pt 1, 15–36.

Smith, D. R., Patterson, R. D., Turner, R., Kawahara, H., & Irino, T. (2005). The processing and perception of size information in speech sounds. *Journal of the Acoustical Society of America*, 117(1), 305–318.

Stein, B. E. & Stanford, T. R. (2008). Multisensory integration: current issues from the perspective of the single neuron. *Nature Reviews Neuroscience*, 9(4), 255–266.

Sugihara, T., Diltz, M. D., Averbeck, B. B., & Romanski, L. M. (2006). Integration of auditory and visual communication information in the primate ventrolateral prefrontal cortex. *Journal of Neuroscience*, 26(43), 11138–11147.

Tian, B., Reser, D., Durham, A., Kustov, A., & Rauschecker, J. P. (2001). Functional specialization in rhesus monkey au
ditory cortex. *Science*, 292(5515), 290–293.

Tsao, D. Y. & Freiwald, W. A. (2006). What's so special about the average face? *Trends in Cognitive Sciences*, 10(9), 391–393.

Tsao, D. Y., Freiwald, W. A., Tootell, R. B., & Livingstone, M. S. (2006). A cortical region consisting entirely of face-selective cells. *Science*, 311(5761), 670–674.

Tsao, D. Y. & Livingstone, M. S. (2008). Mechanisms of face perception. *Annual Review of Neuroscience*, 31, 411–437.

Tsao, D. Y., Schweers, N., Moeller, S., & Freiwald, W. A. (2008). Patches of face-selective cortex in the macaque frontal lobe. *Nature Neuroscience*, 11(8), 877–879.

von Kriegstein, K., Eger, E., Kleinschmidt, A., & Giraud, A. L. (2003). Modulation of neural responses to speech by directing attention to voices or verbal content. *Brain Research. Cognitive Brain Research*, 17(1), 48–55.

von Kriegstein, K. & Giraud, A. L. (2006). Implicit multisensory associations influence voice recognition. *PLoS Biology*, 4(10), e326.

von Kriegstein, K., Kleinschmidt, A., Sterzer, P., & Giraud, A. L. (2005). Interaction of face and voice areas during speaker recognition. *Journal of Cognitive Neuroscience*, 17(3), 367–376.

Wang, X. (2000). On cortical coding of vocal communication sounds in primates. *Proceedings of the National Academy of Sciences of the United States of America*, 97(22), 11843–11849.

Watson, R., Latinus, M., Charest, I., Crabbe, F., & Belin, P. (2014). People-selectivity, audiovisual integration and heteromodality in the superior temporal sulcus. *Cortex*, 50, 125–136.

Werner, S. & Noppeney, U. (2010). Distinct functional contributions of primary sensory and association areas to audiovisual integration in object categorization. *Journal of Neuroscience*, 30(7), 2662–2675.

Wollberg, Z. & Newman, J. D. (1972). Auditory cortex of squirrel monkey: response patterns of single cells to species-specific vocalizations. *Science*, 175(18), 212–214.

Yau, J. M., DeAngelis, G. C., & Angelaki, D. E. (2015). Dissecting neural circuits for multisensory integration and crossmodal processing. *Philosophical Transactions of the Royal Society of London B: Biol Sciences*, 370(1677), 20140203.

Young, A. W. & Bruce, V. (2011). Understanding person perception. *British Journal of Psychology*, 102(4), 959–974.

CHAPTER 16

....

VOICE PERCEPTION
ACROSS SPECIES

....

ATTILA ANDICS AND TAMÁS FARAGÓ

16.1 Voice Production in Vertebrates

16.1.1 Similarities in Voice Production Mechanisms Across Species

The neural architecture for producing vocalizations is highly conserved and shows clear homologies across vertebrates, even if peripheral end organs to create sounds are very different (Newman, 2010). Vocal control relies on a limited number of brain structures. The pathway found in most animals extends from subcortical forebrain regions, namely limbic structures and the hypothalamus, to midbrain regions, in particular the periaqueductal grey matter (PAG). The PAG elicits species-specific vocalizations in many species via excitatory amino acid transmitters (Jürgens, 1994). The homologous region of PAG is even found to be involved in communicating, via electronic signals, in some fish species (Heiligenberg, 1988). The PAG projects to the parvocellular reticular formation of the medulla and pons. The reticular formation is responsible for the patterning of vocal utterances, by controlling basal motor nuclei (Jürgens, 2009). Motor nuclei then project to the larynx and other articulatory structures (Jürgens, 2002; Liebal, 2014). This limbic pathway is thought to account for most emotional vocalizations. The involvement of parallel motor cortical pathways, and of cortical regions in general, is less well understood, and phylogenetically certainly less widespread, although recent findings suggest that in monkeys, just like in humans, voluntarily produced vocalizations are mediated by the prefrontal cortex (Coudé et al., 2011; Hage et al., 2013).

Across tetrapods, the main functional elements of the vocal tract are also conservative, much less variable than bodies (Fitch & Hauser, 2003). Although modifications and additional organs (e.g. vocal sacs, pads, elongations of the vocal tract) are present in some species, the basic mechanisms of vocal production are the same (even in birds which evolved a completely new sound source, the syrinx; Elemans et al., 2015). According to the source-filter framework (Fant, 1960), as the air flows through the respiratory tract during vocalization, specialized myoelastic vibrators (vocal folds or membranes) in the way of the air begin to open and close cyclically to produce a harmonic, complex sound wave, called the source signal. To exit the body through the nose or the mouth, this sound wave travels through the tubes and cavities of the upper respiratory tract (vocal tract), which modifies the frequency structure of the source signal. Filtering out of certain frequency bands (formants) gives the form of the final vocalization (Fant, 1960). The speed of the vocal folds' opening–closing cycles defines the fundamental frequency of the vocalizations, which mainly depends on the form, size, and weight of the folds.

Other vocal characteristics are also linked to the source. For example, the completeness of the closure between the two vocal folds affects the harmonicity of the calls, due to the addition of turbulent noise generated by the escaping air through the incomplete closure. Also, the level of vocal-fold asymmetry or the high tension in them can promote the appearance of non-linear phenomena, causing abrupt changes of pitch and tonality in the calls (Fitch et al., 2002). The filtering of the vocal tract contributes to the timbre of the calls and forms the vowels in human speech. The form of the respiratory tube determines the spectral position of the frequency bands that easily pass through it. More importantly, the average frequency steps between these formants (called formant dispersion) are linked to the length of the vocal tract, so they can provide size cues for the listeners during communication.

16.1.2 Similarities in Inner States Across Species

Early on, Darwin (1872/1965) suggested that human emotional expressions are homologous with animal signals of inner states. Since then, the presence of emotion and its level in animals is still disputed, mainly due to the supply of a wide variety of definitions and concurrent frameworks to model emotions (for a current review, see de Vere & Kuczaj, 2016). The recently emerging approach for studying animal emotions is integrative, attempting to combine classic dimensional and discrete models into a functional framework (Mendl et al., 2010). The primary emotional states (seeking, rage, fear, lust, care, panic/grief, and play—following Panksepp, 2005) are linked homologously to specific neural circuitries in a wide range of taxa. They can be mapped on an at least two-dimensional state space, mainly described by core affects (or emotional primitives), the general valence, and arousal states (Russell, 2003). These core affects can also be linked to given neurological and physiological states of the individual, and measured on a continuous scale.

Triggered by specific stimuli, these neural states (basically the activity of specific neural circuitry) evoke certain expressive behaviours that can act as communicative signals, broadcasting the current emotional state of the individual (Dolan, 2002). Although these behaviours can be ritualized and species-specific, the neural background is homologous across phylogeny, and the core affects seem to be shared across a wide range of species (even in arthropods; Anderson & Adolphs, 2014). For example, an infant animal in separation from its caregiver is in a negatively valenced inner state with a high arousal level which elevates over time. This state can be linked to the activity of panic-involved circuitry in the brain, evoking the use of distress signals. Then, upon the approach of the mother, and receipt of care, the arousal level is lowered, and the valence of the individual's inner state changes to positive, being in comfort and giving contact and bonding signals. On the behavioural level, a functional dimension can be linked to these inner states based on the evoked reaction of the used inner state expressions.

Based on Ehret's categorization, this basic biological meaning of signals can be positioned on the approach–stay–withdraw scale (Ehret, 2005). Staying with the previous example, the cries of an infant during separation have a strong approach-evoking potential, attracting the attention of the mother, while the comfort sounds function to maintain the positive interaction. In contrast, in the case of an intruder, the mother will respond aggressively, with the activation of rage circuitry: it will show agonistic signals to repel the intruder. Such signals can be linked to negative inner states with elevated arousal levels. In this regard, agonistic signals are quite similar to separation calls, but their biological meaning and communicative function are just the opposite.

Vocalizations most probably evolved from simple, involuntary noises, caused by the forced exhalation through a narrowing in the respiratory tract. For example, when an individual tries to evade harm during an attack by quickly jumping away, the sudden contraction of the body muscles could push air out of the lungs, which could produce a sound in the larynx (see for example, frog release calls, Gerhardt, 1994). The quality of this sound is assumably already affected by the neurological, emotional state (negative valence, high arousal) of the individual. Thus, the produced sound and the emotion could be associated by listeners, providing the basis of inner-state cues. Communicative signals could emerge from here, through ritualization (Scott-Phillips et al., 2012), but these still carry the cues of inner states due to the homologies in emotional and voice-production systems.

16.1.3 Acoustic Similarities Across Species in the Vocal Expressions of Inner States

Four decades ago, Eugene Morton had already noticed a recurring pattern in different avian and mammalian vocalizations. Comparing a wide range of taxa, he found that the level of aggression and fear of the caller is reflected in the acoustic structure similarly, regardless of the species (Morton, 1977). According to his findings, lower tonality and pitch is linked to a higher level of aggression, while with increasing fear or submission, pitch and tonality will both rise. Later, August and Anderson (1987) suggested the extension of these simple, so-called motivation-structural rules with a third emotion dimension, friendliness, and to take in consideration the role of temporal patterns too. In sum, these general structural rules suggest that aggressive, dominant calls are low-pitched and broadband, and harsh, fearful calls are high-pitched and tonal, while friendly calls are low-pitched, soft, and rhythmic. Note that these three types of calls fit well into Ehret's biological meaning concepts (Ehret, 2005).

Morton hypothesized that these rules are the result of convergent evolution, driven by the fact that the acoustic structure of calls is strongly linked to body size. He reasoned that in agonistic contexts it is adaptive to use low-pitched calls, as these reflect larger size and possibly have more repellent effect in contest situations, while the opposite applies for fearful signals. However, taking into consideration the homology of neural control mechanisms of sound production, and the presence of the same core affects across species, together with the fact that the basic voice production mechanisms are shared in terrestrial vertebrates (Fant, 1960; Fitch & Hauser, 2003), one can hypothesize that these general patterns can be inherent features of the voice production system. Higher arousal levels result in higher tension in the muscles involved in exhalation, causing longer, louder, and higher-pitched calls, while in the source, the laryngeal muscles stretch the vocal folds more, also leading to higher-frequency vocalizations. In the case of valence, this neuroacoustic link is harder to find, mainly due to the lack of research, and especially because of the relative rarity of clearly positive vocalizations. However, a number of recent studies support the idea of shared acoustic rules for emotion encoding in mammalian vocalizations (for reviews, see Briefer, 2012; Zimmermann et al., 2013). See Figure 16.1 and Audios 16.1, 16.2 and 16.3 for examples of sounds from different species, varying in valence and arousal.

In the time domain, parameters like call length, repetition rate, and inter-call interval play a role in emotion communication. Increase of call length and rate, and shorter inter-call intervals seem to be common indicators of elevated arousal, probably due to the higher tension of respiratory muscles (e.g. pig: Linhart et al., 2015; seal: Collins et al., 2011; baboon: Meise et al., 2011; hyena: Theis et al., 2007; tree shrew: Schehka et al., 2007; cat: Scheumann et al., 2012). In some alarm calls, element repetition reflects urgency and level of danger, suggesting a link of this parameter to the arousal of the caller. Some evidence shows that the call length and the inter-call interval can be linked to the valence of the individual too. For example, in playful contexts, dog growls are shorter and faster-pulsing than in agonistic contexts (Faragó, Pongrácz, Range, et al., 2010; Taylor et al., 2009), and the same is true in general for dog and human vocalizations (Faragó et al., 2014; Taylor et al., 2009). Squirrel monkeys (Fichtel et al., 2001) and rats (Brudzynski, 2007) also use shorter calls in rewarding contexts.

In the spectral domain, both source-related parameters (e.g. fundamental frequency, tonality) and filter-related parameters (e.g. formant frequencies) carry emotional information. High pitch, probably due to the higher tension in the laryngeal muscles and the vocal folds, is strongly linked with elevated arousal (e.g. pig: Linhart et al., 2015; cat: Scheumann et al., 2012; Yeon et al., 2011; baboon: Rendall, 2003; chimpanzee: Slocombe & Zuberbühler, 2007; tree shrew: Schehka et al., 2007). In contrast, the role of pitch is less clear in valence encoding. Indeed, pitch can be linked to several oppositely valenced emotional states. Some results indicate that higher pitch is associated with positive inner states, such as playful contexts (rats: Knutson et al., 2002; dog barks: Pongrácz et al., 2005; Yin & McCowan, 2004; dog growls: Faragó, Pongrácz, Range, et al., 2010), but on a more general level, higher-pitched call types are linked to more negative states. Among pig (Tallet et al., 2013) or elephant (Soltis et al., 2011) vocalizations, the calls linked with comfort and positive inner states are lower-pitched. Also, agonistic calls are characterized by low frequency in general. Thus it seems that pitch can be closer linked to the social proximity (approach-withdrawal) dimension.

The tonality of calls depends mainly on the regularity of the vocal fold movements and can be measured with the harmonic-to-noise ratio (HNR), which is affected by both the pressure of the flowing air in the vocal tract, and the position and tension of the vocal folds (Riede et al., 2001, 2005). This parameter thus seems to be mainly associated with the arousal level of the caller. In meerkats, alarm calls become noisier with the decreasing distance of the predator, reflecting the urgency of the alarm (Manser, 2001). In baboons, the graded bark vocalizations have a tonal subtype used as a contact signal to maintain group cohesion, and a harsh subtype used as an alarm call, assumably linked to elevated arousal (Fischer et al., 2001). Blumstein and Récapet (2009) suggested that the occurrence of non-linear phenomena (NLPs) can be an honest signal of arousal, as their appearance in vocalizations is more probable when the tension is high in the vocal folds. Also, the unpredictable nature of these phenomena cause signals carrying them to be hard to ignore (Fitch et al., 2002).

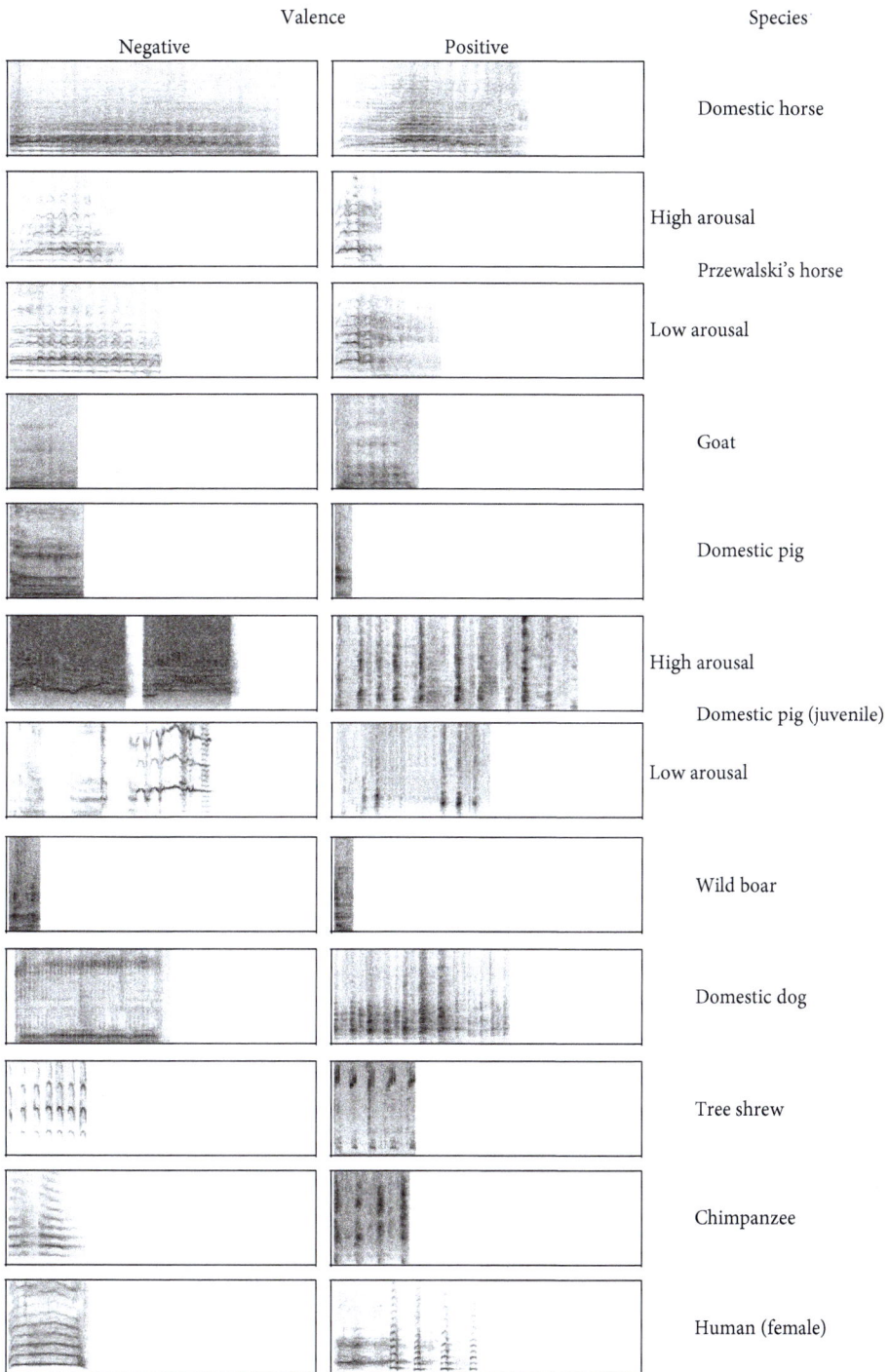

FIGURE 16.1 The general encoding of valence in mammalian vocalizations. Sonograms of vocalization samples from several wild and domesticated mammalian species recorded in negative (agonistic or fear inducing) and positive (affiliative, playful) contexts. Calls linked with positive valence are bouts of short calls with a pulsing, rhythmic structure. All x axes show the time in seconds, the right end representing 3.5 seconds, while all y axes show the frequency scale between 0 and 11 kHz.

This attention-grabbing effect can be highly advantageous in alarm or other distress contexts. Accordingly, meerkats react with higher vigilance and habituate less to alarm calls with NLPs (Karp et al., 2014). Similarly, great-tailed grackles become more vigilant when hearing calls with frequency jumps (Slaughter et al., 2013). However, in some cases we see an opposite pattern, with higher arousal calls carrying less spectral noise or NLPs (macaque aggressive call: Gouzoules et al., 1998; marmot alarm call: Blumstein & Chi, 2011).

The formant frequencies primarily depend on the length and shape of the vocal tract, making it a reliable indexical cue (for a review, see Taylor & Reby, 2010). Formants thus play an important role specifically in mate choice and agonistic encounters (Charlton & Reby, 2016). The vocal tract is more constrained by the anatomy of the individual, and only species with special adaptations (muscles to lower the larynx, proboscis, facial expressions like protruding the lips) are able to actively manipulate it (Fitch & Hauser, 2003). As such, formant frequencies seem to be less important in emotion communication. However, some evidence suggests that higher arousal can cause an upward shift in formants, assumedly due to the decrease of mucus and saliva in the vocal tract, and the constriction of the walls of the respiratory system (pig: Düpjan et al., 2008; baboon: Fischer et al.. 2001; chimpanzee: Slocombe & Zuberbühler, 2007; elephant: Soltis et al., 2011; tree shrew: Schehka & Zimmermann, 2009). Additionally, playful growls in dogs have lower formant dispersion than agonistic growls, suggesting a possible role for formants in valence communication too (Faragó, Pongrácz, Range, et al., 2010).

This link between call structure and the corresponding inner state might be the main reason of the conservativity of certain call types. For example, infant cries and also adult distress calls that are linked to high arousal and strong negative valence, and that evoke an approach reaction from caretakers or group members, share a similar structure across a wide range of taxa (e.g. in birds: Jurisevic & Sanderson, 1998; and for a review, see Lingle et al., 2012). Such calls are loud, high-frequency vocalizations with a rising–constant–falling 'chevron' pattern in their pitch contour, and a clear harmonic structure. Moreover, certain parameters (amplitude, peak frequency, spectral energy) are changed gradually, along with the rise of arousal level of the caller, providing a direct cue of the caller's inner state.

16.2 Voice Perception in Vertebrates

16.2.1 Similarities in Voice-Processing Mechanisms Across Species

Adequate processing of conspecific vocal signals is essential in a number of different situations, including territory disputes, sexual selection, and parental behaviour. The ability and readiness to make inferences about the vocalizer's size, age, sex, group membership, individual identity, and about its actual inner state, to then adjust behaviour accordingly, puts the listener at an obvious advantage. Even though there are differences in how much different species vocalize, the basic motivations and selective forces that make individuals interested in vocalizations are rather similar across species.

The neural pathways that support vocalization processing have been investigated in some Amphibiae (frogs: Kelley, 2004) and reptiles (geckos: Manley & Kraus, 2010), and more extensively in birds, including parental songbirds (canaries: Mello et al., 1992; zebra finches: Hauber et al., 2013; Maul et al., 2009; Mello et al., 1992; Poirier et al., 2009; black-capped chickadees: Avey et al., 2014), brood parasitic songbirds (pin-tailed why-dahs: Louder et al., 2016), and non-songbirds (ring doves: Terpstra et al., 2005), and in a variety of mammalian species, including rodents (mice: Holmstrom et al., 2010; Portfors et al., 2009; rats: Wöhr & Schwarting, 2010; guinea pigs: Šuta, 2003; Šuta et al., 2007, 2013), chiroptera (bats: Pollak, 2013), carnivores (cats: Wang & Kadia, 2001; dogs: Andics et al., 2014), and primates (marmosets: Sadagopan & Wang, 2009; Sadagopan et al., 2015; Wang & Kadia, 2001; rhesus macaques: Gifford et al., 2005; Perrodin et al., 2011; Petkov et al., 2008; Poremba et al., 2004; Rauschecker & Tian, 2000; Tian et al., 2001; chimpanzees: Taglialatela et al., 2009; and humans: Andics et al., 2014; Belin et al., 2000, 2002; Fecteau et al., 2004). A central finding in a majority of these studies is that certain brain regions prefer vocalizations over other sounds in general, or particularly conspecific sounds over both heterospecific sounds and non-vocal sounds.

The neural substrates involved in vocalization processing are apparently highly similar, at least across mammals. Response selectivity for communication sounds appears first in the inferior colliculus (Pollak, 2013), and then, at higher stages of the auditory processing hierarchy (primary auditory cortex; posterior, mid, and anterior portions of the superior temporal gyrus (STG) and superior temporal sulcus (STS); and the anterior temporal pole), neural sensitivity becomes more and more specific to relevant, typically conspecific vocal sounds (e.g. Andics et al., 2014; Sadagopan et al., 2015). The highest selectivity for conspecific vocalizations has been found in the anterior/ventral temporal cortex, particularly the temporal pole, in several primate species, including marmosets (Sadagopan et al., 2015), rhesus macaques (Perrodin et al., 2011; Petkov et al., 2008), chimpanzees (Taglialatela et al., 2009), and humans (Andics et al., 2010, 2014; von Kriegstein et al., 2004). Recently, we demonstrated conspecific preference in the temporal pole of dogs (Andics et al., 2014), extending previous findings to non-primate mammals.

Vocalization processing thus relies on evolutionarily ancient neural pathways, also indicating that conspecific sound preference is based, at least partly, on in-born capacities and sensitivities. However, listener experience (familiarity, expertise) with non-conspecific sound categories may also increase auditory cortex activity (Leech et al., 2009; Liebenthal et al., 2010; Talkington et al., 2012), suggesting an important role for learning. Early experience also shapes vocal neural coding and perception in songbirds (for a review, see Woolley, 2012).

16.2.2 Similarities in the Neural Processing of Acoustic Cues Across Species

A growing body of evidence shows that the basic temporal and spectral acoustic cues of complex communication sounds are processed by parallel brain regions in different species. Sound duration is first coded in the central nucleus of the inferior colliculus, as evidenced in both bats (Covey & Casseday, 1999) and mice (Brand et al., 2000). Sensitivity to call length in vocal sounds has also been found in the auditory thalamus, the medial geniculate body, and also in the near-primary auditory cortex in dogs (Andics et al., 2014).

The tonotopic organization of the cochlea and the auditory pathway up to the primary auditory cortex has been well described in a range of mammals (Merzenich et al., 1976). It has also been shown that tonotopic representations are essential to complex pitch perception (Oxenham et al., 2004). Pitch perception is supported by the specific areas of the auditory cortex. In rhesus monkeys, pitch-selective neurons are found between core and belt auditory cortex (Bendor & Wang, 2005). In humans, pitch sensitivity has been found in an area anterior to Heschl's gyrus (Patterson et al., 2002; for a review, see Bizley & Cohen, 2013). Increased sensitivity to lower pitch in the near-primary auditory cortex has been reported in humans (Norman-Haignere et al., 2013), macaques (Bendor & Wang, 2005), and recently also in dogs (Andics et al., 2014). Pitch-related activity has also been found in non-core auditory cortex in both ferrets (Bizley & King, 2009) and humans (Hall & Plack, 2009; Staeren et al., 2009).

Complex communicative sounds are typically composed from multiple frequencies that are often related harmonically. Harmonic-to-noise ratio (HNR) is an important signal attribute of vocalizations, and the behavioural relevance of sounds with a high HNR motivates the neural preference to harmonically structured sounds. Indeed, harmonicity appears to be a fundamental organizing principle of the auditory cortex. Neurons with multi-peak frequency tuning have been found in various mammalian species (for a review, see Wang, 2013). Increased neural sensitivity to specific combinations of frequencies, and in particular to harmonic complex sounds over inharmonic sounds, has been found in neurons of the auditory cortex or analogous structures in various vertebrates, including zebra finches (Lewicki & Konishi, 1995), bats (Medvedev, 2004), rhesus monkeys (Rauschecker et al., 1995), and recently also marmosets (Feng & Wang, 2017).

The capacity to process spectral peaks and their relations, therefore being sensitive to formant dispersion and timbre in vocalizations, has been demonstrated in vowel-discrimination studies in a number of primate and non-primate mammals, and in several bird species (for a review, see Town & Bizley, 2013). Intensity-independent spectral filtering and integration, a prerequisite to process timbre, occurs first in the inferior colliculus (Egorova & Ehret, 2008).

16.2.3 Similarities in the Neural Processing of Basic Biological Meanings in Vocalizations

Ehret and Kurt (2010) argued that there are general perceptual borders in the mammalian auditory system, supporting the categorization of vocalizations. In the temporal domain, such borders seem to exist across species at 20 ms, 100 ms, and 400 ms. For example, call series with a call repetition rate below 20 ms are perceived as a pitch, between 20 ms and 100 ms the percept is roughness in the sound, while above 100 ms it is heard as a rhythm. The perceptual border is 20–25 ms on the voice onset time (VOT) continuum that separates the perception of /ba/ from /pa/, in both humans (Pisoni & Lazarus, 1974) and chinchillas (Kuhl & Miller, 1975). The same border separates biologically relevant from irrelevant mouse ultrasounds by their mothers (Kuhl & Miller, 1975), and potential prey from other objects during echo-delay evaluation in the moustached bat auditory cortex (Suga et al., 1983). The perceptual border at 100 ms is apparent in humans in the perception of alternating sound frequencies. If the inter-sound interval is shorter than this, then we hear two separate streams, and if longer, then we hear a single stream with alternating frequency (Anstis & Saida, 1985). The 400-ms border is relevant during the loudness summation of click sounds; this summation only happens in the case of inter-sound intervals below 400 ms (Scharf, 1978). Both the 100-ms and 400-ms perceptual borders are also found in mouse mothers processing their pups' wriggling calls (Gaub & Ehret, 2005) and in event-related neural responses recorded in rats (Finlayson, 1999), cats (Calford & Semple, 1995), monkeys (Fishman et al., 2001), and humans (Budd & Michie, 1994).

In the spectral domain, so-called critical bands (CBs) support the processing of spectrally rich sounds, such as vocalizations. CB processing is the basic tool for the categorical perception of sound energy at different frequencies, and therefore for perceiving formants and timbre (Ehret & Kurt, 2010).

Both temporal and spectral perceptual borders may be utilized to separate vocal sounds with different biological meanings. Indeed, these and other general perceptual mechanisms can be used to separate basic biological meanings in vocalizations. Basic biological meanings include attraction, cohesion, and aversion, as also reflected in a functional division of vocalizations from a large variety of mammals (Ehret, 2005), and as characterized by distinct basic behavioural consequences in the perceiver. There is some evidence that the neural distinctions between basic biological meanings, or between emotional categories, also involve similar brain mechanisms in different species. Subcortical regions, especially the amygdala and the basal ganglia, are involved in processing various negative emotions (anger, fear, disgust) expressed during vocal behaviour, and also positive emotions (happiness) in primates (for a review, see Gruber & Grandjean, 2017). In rats, aversive (22 kHz) and affiliative (50 kHz) ultrasonic vocalizations elicited differential limbic system responses (Wöhr & Schwarting, 2010). In bats, distinctive single-neuron responses were found for aggressive and appeasing vocal sequences in the basolateral amygdala (Gadziola et al., 2016). It has also been argued that the amygdala and the limbic system show a general response to high arousal states (Frühholz et al., 2014). In humans, various cortical regions, including the STG, STS, orbitofrontal cortex, inferior frontal cortex (IFC), and prefrontal cortices have also been shown to be involved in processing emotional prosody (Schirmer & Kotz, 2006; Wildgruber et al., 2009).

Comparative evidence for the involvement of cortical regions in vocal emotional processing is scarce, but behavioural studies on lateralization give some indications on differential hemispheric involvement. Similar lateralization patterns are found across all vertebrate classes for emotional processing in general, with a right bias for processing negatively connotated emotions (fear, aggression), and left bias for processing positively connotated emotions (e.g. those elicited by a food reward) (for a review, see Leliveld et al., 2013). For conspecific communication sounds, left hemispheric advantages have been reported in raptors (Palleroni, 2003), starlings (George et al., 2002), mice (Ehret, 1987; Geissler & Ehret, 2004), sea lions (Böye et al., 2005), dogs (Siniscalchi et al., 2008), horses (Basile et al., 2009), and rhesus monkeys (Ghazanfar et al., 2001; Hauser & Andersson, 1994; Hauser et al., 1998), but a right hemispheric advantage was found in vervet monkeys, for differently valenced vocalizations (Gil-da-Costa & Hauser, 2006), suggesting that the advantaged hemisphere may vary across species. The inconsistent coupling of orientating biases and lateralized acoustic processing (Fischer et al., 2009) necessitates more direct measures. In a positron emission tomography (PET) study with rhesus monkeys, Poremba et al. (2004) reported left bias for conspecific sounds in the temporal pole only, and right bias for other, more posterior regions of the STG.

16.3 HETEROSPECIFIC VOICE PERCEPTION

16.3.1 Behavioural Evidence for Heterospecific Voice Processing

In the previous sections, we have argued that motivations to vocalize and to process vocalizations, just like the neural architecture to produce and analyse vocal sounds, are highly similar across species. Vocalizations themselves, and the cues to express specific inner states, are also similar across species acoustically in many respects. These similarities, and also the general ability to learn about vocal sounds, provide a good basis to assume that heterospecific vocalizations, or at least specific cues in these vocalizations, may be efficiently processed. Vocal communication takes place most of the time among conspecifics, but there are various reasons and situations that make heterospecific vocalizations relevant for an individual. Individuals monitor their environment and gather information to behave adaptively in any context, and besides conspecific vocalizations, heterospecific calls are also present in the vicinity. Thus, conspecific vocalizations and heterospecifc calls can be exploited to optimize behaviour. In such cases, the capacity to attend to and adequately process at least part of the encoded information in heterospecific sounds may put the individual at an advantage (Marler, 1955).

The most obvious case of such heterospecific interactions occurs between predators and prey (although it is debated whether these can be considered communicative situations at all; cf. Searcy & Nowicki, 2005). The predator can recognize and locate prey by their calls. There is a strong selection pressure on both parties (although the cost for the caller is higher) leading to an arms race. For the prey, it is advantageous to shift their vocalizations into a frequency range inaudible for the predator, and for the predator it is useful to develop increased sensitivity in the prey's vocalization frequency range. One classic example is how frog-eating bats use the advertisement calls of túngara frogs during hunting (Ryan et al., 1982), although recent findings suggest that predator pressure had lower effect on signal evolution than thought before (Akre et al., 2011). Prey can also eavesdrop on the calls of the predator to avoid attacks. Several moth species use evading tactics when hearing the ultrasonic clicks of a hunting bat, and katydids, when sympatric with bats, alter their song to minimize predation (Belwood & Morris, 1987).

Although in these predator–prey settings the emotional content of the vocalization and the identity of the vocalizer are hardly relevant for the listener, in some cases they can still extract valuable information about their counterparts. A recent study showed that African elephants react to human speech depending on the imposed threat. They are most vigilant at the voice of Maasai men who hunt elephants, compared to Kamba men, and are also able to differentiate men from women and adults from children (McComb et al., 2014). Also, as a special case, certain species can eavesdrop on heterospecific food calls. Japanese sika deer seem to use the calls emitted by Japanese macaques upon discovery of food to locate fruit falls, thus clearly benefiting from eavesdropping (Koda, 2012). In this case, the macaques appear to suffer no disadvantage from deer processing their sounds, but there may well be similar situations when one of two competing species is attracted by the other's food calls and able to usurp and monopolize the food source.

When there is no conflict between the caller and the eavesdropper, and the caller has no or relatively low cost due to the interaction, we talk about interceptive eavesdropping (Peake, 2005). Broadcast signals like alarm and mobbing calls are typical sources of interceptive eavesdropping for sympatric species that share predators but do not compete for the same resources. Accordingly, the most widespread (and well-studied) cases of eavesdropping are when heterospecifics react to alarm calls with fleeing, hiding, or even approaching the predator to engage in repelling behaviours (for a review, see Magrath et al., 2015). Alarm calls seem to broadcast various information, like the presence of a predator, the level of danger, and in some cases even the type of predator. Thus the eavesdropper can have a clear benefit from processing the encoded information on any level.

According to Magrath et al. (2015), several mechanisms can facilitate heterospecific eavesdropping. Acoustic similarities with the eavesdropper's own alarm calls, due to the shared emotional background and voice production mechanisms, can promote a situation of 'lucky confusion' or generalization to the heterospecific call. Key features that evoke the reaction from the responder can be similar across species, and they therefore trigger predation-evading behaviours from bystander species too. Additionally, features like harshness or the presence of non-linear phenomena in alarm calls can be strongly linked to the elevated arousal level (Blumstein & Chi, 2011). During an alarm situation, independently of the caller species, the occurrence of NLPs is an inherent specificity of the voice-production system. Such features can therefore evoke the same alert response from heterospecifics. Moreover, in cases when, due to ecological constraints (noisy environment, high variability of calls), individuals have to be sensitive to a broad range of parameters in the alarm calls, it is advantageous to respond to heterospecific signals that acoustically overlap with their own calls, as missing a true alarm usually has a high cost.

The suggestion that there are shared key features in alarm calls across species is supported by several observations and studies. For example, Aubin used synthetic calls to find such shared features in a playback study with seagulls, crows, and blackbirds (Aubin, 1991). He found that the calls without species-specific features evoked similar alert responses from all test species. Fairy wrens and scrub wrens are found to be mutually responsive to each other's alarm calls. Both species use a similar call structure, and both were found to be sensitive to the urgency encoded in the element repetition number in these calls (Fallow & Magrath, 2010).

Chickadees also encode the urgency in their alarm calls, which is strongly related to the size of the predator. Smaller predators put higher predation risk on small songbirds, and this is reflected in element repetition number within the alarm calls, probably strongly linked to the arousal level of the caller (Templeton et al., 2005). The sympatric nuthatches respond by attacking the predator on these chickadee alarm calls, and even process the level of urgency in these calls. Alarms indicating a smaller predator (which is more dangerous to the nuthatches) evoke stronger mobbing behaviour (Templeton & Greene, 2007). Although the authors suggested that this reaction is a result of learning, as the eavesdropper species' own alarm is acoustically different, the effect of simple arousal-encoding features was not tested and thus cannot be excluded.

The same dilemma between learnt versus innate capacities also stands for recent findings of eavesdropping on alarm calls by solitary or even non-vocal species. One study found that the dik-dik, a non-social ungulate, responds with escape and vigilance behaviours to white-bellied 'go-away' bird alarm calls, but not on a song of another, non-threatening bird (Lea et al., 2008). Similarly, a solitary rodent, the red squirrel, was found to respond to jay alarm calls but not to neutral songs (Randler, 2006). Moreover, non-vocal reptiles also exploit and react to avian alarms with vigilance (Ito & Mori, 2010; Vitousek et al., 2007) or with body-colour change (Ito et al., 2013). All these species have no own alarm-call systems, and live solitarily or have limited social behaviours. One can thus argue that their response is a learnt reaction, the result of association of the call and the attacking predator. However, we cannot exclude the possibility that these species are innately sensitive to emotional cues in these calls (Johnson et al., 2003; Russ et al., 2004) or key features linked to the high arousal level (like repetition rate or the presence of NLP). In these studies, only sympatric, non-alarm songs were used as control sounds. To decide between these two alternate hypotheses, it will be important to use artificially manipulated playbacks or alarm calls of unfamiliar species.

Mobbing is an anti-predator behaviour, where individuals of the potential prey approach and even attack the predator, or an unfamiliar stimulus (Caro, 2005), and it is associated with special signals, including mobbing vocalizations. Upon the detection of the predator, the initiator individual gives mobbing calls that evoke the attention of the nearby conspecifics, and they approach the predator, joining the calling and harassing the predator. Mobbing calls can be considered as special alarm calls. Their acoustic structure seems to be similar across species, with highly salient features (Marler, 1955). Mobbing is associated with a conflicting inner state, with a moderate level of fear that is not high enough to evoke flight response, and also with the motivation to react aggressively to the predator (Lord et al., 2009). Thus, not surprisingly, there are numerous examples of heterospecific reactions to mobbing signals and engagement in anti-predator behaviours (Marler, 1955; chickadee: Hurd, 1996; willow tit and redwing: Forsman & Monkkonen, 2001). Johnson et al. (2003) found that apostlebirds respond to allopatric mobbing calls. Moreover, they showed that these birds also respond to narrow-band noise pulses imitating the time pattern of their own mobbing calls. This suggests that both rhythm and spectral energy distribution are important keys for evoking the mobbing behaviour.

Dog barks confused researchers for a long time, as it was not clear why this call type is so widely used in dogs, while in wolves and other canids it has a specific territory-defence function (for a review, see Pongrácz et al., 2010). It is now believed that dog barks have a general communicative function, their acoustic structure has context-specific variations, and they follow the motivation-structural rules to encode emotions (Pongrácz et al., 2005). Besides, Lord et al. (2009) suggested that based on the acoustic structure, the original function of the dog bark was a call-to-arms signal, basically a mobbing call. It is possible that early humans could eavesdrop on the barks of the proto-dogs living around their encampments and thus be informed about any intruders earlier than otherwise. Then, during the further steps of domestication, they selected for individuals that barked more, and this could be an important factor in the diversification of dog barks.

Infant cries (separation and distress calls) have a strikingly similar acoustic structure across species (Lingle et al., 2012). Consequently, they are possibly capable of evoking reactions not only from the caregiver to whom they were intended, but also from heterospecifics. Nevertheless, approaching a heterospecific vocalizer in distress is, with the exception of a predation context, hardly ever advantageous for any party. Interestingly, Lingle and Riede (2014) found that mule deer and white-tailed deer approached the playback site when hearing an infant cry, regardless of its species, but ignored other calls that fell into the species-specific frequency range, lacking the special structure of a cry. Heterospecific cries may provoke strong reactions, because for a mother, ignoring the cries of her own infant can be much more costly than a false response to a similar, but heterospecific call.

Although it is obvious that different species, sharing the same habitats and competing for the same resources (e.g. food, shelter, territory), have to face conflict situations with each other, to our knowledge very little is known about how they use and understand each other's communicative signals. Vocal signalling in such heterospecific contests should be advantageous as, due to the previously mentioned homologous processes in emotion encoding and shared vocal-production mechanisms, both information transfer and manipulation of the other's behaviour could work. For example, as body size is strongly connected with the individual's resource-holding potential, it would be essential to use size cues in vocalizations to assess the fighting ability of heterospecifics. This seems to be possible, as a growing body of evidence shows that formant dispersion is a widely-used cue for size assessment (for reviews, see Charlton & Reby, 2016; Taylor & Reby, 2010; and e.g. red deer: Reby et al., 2005; koala: Charlton et al., 2012; dog: Faragó, Pongrácz, Miklósi, et al., 2010; Taylor et al., 2011). Furthermore, several experiments have showed that a range of species are sensitive to the formant information in human speech and able to differentiate vowels (reviewed in Bizley & Cohen, 2013; Town & Bizley, 2013). Nevertheless, we know of no studies that directly tested vocalization-based heterospecific size-assessment capacities in non-human listeners. In humans, Taylor et al. (2008) found that listeners are sensitive to the size cue provided by the formant dispersion in aggressive dog growls. Both natural and artificially modified samples were assessed by humans, and they rated the dogs larger if their growls showed larger body size due to lower formant positions.

The family dog is a special species, even among domesticated animals, with regard to the fact that they were selected to live and fit into the human social environment (Miklósi & Topál, 2013). They cooperate and interact with humans on a daily basis, and thus their sociocognitive and communicative abilities have changed dramatically throughout domestication. Accordingly, dogs are able to extract and use important information from human speech or other non-verbal vocalizations during interactions (for an overview, see Miklósi, 2007). They can learn to differentiate numerous words labelling different objects (Kaminski et al., 2004), and can match the gender of a speaker if they have had experience with multiple persons (Ratcliffe et al., 2014). It is also known that dogs show attachment to their owners (Topál et al., 1998) and prefer them over strangers or even other family members (Kerepesi et al., 2015). Thus, we can assume that they are able to differentiate their owners from others by their voice. Indeed, Adachi et al. (2007) found that dogs match the sound of their owners with their faces. Furthermore, they seem to react to human cries with an approach- and empathy-like behaviour suggesting that they process the emotional load of the vocalization (Custance & Mayer, 2012), and they can match dog and human emotional vocalizations with facial expressions. Dog puppies are also responsive to humans using dog-directed speech (Ben-Aderet et al., 2017) that, similarly to human infant-directed speech, is characterized by higher pitch, slower tempo, and clearer articulation of vowels (Gergely et al., submitted).

In sum, there are many different situations when listening to heterospecific sounds has benefits for the listener. It is trivial between predator and prey, but also evident in multispecies communities where one species can use the other's capacities. We have also reviewed examples of true cooperative communicative situations across species. Many of these cases where heterospecific sounds influence behaviour may be based on a mix of inherent capacities to process phylogenetically conserved acoustic cues and capacities to learn about relevant vocal sounds in the environment. Future studies will need to complement existing evidence to better understand the specific contributions of inherited and learnt factors to heterospecific sound processing.

In non-human playback studies, strict control conditions are rarely applied. Therefore, we have extensive evidence showing that cross-species vocal communication sounds may be efficient in influencing behaviour, but how similarly conspecific and heterospecific sounds are processed, and whether the same acoustic and emotional-processing brain mechanisms are used, is much less understood. In the next subsections, we review the findings of heterospecific sound playback studies with humans, and comparative neuroscientific studies on heterospecific sound processing.

16.3.2 Human Behavioural Evidence for Heterospecific Emotional Processing from Voices

It is obvious that humans excel at recognizing conspecific emotions. This recognition capacity has largely culture-independent biological roots, and we are able to assess the emotional load of speech based on prosody, and also recognize non-verbal emotional expressions (Anikin & Persson, 2016; Koeda et al., 2013; Sauter et al., 2015). Furthermore, a growing body of evidence suggests that humans are very talented in recognizing emotions in heterospecific vocalizations.

One of the earliest playback studies showed that humans, without any prior experience, are able to sort macaque vocalizations into emotional categories (e.g. frightened/timid/terrified, submissive/pleading/begging), according to their original contexts (agonistic, submissive, alarm, etc.) (Leinonen et al., 1991). A later study also showed that this ability appears in children during development, along with the ability to recognize conspecific emotions (Linnankoski et al., 1994). This finding suggested that humans might use the same processes to assess non-human animal emotions that they use for human emotions. Further findings in recent years, using mainly domestic animals' vocalizations, seem to support this hypothesis. In these, the human listeners were asked to rate vocalizations of pigs (Tallet et al., 2010) or dog and human emotion expressions (Faragó et al., 2014) on the core-affect level. The results of both studies showed that humans assessed the valence and intensity of conspecific and heterospecific calls according to their contexts. Moreover, it seems that humans use the same simple acoustic rules for this assessment, fitting well with the motivation-structural rules (Morton, 1977). Regardless of the species, call bouts with shorter calls are rated as more positive, while higher call pitch is linked to higher-intensity ratings. This assessment seems to be innate as the rater's personality (Maruščáková et al., 2015) and experience with the given species has minor effect on it.

This assessment ability applies not just across the vocal repertoire of the given species, but within certain vocalization types too. Dog barks (Pongrácz et al., 2005) and growls (Faragó et al., submitted) have a context-specific acoustic variation following the Morton rules, and human listeners attribute emotional states to them accordingly, rating lower-pitched and harsh calls as aggressive, but high-frequency and tonal calls as fearful or playful (Pongrácz et al., 2006). Here again, experience has little effect (Molnár et al., 2009) and, similarly to the results of Linnankoski et al. (1994), the development of human emotion recognition is necessary for proper context associations (Pongrácz et al., 2011). Probably, when the task in such studies is to guess the context of the vocalization, the listeners have to use higher-level cognitive processes to associate the recognized inner state with the possible contexts, and this process requires experience.

However, the picture is not so clear in some other cases. For example, certain other cues can override basic emotion assessment, leading to emotion misattribution. In threatening dog growls, which are poor in temporal information, the combination of pitch and formant cues indicating larger individuals led to rating them as more aggressive (Taylor et al., 2010). Moreover, humans were not able to differentiate threatening and playful single growls, probably due to the lack of distinctive temporal features (Taylor et al., 2009). Similarly, listeners show low accuracy in recognizing the assumed valence or the context of cat meows (Nicastro & Owren, 2003), of a wide range of cat vocalizations (Schötz & Weijer, 2014), and of rhesus macaque calls (Belin et al., 2008). In line with these latter findings, Scheumann et al. (2014) used human infant, dog, chimpanzee, and tree shrew calls from differently valenced contexts and found that experience with these animals had a strong effect on the assessment of emotional load. Moreover, negative human, dog, and chimp calls were all rated according to their context, but only positive human calls were rated as positive.

In sum, humans seem to assess the emotional state of various vocalizing species, suggesting the presence of an acoustic-based general emotion-attributing system. However, the role and the allocation of innate and learned functions in this process, as in the case of non-humans, is still unclear. Albeit, preliminary results show that humans, independently from their cultural background, assess the arousal level of calls from a wide range of taxa similarly (Filippi et al., 2016), suggesting the dominance of innate processes and supporting the use of general rules of acoustic encoding of core affects. On the one hand, further behavioural studies are required, using calls of multiple species recorded from well-controlled contexts to ensure the comparability of the possible emotional backgrounds, and to get a clearer picture of what influences vocal emotion assessment in humans. On the other hand, we have scarce neurological evidence on how this heterospecific emotion processing works in humans and how this is intertwined with the recognition of human emotions.

16.3.3 Neural Capacities for Making Sense of Heterospecific Vocalizations

There have been only a few neuroscientific studies to date that have investigated heterospecific vocalization processing and have compared that not only to conspecific but also to non-vocal control sounds. These include behavioural findings on lateralization, providing indirect evidence for functional hemispheric asymmetries, and also several neuroimaging (fMRI) studies. There are especially few neuroscientific reports on cross-species processing of emotional or referential meanings in vocalizations. In fact, to our knowledge, non-human neuroimaging studies on heterospecific vocal emotional processing have so far only been conducted in dogs (Andics et al., 2014, 2016).

Several lateralization studies investigated head-turning preferences for heterospecific sounds. Japanese macaques showed left-hemisphere dominance for discriminating species-specific calls on the basis of communicative relevance but not for pitch discrimination, while heterospecific monkeys showed no lateralization bias in either tasks (Petersen et al., 1978, 1984). Rhesus monkeys showed a left-hemisphere bias for conspecific and a right bias for heterospecific monkey-call processing (Hauser & Andersson, 1994). Grey mouse lemur males' head turns indicated a left-hemisphere bias for negative conspecific calls, but there was no bias for the sounds of phylogenetically close or distant heterospecific sounds (Scheumann & Zimmermann, 2008). Dogs showed a left-orientating asymmetry, indicating a right-hemisphere advantage, for both cat meows and aggressive dog barks, but no side preference for human words (either nonsense words or the command 'sit') (Reinholz-Trojan et al., 2012). These results suggested lateralized processing in dogs for heterospecific as well as conspecific sounds with a clear biological meaning. Another study also found orientating asymmetries in dogs for processing human sounds—more right turns, indicating a left-hemisphere bias for meaningful segmental cues in human speech, and more left turns, indicating a right-hemisphere bias for prosodic and speaker-related features (Ratcliffe & Reby, 2014). In cats, orientating asymmetries indicated a right-hemisphere bias for the processing of threatening and alarming dog vocalizations, but a left-hemisphere bias for conspecific sounds (Siniscalchi et al., 2015).

These findings together cannot easily be reconciled in a common framework, especially given that the link between orientating asymmetries and actual hemispheric biases is not straightforward (Fischer et al., 2009). Nevertheless, these results confirm that conspecificity is not a single reason behind lateralization, meaningfulness and valence of the sound may also influence hemispheric biases (cf. Leliveld et al., 2013), and these factors in some cases may also apply in heterospecific sound processing.

Several studies have indicated an important role for the middle superior temporal gyri (mSTG) in heterospecific sound processing. The mSTG is a non-primary region of the auditory cortex, preceding the more anterior and ventral temporal pole on the ventral auditory pathway. In a comparative fMRI study, Joly et al. (2012) presented monkey and human sounds to monkeys and humans. They found that the monkey lateral sulcus and STG responded similarly to monkey calls and human vocal sounds, but the human STG and STS clearly preferred human vocalizations. In a human fMRI study, Altmann et al. (2007) observed significantly stronger fMRI responses for recognizable versus spectrotemporally degraded animal vocalizations in the bilateral STG. They also found significant fMRI adaptation effects within the left STG for pairs of identical versus different animal vocalizations. Lewis et al. (2005) demonstrated that in humans, animal vocalizations elicited stronger activity in the bilateral mSTG than hand-manipulated tool sounds, whether the sound was correctly perceived or not. In a later study, Lewis et al. (2009) showed that one of the signal attributes that preferentially activates the mSTG is harmonicity: activity in portions of Heschl's gyri and mSTG increased with a parametric increase in the harmonic structure (HNR) of both natural animal vocalizations and artificially constructed, iterated, rippled noises. Consistently, in a comparative fMRI study with dogs and humans (Andics et al., 2014), we found that the human mSTG, while responding maximally to human vocalizations, also responded stronger to heterospecific (dog) vocalizations than to non-vocal sounds (Figure 16.2A). In contrast, the temporal pole also preferred conspecific sounds, but responded equally to dog and non-vocal sounds (Figure 16.2B).

Taken together, studies that compared heterospecific vocalizations to degraded or non-vocal sounds confirmed that the mSTG has a key role in processing vocalizations, but they also showed that it is not a strictly conspecific-selective part of the auditory processing pathway. Instead, an important function of the mSTG is to distinguish vocal from non-vocal sounds, partly based on the analysis of the overall harmonic structure of the auditory input.

Some human fMRI studies compared the processing of behaviourally relevant cues in both human and animal vocalizations. Von Kriegstein et al. (2007) showed evidence for processing spectral size cues in both conspecific (human) and heterospecific (frog) vocalizations. While the left posterior STG showed neural responses specific to acoustic scale in human voices only, the anterior temporal lobe and the intraparietal sulcus exhibited

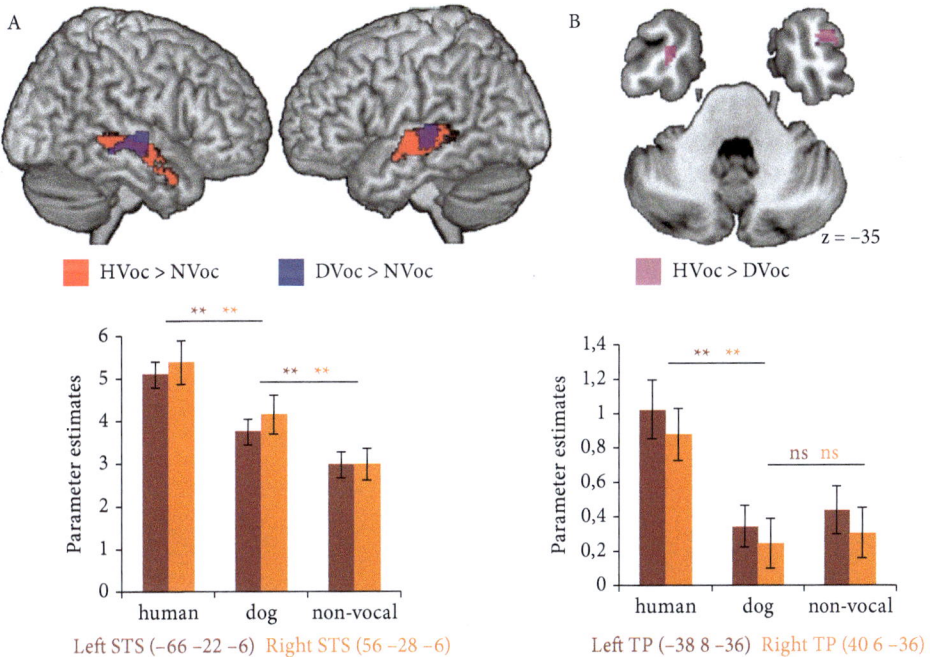

FIGURE 16.2 Human brain responses to human, dog, and non-vocal sounds. (A) Superior temporal sulcus responses, overlaid on a rendered brain. (B) Temporal pole responses, superimposed on an axial slice. Threshold for all contrasts: $p < 0.05$ (FWE-corrected). Bars represent average regional activity per sound type vs silence (beta). Regions: spheres with a 10-mm radius around local maxima of human vs non-vocal. Paired t-tests within region: **: $p < 0.001$. *: $p < 0.05$. ns: not significant. Error bars: S.E. of mean.

HVoc: human vocal, DVoc: dog vocal, NVoc: non-vocal sounds.

Data from Attila Andics, Márta Gácsi, Tamás Faragó, Anna Kis, and Ádám Miklósi, Voice-sensitive regions in the dog and human brain are revealed by comparative FMRI, *Current Biology*, 24 (5), pp. 574–8, 2014.

sensitivity to changes in acoustic scale in both human and heterospecific vocalizations. Belin et al. (2008) found that positively and negatively valenced communication sounds from cats and monkeys elicited different brain responses. This study also reported parallel neural responses to human and animal affective vocalizations in the orbitofrontal cortex, an important component of the limbic system, suggesting that key neural mechanisms involved in processing emotional vocalizations are not conspecific-specific. Belin et al. (2008) also found that humans were not able to differentiate the valence of cat and rhesus macaque vocalizations by overt behavioural responses. However, Faragó et al. (2014) showed that humans excel at rating the valence of dog vocalizations. Together, these findings suggest that the human brain differentiates valence in animal vocalizations, probably using similar acoustic cues for the sounds of different species. However, humans may not be equally good at overtly rating emotional valence from each species, and differences are perhaps based more on social than phylogenetic proximity.

In a direct comparative fMRI study in dogs and humans, we presented identical stimuli (dog vocalizations, human vocalizations, non-vocal sounds) to both species (Andics et al., 2014). We found that dogs and humans recruited similar near-primary auditory regions to process emotional valence in vocalizations, and that the regions responding stronger to more positive valence overlapped for conspecific and heterospecific sounds in each species (Figure 16.3). Furthermore, acoustic analyses revealed that emotional valence processing was based on the processing of simple temporal and spectral cues, call length, and fundamental frequency, and these acoustic cue parameters covaried with the activity in the same near-primary auditory regions.

Finally, in a recent fMRI study, we presented dogs with human speech, namely verbal praise (Andics et al., 2016). We aimed to test how dogs' brains process meaning in human vocalizations. We used the basic meaning of reward because: (1) human verbal rewards (i.e. praise) are relevant to dogs; (2) reward meaning can be expressed both via culturally

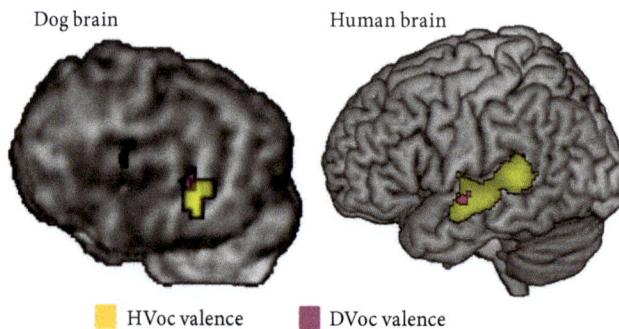

FIGURE 16.3 Dog and human brain responses to emotional valence in dog and human vocal sounds. Activity maps, overlaid on rendered brains, are thresholded at p < 0.005 for dogs and at p < 0.0005 (in clusters of at least 10 voxels) for humans. Positive parametric effects of valence (i.e. more activity for more positive sounds) are shown.

Adapted from *Current Biology*, Volume 24, Issue 5, Attila Andics, Márta Gácsi, Tamás Faragó, Anna Kis, and Ádám Miklósi, 'Voice-Sensitive Regions in the Dog and Human Brain Are Revealed by Comparative fMRI', pp. 574–578, Copyright © 2014 Elsevier Ltd., with permission from Elsevier, https://www.sciencedirect.com/science/article/pii/ S0960982214001237

transmitted (lexical) cues and phylogenetically highly-conserved (emotional intonational) cues; and (3) the primary reward circuitry of the brain is well described (Haber & Knutson, 2010). Dogs exhibited a lateralization bias for learned meaningfulness (i.e. for praise words that were meaningful to them) but not for similarly frequent conjunction words that were meaningless to them. We also demonstrated that a near-primary auditory brain region, the mid ectosylvian gyrus (mESG), is involved in the emotional intonational processing of speech and is directly modulated by fundamental frequency, in line with what we have previously shown for non-speech human sounds (Andics et al., 2014). Furthermore, mESG exhibited stronger functional connectivity to the reward-region caudate nucleus for intonationally marked than unmarked human speech. Also, primary reward regions showed an overall higher activity for praise words in praising intonation than for praise words in neutral intonation or neutral words in praising intonation, demonstrating that both learnt, lexical cues and evolutionarily preserved emotional intonational cues in human vocalizations can be meaningful to dogs. The importance of this study from the perspective of the present review is that, for the first time, it provided direct neural measures of interpreting the perceived meaning of heterospecific emotional vocalizations.

16.4 Conclusions

Adequate processing of heterospecific communication sounds is supported by phylogenetically conserved, anatomically and physiologically determined acoustic regularities in emotional vocalizations. Observational data and behavioural experiments using sound playback in the field or in a laboratory all underscore the claim that cross-species vocal communication sounds can be used to optimize behaviour in a variety of situations, across a wide range of taxa. Existing neuroscientific evidence suggests that heterospecific vocalization processing may work efficiently in many species, and shares the neural substrates involved in the processing of conspecific communication sounds. Nevertheless, research on the perceptual and especially the neural capacities to process basic biological meanings in heterospecific vocalizations is still in its infancy. The social proximity of dogs and humans provides an ideal case for comparative behavioural and neurocognitive investigations of how two evolutionarily distant species can make sense of the vocal communication sounds of the other species. Also, future studies will need to complement existing evidence to better understand the specific contributions of inherited and learnt factors to heterospecific sound processing.

ACKNOWLEDGEMENTS

Both authors contributed equally to this work. The study was supported by the National Research, Development, and Innovation Office (NKFIH PD116181 to AA) and the Hungarian Academy of Sciences through a Bolyai Scholarship to AA, a Premium Postdoctoral Scholarship (460002) of the Office for Research Groups Attached to Universities and Other Institutions of the Hungarian Academy of Sciences to TF, a grant to the MTA-ELTE 'Lendület' Neuroethology of Communication Research Group (95025), and a grant to the MTA-ELTE Comparative Ethology Research Group (F01/031).

REFERENCES

Adachi, I., Kuwahata, H., & Fujita, K. (2007). Dogs recall their owner's face upon hearing the owner's voice. *Animal Cognition*, 10, 17–21.

Akre, K. L., Farris, H. E., Lea, A. M. et al. (2011). Signal perception in frogs and bats and the evolution of mating signals. *Science*, 333, 751–752.

Altmann, C. F., Doehrmann, O., & Kaiser, J. (2007). Selectivity for animal vocalizations in the human auditory cortex. *Cerebral Cortex*, 17, 2601–2608.

Anderson, D. J. & Adolphs, R. (2014). A framework for studying emotions across species. *Cell*, 157, 187–200.

Andics, A., Gabor, A., & Gacsi, M. et al. (2016). Neural mechanisms for lexical processing in dogs. *Science*, 353, 1030–1032.

Andics, A., Gácsi, M., Faragó, T. et al. (2014). Voice-sensitive regions in the dog and human brain are revealed by comparative fMRI. *Current Biology*, 24, 574–578.

Andics, A., McQueen, J. M., Petersson, K. M. et al. (2010). Neural mechanisms for voice recognition. *NeuroImage*, 52, 1528–1540.

Anikin, A. & Persson, T. (2016). Nonlinguistic vocalizations from online amateur videos for emotion research: a validated corpus. *Behaviour Research Methods*. doi: 10.3758/s13428-016-0736-y

Anstis, S. M. & Saida, S. (1985). Adaptation to auditory streaming of frequency-modulated tones. *Journal of Experimental Psychology: Human Perception and Performance*, 11, 257–271.

Aubin, T. (1991). Why do distress calls evoke interspecific responses? An experimental study applied to some species of birds. *Behaviour Processes*, 23, 103–111.

August, P. V. & Anderson J. G. T. (1987). Mammal sounds and motivation-structural rules: a test of the hypothesis. *Journal of Mammalogy*, 68, 1–9.

Avey, M. T., Bloomfield, L. L., Elie, J. E. et al. (2014). ZENK activation in the nidopallium of black-capped chickadees in response to both conspecific and heterospecific calls. *PLoS One*, 9: e100927.

Basile, M., Boivin, S., Boutin, A. et al. (2009). Socially dependent auditory laterality in domestic horses (*Equus caballus*). *Animal Cognition*, 12, 611–619.

Belin, P., Fecteau, S., Charest, I. et al. (2008). Human cerebral response to animal affective vocalizations. *Proceedings of the Royal Society B: Biological Sciences*, 275, 473–481.

Belin, P., Fillion-Bilodeau, S., & Gosselin, F. (2008). The Montreal Affective Voices: a validated set of nonverbal affect bursts for research on auditory affective processing. *Behaviour Research Methods*, 40, 531–539.

Belin, P., Zatorre, R. J., & Ahad, P. (2002). Human temporal-lobe response to vocal sounds. *Brain Research: Cognitive Brain Research*, 13, 17–26.

Belin, P., Zatorre, R. J., Lafaille, P. et al. (2000). Voice-selective areas in human auditory cortex. *Nature* 403, 309–312.

Belwood, J. J. & Morris, G. K. (1987). Bat predation and its influence on calling behavior in neotropical katydids. *Science*, 238, 64–67.

Ben-Aderet, T., Gallego-Abenza, M., Reby, D. et al. (2017). Dog-directed speech: why do we use it and do dogs pay attention to it? *Proceedings of the Royal Society B: Biological Sciences*, 284, 20162429.

Bendor, D. & Wang, X. (2005). The neuronal representation of pitch in primate auditory cortex. *Nature*, 436, 1161–1165.

Bizley, J. K. & Cohen, Y. E. (2013). The what, where and how of auditory-object perception. *Nature Reviews Neuroscience*, 14, 693–707.

Bizley, J. K. & King, A. J. (2009). Visual influences on ferret auditory cortex. *Hearing Research*, 258, 55–63.

Blumstein, D. T. & Chi, Y. Y. (2011). Scared and less noisy: glucocorticoids are associated with alarm call entropy. *Biology Letters*, 8, 189–192.

Blumstein, D. T. & Récapet, C. (2009). The sound of arousal: the addition of novel non-linearities increases responsiveness in marmot alarm calls. *Ethology*, 115, 1074–1081.

Boeckle, M. & Bugnyar, T. (2012). Long-term memory for affiliates in ravens. *Current Biology*, 22, 801–806.

Böye, M., Güntürkün, O., & Vauclair, J. (2005). Right ear advantage for conspecific calls in adults and subadults, but not infants, California sea lions (*Zalophus californianus*): hemispheric specialization for communication? *European Journal of Neuroscience*, 21, 1727–1732.

Brand, A., Urban, R., & Grothe, B. (2000). Duration tuning in the mouse auditory midbrain. *Journal of Neurophysiology*, 84, 1790–1799.

Briefer, E. F. (2012). Vocal expression of emotions in mammals: mechanisms of production and evidence. *Journal of Zoology*, 288, 1–20.

Briefer, E. F., Maigrot, A.-L., Mandel, R. et al. (2015). Segregation of information about emotional arousal and valence in horse whinnies. *Science Report*, 4, 9989.

Briefer, E. F., Tettamanti, F., & McElligott A. G. (2015). Emotions in goats: mapping physiological, behavioural and vocal profiles. *Animal Behaviour*, 99, 131–143.

Brudzynski, S. M. (2007). Ultrasonic calls of rats as indicator variables of negative or positive states: acetylcholine–dopamine interaction and acoustic coding. *Behaviour and Brain Research*, 182, 261–273.

Budd, T. W. & Michie, P. T. (1994). Facilitation of the N1 peak of the auditory ERP at short stimulus intervals. *NeuroReport*, 5, 2513–2516.

Calford, M.B. & Semple M. N. (1995). Monaural inhibition in cat auditory cortex. *Journal of Neurophysiology*, 73(5), 1876–1891.

Caro, T. (2005). *Antipredator Defenses in Birds and Mammals*. Chicago: The University of Chicago Press.

Charlton, B. D., Ellis, W. H., Larkin, R. et al. (2012). Perception of size- related formant information in male koalas (*Phascolarctos cinereus*). *Animal Cognition*. doi: 10.1007/s10071-012-0527-5

Charlton, B. D. & Reby, D. (2016). The evolution of acoustic size exaggeration in terrestrial mammals. *Nature Communication*, 7, 12739.

Collins, K. T., McGreevy, P. D., Wheatley, K. E. et al. (2011). The influence of behavioural context on Weddell seal (*Leptonychotes weddellii*) airborne mother-pup vocalisation. *Behaviour Processes*, 87(3), 286–290.

Coudé, G., Ferrari, P. F., Rodà, F. et al. (2011). Neurons controlling voluntary vocalization in the macaque ventral premotor cortex. *PLoS One*, 6, e26822.

Covey, E. & Casseday, J. H. (1999). Timing in the auditory system of the bat. *Annual Reviews in Physiology*, 61, 457–476.

Custance, D. & Mayer, J. (2012). Empathic-like responding by domestic dogs (*Canis familiaris*) to distress in humans: an exploratory study. *Animal Cognition*, 15, 851–859.

Darwin, C. (1872). *The Expression of the Emotions in Man and Animals*. University of Chicago Press (1965 edn).

Dolan, R. J. (2002). Emotion, cognition, and behavior. *Science*, 298, 1191–1194.

Düpjan, S., Schön, P.-C., Puppe, B. et al. (2008). Differential vocal responses to physical and mental stressors in domestic pigs (*Sus scrofa*). *Applied Animal Behaviour Science*, 114, 105–115.

Egorova, M. & Ehret, G. (2008). Tonotopy and inhibition in the midbrain inferior colliculus shape spectral resolution of sounds in neural critical bands. *European Journal of Neuroscience*, 28, 675–692.

Ehret, G. (1987). Left hemisphere advantage in the mouse brain for recognizing ultrasonic communication calls. *Nature*, 325, 249–251.

Ehret, G. (2005). Infant rodent ultrasounds? A gate to the understanding of sound communication. *Behavior Genetics*, 35, 19–29.

Ehret, G. & Kurt, S. (2010). Selective perception and recognition of vocal signals. In: SM Brudzynski (ed) *Handbook of Mammalian Vocalization: An Integrative Neuroscience Approach* (pp. 125–134). London, UK: Academic Press.

Elemans, C. P. H., Rasmussen, J. H., Herbst, C. T. et al. (2015). Universal mechanisms of sound production and control in birds and mammals. *Nature Communication*, 6, 8978.

Fallow, P. M. & Magrath, R. D. (2010). Eavesdropping on other species: mutual interspecific understanding of urgency information in avian alarm calls. *Animal Behaviour*, 79, 411–417.

Fant, G. (1960). *Acoustic Theory of Speech Production*. The Hague, Netherlands: Mouton & Co.

Faragó, T., Andics, A., Devecseri, V. et al. (2014). Humans rely on the same rules to assess emotional valence and intensity in conspecific and dog vocalizations. *Biology Letters*, 10, 20130926.

Faragó, T., Pongrácz, P., Miklósi, Á. et al. (2010). Dogs' expectation about signalers' body size by virtue of their growls. *PLoS One*, 5, e15175.

Faragó, T., Pongrácz, P., Range, F. et al. (2010). 'The bone is mine': affective and referential aspects of dog growls. *Animal Behaviour*, 79, 917–925.

Fecteau, S., Armony, J. L., Joanette, Y. et al. (2004). Is voice processing species-specific in human auditory cortex? An fMRI study. *NeuroImage*, 23, 840–848.

Feng, L. & Wang, X. (2017). Harmonic template neurons in primate auditory cortex underlying complex sound processing. *Proceedings of the National Academy of Sciences of the United States of America*, 114, E840–848.

Fichtel, C., Hammerschmidt, K., & Jürgens, U. (2001). On the vocal expression of emotion. A multi-parametric analysis of different states of aversion in the squirrel monkey. *Behaviour*, 138, 97–116.

Filippi, P., Congdon, J. V., Hoang, J. et al. (2016). Humans recognize vocal expressions of emotional states universally across species. *Evolution of Language*, 11, 2–4.

Finlayson, P. G. (1999). Post-stimulatory suppression, facilitation and tuning for delays shape responses of inferior colliculus neurons to sequential pure tones. *Hearing Research*, 131, 177–194.

Fischer, J., Metz, M., Cheney, D. L. et al. (2001). Baboon responses to graded bark variants. *Animal Behaviour*, 61, 925–932.

Fischer, J., Teufel, C., Drolet, M. et al. (2009). Orienting asymmetries and lateralized processing of sounds in humans. *BMC Neuroscience*, 10, 14.

Fishman, Y. I., Reser, D. H., Arezzo, J. C. et al. (2001). Neural correlates of auditory stream segregation in primary auditory cortex of the awake monkey. *Hearing Research*, 151, 167–187.

Fitch, W. T. & Hauser, M. D. (2003). Unpacking 'honesty': vertebrate vocal production and the evolution of acoustic signals. In: A. M. Simmons, A. N. Popper, & R. R. Fay (eds) *Acoustic Communication* (pp. 65–137). New York, NY: Springer-Verlag.

Fitch, W. T., Neubauer, J., & Herzel, H. (2002). Calls out of chaos: the adaptive significance of nonlinear phenomena in mammalian vocal production. *Animal Behaviour*, 63, 407–418.

Forsman, J. T. & Monkkonen, M. (2001). Responses by breeding birds to heterospecific song and mobbing call playbacks under varying predation risk. *Animal Behaviour*, 62, 1067–1073.

Frühholz, S., Trost, W., & Grandjean, D. (2014). The role of the medial temporal limbic system in processing emotions in voice and music. *Progress in Neurobiology*, 123, 1–17.

Gadziola, M. A., Shanbhag, S. J., & Wenstrup, J. J. (2016). Two distinct representations of social vocalizations in the basolateral amygdala. *Journal of Neurophysiology*, 115, 868–886.

Gaub, S. & Ehret, G. (2005). Grouping in auditory temporal perception and vocal production is mutually adapted: the case of wriggling calls of mice. *Journal of Comparative Physiology*, 191, 1131–1135.

Geissler, D. B. & Ehret, G. (2004). Auditory perception vs. recognition: representation of complex communication sounds in the mouse auditory cortical fields. *European Journal of Neuroscience*, 19, 1027–1040.

George, I., Cousillas, H., Richard, J.-P. et al. (2002). Song perception in the European starling: hemispheric specialisation and individual variations. *Comptes Rendus Biologies* 325, 197–204.

Gerhardt, H. C. (1994). The evolution of vocalization in frogs and toads. *Annual Review of Ecology, Evolution, and Systematics*, 25, 293–324.

Ghazanfar, A. A., Smith-Rohrberg, D., & Hauser, M. D. (2001). The role of temporal cues in rhesus monkey vocal recognition: orienting asymmetries to reversed calls. *Brain, Behavior and Evolution*, 58, 163–172.

Gifford, G. W., MacLean, K. A., Hauser, M. D. et al. (2005). The neurophysiology of functionally meaningful categories: macaque ventrolateral prefrontal cortex plays a critical role in spontaneous categorization of species-specific vocalizations. *Journal of Cognitive Neuroscience*, 17, 1471–1482.

Gil-da-Costa, R. & Hauser, M. D. (2006). Vervet monkeys and humans show brain asymmetries for processing conspecific vocalizations, but with opposite patterns of laterality. *Proceedings of the Royal Society B: Biological Sciences*, 273, 2313–2318. doi:10.1098/rspb.2006.3580

Gouzoules, H., Gouzoules, S., & Tomaszycki, M. (1998). Agonistic screams and the classification of dominance relationships: are monkeys fuzzy logicians? *Animal Behaviour*, 55, 51–60.

Gruber, T. & Grandjean, D. (2017). A comparative neurological approach to emotional expressions in primate vocalizations. *Neuroscience & Biobehavioral Reviews*, 73, 182–190.

Haber, S. N. & Knutson, B. (2010). The reward circuit: linking primate anatomy and human imaging. *Neuropsychopharmacology*, 35, 4–26.

Hage, S. R., Gavrilov, N., & Nieder, A. (2013). Cognitive control of distinct vocalizations in rhesus monkeys. *Journal of Cognitive Neuroscience*, 25, 1692–1701.

Hall, D. A. & Plack, C. J. (2009). Pitch processing sites in the human auditory brain. *Cerebral Cortex*, 19, 576–585.

Hauber, M. E., Woolley, S. M. N., Cassey, P. et al. (2013). Experience dependence of neural responses to different classes of male songs in the primary auditory forebrain of female songbirds. *Behavioural Brain Research*, 243, 184–190.

Hauser, M. D., Agnetta, B., & Perez, C. (1998). Orienting asymmetries in rhesus monkeys: the effect of time-domain changes on acoustic perception. *Animal Behaviour*, 56, 41–47.

Hauser, M. D. & Andersson, K. (1994). Left hemisphere dominance for processing vocalizations in adult, but not infant, rhesus monkeys: field experiments. *Proceedings of the National Academy of Sciences of the United States of America*, 91, 3946–3948.

Heiligenberg, W. (1988). The neuronal basis of electrosensory perception and its control of a behavioral response in a weakly electric fish. In: *Sensory Biology of Aquatic Animals* (pp. 851–868). New York, NY: Springer.

Holmstrom, L. A., Eeuwes, L. B. M., Roberts, P. D. et al. (2010). Efficient encoding of vocalizations in the auditory midbrain. *Journal of Neuroscience*, 30, 802–819.

Hurd, C. R. (1996). Interspecific attraction to the mobbing calls of black-capped chickadees (*Parus atricapillus*). *Behavioral Ecology and Sociobiology*, 38, 287–292.

Ito, R., Ikeuchi, I., & Mori, A. (2013). A day gecko darkens its body color in response to avian alarm calls. *Current Herpetology*, 32, 26–33.

Ito, R. & Mori, A. (2010). Vigilance against predators induced by eavesdropping on heterospecific alarm calls in a non-vocal lizard *Oplurus cuvieri cuvieri* (Reptilia: Iguania). *Proceedings of the Royal Society B: Biological Sciences*, 277, 1275–1280.

Johnson, F. R., McNaughton, E. J., Shelley, C. D. et al. (2003). Mechanisms of heterospecific recognition in avian mobbing calls. *Australian Journal of Zoology*, 51, 577–585.

Joly, O., Ramus, F., Pressnitzer, D. et al. (2012). Interhemispheric differences in auditory processing revealed by fMRI in awake rhesus monkeys. *Cerebral Cortex*, 22, 838–853.

Jürgens, U. (1994). The role of the periaqueductal grey in vocal behaviour. *Behavioural Brain Research*, 62, 107–117.

Jürgens, U. (2002). Neural pathways underlying vocal control. *Neuroscience & Biobehavioral Reviews*, 26, 235–258.

Jürgens, U. (2009). The neural control of vocalization in mammals: a review. *Journal of Voice*, 23, 1–10.

Jurisevic, M.A. & Sanderson, K. J. K. (1998). A comparative analysis of distress call structure in Australian passerine and non-passerine species: influence of size and phylogeny. *Journal of Avian Biology*, 29, 61–71.

Kaminski, J., Call, J., & Fischer, J. (2004). Word learning in a domestic dog: evidence for 'fast mapping'. *Science*, 304, 1682–1683.

Karp, D., Manser, M. B., Wiley, E. M. et al. (2014). Nonlinearities in meerkat alarm calls prevent receivers from habituating. *Ethology*, 120, 189–196.

Kelley, D. B. (2004). Vocal communication in frogs. *Current Opinion in Neurobiology*, 14, 751–757.

Kerepesi, A., Dóka, A., & Miklósi, Á. (2015). Dogs and their human companions: the effect of familiarity on dog–human interactions. *Behavioural Processes*, 110, 27–36.

Knutson, B., Burgdorf, J., & Panksepp, J. (2002). Ultrasonic vocalizations as indices of affective states in rats. *Psychology Bulletin*, 128, 961–977.

Koda, H. (2012). Possible use of heterospecific food-associated calls of macaques by sika deer for foraging efficiency. *Behavioural Processes*, 91, 30–34.

Koeda, M., Belin, P., Hama, T., Masuda, T., Matsuura, M., & Okubo, Y. (2013). Cross-cultural differences in the processing of non-verbal affective vocalizations by Japanese and Canadian listeners. *Frontiers in Psychology*, 4, 105.

von Kriegstein, K., Giraud, A.-L., Kriegstein, K. V. et al. (2004). Distinct functional substrates along the right superior temporal sulcus for the processing of voices. *NeuroImage*, 22, 948–955.

von Kriegstein, K., Smith, D. R. R., Patterson, R. D. et al. (2007). Neural representation of auditory size in the human voice and in sounds from other resonant sources. *Current Biology*, 17, 1123–1128.

Kuhl, P. K. & Miller, J. D. (1975). Speech perception by the chinchilla: voiced-voiceless distinction in alveolar plosive consonants. *Science*, 190, 69–72.

Lea, A. J., Barrera, J. P., Tom, L. M. et al. (2008). Heterospecific eavesdropping in a nonsocial species. *Behavioral Ecology*, 19, 1041–1046.

Leech, R., Holt, L. L., Devlin, J. T. et al. (2009). Expertise with artificial nonspeech sounds recruits speech-sensitive cortical regions. *Journal of Neuroscience*, 29, 5234–5239.

Leinonen, L., Linnankoski, I., Laakso, M.-L. et al. (1991). Vocal communication between species: man and macaque. *Language & Communication*, 11, 241–262.

Leliveld, L. M. C., Langbein, J., & Puppe, B. (2013). The emergence of emotional lateralization: evidence in non-human vertebrates and implications for farm animals. *Applied Animal Behaviour Science*, 145, 1–14.

Lewicki, M. S. & Konishi, M. (1995). Mechanisms underlying the sensitivity of songbird forebrain neurons to temporal order. *Proceedings of the National Academy of Sciences of the United States of America*, 92, 5582–5586.

Lewis, J. W., Brefczynski, J. A., Phinney, R.E. et al. (2005). Distinct cortical pathways for processing tool versus animal sounds. *Journal of Neuroscience*, 25, 5148–5158.

Lewis, J. W., Talkington, W. J., Walker, N. A. et al. (2009). Human cortical organization for processing vocalizations indicates representation of harmonic structure as a signal attribute. *Journal of Neuroscience*, 29, 2283–2296.

Liebal, K., Waller, B. M., Burrows, A. M., & Slocombe, K. (2014). *Primate Communication: A Multimodal Approach*. Cambridge: Cambridge University Press.

Liebenthal, E., Desai, R., Ellingson, M. M. et al. (2010). Specialization along the left superior temporal sulcus for auditory categorization. *Cerebral Cortex*, 20, 2958–2970.

Lingle, S. & Riede, T. (2014). Deer mothers are sensitive to infant distress vocalizations of diverse mammalian species. *American Naturalist*, 184, 510–522.

Lingle, S., Wyman, M. T., Kotrba, R. et al. (2012). What makes a cry a cry? A review of infant distress vocalizations. *Current Zoology*, 58(5), 698–726.

Linhart, P., Ratcliffe, V. F., Reby, D. et al. (2015). Expression of emotional arousal in two different piglet call types. *PLoS One*, 10, e0135414.

Linnankoski, I., Laakso, M.-L., Aulanko, R. et al. (1994). Recognition of emotions in macaque vocalizations by children and adults. *Language and Communication*, 14, 83–192.

Lord, K., Feinstein, M., & Coppinger, R. P. (2009). Barking and mobbing. *Behavioural Processes*, 81, 358–368.

Louder, M. I. M., Voss, H, U., Manna, T. J. et al. (2016). Shared neural substrates for song discrimination in parental and parasitic songbirds. *Neuroscience Letters*, 622, 49–54.

Magrath, R. D., Haff, T. M., Fallow, P. M. et al. (2015). Eavesdropping on heterospecific alarm calls: from mechanisms to consequences. *Biology Review*, 90, 560–586.

Manley, G. A. & Kraus, J. E. M. (2010). Exceptional high-frequency hearing and matched vocalizations in Australian pygopod geckos. *Journal of Experimental Biology*, 213, 1876–1885.

Manser, M. B. (2001). The acoustic structure of suricates' alarm calls varies with predator type and the level of response urgency. *Proceedings of the Royal Society B: Biological Sciences*, 268, 2315–2324.

Marler, P. (1955). Characteristics of some animal calls. *Nature*, 176, 6–8.

Maruščáková, I. L., Linhart, P., Ratcliffe, V. F. et al. (2015). Humans (*Homo sapiens*) judge the emotional content of piglet (*Sus scrofa domestica*) calls based on simple acoustic parameters, not personality, empathy, nor attitude toward animals. *Journal of Computational Psychology*, 129, 121–131.

Maul, K. K., Voss, H. U., Parra, L. C. et al. (2009). The development of stimulus-specific auditory responses requires song exposure in male but not female zebra finches. *Developmental Neurobiology*, 70(1), 28–40.

McComb, K., Shannon, G., Sayialel, K. N. et al. (2014). Elephants can determine ethnicity, gender, and age from acoustic cues in human voices. *Proceedings of the National Academy of Sciences of the United States of America*, 111(4), 5433–5438.

Medvedev, A. V. (2004). Local field potentials and spiking activity in the primary auditory cortex in response to social calls. *Journal of Neurophysiology*, 92, 52–65.

Meise, K., Keller, C., Cowlishaw, G. et al. (2011). Sources of acoustic variation: implications for production specificity and call categorization in chacma baboon (*Papio ursinus*) grunts. *Journal of the Acoustical Society of America*, 129, 1631.

Mello, C. V., Vicario, D. S. & Clayton, D. F. (1992). Song presentation induces gene expression in the songbird forebrain. *Proceedings of the National Academy of Sciences of the United States of America*, 89, 6818–6822.

Mendl, M. T., Burman, O. H. P. & Paul, E. S. (2010). An integrative and functional framework for the study of animal emotion and mood. *Proceedings of the Royal Society B: Biological Sciences*, 277, 2895–2904.

Merzenich, M. M., Kaas, J. H. & Roth, G. L. (1976). Auditory cortex in the grey squirrel: tonotopic organization and architectonic fields. *Journal of Computational Neurology*, 166, 387–401.

Miklósi, Á. (2007). *Dog Behaviour, Evolution, and Cognition*. Oxford: Oxford University Press.

Miklósi, Á. & Topál, J. (2013). What does it take to become 'best friends'? Evolutionary changes in canine social competence. *Trends in Cognitive Sciences*, 17, 287–294.

Molnár, C., Pongrácz, P. & Miklósi, Á. (2009). Seeing with ears: sightless humans' perception of dog bark provides a test for structural rules in vocal communication. *Quarterly Journal of Experimental Psychology*, 63(5), 1004–1013.

Morton, E. S. (1977). On the occurrence and significance of motivation—structural rules in some bird and mammal sounds. *American Naturalist*, 111, 855–869.

Newman, J. D. (2010). Evolution of the communication brain in control of mammalian vocalization. In: S. M. Brudzynski (ed.) *Handbook of Mammalian Vocalizations* (pp. 23–28). Amsterdam: Elsevier.

Nicastro, N. & Owren, M. J. (2003). Classification of domestic cat (*Felis catus*) vocalizations by naïve and experienced human listeners. *Journal of Computational Psychology*, 117, 44–52.

Norman-Haignere, S., Kanwisher, N., & McDermott, J. H. (2013). Cortical pitch regions in humans respond primarily to resolved harmonics and are located in specific tonotopic regions of anterior auditory cortex. *Journal of Neuroscience*, 33, 19451–19469.

Oxenham, A. J., Bernstein, J. G. W. & Penagos, H. (2004). Correct tonotopic representation is necessary for complex pitch perception. *Proceedings of the National Academy of Sciences of the United States of America*, 101, 1421–1425.

Padilla de la Torre, M., Briefer, E. F., Reader, T. et al. (2015). Acoustic analysis of cattle (*Bos taurus*) mother–offspring contact calls from a source-filter theory perspective. *Applied Animal Behaviour*, 163, 58–68.

Palleroni, A. (2003). Experience-dependent plasticity for auditory processing in a raptor. *Science*, 299, 1195.

Panksepp, J. (2005). Affective consciousness: core emotional feelings in animals and humans. *Conscious Cognition*, 14, 30–80.

Patterson, R. D., Uppenkamp, S., Johnsrude, I. S. et al. (2002). The processing of temporal pitch and melody information in auditory cortex. *Neuron*, 36, 767–776.

Peake, T. M. (2005). Eavesdropping in communication networks. In: P. K. McGregor (ed.) *Animal Communication Networks* (pp. 13–37). New York: Cambridge University Press.

Perrodin, C., Kayser, C., Logothetis, N. K. et al. (2011). Voice cells in the primate temporal lobe. *Current Biology*, 21, 1408–1415.

Petersen, M. R., Beecher, M., Moody, D. et al. (1978). Neural lateralization of species-specific vocalizations by Japanese macaques (*Macaca fuscata*). *Science*, 202, 324–327.

Petersen, M. R., Beecher, M. D., Zoloth, S. R. et al. (1984). Neural lateralization of vocalizations by Japanese macaques: communicative significance is more important than acoustic structure. *Behavioral Neuroscience*, 98, 779–790.

Petkov, C. I., Kayser, C., Steudel, T. et al. (2008). A voice region in the monkey brain. *Nature Neuroscience*, 11, 367–374.

Pisoni, D. B. & Lazarus, J. H. (1974). Categorical and noncategorical modes of speech perception along the voicing continuum. *Journal of the Acoustical Society of America*, 55, 328–333.

Poirier, C., Boumans, T., Verhoye, M. et al. (2009). Own-song recognition in the songbird auditory pathway: selectivity and lateralization. *Journal of Neuroscience*, 29, 2252–2258.

Pollak, G. D. (2013). The dominant role of inhibition in creating response selectivities for communication calls in the brainstem auditory system. *Hearing Research*, 305, 86–101.

Pongrácz, P., Molnár, C., Dóka, A. et al. (2011). Do children understand man's best friend? Classification of dog barks by pre-adolescents and adults. *Applied Animal Behaviour Science*, 135, 95–102.

Pongrácz, P., Molnár, C. & Miklósi, Á. (2006). Acoustic parameters of dog barks carry emotional information for humans. *Applied Animal Behaviour Science*, 100, 228–240.

Pongrácz, P., Molnár, C. & Miklósi, Á. (2010). Barking in family dogs: an ethological approach. *Veterinary Journal*, 183, 141–147.

Pongrácz, P., Molnár, C., Miklósi, Á. et al. (2005). Human listeners are able to classify dog (*Canis familiaris*) barks recorded in different situations. *Journal of Computational Psychology*, 119, 136–144.

Poremba, A., Malloy, M., Saunders, R. C. et al. (2004). Species-specific calls evoke asymmetric activity in the monkey's temporal poles. *Nature*, 427, 448–451.

Portfors, C. V., Roberts, P.D. & Jonson, K. (2009). Over-representation of species-specific vocalizations in the awake mouse inferior colliculus. *Neuroscience*, 162, 486–500.

Randler, C. (2006). Red squirrels (*Sciurus vulgaris*) respond to alarm calls of Eurasian jays (*Garrulus glandarius*). *Ethology*, 112, 411–416.

Ratcliffe, V. F., McComb, K. & Reby, D. (2014). Cross-modal discrimination of human gender by domestic dogs. *Animal Behaviour*, 91, 126–134.

Ratcliffe, V. F. & Reby, D. (2014). Orienting asymmetries in dogs' responses to different communicatory components of human speech. *Current Biology*, 24, 1–5.

Rauschecker, J. P. & Tian, B. (2000). Mechanisms and streams for processing of 'what' and 'where' in auditory cortex. *Proceedings of the National Academy of Sciences of the United States of America*, 97, 11800–11806.

Reby, D., McComb, K., Cargnelutti, B. et al. (2005). Red deer stags use formants as assessment cues during intrasexual agonistic interactions. *Proceedings of the Royal Society B: Biological Sciences*, 272, 941–947.

Reinholz-Trojan, A., Włodarczyk, E., Trojan, M. et al. (2012). Hemispheric specialization in domestic dogs (*Canis familiaris*) for processing different types of acoustic stimuli. *Behavioural Processes*. doi: 10.1016/j.beproc.2012.07.001

Rendall, D. (2003). Acoustic correlates of caller identity and affect intensity in the vowel-like grunt vocalizations of baboons. *Journal of the Acoustical Society of America*, 113, 3390.

Riede, T., Herzel, H., Hammerschmidt, K. et al. (2001). The harmonic-to-noise ratio applied to dog barks. *Journal of the Acoustical Society of America*, 110, 2191.

Riede, T., Mitchell, B. R., Tokuda, I. T. et al. (2005). Characterizing noise in nonhuman vocalizations: acoustic analysis and human perception of barks by coyotes and dogs. *Journal of the Acoustical Society of America*, 118, 514.

Russ, J. M., Jones, G., Mackie, I. J. et al. (2004). Interspecific responses to distress calls in bats (*C hiroptera: Vespertilionidae*): a function for convergence in call design? *Animal Behaviour*, 67, 1005–1014.

Russell, J. A. (2003). Core affect and the psychological construction of emotion. *Psychological Review*, 110, 145–172.

Ryan, M. J., Tuttle, M. D. & Rand, A. S. (1982). Bat predation and sexual advertisement in a neotropical anuran. *American Naturalist*, 119, 136–139.

Sadagopan, S., Temiz-Karayol, N. Z., Voss, H. U. et al. (2015). High-field functional magnetic resonance imaging of vocalization processing in marmosets. *Science Report*, 5, 10950.

Sadagopan, S. & Wang, X. (2009). Nonlinear spectrotemporal interactions underlying selectivity for complex sounds in auditory cortex. *Journal of Neuroscience*, 29, 11192–11202.

Sauter, D. A., Eisner, F., Ekman, P. et al. (2015). Emotional vocalizations are recognized across cultures regardless of the valence of distractors. *Psychological Science*, 26, 354–356.

Scharf, B. (1978). Loudness. In: E Carterette, MP Friedman (eds) *Handbook of Perception. Vol. 4: Hearing* (pp. 187–242). New York: Academic Press.

Schehka, S., Esser, K.-H. Zimmermann, E. (2007) *Acoustical expression of arousal in conflict situations in tree shrews (Tupaia belangeri). Journal of Comparative Physiology A: Neuroethology, Sensory, Neural, and Behavioral Physiology*, 193, 845–852.

Schehka, S. & Zimmermann, E. (2009). Acoustic features to arousal and identity in disturbance calls of tree shrews (*Tupaia belangeri*). *Behavioural Brain Research*, 203, 223–231.

Scheumann, M., Hasting, A. S., Kotz, S. A. et al. (2014). The voice of emotion across species: how do human listeners recognize animals' affective states? *PLoS One*, 9, e91192.

Scheumann, M., Roser, A.-E., Konerding, W. S. et al. (2012). Vocal correlates of sender-identity and arousal in the isolation calls of domestic kitten (*Felis silvestris catus*). *Frontiers in Zoology*, 9, 36.

Scheumann, M. & Zimmermann, E. (2008). Sex-specific asymmetries in communication sound perception are not related to hand preference in an early primate. *BMC Biology*, 6, 3.

Schirmer, A. & Kotz, S. A. (2006). Beyond the right hemisphere: brain mechanisms mediating vocal emotional processing. *Trends in Cognitive Sciences*, 10, 24–30.

Schötz, S. & van de Weijer, J. (2014). *A study of human perception of intonation in domestic cat meows*. Proceedings of Speech Prosody 2014. Dublin, Ireland.

Scott-Phillips, T. C., Blythe, R. A., Gardner, A. et al. (2012). How do communication systems emerge? *Proceedings of the Royal Society B: Biological Sciences*, 279, 1943–1949.

Searcy, W. A. & Nowicki, S. (2005). *The Evolution of Animal Communication: Reliability and Deception in Signaling Systems*. Princeton: Princeton University Press.

Siniscalchi, M., Laddago, S. & Quaranta, A. (2015). Auditory lateralization of conspecific and heterospecific vocalizations in cats. *Laterality*, 678, 1–13.

Siniscalchi, M., Quaranta, A. & Rogers, L. J. (2008). Hemispheric specialization in dogs for processing different acoustic stimuli. *PLoS One*, 3, e3349.

Slaughter, E. I., Berlin, E. R., Bower, J. T. et al. (2013). A test of the nonlinearity hypothesis in great-tailed grackles (*Quiscalus mexicanus*). *Ethology*, 119, 309–315.

Slocombe, K. E. & Zuberbühler, K. (2007). Chimpanzees modify recruitment screams as a function of audience composition. *Proceedings of the National Academy of Sciences of the United States of America*, 104, 17228–17033.

Soltis, J., Blowers., T. E. & Savage, A. (2011). Measuring positive and negative affect in the voiced sounds of African elephants (*Loxodonta africana*). *Journal of the Acoustical Society of America*, 129, 1059.

Staeren, N., Renvall, H., De Martino, F. et al. (2009). Sound categories are represented as distributed patterns in the human auditory cortex. *Current Biology*, 19, 498–502.

Suga, N., O'Neill, W. E., Kujirai, K. et al. (1983). Specificity of combination-sensitive neurons for processing of complex biosonar signals in auditory cortex of the mustached bat. *Journal of Neurophysiology*, 49(6), 1573–1626.

Suta, D. (2003). Representation of species-specific vocalizations in the inferior colliculus of the guinea pig. *Journal of Neurophysiology*, 90, 3794–3808.

Šuta, D., Popelář, J., Burianová, J. et al. (2013). Cortical representation of species-specific vocalizations in guinea pig. *PLoS One*, 8, e65432.

Šuta, D., Popelář, J., Kvašňák, E. et al. (2007). Representation of species-specific vocalizations in the medial geniculate body of the guinea pig. *Experimental Brain Research*, 183, 377–388.

Szipl, G., Boeckle, M., Werner, S. A. B. et al. (2014). Mate recognition and expression of affective state in croop calls of Northern Bald Ibis (*Geronticus eremita*). *PLoS One*, 9, 1–8.

Taglialatela, J. P., Russell, J. L., Schaeffer, J. A. et al. (2009). Visualizing vocal perception in the chimpanzee brain. *Cerebral Cortex*, 19, 1151–1157.

Talkington, W. J., Rapuano, K. M., Hitt, L. A. et al. (2012). Humans mimicking animals: a cortical hierarchy for human vocal communication sounds. *Journal of Neuroscience*, 32, 8084–8093.

Tallet, C., Linhart, P., Policht, R. et al. (2013). Encoding of situations in the vocal repertoire of piglets (*Sus scrofa*): a comparison of discrete and graded classifications. *PLoS One*, 8, e71841.

Tallet, C., Špinka, M., Maruščáková, I. L. et al. (2010). Human perception of vocalizations of domestic piglets and modulation by experience with domestic pigs (*Sus scrofa*). *Journal of Computational Psychology*, 124, 81–91.

Taylor, A. M. & Reby, D. (2010). The contribution of source-filter theory to mammal vocal communication research. *Journal of Zoology*, 280, 221–236.

Taylor, A. M., Reby, D., & McComb, K. (2008). Human listeners attend to size information in domestic dog growls. *Journal of the Acoustical Society of America*, 123, 2903–2909.

Taylor, A. M., Reby, D., & McComb, K. (2009). Context-related variation in the vocal growling behaviour of the domestic dog (*Canis familiaris*). *Ethology*, 115, 905–915.

Taylor, A. M., Reby, D., & McComb, K. (2010). Why do large dogs sound more aggressive to human listeners: acoustic bases of motivational misattributions. *Ethology*, 116, 1155–1162.

Taylor, A. M., Reby, D., & McComb, K. (2011). Cross modal perception of body size in domestic dogs (*Canis familiaris*). *PLoS One*, 6, e17069.

Templeton, C. N. & Greene, E. (2007). Nuthatches eavesdrop on variations in heterospecific chickadee mobbing alarm calls. *Proceedings of the National Academy of Sciences of the United States of America*, 104, 5479–5482.

Templeton, C. N., Greene, E., & Davis, K. (2005). Allometry of alarm calls: black-capped chickadees encode information about predator size. *Science*, 308, 1934–1937.

Terpstra, N. J., Bolhuis, J. J., den Boer-Visser, A. M. et al. (2005). Neuronal activation related to auditory perception in the brain of a non-songbird, the ring dove. *Journal of Computational Neuroscience*, 488, 342–351.

Theis, K. R., Greene, K. M., Benson-Amram, S. R. et al. (2007). Sources of variation in the long-distance vocalizations of spotted hyenas. *Behaviour*, 144, 557–584.

Tian, B., Reser, D., Durham, A. et al. (2001). Functional specialization in rhesus monkey auditory cortex. *Science*, 292, 290–293.

Topál, J., Miklósi, Á., Csányi, V. et al. (1998). Attachment behavior in dogs (*Canis familiaris*): a new application of Ainsworth's (1969) strange situation test. *Journal of Computational Psychology*, 112, 219–229.

Town, S. M. & Bizley, J. K. (2013). Neural and behavioral investigations into timbre perception. *Frontiers in Systems Neuroscience*, 7, 88.

de Vere, A. J. & Kuczaj, S. A. (2016). Where are we in the study of animal emotions? *Wiley Interdisciplinary Reviews: Cognitive Science*, 7, 354–362.

Vitousek, M. N., Adelman, J. S., Gregory, N. C. et al. (2007). Heterospecific alarm call recognition in a non-vocal reptile. *Biology Letters*, 3, 632–634.

Wang, X. (2013). The harmonic organization of auditory cortex. *Frontiers in Systems Neuroscience*, 7. doi: 10.3389/fnsys.2013.00114

Wang, X. & Kadia, S. C. (2001). Differential representation of species-specific primate vocalizations in the auditory cortices of marmoset and cat. *Journal of Neurophysiology*, 86, 2616–2620.

Wildgruber, D., Ethofer, T., Grandjean, D. et al. (2009). A cerebral network model of speech prosody comprehension. *International Journal of Speech and Language Pathology*, 11, 277–281.

Wöhr, M. & Schwarting, R. K. W. (2010). Activation of limbic system structures by replay of ultrasonic vocalization in rats. In: S. M. Brudzynski (ed.) *Handbook of Mammalian Vocalizations* (pp. 113–124). Amsterdam: Elsevier.

Woolley, S. M. N. (2012). Early experience shapes vocal neural coding and perception in songbirds. *Developmental Psychobiology*, 54, 612–631.

Yeon, S.-C., Kim, Y. K., Park, S. J. et al. (2011). Differences between vocalization evoked by social stimuli in feral cats and house cats. *Behavioural Processes*, 87(2), 183–189.

Yin, S. & McCowan, B. (2004). Barking in domestic dogs: context specificity and individual identification. *Animal Behaviour*, 68, 343–355.

Zimmermann, E., Leliveld, L. M. C. & Schehka, S. (2013). Toward the evolutionary roots of affective prosody in human acoustic communication: a comparative approach to mammalian voices. In: E. Altenmüller, S. Schmidt, & E Zimmermann (eds) *Evolution of Emotional Communication: From Sounds in Nonhuman Mammals to Speech and Music in Man* (pp. 116–132). Oxford, UK: Oxford University Press.

CHAPTER 17

EMOTIONAL AND SOCIAL COMMUNICATION IN NON-HUMAN ANIMALS

CHARLES T. SNOWDON

17.1 INTRODUCTION

VOCAL communication can be a highly energetic activity. Birds may sing for several minutes at a time at dawn and dusk; gibbons of both sexes exchange great calls several times a day; the loud and long calls of many primates may travel for up to 3 km with calling occurring many times a day. In addition to the energetic costs of communication, any vocalizing organism is making itself conspicuous not only to conspecific recipients but also to potential predators. Combining the energetic costs of vocal production with the risks of predation makes vocal communication potentially very costly. Why, then, should animals vocalize at all? What are the benefits of vocalizing?

Benefits may occur in several ways. Calls may warn others of predators or of threats from conspecifics; calls may provide information about food or shelter; calls from infants may induce parental care and nurturance; calls can signify play, and can identify and lead to evaluation of potential mates; calls can signify status and can be used to manage social relationships and assess behaviour of others; calls can communicate emotional states or can be used to induce emotional states in others; calls can provide an index of social belongingness by identifying a mate, a preferred social partner, a social group, a population, or species. After a brief introduction to some current theoretical issues with respect to the putative functions of vocal signalling, I will provide a brief review of the emotional and social aspects of vocal communication in non-human animals.

It is difficult to write about emotional communication in non-human animals because humans find emotional states to be highly personal experiences that are not easily communicated to others. If it is difficult for humans to communicate their emotional states through language, how much more difficult is it to study emotional signals in non-verbal, non-human animals? Fortunately, Darwin (1872/1998) paved the way for the comparative study of emotion in human and non-human animals. His work on facial expressions and body postures looked for similarities across species based on the assumption that signals produced in similar contexts must have similar meaning or function. In a continuation of Darwin's paradigm, I will use comparative data from human and animal vocal communication to illustrate how emotional signals share some common properties across species, thereby examining whether there are some universals in vocal signalling of emotions and in the induction of emotional states.

Following the discussion of emotional signals, I then examine how vocal signals are used in social relationships and how social relationships, in turn, affect signal structure and usage. First, I will detail the various levels of identity that are moderated by vocal communication. Then, I will look at how social relationships influence vocal structure and, finally, will examine how animals use vocalizations to influence social relationships.

17.2 THEORETICAL PERSPECTIVES

Researchers have had conflicting views of the benefits of vocal communication in non-human animals. Many researchers have searched for parallels between non-human communication and language and, based on this, have argued that communication is basically about the transfer of information from caller to recipient. Studies have shown that animals can communicate about the presence and quality of food, the type of predator located, the status of a competitor being faced, all classified as functionally referential signals (e.g. Seyfarth et al., 2010), as well as communication of specific information about the caller's emotional or affective state. Even if information transfer is not intended by the caller, listeners can often infer information about the caller's social or emotional status or about the context (predator detection, food location, etc.) of the caller.

In contrast, other researchers have argued that communication has evolved to allow callers to manipulate or manage the behaviour of others (e.g. Rendall et al., 2009). In this view of communication, call structures have evolved that have direct influences on the sensory, physiological, and behavioural processes of recipients. The caller may or may not be providing accurate information about its own state or behaviour. The benefit of calling resides in the effects of calls on others. In the closely related assessment-management theory (Owings & Morton, 1997), communication is considered to be a dynamic process whereby organisms continually assess the behaviour of one another and act to manage each other's behaviour to the advantage of the caller.

Under the informational perspective, callers are expected to provide honest and accurate information about their emotional or behavioural state, whereas under the manipulation or management views, callers use signals that are designed to induce emotional states in others, even if the callers are not experiencing those states themselves. Thus, with an informational perspective, animals communicate about predators, food, dominance status, and internal emotions, and calls can be sorted according to their social function (e.g. alarm, arousal, avoidance, affiliation). With a manipulation or management perspective, calls are sorted according to the effects they have on listeners (e.g. inducing fear, avoidance, approach, soliciting mating).

In reality, the separation of these different functions is often difficult, and it is possible that the same caller might engage in both informative and manipulative calling depending on the social context and on which receivers are present. Alarm calls given by monkeys can be specific to the predator class involved, as in the eagle, leopard, and snake alarm calls of vervet monkeys (*Chlorocebus pygerythrus*) (Seyfarth et al., 1980). Yet, at the same time, there is likely to be an element of fear encoded in the call as well as the potential management of others (e.g. for one's offspring to freeze, for other group members to join in mobbing a predator). Mobbing calls that elicit action toward a predator often have several short, broadband notes that span a broad frequency range, whereas alarm calls that elicit freezing are often long, high-pitched notes that are difficult for predators to localize (i.e. structures that are likely to have direct physiological effects on listeners; Owren & Rendall, 2001). Infant screams may be highly aversive to mothers, who may continue to nurse an infant during the weaning process to reduce the aversion. Screams from a subordinate animal may deter aggression from dominants due to the aversive quality of the calls.

Since the focus of this review is on social and emotional communication, I will not cover the topic of functionally referential calls, but will include both informational and manipulation aspects of vocal signals. Let us first consider how emotions are communicated.

17.3 EMOTIONAL SIGNALS AND INDUCTION OF EMOTIONS

17.3.1 Relationship of Human and Non-Human Emotional Signals

As Darwin made an appeal based on comparative human and non-human similarities in facial and body expressions of emotion, so might a similar comparative approach be a good start for vocal signals. Although humans have a rich language to communicate about emotions, it is in fact our tone of voice (or speech prosody) that is likely to be more accurate than language in communication of emotional state. Furthermore, one function of music is the induction of emotions in listeners, and Juslin and Laukka (2003) have shown a close concordance between emotional communication in music and speech.

Scherer (1995) suggested that sadness is communicated in music by slow tempos, a narrow frequency range, slow rate of articulation, and decreases in pitch. The emotion of joy is expressed in fast tempos, rising pitches that are highly variable, and a rapid rate of articulation. Anger is expressed by an increased fundamental frequency and increased amplitude, whereas fear is communicated by a fast rate of articulation, many high-frequency components, and an increased fundamental frequency. These are the features that Juslin and Laukka (2003) identified as being similar in both speech and music. Bresin and Friburg (2011) experimentally tested Scherer's (1995) hypotheses using twenty trained musicians, who were able to manipulate variables of tempo, intensity, rate of articulation, phrasing, register, timbre, and attack speed in order to alter the same musical piece to communicate different emotions. Happiness was communicated with a fast tempo, staccato articulation, high register, high intensity, and fast attack. Fear was communicated by fast tempo, staccato articulation, low register, and slow attack rate, whereas sadness was communicated with slow tempo, low intensity, legato articulation, and slow attack speeds. Calmness was communicated by a slow

Table 17.1 Structural features of emotional signals

Variable	Calming	Arousing	Fear	Threat
	(Sadness)	(Happy)	(Alarm)	(Anger)
Tempo	Slow	Fast	Fast	Moderate
Pitch	Descending	Ascending	High	Low
Intensity	Low	High	High	Moderate
Rate of articulation	Legato	Staccato	Staccato	Staccato
Register	High	High	Low	Low
Timbre	Harmonic	Harmonic	Dissonant	Dissonant
Attack speed	Slow	Fast	Slow	Fast

Adapted from Scherer (1995), Juslin & Laukka (2003), Bresin & Friburg (2011), and Snowdon & Teie (2013)

tempo, low intensity, legato articulation, high register, and slow attack rate. Thus, professional musicians used the same variables identified by Scherer (1995) to express different emotions within the same piece of music. Table 17.1 summarizes the musical features that communicate different emotions that are also found in animal vocalizations.

In a different type of study, Schwartz et al. (2003) showed that the distribution of harmonics in human vowel sounds showed peaks at frequency ratios that matched the chromatic scale. Subsequently, Bowling et al. (2010) found that in excited speech, vowel sounds matched the major chromatic scale, whereas in subdued speech, vowel sounds matched a minor chromatic scale, showing that even in vowel sounds of speech, humans communicate emotions. However, these studies were done with Western music, Western musicians, and Western speakers. Do these same features generalize to other cultures? Han et al. (2011) showed that the vowel harmonic distributions of Mandarin, Farsi, and Tamil speakers showed the same match to the chromatic scale as English speakers, and when Western listeners with no prior experience with Indian ragas were presented with ragas intended to communicate different emotions, they could discriminate between ragas intended to communicate joy, sadness, and anger, although they failed to discriminate between ragas of sadness and those of peace (calmness) (Balkwell & Thompson, 1999). Thus, despite different language roots and different musical traditions, there appear to be some emotional universals in music.

Can we also find similar universals in the calls of other species? One starting point is to look at signals humans use with non-verbal infants and with pets and working animals. Are there similarities? McConnell (1990, 1991) studied how humans controlled working sheep dogs (*Canus lupus familiaris*) and Fernald (1992) studied how parents communicate with non-verbal human infants. The results were amazingly similar. To arouse or get a dog or baby to become active, short, staccato calls or phrases with a rising-frequency modulation were used. To calm an infant or slow a dog's activity, long, legato notes with descending frequency were used, and to stop an action a sharp, short plosive note was used. Note that the arousing calls are similar to the features used in music to communicate happiness, whereas the calming calls are similar to those used in sad or calming music. These results suggest the same acoustic structures that adult humans use in emotional communication can also induce behavioural change in human infants and in other species. Furthermore, it is likely that humans in both cases are not communicating their own emotional state but rather trying to manage the state of their infants or dogs. These examples are good illustrations of the manipulation or management functions of communication.

If different prosodic features used by humans have similar effects on the behaviour of babies and animals, then it is reasonable to expect that humans should be able to discriminate between the affective states of animal vocalizations. Belin et al. (2008) presented human participants with affective vocalizations from humans, cats (*Felis catus*), and rhesus macaques (*Macaca mulatta*). Although the humans could readily distinguish between positive and negative valence calls from humans, they were unable to discriminate positive and negative affect in cat and macaque vocalizations, suggesting that humans cannot discriminate affective states in animal calls. However, the same participants were presented with the same sets of calls during functional magnetic resonance imaging (fMRI) of their brains and, in contrast to behavioural results, several brain areas responded differentially to the positive and negative vocalizations of all three species. Notably, bilateral regions of the auditory cortex were activated more by negative calls as was the right orbital-frontal cortex. Both sides of the lateral inferior prefrontal cortex were activated more by positive vocalizations from all three species. Thus, although human participants could not consciously discriminate between different affective calls from cats and macaques, their brains could discriminate!

Other studies have suggested that human discrimination of animal calls is a function of experience. Nicastro and Owren (2003) reported that human listeners could not distinguish or identify affective vocalizations in cats, but did find that participants with experience with cats were better at discriminating among calls. Scheumann et al. (2014) tested the ability of humans to discriminate between affiliative and agonistic calls of humans, dogs, chimpanzees (*Pan troglodytes*), and tree shrews (*Tupaia belangeri*) and found that, with greater familiarity with a species, there was better discrimination of affective calls. Thus, experience helps with conscious discrimination of affect in calls, but the fMRI results of Belin et al. (2008) raise the tantalizing notion that within our brains there is a universal ability to distinguish between positive and negative affective calls in other species, as well as in our own species.

In summary, there appear to be some universals of emotional expression in the music and speech of different human cultures, and many of the same cues to human emotion can be used by us to induce emotional or behavioural changes in non-verbal infants and in animals. Furthermore, although experience with different species appears necessary to consciously discriminate between affective calls of other species, our brains appear to be organized to discriminate between affiliative and agonistic vocalizations in other species, an ability that might have had great adaptive advantage to our ancestors.

17.3.2 Are there Affective Universals in Non-Human Animal Calls?

Let me now examine whether there are any affective universals in animal calls. The best known model relating vocal structure to affective state is that of Morton (1977; Owings

& Morton, 1998). Morton evaluated the call structure used by several species of birds and mammals in fear versus threat contexts and suggested that fear calls were characterized by high frequency and narrow bandwidth, with threat or aggressive calls being noisy, with low frequency and high bandwidth. These structures have adaptive parallels in that the sources of high-pitched narrow-band calls are more difficult to localize than low-pitched broad-bandwidth calls. Marler (1955) observed that many songbirds produced high-pitched calls upon sighting a predator, leading other birds (of a variety of species) to freeze, whereas low-pitched, staccato, broad-bandwidth calls were associated with mobbing of a predator.

Owren and Rendall (1997, 2001) suggested that calls with rapidly rising amplitude, sudden onset with a plosive quality induce a startle response in listeners, as confirmed by the short plosive sounds that inhibit actions in dogs and babies. These calls correspond to primate alarm and distress calls. On the other hand, they hypothesized that low-pitched, harmonic calls provide information on sex, age, status, physical quality, and individual signatures.

Snowdon and Teie (2013), based on research on emotional communication in music and how humans use different prosodic structures to influence the behaviour of babies and pets, proposed that staccato notes would be arousing and legato notes calming; that narrow-bandwidth (pure tones) and harmonically structured calls would be more likely to be used in positive, affiliative contexts, whereas dissonant or noisy structures would be associated with negative contexts, paralleling the hypotheses of Owren and Rendall (1997, 2001). Regular rhythms should be associated with positive states, with irregular rhythms associated with negative states. To what extent can these hypotheses be seen in animal vocalizations?

Snowdon and Teie (2013) presented several examples of cotton-top tamarin (*Saguinus oedipus*) vocalizations to professional musicians (Audios 17.1–17.3), asking them to cluster different calls on the basis of articulation, tempo, timbre, and noise or dissonance. The musicians were not aware of the contexts in which the calls were given. Calls with harmonic structure, narrow bandwidth, legato articulation, and ascending frequency were all used in affiliative contexts. Broadband staccato calls with harmonic intervals were associated with contexts of high arousal and threat. Noisy, dissonant, staccato calls were used in fear contexts, and legato calls with harmonic structure were used in confident threat contexts (where threat was not mixed with fear). Harmonic calls with triple metre were used in approach contexts. Can these structures be seen in other species as well?

Making comparisons across a broad range of species is difficult since researchers often use different criteria for classifying vocalizations and behavioural contexts. Nonetheless, some comparative data are available. In rodents, Keesom et al. (2015) studied aggressive behaviour in Siberian hamsters (*Phodopus sungorus*) and found that production of low-pitched, broadband vocalizations (both legato and staccato) were directly correlated with the degree of aggression shown, supporting Morton's (1977) idea that threats are low-pitched, broadband calls. Supporting this are findings in California mice (*Peromyscus californicus*) where short, frequency-modulated, ultrasonic bark-like calls are given during aggressive encounters (Pultorak et al., personal communication). Brudzynski (2013) reported for rats (*Rattus norvegicus*) that lower-frequency ultrasonic calls were used in aversive contexts (alarm and threat) and could be elicited by activity in the mesolimbic cholinergic system, whereas higher-pitched calls were associated with positive appetitive states (affiliative and cooperative) induced by dopamine activity in the ventral tegmental area. Notably, the higher-pitched calls were much shorter in duration, with much frequency modulation, supporting the results on how calls increase arousal in infants and pets.

In courtship contexts, Yang et al. (2013) found that male mice (*Mus musculus*) increased the rate of frequency-modulated, ascending-frequency, ultrasonic calls when they were separated from their mates. Males returned to longer, constant-frequency calls when their mates were returned, as predicted by the use of short-frequency modulated calls to induce arousal and long, constant-frequency calls to indicate calmness.

Soltis (2013) studied African elephants (*Loxodonta africana*) and found that calls given in dominance interactions were associated with increased intensity and duration of calls, and social agitation was associated with increased and more variable fundamental frequency and shorter duration calls. Aggression and mating calls were typically high-pitched, relative to the elephant's repertoire. Although these results do not completely support the predictions, they do provide partial support, with shorter notes and greater bandwidth during contexts of agitation.

Zimmermann et al. (2013) reviewed more than three dozen papers on mammalian vocalizations and reported that increases in call rate were associated with alarm and disturbance, although also associated in some cases with affiliation. Increased call duration and increased fundamental frequency were seen in both alarm and aggressive contexts, in contrast with the clear separation between these contexts reported for songbirds by Marler (1955) and Morton (1977).

Gray mouse lemur (*Microcebus murinus*) calls increase in both pitch and duration with increased arousal. A female rejecting a male mating attempt uses short, broadband calls but courting males use long, frequency-modulated calls. A startled lemur produces short, loud, noisy calls. Infant lemurs produce brief, frequency-modulated calls when threatened and purring-like calls while being groomed (Zimmermann, 2009).

In three species of Old World primates, Lemasson et al. (2012) reported that monkeys produced longer duration, higher-pitched calls in a high-arousal situation, appearing to contradict the predictions made earlier in the chapter. However, it is possible that the high-intensity situation produced fearfulness rather than arousal, and in this case the predictions of fear associated with higher pitches and longer notes would be supported.

Thus, although there seems to be considerable variation in the structure of calls given in various affective contexts across species, undermining a search for universals in acoustic structure, it may be that with more precise definitions of the behavioural contexts and behavioural responses, there would appear to be more consistency in call structure in specific contexts across species. The hypothesis that acoustic structures specify particular functions of calls (Owren & Rendall, 2001) requires that there be some consistency in acoustic structures in specific contexts across a broad range of species.

17.3.3   Can Vocal Signals Induce Affective States?

Owren and Rendall (2001) also proposed that call structures have evolved to induce emotions and/or to alter behaviour in recipients. What evidence is there of emotional contagion in other species? Animal calls frequently induce contagious calling in others. A bird singing induces others of its own and other species to sing, leading to a dawn chorus. A gibbon (*Hylobates sp.*) starts to produce a phrase and its mate adds another phrase and additional calls continue until culmination in a 'great call' involving both mates. Pair-bonded titi monkeys (*Callicebus sp.*) induce each other to call every morning, and neighbours begin calling as well. This joint, contagious calling appears to reinforce social relationships within a pair or group and serves to keep others away. However, this call contagion is not the same as inducing emotional or behavioural changes in others.

I suggested earlier in the chapter that the prosodic structure we use with infants and animals is designed to induce behavioural change, not simply communicate the emotional state of the caller. Can the calls of other species induce emotional states? This is difficult to test directly since animals are likely to have learned relationships between calls and contexts (Owren & Rendall, 1997), and it would be difficult to find naïve subjects to test. However, one test comes from Snowdon and Teie (2010) who presented cotton-top tamarin monkeys with music composed to be in the frequency range and tempo used by tamarins in their vocalizations (Audios 17.4 and 17.5). Music that included staccato notes with high-pitch modulation, dissonance, and noise aroused monkeys and led to increased locomotion, anxious behaviour, and social comforting, whereas music that was harmonic, with more legato notes and a slower tempo, made tamarins calmer and more relaxed. Since the music did not imitate natural monkey calls but used the acoustic principles that are related to emotional expression, we can conclude that the music induced affective changes in the monkeys who had never heard this music before and, thus, could not have learned any associations.

One final note concerns the affective nature of calling itself. In a remarkable experiment, Jürgens (1979) implanted electrodes in the brains of squirrel monkeys (*Saimiri sciureus*) in each of the areas where stimulation was known to induce a monkey to produce a call. He gave the monkeys control over whether they would stimulate these areas or not. If a monkey entered one chamber, stimulation of a vocal area would commence, and if the monkey moved to another chamber, stimulation would cease. Jürgens (1979) examined sixteen different calls organized by functional context—threat and aggression; confirming social bonds; contact seeking and flight, warning, and alarm; and fear and defensiveness. The overall call structures more or less matched the predictions made previously. Threat, aggressive, and defensive calls were broadband, staccato notes with lots of noise. Calls confirming social bonds were also staccato but had clearer harmonic structures. Warning and alarm calls were brief, broadband, single-note calls, and calls involving contact seeking were more tonal and legato than other calls. What was most remarkable was that only one of the vocalizations (involving social bonds) had a positive valence. Five calls were classified as neutral and ten were negative. That is, when the areas in the monkeys' brains associated with vocalization were stimulated, the stimulation was generally aversive to the monkey. This suggests that, for squirrel monkeys, the production of most of their vocalizations is aversive. Only rarely, does it seem, do monkeys find pleasure in vocalizing. This may be related to the point that, for most animals, vocalizations are both costly and risky and thus to be produced only when the benefits outweigh the costs. Let us now turn to the social functions of animal vocalizations.

17.4 SOCIAL ASPECTS AND SOCIAL INFLUENCES ON VOCAL COMMUNICATION

There are a large number of social functions that use vocal communication. Table 17.2 presents a list of these. It would require several chapters to discuss each of these, so for current purposes I will focus on three areas—the use of vocalization for social identification, how social interactions can shape and influence vocal structure, and how for some species vocalizations can be used flexibly according to social and environmental influences.

17.4.1 Social Identification

One principal function of vocal communication is identification. This can be at several different levels—species, subspecies, population, sex, social status, social group, family (or mates), and individuals. Each of these types of identification can be of importance in the social life of animals. For example, in mating, it is important to select a mate of the same species and opposite sex. It may be prudent to avoid mating with a relative, so being able to identify individuals (or at least to discriminate between familiar and unfamiliar individuals or relatives versus non-relatives) can be important. As other examples, if an individual is subordinate it may be valuable to identify the dominant animal in a group; parents may need to identify their own infants so that they do not invest parental care in unrelated infants; and animals with close social relationships may have ways to identify 'friends'.

There are good examples of each of these levels of identification in animal vocalizations. Most birds have distinct species-specific songs (Catchpole & Slater, 2008) and in developmental studies, some birds can readily learn the songs of their own species while being unable to learn songs of closely related species (e.g. Marler, 1970; Marler & Tamura, 1964). However, white-crowned sparrows (*Zonotrichia leuophrys*) can learn the song dialect of a different population if it is exposed to that song, rather than the song of its biological parents, during a sensitive period (Marler, 1970). Marmosets and tamarins, small primates from Central and South America, have species-distinct long calls (Snowdon, 1993) and where there are subspecies, these may have distinct subspecies call types as well (Hodun et al., 1981). Different populations of the pygmy marmoset (*Cebuella pygmaea*), the world's smallest monkey native to the Western Amazon, have been shown to have distinct variants of two of their most commonly used vocalizations (de la Torre & Snowdon, 2009), and these variants cannot be accounted for by differences in habitat acoustics.

Chimpanzees produce long, complex calls known as pant-hoots and different populations in East Africa display differences in the structure of pant-hoots (Mitani et al., 1992, 1999), and Crockford et al. (2004) have reported that males in neighbouring communities in West Africa have distinctly different pant-hoot structures that they hypothesize indicate group membership.

Sex differences are often seen in vocalizations where in most Northern temperate zone songbirds, only males produce song (Catchpole & Slater, 2008). In highly dimorphic

Table 17.2 Social functions of animal vocalizations

Behavioural

Seeking or avoiding interaction

Attack

Escape

Copulation

Association

Locomotion

Monitoring

Begging

Locating food

Predator alarm

Predator mobbing

Distress

Assembly or recruiting

Grooming or grooming invitation

Play or play invitation

Behavioural synchronization

Modifiers

Probability of action

Relative intensity

Relative stability

Direction

Location

Identifiers

Species

Subspecies

Population

Group

Sex

Family

Age

Individual

Reproductive condition

primate species, both the physical differences in body size as well as some specific adaptations lead to sex differences in fundamental frequency and may also lead to sex differences in vocal repertoires. In great apes such as gorillas (*Gorilla sp.*) and orangutans (*Pongo sp.*), males may be twice as large as females and have much lower voices (Dixson, 2009; Mitra Setia & van Schaik, 2007), and in many dimorphic Old World primates, some loud-call types are seen only in males (Gautier & Gautier, 1977). Ungulates also have a high degree of sexual dimorphism and in red deer (*Cervus elaphus*) there is an adaptation to increase the length of the vocal tract to accentuate the low pitch of roars (Fitch & Reby, 2001). Many New World primates are relatively monomorphic but howler monkey (*Alouatta sp.*) males have a specialized hyoid apparatus that not only allows for great amplification of their calls (Schön, 1971; Schön Ybarra, 1986) but also allows production of much lower pitches than predicted by their body size (Dunn et al., 2015). Even monomorphic species such as cotton-top tamarins display sex differences in call structure (Miller et al., 2004) and in call usage during territorial encounters (McConnell & Snowdon, 1986), although a study on the same colony 20 years later found a complete sex reversal in the use of territorial calls (Scott et al., 2006), suggesting that in monomorphic species these sex differences may be labile.

Recognition of one's relatives may be important both for distinguishing a potential ally and to avoid any possible inbreeding. Studies of northern fur seals (*Callorhinus ursinus*) have demonstrated recognition of mother and infant calls up to 4 years after the mothers and infants were together (Insley, 2000), and a study of captive cotton-top tamarins reported that monkeys could discriminate between calls of strangers and those of relatives from which they had been separated for up to 5.5 years (Matthews & Snowdon, 2011). Thus, when memory for calls of relatives has been tested, the memory duration has been impressive.

Dominance status can be signalled by voice. In many species, size and dominance are correlated so that the larger animal is more dominant and, by virtue of larger size, the dominant has a lower-pitched voice than other group members. However, there is an interesting exception to this general rule. In chacma baboons (*Papio hamadryas ursinus*), the dominant male has a higher-pitched bark vocalization than other males in the group, and the male's voice rises in pitch as he gains dominance and lowers again after he is supplanted by another male (Fischer et al., 2004).

Although it seems axiomatic that parents should be able to identify their offspring, the data on vocal recognition of offspring are quite variable. In bank swallows (*Riparia riparia*), infant birds produce complex vocalizations that are individually distinct, but in rough-winged swallows (*Stelgidopteryx ruficollis*), infants produce calls of very simple structures that are not individually distinct (Beecher, 1982). What could account for the difference? The more complex, identifiable calls are produced by young birds in a species that nests communally, with many different nests clustered together, whereas the simpler calls are produced by young in a species that nests alone, far from other nests of the same species. For the colonial species, young of many different nests are close together and distinct individually-specific calls between parents and offspring are necessary, but in the solitary-nesting species, the nest location itself provides a sufficient cue to the location of offspring.

In a study of chacma baboons, Rendall et al. (2009) studied individual differences in infant contact calls and distress screams. Although individual signatures could be seen in both types of calls, there was a greater degree of individuality in contact calls than in distress calls. Furthermore, when mothers were tested in a playback study using calls from their own versus another infant, mothers discriminated between the contact calls, but not the distress screams, in terms of latency of response. Thus, not all the calls in a vocal repertoire are individually distinct to listeners. Mothers responded more quickly to all distress calls and to their own infant's contact calls, compared to contact calls of another infant, suggesting that in a distress context, there may be a high priority on responding quickly, without taking the time to discriminate between individuals.

A final form of identification is between closely affiliated animals. Across many taxa there is evidence that animals in close social relationships either adopt each other's calls or converge to a common call type. Squirrel monkeys produce a 'chuck-call' only between females that have a close social relationship (Smith et al., 1982). Female starlings (*Sturnus vulgaris*) that have close social affinities also show convergence in their song motifs and these shared motifs change when females are moved from one social group to another and develop new affinities (Hausberger et al., 1995). Male indigo buntings returning from migration develop the song variants of the males in the area where they will breed (Payne & Payne, 1993). When black-capped chickadees (*Parus atricapillus*) form flocks in the winter they show convergence in the structure of the D-notes in the 'chick-a-dee' call (Nowicki, 1989). Newly-formed groups of budgerigars (*Melopsittacus undulatus*) converge on common group calls (Farabaugh et al., 1994). Mated goldfinches (*Spinus tristis*) converge on the call types they will use after pairing (Mundinger, 1970). Newly-paired pygmy marmosets change the structure of their trill vocalizations to match that of their mates (Snowdon & Elowson, 1999). Greater spear-nosed bat (*Phyllostomus hastatus)* females show a roost-specific call structure (Boughman, 1997) and group members are moved to new groups, they quickly match their calls to those of the new group (Boughman, 1998). Bottle-nosed dolphin (*Tursiops truncatus*) males form coalitions with other males and, in doing so, they begin producing the signature whistle of their coalition partner (King et al., 2013). Humans, on moving to a new dialect area, adjust their original dialect to converge with the new local dialect (Giles & Smith, 1979). Many other examples could be presented, but many species mark specific social relationships by sharing similar calls.

17.4.2 Social Influences on Vocal Structure

The previous section demonstrated that convergence of call structures is quite common across a broad taxonomic range and that shared vocal signatures appear to be markers of population and group identity, as well as of pair bonds, and of specific social relationships between individuals within a group or population. However, the mechanisms by which this convergence occurs are unclear. Convergence can be quite rapid, within a week in the case of black-capped chickadees (Nowicki, 1989) or within three weeks in newly-mated pygmy marmosets (Snowdon & Elowson, 1999). In goldfinches, males and females retain some of their own calls and acquire some of the calls of their mate (Mundinger, 1970). Bottle-nosed dolphins acquire the signature whistles of their close companions while still retaining their own whistles (King et al., 2013), whereas experimentally rearranged groups of starlings will develop completely new motifs with a new preferred social partner (Hausberger et al., 1995). There appear to be several possible mechanisms that may vary across species.

In a few cases, there is good evidence of how calls are shaped through social inter-actions. In zebra finches (*Taeniopygia guttata*) and white-crowned sparrows (*Zonotrichia leucophrys*), the period for song learning can be extended through the use of live tutors (Baptista & Petrinovich, 1986; Eales, 1985), and in zebra finches, aggressive interactions be-tween adult males and young birds were critical for song learning (Clayton, 1987). Cowbirds (*Molothrus ater*) are interesting because they are brood parasites, laying eggs in nests of other species, and yet males learn song and can alter their dialect to match the dialect of other birds. Very clever experiments have shown that a subtle visual display (wing-stroke) from a female reinforces a male's singing so that it matches the female's preferred song (West & King, 1988).

In pygmy marmosets, Elowson et al. (1998) described long bouts of vocal behaviour that was superficially similar to babbling seen in human infants. One characteristic of this babbling was that parents responded to a babbling infant by interacting with it socially. Young monkeys that babbled more in infancy showed more rapid development toward an adult repertoire (Snowdon & Elowson, 2001) suggesting that social reinforcement by parents may be important in shaping adult calls. An experimental approach with common marmosets (*Callithrix jacchus*) has demonstrated the importance of parental vocal feed-back on shaping calling in young marmosets (Takahashi et al., 2015). Young marmosets produced a variety of vocalizations when separated from their family, but with time, these diverse calls converged to a 'phee' vocalization. Takahashi et al. (2015) showed that this convergence was not due to physical maturation, but rather that parents differed in the degree to which they vocalized with well-formed phee calls to infants. Infants with high-responding parents acquired adult-like phee calls sooner than those with low-responding parents. As with cowbirds, we have direct evidence of a social mechanism that shapes call development.

17.4.3 Flexible Usage of Calls

The previous section illustrated how social factors shape call structure. This section con-siders the influences on call usage. Cotton-top tamarins have two chirp-like (short, frequency-modulated) calls that are used in feeding contexts. Young tamarins give versions of these calls when presented with food, but also produce several other call types that adults do not use when feeding. Curiously, Roush and Snowdon (1994) found no change in call structure or usage over development, with post-pubertal subadults still showing infant vocal responses. However, these are cooperatively-breeding monkeys where subordinate ani-mals are reproductively suppressed. When post-pubertal subadults were removed from the family and given a mate of their own, they rapidly developed adult versions of food chirps and stopped using the other vocalizations, suggesting that the adult use of food calls is, in part, a function of social status (Roush & Snowdon, 1999). Similarly in pygmy marmosets, although much vocal development occurs during juvenile and subadult stages, adult ver-sions of trill vocalizations did not emerge until animals had reached dominant reproductive status (Snowdon & Elowson, 2001).

Adult cotton-top tamarins also use a rapidly repeating version of food chirps during food-sharing bouts with young, and young who receive food from adults at an earlier age are able to feed independently and give their own food calls sooner than others (Joyce &

Snowdon, 2007). When juvenile tamarins, who no longer received food calls or sharing from adults, were presented with a novel foraging apparatus that their parents could solve, the parents again started to use the rapid food calls and engaged in food sharing until the juveniles first solved the novel task on their own (Humle & Snowdon, 2008). After that first success, adults no longer gave food calls or shared food. Thus, adult calling shapes infant vocal development and when juveniles are faced with a new task, adults again begin food calling and food sharing.

When tamarins were faced with a highly-preferred food that was adulterated with white pepper, those animals first sampling the food gave alarm calls in a totally novel context, but the effect was to keep others from sampling the food (Snowdon & Boe, 2003). Captive-born tamarins did not give alarm or mobbing calls when presented with live boa constrictors (a natural predator in the wild) but did give mobbing calls to someone dressed in veterinary garb and to some cage-cleaning materials (Campbell & Snowdon, 2007), suggesting the ability to apply natural calls to the novel contexts of captivity.

As noted in the introduction, vocal communication entails risks of attracting predators and thus it may be adaptive to adjust call structures to minimize predator detection. This is clearly seen in many songbirds that use high-pitched calls with gradual amplitude onsets and offsets in alarm calls and short, rapidly-repeating, frequency-modulated calls during mobbing (Marler, 1955). The former calls are difficult to localize in space, whereas the mobbing calls allow accurate localization and may even alert the predator that it has been seen, deterring predation. Pygmy marmosets adjust call structure to increase cues for sound localization as a function of distance from conspecifics. Calls when marmosets are within 5–10 metres of each other are single, high-pitched calls with relatively little frequency modulation, but with increasing distance from other group members, marmosets give shorter, more frequent notes that cover a broader frequency range, providing increased cues for localizing the caller (de la Torre & Snowdon, 2002).

Calls are also modified in response to environmental noise. The 'Lombard effect', described in humans as an increase in amplitude and duration of speech during noise, has also been seen in calls of common marmosets (Brumm et al., 2004) and cotton-top tamarins (Egnor & Hauser, 2006). De la Torre and Snowdon (2002) found that pygmy marmosets use a frequency range above the frequency of the calls of other animals and that in habitats with different ambient noise spectra, the lower frequency of marmoset calls differed. Thus, some monkeys can modify call structure in response to environmental noise.

17.5 SUMMARY

This chapter has provided a brief and selective review of social and emotional vocal communication in non-human animals. Using the comparative method pioneered by Darwin to understand emotional aspects of visual displays, we have compared vocal communication of emotion in humans with that seen in other species, finding some clear parallels. In accordance with theories that suggest animals use vocal signals to induce emotional states in listeners, we have seen how specific call structures used by humans can induce affective change in babies and working animals, and the same call structures appear in calls of other species.

Although researchers use differing methods and definitions of context, there do appear to be some potential universals of emotional signalling across a range of species. Using music composed in the frequency range and tempo of a species' natural vocalizations and manipulating acoustic structures thought to be related to affect has been successful in inducing affective states in other species.

Beyond communicating or influencing affective state, vocal signals serve other important social functions. Identifiers of species, population, social group, sex, dominance or reproductive status, and individuals are all important in the social lives of animals. Among the more interesting uses of vocalizations is to mark strong social bonds between individuals and to indicate group membership. Experiments with birds and mammals have found rapid changes in vocal structure as animals converge in some aspects of call structure with mates or preferred social partners. Vocal reinforcement from potential mates and from parents can shape vocal structure and usage in others. Non-human animals also display flexibility in the structure and use of vocalizations in response to social variables, to novel ecological niches, such as captivity, and to environmental noise.

REFERENCES

Balkwell, L. L. & Thompson, W.F. (1999). A cross-cultural investigation of the perception of emotion in music: psychophysical and cultural cues. *Music Perception*, 17, 43–64.

Baptista, L. F. & Petrinovich, L. (1986). Song development in the white-crowned sparrow: social factors and sex differences. *Animal Behaviour*, 34, 1359–1371.

Beecher, M. D. (1982). Signature systems and kin recognition. *American Zoologist*, 22, 477–490.

Belin, P., Fecteau, S., Charest, I., Nicastro, N., Hauser, M. D., and Armony, J. L. (2008). Human cerebral response to animal affective vocalizations. *Proceedings of the Royal Society: Series B*, 275, 473–481.

Boughman, J. W. (1997). Greater spear-nosed bats give group distinctive calls. *Behavioral Ecology and Sociobiology*, 39, 50–69.

Boughman, J. W. (1998). Vocal learning by greater spear-nosed bats. *Proceedings of the Royal Society: London B*, 154, 116–122.

Bowling, D. L., Gill, K., Choi, J. D., Prinz, J., & Purves, D. (2010). Major and minor music compared to excited and subdued speech. *Journal of the Acoustical Society of America*, 127, 491–503.

Bresin, R. & Friberg, A. (2011). Emotion rendering in music: range and characteristic values of seven musical variables. *Cortex*, 47, 1068–1081.

Brudzynski, S. M. (2013). Ethotransmission: communication of emotional state though ultrasonic vocalizations in rats. *Current Opinion in Neurobiology*, 23, 310–317.

Brumm, H., Voss, K., Köllmer, I., & Todt, D. (2004). Acoustic communication in noise: regulation of call characteristics in a New World monkey. *Journal of Experimental Biology*, 207, 443–448.

Campbell, M. W. & Snowdon, C. T. (2007). Vocal response of captive-reared *Saguinus oedipus* during mobbing. *International Journal of Primatology*, 28, 257–270.

Catchpole, C. K. & Slater, P. J .B. (2008). *Bird Song: Biological Themes and Variations*. Cambridge: Cambridge University Press.

Clayton, N. S. (1987). Song tutor choice in zebra finches. *Animal Behaviour*, 35, 714–721.

Crockford, C., Herbinger, I., Vigilant, L., & Boesch, C. (2004). Wild chimpanzees produce group specific calls: a case for vocal learning? *Ethology*, 110, 221–243.

Darwin, C. (1872/1988). *The Expression of Emotions in Man and Animals* (definitive edition with commentary by P. Ekman). New York: Oxford University Press.

De la Torre, S. & Snowdon, C. T. (2002). Environmental correlates of vocal communication of wild pygmy marmosets, *Cebuella pygmaea*. *Animal Behaviour*, 63, 847–856.

De la Torre, S. & Snowdon, C. T. (2009). Dialects in pygmy marmosets? Population variation in call structure. *American Journal of Primatology*, 71, 333–342.

Dixson, A. F. (2009). *Sexual Selection and the Origin of Human Mating Systems*. Oxford: Oxford University Press.

Dunn, J. C., Halenar, L. B., Davies, T. G., Cristobal-Azkarate, J., Reby, D., Sykes. D., & Knapp, L. A. (2015). Evolutionary trade-off between vocal tract and testes dimensions in howler monkeys. *Current Biology*, 25, 2839–2844.

Eales, L. A. (1985). Song learning in zebra finches: some effects of song model availability on what is learnt and when. *Animal Behaviour*, 33, 1293–1300.

Egnor, S. E. R. & Hauser, M. D. (2006). Noise-induced vocal modulation in cotton-top tamarins (*Saguinus oedipus*). *American Journal of Primatology*, 68, 1183–1190.

Elowson, A. M., Snowdon, C. T., & Lazaro-Perea, C. (1998). Infant 'babbling' in a nonhuman primate: complex vocal sequences with repeated call types. *Behaviour*, 135, 643–664.

Farabaugh, S. M., Linzenbold, A., & Dooling, R. J. (1994). Vocal plasticity in budgerigars (*Melopsittacus undulatus*): evidence of social factors in the learning of contact calls. *Journal of Comparative Psychology*, 108, 81–92.

Fernald, A. (1992). Human maternal vocalizations to infants as biologically relevant signals: an evolutionary perspective. In: J. Barkow, L. Cosmides, & J. Tooby (eds) *The Adapted Mind* (pp. 391–428). New York: Oxford University Press.

Fischer, J., Kitchen, D. M., Seyfarth, R. M., & Cheney, D. L. (2004). Baboon loud calls advertise male quality: acoustic features and their relation to rank, age, and exhaustion. *Behavioral Ecology and Sociobiology*, 56, 140–148.

Fitch, W. T. & Reby, D. (2001). The descended larynx is not uniquely human. *Proceedings of the Royal Society: B*, 268, 1669–1675.

Gautier, J. P. & Gautier, A. (1977). Communication in Old World monkeys. In: T. A. Sebeok (ed.) *How Animals Communicate* (pp. 890–964). Bloomington, IN: Indiana University Press.

Giles, H. & Smith, P. (1979). Accommodation theory: optimal levels of convergence. In: H. Giles and R. N. St. Clair (eds) *Language and Social Psychology* (pp. 45–65). Oxford: Basil Blackwell.

Han, S., Sundararajan, J., Bowling, D. L., Lake, J., & Purves, D. (2011). Co-variation of tonality in the music and speech of different cultures. *PLoS One*, 6, e20160.

Hausberger, M., Richard, M. A., Henry, L., Lepage, L., & Schmidt, S. (1995) Song sharing reflects the social organization in a captive group of European starlings (*Sturnus vulgaris*). *Journal of Comparative Psychology*, 109, 222–241.

Hodun, A., Snowdon, C. T., & Soini, P. (1981) Subspecific variation in the long calls of the tamarin, *Saguinus fuscicollis. Zeitschrift fur Tierpsychologie*, 57, 97–110.

Humle, T. & Snowdon, C. T. (2008). Socially biased learning in the acquisition of a complex foraging task in juvenile cottontop tamarins (*Saguinus oedipus*). *Animal Behaviour*, 75, 267–277.

Insley, S. J. (2000). Long-term vocal recognition in the northern fur seal. *Nature*, 406, 404–405.

Joyce, S. M. & Snowdon, C. T. (2007). Developmental changes in food transfers in cotton-top tamarins (*Saguinus oedipus*). *American Journal of Primatology*, 28, 257–270.

Jürgens, U. (1979). Vocalization as an emotional indicator: a neuroethological study in the squirrel monkey. *Behaviour*, 69, 88–117.

Jürgens, U. (1982). A neuroethological approach to the classification of vocalization in the squirrel monkey. In: C. T. Snowdon, C. H. Brown, & M. R. Petersen (eds) *Primate Communication* (pp. 50–66). New York: Cambridge University Press.

Juslin, P. N. & Laukka, P. (2003). Communication of emotions in vocal expression and music performance: different channels same code? *Psychological Bulletin*, 129, 770–814.

King, S. L., Sayigh, L. S., Wells, R. S., Fellner, W., & Janik, V. M. (2013). Vocal copying of individually distinct signature whistles in bottlenose dolphins. *Proceedings of the Royal Society: B*, 280, 20130053.

Lemasson, A., Remouf, K., Rossard, A., & Zimmermann, E. (2012). Cross-taxa similarities in affect-induced changes of vocal behavior and voice in arboreal monkeys. *PLoS One*, 7, e45106.

Keesom, S. M., Rendon, N. M., Demas, G. E., & Hurley, L. M. (2015). Vocal behavior during aggressive encounters between Siberian hamsters, *Phodopus sungorus*. *Animal Behaviour*, 102, 85–93.

Marler, P. (1955). Characteristics of some animal calls. *Nature*, 176, 6–8.

Marler, P. (1970). A comparative approach to vocal learning: song development in white crowned sparrows. *Journal of Comparative Psychology*, 71 (Suppl.), 1–25.

Marler, P. & Tamura, M. (1964). Song dialects in three populations of white-crowned sparrows. *Science*, 146, 1483–1486.

Matthews, S. A. & Snowdon, C. T. (2011). Long-term memory for calls of relatives in cotton-top tamarins (*Saguinus oedipus*). *Journal of Comparative Psychology*, 125, 366–369.

McConnell, P. B. (1990). Acoustic structure and receiver response in domestic dogs (*Canis familiaris*). *Animal Behaviour*, 39, 897–904

McConnell, P. B. (1991). Lessons from animal trainers: the effects of acoustic structure on an animal's response. In: P. Bateson & P. Klopfer (eds) *Perspectives in Ethology* (pp. 165–187). New York: Plenum Press.

McConnell, P. B. & Snowdon, C. T. (1986). Vocal interactions between unfamiliar groups of captive cotton top tamarins. *Behaviour*, 97, 273–296.

Miller, C. T., Scarl, J., & Hauser, M. D. (2004). Sensory biases underlie sex differences in tamarin long call structure. *Animal Behaviour*, 68, 713–720.

Mitani, J. C., Hasegawa, T., Gros-Louis, J., Marler, P., & Byrne, R. (1992). Dialects in wild chimpanzees? *American Journal of Primatology*, 27, 233–243.

Mitani, J. C., Hunley, K. L., & Murdoch, M. E. (1999). Geographic variation in the calls of wild chimpanzees: a re-assessment. *American Journal of Primatology*, 47, 133–152.

Mitra Setia, T. & van Shaik, C. P. (2007). The response of adult orang-utans to adult male long-calls: inferences about their function. *Folia Primatologica*, 78, 215–226.

Morton, E. S. (1977). On the occurrence and significance of motivational-structural rules in some bird and mammal sounds. *American Naturalist*, 111, 855–869.

Mundinger, P. C. (1970) Vocal imitation and individual recognition of finch calls. *Science*, 168, 480–482.

Nicastro, N. & Owren, M. J. (2003). Classification of domestic cat (*Felis catus*) vocalizations by naïve and experienced human listeners. *Journal of Comparative Psychology*, 117, 44–52.

Nowicki, S. (1989). Vocal plasticity in captive black-capped chickadees: the acoustic basis and rate of call convergence. *Animal Behaviour*, 37, 64–73.

Owings, D. H. & Morton, E. S. (1998). *Animal Vocal Communication: A New Approach.* Cambridge: Cambridge University Press.

Owren, M. J. & Rendall, D. (1997). An affect-conditioning model of nonhuman primate vocal signaling. In: M. D. Beecher, D. H. Owings, & N. H. Thompson (eds) *Perspectives in Ethology, Volume 12* (pp. 329–346). New York: Plenum Press.

Owren, M. J. & Rendall, D. (2001). Sound on the rebound: returning form and function to the forefront of understanding nonhuman primate signaling. *Evolutionary Anthropology*, 10, 58–71.

Payne, R. B. & Payne L. L. (1993). Song copying and cultural transmission in indigo buntings. *Animal Behaviour*, 46, 1045–1065.

Rendall, D., Notman, H., & Owren, M. J. (2009). Asymmetries in the individual distinctiveness and maternal recognition of infant contact calls and distress screams in baboons. *Journal of the Acoustical Society of America*, 125, 1792–1805.

Rendall, D., Owren, M. J., & Ryan, M. J. (2009). What do animal signals mean? *Animal Behaviour*, 78, 233–240.

Roush, R. S. & Snowdon, C. T. (1994). Ontogeny of food associated calls in cotton-top tamarins. *Animal Behaviour*, 47, 263–273.

Roush, R. S. & Snowdon, C. T. (1999). The effects of social status on food associated calls in captive cotton-top tamarins. *Animal Behaviour*, 58, 1299–1305.

Scherer, K. R. (1995). Expression of emotion in voice and music. *Journal of Voice*, 9, 235–248.

Scheumann, M., Hasting, A. D., Kotz, S. A., & Zimmermann, E. (2014). The voice of emotion across species: how do human listeners recognize animals' affective states? *PLoS One*, 9, e91192.

Schön M. A. (1971). The anatomy of the resonating mechanism in howling monkeys. *Folia Primatologica*, 15, 117–132.

Schön Ybarra, M. A. (1986). Loud calls of adult male red howling monkeys (*Alouatta seniculus*). *Folia Primatologica*, 47, 204–216.

Schwartz, D. A., Howe, C. Q., & Purves, D. (2003). The statistical structure of human speech sounds predicts musical universals. *Journal of Neuroscience*, 23, 7160–7168.

Scott, J. J., Carlson, K. L., & Snowdon, C. T. (2006). Lability of sex differences in long calling in cotton-top tamarins. *American Journal of Primatology*, 68, 153–160.

Seyfarth, R. M., Cheney, D. L., Bergman, T., Fischer, J., Zuberbühler, K., & Hammerschmidt, K. (2010). The central importance of information in studies of animal communication. *Animal Behaviour*, 80, 3–8.

Seyfarth, R. M., Cheney, D. L., & Marler, M. (1980). Monkey responses to three different alarm calls: evidence of predator classification and semantic communication. *Science*, 210, 801–803.

Smith, H. J., Newman, J. D., & Symmes, D. (1982). Vocal concomitants of affiliative behavior in squirrel monkeys. In: C. T. Snowdon, C. H. Brown, & M. R. Petersen (eds) *Primate Communication* (pp. 30–49). New York: Cambridge University Press.

Snowdon, C. T. (1993). A vocal taxonomy of the Callitrichids. In: A. Rylands (ed.) *Marmosets and Tamarins: Systematics Ecology and Behaviour* (pp. 78–94). Oxford: Oxford University Press.

Snowdon, C. T. & Boe, C. Y. (2003). Social communication about unpalatable foods in tamarins (*Saguinus oedipus*). *Journal of Comparative Psychology*, 117, 142–148.

Snowdon, C. T. & Elowson, A. M. (1999). Pygmy marmosets modify call structure when paired. *Ethology*, 105, 893–908.

Snowdon, C. T. & Elowson, A. M. (2001). 'Babbling' in pygmy marmosets: development after infancy. *Behaviour*, 138, 1235–1248.

Snowdon, C. T. & Teie, D. (2010). Affective responses in tamarins elicited by species-specific music. *Biology Letters*, 6, 30–32.

Snowdon, C. T. & Teie, D. (2013). Emotional communication in monkeys: music to their ears? In: E. Altenmüller, S. Schmidt, & d E. Zimmermann (eds) *Evolution of Emotional Communication* (pp. 133–151). Oxford: Oxford University Press.

Soltis, J. (2013). Emotional communication in African elephants (*Loxodonta africana*). In: E. Altenmüller, S. Schmidt, & E. Zimmermann (eds) *Evolution of Emotional Communication* (pp. 105–115). Oxford: Oxford University Press.

Takahashi, D. Y., Fenley, A. R., Teramoto, Y., Narayanan, D. Z., Borjon, J. I., Holmes, P., & Ghazanfar, A. A. (2015). The developmental dynamics of marmoset monkey vocal production. *Science*, 349, 734–738.

West, M. J. & King, A. P. (1988). Female visual displays affect the development of male song in the cowbird. *Nature*, 334, 244–246.

Yang, M., Loureiro, D., Kalikhman, D., & Crawley, J. N. (2013). Male mice emit distinct ultrasonic vocalizations when the female leaves the social interaction arena. *Frontiers in Behavioral Neuroscience*, 7, 159.

Zimmermann, E. (2009). Vocal expression of emotion in a nocturnal prosimian primate group, mouse lemurs. In: S. Brudzynski (ed.) *Handbook of Mammalian Vocalization* (pp. 215–225). Oxford: Academic Press.

Zimmermann, E., Lelivold, L., & Schehka, S. (2013). Toward the evolutionary roots of human prosody in human acoustic communication: a comparative approach to mammalian voices. In: E. Altenmüller, S. Schmidt, & E. Zimmermann (eds) *Evolution of Emotional Communication* (pp. 116–132). Oxford: Oxford University Press.

CHAPTER 18

DUAL STREAM MODELS OF AUDITORY VOCAL COMMUNICATION

JOSEF P. RAUSCHECKER

18.1 INTRODUCTION

VOCAL communication is a feat that has developed in a large number of animal species, most notably in birds and mammals. It has reached its culmination in humans, where it turns into a sophisticated system referred to as speech and, ultimately, language. Neither the end product of this evolution nor its precursors are well understood in neural terms. This chapter summarizes findings from more than twenty years of neurobiological research into the neural bases of central auditory processing and vocal communication in two primate species, macaques and humans. Although the macaque's vocal communication system is much more primitive than that of humans, it is supported by a cerebral cortex that is in many ways similar to that of humans (Rauschecker, 2017).

Not only is the organization of 'early' auditory cortex into core and belt regions astonishingly similar (Chevillet et al., 2011; Leaver & Rauschecker, 2016) but also the organization of higher auditory processing outside the classical auditory cortical areas suggests a very similar grouping into a dual-pathway system in the two primate species (Rauschecker & Scott, 2009; Rauschecker & Tian, 2000)—an anterior-ventral processing stream that encodes and recognizes complex sounds or 'auditory objects', and a dorsal stream that links posterior auditory regions with parietal, premotor, and prefrontal cortices that are involved in the planning and production of vocal communication sounds. Both pathways, in both species, converge onto an inferior frontal region that is commonly referred to as 'Broca's area' in humans, where it supports speech production as well as comprehension. Elucidating the sensorimotor functions of the auditory dorsal stream in non-human primates may be one of the most important tasks for an understanding of language evolution.

Processing and recognizing voices is a very significant portion of vocal communication in both primate species. Voices, as we commonly define them, do not only carry detailed referential or phonetic information (as in speech) but also more general non-verbal cues about the speaker's inner state or intentions. The same vocal apparatus generates both types of information, although they may originate from different parts of the brain. Voices also carry a host of other incidental information about its producer, which can be used for speaker identification and its many ramifications, thus enabling the recognition of gender, size, age, and emotional disposition ('mood') of the speaker. It will be interesting to know whether the many different types of information conveyed by voices are processed by the same or different regions in the brain.

Because they carry so much information about an individual, voices have often been compared with faces. Indeed, much recent research has suggested that a network of specialized voice areas exists in the superior temporal cortex (and other regions) of the brain (Belin & Zatorre, 2003), equivalent to the network of specialized face areas (or patches) in the ventral temporal cortex (Freiwald et al., 2009 ; Tsao et al., 2008). How these voice and face networks interact and are driven by the same processing streams is another interesting topic of current research, and there are clear indications that voice processing (like speech) takes place in segregated ventral and dorsal regions (Frühholz et al., 2015; Sammler et al., 2015).

18.2 VENTRAL-STREAM REGIONS INVOLVED IN VOCAL COMMUNICATION

Early auditory cortex in the macaque is subdivided into core areas, including primary auditory cortex A1 and rostral area R, and belt regions on the lateral and medial side of the core (Kaas & Hackett, 2000; Morel et al., 1993). While neurons in the core respond well to pure tones, neurons in belt areas and beyond (parabelt) prefer complex natural sounds (Rauschecker, 1997, 1998a; Rauschecker et al., 1995). Rostral (anterolateral) belt area AL has been shown to contain neurons highly selective for different types of species-specific vocalizations in the rhesus monkey (Figure 18.1; Tian et al., 2001; Audio 18.1). Area AL projects anteriorly to ventrolateral prefrontal cortex (Romanski et al., 1999), and this ventral auditory pathway carries mostly non-spatial information (Cohen et al., 2009), including information about pitch (Bendor & Wang, 2005).

Whether area AL is the endpoint of vocalization processing is doubtful, to say the least. It is more likely that neurons become even more specific at higher levels of a hierarchically organized ventral processing pathway. Selectivity along the antero-ventral stream increases further towards more anterior locations (Kikuchi et al., 2010, 2014). This trend extends all the way to the temporal pole, which is auditorily activated in the macaque and shows a hemispheric difference for species-specific communication sounds (Poremba et al., 2003, 2004). The decisive initial step at the belt level seems to be that neurons there prefer complex sounds over pure tones, thus implementing the first step of integration in the frequency domain. This integration occurs in a highly selective manner, rendering neurons specific to, for example, spectral bandwidth, as described in the following.

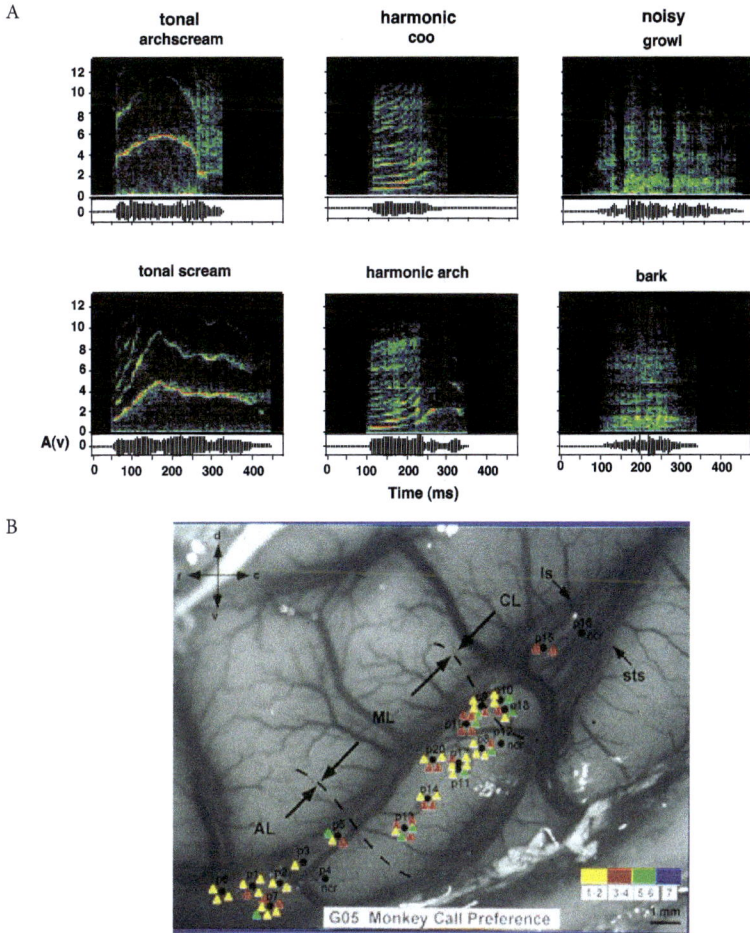

FIGURE 18.1 Selectivity of lateral belt neurons for species-specific calls in macaques. (A) Spectrograms of vocalizations and (B) selectivity of recording sites for these vocalizations in lateral belt cortex. Yellow symbols represent recording sites that responded to only one or two calls. They were concentrated in more anterior regions of the lateral belt.

(A) Reprinted from *Current Opinion in Neurobiology*, Volume 8, Issue 4, Rauschecker J.P., 'Cortical processing of complex sounds', pp. 516–521, Copyright © 1998 Elsevier Ltd., with permission from Elsevier, http://www.sciencedirect.com/science/article/pii/S0959438898800408?via%3Dihub
(B) From Tian B. et al., 'Functional Specialization in Rhesus Monkey Auditory Cortex', *Science,* Volume 292, Issue 5515, Copyright © 2001, doi: 10.1126/science.1058911. Reprinted with permission from AAAS.

18.2.1 Selectivity for Band-Passed Noise

One fundamental finding that was secured in initial studies (Rauschecker et al., 1995) and confirmed in detail later (Rauschecker & Tian, 2004), was the enhanced response of lateral belt (LB) neurons to band-passed (BP) noise compared to pure tones (Figure 18.2A,B; Audio 18.2). This demonstrated the ability of LB neurons to integrate over a finite frequency spectrum in a facilitatory fashion. By comparison, this integrative ability is largely absent in A1 neurons, a significant difference that we will return to later.

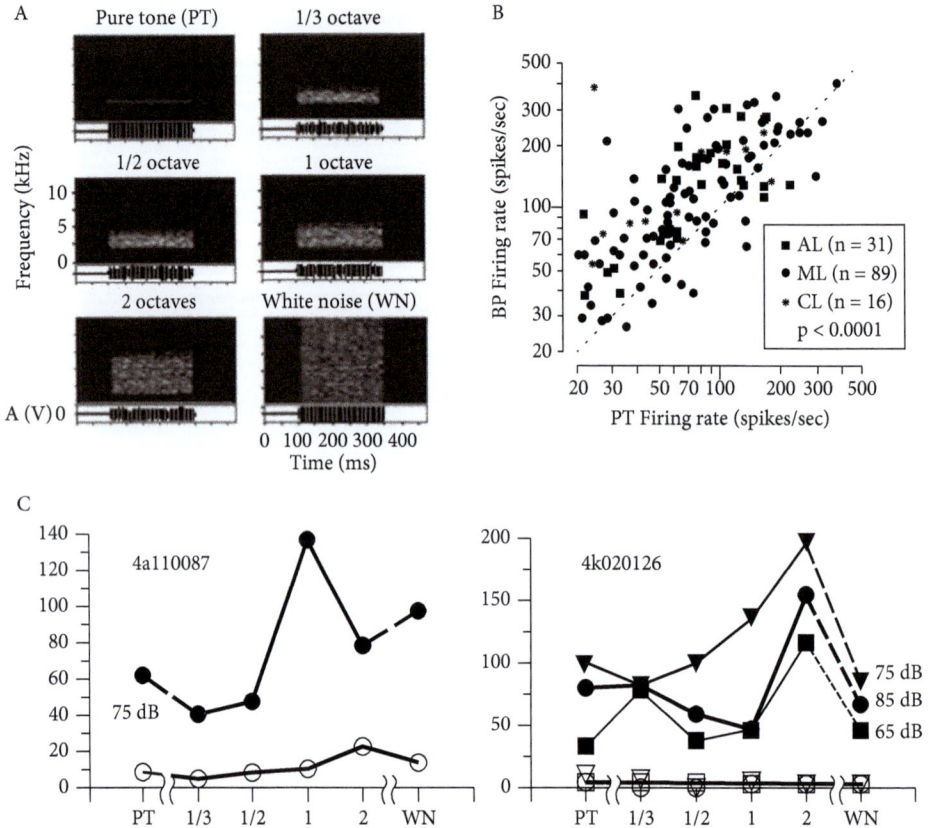

FIGURE 18.2 Selectivity of neurons in lateral auditory belt cortex of the macaque for band-passed noise bursts. (A) Band-passed noise stimuli of varying bandwidth from pure tones (PT) to white noise (WN). (B) Facilitation of responses (in spikes/sec) to band-passed (BP) noise bursts compared to PT. (C) Tuning selectivity to BP noise bursts of different band-width (in octaves).

Adapted from Rauschecker J.P., Tian B., & Hauser M., 'Processing of complex sounds in the macaque nonprimary auditory cortex', Science, Volume 268, Issue 5207, pp. 111–114, Copyright © 1995, doi: 10.1126/science.7701330. Reprinted with permission from AAAS.

Band-passed noise (BPN) bursts have a clearly defined centre frequency as well as a defined spectral bandwidth. Mapping of the LB along the rostro-caudal dimension revealed a smooth gradient for best centre frequency with two reversals (Rauschecker et al., 1995). This suggests that three cochleotopically organized areas exist within the LB, which have been termed the anterolateral (AL), middle lateral (ML), and caudolateral (CL) areas (Rauschecker et al., 1995).

LB neurons integrate over frequency in a way that produces the best response at a specific 'best bandwidth' (BBW) (Figure 18.2C), as a result of interactions between excitatory and inhibitory inputs. When tested in the LB, there was a clear trend for BBW to increase from core towards belt (Rauschecker & Tian, 2004). The same was later found for medial belt (Kusmierek & Rauschecker, 2009).

Neurons with selectivity for the centre frequency and bandwidth of BPN bursts are ideally suited to participate in the decoding of communication sounds, for which BPN bursts constitute ubiquitous ingredients in many species (Wang, 2000), including humans (see Figure 18.1A). BPN detectors, therefore, must be included in the repertoire of feature detectors dealing with communication sounds. Such feature detectors would have to preserve their selectivity regardless of sound intensity. Indeed, centre and bandwidth selectivity of LB neurons is generally invariant against changes in intensity (Figure 18.2C).

18.2.2 Selectivity for Frequency-Modulated Sweeps

Other features that are highly typical for communication sounds in most species are changes in frequency over time ('frequency-modulated sweeps'), also sometimes referred to as chirps or glides. Frequency-modulated (FM) sweeps are characterized by two parameters—FM rate and direction. Neurons in the LB are highly selective for both parameters (Tian & Rauschecker, 2004): over 90% of LB neurons respond to FM stimuli in at least one direction. Following a common criterion, a neuron is considered direction-selective when the response in one FM direction is at least twice as large as that in the other direction. About 60% of LB neurons are direction-selective on the basis of this criterion, with roughly equal proportions of neurons preferring upward and downward directions (Tian & Rauschecker, 2004). An example is shown in Figure 18.3.

Even more striking was the selectivity of LB neurons for FM rate. Various types of FM-rate tuning can be discerned in the LB, including high-pass, low-pass, and band-pass tuning (Tian & Rauschecker, 2004). Neurons tuned to both FM direction and FM rate, like the neuron in Figure 18.3, are ideal candidates for the extraction of communication-sound features, such as formant transitions in human speech. Preferred FM rate differed markedly between LB areas. AL neurons preferred FM rates below 64 Hz/ms. CL neurons, in contrast, preferred higher FM rates (above 64 Hz/ms, with medians of 160 Hz/ms for both directions). According to these findings, AL neurons are best suited to participate in the decoding of species-specific vocalizations, for which FM rates range mostly between 8 and 50 Hz/ms (Hauser, 1996; Rauschecker, 1998b). Only some of the 'screams' contain FM rates above 100 Hz/ms, and it is noteworthy that screams play an important role as alarm calls, which have to be clearly localizable by members of the same species. This is compatible with the presumed involvement of the caudal belt (and specifically area CL) in sound localization.

18.2.3 Selectivity for Species-Specific Vocalizations

LB neurons also respond differentially to different types of monkey calls (Figure 18.4). This may be a consequence of their tuning to the various lower-order features discussed in the previous paragraphs, like selectivity for the bandwidth of a BPN burst or for the direction and/or rate of an FM sweep. However, it could also be an emergent property resulting from the combination of these features. Although calls often have the same or comparable bandwidths, neuronal responses differ. Response selectivity, therefore, must

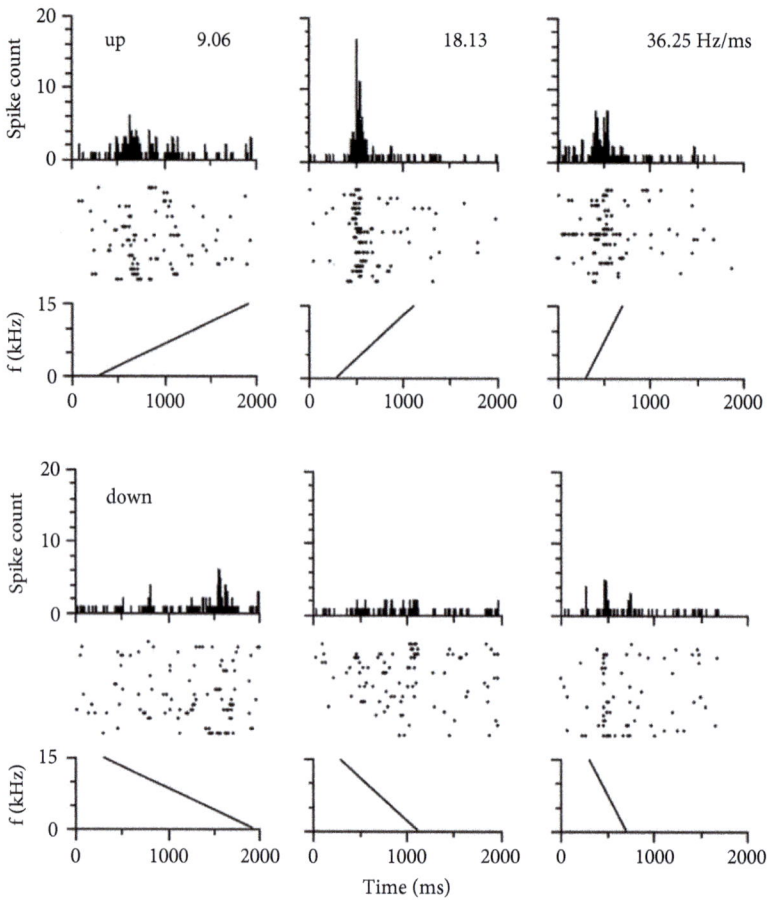

FIGURE 18.3 Selectivity of lateral belt neurons to frequency-modulated (FM) sweeps with varying speed and direction. Results of single-unit recording are shown as pairs of peri-stimulus time histograms (top) and dot-raster displays (bottom). Corresponding FM sweeps are shown below each pair.

Reproduced from Tian B. & Rauschecker J.P., 'Processing of Frequency-Modulated Sounds in the Lateral Auditory Belt Cortex of the Rhesus Monkey', *Journal of Neurophysiology*, Volume 92, Issue 5, pp. 2993–3013, Copyright © 2004 American Physiological Society, doi: 10.1152/jn.00472.2003.

be based on features contained in the phonetic fine structure of the calls, and it is a particular combination of features that causes a cell to respond to a specific type of call and not to others. Indeed, two fundamental mechanisms were identified as causing neuronal selectivity—non-linear summation in the spectral domain ('spectral facilitation', SFA) and non-linear summation in the temporal domain ('temporal facilitation', TFA), which have also been referred to as spectral and temporal combination sensitivity (CS), respectively, borrowing a term from neuroethological work (Margoliash & Fortune, 1992; Suga et al., 1978).

In spectral CS or SFA, inputs from lower-order neurons, such as band-pass-selective neurons, are combined in the frequency domain. In temporal CS or TFA, inputs are

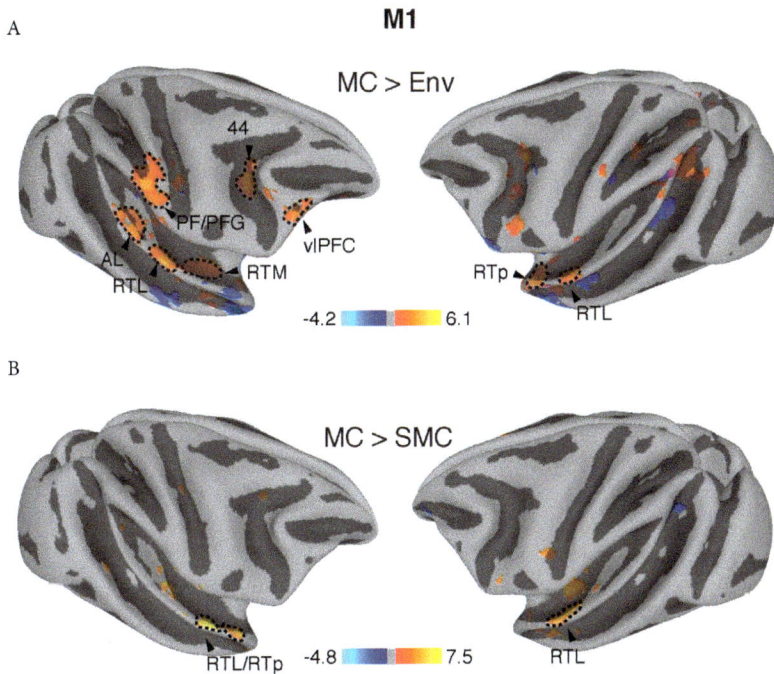

FIGURE 18.4 Cortical regions specifically activated by species-specific vocalizations as demonstrated by functional magnetic resonance imaging (fMRI) in awake monkeys. (A) Location of vocalization-sensitive regions is shown by comparison between the effects of monkey calls (MC) and environmental sounds (Env) in one monkey (M1). Activation maps were displayed on a semi-flattened surface of the macaque template. Active regions were found along the auditory ventral stream in the anterolateral area (AL), lateral and medial rostrotemporal areas (RTL, RTM), rostrotemporal pole (RTp), and ventrolateral prefrontal cortex (vlPFC). In addition, inferior parietal areas (PF and PFG) and the homologue of area 44 were activated more strongly by MC than Env. (B) Regions most strongly activated by monkey calls in comparison to *scrambled* monkey calls (SMC) are essentially restricted to areas in the anterior STG and RTL/RTp. Red/orange: significantly higher activation by MC than by control sounds (Env or SMC); blue: significantly higher activation by Env or SMC than by MC.

Reproduced from Ortiz-Rios M., 'Functional MRI of the vocalization-processing network in the macaque brain', *Frontiers in Neuroscience*, Volume 9, Issue 113, Copyright © 2015 Ortiz-Rios et al., doi: 10.3389/fnins.2015.00113, under the terms of the Creative Commons Attribution Licence (CC BY 4.0).

combined in the time domain. However, both mechanisms are based on the same principle—coincidence detection with a relatively high threshold (i.e. a logical *AND* gate principle). Only when all inputs are present simultaneously is a response evoked; with one input alone, no response follows. This explains why single components (or syllables) within a call are usually not sufficient to elicit a response. Temporal summation is accomplished by introducing staggered delays in the input pathways transmitting the early components, so all inputs eventually arrive simultaneously at the higher-order target neuron (Rauschecker, 2012).

One of the most striking differences between core and belt areas identified so far is the difference in their ability to non-linearly integrate information both in the spectral and time domain. While more than half of the neurons in LB show some form of non-linear interaction, only ~10% (or less) of the neurons in A1 or R display the same form of behaviour. This demonstrates a quantum leap in the processing characteristics of auditory cortex and is one of the strongest arguments for a hierarchical organization in auditory cortex.

These kinds of operations, convincingly demonstrated in anterior belt of rhesus monkey auditory cortex, are very likely the early building blocks in the evolution of phonological processing in human speech. It was reassuring, therefore, when an extensive meta-analysis of human imaging data of speech processing showed that areas in anterior superior temporal cortex (STC) are most selective to phonemes, words, and short phrases (DeWitt & Rauschecker, 2012; Figure 18.5). Regions were lined up from a

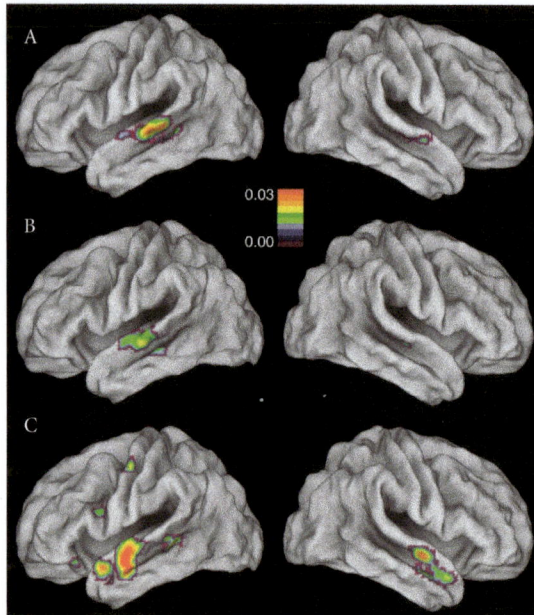

FIGURE 18.5 Regions of anterior superior temporal cortex in humans selective for phonemes, words, and short phrases. Cortical regions selective for speech sounds of increasing complexity are lined up from a mid superior temporal region anterior-lateral to Heschl's gyrus (selective for phonemes, shown in A) to regions in far-anterior superior temporal cortex (selective to phrases, shown in C) with word representations in between (B). These results of an extensive meta-analysis of human imaging data correspond extremely well with the hierarchical model of auditory processing in the macaque. Both species show activation along the auditory ventral stream by species-specific vocal sounds.

Reproduced from DeWitt I. & Rauschecker J.P., 'Phoneme and word recognition in the auditory ventral stream', *Proceedings of the National Academy of Sciences*, Volume 109, Issue 8, E505–E514, Copyright © 2011 DeWitt& Rauschecker, doi: 10.1073/pnas.1113427109

mid superior temporal region anterior-lateral to Heschl's gyrus (selective for phonemes) to regions in far-anterior superior temporal cortex (selective to phrases) with word representations in between. While matching the hierarchical monkey model almost perfectly, the finding was surprising with regard to the classical notion of a 'Wernicke's area' selective for speech processing in posterior superior temporal cortex. We will discuss this discrepancy next.

18.3 ROLE OF DORSAL-STREAM REGIONS IN VOCAL COMMUNICATION

Posterior regions of superior temporal cortex (PST) are, by definition, part of the dorsal auditory processing pathway, because they are situated behind primary auditory cortex (in Heschl's gyrus) and thus constitute the beginning of the dorsal stream with its anatomical projections to inferior parietal cortex, premotor cortex, and dorsolateral prefrontal cortex (DLPFC). In order to make this clearer, we sometimes refer to the dorsal stream as posterodorsal. A common mistake is to include PST (implicitly or explicitly) in the ventral processing stream merely on the basis of its location on the ventral bank of the sylvian fissure, without regard for PST's functional-anatomical connections. On the other hand, assigning PST to the dorsal stream poses the problem that a cortical region ('Wernicke's area') supposedly pertinent to 'speech perception' in humans exists outside the auditory ventral stream and, thus, seems to contradict the non-human primate model.

The solution to this apparent paradox, which has led some authors to doubt the validity of the monkey model for speech processing, is quite obvious: PST (or 'Wernicke's area') is, in fact, not a speech perception area in the sense of extracting and decoding acoustic-phonetic or 'perceptual' information from speech. This role has now consistently been assigned to anterior superior temporal (AST) cortex in both primate species (see Section 18.2). PST, by contrast, has been shown to play a role in audio-motor integration and control (Rauschecker, 2011; Rauschecker & Scott, 2009). As such, the auditory dorsal stream ties auditory representations to articulatory representations, setting up internal models that can be run in forward or inverse mode. This function includes the traditional, established role of the dorsal stream in spatial processing, which can also be considered a primarily sensorimotor function.

Data from both monkeys and humans have also advocated a role of the dorsal stream in temporal processing and in creating the ability to process temporal sequences (humans: Green et al., 2018; Leaver et al., 2009; Rauschecker, 2014 (Figure 18.6); monkeys: Artchakov et al., 2012; Camalier et al., 2012; Kusmierek & Rauschecker, 2014). Like spatial processing, temporal processing is an integral part of the sensorimotor function of the dorsal stream. Just as motion-in-space is the temporal derivative of space, spectral motion is the change of frequency content over time. While the former can be used as an error signal for fixation and sensory-guided movement, the latter is essential for speech and voicing.

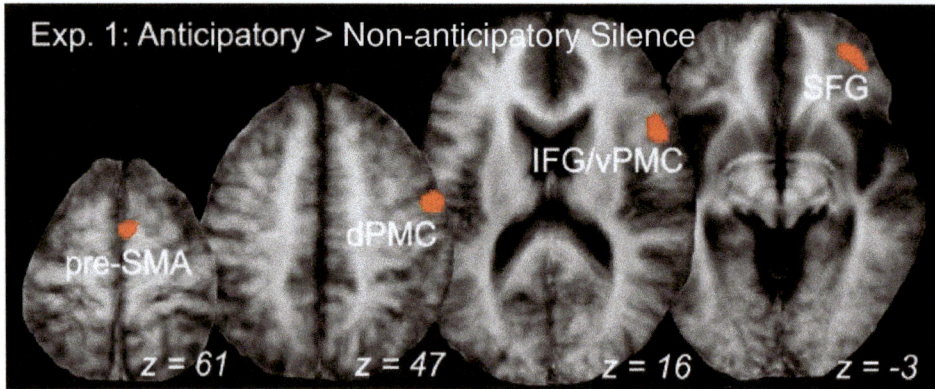

FIGURE 18.6 Sequence processing in the auditory dorsal stream of humans. Activation of brain areas during anticipatory imagery of familiar musical melodies was studied. In Experiment 1 (Exp. 1), stimuli consisted of the final seconds of familiar or unfamiliar tracks from a compact disk (CD), followed by 8 s of silence. During the silent period following familiar tracks (anticipatory silence), subjects (Ss) reported experiencing anticipatory imagery for the subsequent track. Stimuli presented during unfamiliar trials consisted of music that the Ss had never heard before. During this condition, Ss could not anticipate the onset of the following track (non-anticipatory silence, NS). While in the MRI scanner, Ss were instructed to attend to the stimulus being presented and to imagine, but not vocalize, the subsequent melody where appropriate. Activated brain regions were found in frontal regions, including inferior and superior frontal gyrus (IFG, SFG), pre-supplementary motor area (pre-SMA), as well as dorsal and ventral premotor cortex (dPMC, vPMC). This result first demonstrated the involvement of areas in the auditory dorsal stream during processing of familiar auditory sequences.

Reproduced from Leaver A.M. et al., 'Brain Activation during Anticipation of Sound Sequences', *Journal of Neuroscience*, Volume 29, Issue 8, pp. 2477–85, Copyright © 2009 Society for Neuroscience, doi: 10.1523/JNEUROSCI.4921-08.2009, by permission of the Society for Neuroscience.

18.4 Voice Regions, Vocalizations, and the Evolution of Language

Belin et al. (2000; Belin & Zatorre, 2002, 2003) were the first to describe regions in human auditory cortex, specifically in AST cortex, selectively responding to human voices. These regions did not primarily respond to phonological information, but were activated by human voices making non-verbal sounds like laughing, weeping, or coughing. Around the same time, two other studies demonstrated that identification of human speech sounds also activated AST (and not PST, as had classically been postulated) (Binder et al., 2000; Scott et al., 2000).

These three discoveries were of fundamental importance because they demonstrated for the first time that human auditory cortex was organized hierarchically like auditory cortex of non-human primates, with more complex sounds being processed farther away from core than simpler sounds. In the case of voice processing, this hierarchy furthermore culminated in the representation of ethologically essential information. The findings also opened a new perspective in neurolinguistic research in that non-verbal voice information may be considered a precursor signal for phonological processing. Although non-verbal voice signals contain less detailed information than the speech signal, voices do contain semantic meaning, for instance about emotions, and use acoustic information not unrelated to prosody in language (Rauschecker, 2013). In any event, both classes of signals fall under the rubric of auditory objects (Griffiths & Warren, 2004; Scott, 2005) that are typically processed in AST and the ventral stream.

Petkov et al. (2008) and Perrodin et al. (2011) later extended the concept of a voice area to rhesus monkeys. Microstimulation of voice-sensitive cortex engages a whole network of regions in the ipsilateral temporal lobe (Petkov et al., 2015). These studies were highly relevant because they demonstrated, directly, the homology between human and non-human primates in this domain. Although old-world monkey vocalizations had been studied extensively at the behavioural level (Hauser & Marler, 1993; Seyfarth et al., 1980), the distinction between different forms of vocal communication (call versus voice), let alone neurophysiological studies of their neural representations, had not been made until that point.

Voice representations can be discussed together in the context of dual processing streams. Voice sounds have a lot in common with speech, despite the fact that they do not possess phonological content. First of all, they are complex sounds with semantic meaning. As such one expects the acoustic and semantic content of voices to be represented in the temporal lobe, more specifically in anterior temporal cortex. This is indeed the case and resembles the face patch system in vision (Tsao et al., 2008). However, voice sounds commonly also contain temporal sequences and have audio-motor character, as they are self-produced doable sounds. For this reason, it is very plausible that activation can also be found in the auditory dorsal stream (Frühholz & Grandjean, 2012).

A fundamental question with regard to the evolution of auditory cortex, which culminates in the evolution of speech, language, and music in humans, is whether human and monkey brains show principal differences in their organization (e.g. new pathways or new areas appearing perhaps as the result of a genetic mutation), or whether these differences are largely of a quantitative nature. There is little doubt about a similar role of the ventral auditory pathway (anterolateral STC to ventral inferior frontal cortex) in both humans and monkeys in the decoding of spectrally complex sounds, which some authors have referred to as auditory object recognition (Griffiths & Warren, 2004; Scott, 2005). This function includes the decoding of vocalizations and speech sounds ('speech perception') and their ultimate linking to meaning ('semantics'), but it also includes the perception and interpretation of voice sounds, as discussed in this chapter.

The role of the auditory dorsal pathway (posterior STC to inferior parietal cortex and on to premotor and dorsal prefrontal regions) was originally presumed to lie in spatial processing, by analogy to the visual dorsal pathway (Rauschecker & Tian, 2000). While this function has been confirmed many times over by studies in humans (Arnott et al., 2004; Rauschecker, 2007) as well as monkeys (Ortiz-Rios et al., 2017; Woods et al., 2006), it has been expanded into one of sensorimotor integration and control. This concept still includes the processing of space and motion but now extends to the processing of sequences in space and time. Thus it seems that at least the basic layout of auditory cortex in humans and non-human primates is quite similar, although some quantitative refinement in one or several of these structures and their connectivity seems likely (Bornkessel-Schlesewsky et al., 2015).

18.5 CONCLUSIONS

The purpose of this chapter was two-fold. First and foremost, the goal was to demonstrate that the use of natural complex sounds, such as species-specific vocalizations, is a useful and viable approach for stimulation and testing of auditory cortical neurons. At the same time, breaking down these acoustically complex vocalizations into their constituent elements allows us to test various parameter domains (e.g. spectral bandwidth or change of frequency over time) more systematically and leads to a hierarchical model of auditory processing. Secondly, a comparative approach, in which data from humans and non-human primates inform each other, is particularly promising, as it yields valuable information about the evolution of communication systems and, ultimately, language. The existence of dual processing streams in both species, for instance, is a strong indication that common principles of functional organization govern auditory communication systems in monkeys and humans. How these processing streams interact, and how auditory and visual information is integrated in the processing of vocalizations and voices are major issues for future research (see Figure 18.7).

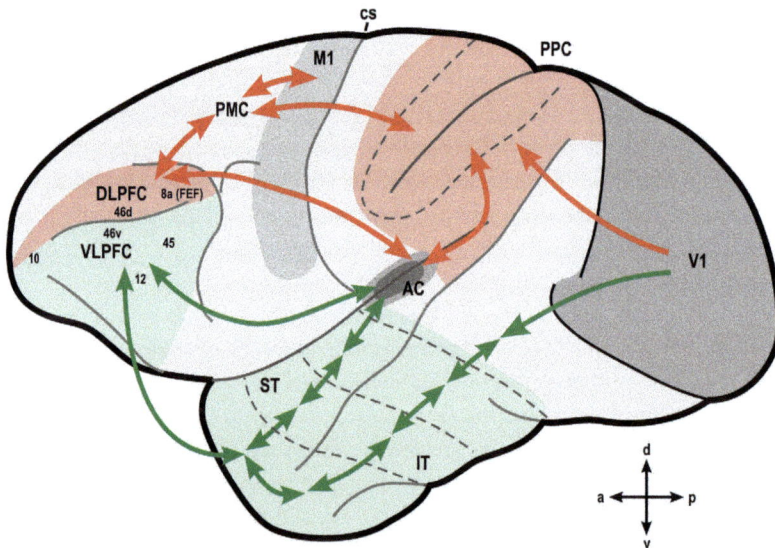

FIGURE 18.7 Dual processing streams for audition and vision in the macaque. Brain regions in green are part of the ventral stream for the identification of objects; areas in red are part of the expanded dorsal stream for sensorimotor integration and control.

IT; inferotemporal cortex; ST: superior temporal cortex; V1: primary visual cortex; AC: auditory cortex (core regions in dark grey, surrounding belt regions in lighter grey); M1: primary motor cortex; PPC: posterior parietal cortex; PMC: premotor cortex; DLPFC, VLPFC: dorsolateral, ventrolateral prefrontal cortex; FEF: frontal eye fields; d: dorsal; v: ventral; a: anterior; p: posterior. Numbers refer to Brodmann areas.

Adapted from Rauschecker J.P., 'Auditory and visual cortex of primates: a comparison of two sensory systems', *European Journal of Neuroscience*, Volume 41, Issue 5, pp. 579–85, Copyright © 2015 Federation of European Neuroscience Societies and John Wiley & Sons Ltd., doi: 10.1111/ejn.12844

ACKNOWLEDGEMENTS

The research summarized here was supported by grants from the National Science Foundation (BCS-0519127 and OISE-0730255) and the National Institutes of Health (R01DC03489, R01NS052494, and R01DC014989). The manuscript was prepared with partial support from the Technische Universität München—Institute for Advanced Study, funded by the German Excellence Initiative and the European Union Seventh Framework Programme under grant agreement n° 291763 (JPR).

This chapter is an updated synthesis of prior publications by the author (Rauschecker, 2012, 2013, 2017).

REFERENCES

Arnott, S. R., Binns, M. A., Grady, C. L., & Alain, C. (2004). Assessing the auditory dual-pathway model in humans. *NeuroImage*, 22, 401–408.

Artchakov, D., Ortiz, M., Kusmierek, P., Cui, D., VanMeter, J., Jääskeläinen, I., Sams, M., & Rauschecker, J. P. (2012). Representation of sound sequences in the auditory dorsal stream after sensorimotor learning in the rhesus monkey. *Society for Neuroscience Abstract*, 368.04.

Belin, P. & Zatorre, R. J. (2003). Adaptation to speaker's voice in right anterior temporal lobe. *NeuroReport* 14(16), 2105–2109.

Belin, P., Zatorre, R. J., & Ahad, P. (2002). Human temporal-lobe response to vocal sounds. *Brain Research: Cognitive Brain Research*, 13(1), 17–26.

Belin, P., Zatorre, R. J., Lafaille, P., Ahad, P., & Pike, B. (2000). Voice-selective areas in human auditory cortex. *Nature*, 403(6767), 309–312.

Bendor, D. & Wang, X. (2005). The neuronal representation of pitch in primate auditory cortex. *Nature*, 436, 1161–1165.

Binder, J. R., Frost, J. A., Hammeke, T. A., Bellgowan, P. S. F., Springer, J. A., Kaufman, J. N., & Possing, E. T. (2000). Human temporal lobe activation by speech and nonspeech sounds. *Cerebral Cortex*, 10, 512–528.

Bornkessel-Schlesewsky, I., Schlesewsky, M., Small, S. L., & Rauschecker, J. P. (2015). Neurobiological roots of language in primate audition: common computational properties. *Trends in Cognitive Sciences*, 19(3), 142–150.

Camalier, C. R., D'Angelo, W. R., Sterbing-D'Angelo, S. J., de la Mothe, L. A., & Hackett, T. A. (2012). Neural latencies across auditory cortex of macaque support a dorsal stream supramodal timing advantage in primates. *Proceedings of the National Academy of Sciences of the United States of America*, 109, 18168–18173.

Chevillet, M., Riesenhuber, M., & Rauschecker, J. P. (2011). Functional correlates of the anterolateral processing hierarchy in human auditory cortex. *Journal of Neuroscience*, 31(25), 9345–9352.

Cohen, Y. E., Russ, B. E., Davis, S. J., Baker, A. E., Ackelson, A. L., & Nitecki, R. (2009). A functional role for the ventrolateral prefrontal cortex in non-spatial auditory cognition. *Proceedings of the National Academy of Sciences of the United States of America*, 106(47), 20045–20050.

DeWitt, I. & Rauschecker, J. P. (2012). Phoneme and word recognition in the auditory ventral stream. *Proceedings of the National Academy of Sciences of the United States of America*, 109(8), E505–514.

Freiwald, W., Tsao, D., & Livingstone, M. (2009). A face feature space in the macaque temporal lobe. *Nature Neuroscience*, 12, 1187–1196.

Frühholz, S. & Grandjean, D. (2012). Towards a fronto-temporal neural network for the decoding of angry vocal expressions. *NeuroImage*, 62, 1658–1666.

Frühholz, S., Gschwind, M., & Grandjean, D. (2015). Bilateral dorsal and ventral fiber pathways for the processing of affective prosody identified by probabilistic fiber tracking. *NeuroImage*, 109, 27–34.

Green, B., Sams, M., Jääskeläinen, I. P., & Rauschecker, J. P. (2018). Distinct brain areas process novel and repeating sound sequences. *Brain & Language* (in prep.)

Griffiths, T. D. & Warren, J. D. (2004). What is an auditory object? *Nature Reviews Neuroscience*, 5(11), 887–892.

Hauser, M. D. (1996). *The Evolution of Communication*. MIT Press.

Hauser, M. D. & Marler, P. (1993). Food-association calls to rhesus macaques (*Macaca mulatta*). I. Sociological factors. *Behavioral Ecology*, 4, 194–205.

Kaas, J. H. & Hackett, T. A. (2000). Subdivisions of auditory cortex and processing streams in primates. *Proceedings of the National Academy of Sciences of the United States of America*, 97, 11793–11799.

Kikuchi, Y., Horwitz, B., & Mishkin, M. (2010). Hierarchical auditory processing directed rostrally along the monkey's supratemporal plane. *Journal of Neuroscience*, 30(39), 13021–13030.

Kikuchi, Y., Horwitz, B., Mishkin, M., & Rauschecker, J. P. (2014). Processing of harmonics in the lateral belt of macaque auditory cortex. *Frontiers in Neuroscience*, 8, 204. doi: 10.3389/fnins.2014.00204

Kusmierek, P. & Rauschecker, J. P. (2009). Responses of rhesus monkey rostral and middle medial belt neurons to tones, noises, and natural sounds *Journal of Neurophysiology*, 102(3), 1606–1622.

Kusmierek, P. & Rauschecker, J. P. (2014). Selectivity for space and time in early areas of the auditory dorsal stream in the rhesus monkey. *Journal of Neurophysiology*, 111(8), 1671–1685.

Leaver, A. M., Van Lare, J. E., Zielinski, B. A., Halpern, A., & Rauschecker, J. P. (2009). Brain activation during anticipation of sound sequences. *Journal of Neuroscience*, 29(8), 2477–2485.

Leaver, A. M. & Rauschecker, J. P. (2016). Functional topography of human auditory cortex. *Journal of Neuroscience*, 36(4), 1416–1428.

Margoliash, D. & Fortune, E. S. (1992). Temporal and harmonic combination-sensitive neurons in the zebra finch's HVc. *Journal of Neuroscience*, 12, 4309–4326.

Morel, A., Garraghty, P. E., & Kaas, J. H. (1993). Tonotopic organization, architectonic fields, and connections of auditory cortex in macaque monkeys. *Journal of Computational Neurology*, 335(3), 437–459.

Ortiz-Rios, M., Azevedo, F. A. C., Kuśmierek, P., Balla, D. Z., Munk, M. H., Keliris, G. A., Logothetis, N. K., & Rauschecker, J. P. (2017). Opponent signals and posterior specialization represent sound location in macaque auditory cortex. *Neuron*, 93(4), 971–983.

Ortiz-Rios, M., Kusmierek, P., DeWitt, I., Archakov, D. A., Azevedo, F. A. C., Sams, M., Keliris, G. A., & Rauschecker, J. P. (2015). Functional MRI of the vocalization-processing network in the macaque brain. *Frontiers in Neuroscience*, 9, 113. doi: 10.3389/fnins.2015.00113

Petkov, C. I., Kayser, C., Steudel, T., Whittingstall, K., Augath, M., & Logothetis, N. K. (2008). A voice region in the monkey brain. *Nature Neuroscience*, 11, 367–374.

Petkov, C. I., Kikuchi, Y., Milne, A., Mishkin, M., Rauschecker, J. P., & Logothetis, N. K. (2015). Different forms of effective connectivity in primate frontotemporal pathways. *Nature Communications*, 6, 6000. doi: 10.1038/ncomms7000

Perrodin, C., Kayser, C., Logothetis, N. K., & Petkov, C. I. (2011). Voice cells in the primate temporal lobe. *Current Biology*, 21, 1408–1415.

Poremba, A., Malloy, M., Saunders, R. C., Carson, R. E., Herscovitch, P., & Mishkin, M. (2004). Species-specific calls evoke asymmetric activity in the monkey's temporal poles. *Nature*, 427(6973), 448–451.

Poremba, A., Saunders, R. C., Crane, A. M., Cook, M., Sokoloff, L., & Mishkin, M. (2003). Functional mapping of the primate auditory system. *Science*, 299(5606), 568–572.

Rauschecker, J. P. (1997). Processing of complex sounds in the auditory cortex of cat, monkey and man. *Acta Otolaryngologica (Stockholm)*, Suppl. 532, 34–38.

Rauschecker, J. P. (1998a). Cortical processing of complex sounds. *Current Opinion in Neurobiology*, 8, 516–521.

Rauschecker, J. P. (1998b). Parallel processing in the auditory cortex of primates. *Audiology and Neurootology*, 3, 86–103.

Rauschecker, J. P. (2007). Cortical processing of auditory space: pathways and plasticity. In: F. Mast & L. Jäncke (eds) *Spatial Processing in Navigation, Imagery, and Perception* (pp. 389–410). New York: Springer-Verlag.

Rauschecker, J. P. (2011). An expanded role for the dorsal auditory pathway in sensorimotor integration and control. *Hearing Research*, 271, 16–25.

Rauschecker, J. P. (2012). Processing streams in the auditory cortex. In: Y. Cohen, R. R. Fay, & A. N. Popper (eds) *Neural Correlates of Auditory Cognition. Springer Handbook of Auditory Research* (pp. 7–44). New York: Springer.

Rauschecker, J. P. (2013). Brain networks for the encoding of emotions in communication sounds of human and nonhuman primates. In: E. Altenmüller, S. Schmidt, & E. Zimmermann (eds) *The Evolution of Emotional Communication* (pp. 49–60). Oxford, UK: Oxford University Press.

Rauschecker, J. P. (2014). Is there a tape recorder in your head? How the brain stores and retrieves musical melodies. *Frontiers in Systems Neuroscience*, 8, 149. doi: 10.3389/fnsys.2014.0014928

Rauschecker, J. P. (2015). Auditory and visual cortex of primates: a comparison of two sensory systems. *European Journal of Neuroscience*, 41(5), 579–585. doi: 10.1111/ejn.12844

Rauschecker, J. P. (2017). The evolution of auditory cortex in humans. In: J. Kaas (ed) *Evolution of Nervous Systems, vol. 4* (2nd edn) (pp. 293–299). Oxford: Elsevier.

Rauschecker, J. P. & Scott, S. K. (2009). Maps and streams in the auditory cortex: nonhuman primates illuminate human speech processing. *Nature Neuroscience*, 12, 718–724.

Rauschecker, J. P. & Tian, B. (2000). Mechanisms and streams for processing of 'what' and 'where' in auditory cortex. *Proceedings of the National Academy of Sciences of the United States of America*, 97, 11800–11806.

Rauschecker, J. P. & Tian, B. (2004). Processing of band-passed noise in the lateral auditory belt cortex of the rhesus monkey. *Journal of Neurophysiology*, 91(6), 2578–2589.

Rauschecker, J. P. Tian, B., & Hauser, M. (1995). Processing of complex sounds in the macaque nonprimary auditory cortex. *Science*, 268, 111–114.

Romanski, L. M., Tian, B., Fritz, J., Mishkin, M., Goldman-Rakic, P. S., & Rauschecker, J. P. (1999). Dual streams of auditory afferents target multiple domains in the primate prefrontal cortex. *Nature Neuroscience*, 2, 1131–1136.

Sammler, D., Grosbras, M. H., Anwander, A., Bestelmeyer, P. E. G., & Belin, P. (2015). Dorsal and ventral pathways for prosody. *Current Biology*, 25, 3079–3085.

Scott, S. K. (2005) Auditory processing–speech, space and auditory objects. *Current Opinion in Neurobiology*, 15(2), 197–201.

Scott, S. K., Blank, C. C., Rosen, S., & Wise, R. J. (2000). Identification of a pathway for intelligible speech in the left temporal lobe. *Brain*, 123(Pt 12), 2400–2406.

Seyfarth, R. M., Cheney, D. L., & Marler, P. (1980). Monkey responses to three different alarm calls: evidence of predator classification and semantic communication. *Science*, 210(4471), 801–803.

Suga, N., O'Neill, W. E., & Manabe, T. (1978). Cortical neurons sensitive to combinations of information-bearing elements of biosonar signals in the mustache bat. *Science*, 200, 778–781.

Tian, B. & Rauschecker, J. P. (2004). Processing of frequency-modulated sounds in the lateral auditory belt cortex of the rhesus monkey. *Journal of Neurophysiology*, 92(5), 2993–3013.

Tian, B., Reser, D., Durham, A., Kustov, A., & Rauschecker, J. P. (2001). Functional specialization in rhesus monkey auditory cortex. *Science*, 292, 290–293.

Tsao, D., Moeller, S., & Freiwald, W. (2008). Comparing face patch systems in macaques and humans. *Proceedings of the National Academy of Sciences of the United States of America*, 105, 19514–19519.

Wang, X. (2000). On cortical coding of vocal communication sounds in primates. *Proceedings of the National Academy of Sciences of the United States of America*, 11843–11849.

Woods, T. M., Lopez, S. E., Long, J. H., Rahman, J. E., & Recanzone, G. H. (2006). Effects of stimulus azimuth and intensity on the single-neuron activity in the auditory cortex of the alert macaque monkey. *Journal of Neurophysiology*, 96, 3323–3337.

PART IV

EMOTIONAL AND
MOTIVATIONAL
VOCAL EXPRESSION

CHAPTER 19

THE NEURAL NETWORK UNDERLYING THE PROCESSING OF AFFECTIVE VOCALIZATIONS

SASCHA FRÜHHOLZ AND LEONARDO CERAVOLO

19.1 INTRODUCTION

OUR daily life is rich in affective information that appears both in natural and social environments. Some of these events can frighten us, such as the barking of a dog, or the aggressive face of another individual. Other events are more pleasurable, such as the laughing of another individual, the sound of music, or the smell of flowers. These examples demonstrate that affective information can be conveyed by different types of sensory channels (visual, auditory, olfactory, etc.) and by different means of signal transmission (natural events, social interactions, telecommunication, etc.).

Concerning auditory social signals, the human voice is a rich source of affective information and it can convey relevant information about the emotional state of the speaker. It is not only the linguistic dimension that speakers use to convey and that listeners use to recognize social information, by expressing and hearing inner emotional states in words (Kissler, 2013), but it is also the paralinguistic dimension of these vocalizations, in terms of the tone, loudness, timbre, and melody, which carries a wealth of information about the emotional state.

This information is encoded in specific acoustic properties and modulations of the speaker's voice (Banse & Scherer, 1996; Patel et al., 2011) (see Scherer, this volume). These acoustic properties relate to specific acoustic features as well as the more global voice quality of affective vocalizations, and they concern different types of affective modulations of the paralinguistic dimension of vocalizations. These types refer to vocal intonations that are part of several types of vocal utterances, such as non-verbal affect bursts (Scherer, 1994), intonation during speaking (referred to as affective prosody) (Hammerschmidt & Jurgens, 2007), and partly also singing (Weninger et al., 2013). Non-verbal affective vocalizations especially are a medium of expressing inner emotional states that are mainly shared with close relatives of humans, such as non-human primates (Zimmermann et al., 2013), pointing to an evolutionary trajectory for vocal expressions. It was even proposed that affective intonations superimposed on speech are derived from older types of non-verbal affective intonation (Scherer, 1994).

The primate brain has developed specific neural mechanisms for the perception and the decoding of these acoustically encoded emotional signals. Accordingly, these acoustic cues receive a cascade of signal transmissions and signal decoding in the neural auditory brain system and associated areas. This chapter will describe the distributed neural processing of affective vocalizations by mainly referring to the recent neuroimaging literature and also to studies including brain-lesioned patients.

There are four major questions that hopefully will be answered while reading this chapter. First, how do we perceive and how does the brain process the acoustic quality of affective voices both in terms of tonal and temporal information? Second, how do we perceive and how does the brain process the affective meaning conveyed by these voices and voice features? Third, how do we evaluate the emotional and social significance of these affective voices? Finally fourth, what is good about the fact that the human neurocognitive system is highly sensitive to the affective meaning conveyed by voices; more specifically, does this sensitivity have an influence on other cognitive functions?

19.2 Early Evidence from Brain-Lesioned Patients

Early evidence on the neural mechanisms of processing affective voices comes from studies including patients with focal, but still large, brain lesions due to cerebral stroke (Lalande et al., 1992; Ross, 1981). These studies were mainly concerned with a dominant and recurrent question in the affective neurosciences about the brain lateralization of emotional processing (Borod et al., 1998; Davidson et al., 1990), which is still under debate (Frühholz, Hofstetter, et al., 2015). These early studies have pointed to a predominance of the right hemisphere, and especially of the right auditory cortex (AC), in processing affective voices, such that right-lateralized brain lesions lead to pervasive difficulties in understanding affect from the tonal information in voices and speech (Figure 19.1A). These findings seemed to be in accordance with the general view that the right, compared with the left, hemisphere is predominantly sensitive to the affective meaning of stimuli (Borod et al., 1998).

These early data seem to be confirmed by more recent studies, including studies of brain-lesioned patients, that however do not point to an exclusive role of the right hemisphere in understanding affective meaning from voices (Kucharska-Pietura et al., 2003; Pell, 2006b; Ross & Monnot, 2008, 2011). Some left brain lesions can also have effects on affective voice understanding that seem more subtle and less severe (e.g. Kucharska-Pietura et al., 2003). Left hemisphere lesions can lead to difficulties in understanding of affective prosody as the paralinguistic dimension of speech. Specifically, these patients have difficulties in using this paralinguistic dimension (i.e. 'how' something is said) for a better understanding of the linguistic dimension (i.e. 'what' is said) (Pell, 2006a).

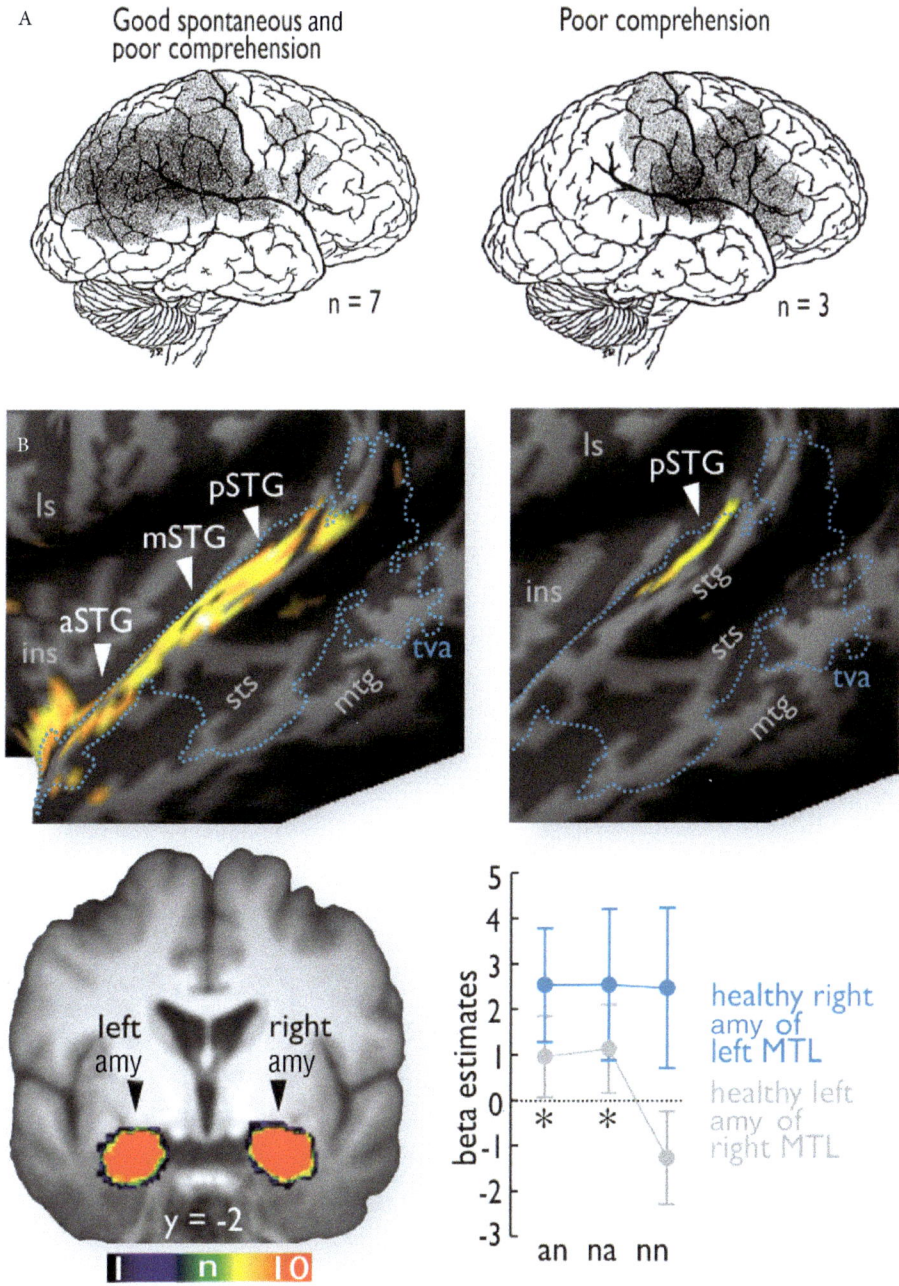

FIGURE 19.1 Affective voice processing in brain-lesioned patients. (A) Studies including patients with different focal brain lesions indicate that especially lesions in the right superior temporal lobe lead to impairments in understanding the affective intonation in speech, while the spontaneous production of such affective intonated speech seems unimpaired (left panel). Especially lesions in the right temporal planum seem to lead to considerable impairments in the processing of affective prosody. (B) Lesions in the left amygdala can lead

These studies provided the first evidence, at least in terms of hemispheric lateralization, of brain functions underlying the recognition of affective meaning from voices, although the partly largely extended size of the lesions—that were focal, but extended into neighbouring regions and brain lobes—made it difficult to precisely identify the brain areas important for affective voice processing. More recent studies thus investigated patients with more localized brain lesions in certain brain areas. For example, localized lesions in the basal ganglia (BG) (e.g. Ariatti et al., 2008; Calder et al., 2004; Dara et al., 2008; Paulmann et al., 2009; Schroder et al., 2006) and the amygdala (e.g. Brierley et al., 2004; Milesi et al., 2014) can lead to impairments in the cognitive and neural decoding of affective voices (Figure 19.1B). The latter results about the influence of amygdala lesions, however, show some inconsistency across studies (e.g. Adolphs & Tranel, 1999; Bach et al., 2013).

19.3 NEURAL SYSTEMS AND NETWORK

The aforementioned patient studies provided the first evidence about the potential neural network involved in processing affective voices and the supposed underlying functional mechanisms. If we think more precisely about the most necessary brain networks and functions for decoding the affective meaning from voices under normal conditions, we could think of two core functions: (1) there needs to be some acoustic analysis of the voices to extract relevant vocal cues and features, and (2) there needs to be some kind of decoding and classification of the affective quality of those voices. Both functions seem initially sufficient for a proper decoding of the affective meaning from voices. Recent neuroimaging studies pointed to a distributed large-scale neural network underlying these different functional processes.

19.3.1 The Large-Scale Neural Network

Given that the functional processes just described are quite different, it seems plausible that different brain regions support them. We will highlight especially the functional roles of the AC, the amygdala, and the inferior frontal cortex (IFC). These regions represent the core of the large-scale network (Figure 19.2).

---

to impaired processing of affective prosody in the auditory cortex, especially in the voice-sensitive superior temporal gyrus (blue outline). While patients with right amygdala lesions show normal patterns of AC activity and activity of their healthy left amygdala, no such patterns were observed with left medial temporal lobe (MTL) patients.

Abbreviations: a/m/pSTG: anterior/mid/posterior superior temporal gyrus; amy: amygdala; an: anger attended trials; na: anger unattended trials; nn: neutral trials.

In terms of an acoustic decoding of affective voices, the AC has obviously received a lot of attention in neuroimaging studies (Figure 19.1A,B). The primate auditory cortex is located in the superior part of the temporal cortex, with large parts of its primary and secondary fields hidden inside the lateral sulcus, whereas higher-level auditory association cortex is located in the lateral surface (Hackett, 2011). Almost all neuroimaging studies about affective voice processing show large activations in the AC (Frühholz & Grandjean, 2013b; Grandjean et al., 2005). These activations are predominantly located within the lateral AC that is generally sensitive to conspecific voices (Belin & Zatorre, 2000) and has been supposed to be a specific area for affective voice processing (Ethofer et al., 2012). Besides neuroimaging studies that show enhanced activity in the AC in response to affective voices, studies using transcranial magnetic stimulation (TMS) showed that temporarily inhibiting the AC impairs behavioural classification of these voices, especially for vocal expressions of fear and sadness (Hoekert et al., 2008).

Given that these functional activations usually extend over low-level (primary and secondary AC) and higher-level auditory regions (auditory associations areas), the functional meaning of the auditory cortical activation has been interpreted in two ways. First, specific activity in low-level auditory regions might be involved in an acoustic decoding of relevant cues and features in affective voices that support their classification. This acoustic decoding might be especially relevant for affective relative to neutral voices, since the former includes several static and dynamic acoustic modulations of voice features that are used by listeners to infer the affective state of the speaker (Banse & Scherer, 1996).

Second, given that affective voices activate the same regions as neutral voices, but usually to a higher degree, this increased activation also points to some kind of vocal affective-meaning processing in the AC beyond a simple acoustic analysis. Again, this increased activation for affective voices could be interpreted two ways, either as generic affective processing in the AC (Frühholz et al., 2014) or enhanced decoding of emotionally relevant acoustic cues of these voices, and this enhancement is remotely driven by activity in other brain areas, such as the limbic system (Frühholz, Hofstetter, et al., 2015). The latter hypothesis mainly receives confirmation by studies of patients with lesions especially to the limbic system (Frühholz, Hofstetter, et al., 2015; Vuilleumier et al., 2004) (Figure 19.1B), while the former hypothesis might be especially indicated by studies that show increased auditory cortical activation to affective voices that is unaccompanied by activity in the limbic system, especially in the amygdala (e.g. Alba-Ferrara et al., 2011; Beaucousin et al., 2011; Ethofer, Anders, Erb, et al., 2006; Kotz et al., 2013; Mitchell, 2007; Warren et al., 2006; Wiethoff et al., 2008).

This discussion about what drives the enhanced activity in the AC in response to affective voices points to the second meaningful brain system that has been extensively discussed for processing emotional stimuli in general and of affective voices specifically. The limbic brain regions have been associated with emotional processing for several decades, and many neuroimaging studies point to activity especially in the amygdala in response to affective voices (Fecteau et al., 2007; Frühholz et al., 2014; Wiethoff et al., 2009). The amygdala is an almond-shaped grey-matter structure located in the anterior part of the medial temporal cortex (Zald, 2003), and it is composed of several subnuclei (Amunts et al., 2005). As it has been suggested for the processing of emotional stimuli in general, the amygdala seems also sensitive to the affective meaning conveyed by voices. However, the amygdala does not always show enhanced activity to the affective meaning of voices in neuroimaging studies, and

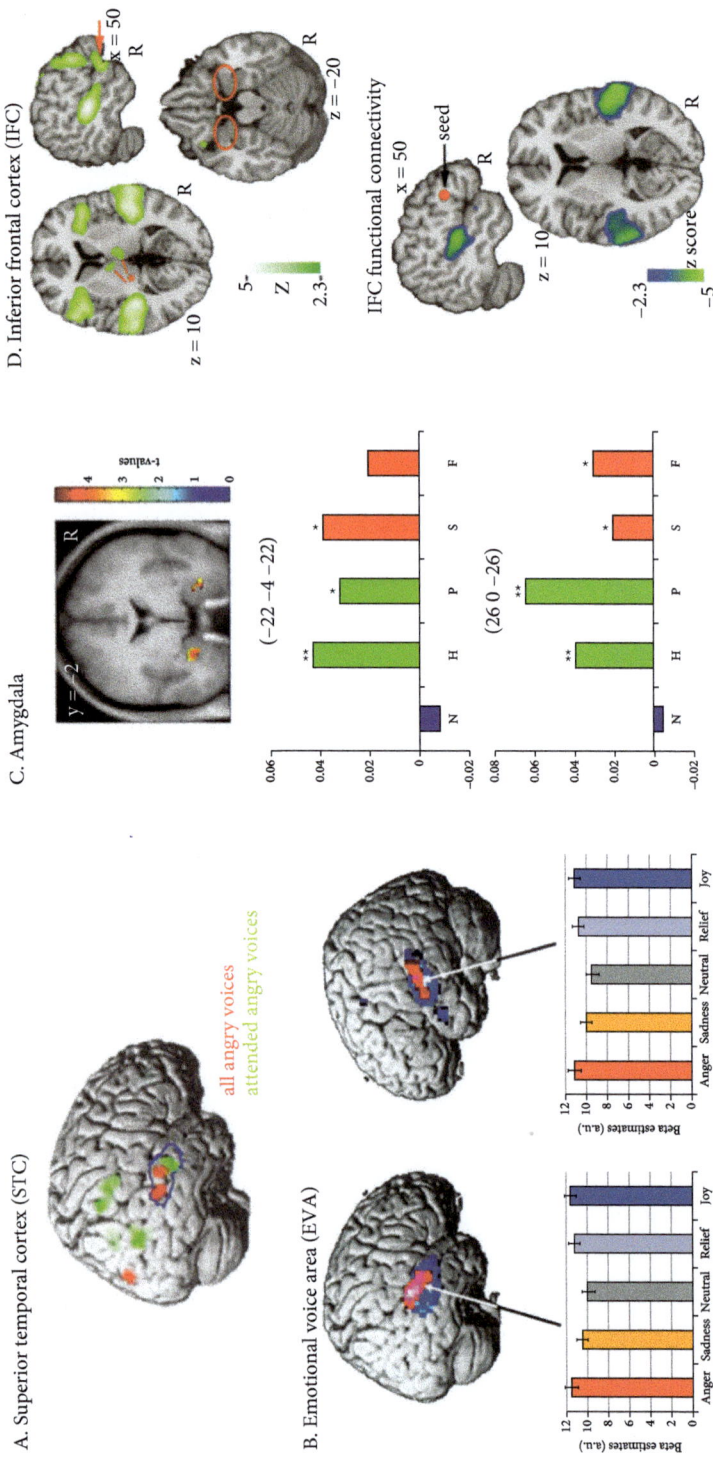

FIGURE 19.2 The neural large-scale network for decoding the affective meaning from voices. (A) Affective voices and especially angry voices elicit enhanced activity in the superior temporal cortex (STC) as part of the voice-sensitive auditory cortex (blue outline). Different peak locations of activity can be observed when listening to all angry voices (red), or when listening to angry voices that are in the spatial focus of attention (green) in conditions when different voices are presented to both ears. (B) Given the high consistency of AC activity in response to affective voices, a uniform bilateral 'emotional voice area' (EVA) has been recently proposed, that responds to all kinds of emotions conveyed by voices (H: happy; P: sexual pleasure; S: sad; F: fear) compared to neutral voices (N). (C) Like the AC, the bilateral amygdala also responds to different emotions

conveyed by voices. **(D)** Consistent activity for affective voices is also found in bilateral inferior frontal cortex (IFC; upper panel), and right IFC activity is functionally linked to activity in bilateral AC during processing of voices that are less clear in their acoustic cues that are relevant for an affect classification of these voices (lower panel).

some studies, including those of patients with lesions in the amygdala, have not reported any kind of impairments in processing the affective meaning of voices (e.g. Adolphs & Tranel, 1999; Bach et al., 2013). Thus, the literature on the role of the amygdala in processing affective voices seems largely inconsistent. Until now it is unclear what causes this high variability in amygdala responses to affective voices. It could be that certain stimulus- and context-specific conditions influence if and how the amygdala responds to affective voices (see following text).

So far we have outlined the functional roles of the AC and the amygdala, which both might contribute to the two main functions mentioned before—acoustic analysis and affective analysis of voice. However, the brain network underlying affective voice processing still seems to involve more brain regions that might contribute additional functions to the processing. For example, the inferior frontal cortex (IFC) (Figure 19.2D) shows some consistent activity in response to affective voices (Frühholz & Grandjean, 2013c). The IFC covers large parts of the lateral inferior frontal lobe (i.e. inferior frontal gyrus and inferior frontal sulcus), but it also extends into the lateral sulcus covering parts of the frontal operculum and the orbitofrontal cortex (Frühholz & Grandjean, 2013c; Petrides, 2005). The IFC is a brain region usually not restricted to affective processing, but it has been supposed to be generally involved in many types of social processing (Norris & Cacioppo, 2007).

The consistency of IFC activity in response to affective voices was mostly found when participants were asked to provide judgements on these voices in terms of different tasks. This led to the suggestion that the IFC is involved in a cognitive evaluation of affective voices to support an accurate judgement on these voices (Schirmer & Kotz, 2006). This judgement function is beyond the functions of an acoustic and affective analysis of voices, and it seems especially relevant when the processing of affective voices becomes more challenging, either when relevant voice features are less acoustically clear (Leitman et al., 2010) or when confronted with additional competing voice information, such as in the linguistic dimension of vocalizations (Schirmer et al., 2004). Thus, the IFC might accompany activity in the AC and/or the amygdala under conditions that require increased cognitive evaluation of voices for a proper affective classification. Enhanced IFC activity and connectivity was also found in conditions where participants were asked to reappraise the affective meaning of voices, either by enhancing or suppressing the emotional contagion to these voices (Korb et al., 2015). IFC activity and its connectivity underlying the cognitive evaluation can also be changed by training affect voice classification (Rota et al., 2011). Furthermore, temporarily inhibiting the function of the IFC, using TMS, can also lead to impaired behavioural responses to these voices (Hoekert et al., 2008, 2010; van Rijn et al., 2005).

The latter studies point to the important fact that the regions mentioned so far, that is, the AC, the amygdala, and the IFC, do not function in isolation but, rather, show functional connectivity to accomplish the task of classifying voices according to their affective meaning. Several studies found a functional connectivity between the AC and the IFC (Ethofer et al., 2012; Frühholz & Grandjean, 2012; Leitman et al., 2010), which is based on a structural connectivity (i.e. neural fibre bundles belonging to brain white matter) between these regions (Ethofer et al., 2012; Frühholz, Gschwind, et al., 2015). Similarly, the amygdala seems also functionally connected to the IFC (Frühholz et al., 2015b). The IFC thus seems to integrate both acoustic information primarily provided by the AC and affective information provided both by the amygdala and the AC that support a proper cognitive evaluation and classification by the IFC. This afferent functional connectivity to the IFC has been summarized also in recent neural network models of affective voice processing (Schirmer & Kotz, 2006; Wildgruber et al., 2009).

The previous paragraphs described the core of the large-scale neural network underlying affective voice processing. This network indicates distributed functional processes that need to be accomplished for decoding the affective meaning from voices.

19.3.2 Recent Evidence for Local Neural Subnetworks

Besides these major functional processes represented by the large-scale network, each of these functions seems to also imply several subfunctions. For example, the acoustic analysis of affective voices requires not only the decoding of single acoustic features and cues, such as the mean of the vocal pitch or the vocal intensity (i.e. loudness). To make meaning out of these features, they have to be integrated into an auditory percept of the voice as a whole; that is, single features are only meaningful when perceived as belonging to the voice as an auditory object (i.e. the mean of pitch is part of several meaningful voice features). Furthermore, important subfunctions of emotional processing are the detection of the beginning and the end of an emotional event. Accordingly, recent studies also point to local neural networks within the major regions of the large-scale network that might support these proposed important subfunctions (Figure 19.3).

Concerning the acoustic analysis of voices in the AC, it has been proposed that the AC supports both the decoding of emotionally relevant voice features and cues as well as the integration of these voice features into an auditory percept. A recent study identified several subareas in the voice-sensitive AC, especially in the right AC (Figure 19.3B). These subregions were sensitive to central voice features, such as the mean and the variation of the pitch and the intensity, while other subregions of the AC were insensitive to these features (Frühholz et al., 2012). Feature-sensitive areas were located in the posterior superior temporal cortex (STC), while more mid to anterior STC showed feature insensitivity indicative of an auditory representation of voices that is already beyond single-voice features. This points to a posterior-to-anterior gradient for the proposed subfunctions such that posterior AC regions decode important voice features that are integrated in the anterior AC (Frühholz et al., 2016).

This indicates that neural responses in the AC to affective voices are not uniform and point to a diversity of processing-related neural subfields in the AC. Similarly, the amygdala is not a uniform brain region. The amygdala is actually composed of several subnuclei (Amunts et al., 2005). On the most general level, the amygdala can be divided in three major subregions that are termed laterobasal (LB) complex, centromedian complex (CM), and superficial (SF) complex. These subnuclei support different affective functions, such as the affective evaluation of sensory stimuli mainly accomplished by the laterobasal complex, but also the shaping of emotional output behaviour mainly accomplished by the centromedian complex (LeDoux, 2012). A recent study used high spatial resolution scanning of the amygdala and found several clusters of activations in the LB and SF complex of the amygdala in response to affective voices (Frühholz & Grandjean, 2013a) (Figure 19.3C).

This multitude of functional clusters of activations in the amygdala also showed differential responses according to different time windows of an emotional event. In general,

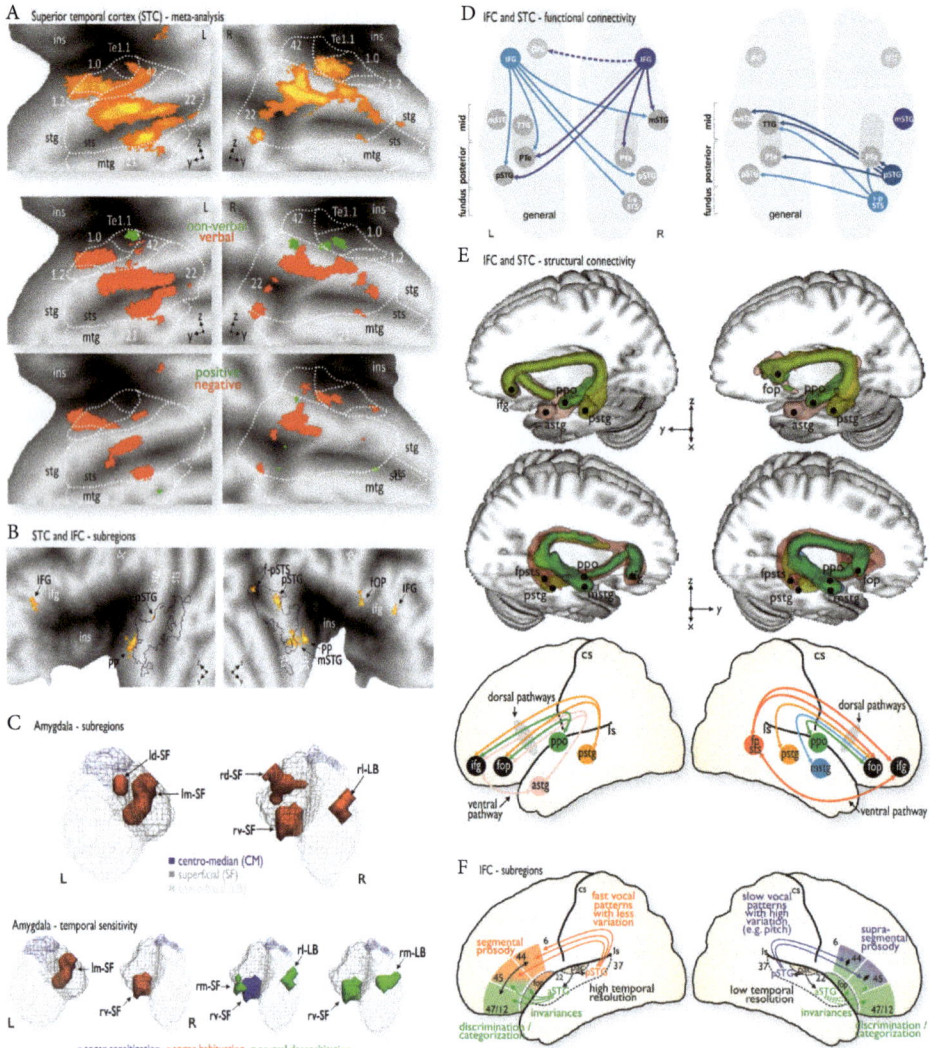

FIGURE 19.3 The local neural network as well as the inter-regional functional and structural network for decoding affective meaning from voices. (A) A recent meta-analysis of functional activity reported across several recent neuroimaging studies revealed widespread and distributed auditory cortical activity in response to affective voices (upper panel). Activity was located in primary (Te1.0, Te1.1, and Te1.2), secondary (BA 42), and higher-level (BA 21–22) auditory cortex. Different patterns of activity emerged for the comparison of verbal and non-verbal vocal expressions (middle panel), and for positive and negative affective voices (lower panel). (B) More specifically, a recent fMRI study with spatial high-resolution scanning of the auditory cortex and the inferior frontal cortex, revealed local patterns of activity in response to affective voices. The right AC and IFC in particular showed activity in four and two local subregions, respectively. (C) Like the AC and the IFC, the amygdala also shows local patterns of activity in response to affective voices in two of its major subregions (upper panel), that is, the superficial complex (SF) and the latero-basal complex (LB). These amygdala subregions were differentially sensitive to the temporal order of affective

an emotional event or an emotional period is represented by the onset of the emotional event, by its duration, and by the end of the emotional event. Each of these event parts has its functional significance to provide adaptive responses in terms of engaging and releasing neural and cognitive processing resources. The previously mentioned study (Frühholz & Grandjean, 2013a) accordingly found that the right SF complex signals the onset of an emotional event, while the right SF and right LB complex signal the end of an emotional event. The bilateral SF complex also signifies the duration and the ongoing state of an emotional event by responding with signal habituation to a continuous stimulation with affective voices. Thus instead of a uniform response of the whole amygdala to an emotional event, the subregions of the amygdala respond differentially to the different time parts of an emotional event, pointing to a local distribution of several functions in the amygdala.

So far we have described the local subnetwork for the AC and the amygdala, but there is also reason to believe that the IFC is not a uniform brain region in terms of its functional responses to affective voices (Frühholz & Grandjean, 2013c) (Figure 19.3B). Recent studies

---

voices (lower panel), showing either sensitivity to the first appearance of affective voices (i.e. sensitization), to the repetition of affective voices (i.e. habituation), or to the offset of affective voices (i.e. desensitization). (D) Besides the diversity of local neural network activity in the AC and the IFC, both regions also show strong functional inter-connectivity, with connections from and to low- and high-level AC regions. (E) The functional AC–IFC connectivity is based on multiple structural connections between both regions as determined by probabilistic fibre tracking. This fibre tracking highlights a predominance of dorsal fibre pathways between both functional areas. (F) Given the multitude of functional and structural connections between the AC and the IFC, it was recently also hypothesized that there exist different functional subregions in the left and right IFC, which support the decoding of temporal sound features of voices at different temporal levels (i.e. dorsal pathways), and the classification of these affective voices (i.e. ventral pathway). Numbers correspond to Brodmann areas.

Abbreviations: a/m/pSTG: anterior/mid/posterior superior temporal gyrus; cs: central sulcus; fOP: frontal operculum; (f-p)STS: (posterior fundus) superior temporal sulcus; IFG: inferior frontal gyrus; Ins: insula; ld-/lm-/rd-/rv-SF left-dorsal/left-mid/right-dorsal/right ventral superficial complex of the amygdala; ls: lateral sulcus; MTG: middle temporal gyrus; OFC: orbitofrontal cortex; PP/PPo: planum polare; rl-/rm-LB: right-lateral/right-mid latero-basal complex of the amygdala.

reported activity that broadly extends over the IFC (Beaucousin et al., 2007; Leitman et al., 2010; Szameitat et al., 2010; Wildgruber et al., 2004), or is located either in the posterior (Beaucousin et al., 2007; Ethofer, Anders, Erb, et al., 2006; Wildgruber et al., 2005) or anterior IFC (Beaucousin et al., 2011; George et al., 1996). This distribution of peak activations again suggests a local subnetwork in the IFC that supports different subfunctions. A recent meta-analysis (Frühholz & Grandjean, 2013c) on functional activations reported in the IFC indicated that this posterior-to-anterior distribution in the IFC might follow different demands that are imposed by different tasks during the classification of affective voices (Figure 19.3F). More simple tasks, such as simply determining the presence or absence of a specific vocal emotion (e.g. an angry voice or not), should activate the anterior IFC, while more complex tasks, such as deciding between many different classification options (e.g. between an angry, a happy, or a fearful voice), should more involve the posterior IFC.

This posterior-to-anterior distinction also follows the cerebral pathways that connect the different subregions of the IFC with the AC (Figure 19.3D–F). The AC–IFC connections could either take ventral or dorsal fibre pathways, termed 'ventral stream' and 'dorsal stream' respectively (Rauschecker, 2012). These different streams are supposed to provide different types of auditory object information to the IFC. While the ventral stream mainly provides sound-identity information, the dorsal stream seems to provide information about the dynamic variability of sounds. Processing affective meaning from sounds shows a predominance of the dorsal streams, indicating that feedforwarding dynamic voice-feature information to the IFC is relevant for their correct classification (i.e. complex categorization) among several choice options (Frühholz et al., 2015a). Ventral stream information mainly targets the anterior IFC that supports more simple decisions about detecting specific affective voices (i.e. simple discrimination) (Frühholz & Grandjean, 2013c).

Taken together, these data point to a large-scale network consisting of the AC, the amygdala, and the IFC. Each of these regions seems to host a local subnetwork of at least two subregions that are associated with different subfunctions during the processing of affective voices. Both the AC and the IFC show a posterior-to-anterior gradient and this gradient reflects aforementioned subfunctions, consisting of sensory decoding and sensory integration as well as affect categorization and discrimination, respectively. Furthermore, different subregions of the amygdala are associated with the subfunctions of signifying the beginning, the duration, and the end of an emotional event.

19.3.3 So-Far Neglected Regions

Previously we described the large-scale neural network and its local subnetworks for the processing of affective voices. This network consists of the AC, the amygdala, and the IFC. However, the neural processing of affective voices is not restricted to these brain areas which, however, have so far showed the most consistent activity. Besides this core network, recent studies also reported activity in other brain regions, which have been proposed to play additional important roles during the processing of affective voices. Different regions have different functional roles which are not exclusive and show some overlap between regions. These additional brain regions are the hippocampus, the medial frontal cortex (MFC), and the basal ganglia (BG).

The BG is a neural complex of deep brain grey-matter nuclei composed of the BG proper and also of the subthalamic nucleus (STN) (Peron et al., 2013) (Figure 19.4A,B). The STN is sensitive to affective voices and shows functional and structural connectivity to the amygdala, the AC, and the BG proper (Peron et al., 2013, 2016). Accordingly, studies also report activity in the BG especially for affective prosody processing (Bach et al., 2008; Beaucousin et al., 2011; Frühholz et al., 2012; Leitman et al., 2010). Given that the BG are assumed to provide temporal decoding and temporal prediction (Kotz et al., 2009), their role in affective voice processing might be related to tracking the temporal evolvement of affective vocalizations.

This temporal evolvement of several features, such as the pitch envelope, the glottal waveform, speech rate, and pause proportions, is commonly a strong cue to the affective meaning of voices (Juslin & Laukka, 2003). The decoding of this temporal evolvement of vocalization might be the underlying deficit of the impairments of BG-lesion patients for the decoding of the affective meaning of voices (e.g. Calder et al., 2004; Dara et al., 2008; Paulmann et al., 2009; Pell & Leonard, 2003). This concerns tempo and speed cues in vocalizations (Breitenstein et al., 2001) as well as more subtle affective vocalizations (Buxton et al., 2013) that probably require an enhanced decoding of temporal information.

Unlike the temporal decoding in the BG, the MFC supports more higher-level social and emotional functions related to interpersonal communication and understanding (Amodio & Frith, 2006). Activity in the MFC has been found in a recent study about the neural mechanisms of perceiving human laughter (Szameitat et al., 2010) (Figure 19.4C). The authors found increased MFC activity when comparing emotional laughter relative to tickling laughter. Emotional laughter is a socially and acoustically more complex type of laughter that might be specific to human primates. Given this complexity of emotional laughter, activity in the MFC might reflect the more demanding decoding mechanisms for this type of laughter that also receives enhanced decoding on the AC (Szameitat et al., 2010).

Thus, the functional role of the MFC might be similar to that of the IFC as described before. However, there might be functional differences in terms of the complexity of the cognitive evaluation of voices. The IFC is usually only involved in explicit voice evaluations and what we will call 'first-order' evaluations. These first-order evaluations concern evaluations of the stimulus itself. The MFC seems more involved in 'second-order' evaluations that concern the inference from the stimulus to the mind of the other person. Accordingly, many studies investigating the neural decoding of affective prosody as a socially more complex type of affective expression found activity in the MFC (Alba-Ferrara et al., 2011; Bach et al., 2008; Frühholz et al., 2012; Kotz et al., 2013; Leitman et al., 2010).

A final brain region that has received only limited attention in neuroimaging studies on affective voice processing is the hippocampus. Many studies focused on the functional role of the amygdala during the processing of affective voices, given the general importance of the limbic system in emotional processing. However, the amygdala is in close neighbourhood and close connectivity with the hippocampus (Frühholz et al., 2014), and some emotional processes seem to necessarily imply co-activation of the hippocampus, especially during emotional learning (Buchel et al., 1999). The hippocampus shows considerable activity in response to these voices (e.g. Beaucousin et al., 2007; Leitman et al., 2010; Szameitat et al., 2010; Wiethoff et al., 2008) (Figure 19.4D,E). The specific functional role of the hippocampus might be to retrieve emotional and memory associations possibly related to the

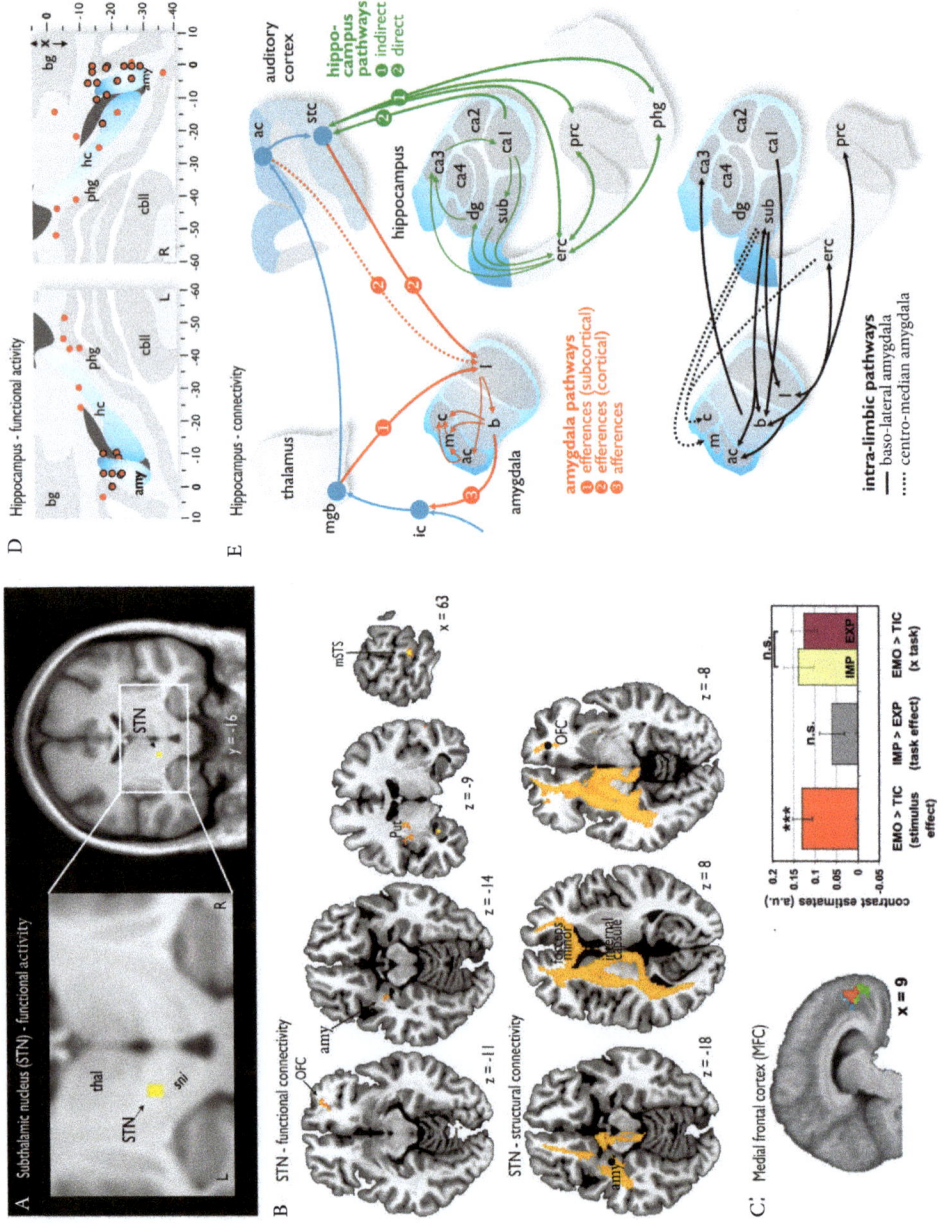

FIGURE 19.4 Other brain systems for processing affective voices. (A) The subthalamic nucleus (STN) is part of the basal ganglia brain system, and is responsive to affective voices. (B) The STN also shows functional connections to the OFC, the amygdala, the BG, and the AC during

affective voice processing (upper panel), and these functional connections are also based on structural brain connections to the amygdala and the OFC (lower panel). (C) The medial frontal cortex is involved in processing complex emotion in voices, such as in emotional compared with tickling laughter. (D) As indicated by a recent meta-analysis, the hippocampus shows activity to affective voices next to activity in the amygdala. (E) This hippocampus (and amygdala) activity might be elicited by a close connection of both brain system to the auditory brain system at different levels and by a close inter-connection between the hippocampus and the amygdala.

expression of a certain vocal emotion or type of expression linked to specific previous episodic life events (Frühholz et al., 2014). Furthermore, more ambiguous vocal expression of voices might be enriched by memory information that supports their proper classification (Leitman et al., 2010).

Let us quickly summarize what we have learned so far about the neural processing of affective voices. First, early neuroimaging studies identified a large-scale neural network (AC, amygdala, and IFC) that responds to affective voices. Second, this core network hosts local subnetworks with specific subfunctions. Third, there is an extended network of brain regions that only came into focus recently (BG, hippocampus, MFC), but this network adds important function during affective voice processing. This complex neural network hosts a diversity of global functions (acoustic analysis, affective analysis, cognitive evaluation, social perception, memory associations, temporal prediction) and subfunctions (feature decoding/feature integration, emotional timing, categorizations/discrimination), that partly overlap across brain regions.

19.4 STIMULUS AND TASK FACTORS THAT INFLUENCE THE NEURAL PROCESSING OF AFFECTIVE VOICES

The neural activity described so far is reported across recent neuroimaging studies with some consistency, but there is also some variability with regard to if and how these regions show activity in response to affective voices. This variability could be due to stimulus- and context-specific conditions. Stimulus-specific conditions concern the acoustic distinctiveness, medium, valence/arousal, and social complexity of affective voices. On the other hand, context-specific conditions are related to personality factors and to how much attention is paid to processing of these voices. These factors and their influence on the neural processing of affective voices will be briefly discussed in the next paragraphs.

19.4.1 Arousal, Valence, and Social Complexity of Affective Voices

Affect in voices can be expressed with different levels of intensity, which strongly depend on the bodily arousal that underlies these vocalizations. Bodily arousal depends on the intensity of the emotional event or situation and on individual predisposition in responding to such events. Bodily arousal influences the different vocal tract parameters, such as the subglottal air pressure, that determine the acoustic quality of the produced affective voices. For example, vocal happiness can be expressed in different levels of intensity, resulting perhaps in mild expressions and vocalizations of happiness, or strong expressions of happiness and vocalizations of joyful elation (Banse & Scherer, 1996).

To date, only a few studies have investigated the perception of the vocal arousal level (Ethofer, Anders, Wiethoff, et al., 2006; Warren et al., 2006; Wiethoff et al., 2008). The intensity of affective voices correlated with activity in premotor areas (Warren et al., 2006) or in bilateral AC (Ethofer, Anders, Wiethoff, et al., 2006; Wiethoff et al., 2008). Especially the latter result indicates that the AC not only is involved in an acoustic and affective analysis of voices, but more specifically it also decodes the level of intensity of affect expressed in voices. The arousal-sensitive region was located in the posterior AC that also shows sensitivity to central voice features. Vocal arousal is encoded in specific voice features, and the brain decodes the intensity of affective voices from certain voice features, such as the level of vocal pitch or the level of vocal intensity (Wiethoff et al., 2008).

Besides the arousal level or intensity of affective voices, another important question concerns the specificity of brain activations for vocal expressions of a certain valence. More specifically, the question is if specific emotions can be consistently localized in certain brain areas. This is a highly debated topic in the affective neurosciences in general, with researchers providing evidence for brain specificity (Murphy et al., 2003; Phan et al., 2002) or against it (Lindquist et al., 2012). While studies including patients with lesions in certain brain areas indicate the amygdala might be specifically sensitive to vocal fear and anger (Scott et al., 1997; Sprengelmeyer et al., 1999), the BG/insula for vocal disgust (Calder et al., 2000; Sprengelmeyer et al., 1996), and the ventromedial MFC to vocal sadness and anger (Hornak et al., 2003), neuroimaging studies including healthy participants are few (Phillips et al., 1998). They report activity in the AC for disgust and in the AC, the hippocampus, and the amygdala for fear (Phillips et al., 1998). The latter results might support the notion of the amygdala as a 'fear module' (Ohman & Mineka, 2001). However, other neuroimaging studies also report amygdala activity in response to vocal anger (Ethofer et al., 2009; Frühholz & Grandjean, 2013a; Grandjean et al., 2005; Mothes-Lasch et al., 2011; Schirmer et al., 2008) and vocal sadness (Sander & Scheich, 2005). This example regarding amygdala activity should demonstrate that there is no simple mapping between certain emotions and localized processing in certain brain areas. Rather, there would be a neural network of distributed brain regions involved in processing the affective meaning from voices. This is highlighted in this chapter by a multiregional and multifunctional theoretical approach.

Similar to the question of a regional specificity of certain emotions in the brain is the question of whether the brain neurally processes complex vocal expressions in a similar way as for simple vocal expressions of emotions. These more complex emotions include *pride, guiltiness, boredom* (Alba-Ferrara et al., 2011), *irony*, and *doubt* (Beaucousin et al., 2007). Complex vocal emotions elicit activity in the AC and the MFC indicative of enhanced acoustic analysis and social processing of these voices, but they also elicit activity in the hippocampus (Alba-Ferrara et al., 2011). The latter region has been recently implicated in encoding and decoding affective meaning from more complex sounds in general by specifically providing relevant memory and affective associations that might also be relevant for proper socioaffective recognition of voices (Frühholz et al., 2014).

19.4.2 The Medium of Vocalizations

Vocal expressions of emotions usually appear in two different forms, that is, either as nonverbal expressions or as vocal intonations superimposed on speech (i.e. affective prosody). This distinction refers to the medium of affective vocalizations. The major difference between these two media of affective vocalizations is that affective prosody includes a linguistic dimension besides the paralinguistic or non-verbal dimension. This difference might lead to a hemispheric difference in processing non-verbal expressions and affective prosody, given that the left hemisphere might respond more strongly to the linguistic dimension of vocalizations. This explanation might be also valid for the superimposed paralinguistic dimension for affective prosody.

Although the neural processing of affective prosody and non-verbal expression has not been compared directly yet, a recent meta-analysis of AC activity provides some evidence. This meta-analysis showed some differential lateralization at the level of the AC (Figure 19.3A). Non-verbal expressions were associated with activity in bilateral primary AC and right STC, while affective prosody consistently elicited activity in left low-level AC and bilateral STC (Frühholz & Grandjean, 2013b). While activity in low-level AC for both vocalizations might indicate in-depth acoustic analysis of relevant acoustic cues to the affective meaning of voices, the right-hemispheric STC activity for non-verbal expression points to the right-hemisphere predominance for non-speech voice cues (Zatorre et al., 2002), while bilateral STC activity for affective prosody might point to a processing of relevant speech and non-speech cues in voices to infer their emotional meaning.

Besides the auditory cortex, the amygdala might also be involved in processing affective voices from either affective prosody or from non-verbal expressions. A patient with lesions in the amygdala showed problems in identifying sadness, fear, and anger in affective prosody, and in identifying fear and anger in non-verbal expressions (Scott et al., 1997). This suggests that the neural processing of affective voices in the amygdala is mostly impaired for vocal fear and anger, independent of whether expressed in speech or non-speech.

19.4.3 Attentional Levels of Processing Imposed by Different Tasks

So far we have discussed how stimulus-specific conditions could influence the neural processing of affective voices. There are also context-specific conditions, such as different levels of processing affective voices that influence how we process the affective meaning in voices. This level of processing mainly refers to different attentional attitudes towards the affective meaning of voices.

In general, we can distinguish two different task conditions—either participants could be asked to explicitly focus on the emotional meaning conveyed by the tone of voices, or they could be asked to focus on another non-emotional attribute of voices. For the former, participants are usually asked to provide explicit judgements about the affective tone of a voice, while in the latter case participants are, for example, asked to discriminate the gender of the voice's speaker. The latter case is often termed 'implicit' processing of the affective meaning of a voice. Although participants focus on another non-emotional feature of voices, the affective meaning should still be processed on an implicit level given its relevance for the listener.

The IFC, MFC, BG, and AC have been found to be consistently involved in explicit evaluation of voices (Bach et al., 2008; Ethofer et al., 2009; Szameitat et al., 2010). Contrarily, activity in the amygdala has been predominantly found during implicit processing (Bach et al., 2008; Ethofer et al., 2009), pointing to their functional role of detecting relevant emotional information, when presented outside the focus of attention (Vuilleumier, 2005). These results point to separate brain systems that either explicitly evaluate the affective meaning of voices or implicitly register the affective meaning.

The previously mentioned studies, however, only compared the global effects of different attentional conditions during voice processing, while largely neglecting the emotional dimension. Results of a recent study provide a slightly more complex picture about the neural system in the explicit and implicit processing of the affective meaning of voices (Frühholz et al., 2012). By directly comparing processing of the affective meaning (i.e. emotional versus neutral voices) for explicit and implicit tasks, posterior AC and left IFC activity was not influenced by the attentional conditions, the amygdala and the anterior AC were more active during the explicit processing, and the right IFC showed activity during implicit processing, (Frühholz et al., 2012). Additionally, the low-level AC seems to be more consistently active during implicit processing of the affective meaning of voices (Frühholz & Grandjean, 2013b). This increased activity in the low-level AC and the right IFC points to increased acoustical decoding and cognitive evaluation of voices during the more challenging task of processing the affective meaning of voices when presented outside the focus of attention. This is also indicated by an increased IFC–AC coupling during the more challenging implicit-processing task (Frühholz & Grandjean, 2012), similar to the previously mentioned increased IFC–AC coupling during the more challenging processing of affective voices with degraded acoustic cues (Leitman et al., 2010).

19.5 BENEFITS OF PRIORITIZED PROCESSING OF AFFECTIVE VOICES

Because cues related to the affective tone of the voice are biologically relevant for humans, they seem to be prioritized during processing, especially when they impose a potential threat to the listener, or when they are positively valenced. This prioritization of affective voices might not only be beneficial for their own processing but might also facilitate other cognitive functions, such as (spatial) attentional orientating or the remembering of important environmental events.

Concerning the former, the posterior parietal cortex (PPC) has been involved in the voluntary control of spatial and non-spatial attention in the auditory domain (Shomstein & Yantis, 2006). The PPC is also involved in auditory spatial localization and is directly involved in auditory attention (At et al., 2011; Lewald & Guski, 2004) together with the STC (Lewald et al., 2004). Interestingly, the middle part of the STC (Frühholz et al., 2011; Grandjean et al., 2005) and the amygdala (Sander et al., 2005) were shown to respond to angry compared with neutral vocal stimuli when attention was not directed to the affective meaning of the voice. In the case of voluntary attention to the affective meaning of a voice, a modulation of the OFC was observed (Sander et al., 2005). Emotional voices were also shown to facilitate the detection of a visual target when presented at the same spatial position (Brosch et al., 2008).

The latter results were replicated in a unimodal auditory paradigm involving an auditory target preceded by angry voices, showing a crucial implication of the AC and the amygdala in an attentional modulation by emotional voices (Ceravolo et al., 2016a) and of the AC in the implicit processing of affective voices in space (Ceravolo et al., 2016b) (Figure 19.5A,B). Affective voice processing hence allows for an attentional advantage over neutral vocal content that some authors have named 'emotional attention' (Vuilleumier, 2005), such mechanisms being supported by the amygdala, AC, and parietal brain regions.

Affective voices might also influence memory functions. This interactive process between emotion and memory has been termed 'emotional memory' (LaBar & Cabeza, 2006). Research on the influence of affective voices on memory has highlighted a change in representations of 'to-be-retrieved' words spoken in an affective tone, showing an indirect impact of affective voices on memory (Schirmer, 2010). Emotional vocal stimuli were also shown to impact on memory when played as distractors during a memory span task, leading to improved incidental verbal memory of the (outside the focus of attention) sentence for the heavy memory load condition (Kitayama, 1996). This result was significant most notably for

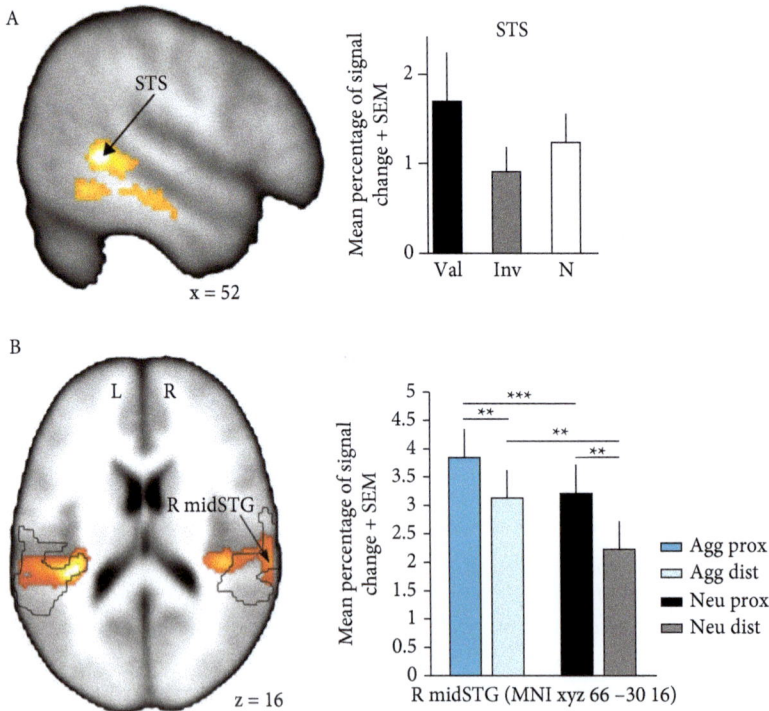

FIGURE 19.5 The benefits of a prioritized processing of affect in voices. (A) Auditory spatial attention is modulated by angry voices cueing in an exogenous attention task with underlying activity in the mid STG. (B) Perceiving the spatial distance of auditory threat relies on the right mid STG, which is more strongly activated for aggressive than neutral voices.

negative voices and it provides evidence for divided attentional mechanisms taking place when survival-related, relevant affective voices are present even when not in the focus of attention and task-irrelevant (Kitayama, 1996).

Using auditory priming (Schacter & Church, 1992), other studies have emphasized an impact of voice intonation and fundamental frequency changes between encoding and testing on subsequent implicit memory for voices (Church & Schacter, 1994). This result further emphasizes the automatic attentional capture of affective/intonation-related voices that leads to an impact on memory systems. Rämä and colleagues (2001) identified brain regions underlying such memory mechanisms. The most consistently activated area they found was in the IFC, in addition to parietal and temporal brain regions (Rämä et al., 2001).

Finally, the prioritized processing of affective emotions in voices can be evaluated in order to reduce its impact on subjective emotional feeling, for instance, and such a field relates to emotional regulation. As a top–down mechanism able to influence our emerging feelings when exposed during an emotional situation, reappraisal of the event to reduce/increase one's emotion has been studied in the literature, and such a mechanism seems to depend on the frontal cortex when reappraising to increase emotional response to angry prosody (Korb et al., 2015). On the other hand, activity in the medial frontal and PPC was shown to underlie reappraisal mechanisms when decreasing the emotional response to angry prosody (Korb et al., 2015; Ochsner et al., 2004). Taken together, these data highlight an automatic, prioritized processing of affective voices being down- or up-regulated by a top–down cognitive process of emotional regulation through reappraisal of affective events.

19.6 Conclusions

In this chapter we have outlined the large-scale network and several local neural networks for processing affective voices. The processing of affective voices is not accomplished in single brain regions, nor does it involve some simple acoustic and emotional decoding that is restricted to the AC and the amygdala, respectively. Rather, the neural processing of affective voices depends on a widespread neural network across many brain regions that provide different but also partly overlapping functional contributions to the understanding of affective voices. These functions are not only distributed across the large-scale network but also across recently discovered local subnetworks in the AC, the amygdala, and the IFC. In humans, the neural processing of affective voices thus involves a distributed neural network. Evidence for this neural processing of affective voices also comes from recent research in non-human primates (see Part III, this volume) and from human studies including psychiatric patients (see Part VII, this volume).

Acknowledgements

We thank many of our colleagues and collaborators for many fruitful discussions and for our joint scientific achievements over the past years—Patrik Vuilleumier, Didier Grandjean, Markus Gschwind, Wiebke Trost, Andy Christen, Julie Peron, Wietske Van Der Zwaag, and Valerie Milesi. We also acknowledge the funding provided by the Swiss

National Science Foundation (SNSF PP00P1_157409), which supported and supports many of our research projects.

References

Adolphs, R. & Tranel, D. (1999). Intact recognition of emotional prosody following amygdala damage. *Neuropsychologia*, 37, 1285–1292.

Alba-Ferrara, L., Hausmann, M., Mitchell, R. L., & Weis, S. (2011). The neural correlates of emotional prosody comprehension: disentangling simple from complex emotion. *PLoS One*, 6, e28701.

Amodio, D. M. & Frith, C. D. (2006). Meeting of minds: the medial frontal cortex and social cognition. *Nature Reviews Neuroscience*, 7, 268–277.

Amunts, K., Kedo, O., Kindler, M., Pieperhoff, P., Mohlberg, H., Shah, N. J., ... Zilles, K. (2005). Cytoarchitectonic mapping of the human amygdala, hippocampal region and entorhinal cortex: intersubject variability and probability maps. *Anatomy and Embryology*, 210, 343–352.

Ariatti, A., Benuzzi, F., & Nichelli, P. (2008). Recognition of emotions from visual and prosodic cues in Parkinson's disease. *Neurological Sciences*, 29, 219–227.

At, A., Spierer, L. & Clarke, S. (2011). The role of the right parietal cortex in sound localization: a chronometric single pulse transcranial magnetic stimulation study. *NeuropsychologiaI*, 49, 2794–2797.

Bach, D. R., Grandjean, D., Sander, D., Herdener, M., Strik, W. K., & Seifritz, E. (2008). The effect of appraisal level on processing of emotional prosody in meaningless speech. *NeuroImage*, 42, 919–927.

Bach, D. R., Hurlemann, R., & Dolan, R. J. (2013). Unimpaired discrimination of fearful prosody after amygdala lesion. *Neuropsychologia*, 51, 2070–2074.

Banse, R. & Scherer, K. R. (1996). Acoustic profiles in vocal emotion expression. *Journal of Personality and Social Psychology*, 70, 614–636.

Beaucousin, V., Lacheret, A., Turbelin, M.-R., Morel, M., Mazoyer, B., & Tzourio-Mazoyer, N. (2007). FMRI study of emotional speech comprehension. *Cerebral Cortex*, 17, 339–352.

Beaucousin, V., Zago, L., Hervé, P.-Y., Strelnikov, K., Crivello, F., Mazoyer, B., & Tzourio-Mazoyer, N. (2011). Sex-dependent modulation of activity in the neural networks engaged during emotional speech comprehension. *Brain Research*, 1390, 108–117.

Belin, P. & Zatorre, R. J. (2000). Voice-selective areas in human auditory cortex. *Nature*, 403, 309.

Borod, J. C., Cicero, B. A., Obler, L. K., Welkowitz, J., Erhan, H. M., Santschi, C., ... Whalen, J. R. (1998). Right hemisphere emotional perception: evidence across multiple channels. *Neuropsychology*, 12, 446–458.

Breitenstein, C., Van Lancker, D., Daum, I., & Waters, C. H. (2001). Impaired perception of vocal emotions in Parkinson's disease: influence of speech time processing and executive functioning. *Brain and Cognition*, 45, 277–314.

Brierley, B., Medford, N., Shaw, P., & David, A. S. (2004). Emotional memory and perception in temporal lobectomy patients with amygdala damage. *Journal of Neurology, Neurosurgery and Psychiatry*, 75, 593–599.

Brosch, T., Grandjean, D., Sander, D., & Scherer, K. R. (2008). Behold the voice of wrath: cross-modal modulation of visual attention by anger prosody. *Cognition*, 106, 1497–1503.

Buchel, C., Dolan, R. J., Armony, J. L., & Friston, K. J. (1999). Amygdala-hippocampal involvement in human aversive trace conditioning revealed through event-related functional magnetic resonance imaging. *Journal of Neuroscience*, 19, 10869–10876.

Buxton, S. L., MacDonald, L., & Tippett, L. J. (2013). Impaired recognition of prosody and subtle emotional facial expressions in Parkinson's disease. *Behavioral Neuroscience*, 127, 193–203.

Calder, A. J., Keane, J., Lawrence, A. D., & Manes, F. (2004). Impaired recognition of anger following damage to the ventral striatum. *Brain*, 127, 1958–1969.

Calder, A. J., Keane, J., Manes, F., Antoun, N., & Young, A. W. (2000). Impaired recognition and experience of disgust following brain injury. *Nature Neuroscience*, 3, 1077–1078.

Ceravolo, L., Frühholz, S., & Grandjean, D. (2016a). Modulation of auditory spatial attention by angry prosody: an fMRI auditory dot-probe study. *Frontiers in Neuroscience*, 10, 216.

Ceravolo, L., Frühholz, S., & Grandjean, D. (2016b). Proximal vocal threat recruits the right voice- sensitive auditory cortex. *Social Cognitive and Affective Neuroscience*, 11, 793–802.

Church, B. A. & Schacter, D. L. (1994). Perceptual specificity of auditory priming: implicit memory for voice intonation and fundamental frequency. *Journal of Experimental Psychology: Learning, Memory, and Cognition*, 20, 521–533.

Dara, C., Monetta, L., & Pell, M. D. (2008). Vocal emotion processing in Parkinson's disease: reduced sensitivity to negative emotions. *Brain Research*, 1188, 100–111.

Davidson, R. J., Ekman, P., Saron, C. D., Senulis, J. A., & Friesen, W. V. (1990). Approach-withdrawal and cerebral asymmetry: emotional expression and brain physiology. I. *Journal of Personality and Social Psychology*, 58, 330–341.

Ethofer, T., Anders, S., Erb, M., Herbert, C., Wiethoff, S., Kissler, J., Grodd, W., & Wildgruber, D. (2006). Cerebral pathways in processing of affective prosody: a dynamic causal modeling study. *NeuroImage*, 30, 580–587.

Ethofer, T., Anders, S., Wiethoff, S., Erb, M., Herbert, C., Saur, R., Grodd, W., & Wildgruber, D. (2006). Effects of prosodic emotional intensity on activation of associative auditory cortex. *NeuroReport*, 17, 249–253.

Ethofer, T., Bretscher, J., Gschwind, M., Kreifelts, B., Wildgruber, D., & Vuilleumier, P. (2012). Emotional voice areas: anatomic location, functional properties, and structural connections revealed by combined fMRI/DTI. *Cerebral Cortex*, 22, 191–200.

Ethofer, T., Kreifelts, B., Wiethoff, S., Wolf, J., Grodd, W., Vuilleumier, P., & Wildgruber, D. (2009). Differential influences of emotion, task, and novelty on brain regions underlying the processing of speech melody. *Journal of Cognitive Neuroscience*, 21, 1255–1268.

Fecteau, S., Belin, P., Joanette, Y., & Armony, J. L. (2007). Amygdala responses to nonlinguistic emotional vocalizations. *NeuroImage*, 36, 480–487.

Frühholz, S., Ceravolo, L., & Grandjean, D. (2012). Specific brain networks during explicit and implicit decoding of emotional prosody. *Cerebral Cortex*, 22(5), 1107–1117.

Frühholz, S. & Grandjean, D. (2012). Towards a fronto-temporal neural network for the decoding of angry vocal expressions. *NeuroImage*, 62, 1658–1666.

Frühholz, S. & Grandjean, D. (2013a). Amygdala subregions differentially respond and rapidly adapt to threatening voices. *Cortex*, 49, 1394–1403.

Frühholz, S. & Grandjean, D. (2013b). Multiple subregions in superior temporal cortex are differentially sensitive to vocal expressions: a quantitative meta-analysis. *Neuroscience and Biobehavioral Reviews*, 37, 24–35.

Frühholz, S. & Grandjean, D. (2013c). Processing of emotional vocalizations in bilateral inferior frontal cortex. *Neuroscience and Biobehavioral Reviews*, 37, 2847–2855.

Frühholz, S., Gschwind, M., & Grandjean, D. (2015). Bilateral dorsal and ventral fiber pathways for the processing of affective prosody identified by probabilistic fiber tracking. *NeuroImage*, 109, 27–34.

Frühholz, S., Hofstetter, C., Cristinzio, C., Saj, A., Seeck, M., Vuilleumier, P., & Grandjean, D. (2015). Asymmetrical effects of unilateral right or left amygdala damage on auditory cortical processing of vocal emotions. *Proceedings of the National Academy of Sciences of the United States of America*, 112, 1583–1588.

Frühholz, S., Trost, W., & Grandjean, D. (2014). The role of the medial temporal limbic system in processing emotions in voice and music. *Progress in Neurobiology*, 123, 1–17.

Frühholz, S., van der Zwaag, W., Seanz, M., Belin, P., Schobert, A.-K., Vuilleumier, P., & Grandjean, G. (2016). Neural decoding of discriminative auditory object features depends on their socio-affective value. *Social Cognitive and Affective Neuroscience*, 11(10), 1638–1649.

George, M. S., Parekh, P. I., Rosinsky, N., Ketter, T. A., Kimbrell, T. A., Heilman, K. M., Herscovitch, P., & Post, R. M. (1996). Understanding emotional prosody activates right hemisphere regions. *Archives of Neurology*, 53, 665–670.

Grandjean, D., Sander, D., Pourtois, G., Schwartz, S., Seghier, M. L., Scherer, K. R., & Vuilleumier, P. (2005). The voices of wrath: brain responses to angry prosody in meaningless speech. *Nature Neuroscience*, 8, 145–146.

Hackett, T. A. (2011). Information flow in the auditory cortical network. *Hearing Research*, 271, 133–146.

Hammerschmidt, K. & Jurgens, U. (2007). Acoustical correlates of affective prosody. *Journal of Voice*, 21, 531–540.

Hoekert, M., Bais, L., Kahn, R. S., & Aleman, A. (2008). Time course of the involvement of the right anterior superior temporal gyrus and the right fronto-parietal operculum in emotional prosody perception. *PLoS One*, 3, e2244.

Hoekert, M., Vingerhoets, G., & Aleman, A. (2010). Results of a pilot study on the involvement of bilateral inferior frontal gyri in emotional prosody perception: an rTMS study. *BMC Neuroscience*, 11, 93.

Hornak, J., Bramham, J., Rolls, E. T., Morris, R. G., O'Doherty, J., Bullock, P. R., & Polkey, C. E. (2003). Changes in emotion after circumscribed surgical lesions of the orbitofrontal and cingulate cortices. *Brain*, 126, 1691–1712.

Juslin, P. N. & Laukka, P. (2003). Communication of emotions in vocal expressions and music performance: different channels, same code? *Psychological Bulletin*, 129, 770–814.

Kissler, J. (2013). Love letters and hate mail: cerebral processing of emotional language content. In: J. Armony & P. Vuilleumier (eds) *Human Affecive Neuroscience* (pp. 304–328). Cambridge: Cambridge University Press.

Kitayama, S. (1996). Remembrance of emotional speech: improvement and impairment of incidental verbal memory by emotional voice. *Journal of Experimental Social Psychology*, 32, 289–308.

Korb, S., Frühholz, S., & Grandjean, D. (2015). Reappraising the voices of wrath. *Social Cognitive and Affective Neuroscience*, 10(12), 1644–1660.

Kotz, S. A., Kalberlah, C., Bahlmann, J., Friederici, A. D., & Haynes, J. D. (2013). Predicting vocal emotion expressions from the human brain. *Human Brain Mapping*, 34, 1971–1981.

Kotz, S. A., Schwartze, M., & Schmidt-Kassow, M. (2009). Non-motor basal ganglia functions: a review and proposal for a model of sensory predictability in auditory language perception. *Cortex*, 45, 982–990.

Kucharska-Pietura, K., Phillips, M. L., Gernand, W., & David, A. S. (2003). Perception of emotions from faces and voices following unilateral brain damage. *Neuropsychologia*, 41, 1082–1090.

LaBar, K. S. & Cabeza, R. (2006). Cognitive neuroscience of emotional memory. *Nature Reviews Neuroscience*, 7, 54–64.

Lalande, S., Braun, C. M., Charlebois, N., & Whitaker, H. A. (1992). Effects of right and left hemisphere cerebrovascular lesions on discrimination of prosodic and semantic aspects of affect in sentences. *Brain and Language*, 42, 165–186.

LeDoux, J. (2012). Rethinking the emotional brain. *Neuron*, 73, 653–676.

Leitman, D. I., Wolf, D. H., Ragland, J. D., Laukka, P., Loughead, J., Valdez, J. N., . . . Gur, R. C. (2010). 'It's not what you say, but how you say it': a reciprocal temporo-frontal network for affective prosody. *Frontiers in Human Neuroscience*, 4, 1–13.

Lewald, J. & Guski, R. (2004). Auditory-visual temporal integration as a function of distance: no compensation for sound-transmission time in human perception. *Neuroscience Letters*, 357, 119–122.

Lewald, J., Meister, I. G., Weidemann, J., & Topper, R. (2004). Involvement of the superior temporal cortex and the occipital cortex in spatial hearing: evidence from repetitive transcranial magnetic stimulation. *Journal of Cognitive Neuroscience*, 16, 828–838.

Lindquist, K. A., Wager, T. D., Kober, H., Bliss-Moreau, E., & Barrett, L. F. (2012). The brain basis of emotion: a meta-analytic review. *Behavioral and Brain Sciences*, 35, 121–143.

Milesi, V., Cekic, S., Peron, J., Frühholz, S., Cristinzio, C., Seeck, M., & Grandjean, D. (2014). Multimodal emotion perception after anterior temporal lobectomy (ATL). *Frontiers in Human Neuroscience*, 8, 275.

Mitchell, R. L. (2007). fMRI delineation of working memory for emotional prosody in the brain: commonalities with the lexico-semantic emotion network. *NeuroImage*, 36, 1015–1025.

Mothes-Lasch, M., Mentzel, H. J., Miltner, W. H., & Straube, T. (2011). Visual attention modulates brain activation to angry voices. *Journal of Neuroscience*, 31, 9594–9598.

Murphy, F., Nimmo-Smith, I., & Lawrence, A. (2003). Functional neuroanatomy of emotions: a meta-analysis. *Cognitive, Affective, and Behavioral Neuroscience*, 3, 207–233.

Norris, C. J. & Cacioppo, J. T. (2007). I know how you feel. Social and emotional information processing in the brain. In: E. Harmon-Jones & P. Winkielman (eds) *Social Neuroscience: Integrating Biological and Psychological Explanations of Social Behavior* (pp. 84–105). New York: The Guilford Press.

Ochsner, K. N., Ray, R. D., Cooper, J. C., Robertson, E. R., Chopra, S., Gabrieli, J. D., & Gross, J. J. (2004). For better or for worse: neural systems supporting the cognitive down- and up-regulation of negative emotion. *NeuroImage*, 23, 483–499.

Ohman, A. & Mineka, S. (2001). Fears, phobias, and preparedness: toward an evolved module of fear and fear learning. *Psychological Review*, 108, 483–522.

Patel, S., Scherer, K. R., Bjorkner, E., & Sundberg, J. (2011). Mapping emotions into acoustic space: the role of voice production. *Biological Psychology*, 87, 93–98.

Paulmann, S., Pell, M. D., & Kotz, S. A. (2009). Comparative processing of emotional prosody and semantics following basal ganglia infarcts: ERP evidence of selective impairments for disgust and fear. *Brain Research*, 1295, 159–169.

Pell, M. D. (2006a). Cerebral mechanisms for understanding emotional prosody in speech. *Brain and Language*, 96, 221–234.

Pell, M. D. (2006b). Judging emotion and attitudes from prosody following brain damage. *Progress in Brain Research*, 156, 303–317.

Pell, M. D. & Leonard, C. L. (2003). Processing emotional tone from speech in Parkinson's disease: a role for the basal ganglia. *Cognitive, Affective, and Behavioral Neuroscience*, 3, 275–288.

Peron, J., Frühholz. S., Ceravolo, L., & Grandjean, D. (2016). Structural and functional connectivity of the subthalamic nucleus during vocal emotion decoding. *Social Cognitive and Affective Neuroscience*, 11, 349–356.

Peron, J., Frühholz, S., Verin, M., & Grandjean, D. (2013). Subthalamic nucleus: a key structure for emotional component synchronization in humans. *Neuroscience and Biobehavioral Reviews*, 37, 358–373.

Petrides, M. (2005). Lateral prefrontal cortex: architectonic and functional organization. *Philosophical Transactions of the Royal Society of London. Series B, Biological Sciences*, 360, 781–795.

Phan, K. L., Wager, T., Taylor, S. F., & Liberzon, I. (2002). Functional neuroanatomy of emotion: a meta-analysis of emotion activation studies in PET and fMRI. *NeuroImage*, 16, 331–348.

Phillips, M. L., Young, A. W., Scott, S. K., Calder, A. J., Andrew, C., Giampietro, V., … Gray, J. A. (1998). Neural responses to facial and vocal expressions of fear and disgust. *Proceedings of the Royal Society B: Biological Sciences*, 265, 1809–1817.

Rämä, P., Martinkauppi, S., Linnankoski, I., Koivisto, J., Aronen, H. J., & Carlson, S. (2001). Working memory of identification of emotional vocal expressions: an fMRI study. *NeuroImage*, 13, 1090–1101.

Rauschecker, J. P. (2012). Ventral and dorsal streams in the evolution of speech and language. *Frontiers in Evolutionary Neuroscience*, 4, 7.

Ross, E. D. (1981). The aprosodias: functional-anatomic organization of the affective components of language in the right hemisphere. *Archives of Neurology*, 38, 561–569.

Ross, E. D. & Monnot, M. (2008). Neurology of affective prosody and its functional– anatomic organization in right hemisphere. *Brain and Language*, 104, 51–74.

Ross, E. D. & Monnot, M. (2011). Affective prosody: what do comprehension errors tell us about hemispheric lateralization of emotions, sex and aging effects, and the role of cognitive appraisal? *Neuropsychologia*, 49, 866–877.

Rota, G., Handjaras, G., Sitaram, R., Birbaumer, N., & Dogil, G. (2011). Reorganization of functional and effective connectivity during real-time fMRI-BCI modulation of prosody processing. *Brain and Language*, 117, 123–132.

Sander, D., Grandjean, D., Pourtois, G., Schwartz, S., Seghier, M. L., Scherer, K. R., & Vuilleumier, P. (2005). Emotion and attention interactions in social cognition: brain regions involved in processing anger prosody. *NeuroImage*, 28, 848–858.

Sander, K. & Scheich, H. (2005). Left auditory cortex and amygdala, but right insula dominance for human laughing and crying. *Journal of Cognitive Neuroscience*, 17, 1519–1531.

Schacter, D. L. & Church, B. A. (1992). Auditory priming: implicit and explicit memory for words and voices. *Journal of Experimental Psychology: Learning, Memory, and Cognition*, 18, 915.

Scherer, K. R. (1994). Affect bursts. In: S. van Goozen, N. E. van de Poll, & J. A. Sergeant (eds) *Emotions: Essays on Emotion Theory* (pp. 161–196). Hillsdale, NJ: Erlbaum.

Schirmer, A. (2010). Mark my words: tone of voice changes affective word representations in memory. *PLoS One*, 5, e9080.

Schirmer, A., Escoffier, N., Zysset, S., Koester, D., Striano, T., & Friederici, A. D. (2008). When vocal processing gets emotional: on the role of social orientation in relevance detection by the human amygdala. *NeuroImage*, 40, 1402–1410.

Schirmer, A. & Kotz, S. A. (2006). Beyond the right hemisphere: brain mechanisms mediating vocal emotional processing. *Trends in Cognitive Sciences*, 10, 24–30.

Schirmer, A., Zysset, S., Kotz, S. A., & Yves von Cramon, D. (2004). Gender differences in the activation of inferior frontal cortex during emotional speech perception. *NeuroImage*, 21, 1114–1123.

Schroder, C., Mobes, J., Schutze, M., Szymanowski, F., Nager, W., Bangert, M., Munte, T. F., & Dengler, R. (2006). Perception of emotional speech in Parkinson's disease. *Movement Disorders*, 21, 1774–1778.

Scott, S. K., Young, A. W., Calder, A. J., Hellawell, D. J., Aggleton, J. P., & Johnson, M. (1997). Impaired auditory recognition of fear and anger following bilateral amygdala lesions. *Nature*, 385, 254–257.

Shomstein, S. & Yantis, S. (2006). Parietal cortex mediates voluntary control of spatial and nonspatial auditory attention. *Journal of Neuroscience*, 26, 435–439.

Sprengelmeyer, R., Young, A. W., Calder, A. J., Karnat, A., Lange, H., Homberg, V., Perrett, D. I., & Rowland, D. (1996). Loss of disgust. Perception of faces and emotions in Huntington's disease. *Brain*, 119 (Pt 5), 1647–1665.

Sprengelmeyer, R., Young, A. W., Schroeder, U., Grossenbacher, P. G., Federlein, J., Buttner, T., & Przuntek, H. (1999). Knowing no fear. *Proceedings of the Royal Society B: Biological Sciences*, 266, 2451–2456.

Szameitat, D. P., Kreifelts, B., Alter, K., Szameitat, A. J., Sterr, A., Grodd, W., & Wildgruber, D. (2010). It is not always tickling: distinct cerebral responses during perception of different laughter types. *NeuroImage*, 53, 1264–1271.

van Rijn, S., Aleman, A., van Diessen, E., Berckmoes, C., Vingerhoets, G., & Kahn, R. S. (2005). What is said or how it is said makes a difference: role of the right fronto-parietal operculum in emotional prosody as revealed by repetitive TMS. *European Journal of Neuroscience*, 21, 3195–3200.

Vuilleumier, P. (2005). How brains beware: neural mechanisms of emotional attention. *Trends in Cognitive Sciences*, 9, 585–594.

Vuilleumier, P., Richardson, M. P., Armony, J. L., Driver, J., & Dolan, R. J. (2004). Distant influences of amygdala lesion on visual cortical activation during emotional face processing. *Nature Neuroscience*, 7, 1271–1278.

Warren, J. E., Sauter, D. A., Eisner, F., Wiland, J., Dresner, M. A., Wise, R. J., Rosen, S., & Scott, S. K. (2006). Positive emotions preferentially engage an auditory-motor 'mirror' system. *Journal of Neuroscience*, 26, 13067–13075.

Weninger, F., Eyben, F., Schuller, B. W., Mortillaro, M., & Scherer, K. (2013). On the acoustics of emotion in audio: what speech, music, and sound have in common. *Frontiers in Psychology*, 4, 1–12.

Wiethoff, S., Wildgruber, D., Grodd, W., & Ethofer, T. (2009). Response and habituation of the amygdala during processing of emotional prosody. *NeuroReport*, 20, 1356–1360.

Wiethoff, S., Wildgruber, D., Kreifelts, B., Becker, H., Herbert, C., Grodd, W., & Ethofer, T. (2008). Cerebral processing of emotional prosody—influence of acoustic parameters and arousal. *NeuroImage*, 39, 885–893.

Wildgruber, D., Ethofer, T., Grandjean, D., Kreifelts, B. (2009). A cerebral network model of speech prosody comprehension. *International Journal of Speech-Language Pathology*, 11, 277–281.

Wildgruber, D., Hertrich, I., Riecker, A., Erb, M., Anders, S., Grodd, W., & Ackermann, H. (2004). Distinct frontal regions subserve evaluation of linguistic and emotional aspects of speech intonation. *Cerebral Cortex*, 14, 1384–1389.

Wildgruber, D., Riecker, A., Hertrich, I., Erb, M., Grodd, W., Ethofer, T., & Ackermann, H. (2005). Identification of emotional intonation evaluated by fMRI. *NeuroImage*, 24, 1233–1241.

Zald, D. H. (2003). The human amygdala and the emotional evaluation of sensory stimuli. *Brain Research: Brain Research Reviews*, 41, 88–123.

Zatorre, R. J., Belin, P., & Penhune, V. B. (2002). Structure and function of auditory cortex: music and speech. *Trends in Cognitive Sciences*, 6, 37–46.

Zimmermann, E., Leliveld, L., & Schehka, S. (2013). Toward the evolutionary roots of affective prosody in human acoustic communication: a comparative approach to mammalian voices. In: E. Altenmuller, S. Schmidt, & E. Zimmermann (eds) *Evolution of Emotional Communication: From Sounds in Nonhuman Mammals to Speech and Music in Man.* Oxford: Oxford University Press.

CHAPTER 20

THE ELECTROPHYSIOLOGY AND TIME COURSE OF PROCESSING VOCAL EMOTION EXPRESSIONS

SILKE PAULMANN AND SONJA A. KOTZ

20.1 INTRODUCTION

'EVERYTHING becomes a little bit different as soon as it is spoken out loud' (Hermann Hesse)—quotes like these nicely illustrate the power of prosody (or tone of voice). By modifying vocal characteristics such as vocal pitch (high/low), loudness (loud/silent), tempo (fast/slow), or voice quality (clear/harsh), we give meaning to 'simple' words. It helps listeners understand how we feel (e.g. happy, sad, nervous, pleasantly excited) and allows them to respond in a socially acceptable manner. In fact, the listener benefits from grasping our emotional state of mind quickly—interpreting emotional vocal signals accurately helps them distinguish friend and foe. This chapter reviews past and current research on how and when emotional vocal signals are recognized and outlines our present understanding of the neurocognitive architecture underlying vocal emotion expressions.

As just mentioned, we often give emotional colouring to the words we use—sometimes the words themselves convey emotional meaning (e.g. 'love', 'hate', 'fear'); at other times, seemingly neutral words will be perceived as emotionally meaningful, simply because of the tone of voice and the voice quality used to express these words (e.g. 'I walked through the snow' spoken with pure joy or with annoyance). Not surprisingly, humans are not the only species that are argued to express their feelings through vocal parameters. For instance, it has been reported that animals from different mammalian groups such as bats (Bastian & Schmidt, 2008), silver foxes (Gogoleva et al., 2010), and tree shrews (Schehka & Zimmermann, 2009) all display similar vocal changes to their voice when expressing agonistic or affiliate behaviour (see Scheumann et al., 2014). In fact, as early as 1872, Darwin already suggested that emotional vocal expressions are the result of innate production mechanisms, and that human emotional vocal expressions have evolved from emotional animal sounds (Darwin, 1872). In other words, humans are argued to rely on similar emotion expression strategies as animals.

Building on this assumption, Morton (1977) reported that animals tend to modify their pitch and voice quality use according to two relatively simple strategies: high-pitched, pure tones are used to show submissive and friendly behaviour, while low pitch and harsh tones are used when expressing anger or aggression. Ohala (1984) then extended this framework and argued that humans rely on the same emotional production mechanisms: namely, high-pitched, rhythmic voices are linked to friendliness, while low pitch and rough voice quality are linked to aggressive behaviour. These production mechanisms are arguably also linked to physiological constraints—a smile during a friendly conversation will lead to lip spreading, which causes vocal tract shortening, leading to heightened formant frequencies. The resulting change in resonance is associated with brighter-sounding expressions. Crucially, short vocal tract length is linked to signalling smaller body size (i.e. less threatening). It has also been argued that pitch is raised during smiles, again making the sound appear more pleasant (see, for example, Noble & Xu, 2011; Xu et al., 2013). Conversely, the open mouth often displayed during aggressive interactions (e.g. shouting) automatically lengthens the vocal tract of the speaker, resulting in lowered formant frequencies. Hence, physiological constraints impact on emotional vocal expression production and these constraints seem to be shared across species (cf. Ohala, 1984).

There is not only evidence that emotional vocal expression *production* has evolved through natural selection, but the same has been argued for emotional vocal expression *recognition*. Obviously, recognizing both positive and negative emotional vocal expressions quickly will be beneficial for the listener. For instance, hearing a happy vocal expression means that the expresser is friendly and approachable, while hearing a frightened voice signals that danger is near. Whether or not positive and negative emotion recognition needs to follow the same time course, however, is still under debate. Some findings suggest that positive and negative vocal expressions are rapidly distinguished from neutral stimuli, as evidenced through the use of electrophysiological methods (e.g. Paulmann & Kotz, 2008; Sauter & Eimer, 2010). In contrast, behavioural findings have revealed that listeners take longer to recognize happy vocalizations as opposed to angry vocalizations (e.g. Pell & Kotz, 2011; Rigoulot et al., 2013). Part of the discrepancy between the on-line (electrophysiological) and off-line (behavioural) results may stem from accentuating different stages of the emotion recognition process. Recent sociocognitive neuroscience models on vocal emotion processing have proposed that the recognition of emotional intonation in speech is a multi-layered process mediated by a diverse brain network (e.g. Kotz & Paulmann, 2011; Schirmer & Kotz, 2006; Wildgruber et al., 2009).

In such models, three relatively broad processing stages have been suggested. First, features inherent to emotional vocal expressions (e.g. pitch, loudness, voice quality, tempo, rhythm of vocal signal) are assessed in an early sensory analysis. This evaluation has been ascribed to include left and right primary and secondary auditory cortices. Second, emotionally relevant acoustic patterns are considered to assess their motivational and emotional relevance; this early characterization and identification of emotionally relevant signals is paramount for further processing, and argued to engage the right anterior superior temporal sulcus/anterior superior temporal gyrus. Third, amodal evaluation (i.e. integrating information from different sources such as lexical semantics and prosodic information, as well as broader context information) has been linked to the bilateral inferior frontal and orbito-frontal cortex. This later, often called more fine-grained, analysis of emotional vocal expressions is tied to enhanced cognitive evaluation of emotional associative details.

This chapter aims to review evidence from behavioural and electrophysiological investigations on how emotions are communicated through voice and tone of voice. We will present research on two different types of emotional vocal expressions—namely, non-linguistic emotional vocalizations and emotional intonation in speech. The evidence presented will support the view that prosody processing entails multi-step evaluations of emotional vocal signals.

20.2 EVIDENCE ON VOCAL EMOTION PROCESSING: NON-LINGUISTIC EMOTIONAL VOCALIZATIONS

Non-verbal vocalizations such as laughs, cries, or moans play an important role in human affective interactions, especially when verbal communication is limited. For instance, infants can successfully signal their needs (hunger, discomfort, comfort) with non-verbal vocalizations. Similarly, someone at a dinner party who does not speak the host's native language will still be able to signal friendliness through a shy laugh. Moreover, non-verbal vocalizations have been argued to 'travel the distance' (i.e. they are accessible even when sight is limited) (e.g. Hawk et al., 2009).

The crucial difference between emotions expressed by non-verbal (non-linguistic) vocalizations and emotions expressed in speech is the way in which articulators (e.g. larynx, pharynx, tongue, lips) can move. While emotional speech is governed by the (supra)-segmental structure of any given language, non-verbal vocalizations are argued to be 'pure' examples of emotional expressions, given the lack of constraints on the articulators (e.g. Sauter et al., 2010). This, in turn, should lead to more variation in expressing non-verbal emotional vocalizations when compared to emotional speech (cf. Jessen & Kotz, 2011). For instance, cries can be expressed by using a high-pitched, shrill, and loud voice, or by using a 'normal'-pitched, quiet, sobbing voice. Still, despite this possible variation in acoustic cue use, emotions expressed through non-verbal vocalizations are generally well recognized (e.g. Belin et al., 2008; Lima et al., 2013; Sauter & Scott, 2007; Sauter et al., 2010; Schröder, 2003). Some of the research investigating the ease with which non-verbal emotional vocalizations are recognized will now be presented.

20.2.1 Behavioural Findings

Several studies have explored the ease with which non-verbal vocalizations are recognized (e.g. Belin et al., 2008; Lima et al., 2013; Sauter & Scott, 2007; Sauter et al., 2010; Schröder, 2003). For instance, Schröder (2003) presented 'affect bursts' (e.g. laughter, sobbing, sneezes) expressed by German speakers and asked participants to recognize them in a forced-choice task, in which participants had ten response alternatives. Results showed that overall recognition rates were close to 90% accuracy, suggesting that listeners found it relatively easy to recognize the emotional connotation of the stimuli. Similarly, Belin et al. (2008) investigated affect bursts spoken in eight different emotions and neutral, expressed by ten different actors. Again, results showed overall good recognition rates of stimuli (mean of 68%); however, results also revealed that expressions produced by female actors were more easily recognized than those produced by male actors, suggesting that women may be better at expressing emotions through prosody than men.

In another study by Lima and colleagues (2013), more than 120 different vocalizations spoken by two female and two male Portuguese speakers were tested. Here, participants were asked to categorize the stimuli into one of eight (rather than ten) response alternatives. Average recognition rates were comparable to the ones reported in Schröder (2003)—that is, more than 85% of their stimuli were categorized successfully. Slightly lower recognition rates, but still significantly better than chance performance, were reported by Szameitat and colleagues (2009) for different types of laughter (namely tickling, joyous, taunting laughter, and Schadenfreude). Together, these data indicate that emotional recognition for so-called 'pure' signals is a relatively easy task for participants, at least when stimuli are expressed by speakers of their own language.

Based on observations that these non-linguistic expressions are not only recognized easily, but also elicit haemodynamic brain responses similar to expressions that contain lexical content, researchers have been prompted to hypothesize that 'interjections might trace back to proto-speech vocalizations of an early stage of language evolution' (Dietrich et al., 2008).

Whether these non-verbal emotional signals can be recognized pan-culturally was first addressed by Sauter and Scott (2007), who presented British and Swedish participants with vocalizations spoken by British speakers expressing positive (e.g. amusement, content) emotions only. Indeed, participants from both language groups were better than expected by chance in categorizing stimuli; interestingly, Sauter and Scott (2007) report an in-group advantage though. Specifically, it was found that British listeners outperformed Swedish listeners when judging the different positive emotions. Similarly, Koeda et al. (2013) report recognition differences between Canadian and Japanese listeners who were tested with the Montreal Affective Voices (MAVs). Japanese listeners judged angry-, disgusted-, and fearful-sounding voices as less negative, and pleasant outbursts as less positive, than Canadian listeners; interestingly, the non-native listeners also judged stimuli as sounding less intense. The latter finding could imply that emotion *production* differs across cultures and is guided by culturally accepted norms. Non-native listeners might not be sensitive enough to all cues and thus judge materials expressed by speakers from a different cultural group as less intense.

However, given that these studies did not employ a fully-balanced design (i.e. present both listener groups with stimuli spoken by speakers of both language groups), the implications for pan-cultural emotional-recognition abilities remained inconclusive. This point was followed up by Sauter and colleagues a few years later (2010). This time, they presented both Himba and English listeners with non-verbal vocalizations expressed by both English and Himba speakers. Results showed that non-verbal vocalizations expressing basic emotions were recognized above chance level in both listener groups, irrespective of speaker language. These findings then indicate that emotional vocalizations can even be recognized cross-culturally.

While these behavioural studies are informative as they highlight listeners' abilities to recognize emotions from non-verbal vocalizations, they do not allow comment on how recognition unfolds in time. All studies reviewed here reported recognition rates for emotions only. No information about the time it took listeners to make an emotional decision was provided. Thus, nothing is known about the time it took them to recognize the emotional category of a stimulus. In fact, in some studies (e.g. Schröder, 2003) participants were even allowed to listen to the stimuli as often as they liked. This makes it difficult to assess whether the emotional meaning of the presented expressions were easily *and* rapidly detected.

20.2.2 Event-Related Potential Findings

As described in the introduction, it has been argued repeatedly that emotional information needs to be detected *rapidly*. The need for speed is often linked to evolutionary, survival reasons (fight/flight/freeze). As a first step, a differentiation between affective and non-affective signals is crucial for this survival mechanism. In particular, research has explored how quickly (and reliably) emotional stimuli can be distinguished from non-emotional stimuli. In addition, it has been investigated at what point in time the extracted information is combined to fully recognize emotional meanings of stimuli. To this end, event-related potentials (ERPs) have proven to be particularly useful.

So-called early processing stages (i.e. extraction of salient acoustic features that signal emotionality) have been explored by several authors using non-verbal vocalizations (Belin 2009; Charest et al., 2009; Pell et al., 2015; Sauter & Eimer, 2010). For example, Charest et al. (2009) reported a differentiation of short voice (e.g. laughter, gargle, yawn), bird, and environmental sounds as early as 164 ms after stimulus onset. This effect was found even though participants did not have an explicit task to discriminate between the different sound categories, suggesting that this early differentiation is involuntary. Given that the goal of Charest and colleagues was to explore the time course underlying human vocalization, these findings do not allow for comment on the influence of emotions on this process. While the majority of the stimuli will have had explicit emotional connotations (e.g. laughter representing happiness), some of them (e.g. yawn) might not.

Sauter and Eimer (2010) specifically focused on the early detection of emotions from non-verbal signals. In the second experiment of their study, participants were presented with different emotional vocalizations (e.g. screams, laughter), which were compared to neutral vocalizations as well as spectrally rotated (i.e. non-emotional) sounds. Task demands were not focused on the emotionality of the stimuli as participants performed a beep-detection task. Results revealed that emotional vocalizations were distinguished from neutral vocalizations around 150 ms after stimulus onset, as reflected in an enhanced frontal positive ERP component for emotional but not neutral stimuli. This suggests rapid detection of emotionally relevant auditory cues from non-verbal vocalizations.

A similar early detection of emotionally relevant auditory cues was observed by Jessen and Kotz (2011). They report differentiation between emotional (anger, fear) and neutral stimuli shortly after the onset of their vocalizations (~120 ms post-stimulus) (for similar evidence, see Ho et al., 2015; Kokinous et al., 2015). Similarly, Liu and colleagues (2012) report enhanced P200 amplitudes in response to happy (laughter) and angry ('humph') vocalizations when compared to neutral ('mmm') ones, highlighting once more that emotional vocalizations are rapidly assessed with regard to their emotional salience. In a recent study, similar findings have been reported when looking at individual participants rather than at group-level perception (Salvia et al., 2014). In this MEG study, three participants were presented with over 6,000 affective non-verbal vocalizations (vowel /a/) representing three emotional categories (anger, fear, pleasure). Results revealed that early emotion effects (~100ms after sound onset) could be found in all three participants; however, the authors also report that these effects nearly disappear when the impact of acoustic properties of stimuli is taken into account in the statistical model used to explore these effects. In other words, this study shows that very early effects are predominantly driven by dominant acoustic features.

In addition to early emotion effects, research has also looked at more fine-tuned emotional processing. For instance, in a classic passive oddball paradigm, Bostanov and Kotchoubey (2004) presented participants with positive exclamations ('Yeah', 'Heey', 'Wow', and 'Oooh') as standards and a negative exclamation ('Ooh') serving as a deviant. Recognition of deviant vocalizations led to an enhanced N300 ERP response, suggesting that emotional meaning of vocalizations was extracted around 300 ms after stimulus onset. However, one of the limitations of an oddball paradigm is that it is unclear how far vocalizations were recognized accurately—after all, the N300 response could merely be discrimination between positive and negative signals. Thus, in a second experiment, the authors employed a priming paradigm, in which non-verbal vocalizations were preceded by contextually (i.e. emotional) appropriate or inappropriate words. For this study, the authors also report an enhanced N300 in response to incongruous prime-target pairs, emphasizing that emotional (prosodic) meaning extraction occurs within 300 ms after stimulus onset (Bostanov & Kotchoubey, 2004).

Recently, Pell and colleagues (2015) have explored early and late emotional-processing stages in one experimental design. Specifically, the authors looked at the P200 and late positive component elicited in response to vocalizations expressing anger, sadness, or happiness. They report enhanced P200 responses for angry and happy vocalizations when compared to sad vocalizations. Anger also differentiated from happy and sad in the late positive component. The authors claimed that this later effect is linked to a more fine-grained analysis of stimulus properties expressing anger. They argued that anger is linked to threat and aggression (cf. Öhman, 1987), and thus requires enhanced attention. In fact, Jessen and Kotz (2011) report this late positive component (LPC) differentiation between neutral and emotional vocalizations for fearful and angry expressions, lending support to the idea that survival-related emotions undergo additional evaluation processes.

Taken together, these results suggest at least two different stages of emotional vocalization processing: a first initial salience detection occurring approximately 150 ms after stimulus onset, followed by a more elaborate emotional analysis starting as early as 300 ms after vocalization onset depending on paradigm and stimuli used. These findings are in line with recent time-course-orientated neurocognitive models on emotional speech processing (cf. Kotz & Paulmann, 2011; Schirmer & Kotz, 2006).

20.3 EVIDENCE ON VOCAL EMOTION PROCESSING: EMOTIONAL SPEECH INTONATION

Listening to the 'melody' of speech is crucial in daily interactions—listeners always have to pay attention to the controlled modulations of pitch, tempo, and loudness as these cues signal how the speaker feels. The acoustic cues used to express emotional prosody are modulated over time. For instance, someone yelling 'Come back and tidy up now' may put particular emphasis (e.g. through high pitch) on the start of that sentence, but the same cues are less prominent towards the end of the utterance (e.g. at this point loudness is accented more). This pattern can further differ between long ('Come back and tidy up now') and shorter utterances ('Come back now'). Finally, as previously mentioned, emotional speech prosody is governed by phonemic properties of utterances (i.e. there are constraints on the articulators when expressing emotions through speech). Thus, although there are some commonalities between emotional speech prosody and non-verbal vocalizations, the two cannot be considered identical twins and, not surprisingly, these two types of emotional vocal expressions have, for the most part, been investigated separately. In the following paragraphs, we will summarize the findings underlying the time course of emotional intonation in speech.

20.3.1 Behavioural Findings

In contrast to work on emotional vocalizations, several studies have employed behavioural measures to investigate the time course of emotional speech prosody recognition. One paradigm is argued to be particularly helpful when estimating how much information listeners need before they recognize the emotional meaning of a sentence due to its temporal sensitivity—namely, the so-called 'gating paradigm'. In a typical emotional prosody gating study, participants are presented with successively building fragments of pseudo-sentences (i.e. sentences that contain no lexical-semantic emotional information) (e.g. 'Frisk the dult lantery') (see Audios 20.1–20.3 for some examples), and after each fragment they are asked to indicate which emotion the speaker tried to convey. Often, this emotional prosody recognition task is accompanied by a confidence rating. The idea behind this paradigm is as follows: (a) experimenters can control how much auditory information participants are presented with, and (b) experimenters can investigate at which point in time listeners do not change their evaluation of the stimulus any longer—the point that researchers refer to as 'recognition point'.

To our knowledge, the first study that used the gating paradigm to explore the time course of emotional speech recognition was conducted by Cornew et al. (2010). They presented happy, angry, and neutral sentences, and reported that listeners recognized neutral prosody more quickly (and more confidently) than emotional sentences. These results were taken as evidence for a neutral bias, a finding in stark contrast to the emotional (or negativity) bias reported in studies that did not focus on the time course of emotional prosody processing. While surprising that neutral prosody was recognized more quickly than happy or angry prosody, results also showed that angry prosody was recognized earlier than happy prosody. The latter result is in line with the idea that potentially-relevant stimuli (e.g. anger, fear) lead to facilitated processing (see previous text).

In an attempt to replicate and expand these findings, Pell and Kotz (2011) conducted a similar gating experiment, this time testing five emotions (anger, disgust, fear, sadness, happiness) and neutral. Their results confirmed that it takes longest to recognize happy prosody (mean recognition point: 977 ms); however, while neutral prosody (510 ms) was significantly faster recognized than happy, angry (710 ms), and disgust (1486 ms) prosody, its recognition point did not differ from fear (517 ms) or sadness (576 ms). Thus, when presenting more than two emotions and neutral prosody simultaneously, the neutral bias could not be replicated. The latter time-course results were somewhat replicated by Jiang et al. (2015) in a cross-cultural study. For English speakers listening to English gated materials, only minor differences were found to Pell and Kotz (2011). In particular, looking at recognition-point means, it was shown that anger was more quickly recognized than sadness or fear. Still, results suggest that salient, negative emotions are more quickly evaluated than positive emotions. Interestingly, while English listeners were also slow to recognize happiness from Hindi stimuli, the same was not found for Hindi listeners when listening to Hindi materials. This may suggest that the relative advantage for happiness found in previous studies was material- and/or speaker-dependent. Naturally, materials between languages differed with regard to phonological properties. However, some recent evidence suggests that phonological iconicity plays a role when determining emotional saliency (Aryani et al., 2013). Thus, it can be hypothesized that, at least for speech intonation, the speed with which emotional categories are determined may also depend on phonemic structure.

Finally, Rigoulot et al. (2013) also explored emotional recognition points, but this time presented the materials used in Pell and Kotz (2011) gated from sentence *offset* rather than onset. This 'backwards' gating was used to explore whether the recognition time differences between different emotions was related to the amount of speech heard by the listeners, or whether it was linked to the position of relevant acoustic cues in the material. Again, Rigoulot et al.'s results suggest that, at least for some emotions (e.g. happiness), the position of emotionally-relevant cues is tightly linked to recognition speed. In short, emotional prosody gating studies suggest that offline recognition of different emotions follows a distinct time course.

20.3.2 Event-Related Potential Findings

In addition to the evidence from gating studies, there is a wealth of data on the underlying time course of emotional speech prosody processing (both at the sentence and word levels). Similar to non-linguistic vocal expressions, several early (N100, P200) and late (P300, N400, LPC) ERP components have been shown to be of particular relevance. Extraction of acoustic cues (i.e. processing of pitch, tempo, and loudness) has been linked to the N100 component. There is some debate as to whether the N100 is influenced by emotional characteristics of stimuli or whether it reflects a pure sensory-processing response. Recently, however, some studies have reported emotional effects on this early component. For example, Pinheiro and colleagues (2013) presented participants with semantically-neutral sentences spoken in neutral, angry, or happy prosody. They reported enhanced N100 components for neutral when compared to angry prosody, an effect which authors attribute to listeners' emotional evaluation of incoming sensory information (see also Kokinous et al., 2015). In the same study, Liu et al. (2012) also compared ERP responses to emotional and neutral stimuli when semantic content was unintelligible. In this 'pure' prosody condition, they report enhanced N100 components for neutral when compared to both angry and happy prosody. Given the differences found between the different conditions, it seems as if the emotionality evaluation at this early stage is predominantly driven by salient acoustic cues. In other words, this component is particularly modulated by sensory cues, which may (but do not have to) be influenced by emotional connotations of stimuli.

The N100 is generally followed by a fronto-centrally distributed positive component peaking 200 ms after stimulus onset (i.e. the P200). The component has been linked to both emotional prosodic (e.g. Paulmann & Kotz, 2008; Schirmer et al., 2013) and arousal (Paulmann et al., 2013) characteristics of speech stimuli. While the direction of the P200 effect is known to vary between studies, probably due to different acoustic and arousal attributes of stimuli across studies, there is relatively high agreement that neutral stimuli can be distinguished from different emotional prosodies (e.g. Paulman & Kotz, 2008; Pell et al., 2015; Schirmer et al., 2013) at this point in time. Some studies (e.g. Paulmann et al., 2013) have also reported that different basic emotions (anger, disgust, fear, sadness, happiness, pleasant surprise) can be distinguished from one another within 200 ms of stimulus onset.

Compared to vocalizations, emotional prosodic stimuli used in these P200 studies have been of relatively long duration (up to 3 seconds long). Still, emotional characteristics of the stimuli used in speech prosody studies have been extracted far before a sentence is completed, suggesting that even sentence prosody (which develops over time) is routinely scanned for saliency. So far, however, it is unclear which specific acoustic parameter combinations are used (and/or needed) by listeners to detect the emotionality of a stimulus. Similar to the N100, the P200 is sensitive to both loudness (Picton et al., 1977) and pitch (Pantev ct al., 1996) variations, and both cues are likely candidates to play a leading role in this early saliency detection process.

Next to the P200 component, which is elicited under attentive processing conditions, with or without task instructions focusing on emotional aspects of stimuli, there is also evidence that emotions are detected pre-attentively as reflected in the mismatch negativity (MMN) component (e.g. Schirmer et al., 2005). The MMN has been argued to reflect pre-attentive auditory change detection. In a typical MMN paradigm, participants engage in a task which distracts them from processing auditory stimuli explicitly. For instance, Schirmer and Escoffier (2010) asked participants to watch a silent movie while simultaneously presenting them with angry and neutral voices, of which one category served as standard (presented frequently) and the other as deviant (presented infrequently). In their study, the authors could not only show that listeners detect auditory change pre-attentively (i.e. while watching a movie) but also that listeners' heartbeat and state anxiety correlated with the MMN which was elicited in response to angry deviants (i.e. when the change detection was 'emotional' in nature). Results suggest that pre-attentively processed emotional voices activate the sympathetic nervous system. This finding goes well with suggestions that this component—similar to the P200—has been linked to an early emotional appraisal or evaluation stage (e.g. Kotz & Paulmann, 2011; Schirmer & Kotz, 2006).

As previously mentioned, according to multi-stage models on emotional prosody perception (e.g. Kotz & Paulmann, 2011; Schirmer & Kotz, 2006; Wildgruber et al., 2009), an early emotional salience detection mechanism must be followed by a more effortful approach to evaluate emotional meaning. Later ERP components such as the P300 (e.g. Wambacq & Jerger, 2004), N400 (e.g. Paulmann & Pell, 2010; Schirmer & Kotz, 2003; Schirmer et al., 2002, 2005), and the late positive complex (LPC) (Paulmann et al., 2013; Schirmer et al., 2013) have been associated with this more enhanced processing of emotional details.

For instance, Schirmer and Kotz (2003) presented participants with prosodically and semantically matching (e.g. 'joy' spoken in a happy tone) or mismatching words (e.g. 'joy' spoken in an angry tone). They reported enhanced N400 amplitudes in response to mismatching stimuli when compared to matching stimuli, suggesting that listeners detect prosodic and semantic valence mismatch at this emotional meaning evaluation processing stage. Following this, Paulmann and Pell (2010) investigated this processing stage further. They specifically explored how *much* prosodic information listeners need to recognize emotional meaning. To this aim, participants were presented with sentence fragments of different length (200 ms or 400 ms long). The emotional prosodic snippets were used as primes before participants were presented with emotionally congruent or incongruent facial expressions. The authors report N400-like priming effects in response to emotionally mismatching prime-target pairs, albeit extremely short sentence fragments (200 ms long) led to a reversed priming effect.

Next to the N400, another 'late' component has repeatedly been linked to more cognitively-driven emotional meaning evaluation—namely, the LPC. Specifically, Paulmann et al. (2013) report differently-modulated LPC amplitudes in response to different emotional prosody categories (anger, disgust, fear, sadness, happiness, surprise). They argue that the LPC modulations reflect enhanced processing of emotional attributes (e.g. mapping of emotional attributes and emotional memory representations). Similarly, Schirmer et al. (2013) reported differently-modulated LPCs in response to different emotional prosodies. Interestingly, this group also showed that modulations of early ERP effects (e.g. P200) can predict the variation of the LPCs that followed these early effects. The latter finding nicely demonstrates that the individual processing steps are not isolated processes; rather, the different processing steps involved are well-orchestrated subprocesses needed to process emotional prosody quickly and effectively.

20.4 Summary

The findings reviewed here confirm the idea that processing emotions from non-verbal vocalizations, or speech prosody, comprises several subprocesses including rapid early emotional appraisal and cognitive evaluation of emotional meaning in speech comprehension. It seems as if these early steps are not directly linked to the attention focus of listeners, suggesting that they occur involuntarily. However, reported results also reveal that electrophysiological correlates are modulated by changes in task demand, stimulus quality, and experimental design, leading to differences in polarity and timing of effects.

Interestingly, when comparing findings for non-verbal expressions and emotional sentence prosody, findings suggest that vocalizations elicit slightly earlier responses (consistently) than emotional sentences. The difference in timing of effects might be linked to the complexity of stimuli, as well as the fact that sentence prosody can develop over time whereas vocalizations or affect bursts are short-lived in nature. Thus, speakers have more chances to modulate voice parameters during sentence production than during spontaneous exclamations. Moreover, as argued here, parameter changes for sentence prosody are more closely constrained by articulator movements, making it at times more difficult for speakers to express their emotions with an emphasis comparable to vocal expression production. Taken together, this may mean that detecting emotions from tone of voice is governed by stimulus properties.

We believe that in addition to these factors, individual differences, or social-psychological factors, will also contribute to effects. So far, the majority of research has

- Routine scanning for emotional saliency
- Combining salient acoustic cues to form an emotional Gestalt
- Enhanced attention to emotional and arousing attributes leading to preferential processing

- Extraction of acoustic cues (pitch, tempo, loudness)
- Early emotional evaluation of incoming sensory information
- Forming and maintaining a memory trace

- Integration of emotionally relevant cues across channels (e.g. semantics/prosody)
- Emotional meaning evaluation
- Enhanced processing of emotional attributes (e.g. mapping of emotional attributes and emotional memory representations)

- Continued monitoring of emotional features
- Build-up of an emotional representation
- 2nd pass of emotional analysis
- Linguistic labelling

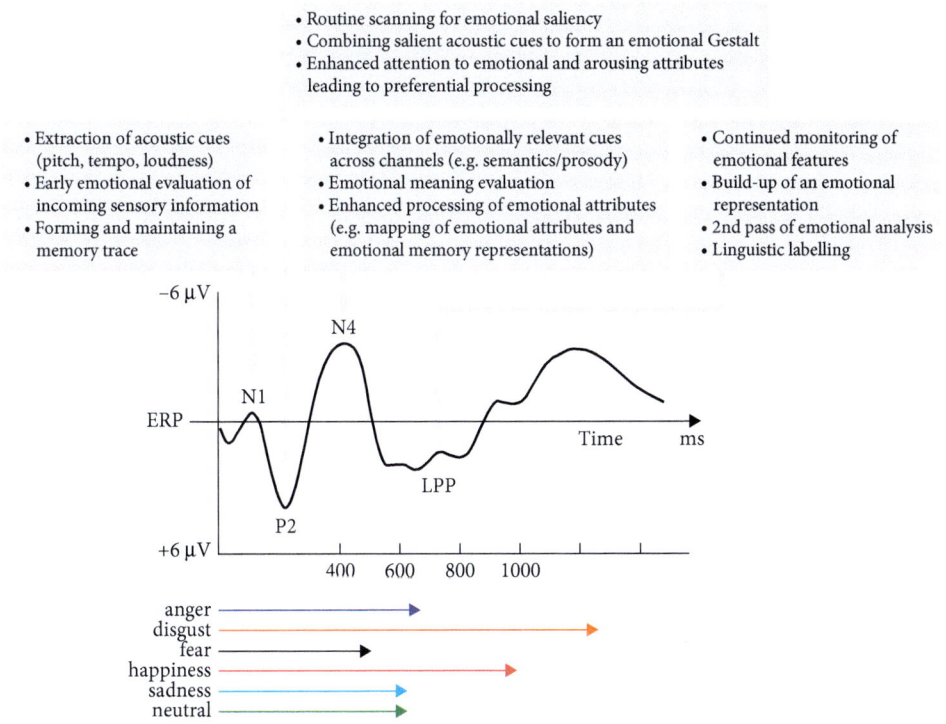

FIGURE 20.1   A visual summary of ERP and behavioural findings as described in Paulmann and Kotz (this volume).

concentrated on exploring differences in emotional intonation processing as a function of sex (e.g. Schirmer et al., 2002, 2003, 2005), age (e.g. Mitchell & Kingston, 2014; Paulmann et al., 2008), or cultural and language background (e.g. Jiang et al., 2015; Pell et al., 2009; Scherer et al., 2001). Very recently, the impact of social power (e.g. Uskul et al., 2016), as well as stress level of listeners (e.g. Paulmann et al., 2016), have also been explored.

This review also highlights that online and offline results do not always go 'hand in hand' (see Figure 20.1). For instance, behavioural findings suggest that neutral is recognized more quickly than angry prosody (e.g. Pell & Kotz, 2011). Yet, the two categories are first differentiated within 100 ms, suggesting that an early appraisal may be emotion-category independent. Thus, early stages of affective voice processing are more driven by factors that signal saliency, importance, motivational relevance, or similar non-emotion category-specific details. Only later (between 200—300 ms) are specific category details evaluated more specifically (see, for example, Paulmann & Pell, 2010), before accumulated affective details are processed more deeply. Depending on the clarity and unambiguity of the processed details, different recognition points can be found for different emotional and affective categories. For instance, an emotion such as anger might still be more easily confused with fear than with neutral, leading to earlier offline recognition for neutral as opposed to specific emotional categories.

Combined, this research highlights that more fine-tuned, current, social-cognitive neuroscientific models of emotional vocal expression processing will not only have to continue to understand emotional vocalizations and prosody processing as a multi-layered process, but will also have to start modelling effects of socio-psychological variables on these processes.

References

Aryani, A., Jacobs, A. M., & Conrad, M. (2013). Extracting salient sublexical units from written texts: 'Emophon,' a corpus-based approach to phonological iconicity. *Frontiers in Psychology*, 4(654).

Bastian, A. & Schmidt, S. (2008). Affect cues in vocalizations of the bat, *Megaderma lyra*, during agonistic interactions. *The Journal of the Acoustical Society of America*, 124(1), 598–608.

Bostanov, V. & Kotchoubey, B. (2004). Recognition of affective prosody: continuous wavelet measures of event-related brain potentials to emotional exclamations. *Psychophysiology*, 41(2), 259–268.

Charest, I., Pernet, C. R., Rousselet, G. A., Quiñones, I., Latinus, M., Fillion-Bilodeau, S., ... Belin, P. (2009). Electrophysiological evidence for an early processing of human voices. *BMC Neuroscience*, 10(1), 127.

Cornew, L., Carver, L., & Love, T. (2010). There's more to emotion than meets the eye: a processing bias for neutral content in the domain of emotional prosody. *Cognition and Emotion*, 24(7), 1133–1152.

Darwin, C. (1872). *The Expression of Emotion in Animals and Man*. London: Methuen.

Darwin, C. (1877). A biographical sketch of an infant. *Mind*, 2, 285–294.

Dietrich, S., Hertrich, I., Alter, K., Ischebeck, A., & Ackermann, H. (2008). Understanding the emotional expression of verbal interjections: a functional MRI study. *NeuroReport*, 19(18), 1751–1755.

Gogoleva, S. S., Volodina, E. V., Volodin, I. A., Kharlamova, A. V., & Trut, L. N. (2010). The gradual vocal responses to human-provoked discomfort in farmed silver foxes. *Acta Ethologica*, 13(2), 75–85.

Hawk, S. T., Van Kleef, G. A., Fischer, A. H., & Van Der Schalk, J. (2009). 'Worth a thousand words': absolute and relative decoding of nonlinguistic affect vocalizations. *Emotion*, 9(3), 293.

Ho, H. T., Schröger, E., & Kotz, S. A. (2015). Selective attention modulates early human evoked potentials during emotional face–voice processing. *Journal of Cognitive Neuroscience*, 27(4), 798–818.

Jessen, S. & Kotz, S. A. (2011). The temporal dynamics of processing emotions from vocal, facial, and bodily expressions. *NeuroImage*, 58(2), 665–674.

Jiang, X., Paulmann, S., Robin, J., & Pell, M. D. (2015). More than accuracy: nonverbal dialects modulate the time course of vocal emotion recognition across cultures. *Journal of Experimental Psychology: Human Perception and Performance*, 41(3), 597.

Koeda, M., Belin, P., Hama, T., Masuda, T., Matsura, M., & Okubo, Y. (2013). Cross-cultural differences in the processing of non-verbal affective vocalizations by Japanese and Canadian listeners. *Frontiers in Psychology*, 4, 105.

Kokinous, J., Kotz, S. A., Tavano, A., & Schröger, E. (2015). The role of emotion in dynamic audiovisual integration of faces and voices. *Social, Cognitive, and Affective Neuroscience*, 10(5), 713–720.

Kotz, S. A. & Paulmann, S. (2011). Emotion, language, and the brain. *Language and Linguistics Compass*, 5(3), 108–125.

Lima, C. F., Castro, S. L., & Scott, S. K. (2013). When voices get emotional: a corpus of nonverbal vocalizations for research on emotion processing. *Behavior Research Methods*, 45(4), 1234–1245.

Liu, T., Pinheiro, A. P., Deng, G., Nestor, P. G., McCarley, R. W., & Niznikiewicz, M. A. (2012). Electrophysiological insights into processing nonverbal emotional vocalizations. *NeuroReport*, 23(2), 108–112.

Mitchell, R. L. & Kingston, R. A. (2014). Age-related decline in emotional prosody discrimination. *Experimental Psychology*, 61(3), 215–223.

Morton, E. S. (1977). On the occurrence and significance of motivation-structural rules in some bird and mammal sounds. *American Naturalist*, 855–869.

Noble, L. & Xu, Y. (2011). *Friendly speech and happy speech—are they the same?* In: Proceedings of the 17th International Congress of Phonetic Sciences, Hong Kong (pp. 1502–1505).

Ohala, J. J. (1984). An ethological perspective on common cross-language utilization of F0 of voice. *Phonetica*, 41(1), 1–16.

Öhman, A. (1987). The psychophysiology of emotion: an evolutionary-cognitive perspective. *Advances in Psychophysiology*, 2(79), 127.

Pantev, C., Elbert, T., Ross, B., Eulitz, C., & Terhardt, E. (1996). Binaural fusion and the representation of virtual pitch in the human auditory cortex. *Hearing Research*, 100(1), 164–170.

Paulmann, S., Bleichner, M., & Kotz, S. A. (2013). Valence, arousal, and task effects in emotional prosody processing. *Frontiers in Psychology*, 4, 345. doi: 10.3389/fpsyg.2013.00345

Paulmann, S. & Kotz, S. A. (2008). Early emotional prosody perception based on different speaker voices. *NeuroReport*, 19(2), 209–213.

Paulmann, S. & Pell, M. D. (2010). Contextual influences of emotional speech prosody on face processing: how much is enough? *Cognitive, Affective, & Behavioral Neuroscience*, 10(2), 230–242.

Pell, M. D. & Kotz, S. A. (2011). On the time course of vocal emotion recognition. *PLoS One*, 6(11), e27256.

Pell, M. D., Monetta, L., Paulmann, S., & Kotz, S. A. (2009). Recognizing emotions in a foreign language. *Journal of Nonverbal Behavior*, 33(2), 107–120.

Pell, M. D., Rothermich, K., Liu, P., Paulmann, S., Sethi, S., & Rigoulot, S. (2015). Preferential decoding of emotion from human non-linguistic vocalizations versus speech prosody. *Biological Psychology*, 111, 14–25.

Picton, T. W., Woods, D. L., Baribeau-Braun, J., & Healey, T. M. (1977). Evoked potential audiometry. *Journal of Otolaryngology*, 6(2), 90–119.

Pinheiro, A. P., Del Re, E., Mezin, J., Nestor, P. G., Rauber, A., McCarley, R. W., … Niznikiewicz, M. A. (2013). Sensory-based and higher-order operations contribute to abnormal emotional prosody processing in schizophrenia: an electrophysiological investigation. *Psychological Medicine*, 43(03), 603–618.

Rigoulot, S., Wassiliwizky, E., & Pell, M. D. (2013). Feeling backwards? How temporal order in speech affects the time course of vocal emotion recognition. *Frontiers in Psychology*, 4, 367. doi: 10.3389/fpsyg.2013.00367

Salvia, E., Bestelmeyer, P. E., Kotz, S. A., Rousselet, G. A., Pernet, C. R., Gross, J., & Belin, P. (2014). Single-subject analyses of magnetoencephalographic evoked responses to the acoustic properties of affective non-verbal vocalizations. *Frontiers in Neuroscience*, 8, 422.

Sauter, D. A. & Eimer, M. (2010). Rapid detection of emotion from human vocalizations. *Journal of Cognitive Neuroscience*, 22(3), 474–481.

Sauter, D. A., Eisner, F., Ekman, P., & Scott, S. K. (2010). Cross-cultural recognition of basic emotions through nonverbal emotional vocalizations. *Proceedings of the National Academy of Sciences*, 107(6), 2408–2412.

Sauter, D. A. & Scott, S. K. (2007). More than one kind of happiness: can we recognize vocal expressions of different positive states? *Motivation and Emotion*, 31(3), 192–199.

Schehka, S. & Zimmermann, E. (2009). Acoustic features to arousal and identity in disturbance calls of tree shrews (*Tupaia belangeri*). *Behavioural Brain Research*, 203(2), 223–231.

Scherer, K. R., Banse, R., & Wallbott, H. G. (2001). Emotion inferences from vocal expression correlate across language and cultures. *Journal of Cross-Cultural Psychology*, 32(1), 76–92.

Scheumann, M., Hasting, A. S., Kotz, S. A., & Zimmermann, E. (2014). The voice of emotion across species: how do human listeners recognize animals' affective states? *PloS One*, 9(3), e91192.

Schirmer, A., Chen, C. B., Ching, A., Tan, L., & Hong, R. Y. (2013). Vocal emotions influence verbal memory: neural correlates and inter-individual differences. *Cognitive, Affective, & Behavioral Neuroscience*, 13(1), 80–93.

Schirmer, A. & Escoffier, N. (2010). Emotional MMN: anxiety and heart rate correlates with the ERP signature for auditory change detection. *Clinical Neurophysiology*, 121(1), 53–59.

Schirmer, A. & Kotz, S. A. (2006). Beyond the right hemisphere: brain mechanisms mediating vocal emotional processing. *Trends in Cognitive Sciences*, 10(1), 24–30.

Schirmer, A. & Kotz, S. A. (2003). ERP evidence for a sex-specific Stroop effect in emotional speech. *Journal of Cognitive Neuroscience*, 15(8), 1135–1148.

Schirmer, A., Kotz, S. A., & Friederici, A. D. (2002). Sex differentiates the role of emotional prosody during word processing. *Cognitive Brain Research*, 14(2), 228–233.

Schirmer, A., Kotz, S. A., & Friederici, A. D. (2005). On the role of attention for the processing of emotions in speech: sex differences revisited. *Cognitive Brain Research*, 24(3), 442–452.

Schirmer, A., Striano, T., & Friederici, A. D. (2005). Sex differences in the preattentive processing of vocal emotional expressions. *NeuroReport*, 16(6), 635–639.

Schröder, M. (2003). Experimental study of affect bursts. *Speech Communication*, 40(1), 99–116.

Szameitat, D. P., Alter, K., Szameitat, A. J., Darwin, C. J., Wildgruber, D., Dietrich, S., & Sterr, A. (2009). Differentiation of emotions in laughter at the behavioral level. *Emotion*, 9(3), 397.

Uskul, A. K., Paulmann, S., & Weick, M. (2016). Social power and recognition of emotional prosody: high power is associated with lower recognition accuracy than low power. *Emotion*, 16(1), 11–15.

Wambacq, I. J. & Jerger, J. F. (2004). Processing of affective prosody and lexical-semantics in spoken utterances as differentiated by event-related potentials. *Cognitive Brain Research*, 20(3), 427–437.

Wildgruber, D., Ethofer, T., Grandjean, D., & Kreifelts, B. (2009). A cerebral network model of speech prosody comprehension. *International Journal of Speech-Language Pathology*, 11(4), 277–281.

Xu, Y., Lee, A., Wu, W.-L., Liu, X., & Birkholz, P. (2013). Human vocal attractiveness as signaled by body size projection. *PLoS One*, 8, e62397.

CHAPTER 21

AMYGDALA PROCESSING OF VOCAL EMOTIONS

JOCELYNE C. WHITEHEAD AND
JORGE L. ARMONY

21.1 INTRODUCTION

As a multimodal structure, the amygdala plays a prominent role in processing emotional information across the senses. It receives stimulus information from the surrounding environment via a number of sensory modalities (LeDoux, 2007). The sensory information is then interpreted, and in return, elicits an emotional response (Armony & LeDoux, 1997). The primitive rationalization for these emotional reactions was to avoid threat, and to ensure the survival of oneself and one's conspecifics (Darwin, 1872). In today's society, emotions have a more socially relevant use, as they aid our ability to communicate with one another, and ultimately achieve long-standing social objectives (Britton, 2006).

Most emotional information is relayed through visual and auditory channels. Unlike the visual system, auditory information can be detected at long range, and is pervious to environmental barriers. It can be quickly transmitted through the nervous system, triggering a redirection of attention and consequently, a rapid response to a threatening stimulus. This innate responsive action aligns with the notion that processing acoustic emotional information is universal, being that all humans have the same evolutionary predisposition to respond to these low-level cues of emotion for survival purposes (Darwin, 1872). Cultural differences have, however, been identified within the human population (Liu et al., 2015).

A significant amount of information can be conveyed through the voice, irrespective of the semantics. Acoustic variation of the voice, including changes in pitch, loudness, and rhythm, can each contribute to how an explicit emotion is perceived. For example, anger and fear can both be catalogued by a fast speech rate and an increasing intensity and pitch; however, anger tends to be perceived as having more variable pitches (Banse & Scherer, 1996). These modulations in vocal quality arise from physiological changes that coincide with the subject's emotional state, in which the brain executes a number of top–down commands through the somatic and autonomic nervous systems as to produce a response. This manipulation of the voice could be in the form of increased laryngeal tension and subglottic air pressure, as to bear a greater intensity in the presence of an imposing threat (Scherer, 1989).

Functional neuroimaging research has improved our understanding of what is happening, in real time, to the listener's brain as they decode and process the emotional vocal characteristics emitted by the speaker. In contrast to processing emotionally neutral speech, the brain's neural activity tends to intensify in response to emotionally salient auditory stimuli (reviewed in Brück et al., 2013). Interestingly, comparable neural activation is observed in response to emotional music (Koelsch, 2006). The recognition of common neural circuits between music and speech perception has initiated debate, specifically, on whether this circuitry can be characterized as 'neural sharing' or, rather, as independent and separable 'neural overlap' (Peretz et al., 2015). This chapter will address these conflicting perspectives and the literature that supports their relevance to emotional processing.

Exploration into the neural correlates of affective perception has extended to encompass structures that decode information across modalities, such as the amygdala (Adolphs et al., 1995). In this chapter, we aim to synchronize the current findings of acoustic processing with the already well-researched area of visual perception of emotion, specifically facial expressions, to emphasize the contribution of multimodal structures in processing affective information. A majority of the literature focuses on the expression of fearful emotions and their ability to evoke an amygdala response, yet studies have now demonstrated that the amygdala has the capacity to respond to a range of positive and negative emotions, including happiness, sadness, anger, and disgust, as seen in the visual modality (Sergerie et al., 2008). These findings have led to a re-evaluation of the nature of the amygdala, from its role in fear detection, to alternatively acting as a novelty detector, irrespective of task relevance (reviewed in Armony, 2013). The chapter will help provide support for this proposed function and will draw conclusions from the field on its relevance to processing multisensory information.

21.2 EMOTION IN THE VOICE

Similar to facial expressions, the voice provides us with cues for identifying individuals and the emotions that they express. The voice has a number of physically defining attributes, and modulation of these attributes form patterns that are used for interpreting emotion in the voice (reviewed in Belin et al., 2004). Studies of vocal affective processing often involve attending to non-linguistic vocalizations or speech without content (audio 21.1; Armony et al., 2007; Aubé et al., 2013; Fecteau et al., 2005, 2007). Non-linguistic vocalizations ('vocalizations' hereafter) are innate sounds that are produced to convey one's emotional state, such as laughing, screaming, or crying. These vocalizations have been equated to the facial features that are commonly attributed to the same respective emotions of joy, fear, and sadness (reviewed in Belin et al., 2004). As language has advanced from the grunts and groans of our evolutionary predecessors, it is still the various intonations and changes in prosody that give us most of our information for social communication. Regardless of the semantics, much can be conveyed through the pace and pause duration of the speech (reviewed in Banse & Scherer, 1996). Pseudo-utterances are commonly used to illustrate these qualities of vocal emotional expression when conducting research. The pseudo-utterances sound like real words and can be structured into sentences, yet are non-existent words without meaning (audio 21.2; Pell et al., 2009).

Prosody and vocalizations are found to recruit varying neural structures and to differing degrees, such that more primal vocal expressions tend to rely on the involvement of the amygdala and anterior insula, while increased activity is typically seen in the right temporal lobe and right inferior prefrontal cortex in response to emotional prosody (reviewed in Belin et al., 2004). These differences are consistent with the notion that higher-order structures are required for decoding and processing more sophisticated emotional communication (i.e. speech). Research by Hawk et al. (2009) identified that individuals can more accurately decode emotion in facial expressions and vocalizations than prosody, for both positive and negative emotions. An electroencephalography (EEG) study using event-related brain potentials (ERPs) identified that emotion in vocalizations is recognizable prior to emotion in speech. The authors attributed this finding to differences in arousal, as seen between vocalizations and speech (Pell et al., 2015).

21.3 FEAR CONDITIONING

Most of our understanding about the neurobiology of auditory emotional processing comes from studying fear conditioning—a form of Pavlovian conditioning. We have been able to gain insight into how organisms learn from past experiences and how they apply said knowledge to predict oncoming danger in their environment. During the fear-conditioning paradigm, the subject is exposed to a conditioned stimulus (CS), such as a neutral tone that does not contain emotional content. The CS is then paired in presentation with a noxious unconditioned stimulus (US), such as an electric shock. The shock innately evokes a defensive response in the subject (e.g. a freezing behaviour in rodents), and after repeated pairings of the CS with the US, the defensive response becomes conditioned to occur when the subject is exposed to the neutral tone alone. The fear-conditioning paradigm is a reliable and methodological way of studying the fear response across species. Neural structures and circuitry recruited during fear conditioning are evolutionarily conserved across species, allowing for us to study the functional mechanisms of the behaviour via the use of animal models, and ultimately translate the acquired knowledge to humans (Armony & Dolan, 2001; reviewed in Armony, 2013).

The fear response in humans can be measured through various changes in the sympathetic nervous system, including blood pressure and regional blood flow, pupil dilation, heart rate, breathing rate, and electrodermal activity (see Winters et al., 2002). Fear conditioning is a simple, yet powerful paradigm, as it allows for conclusions to be drawn from observing subjects' reactions to the same, unchanged stimulus prior to and after the pairing. Investigating how fear is both acquired and extinguished provides valuable insight into neural abnormalities that arise in clinical disorders of fear such as post-traumatic stress disorder (PTSD), phobias, and anxiety (Mahan & Ressler, 2012). The amygdala, hippocampus, and prefrontal cortex are three limbic structures that tend to function irregularly in patients with PTSD. Reduced top–down regulation from the hippocampus and the prefrontal cortex may be responsible for triggering hyperactivation in the amygdala and insula during anxiety disorders, phobias, and PTSD, which in return translates to an overgeneralization of the conditioned fear or sensitization to stress (Etkin & Wager, 2007).

21.3.1 The Amygdala and Fear Conditioning

The amygdala is a small, almond-shaped structure, located deep within the medial part of the temporal lobe (see Figure 21.1). Burdach was the first to identify the small mass of grey matter during the nineteenth century, now referred to as the basolateral complex, one of the three major groups comprising the amygdaloid complex. The centromedial group and the superficial group make up the remaining two major divisions, while additional nuclei have been identified including the amygdalohippocamal area and the intercalated cell masses. The amygdaloid complex is comprised of a collection of approximately thirteen nuclei that fit into the aforementioned clusters, yet their definitive partitioning and categorization is still under debate and remains a general approximation, as investigation in the field continues. The nuclei are further divided into smaller subnuclei that are also characterized by their specific histochemistry and cytoarchitecture (see Sah et al., 2003).

Injecting anterograde and retrograde tracers into various neural regions has enabled the visualization of afferent and efferent connections, spanning between the amygdala and associated structures in the cortical and subcortical layers. Each amygdaloid nucleus sends and receives distinct connections that contribute to their defining role in the overarching processes of the amygdala (see Sah et al., 2003).

During auditory fear conditioning, the initial input signal produced by the CS is received at the cochlear receptors, and is then transmitted to the medial geniculate body (MGB) in the thalamus via the brainstem. Projections from the MGB to the amygdala consist of both a direct and indirect route, in which the direct route typically commences in the medial MGB (MGm) and the posterior intralaminar nucleus (PIN) (LeDoux, 1996). The indirect path originates in various areas throughout the MGB and travels to the auditory cortex, making a number of cortical connections along the way. Input from both the thalamic and cortical

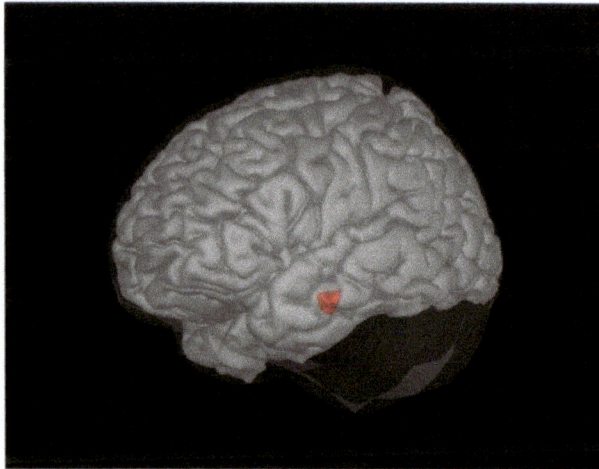

FIGURE 21.1 Sagittal view of 3-D reconstruction of the amygdala in the left hemisphere.

Adapted from Armony J.L. & LeDoux J.E., 'Emotional responses to auditory stimuli', Palmer A.R. & Rees A. (eds), *The Oxford Handbook of Auditory Science: The Auditory Brain*, Copyright © 2010, doi: 10.1093/oxfordhb/9780199233281.013.0019, by permission of Oxford University Press.

paths go to the lateral nucleus of the amygdala (LA) where the paths converge and information from both the US and CS is integrated at a cellular level (Romanski & LeDoux, 1993; Romanski et al., 1993). The complex intra-amygdaloid circuitry facilitates an integration of inputs from functionally diverse amygdaloid nuclei to converge and consolidate information at the central nucleus (CE) (Pitkänen et al., 1997). Efferent fibres travel from the CE, out of the amygdala, and through to the brainstem and the hypothalamus, ultimately to evoke a behavioural response to the stimulus (see Figure 21.2).

During auditory fear conditioning, neural connections within the amygdala, as well as the external network projecting to and from the amygdala, all rely on a strengthening of synapses at their junctions. An essential site for synaptic plasticity occurs at the LA, where synapses are strengthened when the input fibres carrying the acoustic signal and those carrying the somatosensory information converge. When the CS is then presented alone, it is able to elicit a stronger conditioned fear response. The degree of plasticity in the LA during fear conditioning is relative to the rate and temporal accuracy of firing from the thalamus. Synaptic plasticity relies on long-term potentiation (LTP), which occurs when presynaptic activity precedes postsynaptic activity to the degree of milliseconds, also known as *spike-timing-dependent synaptic plasticity*. The postsynaptic N-methyl-D-aspartate (NMDA) receptors act as coincidence detectors, correlating the timing of the presynaptic release of glutamate with the depolarization of the postsynaptic cell. The postsynaptic NMDA receptors bind glutamate and allow for an influx of calcium to occur. This process is only apparent for synaptic plasticity in the LA with inputs coming from the thalamus; LA plasticity from the cortex instead relies on a synchronous pairing of thalamic and cortical presynaptic inputs (for review, see Pape & Paré, 2010).

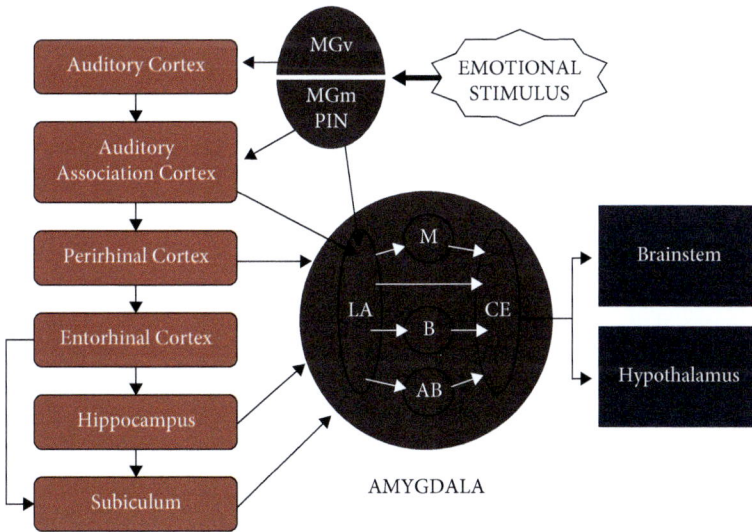

FIGURE 21.2 A basic schematic of the neural circuitry involved in emotional processing of auditory emotional information.

LA: lateral nucleus of the amygdala; CE: central nucleus of the amygdala

Adapted from Armony J.L. & LeDoux J.E., 'Emotional responses to auditory stimuli', Palmer A.R. & Rees A. (eds), *The Oxford Handbook of Auditory Science: The Auditory Brain*, Copyright © 2010, doi: 10.1093/oxfordhb/9780199233281.013.0019, by permission of Oxford University Press.

The role of the LA in fear conditioning is critical, and if lesioned prior to training or if transiently inactivated, can inhibit the fear acquisition entirely. Similar findings have been found for the CE and its role in plasticity during fear conditioning (for review, see Paré et al., 2004). LeDoux (2000) proposed that the LA and CE play the most prominent part in fear conditioning, in which the LA is required for integrating sensory information, while the CE drives the motor response.

Lesion studies have helped shape our understanding of fear conditioning in the amygdala. Most lesion studies are done using non-human primates and rodent models, as the neural structures and functions are highly translatable to humans. Antoniadis et al. (2007) conducted a study with rhesus monkeys, in which they identified that through lesioning the bilateral amygdala, they could inhibit the acquisition of the fear startle-response provoked by a noxious air puff (US) that had been paired with a light presentation (CS). The study also identified that the retention of the fear startle-response could be spared if the amygdala was lesioned post conditioning. This behavioural deficit has been similarly illustrated in rats, in which the fear response of freezing was significantly decreased when the rats had undergone bilateral amygdala lesions (Blanchard & Blanchard, 1972). Lesioning the contralateral auditory cortex and the unilateral medial geniculate body in the thalamus of rats, after training in an auditory fear-conditioning paradigm, can lead to a complete abolition of the freezing behaviour. However, if the auditory cortex remains intact, and if instead the MGm is lesioned, small traces of the fear response can be conserved (Boatman & Kim, 2006). These findings stress the integral involvement of varied neural structures along the processing pathway and the degree of contribution that each provides to processing auditory emotional information.

21.4 HUMAN LESION STUDIES

Using human lesion studies to explore the function of the amygdala during emotional processing of acoustic information has proven difficult, with a number of inconsistent findings. Patients with bilateral or unilateral damage to the amygdala do not always present deficits while processing said information. It was suggested that other extra-amygdala structures in the right hemisphere, such as the basal ganglia, may play a more pertinent role during this processing (Adolphs & Tranel, 1999; Anderson & Phelps, 2002). However, as research in the field continues, we are finding that these incongruities are more likely to be attributed to variation in the severity and expanse of damage across patients, as many of the lesions extend beyond the boundaries of the amygdala (Adolphs & Tranel, 1999).

The first study to identify positive results for amygdala involvement was conducted by Scott et al. (1997), in which a patient with bilateral damage to the amygdala was incapable of perceiving varied intonations in human speech, hindering their capacity to comprehend emotion, as portrayed through the voice. The patient's damage extended only to the recognition of fear and anger, as they were able to understand expressions of positive affect, such as happiness. The deficit in their vocal perception was comparable to their visual deficit, specifically to emotions expressed via faces. Sprengelmeyer et al. (1999) further replicated these results with a patient having more extensive damage, encompassing the bilateral amygdala and part of the left thalamus. This patient was unable to recognize fear as expressed through faces, body postures, and non-verbal auditory emotion, yet was not inhibited when perceiving anger.

Surrounding limbic structures are a source of frequent inquiry, as lesions of the amygdala largely spill over to encompass these neighbouring regions. The hippocampus is one of these nearby structures, with strong connections to the amygdala, and is cohesive in nature as pertaining to emotional processing. Bechara et al. (1995) made efforts to parse apart the role of the amygdala and hippocampus during fear conditioning by contrasting the behavioural results of three patients with varying lesion compositions of the amygdala and hippocampus. The first, a patient with bilateral damage to the amygdala, yet intact hippocampus, did not produce an elevated autonomic response (skin conductance response) when the US (a noxious sound) was paired with the CS (tone). Conversely, the patient was able to gain declarative facts about the CS. The second patient, with exclusively bilateral hippocampal damage, could not gain declarative facts, but was conditioned to the tone. The final participant, with bilateral lesions to both the amygdala and hippocampus, could neither acquire the conditioning nor the declarative facts.

These findings suggest that the amygdala may be critical for forming associations between external cues and internal affect, while the hippocampus may have more involvement in creating connections among external cues. The amygdala has been proposed to make a greater contribution to the crude processing of emotion in voice, while the involvement of the hippocampus is attuned to more complicated deconstruction of the stimulus, integrating contextual information and associated memories. Increased neural activation is seen in the hippocampus in response to both positive and negative forms of laughter, supporting the notion that contextual information, critical for understanding the intent behind the laughter, may be integrated at the level of the hippocampus (for review, see Frühholz et al., 2014).

Beyond demarcating functional boundaries within the limbic system, lesion studies have also allowed for the investigation of lateralization in regards to emotional processing. Kucharska-Pietura et al. (2003) studied patients with unilateral lesions, to identify if lateralization was evident during the processing of emotional expressions presented via faces or voices. The location and extent of the damage varied across participants, but was limited to a single hemisphere. Patients with left-hemispheric lesions performed worse than controls during a prosodic emotion-recognition task, and relatively equivalent to controls when processing facial expressions. This observed difference of processing in the left hemisphere maintains the notion that it may have a more pertinent role in processing emotions acoustically, rather than visually, at least in regards to speech. Interestingly, individuals with right-hemispheric damage performed significantly worse at the emotion-recognition task, regardless of the modality. This prominent deficit seen in individuals with specifically right-hemispheric lesions, is consistent with the findings of a lesion study consisting of sixty-six patients with focal brain damage in varying regions throughout the brain. The lesioned areas were mapped and correlated with the participants' performances on an emotion-recognition task using auditory stimuli. The documented overlap across participants illustrated the involvement of an extensive neural network for processing emotional prosody, including the frontal lobe and parietal lobe in the right hemisphere (Adolphs et al., 2002).

Lesion studies have provided the groundwork for cataloguing functional differences across limbic structures, and for acknowledging a congruency between lesion size and the magnitude of impairment during affective processing. The development of neuroimaging tools has allowed for this knowledge to be translated to healthy populations, where investigative questions can be moulded with respect to the precise structure and function of interest. The assessments can be replicated extensively within and across subjects, ensuring reliability of the observations and allowing for a more comprehensive outlook on emotional processing.

21.5 NEURAL CONNECTIVITY AND NEUROIMAGING

The greater involvement of the right hemisphere during processing emotional prosody has been refuted via a model developed by Schirmer and Kotz (2006) that proposes the engagement of more intricate hierarchical processing. The model provides a rationalization for the variability in neural activation depicted across the literature and accounts for the variation of task requirements, the context, and individual differences of the participant.

The model consists of three hierarchical steps, where the first level is ascribed to the crude processing of auditory information—deconstructing the sound into its rudimentary acoustical properties. This process has been suggested to take place in the primary auditory cortex and, to some extent, the secondary auditory cortex. The secondary auditory cortex is suggested to have a more extensive role at the subsequent level, where it continues to break the sound down into more complex features. It categorizes and integrates the information from a series of inputs, and forms defined acoustic entities that are representative of specific emotions. The superior temporal sulcus (STS) has been recognized as the voice-sensitive region of the auditory cortex. Specifically, the bilateral upper region of the central part of the STS has shown an elevated neural response to vocal sounds (speech or vocalizations) as compared to non-verbal environmental sounds (Belin et al., 2000).

The final step of the model involves higher-order cognition in anterior areas, including the inferior frontal areas and the orbitofrontal cortex (OFC). This level of processing has strong influences of top–down control, integrating information from the task and the context as to modify the individuals' subjective perceptions. It is proposed that evaluative judgements about the prosodic emotions are made in the right inferior frontal gyrus (IFG) and OFC. Such judgements also suggest that language processing and information from the emotional voice are integrated within the left IFG (for review, see Schirmer & Kotz, 2006).

This model does not include involvement of the amygdala; however, recent findings obtained through advanced methodology and with the use of appropriate controls have justified the need to incorporate amygdala involvement into the model. Interestingly, individuals with schizophrenia, a disorder presenting deficits of emotional interpretation, present abnormalities in the neural fibres between the MGB and the auditory cortex, and from the auditory cortex to temporal and inferior frontal areas (the ventral and dorsal auditory streams), as seen with diffusion tensor MRI fractional anisotropy. These deficits are also highly correlated with irregularities in white matter clusters lateral to the amygdala. Thus, the alternative method of exploring structure and function within white-matter tracts provides additional evidence for the involvement of auditory and amygdala pathways in the processing of acoustic emotional information (Leitman et al., 2007).

21.5.1 The Amygdala

Analogous to lesion studies, functional neuroimaging research has produced a number of mixed results regarding the role of the amygdala in processing auditory emotional information. Phillips et al. (1998) conducted an fMRI study, observing bilateral activation in response to both fearful faces and vocalizations, in comparison to moderately happy faces and voices. In contrast to these findings, Morris et al. (1999) completed a positron emission tomography (PET) study, in which they saw a decreased response to fearful vocalizations compared to voices expressing happiness, sadness, or neutrality. There are a number of theories proposed as to explain these incongruities, yet the amygdala remains an area of constant investigation.

The inconsistent findings can be attributed to a number of confounding factors, such as individual differences, unaccounted for adaptation effects, or inefficient controls. Most studies use a control condition through a subtractive approach, in which the emotional stimulus is compared to the control, as to isolate neural regions that are responsive to solely that emotion (reviewed in Armony & LeDoux, 2010). Sergerie et al. (2008) conducted a quantitative meta-analysis of functional neuroimaging studies that investigated the role of the amygdala, in response to visual emotional information. In this analysis they recognized that the amygdala is particularly dependent on the type of control condition that is used, as this choice has a direct impact on whether the effects reach statistical significance. For studies of acoustic emotional processing, these controls have been seen to vary from neutral prosody to silence. It is also highly likely that the salience of the stimuli and the level of attention required for the task, both control and experimental, would influence the neural response of the subject (Bach, Grandjean, et al., 2008; Leitman et al., 2010).

These shortcomings are seen in the early fear-conditioning literature, which have dispensed a biased understanding of the amygdala's function, encouraging the widespread acceptance of its role as a 'fear detector'. Its consistent involvement in processing faces and voices with negative affect in these studies has discouraged the possibility of its impartiality to emotional valence. This ideology has more recently transformed, as there has been greater investigation into the valence of emotion when processing the voice. An fMRI study conducted by Fecteau et al. (2007) looked at the neural response to positive, negative, and neutral vocalizations (e.g. laughing, crying, screaming). The study used appropriate controls, in which the stimuli were taken from a previously validated database, where neutral vocalizations were used as the control condition, and the vocalizations were produced by a number of different speakers. In addition, the presentation order of the stimuli was pseudo-randomized, as to reduce habituation and expectancy effects. Fecteau and colleagues (2007) observed bilateral activation in the amygdala for both positive and negative emotional vocalizations (see Figure 21.3).

Since then, similar findings have been replicated, in which bilateral activation of the amygdala occurred in response to the emotional voice (Wiethoff et al., 2009). One fMRI study required the participants to listen to a 19-minute audio drama that expressed varied emotions in the form of narrations, dialogue, as well as non-speech environmental sounds.

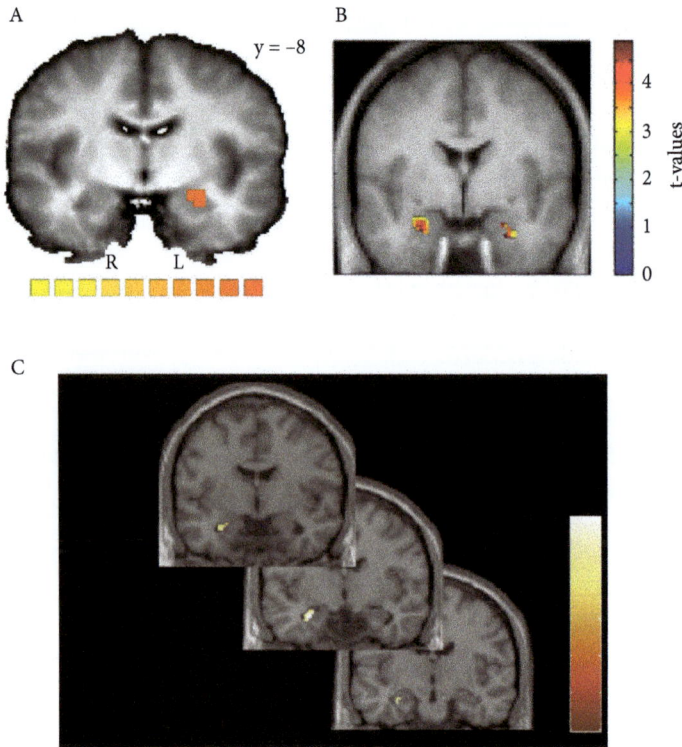

FIGURE 21.3 (A) Left amygdala activation, with the main effect of emotional–neutral ([−2, −10, −21], $F_{(1,19)}$ = 31.8). (B) Bilateral amygdala activation, with the main effect of emotional–neutral vocalizations ([−22 4 −22], Z = 3.51; [26 0 −26], Z = 4.24). (C) Activation clusters in the left amygdala, with the main effect of fearful–neutral emotional expression across faces, voices, and music ([−28 −8 −22], Z = 4.79).

(A) Reproduced from Mothes-Lasch M., Becker M.P.I., Miltner W.H.R, & Straube T., 'Neural basis of processing threatening voices in a crowded auditory world', *Social Cognitive and Affective Neuroscience*, Volume 11, Issue 5, pp. 821–8, Copyright © 2016, doi: 10.1093/scan/nsw022, by permission of Oxford University Press.

(B) Reprinted from *NeuroImage*, Volume 36, Issue 2, Fecteau S., Belin P., Joanette Y., & Armony J.L., 'Amygdala responses to nonlinguistic emotional vocalizations', pp. 480–7, Copyright © 2007 Elsevier Inc., with permission from Elsevier, http://www.sciencedirect.com/science/article/pii/S1053811907001656.

(C) Reprinted from Aubé W., Angulo-Perkins A., Peretz I., Concha L., & Armony J.L., 'Fear across the senses: brain responses to music, vocalizations and facial expressions', *Social Cognitive and Affective Neuroscience*, Volume 10, Issue 3, pp. 399–407, Copyright © 2014, doi: 10.1093/scan/nsu067, by permission of Oxford University Press.

The audio drama produced an increased activation in temporal, parietal, and frontal lobes, as well as the cingulate cortex and the amygdala. An intersubject-correlation map identified a strong synchronization across subjects in the amygdala in response to the emotion portrayed throughout the dialogue (Boldt et al., 2013).

Sander et al. (2005) identified activation in the right amygdala and bilateral STS in response to pseudo-utterances expressed with anger, regardless of whether the participants were attending to the sounds or not. The level of attention directed towards the emotional auditory cue can significantly alter the magnitude of response. This was illustrated with observable heightened activation in the OFC and cuneus of the medial occipital cortex, when focus was brought to the stimulus.

21.5.1.1 *Implications of Attention in Emotional Processing*

Variations in experimental design can significantly impact the data acquired during neuroimaging studies, when the emotional information can be processed either with or without conscious awareness. Neuroimaging studies of emotional processing may require the participants' complete attention for the duration of the task, while others may only need the participant to be passively observing the emotional stimulus, or even ignoring it entirely. A number of studies have investigated appraisal processing with emotional cues (i.e. the subjective evaluation of one's emotional reaction to an event), and whether the neural response differs when necessitating explicit or implicit attention to the task.

Bach, Grandjean, et al. (2008) conducted an fMRI study that used an implicit (low-level appraisal) task, instructing the participant to attend to and discriminate the gender of the speaker, and an explicit (high-level appraisal) task that required the participant to label the emotion expressed by the speaker via their vocal prosody. Irrespective of attention, the superior temporal gyrus (STG), bilateral anterior cingulate, left IFG, insula, and bilateral putamen showed greater activation in response to emotional (anger and fear) versus neutral prosody (pseudo-speech). Interestingly, there was significantly greater bilateral activation in the amygdala, the left STS, and areas within the right parietal lobe during the implicit processing task, while the explicit processing task produced observable differences in the left IFG, bilateral parietal, anterior cingulate, and supplementary motor areas. During the explicit processing task, emotional prosody evoked a greater response in the basal ganglia and right anterior cingulate, than neutral prosody. These findings support the existence of an amygdala–prefrontal–cingulate network for varying appraisal levels, in which high-level appraisal processing occurs in the frontal and cingulate regions, while the amygdala is recruited for low-level appraisal processing. This pattern may be a reflection of top–down control of the prefrontal cortex over the amygdala.

Ethofer et al. (2009) conducted an fMRI study in which they gave the task of judging the emotional prosody as being either negative or neutral (explicit), or of classifying words into adjectives or nouns (implicit). Consistent with the previous study, neural activation was stronger in response to angry versus neutral prosody in the amygdala, insula, and mediodorsal thalami, regardless of the task. The right middle temporal gyrus and bilateral OFC demonstrated greater activation during the emotional task than the word classification. These results align with the notion that low-level processing of emotional information occurs in regions such as the posterior STS and the amygdala, while explicit processing recruits higher-level processing areas, including the OFC and IFG.

Interestingly, recent studies have demonstrated opposing results in which, when attention is paid to the affect expressed through the voice, there is a stronger observable neural response in the amygdala than when one does not focus on the emotion. This was identified in an fMRI study conducted by Mothes-Lasch et al. (2016), in which the participants were required to attend to angry and neutral prosody that were played concurrently with complex non-speech background sounds, as to reflect a natural auditory environment. They identified that, regardless of the background complexity, the amygdala and the anterior superior temporal cortex demonstrated a greater neural response to angry versus neutral prosody (see Figure 21.3). In contrast, when the level of attention paid to the emotional prosody was lowered, the observable difference between angry and neutral prosody diminished (Mothes-Lasch et al., 2016).

A similar study looked at the neural response to angry and neutral prosody, but, rather, using a visual distractor, as to determine whether there were effects of attentional demand across modalities, while processing emotional prosody. The findings demonstrated that, similar to the auditory-only task, there was greater activation in the amygdala and the auditory cortex in response to angry versus neutral prosody when attention was paid to the prosody, but not when the attention was placed on the visual stimulus (Mothes-Lasch et al., 2011).

These experimental designs differ from the earlier studies, as they require the participant to process two types of stimuli simultaneously, rather than attending to separate attributes of the same stimulus. It is plausible that there is different neural circuitry involved during these two types of tasks that could explain why, unlike the earlier studies, the latter were able to elicit an increased activation in the amygdala in response to angry prosody.

21.5.1.2 *Individual Differences*

There are a number of factors, both inherent and learned, that could influence one's capacity to detect and process emotional information. Examples of these considerations include one's sex, degree of emotional intelligence, level of neuroticism or anxiety, and cultural background. It is essential that there is a high variability in the pool of stimuli as to avoid participant bias, as a particular stimulus may be meaningful to some and novel and/or irrelevant to others. It is plausible that the neural responses are influenced by these personal biases, which emphasizes the importance of appropriate controls and variation within the design.

Gender differences have been identified in an EEG experiment, in which the participants were required to recognize changes in the emotional tone of a voice while attending to another stimulus. The mismatch negativity (MMN), a neural correlate that detects preattentive change to the auditory emotional stimuli, was much larger in women than men, in response to emotional versus neutral prosody excerpts. Both sexes were able to identify changes in the voice, yet only women were able to identify the specific change of emotional valence in the voice (Schirmer et al., 2005).

Emotional processing of affective prosody can also vary across individuals based on their social orientation, defined by Schirmer et al. (2008) as a way of quantifying an individual's awareness and concern for others. Schirmer and colleagues implemented an fMRI study that uncovered differences across participants with varying social orientations. Emotional prosody elicited greater activation in the right amygdala and bilateral OFC than neutral prosody, and was positively correlated with one's social-orientation score. Individuals with a higher social-orientation score were more attuned to subtle fluctuations in the emotional vocalizations. It can therefore be suggested that greater involvement of the amygdala and higher-order structures are required during the recognition and processing of emotions.

Similar findings were observed in individuals who scored highly for neuroticism on a standardized self-report questionnaire about personality traits. A positive correlation was identified between the degree of neuroticism and the haemodynamic response in the right amygdala, left post-central gyrus, and structures in the frontal lobe (Brück et al., 2011). Individuals expressing traits of anxiety also tend to have a more heightened perception of emotional content. An EEG experiment studied participants' heart rate acceleration and their MMN, and compared this data to their individual anxiety states. A positive correlation was detected between the large MMN in the right frontal regions to angry voice deviants and an acceleration in heart rate, which were both further elevated with a high state of anxiety (Schirmer & Escoffier, 2010).

More extensively, collective differences in the processing of acoustic emotions have been recognized between populations. East-Asian cultures are more influenced by vocal emotional cues during social communication than individuals in a Western culture (Liu et al., 2015). These disparities across participants, based on their personality, gender, or cultural background, each emphasize the importance of having a diverse and controlled study population when investigating emotional perception.

21.5.1.3 *Emotional Salience and Intensity*

A study conducted by Leitman et al. (2010) using fMRI techniques investigated the saliency of acoustic cues reflective of natural emotional communication. As noted previously, there are a number of attributes of vocal expression that allow us to categorize different expressed emotions, including the quality of the voice, the pitch, and the intensity. Therefore, high-salient affective cues are ones that are clearly defined and easily distinguishable, being rich in relevant information. Low-salient cues tend to be ambiguous and contain qualities that may be conflicting or irrelevant, preventing the categorization of emotions. This study varied the level of saliency for each of the emotions—happiness, fear, anger, and neutrality. Saliency was modified through increasing or decreasing the acoustic attribute that best correlated with each emotion, as determined during an emotion-identification task. The neural activation in response to these changes was observed. The most identifiable and discriminatory cue for happiness and fear was the variability in pitch (fundamental frequency), while the proportion of high-frequency spectral energy is the most recognizable characteristic for anger. In response to saliently rich cues, there was a stronger activation in the STC, specifically the planum temporale, the posterior STG, and the posterior middle gyrus, as well as the amygdala. Low-salient stimuli were correlated with activation in the inferior frontal and temporo-frontal areas.

The increased activation in the amygdala and temporal cortex suggests that there may be increased sensory integration with acoustic cues that are rich in emotional information. Acoustic cues that are not highly salient require greater recruitment of these neural structures, such as the IFG and its connections to the STG. The strength of the IFG–STG connection is inversely correlated with the saliency level of the emotional stimulus, as determined by a psychophysiological interaction (PPI) functional connectivity analysis (Friston et al., 1997; Leitman et al., 2010). These findings are in support of the model devised by Schirmer and Kotz (2006), where lower sensory processing occurs, proceeded by the decoding and integration of salient acoustic attributes as to form an emotional acoustic entity. The acoustic object is then received at the level of the IFG, which is suggested to play a role in more effortful higher-order evaluations of emotional information.

Further to acknowledging the significance of stimulus saliency, the rising intensity of auditory cues can act as an efficient way of detecting threat, as it triggers an autonomic orientating reflex and quicker reaction times for reallocating attention. It elicits increased activation in the right amygdala and right intraparietal sulcus, left STS, and left temporal plane—structures commonly identified in the emotional processing circuit. These findings are cohesive with evolutionary rationalization, in which sounds with a rising intensity would signify an approaching threat, while a falling intensity may portray a retreating threat (Bach, Schachinger, et al., 2008).

21.5.1.4 *Adaptation Effects*

When designing a study that investigates emotional processing, it is imperative to account for the behaviour of the blood oxygen level dependent (BOLD) signal, which reflects an accumulation of the neural activity in response to a given stimulus. Neuronal adaptation can be observed when the same, or a similar stimulus is presented successively. The neurons are expected to habituate to the stimulus, which consequently reduces the observed BOLD signal. Neural habituation in the amygdala was originally observed in the visual domain, with participants demonstrating adaptation to both fearful and neutral facial expressions (Breiter et al., 1996). This behaviour has since been seen in studies using emotional prosody that explore adaptation effects via an expansive range of vocal emotions, including anger, fear, happiness, eroticism, and neutrality. Neutral words without meaning were spoken in these varying emotions, and all but happy prosody produced a reduced BOLD response, depictive of neural repetition suppression. Habituation to angry and erotic prosody was identified within the bilateral amygdala (Wiethoff et al., 2009).

In recognizing the effects of neural adaptation during processing of emotional prosody, neuroimaging paradigms have been strategically developed to encompass these changes. Bestelmeyer et al. (2010) employed an adaptation paradigm to identify the occurrence of vocal emotional after-effects, in which the vocalizations were presented on an anger–fear morph continuum. The stimulus attributes were synthetically manipulated to vary in the degree in which they could be distinguished as either fear or anger. The results confirmed that when participants are exposed to a repeated presentation of a single emotion, they will habituate to this emotion. The boundary, at which they perceive the stimulus as 'affectively ambiguous', shifts or recalibrates in the direction of the repeated stimulus. For example, after habituating to the presentation of angry vocalizations, the participant will perceive the ambiguous stimulus as being more fearful than it actually is, and vice versa. Thus, this habituation behaviour can complicate studies that attempt to parse apart the neural structures responsive to various emotions, and must be accounted for in the design to ensure accuracy of the results.

An additional fMRI study conducted by Bestelmeyer and colleagues employed a similar continuous carry-over design using the vocalizations from the anger–fear morph continuum. The continuous carry-over design involves a consecutive presentation of stimuli, whose sequence has been pseudo-randomized and counterbalanced, as to study the effect that one stimulus may have on the following presented stimulus (Aguirre, 2007). The analysis allowed for the adaptation effects of the emotional vocalizations to be dissociated, as to isolate the neuronal habituation in response to the acoustic attributes versus the changes in affect. Adaptation effects for the 'physical' acoustic attributes were observed in the right amygdala and in the bilateral STS and STG, while habituation to the 'perceived' emotional information was more dispersed, as seen in the bilateral anterior insula, precentral gyrus, medial superior frontal cortex, and other subcortical regions. This is consistent with the earlier literature that depicts auditory regions and the amygdala to be associated with primary processing stages of the acoustic stimuli, while frontal regions are more involved in the complex perception of emotions (Bestelmeyer et al., 2014).

21.5.1.5 *Amygdala Subnuclei*

The amygdala consists of a number of functionally diverse subnuclei, each with a unique network of connections. In recent years, there has been a growing curiosity as to whether these distinctions underwrite the inconsistencies seen in research concerning emotional processing of the voice. *In vivo* tractography has allowed for the amygdala to be grouped into two subregions based on their cortical connections. Strong networks are seen between superficial amygdala nuclei (e.g. centromedial and cortical) and the lateral orbitofrontal cortex, while deep amygdala nuclei (e.g. basolateral) have more connections with multimodal temporal regions (Bach et al., 2011).

Retrograde tracing in the amygdala has demonstrated that the basolateral group acts as the main source of direct input for emotional sensory information. It consists of the LA, the basal (B) nucleus located ventral to the LA, and the accessory basal (AB) nucleus. The prefrontal cortex provides extensive cortical input to the amygdala, as it receives sensory information from a number of modalities. These projections from the prefrontal cortex typically arrive in the basal nucleus, but also go to the LA, accessory basal, central, and medial (M) nuclei. Long-term declarative memory involves the input to the amygdala from the perirhinal cortex, the entorhinal cortex, the hippocampus, and the parahippocampal cortex (for review, see Sah et al., 2003).

A high-resolution fMRI study conducted by Frühholz and Grandjean (2013) used threatening voices to assess adaptation and sensitivity to certain subregions of the amygdala. The bilateral superficial (SF) complex, and the right laterobasal (LB) complex demonstrated the largest BOLD response when presented with emotional prosody. The results were amplified when attention was explicitly directed towards the emotional quality of the stimulus, particularly in the right LB complex. Neural adaptation was observed in the bilateral SF complexes when the participant was exposed to the repeated presentation of an emotional stimulus (threatening voice preceded by a threatening voice). Sensitization to the fearful stimulus was detected in the right SF complexes when a threatening voice was preceded by a neutral voice, while a decrease in activation occurred within the right SF and LB when a neutral voice was preceded by a threatening voice, illustrating desensitization to the fearful voice. The observable differences of the BOLD response between the SF and the LB, demonstrate functional variation across subnuclei. These dissimilarities illustrate that the subnuclei may be 'learning' differently and that the novelty of the stimulus can have implications for the behaviour of the subnuclei. Thus, this data supports the role of the amygdala as a novelty detector and proposes that the SF complex may be responsible for decoding the emotional attributes of a stimulus. The LB complex is highly connected to sensory cortices (particularly the LB in the right amygdala) and may be involved in decoding acoustic patterns of the voice (Frühholz & Grandjean, 2013). These findings emphasize the importance of high spatial resolution in neuroimaging, as to account for the functional heterogeneity of underlying structures that are responsive to emotional prosody.

An alternative approach has been to use single-neuron recordings with non-human primates, which has allowed for the identification of differences in the amygdala in response to emotional faces versus voices. Kuraoka and Nakamura (2007) found that 77% of neurons responded to faces alone, while 20% responded to both faces and voices, and 1% to solely voices. The neurons demonstrating supramodal responses were located in the central nucleus, the receiving site for the other amygdala subnuclei. It is plausible that the information acquired by the voice, such as a threatening scream, requires the monkey to respond more rapidly than to a visual stimulus alone. Thus the central nucleus would output the emotional information directly to subcortical structures, such as the thalamus, hypothalamus, or brainstem.

21.5.2 The Voice and Music

In addition to auditory perception of vocalizations and prosody, music is an auditory stimulus that can evoke emotion in the listener, without contextual information (Vieillard et al., 2008). Music maintains much interest in the field of affective acoustic processing, as there is no known evolutionary basis for its presence. Similarly to vocal intonations, changes in tempo or mode (minor or major) can alter one's emotional perception of the music, and moreover elicit activation in the associated neural regions (Khalfa et al., 2005). An fMRI study, where participants were required to listen to consonant (pleasant) and dissonant (unpleasant) music, demonstrated increased activation within the amygdala, as well as connecting structures, including the hippocampus, parahippocampus, and temporal poles (Koeslch, 2006).

Much of the affective acoustic processing literature circles around regions of the brain that are responsive to both music and speech, such as the bilateral superior temporal lobe. This is likely due to the similarities in acoustic structure of the sounds, and the need for hierarchical deconstruction and processing. Novel imaging techniques have allowed us to identify whether this observed sharing of neural structures that are involved in music and vocal processing may actually be representative of neural overlap occurring in response to these subsets of auditory stimuli (Peretz et al., 2015). These findings are depicted in recent literature that employed an adaptation-fMRI paradigm with the objective of spatially separating the neural response to music and voice. Interestingly, an area within the anterior STG was found to respond more robustly to music than to voice. This adaptation effect was exposed by contrasting the amplitude of the BOLD signal that reflected the neuronal response to a music stimulus preceded by a music stimulus, versus music preceded by voice (Armony et al., 2015). Our group is currently employing this paradigm to the use of emotional stimuli, as to identify if emotional prosody and music can produce similar findings of neural specificity.

Alternative analysis techniques devised for use in concert with functional neuroimaging practices, such as multivoxel pattern analysis (MVPA), have identified similar findings. Rogalsky et al. (2011) utilized MVPA and found differences in activation patterns in response to music and speech within the anticipated overlapping region of the STG. Additionally, they distinguished that prosody was processed in more ventrolateral regions of the auditory cortex, while music produced a greater response in the dorsomedial regions and into the parietal lobe.

Beyond the similarities of neural activity elicited from musical and vocal emotional information, further studies have found common patterns of activation across modalities.

A recent fMRI study explored the response to emotional stimuli of varying modalities that were presented independently of one another. Exposure to emotional faces, music, and voices produced a shared activation in the posterior amygdala, anterior hippocampus, and posterior insula (see Figure 21.3). This response was particular to fearful stimuli, as happy, sad, and neutral stimuli did not produce activation to the same effect (Aubé et al., 2015).

A similar fMRI study used MVPA to find parallels in the neural response to emotional information conveyed through facial expressions, body language, and voice. This study presented auditory and visual stimuli simultaneously to reflect a characteristic natural environment. They found that regardless of the modality in which the information was portrayed, significant activation was identified in the medial prefrontal cortex (Peelen et al., 2010). Through integrating the simultaneous presentation of auditory and visual information, the ability to correctly classify the emotions increased significantly. The more sensory information that is provided, the easier it is to depict the emotion that is being expressed. The participants demonstrated an increase in activation within the bilateral posterior STG and the right thalamus when presented with the audiovisual stimuli, in comparison to the emotion presented unimodally. There were also observable connections that were strengthened between the auditory processing regions (STG) and the ipsilateral fusiform gyrus (visual processing), with the pSTS (adjacent to the pSTG), signifying the possibility of audiovisual integration (Kreifelts et al., 2007).

21.6 Conclusion

Our voice is a critical tool for social communication with our peers, allowing for an improved understanding of others' intentions and thus, the strengthening of interpersonal relationships. Individuals with affective disorders typically have difficulties accurately depicting and processing emotions, and therefore struggle to find the appropriate social response. These challenges may even cause individuals to isolate themselves, which can further intensify their impairments. Our understanding of how we interpret vocal cues and the concomitant underlying neural structures can assist us in targeting specific regions for intervention, as well as to provide a more comprehensive outlook on the functionality of the emotional processing network and its unified parts.

Vocalizations parallel emotion conveyed through the face, and prompt similar neural pathways throughout the brain. These vocalizations are more innate than speech, and may require more low-level processing, similar to that of our evolutionary predecessors. Comparatively, prosody provides us with a more complex understanding of the individual's intentions. The patterns formed through fluctuations in pitch, quality, rhythm, and volume allow for the categorization of the speech into a specific emotion, regardless of the actual dialogue. This decoding and processing has proven to involve higher-order structures that integrate information about context and that from our working memory. Thus the involved cerebral network is extensive, branching to include a number of cortical and subcortical structures. The amygdala and its functionally diverse subnuclei reflect the complexity involved in processing emotional information.

The controversy around the contribution of the amygdala appeared after numerous lesion and neuroimaging studies had acquired mixed results. Much of the discrepancies have been identified through variation in experimental design, such as the task, the controls used, the stimuli selected, or the diverse ensemble of participants in the testing population. It is important to control for these parameters that are commonly disregarded, and to design the experiment using a rigorous and methodical approach (Armony & LeDoux, 2010). The deviation in experimental design, as seen in the current literature, provides a platform for recognizing factors that may affect the interpretation of the results, specific to the research questions posed in the study.

The involvement of the amygdala in a complex emotional-processing network, formed by several hierarchical levels, is reinforced when the aforementioned technical issues are accounted for. Its strong connections and correlated activity with the auditory cortex, surrounding limbic structures, and frontal regions, during auditory emotional processing, supports the notion of its role as a novelty or relevance detector. The functionality of the amygdala extends beyond processing fearful information, to processing emotions of both positive and negative valence that are significantly relevant for learning about and adapting to one's social environment. Auditory emotional information portrayed through the voice has significant social benefits when it is accurately processed and perceived by the receiving party. Its similar processing pathway to that of musical information encourages the idea that music may make a more sophisticated contribution to social communication than what is currently projected.

REFERENCES

Adolphs, R., Damasio, H., & Tranel, D. (2002). Neural systems for recognition of emotional prosody: a 3-D lesion study. *Emotion*, 2(1), 23–51.

Adolphs, R. & Tranel, D. (1999). Intact recognition of emotional prosody following amygdala damage. *Neuropsychologia*, 37(11), 1285–1292.

Adolphs, R., Tranel, D., Damasio, H., & Damasio, A. R. (1995). Fear and the human amygdala. *The Journal of Neuroscience*, 15(9), 5879–5891.

Aguirre, G. K. (2007). Continuous carry-over designs for fMRI. *NeuroImage*, 35(4), 1480–1494.

Anderson, A. K. & Phelps, E. A. (2002). Is the human amygdala critical for the subjective experience of emotion? Evidence of intact dispositional affect in patients with amygdala lesions. *Journal of Cognitive Neuroscience*, 14(5), 709–720.

Antoniadis, E. A., Winslow, J. T., Davis, M., & Amaral, D. G. (2007). Role of the primate amygdala in fear-potentiated startle: effects of chronic lesions in the rhesus monkey. *The Journal of Neuroscience*, 27(28), 7386–7396.

Armony, J. L. (2013). Current emotion research in behavioural neuroscience: the role(s) of the amygdala. *Emotion Review*, 5(1), 104–115.

Armony, J. L., Aubé, W., Angulo-Perins, A., Peretz, I., & Concha, L. (2015). The specificity of neural responses to music and their relation to voice processing: an fMRI-adaptation study. *Neuroscience Letters*, 593, 35–39.

Armony, J. L., Chochol, C., Fecteau, S., & Belin, P. (2007). Laugh (or cry) and you will be remembered: influence of emotional expression on memory for vocalizations. *Psychology Science*, 18(12), 1027–1029.

Armony, J. L. & Dolan, R. J. (2001). Modulation of auditory neural responses by a visual context in human fear conditioning. *NeuroReport*, 12(15), 3407–3411.

Armony, J. L. & LeDoux, J. E. (2010). Emotional response to auditory stimuli. In: A. Palmer & A. Rees (eds) *Oxford Handbook of Auditory Science: The Auditory Brain* (pp. 479–505). Oxford, UK: Oxford University Press.

Armony, J. L. & LeDoux, J. E. (1997). How the brain processes emotional information. *Annals of the New York Academy of Sciences*, 821, 259–270.

Aubé, W., Angulo-Perkins, A., Peretz, I., Concha, L., & Armony, J. L. (2015). Fear across the senses: brain responses to music, vocalizations and facial expressions. *Social Cognitive and Affective Neuroscience*, 10(3), 399–407.

Aubé, W., Peretz, I., & Armony, J. L. (2013). The effects of emotion on memory for music and vocalisations. *Memory*, 21(8), 981–990.

Bach, D. R., Behrens, T. E., Garrido, L., Weiskopf, N., & Dolan, R. J. (2011). Deep and superficial amygdala nuclei projections revealed *in vivo* by probabilistic tractography. *The Journal of Neuroscience*, 31(2), 618–623.

Bach, D. R., Grandjean, D., Sander, D., Herdener, M., Strik W. K., & Selfrtiz, E. (2008). The effect of appraisal level on processing of emotional prosody in meaning speech. *NeuroImage*, 42(2), 919–927.

Bach, D. R., Schachinger, H., Neuhoff, J. G., Esposito, F., Di Salle, F., Lehmann, C., ... Seifritz, E. (2008). Rising sound intensity: an intrinsic warning cue activating the amygdala. *Cerebral Cortex*, 18(1), 145–150.

Banse, R. & Scherer, K. R. (1996). Acoustic profiles in vocal emotion expression. *Journal of Personality and Social Psychology*, 70(3), 614–636.

Bechara, A., Tranel, D., Damasio, H., Adolphs, R., Rockland C., & Damasio, A. R. (1995). Double dissociation of conditioning and declarative knowledge relative to the amygdala and hippocampus in humans. *Science*, 269(5227), 1115–1118.

Belin, P., Fecteau, S., & Bedard, C. (2004). Thinking the voice: neural correlates of voice perception. *Trends in Cognitive Sciences*, 8(3), 129–135.

Belin, P. & Zatorre, R. J. (2000). Voice-selective areas in human auditory cortex. *Nature*, 309.

Bestelmeyer, P. E., Maurage, P., Rouger, J., Latinus, M., & Belin, P. (2014). Adaptation to vocal expressions reveals multistep perception of auditory emotion. *The Journal of Neuroscience*, 34(24), 8098–8105.

Bestelmeyer, P. E., Rouger, J., DeBruine, L. M., & Belin, P. (2010). Auditory adaptation in vocal affect perception. *Cognition*, 117(2), 217–223.

Blanchard, C. D. & Blanchard, R. J. (1972). Innate and conditioned reactions to threat in rats with amygdaloid lesions. *Journal of Comparative and Psychological Psychology*, 81(2), 281–290.

Boatman, J. A. & Kim, J. J. (2006). A thalamo-cortico-amygdala pathway mediates auditory fear conditioning in the intact brain. *European Journal of Neuroscience*, 24(3), 894–900.

Boldt, R., Malinen, S., Seppä, M., Tikka, P., Savolainen, P., & Hari, R. (2013). Listening to an audio drama activates two processing networks, one for all sounds, another exclusively for speech. *PloS One*, 8(5), e64489.

Breiter, H. C., Etcoff, N. L., Whalen, P. J., Kennedy, W. A., Rauch, S. L., Buckner, R. L., ... Rosen, B. R. (1996). Response and habituation of the human amygdala during visual processing of facial expression. *Neuron*, 17(5), 875–887.

Britton, J. C., Phan, K. L., Taylor, S. F., Welsh, R. C., Berridge, K. C., & Liberzon, I. (2006). Neural correlates of social and non-social emotions: an fMRI study. *NeuroImage*, 31(1), 397–409.

Brück, C., Kreifelts, B., Ethofer, T., & Wildgruber, D. (2013). Emotional voices: the tone of (true) feelings. In: J. L. Armony & P. Vuilleumier (eds) *The Cambridge Handbook of Human Affective Neuroscience* (pp. 265–285). New York, NY: Cambridge University Press.

Brück, C., Kreifelts, B., Kaza, E., Lotze, M., & Wildgruber, D. (2011). Impact of personality on the cerebral processing of emotional prosody. *NeuroImage*, 58(1), 259–268.

Darwin, C. (1872/1998). *The Expression of Emotions in Man and Animals* (3rd edn). London: HarperCollins.

Ethofer, T., Kreifelts, B., Wiethoff, S., Wolf, J., Grodd, W., Vuilleumier, P., & Wildgruber, D. (2009). Differential influences of emotion, task, and novelty on brain regions underlying the processing of speech melody. *Journal of Cognitive Neuroscience*, 21(7), 1255–1268.

Etkin, A. & Wager, T. D. (2007). Functional neuroimaging of anxiety: a meta-analysis of emotional processing in PTSD, social anxiety disorder, and specific phobia. *The American Journal of Psychiatry*, 164(10), 1476–1488.

Fecteau, S., Armony, J. L., Joanette, Y., & Belin, P. (2005). Judgement of emotional nonlinguistic vocalization: age-related differences. *Applied Neuropsychology*, 12(1), 40–48.

Fecteau, S., Belin, P., Joanette, Y., & Armony, J. L. (2007). Amygdala response to nonlinguistic emotional vocalizations. *NeuroImage*, 36(2), 480–487.

Friston, K. J., Buchel, C., Fink, G. R., Morris, J., Rolls, E., & Dolan, R. (1997). Psychophysiological and modulatory interactions in neuroimaging. *NeuroImage*, 6(3), 218–229.

Frühholz, S. & Grandjean, D. (2013). Amygdala subregions differentially respond and rapidly adapt to threatening voices. *Cortex*, 49(5), 1394–403.

Frühholz, S., Trost, W., & Grandjean, D. (2014). The role of the medial temporal limbic system in processing emotions in voice and music. *Progress in Neurobiology*, 123, 1–17.

Hawk, S. T., van Kleef, G. A., Ficher, A. H., & van der Schalk, J. (2009). 'Worth a thousand words': absolute and relative decoding of nonlinguistic affect vocalizations. *Emotion*, 9(3), 293–305.

Kucharska-Pietura, K., Phillips, M. L., Gernand, W., & David, A. S. (2003). Perception of emotions from faces and voices following unilateral brain damage. *Neuropsychologia*, 41(8), 1082–1090.

Khalfa, S., Schon, D., Anton, J. L., & Liégeois-Chauvel, C. (2005). Brain regions involved in recognition of happiness and sadness in music. *NeuroReport*, 16(18), 1981–1984.

Koelsch, S. (2006). Investigating emotion with music: an fMRI study. *Human Brain Mapping*, 27(3), 239–250.

Kreifelts, B., Ethofer, T., Grodd, W., Erb, M., & Wildgruber, D. (2007). Audiovisual integration of emotional signals in voice and face: an event-related fMRI study. *NeuroImage*, 37(4), 1445–1456.

Kuraoka, K. & Nakamura, K. (2007). Responses of single neurons in monkey amygdala to facial and vocal emotions. *Journal of Neurophysiology*, 97(2), 1379–1387.

LeDoux, J. E. (2007). The amygdala. *Current Biology*, 17(20), R868–874.

LeDoux, J. E. (2000). Emotion circuits in the brain. *Annual Review of Neuroscience*, 23, 155–184.

LeDoux, J. E. (1996). *The Emotional Brain: The Mysterious Underpinnings of Emotional Life*. New York: Simon & Schuster.

Leitman, D. I., Hoptman, M. J., Foxe, J. J. et al. (2007). The neural substrates of impaired prosodic detection in schizophrenia and its sensorial antecedents. *The American Journal of Psychiatry*, 164(3), 474–482.

Leitman, D. I., Wolf, D. H., Ragland, J. D. et al. (2010). 'It's not what you say, but how you say it': a reciprocal temporo-frontal network for affective prosody. *Frontiers in Human Neuroscience*, 4(19), 1–13.

Liu, P., Rigoulot, S., & Pell, M. D. (2015). Cultural differences in on-line sensitivity to emotional voices: comparing East and West. *Frontiers in Human Neuroscience*, 9(311). doi:10.3389/fnnhum.2014.00311

Mahan, A. L. & Ressler, K. J. (2012). Fear conditioning, synaptic plasticity, and the amygdala: implications for posttraumatic stress disorder. *Trends in Neurosciences*, 35(1), 24–35.

Morris, J. S., Scott, S. K., & Dolan, R. J. (1999). Saying it with feeling: neural responses to emotional vocalizations. *Neuropsychologia*, 37(10), 1155–1163.

Mothes-Lasch, M., Becher, M. P. I., Miltner, W. H. R., & Straube, T. (2016). Neural basis of processing threatening voices in a crowded auditory world. *Social Cognitive and Affective Neuroscience*, 11(5), 821–828. doi: 10.1093/scan/nsw022

Mothes-Lasch, M., Mentzer, H-J., Miltner, W. H. R., & Straube, T. (2011). Visual attention modulates brain activation in angry voices. *The Journal of Neuroscience*, 31(26), 9594–9598.

Pape, H.-C. & Paré, D. (2010). Plastic synaptic networks of the amygdala for the acquisition, expression, and extinction of conditioned fear. *Physiological Reviews*, 90(2), 419–463.

Paré, D., Quirk, G. J., & LeDoux, J. E. (2004). New vistas on amygdala networks in conditioned fear. *Journal of Neurophysiology*, 92(1), 1–9.

Peelen, M. V., Atkinson, A. P., & Vuilleumier, P. (2010). Supramodal representation of perceived emotions in the human brain. *The Journal of Neuroscience*, 30(30), 10127–10134.

Pell, M. D., Paulmann, S., Dara, C., Alasseri, A., & Kotz, S. A. (2009). Factors in the recognition of vocally expressed emotions: a comparison of four languages. *Journal of Phonetics*, 37(4), 417–335.

Pell, M. D., Rothermich, K., Liu, P., Paulmann, S., Sethi, S., & Rigoulot, S. (2015). Preferential decoding of emotion from human non-linguistic vocalizations versus speech prosody. *Biological Psychology*, 111(2015), 14–25.

Peretz, I., Vuvan, D., Lagrouis, M. É., & Armony, J. L. (2015). Neural overlap in processing music and speech. *Philosophical Transactions of the Royal Society B: Biological Sciences*, 370(1664). doi:10.1098/rstb.2014.0090

Phillips, M. L., Young, A. W., Scott, S. K. et al. (1998). Neural responses to facial and vocal expressions of fear and disgust. *Proceedings of the Royal Society of London. B: Biological Sciences*, 265(1408), 1809–1817.

Pitkänen, A., Savander, V., & LeDoux, J. (1997). Organization of intra-amygdaloid circuitries in the rat: an emerging framework for understanding functions of the amygdala. *Trends in Neuroscience*, 20(11), 517–523.

Rogalsky, C., Rong, F., Saberi, K., & Hickok, G. (2011). Functional anatomy of language and music perception: temporal and structural factors investigated using functional magnetic resonance imaging. *The Journal of Neuroscience*, 31(10), 3843–3852.

Romanski, L. M., Clugnet, M. C., Bordi, F., & LeDoux, J. E. (1993). Somatosensory and auditory convergence in the lateral nucleus of the amygdala. *Behavioural Neuroscience*, 107(3), 444–450.

Romanski, L. M. & LeDoux, J. E. (1993). Information cascade from primary auditory cortex to the amygdala: corticocortical and corticoamygdaloid projections of temporal cortex in the rat. *Cerebral Cortex*, 3(6), 515–532.

Sah, P., Faber, E. S. L., Lopez De Armentia, M., & Power, J. (2003). The amygdaloid complex: anatomy and physiology. *Physiological Reviews*, 83(3), 803–834.

Sander, D., Grandjean, D., Pourtois, G. et al. (2005). Emotion and attention interactions in social cognition: brain regions involved in processing anger prosody. *NeuroImage*, 28(4), 848–858.

Scherer, K. R. (1989). Vocal correlates of emotional arousal and affective disturbance. In: H. Wagner & A. Manstead (eds) *Handbook of Social Psychophysiology* (pp. 165–197). New York: Wiley.

Schirmer, A. & Escoffier, N. (2010). Emotional MMN: anxiety and heart rate correlate with the ERP signature for auditory change detection. *Clinical Neurophysiology*, 121(1), 53–59.

Schirmer, A., Escoffier, N., Zysset, S., Koester, D., Striano, T., & Friederici, A. D. (2008). When vocal processing gets emotional: on the role of social orientation in relevance detection by the human amygdala. *NeuroImage*, 40(3), 1402–1410.

Schirmer, A. & Kotz, S. A. (2006). Beyond the right hemisphere: brain mechanisms mediating vocal emotion processing. *Trends in Cognitive Sciences*, 10(1), 24–30.

Schirmer, A., Striano, T., & Friederici, A. D. (2005). Sex differences in the preattentive processing of vocal emotional expressions. *NeuroReport*, 16(6), 635–639.

Scott, S. K., Young, A. W., Cader, A. J., Hellawell, D. J., Aggleton, J. P., & Johnson, M. (1997). Impaired auditory recognition of fear and anger following bilateral amygdala lesions. *Nature*, 385(6613), 254–257.

Sergerie, K., Chochol, C., & Armony, J. L. (2008). The role of the amygdala in emotional processing: a quantitative meta-analysis of functional neuroimaging studies. *Neuroscience and Biobehavioural Reviews*, 32(4), 811–830.

Sprengelmeyer, R., Young, A. W., Schoreder, U., Grossenbacher, P. G., Federlein, J., Buttner, T., & Przuntek, H. (1999). Knowing no fear. *Proceedings of the Royal Society of London. Series B: Biological Sciences*, 266(1437), 2451–2456.

Vieillard, S., Peretz, I., Gosselin, N., Khalfa, S., Gagnon, L., & Bouchard, B. (2008). Happy, sad, scary and peaceful musical excerpts for research on emotions. *Cognition and Emotion*, 22(4), 720–752.

Wiethoff, S., Wildgruber, D., Grodd, W., & Ethofer, T. (2009). Response and habituation of the amygdala during processing of emotional prosody. *NeuroReport*, 20(15), 1356–1360.

Winters, R. W., McCabe, P. M., & Schneiderman, N. (2002). Functional utility and neurobiology of conditioned autonomic responses. In: J. W. Moore (ed.) A *Neuroscientist's Guide to Classical Conditioning*. New York: Springer Publishing Company.

CHAPTER 22

LAUGHING OUT LOUD! INVESTIGATIONS ON DIFFERENT TYPES OF LAUGHTER

KAI ALTER AND DIRK WILDGRUBER

22.1 Introduction

LAUGHTER is an essential part of human communication occurring in social interactions. Laughter is related to social bonding, affection, and dynamics of group hierarchy. Laughter is also considered to be an expression of emotion (Meyer et al., 2007; Scott et al., 2014; Szameitat et al., 2009a, 2010; Wildgruber et al., 2013). Laughter production is fairly easy to achieve by means of air-flow control such as in breathing. Laughter may contain speech-like components such as vowels and nasal consonants. In this chapter, we want to point out findings from our own research and from other teams working on the production and perception of different types of laughter. A distinction of different types of laughter will be proposed from both a phonological and phonetic point of view. Moreover, some recent findings on the perception and cerebral processing of different types of laughter will be briefly summarized.

22.2 Why Do We Laugh?

Laughter is a phylogenetically very old communicational expression that has been observed in several non-human primates (e.g. bonobos, chimpanzees, gorillas, orangutans) (Davila-Ross et al., 2009) and rodents (e.g. rats) (Panksepp, 2005). Charles Darwin was the first researcher to report on the remarkable similarities between laughter in apes and man. He revealed his observations in his book *The Expressions of the Emotions in Man and Animals*, published in 1872.

In non-human primates and rats, the typical triggering situation is a direct somatosensory stimulation of the body, usually occurring during playful behaviour among animals. It is interesting to note that this reflex-like laughter can also be evoked in these animals by tickling, in much the same way as we know it from humans (Davila-Ross et al., 2011; Panksepp, 2005). However, in humans there are many more diverse triggering situations where laughter is expressed. For example, humans produce laughter in specific social situations (e.g. an inviting or friendly laugh to welcome someone, a shy laugh or giggle as a signal of excuse, a mean taunting laugh as a signal of rough rejection). Moreover, humans display laughter as a response to humour and jokes that require a high level of cognitive processing instead of bodily contact.

Regarding the underlying biological function, laughter in animals is assumed to increase bonding between the participating individuals through induction of positive emotions, and might represent a reward for playing with the young ones, thereby increasing fitness and survival probabilities (Meyer et al., 2007). Humans also laugh mostly in positive social situations, establishing and reinforcing social bonding, as pointed out by Provine (2004). This effect is further increased by a contagious reaction, since humans also laugh in situations when other people are laughing.

However, there are also less positive situations when people or, rather, one person laughs. This is often the case of 'schadenfreude' laughter (i.e. laughing about somebody else's misfortune) or even so-called 'devil's laughter', such as taunting laughter. In these situations, usually one person wants to demonstrate his/her predominant position in the social hierarchy and uses laughter as an expression of superiority. At the same time, the person laughed at often feels submissive and vulnerable. In those situations, people laughed at may express their embarrassment by a kind of giggle, or another type of shy laughter (Beermann & Ruch, 2011).

Furthermore, laughter has also been described as serving as a sexual advertisement, signalling cognitive and physical fitness of individuals to attract possible mating partners, thus increasing the probability of reproduction (Mehu & Dunbar, 2008).

Regarding humour, Wild et al. (2003) proposed that our reaction to humour may elicit laughter by 'violating social expectations in novel ways'; by 'nonsense humor', 'which is funny only because it makes no sense'; by 'sexual humor', which may often be offensive; or by breaking taboos. All these violations of social expectations, however, can be perceived as potential threats to group coherence. In this context, it is interesting to note that the French philosopher Henry Bergson (who received the Nobel Prize for Literature in 1927) characterized laughter as a 'social gesture' that is used to indicate the violation of social rules in human interaction, thereby allowing for a correction of social behaviour. In this sense, laughter serves as a 'corrective instrument' in society (Bergson, 1900). The evoked laughter in these instances is proposed to draw attention to the preceding violation of social rules, as well as signalling the willingness to reintegrate the addressee within the group. If the involved individuals realize that the respective violation of social expectations means no serious harm to the well-being of the group, and the violator has been reintegrated, the coherence of the group is further strengthened by laughing together.

The more diverse types of laughter in humans thus allow for a much more complex regulation of bonding and group coherence by expressing inclusion or rejection of individuals, thereby providing an even stronger increase in survival probability as compared to the more reflex-like laughter in animals. An overview of the observed similarities in animals and

evolution of laughter

	animals (rats, apes)	humans	
trigger	somatosensory (playing)	somatosensory cognitive intentional	(playing, tickling) (humour = brain tickling) (friendly, excusing, hostile)
emotion	positive for laugher & receiver	pos./pos. neg./pos. pos./neg.	(tickling, humour, friendly) (apologizing) (taunting)
function	reinforces bonding & playing	reinforces bonding & playing improves group coherence rejection of troublemakers	(tickling) (humour, friendly) (taunting)
	⬇	⬇	
	increase of survival probability	diversification of laughter types allows for stronger increase of survival probability	

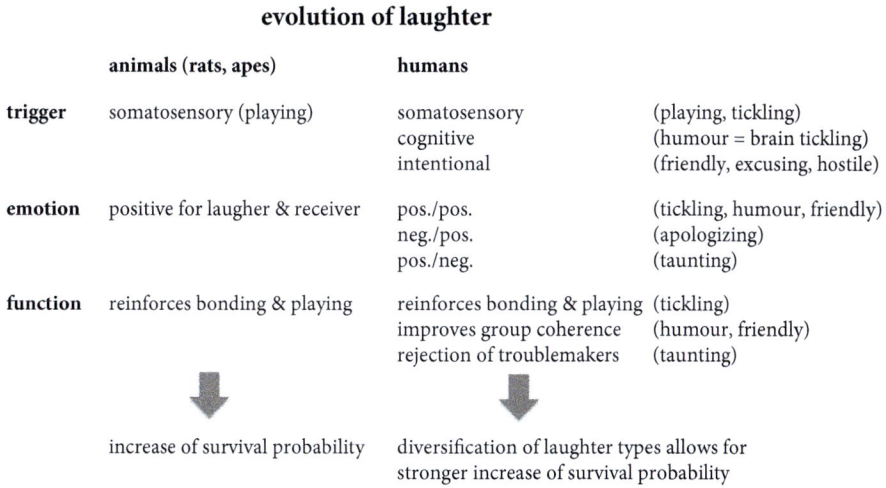

FIGURE 22.1 Phylogenetic diversification of laughter. The figure shows a comparison between animal laughter and human laughter with respect to the trigger, emotional state of the laugher and receiver, as well as social function. The main difference between human and non-human primates/rodents is the human ability to encode a richer diversity of emotional states and social intentions in laughter. Only humans seem to be able to encode both positive and negative emotions in laughter.

humans, as well as the proposed diversification of laughter throughout the course of evolution is shown in Figure 22.1.

22.3 Semiotics of Laughter

Laughter can be characterized as a social signal allowing for the expression of various distinct emotions and intentions without saying a word. Audio 22.1 includes examples of several different types of laughter. These auditory examples have been chosen to further illustrate the description of distinct types of laughter and specific features of laughter.

As mentioned in Section 22.2, laughter is not always connected to positive emotions. Some types of laughter, such as 'schadenfreude' laughter (Audio 22.1d) and taunting laughter (Audio 22.1b), can induce negative emotions in the receiver (i.e. the person being laughed at). In a series of laughter production and perception studies (Szamaitat et al., 2009a,b, 2010, 2011a,b), these two negative laughter types have been compared to two types of positive laughter—friendly/joyful laughter (Audio 22.1h) and tickling laughter (Audio 22.1a). (Please note that friendly and joyful laughter are considered to belong to the same category here.) All four types can be clearly differentiated by the social context and the triggering situations.

Friendly laughter is a signal of invitation, welcomeness, inclusion, or acceptance. Tickling laughter, in contrast, is bound to a very specific social interaction and requires physical or body contact. Being tickled can induce laughter especially when the relation between the participants is a friendly and trustful one. However, this relationship is quite subtle. Without doubt, most of us do not want to be tickled by a person we do not have a close relationship or partnership with, such as someone we meet for the first time. However, a parental relationship (e.g. between father and son, or mother and daughter) or relationship between close friends is the ideal background for a frenzied tickling session. Regarding the link between physical stimulation, joy, and laughter, it is important to note that the feeling of being tickled can at some point become quite unpleasant if the tickling is overdone. Tickling can cause pain, and has been used as a means of torture (Yamey, 2001). In these particular cases, body contact was not achieved between humans, but between animals and sensitive parts of the human body, such as the feet dipped in brine.

Another specific characteristic of laughter is that all types of laughter can become contagious. This often happens in situations when members of a group share positive emotions. Those positive emotions can be induced by external events (e.g. sharing unexpected news or joyful events) and are often related to funny stories or jokes, as well as trustful tickling situations. However, the dark side of contagious laughter may become obvious in situations of 'schadenfreude' laughter (i.e. laughing about somebody's misfortune), a widespread phenomenon in some cultures. Communication may then turn from group laughter into a laughter that focuses on one person. In these situations, members of the group just starting to laugh can prime further laughter and thus reaffirm bonding between in-group members and, at the same time, express the exclusion of the person laughed at.

22.4 How Do We Laugh?

So far, an unequivocal phonological 'grammar' of laughter production does not exist. Therefore, the approach employed in this section is rather preliminary, to cope with the heterogeneous data from acoustic analysis of laughter. It provides an overview of common patterns in laughter. From a phonological point of view, the mode of laughter articulation and the place of articulation can be distinguished.

The mode of articulation is related to the type of phonation. More generally, the type of phonation in laughter production is clearly related to breathing and vocalization. The airstream is essential to speech production and laughter production. However, in laughter, the direction of the airstream varies as both exhalation and inhalation can be used (Audio 22.1j). The airstream can pass through the vocal tract (mouth) or through the nasal cavity (Audio 22.1e). In addition, if the airstream passes the vocal tract, the vocal cords can vibrate with the airstream going in both directions. During exhalation, the laughter can become voiced, and vowel-like sounds are produced. When the airstream is reversed during a laughter sequence, an inhalation can be voiced as well (Audio 22.1i).

A second important phonological feature is the 'place of articulation', indicating which articulators can be used during sound production. Almost the same articulators that are used in speech production can be used in laughter production (Kohler, 2008). Those articulators are the pulmonary system, larynx, and the oral cavity, with modification of articulation

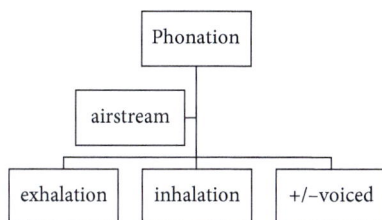

FIGURE 22.2 Phonation during laughter production. Basic features are the direction of the airstream and the use of vocal cords resulting in voiced segments of laughter or, if not in use, resulting in unvoiced segments of laughter. Examples of voiced segments are vowel-like sounds such as in 'ha-ha-ha' or 'hi-hi-hi'; unvoiced segments are often fricatives like 'fff-fff-fff' (Audio 22.1k).

points such as the position of tongue, jaw, and lip. In some instances also, the involvement of the nasal cavity has been observed (e.g. in cases of 'snoring' sounds with an ingressive airstream). An overview of the most important phonological features of laughter production is provided in Figure 22.2 and Table 22.1.

However, such parallels between speech and laughter production do not necessarily mean that laughter is speech-like. Rather, laughter should be seen as a fairly simple glottal and supraglottal modification of the incoming or outgoing pulmonary airstream. Even the vowel-like sounds, which are often paraphrased in balloons in comics, can be roughly described as close-open (e.g. /u/ versus /a/) and front-back (e.g. /i/ versus /o/) (Szameitat et al., 2009b, 2011a). The vowel-like sounds used in laughter are similar to those used in the phonological system of a given language.

Supraglottal features in laughter utilize the oral or nasal cavity and some coronal, labio-dental, and labial constrictions, resulting in different types of fricative-like sounds such as /sss/ and /fff/ (Audio 22.1k). Nasal consonants such as /m/ are also used in laughter, with the oral cavity closed and the nasal cavity open (Audio 22.1f). However, the most important feature, which can be seen as a carrier of laughter sounds, is the pulmonary airstream in both directions.

Table 22.1 Supraglottal features involved in laughter production

Supraglottal modification	
Oral	**Nasal**
Vowel	Consonant
Fricatives	Vowel (?)

Please note that there are no reports, so far, of nasal vowels used in laughter. However, this possibility still exists.

Therefore, at a phonological level, laughter is characterized by fairly simple mechanisms of sound production, and can be compared to breath-control events such as coughing (Audio 22.1l), sneezing, hiccoughing, sniffing (Audio 22.1c), and even snoring.

22.5 ACOUSTICS OF LAUGHTER

Laughter is produced by means of different articulatory mechanisms. Laughter frequently contains a sequence of vocalic segments which are often vowel-like elements. However, as previously stated, they may also be unvoiced in cases when there is no glottal activation. The result is then a sequence of unvoiced elements, such as fricatives like /sss/, or simply noisy expiration. Those segments form larger, phrase-like units called 'laugh phrases', which are marked by a beginning and an end. They are similar to intonational phrases in speech. The beginning often starts with a perceivable inhalation that allows the pulmonary airstream to be exhaled with or without glottal activation. The end of laugh phrases is often marked by silence.

If the laughter outburst is very long (i.e. exceeding the air-volume intake) and necessitates a new breathing cycle, the following phrase starts again with an inhalation. This is often a marker for breathing and signals the beginning of a new laughter phrase (see Figure 22.3). In an analogy to speech, this boundary can be called an 'intonational phrase boundary'. In written sentences, commas may indicate such boundaries which may be a sign to make a break, to inhale, and to restart a new phrase. Thus, a phrase indicates a break, followed by a reset. Vocalic segments are equal to syllables such as 'ha-ha-ha'. A sequence in laughter is comparable to speaking a very long sentence divided by phrases/breaks. In laughter, instead of using comma intonation (i.e. raising the pitch at the end of an intonational phrase followed by a break), the onset of the new laughter phrase is marked by inhalation. This type of laughter sequencing is mostly governed by air-volume capacity, rather than syntactic and phonological structures as in speech.

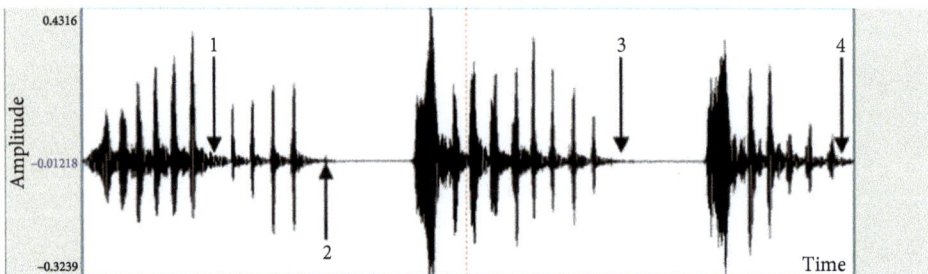

FIGURE 22.3 Time-wave form of a large laughter sequence with three audible exhalations and one audible inhalation: arrow 1—the end of first laughter phrase, arrow 2—beginning of audible inhalation, arrow 3—end of second laughter phrase, arrow 4—end of third laughter phrase (Audio 22.1g).

The rhythmical structure is another important characteristic of laughter. There is little variation in the temporal distance between the laughter segments, and laugh phrases have a very consistent duration. This again is dependent on the pulmonary force of each individual. The following section will discuss some important acoustic features of laughter.

The following data are an extract of a large corpus of laughter data (Szamaitat et al., 2009b, 2011a). Eight professional actors were asked to produce four types of laughter—friendly-joyful, tickling, schadenfreude, and taunting. Laughter was recorded following a specific procedure (see Szamaitat, 2009b), digitized at a sampling rate of 48 kHz and 16 bits, and cut into individual laughter sequences. Each sequence was then classified by thirty-six volunteers in a behavioural study according to the underlying laughter type. An exhaustive acoustic analysis was achieved on a final set of 127 laughter sequences. Overall, forty-three acoustic parameters were analysed. A set of twenty-three parameters showed significant differences between the four types of laughter. A set of acoustic features related to the basic mechanism of laughter—breathing control and phonation—were selected based on discriminant analyses (see Figures 22.2 and 22.3; see also Tables 22.2 and 22.3).

Overall, the data show that tickling laughter was rapid and high-pitched, had the shortest segment duration and inter-phrasal duration, as well as the highest laugh rate and number of phrases. Joyful laughter had the longest time between phrases and a low peak frequency. However, it had a high proportion of harmonic energy (harmonic-to-noise ratio, HNR). Schadenfreude laughter did not show any outstanding characteristics (i.e. most of its parameters were in the middle range) and had a low HNR. Taunting laughter had the lowest fundamental frequency and the highest peak frequency, having a low amount of harmonic energy. Moreover, it showed a high segment duration, which makes it comparable to schadenfreude laughter.

Table 22.2 Selection of acoustic parameters related to phonation and selected based on discriminant analysis. Most are related to vocal–cord activations

Acoustic parameter	Definition
Segment duration	Average duration of a segment
Laugh rate	Average number of segments per second
Number of phrases	Number of laugh phrases separated by inhalation
Inter-phrasal duration	Average duration between phrases
F0 mean	Average fundamental frequency measured across vocalic segments
Peak frequency (mean)	Average peak frequency measured across vocalic segments
% voiced elements	Percentage of segments with a clear harmonic structure

Table 22.3 Selection of acoustic parameters (Szameitat et al., 2009a,b). Pair-wise t-tests were calculated for all combinations of laughter types

	Joy	Tickle	Schadenfreude	Taunt
Segment duration		<	>	>
Laugh rate		>>		
Number of phrases		>>		
Inter-phrasal duration	>>	<<		
FO (mean)		>>		<<
Peak frequency (mean)	<<	<	>	>>
% voiced elements	>	>	<	<
HNR	>>	>	<	<<

Left arrows (<) indicate a significantly smaller mean value for the respective laughter type as compared to at least one of the other laughter types; right arrows (>) indicate significantly higher mean values as compared to at least one other laughter type. (<, >) $p < 0.05$; (<<, >>) $p < 0.01$

22.6 AUDITORY DISTINCTION OF LAUGHTER—BEHAVIOURAL EVIDENCE

The question arises of whether these different types of laughter can be recognized and discriminated solely from the acoustic signal of the laughter recording, without any further contextual knowledge. To answer this question, a selection of laughter recordings were presented to healthy subjects (Szamaitat et al., 2009a,b). The laughter stimuli were recorded by actors, instructed to put themselves into the appropriate emotional state using a script-based auto-induction method and to laugh freely without thinking about the expression of the laughter (for details, see Szameitat et al., 2009a). Overall, 429 sequences were used in this study. Participants (n = 72) listened to each laughter sequence and had to judge whether the sequence was joyful, tickling, schadenfreude, or taunting laughter (four-choice classification paradigm). Each of the four different types of laughter were recognized and discriminated well above chance level. The mean identification accuracy across all four categories was 45% (see Figure 22.4).

In a follow-up study (Szamaitat et al., 2010), the emotional connotation of laughter sounds was evaluated in the framework of four emotional dimensions—arousal, dominance, sender's valence, and receiver-directed valence. Of the 429 sequences previously described (Szamaitat et al., 2009a), only those recordings were used which were correctly rated for the different laughter categories (p = 0.05, two-tailed). The final stimulus set for the study consisted of 123 laughter sequences (n = 49 for male speakers, 10–22 sequences per speaker, 21–36 per laughter type).

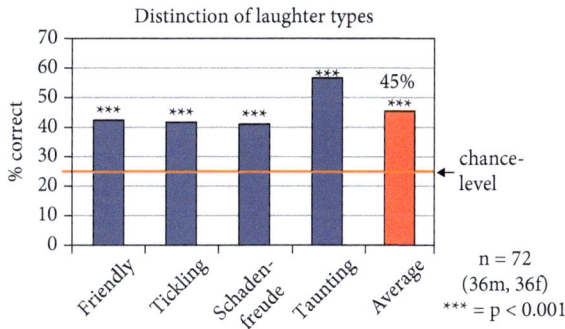

FIGURE 22.4 Percentage of correct answers for the classification of the four types of laughter (friendly, tickling, schadenfreude, taunting). All four categories of laughter were identified significantly above chance level just by listening to the sound files, without any further contextual knowledge.

Each laughter sequence was classified with respect to the aforementioned four emotional dimensions—arousal (physically excited versus calm), dominance (dominant versus submissive), sender's valence (sender being in a pleasant versus unpleasant state), receiver-directed valence (sender feeling pleasant versus unpleasant towards the receiver). These dimensions were selected according to Wilhelm Wundt's work on emotional dimensions (Wundt, 1900). For each laughter sequence, the listener rated the emotional state of the sender (and not his/her own state), that is, the listener evaluated how excited the sender was, how dominant the sender was, whether the sender was in a pleasant state, or whether the sender was pleasant towards the listener.

Each emotional dimension was tested in an individual experiment (including all 123 laughter stimuli) by independent samples of twenty-four (twelve male) participants each (in total, ninety-six native English-speaking participants, mean age 22 years). Accordingly, each of the 123 laughter sequences was evaluated by twenty-four participants per emotional dimension (Szameitat et al., 2009a). For the classification, participants had to evaluate how strongly they found the investigated dimension to be expressed on a four-point rating scale. The participants were not aware of the four laughter types included.

In summary, it was observed that the four different laughter types were associated with specific emotional dimensions (see Figure 22.5 for a more detailed presentation of the results). This is in accordance with the hypothesis that non-verbal vocalizations are powerful means of communicating emotional states to listeners. More specifically, participants perceived high arousal cues in tickling and taunt laughter, and taunt laughter was clearly perceived negatively in the receiver-directed valence rating.

Most interestingly, there were significant negative correlations between dominance and receiver-directed valence ($R = -0.74$, $p < 0.001$), for dominance and arousal ($R = -0.33$, $p < 0.001$), as well as for dominance and valence of the sender ($R = -0.26$, $p < 0.001$), across all laughter types. A positive correlation was observed for arousal and valence of the sender ($R = 0.59$, $p < 0.001$).

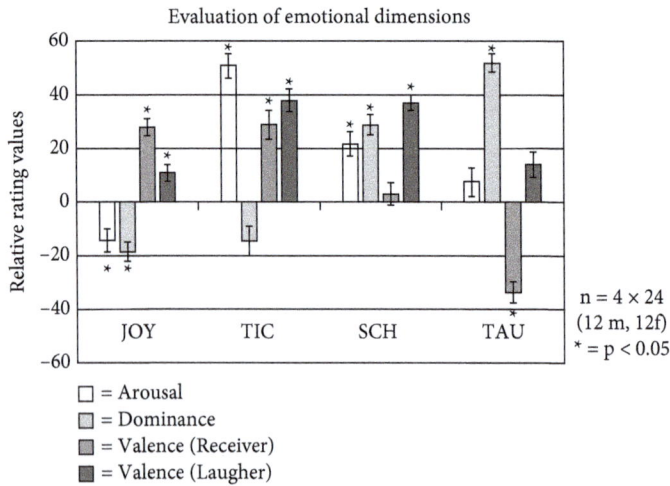

FIGURE 22.5 The different emotional dimensions encoded in distinct types of laughter according to listeners' ratings for arousal, dominance, valence of the laughter, and receiver-directed valence.

JOY: joyful friendly laughter; TIC: tickling laughter: SCH: schadenfreude laughter; TAU: taunting laughter.

Again, during this study only auditory information was presented and differentiation of distinct laughter types regarding emotional dimensions was carried out in the absence of any further contextual cues.

22.7 Perception of Audiovisual Laughter

Aiming to evaluate modality-dependent effects on the accuracy of laughter identification, Ritter (2018) presented laughter stimuli to fourteen healthy participants (seven male, seven female, mean age 24.6 ± 2.4 years) either unimodally auditory (A), unimodally visual (V), or bimodally (AV). The participants were asked to perform a categorical discrimination task (forced choice between three alternatives—friendly, tickling, or taunting). The stimuli (n = 187) were recorded by eight actors (four female, four male) using a script-based self-induction method for each emotional state. The recordings were edited with respect to alignment of the size of portrayed faces, vertical facial symmetry axis, as well as normalization of sound intensity.

In accordance with the well-known facilitation effects of audiovisual integration, the highest identification rates were observed for audiovisual stimuli (AV: 68%) as compared to unimodal stimuli. It is interesting to note, however, that auditory presentation (A: 65%) of laughter sequences yielded significantly higher accuracy rates as compared to visual presentation (V: 59%). The opposite pattern of modality-dependent effects, with higher accuracy ratings during visual presentation of non-verbal emotional cues as compared to auditory presentation of non-verbal emotional cues, has been reported very consistently in the literature regarding perception of facial expressions and speech melody (Lambrecht et al., 2014).

Moreover, evaluation of laughter-type specific modality effects revealed lower identification rates during visual presentation of taunting laughter, whereas joyful laughter and tickling laughter, in contrast, showed similar accuracy rates for visual and auditory presentation (Ritter et al., 2015).

These results indicate an overall higher reliability of the acoustic signal as compared to the visual signal when decoding the emotional states and intention of the laugher. This effect is predominantly driven by misattributions of visually-presented taunting laughter.

22.8 NEUROBIOLOGICAL CORRELATES OF LAUGHTER PERCEPTION

The neurobiological correlates of laughter perception have been evaluated in several studies using functional magnetic resonance imaging. These studies revealed activation of a bilateral network of brain regions including the fronto-temporal cortex and the amygdala during laughter perception (Meyer et al., 2005, 2007; Sander & Scheich, 2001; Szameitat et al., 2010; Wildgruber et al., 2013). Considering specific patterns of cerebral responses depending on distinct types of laughter, a double-dissociation of haemodynamic activation has been observed during perception of tickling laughter and both types of social-intentional laughter (friendly, taunting). Perception of tickling laughter showed a stronger activation within right superior temporal regions, including primary and secondary acoustic areas, presumably linked to its higher acoustic complexity, whereas presentation of friendly and taunting laughter yielded increasing responses within the anterior-rostral medial frontal cortex, presumptively reflecting higher demands on social cognition (Szameitat et al., 2010).

Moreover, the distinct types of laughter were observed to modulate connectivity within the social perception network differently (Wildgruber et al., 2013). Tickling laughter induced stronger increases of connectivity between the auditory association cortex and the lateral prefrontal cortex, most likely reflecting specific demands on acoustic analysis due to increased density of auditory information. In contrast, friendly and taunting laughter were linked to stronger increases of connectivity between auditory association cortices and medial frontal as well as occipital areas. Additionally, it is interesting to note that friendly and taunting laughter were linked to dissociable changes in connectivity when compared directly (see Figure 22.6). Friendly laughter yielded a stronger increase of connectivity between the auditory and visual association areas within the occipital lobe. This effect might be linked to visual imagery supporting the formation of inferences about the intentions of our social counterparts. Taunting laughter, on the other hand, induced stronger increases in connectivity between auditory association areas and the anterio-rostral medial frontal cortex, presumably supporting mentalizing processes required to decode the highly important social information conveyed by taunting laughter.

These laughter-type specific effects at the neurobiological level provide further support for the proposed phylogenetic diversification of human laughter from an unequivocally positive bonding signal, triggered by somatosensory stimulation, to laughter with distinct social-intentional connotations, subserving complex social functions (Wildgruber & Kreifelts, 2015).

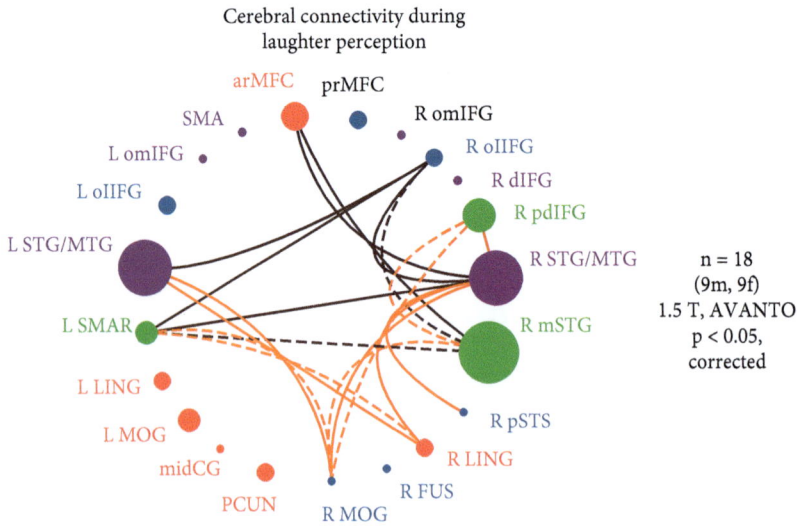

FIGURE 22.6 Cerebral connectivity during perception of joyful and taunting laughter. Increased connectivity during perception of joyful laughter as compared to taunting laughter (joyful > taunting) is represented as orange connections. Increased connectivity during perception of taunting laughter as compared to joyful laughter (taunting > joyful) is represented as dark brown connections. Continuous lines show modulations of connectivity which survive correction for multiple comparisons within the target ROI and additional Bonferroni correction for the number of investigated connections (300). Broken lines represent modulations which survive correction for multiple comparisons within the target ROI but not Bonferroni correction. Brain regions with significantly increased responses to both types of social-intentional laughter as compared to tickling (joyful or taunting > tickling) are shown as red areas. Brain regions with significantly increased responses to tickling laughter as compared to both types of social-intentional laughter (tickling > joyful or taunting) are shown as green areas. Brain regions with significantly increased responses during explicit evaluation of laughter types as compared to implicit processing (task effect: evaluation of laughter types > counting of laughter phrases) are shown as blue areas. Brain regions with common activation under all experimental conditions (conjunction analysis) are shown as purple areas.

Red areas: arMFC = anterio-rostral medial frontal cortex; R LING = right lingual gyrus; L LING = left lingual gyrus; midCG = middle cingulum; PCUN = precuneus; L MOG = left middle occipital gyrus

Green areas: R pdIFG = right inferior frontal gyrus; R mSTG = right superior temporal gyrus/middle part; L SMAR = left supramarginal gyrus/Rolandic operculum

Blue areas: R olIFG = right inferior frontal gyrus/pars triangularis, opercularis; L olIFG = left inferior frontal gyrus/pars orbitalis and triangularis; R pSTS = right superior temporal sulcus/posterior part; R MOG = right middle occipital gyrus; prMFC = posterior-rostral medial frontal cortex; R FUS = right fusiform gyrus

Purple areas: R STG/MTG = right superior temporal gyrus and middle temporal gyrus; L STG/MTG = left superior temporal gyrus and middle temporal gyrus; R omIFG = right orbitomedial IFG; L omIFG = left orbitomedial IFG; SMA = supplementary motor area; R dIFG = right inferior frontal gyrus/dorsal part

Adapted from Wildgruber D. et al., 'Different Types of Laughter Modulate Connectivity within Distinct Parts of the Laughter Perception Network', *PLoS One*, Volume 8, Issue 5, e63441, Copyright © 2013 Wildgruber et al., doi: 10.1371/journal.pone.0063441, under the terms of the Creative Commons Attribution License (CC BY 4.0).

22.9 PERSPECTIVE OF THE SELF DURING LAUGHTER PROCESSING

Since laughter conveys crucial cues about social acceptance or rejection, it is highly important for us to know who the addressee is. The social consequences differ dramatically if the laughter is directed at oneself or at someone else. To evaluate the effects of perspective taking during laughter perception, we carried out an experiment in which we asked the participants to imagine they were directly addressed by the laughter during one session (SELF), whereas they were instructed to imagine that another person was being addressed during the control condition (OTHER). Sixty participants (thirty female, thirty male) took part in a behavioural study, and twenty-six individuals (thirteen female, thirteen male) participated in an fMRI study (3T, Siemens Prisma). Using this approach, joyful laughter was rated as the most inclusive, and taunting as the most exclusive laughter type under both conditions. Under the SELF condition, the difference between laughter types decreased as compared to the OTHER condition (Ritter at al., 2015).

At the neurobiological level, an interaction effect (task × laughter type), with stronger responses during SELF-directed taunting laughter (versus friendly) as compared to OTHER-directed laughter, emerged within the bilateral amygdalae, most likely reflecting the much higher emotional relevance of cues expressing social rejection if these are directed at oneself (Wildgruber et al., 2016). The activation pattern of the amygdalae is shown in Figure 22.7.

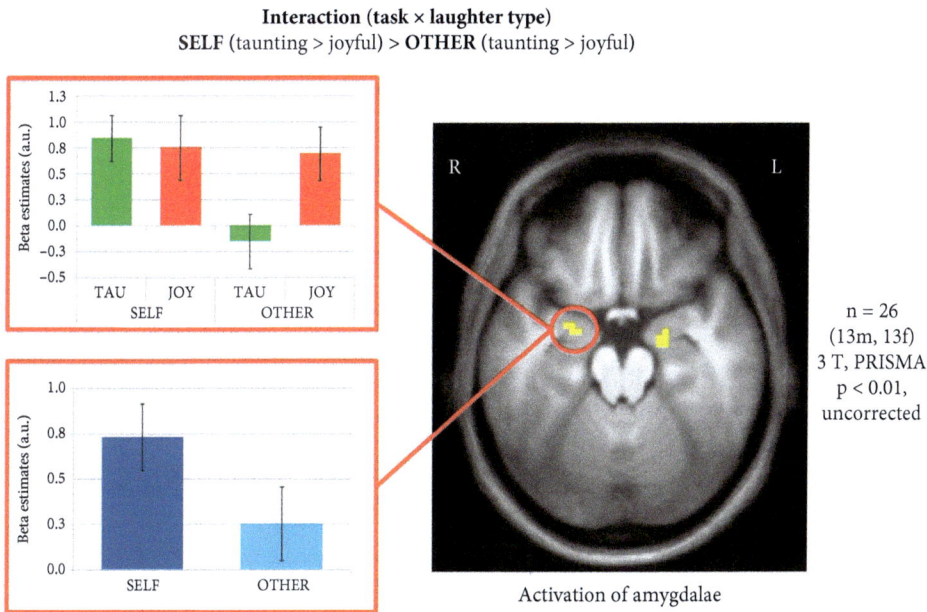

Interaction (task × laughter type)
SELF (taunting > joyful) > **OTHER** (taunting > joyful)

Activation of amygdalae

n = 26
(13m, 13f)
3 T, PRISMA
$p < 0.01$,
uncorrected

FIGURE 22.7 Interaction of task (SELF-directed laughter vs. OTHER-directed laughter) and laughter type (TAU = taunting vs. JOY = joyful). Bilateral amygdalae showed stronger activation during SELF-directed taunting laughter as compared to OTHER-directed taunting laughter, whereas responses to joyful laughter did not differ between task conditions.

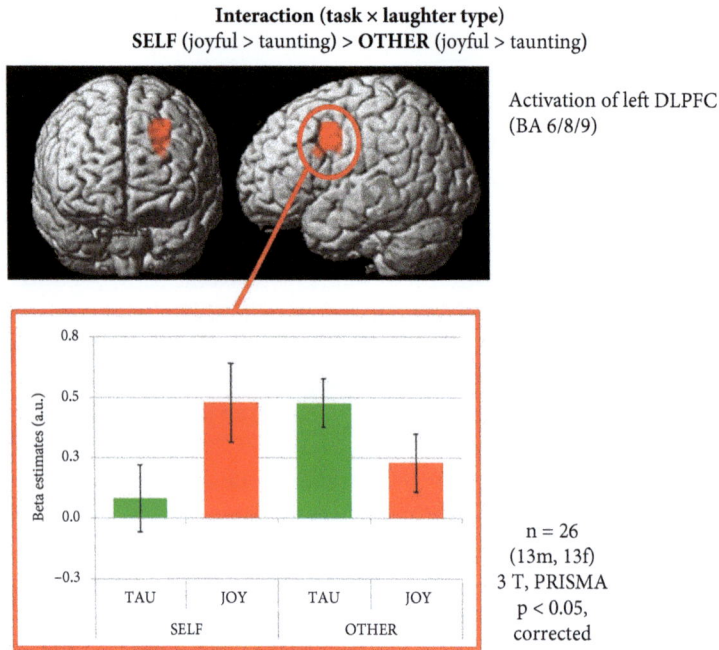

Interaction (task × laughter type)
SELF (joyful > taunting) > **OTHER** (joyful > taunting)

Activation of left DLPFC
(BA 6/8/9)

n = 26
(13m, 13f)
3 T, PRISMA
p < 0.05,
corrected

FIGURE 22.8 Interaction of task (SELF-directed laughter vs. OTHER-directed laughter) and laughter type (TAU = taunting vs. JOY = joyful). The left dorsolateral prefrontal cortex (DLPFC) showed decreased activation during SELF-directed taunting laughter as compared to OTHER-directed taunting laughter, whereas responses to joyful laughter did not differ significantly between task conditions.

In contrast, stronger responses during OTHER-directed taunting laughter (versus friendly) as compared to SELF-directed laughter were observed within the left dorsolateral prefrontal cortex (Brodmann areas 6, 8, and 9) that might be linked to higher degrees of cognitive control or stronger engagement of the mirror neuron system if social cues of rejection are directed at other persons (see Figure 22.8).

These findings highlight the usefulness of laughter as a highly relevant social signal for research on the interrelations of social cue perception and perspective taking (Wildgruber & Kreifelts, 2015).

22.10 GELOTOPHOBIA AND PERCEPTION OF LAUGHTER IN PSYCHIATRIC DISORDERS

About 2–10% of otherwise healthy subjects exhibit a specific fear of being laughed at that can be identified using a questionnaire developed by Ruch and Proyer (2008). This condition has been termed 'gelotophobia' (Ruch, 2009) and has been observed in many different cultures all over the world (Proyer et al., 2009). It is still under debate, however, if gelotophobia can be considered a specific phobia, just like a spider phobia or height phobia, independently of other symptoms, and if it can be clearly differentiated from social phobia, since there is a considerable overlap of both concepts (Ruch et al., 2013). Moreover, a strongly increased rate of gelotophobia has been observed in various psychiatric disorders such as autism spectrum disorder (45%; Samson et al., 2011), schizophrenia (50%; Forabosco, 2009), affective disorders (19%; Forabosco, 2009), and borderline-personality disorder (87%; Brück et al., 2018). With respect to neurobiological correlates of gelotophobia, a first study observed positive associations between gelotophobia scores and path length in the brain's white-matter network (Wu et al., 2016).

In subjects with social anxiety, a negative laughter-interpretation bias has been observed, as well as an attention bias that is characterized by decreased response times towards taunting laughter (Ritter et al., 2015). Moreover, at the neurobiological level, it has been observed that haemodynamic responses within the left dorsolateral frontal attention network are linked to this negative attention bias in patients with social phobia (Kreifelts et al., 2014). Based on this finding, it is promising to evaluate the possibility of modulating cognitive biases in laughter perception by neuropsychological training, non-invasive brain stimulation, or neural feedback-training in further research projects.

22.11 SUMMARY

Laughter is a non-verbal vocalization that serves to express various emotional states and intentions. Laughter is easy to produce given its relatively simple phonetic structure and can even be produced in a prelanguage stage by four-month-old infants. Laughter is not simply a common expression of positive emotions. Positive emotional expressions have been found in both human and non-human primates when related to play behaviour and tickling, but laughter can also have hostile connotations. In the studies cited in this chapter, negative laughter expressions comprise 'schadenfreude' laughter and taunt. Whilst they share some commonalities with the positive laughter types, they also show distinctive acoustic patterns. Follow-up behavioural discrimination and classification tasks revealed that they can be discriminated at acoustic, perceptual, and neurobiological levels.

Laughter is a powerful social signal which can convey social rejection or acceptance even in the absence of further contextual information. It is well suited to evaluate the neurobiological underpinning of social-emotional communication and specific differences in patients with psychiatric disorders

Future research shall reveal how further types of laughter are produced and perceived, and how they fit into a system that is capable of expressing emotions without saying a word.

REFERENCES

Beermann, U. & Ruch, W. (2011). Can people really 'laugh at themselves?'—experimental and correlational evidence. *Emotion*, 11(3), 492–501.

Bergson, H. (1900). *Laughter: An Essay on the Meaning of Comic*. London: Rothwell.

Brück, C., Derstroff, S., Ruch, W., & Wildgruber, D. (2018). Fear of being laughed at in border-line personality disorder. *Frontiers in Psychology*, 9, 4. doi: 10.3389/fpsyg.2018.00004

Davila-Ross, M., Allcock, B., Thomas, C., & Bard, K. A. (2011). Aping expressions? Chimpanzees produce distinct laugh types when responding to laughter of others. *Emotion*, 11(5), 1013–1020.

Davila-Ross, M., Owren, M. J., & Zimmermann, E. (2009). Reconstructing the evolution of laughter in great apes and humans. *Current Biology*, 19, 1106–1111.

Forabosco, G., Ruch, W., & Nucera, P. (2009). The fear of being laughed at among psychiatric patients. *Humor: International Journal of Humor Research*, 22(1–2), 233–251.

Kohler, K. J. (2008). 'Speech-smile', 'speech-laugh', 'laughter' and their sequencing in dialogic interaction. *Phonetica*, 28, 65(1–2), 1–18.

Kreifelts, B., Brück, C., Ritter, J., Ethofer, T., Domin, M., Lotze, M., ... Wildgruber, D. (2014). They are laughing at me: cerebral mediation of cognitive biases in social anxiety. *PLos One*, 9, e99815. doi: 10.1371/journal.pone.0099815

Lambrecht, L., Kreifelts, B., & Wildgruber, D. (2014). Gender differences in emotion recognition—impact of sensory modality and emotional category. *Cognition and Emotion*, 28, 452–469.

Mehu, M. & Dunbar, R. I. M. (2008). Naturalistic observations of smiling and laughter in human group interactions. *Behaviour*, 145, 1747–1780.

Meyer, M., Baumann, S., Wildgruber, D., & Alter, K. (2007). How the brain laughs: comparative evidence from behavioural, electrophysiological and neuroimaging studies in human and monkey. *Behavioral Brain Research*, 182, 245–260.

Meyer, M., Zysset, S., von Cramon, D. Y., & Alter, K. (2005). Distinct fMRI responses to laughter, speech and sounds along the human peri-sylvian cortex. *Cognitive Brain Research*, 24, 291–306.

Panksepp, J. (2005). Beyond a joke: from animal laughter to human joy? *Science*, 308, 62–63.

Provine, R. R. (2004). Laughing, tickling, and the evolution of speech and self. *Current Directions in Psychological Science*, 13, 215–218.

Proyer, R. T., Ruch, W., Ali, N. S. et al. (2009). Breaking ground in crosscultural research on the fear of being laughed at (gelotophobia): a multi-national study involving 73 countries. *Humor: International Journal of Humor Research*, 22, 253–279.

Ritter, J. (2018). *Laughter Perception in Social Anxiety*. Doctoral thesis, University of Tuebingen. https://Publikationsmöglichkeit/xmlui/bitstream/handle/10900/83370/diss_ jmritter.pdf

Ritter, J., Brück, C., Jacob, H., Wildgruber, D., & Kreifelts, B. (2015). Laughter perception in social anxiety. *Journal of Psychiatric Research*, 60, 178–184.

Ruch, W. (2009). Fearing humor? Gelotophobia: the fear of being laughed at. Introduction and overview. *Humor: International Journal of Humor Research*, 22(1–2), 1–25.

Ruch, W., Hofmann, J., Platt, T., & Proyer, R. (2013). The state-of-the art in gelotophobia research: a review and some theoretical extensions. *Humor: International Journal of Humor Research*, 27, 23–45.

Ruch, W. & Proyer, R. T. (2008). Who is gelotophobic? Assessment criteria for the fear of being laughed at. *Swiss Journal of Psychology*, 67(1), 19–27.

Samson, A., Huber, O., & Ruch, W. (2011). Teasing, ridiculing and the relation to the fear of being laughed at in individuals with Asperger's syndrome. *Journal of Autism and Developmental Disorders*, 41(4), 475–483.

Sander, K. & Scheich, H. (2001). Auditory perception of laughter and crying activates human amygdala regardless of attentional state. *Cognitive Brain Research*, 12, 181–198.

Scott, S. K., Lavan, N., Chen, S., & McGettigan, C. (2014). The social life of laughter. *Trends in Cognitive Sciences*, 18(12), 618–620.

Szameitat, D. P., Alter, K., Szameitat, A. J., Darwin, C. J., Wildgruber, D., Dietrich, S., & Sterr, A. (2009a). Differentiation of emotions in laughter at the behavioral level. *Emotion*, 9(3), 397–405.

Szameitat, D. P., Alter, K., Szameitat, A. J., Wildgruber, D., Sterr, A., & Darwin, C. J. (2009b). Acoustic profiles of distinct emotional expressions in laughter. *Journal of the Acoustical Society of America*, 126(1), 354–366.

Szameitat, D. P., Darwin, C. J., Wildgruber, D., Alter, K., & Szameitat, A. J. (2011a). Acoustic correlates of emotional dimensions in laughter: arousal, dominance, and valence. *Cognition & Emotion*, 25(4), 599–611.

Szameitat, D. P., Darwin, C. J., Szameitat, A. J., Wildgruber, D., Sterr, A., Dietrich, S., & Alter, K. (2011b). Formant characteristics of human laughter. *Journal of Voice*, 25, 32–37.

Szameitat, D. P., Kreifelts, B., Alter, K., Szameitat, A. J., Sterr, A., Grodd, W., & Wildgruber, D. (2010). It is not always tickling: distinct cerebral responses during perception of different laughter types. *NeuroImage*, 53(4), 1264–1271.

Wild, B., Rodden, F. A., Grodd, W., & Ruch, W. (2003). Neural correlates of laughter and humour. *Brain*, 126(Pt 10), 2121–2138.

Wildgruber, D. & Kreifelts, B. (2015). Evolutionary perspectives on emotions and their link to intentions, dispositions and behavior. *Physics of Life Reviews*, 13, 89–91.

Wildgruber, D., Ritter, J., Weigel, L., Jacob, H., & Kreifelts, B. (2016). *Perspective of the Self in Laughter Perception*. ESCAN Conference 2016, Porto, Book of Abstracts, 46.

Wildgruber, D., Szameitat, D. P., Ethofer, T., Brück, C., Alter, K., Grodd, W., & Kreifelts, B. (2013). Different types of laughter modulate connectivity within distinct parts of the laughter perception network. *PLoS One*, 8, e63441.

Wu, C. L., Zhong, S. Y., Chan, Y. C., Chen, H. C., Gong, G. L., He, Y., & Li, P. (2016). White-matter structural connectivity underlaying human laughter-related traits processing. *Frontiers in Psychology*, 7, Article 1637.

Wundt, W. (1900). *Völkerkunde. Eine Untersuchung der Entwicklungsgesetze von Sprache, Mythos und Sitte (Die Sprache, Band 1)*. [Ethnology. An Investigation of the Development of Language, Myth, and Custom (Language, Vol.1).] Leipzig: Kröner.

Yamey, G. (2001). Torture: European instruments of torture and capital punishment from the Middle Ages to present. *British Medical Journal*, 323(7308), 346.

PART V

VOCAL IDENTITY, PERSONALITY, AND THE SOCIAL CONTEXT

....

CHAPTER 23

RECOGNIZING SPEAKERS ACROSS LANGUAGES

....

TYLER K. PERRACHIONE

23.1 INTRODUCTION

....

SOME talkers are more or less memorable because of distinctive acoustic properties of their voice—a particularly low pitch, a notable voice quality, or an unusual mismatch between fundamental frequency and formant dispersion. However, some talkers are more or less memorable not because of anything inherent to their voice, but because of something in the mind of the listener—whether the listener and speaker share a common language. Over the last three decades, one of the most reliable observations in studies of voice perception and talker identification has been that listeners are more accurate at identifying voices in their native language compared to a second or foreign language. This phenomenon, called the *language-familiarity effect* in talker identification, has been reported in numerous studies using diverse methodologies and a wide range of language pairings. The language-familiarity effect has been the subject of increasing scientific interest in the past decade, not only because of its importance for developing robust models of voice perception, but also because of the ways this phenomenon can provide new insights into models of speech perception, auditory plasticity, and even developmental disorders of language and communication.

My interest in the language-familiarity effect began in a café in Paris one rainy March afternoon, where I was struck by how much the voice of my waitress sounded like the recorded voice of the announcer at the train station, and even like the voices of some new friends I had met the day before. Surely speakers of French did not sound more alike one another than speakers of English? Yet this was my distinct impression. I returned from my trip to the laboratory of Patrick Wong with a pair of what I thought at the time were relatively simple questions: Does our native language affect our ability to recognize voices speaking other languages, and if so, why? It turns out that the answer to the first question is a resounding 'yes', as many researchers had noted before (Goggin et al., 1991; Hollien et al., 1982; Köster & Schiller, 1997; Sullivan & Schlichting, 2000; Thompson, 1987), and that finding the answer to the second question is not nearly as straightforward as I had hoped.

In this chapter, I review the extant and emerging research on the language-familiarity effect in talker identification, with a particular interest in addressing the question of what it is exactly that a listener knows about a language that helps them more accurately recognize voices speaking that language. It is worth starting out by noting that there is no a priori reason to assume that competence in a language should contribute to the ability to identify voices; indeed, the vast majority of studies of voice distinctiveness have revealed that obviously non-linguistic acoustic features such as pitch, voice quality, and vocal tract length by themselves provide robust dissociation of individual voices (Bachorowski & Owren, 1999; Baumann & Belin, 2008; Carrell, 1984; Latinus & Belin, 2011b; Latinus et al., 2013; Lavner et al., 2001; Remez et al., 2007; Schweinberger et al., 2014). Yet, studies of the effect of language on memory for voices routinely show a substantial improvement in talker identification when listening to a native versus foreign language, regardless of whether the speech is isolated words, short sentences, or longer samples.

It is not surprising that, in any task as behaviourally important as the social obligation to quickly and accurately recognize other individuals, the brain would seek to maximize the availability of potential sources of information. Indeed, there is an enormous amount of inter-talker variability in the phonetic information in speech, which remains relatively consistent for a given talker (Hillenbrand et al., 1995; Theodore et al., 2009) and to which listeners are decidedly sensitive during speech perception (Theodore & Miller, 2010). It stands to reason that listeners would also be able to use consistent inter-talker variation in speech phonetics not only to facilitate speech perception, but also to recognize individual talkers (Francis & Driscoll, 2006; Remez et al., 1997). Languages obviously differ in their phoneme inventories and, thereby, distributions of phonetic features. Correspondingly, the phonetic dimensions along which variation will meaningfully convey phonemic versus idiolectic identity will be different across languages, and listeners' attention or inattention to the relevant dimensions will help or hinder their ability to detect the individuating phonetic features of different talkers' speech and vocal identity.

However, at present, a number of key questions about the role of language processing in talker identification remain only poorly understood. Foremost among these is the question of what information, exactly, a listener gains access to by having competence in a language. Although the answer may trivially seem to be 'everything', a more specific understanding of the language-familiarity effect hinges on how much and what kinds of linguistic competence are required for improved talker-identification abilities. Is passive exposure to the statistical distributions of phonetic features in native- or foreign-language speech sufficient? Do listeners require access to higher-level linguistic processing, such as memory for words or even speech comprehension, to gain the full range of linguistic benefits that support enhanced talker identification? Or is the contribution of linguistic processing to talker identification more like language learning itself, in that it depends not only on exposure, but also on socially-relevant exposure in order to make its fullest contribution (Kuhl et al., 2003)?

In the following sections, I explore what we know about the language-familiarity effect in talker identification. I first briefly survey the extensive literature showing the reverse side of this phenomenon, that talker-specific variability affects speech processing. Then, I describe the various studies that have investigated how listeners are able to recognize voices speaking a foreign language. I consider whether and how foreign-language learning or exposure affect the ability to identify voices speaking an unfamiliar language, as well as how early language exposure appears to establish a nascent language-familiarity effect in infants and children.

Finally, I review the very limited evidence about the brain bases of the language-familiarity effect and describe how these numerous lines of evidence are beginning to converge on alternative psychological models of voice processing that account for the role of language abilities and experiences in talker identification.

23.2 Integration of Indexical and Phonological Processing in Speech Perception

Variability in speech acoustics due to differences across talkers incurs a cognitive cost during speech perception. Listeners are faster to make decisions about the content of speech when listening to a single consistent talker compared to multiple different talkers (Green et al., 1997; Magnuson & Nusbaum, 2007; Mullennix & Pisoni, 1990). Listeners have better memory for words when they hear them spoken again by the same talker than when they are spoken by a new talker (Bradlow et al., 1999; Palmeri et al., 1993). Likewise, in a phenomenon known as the familiar-talker advantage, prior exposure to a talker's voice improves listeners' ability to perceive speech from that voice compared to an unfamiliar talker, particularly in adverse listening conditions like noise (Johnsrude et al., 2013; Newman & Evers, 2007; Nygaard & Pisoni, 1998; Nygaard et al., 1994), and listeners' expectations about talker identity influence speech processing in real time (Creel et al., 2008; K. Johnson, 1990). Listeners' ability to extract the idiosyncratic but consistent source, filter, and dynamic phonetic features of a talker's voice to improve speech perception (Kleinschmidt & Jaeger, 2015) raises the possibility that our mental representations of speech and voice are indeed closely integrated (Kuhl, 2011), such that any information about one aids substantially in perceiving and remembering the other.

23.3 The Language-Familiarity Effect in Talker Identification

Just as familiarity with a talker improves speech recognition, so too does familiarity with speech improve talker recognition. In the language-familiarity effect, listeners are more accurate at distinguishing voices when listening in their native language than when listening in a foreign language (Figure 23.1). This effect is obtained across a host of different experimental design considerations—how many voices are included, the languages spoken by talkers and listeners, whether listeners are asked to identify or discriminate voices, how much exposure listeners have to the target voices, how long between exposure and test, and whether the speech content is the same at exposure and test. In a time of increasing concern over reproducibility in psychological research (Open Science Collaboration, 2015), the language-familiarity effect remains one of the most robust and highly replicable phenomena in the psychology of voice processing. The reliability of this effect notwithstanding,

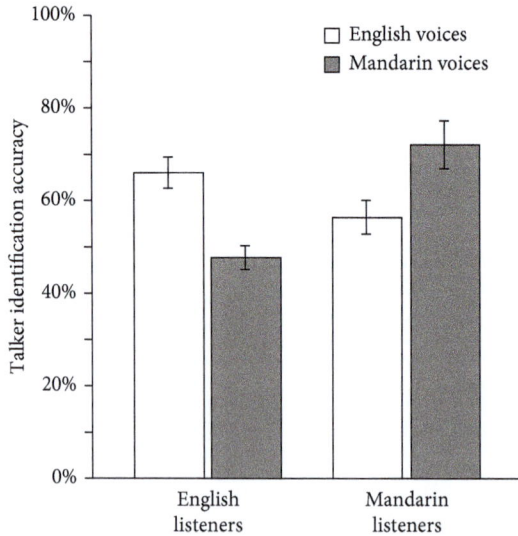

FIGURE 23.1 The language-familiarity effect in talker identification. People identify voices more accurately when listening to their native language than an unfamiliar foreign language. These data (redrawn from Perrachione & Wong, 2007) show that native English-speaking listeners are better at identifying English-speaking voices, whereas native Mandarin-speaking listeners are better at identifying Mandarin-speaking voices. This language-familiarity effect in talker identification has been observed for a wide range of language pairings and task designs.

Reprinted from *Neuropsychologia*, Volume 45, Issue 8, Perrachione T.K. & Wong P.C.M., 'Learning to recognize speakers of a non-native language: Implications for the functional organization of human auditory cortex', pp. 1899–910, Copyright © 2006 Elsevier Ltd, with permission from Elsevier, http://www.sciencedirect.com/science/article/pii/S0028393206004611

a comprehensive model of voice recognition that parsimoniously integrates the potential cognitive, perceptual, and mnemonic bases for this effect has remained elusive.

Most contemporary researchers refer to the work of Judith Goggin and Charles Thompson (Goggin et al., 1991; Thompson, 1987) as the first to investigate how listeners are able to identify voices speaking another language; however, the observation of the language-familiarity effect in talker identification appears to have been originally described in a paper by Harry Hollien and colleagues (Hollien et al., 1982), and reported many years earlier in an abstract at the Acoustical Society of America (Hollien et al., 1974). In that study, Polish-speaking listeners were significantly less accurate at identifying English-speaking voices than were English-speaking listeners. Although it has passed mostly unnoticed in the small field of language and voice, the Hollien study actually presaged many of the observations and approaches that have become standard today. Whereas the intervening years would see most research on the role of language in talker identification conducted using voice line-ups, the Hollien study explicitly trained listeners to identify talkers—the predominant method for studying the language-familiarity effect today. Additionally, Hollien and colleagues not only observed a similar magnitude for the effect of language familiarity to what we find today, they also noted that phonetic manipulations have a much smaller effect on talker identification by foreign-language listeners—an observation in accord with contemporary views of which features of speech are used by listeners to recognize native- versus foreign-language voices.

23.3.1 Identifying Speakers of Other Languages in Voice Line-Ups

Without a doubt, though, the experiments of Goggin and colleagues (1991), following the earlier report of Thompson (1987), represent one of the most comprehensive investigations of the role of language in talker identification. In a series of four experiments utilizing voice line-ups with paragraph-length recordings, Goggin and colleagues found that monolingual English listeners identified talkers' voices better when they were speaking English than German, but that monolingual German listeners showed the opposite effect from the same voices[1]. English monolinguals were also more accurate at identifying voices when they spoke English than Spanish—replicating Thompson (1987)—but English-Spanish bilinguals were equally accurate regardless of which of those languages was being spoken.

Goggin and colleagues' (1991) fourth experiment was particularly clever: they examined talker-identification accuracy as the sampled speech was made increasingly unlike English. They first recorded their talkers reading a paragraph in English; second, they read a paragraph consisting of the same words, but with their order randomized to produce nonsense; third, they read a paragraph consisting of the same syllables, but with their order again randomized to produce nonsense pseudo-English; fourth, they time-reversed the natural English recordings to produce incomprehensible backwards speech. Listeners' ability to accurately identify the target voice in the line-up fell with each manipulation, such that the less the target speech resembled English, the more poorly voices were identified.

The sum of these results was interpreted as suggesting that memories for voices were encoded via 'schemata' that consisted of 'norms for all aspects of a language, including its syntax, lexicon, and phonology', which were 'learned through exposure to voices in a local area' (Goggin et al., 1991). This interpretation, although less formal, is perhaps not so unalike contemporary models of talker identification that posit prototype-based coding (Latinus & Belin, 2011a; Lavner et al., 2001). Furthermore, while no contemporary models—even those that are most assertive about a role for high-level linguistic processing as a basis for the language-familiarity effect (see the following)—would suggest that syntactic processing plays a role in talker identification, there is evidence that listeners do learn talkers' idiosyncratic preferences for certain syntactic structures (Kamide, 2012).

Subsequent studies testing listeners' ability to identify foreign-language voices in voice line-ups (Table 23.1) tended not to compare performance against a native-language condition, but between listeners of different proficiency levels (Köster & Schiller, 1997; Sullivan &

---

[1] This design consideration, to test native listeners of both languages on the same voices, is particularly important, given how stimulus factors can easily contribute to either Type I or Type II errors in studies of the language-familiarity effect. One set of voices may be inherently more distinctive than the other, or bilingual speakers may be inherently more distinctive in one language than the other. Many contemporary studies employ such a reciprocal design to avoid these statistical errors (Bregman & Creel, 2014; Fleming et al., 2014; Perrachione et al., 2009; Perrachione & Wong, 2007; Xie & Myers, 2015); however, many do not (Johnson et al., 2011; Kadam et al., 2016; Orena et al., 2015; Zarate et al., 2015).

Table 23.1 The language-familiarity effect in voice line–ups

Study	Native language	Foreign language	Effect size (d) of LFE	Participants
Thompson, 1987	English	Spanish	*	Control
Goggin et al., 1991	English	German	*	Control
		Spanish		
	German	English	*	Control
Köster & Schiller, 1997	Spanish	German	* †	
	Chinese			
Sullivan & Schlichting, 2000	English	Swedish	* †	Control
Sullivan & Kügler, 2001	English	Swedish	* †	Control
Philippon et al., 2007	English	French	*	Control
Johnson et al., 2011	English	Dutch	0.876	Control
		Japanese	0.827	
		Italian	0.125	

If studies reported multiple experiments, only the first experiment or only those testing the basic effect of language on talker identification are included here. 'Control' participant groups were those selected in experiments that did target a specific population (e.g. musicians) or did not manipulate a between-group difference besides native-language background. Effect sizes are calculated as Cohen's d from summary statistics reported in the papers or obtained from the authors.
* The type of data collected does not allow for calculation of the Cohen's d effect-size statistic.
† Listeners were only tested in the foreign language.
LFE: language-familiarity effect

Kügler, 2001; Sullivan & Schlichting, 2000). These studies are considered in greater detail in Section 23.4. However, two more recent studies did test listeners in multiple-language conditions and found converging results. When tested on line-ups of French-speaking voices, English-speaking listeners were more likely to select the incorrect target voice (more false alarms) than when tested on line-ups of English-speaking voices (Philippon et al., 2007). Likewise, English-speaking listeners were less accurate at identifying Japanese- or Dutch-speaking voices in a line-up than they were English-speaking voices (E. K. Johnson et al., 2011); however, interestingly, the same listeners were not impaired in their ability to identify Italian-speaking voices.

23.3.2 Discriminating Speakers of Other Languages

A relatively less-frequently used technique to explore the language-familiarity effect is the discrimination paradigm, in which listeners hear pairs of voices and decide whether they are the same or different. There are a variety of reasons why discrimination paradigms may be less preferred for studying the role of language in voice processing. For one, listeners' voice discrimination abilities tend to be very good, such that ceiling effects may obfuscate differences between conditions. Additionally, in discrimination paradigms, there is reason to believe that listeners may be attending to different features of the voices, including particularly placing greater emphasis on low-level acoustic differences between pairs of stimuli, which may not accurately represent the psychological processes that are contributing to more ecological voice recognition behaviours (Perrachione et al., 2014; Van Lancker & Kreiman, 1987).

Nonetheless, several experiments have shown an influence of listeners' native language on their ability to discriminate pairs of talkers (Table 23.2). Native English-speaking listeners are more accurate at discriminating pairs of voices speaking English than when the same voices speak in German (Winters et al., 2008). Interestingly, performance falls even further when listeners are required to make the discrimination decision across the two languages. Discrimination performance also improves with explicit prior training on the voices, but there is no interaction between the language spoken during training and that during test, further suggesting that the acoustic features used in voice discrimination are based more on stimulus-specific acoustic features than those that contribute to memory for voices. Similar results have also been obtained for English-speaking listeners discriminating not only English- and German-, but also Finnish- and Mandarin-speaking voices (Wester, 2012), including especially reduced performance for across-language voice discrimination. More recently, Levi and Schwartz (2013) have reported a substantially larger difference between English-speaking listeners' ability to discriminate voices when listening to English speech compared to German.

In an interesting departure from the usual binary response of discrimination paradigms, Fleming and colleagues (2014) conducted a study in which native English- and native Mandarin-speaking listeners rated the subjective similarity of native-, foreign-, and across-language voice pairs. Critically, all speech samples in this experiment were time-reversed, rendering them incomprehensible to listeners regardless of which language was

Table 23.2 The language–familiarity effect in studies of talker discrimination

Study	Native language	Foreign language	Effect size (d) of LFE	Participants
Winters et al., 2008	English	German	*	Control
E. K. Johnson et al., 2011	Dutch	Japanese	*	Infants
		Italian		
Wester, 2012	English	German	*	Control
		Finnish		
		Mandarin		
Levi & Schwartz, 2013	English	German	1.60	Adults
	English	German	0.33	Children
Fleming et al., 2014	English	Mandarin	0.306	Control
	Mandarin	English	0.153	Control

Studies and effect sizes reported as in Table 23.1.

* Effect sizes could not be calculated because the necessary descriptive summary statistics were not available.

LFE: language-familiarity effect

being spoken. Both native English- and Mandarin-speaking listeners rated pairs of voices in their native language as sounding more distinct than pairs of voices in the foreign language, despite never being able to comprehend the speech. These results accord well with the confidence ratings from studies using voice line-ups, in which listeners are more confident in their ability to detect target voices speaking their native language than a foreign one (Goggin et al., 1991; Thompson, 1987; cf. Philippon et al., 2007). Interestingly, listeners also judged across-language voice pairs as sounding significantly more distinct than either within-language pairing—a result curiously at odds with listeners' poor performance discriminating across-language voice pairs (Wester, 2012; Winters et al., 2008). However, the effect size of language familiarity in similarity judgements of time-reversed speech is very small compared to studies in which listeners explicitly identify voices.

23.3.3 Training Listeners to Identify Speakers of Other Languages

The most common method for studying the effect of language on voice recognition—and the one that produces the most consistent and largest effects of language—is to explicitly train listeners to identify talkers speaking in a known and unknown language (Table 23.3). Training explicit talker identification, in which listeners learn to associate different voices with a corresponding label (e.g. name, number, photo, avatar), has the advantage of being more similar to ecological voice-recognition behaviours, as well as incorporating the full range of factors that may contribute to differences in talker-identification abilities, including perception, learning, and memory of voices.

The earliest experiment in which listeners were trained to explicitly identify a slate of talkers found that Polish-speaking monolinguals identified English-speaking voices less accurately than did native English speakers (Hollien et al., 1982). More recently, native speakers of English have been found to be more accurate at explicitly identifying voices speaking English than those speaking Mandarin, whereas native Mandarin speakers are more accurate for Mandarin-speaking voices than English-speaking ones (see Figure 23.1) (Perrachione & Wong, 2007). This latter study further demonstrated that the language-familiarity effect is robust to training when listeners have no knowledge of the foreign language: monolingual English speakers improve in their ability to recognize both English and Mandarin voices across six days of explicit talker-identification training, but are always better at identifying voices speaking English than those speaking Mandarin. Native Mandarin speakers who have some competence in English, however, show a different pattern: although they are initially more accurate identifying Mandarin-speaking voices, after six days of explicit training on both Mandarin- and English-speaking voices, the effect of language disappears for these bilingual listeners. These results have been interpreted to mean that some sort of linguistic competence, not mere exposure, is critical for the enhanced talker-identification accuracy associated with the language-familiarity effect.

Numerous design considerations come into play in developing talker-identification training paradigms. How many voices will be trained? How much training will listeners receive? How should voices be labelled? Interestingly, although some researchers prefer one alternative over another, none of these design considerations appears to meaningfully

Table 23.3 The language–familiarity effect in studies that train talker identification

Study	Native language	Foreign language	Effect size (*d*) of LFE	Participants
Hollien et al., 1982	Polish	English	*	Control
Perrachione & Wong, 2007	English	Mandarin	1.585	Control
	Mandarin	English	0.970	Control
Winters et al., 2008	English	German	*	Control
Perrachione et al., 2009	English	Mandarin	0.902	Control
	Mandarin	English	1.827	Control
Perrachione et al., 2011	English	Mandarin	1.153	Typical readers
	English	Mandarin	–0.091	Readers with dyslexia
Bregman & Creel, 2014	English	Korean	0.922	Monolinguals
	Korean	English	0.449	Bilinguals
Orena et al., 2015	English	French	*	High and low L2 contact groups
Xie & Myers, 2015a	English	Mandarin	1.474	Musicians
		Spanish	0.976	
	English	Mandarin	1.802	Non-musicians
		Spanish	1.671	
	Mandarin	English	1.587	Control
		Spanish	1.949	
Zarate et al., 2015	English	Mandarin	*	Control
		German		
Kadam et al., 2016	English	French	1.743	Average and advanced readers

Studies and effect sizes reported as in Table 23.1.
* Effect sizes could not be calculated because the necessary descriptive summary statistics were not available.
LFE: language-familiarity effect

affect the observation of the language-familiarity effect in talker-identification studies. Experiments training four (Bregman & Creel, 2014; Kadam et al., 2016; Orena et al., 2015) or five voices (Perrachione et al., 2011, 2009; Perrachione & Wong, 2007; Xie & Myers, 2015a; Zarate et al., 2015) do not produce wildly different estimates of the magnitude of the language-familiarity effect. Similar effects of language familiarity are also seen in studies that give all listeners a fixed amount of training (Perrachione et al., 2011, 2009; Perrachione & Wong, 2007; Xie & Myers, 2015a; Zarate et al., 2015) and those in which listeners are trained to a particular level of performance before a generalization test (Bregman & Creel, 2014; Kadam et al., 2016; Orena et al., 2015). Finally, there does not appear to be any difference in listeners' ability to learn voices—or to learn voices better in their native language—when the trained voices are paired with names (Perrachione & Wong, 2007), numbers (Perrachione et al., 2009; Xie & Myers, 2015a), or cartoon avatars (Bregman & Creel, 2014; Kadam et al., 2016; Orena et al., 2015; Perrachione et al., 2011; Zarate et al., 2015).

The numerous studies of talker identification that have confirmed a reliable presence and magnitude of the language-familiarity effect have also pushed forward our understanding of the sources of and factors affecting this phenomenon. Several have investigated how second-language learning and exposure impact the language-familiarity effect (Bregman & Creel, 2014; Orena et al., 2015) and will be addressed in greater detail later. Others have investigated how individual differences in cognitive and perceptual abilities affect native- and foreign-language talker identification. For instance, better native-language phonological skills appear to endow listeners with superior foreign- (but not native-) language talker-identification abilities (Kadam et al., 2016). Moreover, individuals with superior pitch-perception abilities—whether because they are musicians or speakers of a tone language like Mandarin—also have enhanced foreign- (but not native-) language talker-identification abilities (Xie & Myers, 2015a). Still other studies have investigated the contribution of stimulus factors to the language-familiarity effect: Zarate and colleagues (2015) found that the language-familiarity effect was greater for native English speakers when identifying voices speaking Mandarin—a language with a very different phonology compared to English—and smaller when identifying voices speaking German, with its more similar phonology (however, cf. E. K. Johnson et al., 2011; Köster & Schiller, 1997; Xie & Myers, 2015b).

23.4 How Foreign-Language Learning Affects Foreign-Language Talker Identification

To what extent is the language-familiarity effect fixed, the result of some 'critical period' in the early development of voice perception, or to what extent is it plastic to experience with new voices in adulthood? Also, if the contribution of language skills to talker identification is plastic, what kinds of exposure or expertise are necessary to improve foreign-language talker-identification abilities? Although many researchers have taken advantage of natural experiments or designed carefully constructed laboratory studies to address these questions, our poor understanding of how foreign-language talker identification can be improved with experience or training reaffirms how little we understand about the cognitive processes that underlie this effect in the first place.

There is some evidence that the kinds of foreign-language competence one acquires in the usual course of second-language study can improve talker-identification abilities in the second language. Native Chinese-speaking students studying in the United States were found to be able to recognize English-speaking voices in a voice line-up with accuracy equal to that of native English-speaking students (Goldstein et al., 1981). Native speakers of Chinese or Spanish who had completed foreign-language study in German were also more accurate at identifying German-speaking voices than were Chinese or Spanish speakers without any prior German knowledge (Köster & Schiller, 1997). Likewise, native English speakers who had studied Swedish were more accurate than English speakers with no knowledge of Swedish at identifying Swedish-speaking voices in a voice line-up, but advanced students of Swedish did not outperform novices (Sullivan & Kügler, 2001; Sullivan & Schlichting, 2000).

However, more recent studies using explicit talker-identification training may temper our enthusiasm for automatic gains in foreign-language talker-identification abilities following foreign-language study. In similarly obtained samples of native Mandarin-speaking students who had gained satisfactory proficiency in English to study abroad at American universities, Mandarin L1 listeners nonetheless were found to have significantly poorer identification of English-speaking voices compared to either Mandarin-speaking voices or performance by English-speaking listeners (Perrachione et al., 2009; Perrachione & Wong, 2007; Xie & Myers, 2015a). The persistence of the language-familiarity effect in these listeners can, however, be diminished and even eliminated with further explicit training on foreign-language talker identification (Perrachione & Wong, 2007). There is also some preliminary evidence to suggest that foreign-language learners who seek more immersive second-language experiences may overcome the language-familiarity effect to a greater degree than those who still predominately use their native language while abroad (Dougherty & Perrachione, 2016).

Instead of second-language skills acquired in adulthood, Bregman and Creel (2014) investigated whether earlier exposure in childhood to a second language was associated with improved second-language talker-identification skills. They found that, for adult Korean L1, English L2 bilinguals, the younger the age of their English exposure, the faster they were able to learn to identify English-speaking voices and the smaller their relative language-familiarity effect for Korean-speaking voices. These results suggest that earlier acquisition of (or potentially greater lifelong experience with) a second language can improve individuals' ability to recognize voices speaking in that language.

Others have gone further to suggest that lifelong exposure to a foreign language need not involve any actual competence in that language to improve talker-identification abilities: monolingual English-speaking adults from Montreal are faster and more accurate at learning French-speaking voices than are monolingual English-speaking adults from Connecticut (Orena et al., 2015). These results suggest that merely being in an environment in which one regularly hears a foreign language, even without being able to speak it oneself, can improve talker-identification abilities in that language—a result consistent with Goggin and colleagues' (1991) idea of voice schemata based on the local environment.

However, these results also raise the question of how much passive exposure one can have in a language without gaining some degree of linguistic knowledge, and, furthermore, what that knowledge might be and how it might contribute to improved talker-identification skills. Johnson and colleagues (2011) reported a similar observation, that adult listeners' mere familiarity with a language—even in the alleged absence of any particular linguistic competence—may reduce the magnitude of the native-language advantage. However, in contrast, even explicit and extended training on foreign-language talker identification in a controlled laboratory setting failed to diminish the language-familiarity effect for native English speakers attempting to identify Mandarin-speaking voices (Perrachione & Wong, 2007).

Briefly, this small collection of mostly equivocal results has left unanswered many important questions about how listeners learn to deploy second-language skills and knowledge in the service of talker identification, and even what these skills and knowledge consist of.

23.5 THE ROLE OF LANGUAGE IN THE DEVELOPMENT OF VOICE-RECOGNITION ABILITIES

Voice-recognition abilities emerge early in development (Blasi et al., 2011; Grossmann et al., 2010; Kisilevsky et al., 2003; Mehler et al., 1978), paralleling early development of language-specific processing and representations (Kuhl, 2004; Kuhl et al., 1992; Stager & Werker, 1997). It is therefore interesting to consider what role early language experience has on the development of voice-recognition abilities, and what this tells us about the cognitive or mnemonic bases of the language-familiarity effect.

In an ambitious study, and the only one of its kind to date, infants as young as 7 months were found to be more sensitive to a change in talker when listening to speech in their (emerging) native language than when listening to speech in an unfamiliar foreign language or time-reversed speech (E. K. Johnson et al., 2011). This remarkable result suggests that there is a language-familiarity effect in voice perception even in infants who putatively know few words (cf. Bergelson & Swingley, 2012) and who are still learning the phonemic and phonotactic distribution of sounds in their native language. Given the limited linguistic knowledge or experience of these infants, it is a fascinating question to speculate on what distinctive features attract their attention to changing voices in their native language, but not in a foreign language. A lack of attention to foreign-language speech alone does not account for these observations, since infants in that study were just as likely to notice a change from one foreign language to another.

The role that language abilities play in voice recognition is unfortunately no better understood as children get older. In the only study to date of the role of language in voice processing by children, young English-speaking children aged 7–9 years were significantly more accurate at discriminating voices when listening to English speech than German speech (Levi & Schwartz, 2013). Adults in the study also showed this language-familiarity effect in talker discrimination. However, older English-speaking children aged 10–12 years showed no difference in their ability to discriminate German- or English-speaking voices. Why and how do foreign-language voice-discrimination abilities develop across childhood, only to fall off again in adulthood? More work is clearly needed to understand the contribution of language abilities to talker identification across development.

Interestingly, the same study found that neither younger nor older children with specific language impairment (SLI) showed a language-familiarity effect in talker discrimination, and that children with SLI did not underperform in talker discrimination compared to children with typical language abilities. This observation stands in partial contrast to a study of the language-familiarity effect in language-impaired adults. Specifically, adults with dyslexia—a phonologically based disorder of reading development—also do not exhibit a language-familiarity effect in talker identification (Perrachione et al., 2011). This is because adults with dyslexia do not appear to gain the typical advantage for talker identification in a native language compared to a foreign one, even though they are not impaired in foreign-language talker identification compared to adults with typical reading abilities. The parallel between the cognitive processes that underlie reading, such as phonological awareness, and improved ability in talker-identification skills has also been observed by others (Kadam et al., 2016).

Together, these results suggest that the early development of linguistic skills unfolds in parallel with the development of voice-recognition abilities, and that early exposure to voices speaking a particular language yields listeners who are more sensitized to talker-specific differences in that language (Bregman & Creel, 2014; E. K. Johnson et al., 2011). However, the existence of the language-familiarity effect is poorly attested in children, mostly because the only study in this age range used a talker-discrimination paradigm, which, as already discussed, is known to be less sensitive to the role of language in voice processing due to ceiling effects and differences in task demands. More research into how the talker-identification abilities of children are shaped by language experience is clearly necessary.

23.6 NEURAL INTEGRATION OF SPEECH AND VOICE PROCESSING

Although there is a growing understanding of the neural bases of voice processing (Belin et al., 2002, 2000; Latinus et al., 2013; Pernet et al., 2015; von Kriegstein et al., 2003; von Kriegstein & Giraud, 2004), as well as the dynamic integration of representations of voice and speech information (Chandrasekaran et al., 2011; Formisano et al., 2008; Kaganovich et al., 2006; Kreitewolf et al., 2014; Perrachione et al., 2016; Sjerps et al., 2011; von Kriegstein et al., 2010; Wong et al., 2004; Zhang et al., 2016), there has been disappointingly little research into the brain bases of the language-familiarity effect in talker identification. However, given the aforementioned results, we can postulate how neural systems for speech and voice perception might align to facilitate native-language talker identification.

Although voice recognition is generally associated with auditory areas predominately in the right hemisphere (Belin et al., 2011, 2000; von Kriegstein & Giraud, 2004), there is reason to hypothesize that linguistically-derived representations of talker identity may reflect increased bilateral integration between the right and left hemispheres. Evidence from patients with brain injuries suggests that, while the right hemisphere is important for recognizing familiar voices, the left hemisphere plays a role in distinguishing new and unfamiliar voices (Van Lancker & Kreiman, 1987), similar to the important role of language in learning new voice identities. Likewise, although there is an overall left-ear/right-hemisphere bias for talker identification, there appears to be increased recruitment of the left hemisphere specifically in native- compared to foreign-language talker-identification tasks (Perrachione et al., 2009), consistent with neuroimaging evidence for increased left-right integration during processing of talker-specific information in speech (Kreitewolf et al., 2014; von Kriegstein et al., 2010).

Neural representations of speech and voice information also overlap in auditory areas of both hemispheres (Formisano et al., 2008), suggesting that integration of both speech content and talker identity is likely to occur bilaterally. Furthermore, individuals with dyslexia are impaired in their ability to identify native- but not foreign-language voices (Perrachione et al., 2011), and the brains of these individuals show attenuated neural adaptation to the repetition of native-language voices in both the left and right hemispheres compared to controls, but only in the left hemisphere for the repetition of speech content (Perrachione et al., 2016).

Despite these inferences and tangential data, there has been no targeted investigation of the brain bases of native- versus foreign-language talker identification to date. The acquisition paradigms and statistical analysis tools are now in place to ascertain how neural systems integrate speech and voice information in a more sophisticated way than was previously possible using classical cognitive subtractions (Fristen, 1997), and the time is right to make good on decades-old speculation about the brain bases of the language-familiarity effect (Perrachione & Wong, 2007).

23.7 THEORIES AND MODELS OF THE LANGUAGE-FAMILIARITY EFFECT

Based on the converging evidence from voice line-ups, talker discrimination, talker-identification training, foreign-language learning, development, and neuroscience, do we now have sufficient evidence to build a psychological model of voice processing that accurately accounts for the contribution of language to talker identification? Although a dominant model has not emerged, we are closer today than ever before.

Prior explanations for why voices were more identifiable in a familiar language relied on broadly-defined 'schemata' based on the sum of one's experience with voices (Goggin et al., 1991). While this interpretation has held up remarkably well to much of the new evidence collected over the subsequent twenty-five years, it nonetheless falls short of explanatory adequacy in several ways. For one, it borders on tautological to assert that the reason voices are identified more accurately in a native language is because one is more familiar with such voices. What features in particular are more familiar, and what exactly does one know about the language that makes perception of, or memory for, those features more accessible? Additionally, there are some data for which a schema-based model cannot satisfactorily account: it is so far equivocal whether exposure without competence supports foreign-language talker identification (Dougherty & Perrachione, 2016; E. K. Johnson et al., 2011; Orena et al., 2015; Perrachione & Wong, 2007), even though a schema-based model predicts unequivocally that only exposure should matter. Furthermore, the developmental trajectory of talker identification seems to be more complicated than an exposure-only model would predict (Bregman & Creel, 2014; E. K. Johnson et al., 2011; Levi & Schwartz, 2013); likewise, an exposure-only model that does not distinguish the relevant underlying features cannot account for impaired native-, but not foreign-language, talker identification in disorders like dyslexia (Perrachione et al., 2011).

Contemporary researchers have, either implicitly or explicitly, begun to converge on two different descriptive models that go further in explaining how particular features of familiar and native-language speech may contribute to talker identification (Figure 23.2). The first of these—which I will call the *phonetic familiarity hypothesis*—is the idea that talker-identification abilities take advantage of listeners' increased familiarity with the statistical distributions of phonetic features in their native language, including how variations in these features meaningfully reveal phonemic versus idiolectial identity (Fleming et al., 2014; E. K. Johnson et al., 2011; Orena et al., 2015; Zarate et al., 2015). A highly congruent model—which I will call the *linguistic processing hypothesis*—incorporates the role of familiar phonetics from the first model, but goes further in suggesting that a major source of improved talker-identification accuracy in one's native language results from higher-level linguistic processing, such as recognition of words and comprehension of speech content, that depends on linguistic competence (Bregman & Creel, 2014; Perrachione et al., 2015; Perrachione & Wong, 2007). The principal questions in adjudicating between or synthesizing these models are—what linguistic factors contribute

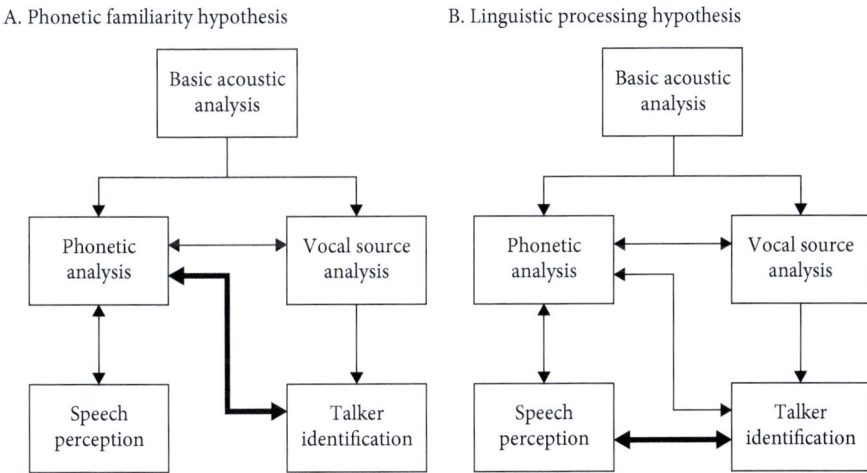

FIGURE 23.2 Psychological models of the language-familiarity effect posit different roles for linguistic processing and representations. Although the phenomenon of superior talker-identification abilities in one's native language has been extensively documented, the psychological bases for this effect remain a matter of active research. (**A**) Familiarity with the phonetics and phonotactics of one's native language is a likely source for the language-familiarity effect. A growing body of evidence demonstrates that increasing familiarity with the phonetic features, phoneme inventory, and phonotactic distributions of a language plays a role in accurate talker identification. (**B**) Other evidence suggests that passive or statistical familiarity with the sound patterns of a language does not explain the full extent of the native-language advantage in talker identification. Beyond phonetics, higher-level linguistic processes, such as recognizing and remembering words and phrases, may also play a role in enhancing listeners' ability to identify voices speaking a familiar language.

to talker identification, and how much do the various factors contribute independently versus depend on one another?

23.7.1 A Phonetic Familiarity Model

The idea that the language-familiarity effect in talker identification arises due to increased familiarity with the phonological system of one's native language is supported by a number of converging lines of evidence. First, a language-familiarity effect has been found in infants at 7 months (E. K. Johnson et al., 2011), well before they have had the opportunity to establish higher-level linguistic representations such as words, but at an age when native-language phonological skills are also beginning to emerge (Kuhl, 2004). Second, listeners judge time-reversed native-language voices to sound more distinct than time-reversed foreign-language voices (Fleming et al., 2014), suggesting that familiar phonetic patterns, such as the vowel space, may contribute to voice processing even in the absence of comprehensible speech. Third, a larger-magnitude language-familiarity effect has been reported between more phonologically dissimilar languages compared to more phonologically similar ones (Zarate et al., 2015), suggesting that the degree to which foreign-language speech can be mapped onto native-language phonological representations may facilitate talker identification. Fourth, the magnitude of the language-familiarity effect has been reported to diminish with increased exposure to a foreign language, even allegedly without any linguistic competence in that language (Orena et al., 2015). Together, these lines of research provide important and convincing evidence of a role for familiarity with language-specific phonetic patterns in enhancing voice processing.

However, there are alternative interpretations of or inconsistencies with the aforementioned results. Although infants exhibit a language-familiarity effect that presumably cannot be based on higher-level linguistic processing, it need not be the case (nor is it even likely) that language-familiarity effects in infants and adults arise from identical mechanisms. Additionally, although listeners rate time-reversed native-language voice pairs as sounding more distinct, we have just seen that the results of paradigms in which listeners discriminate voices do not always map cleanly onto the results of tasks in which they identify talkers. Indeed, more recent evidence has suggested that when asked to learn and identify voices from time-reversed speech, listeners exhibit no language-familiarity effect whatsoever (Perrachione et al., 2015).

Evidence for enhanced talker identification due to phonological similarity between languages is likewise equivocal, with some studies finding a reduced language-familiarity effect when two languages are more typologically similar (Zarate et al., 2015), whereas others that looked for such an effect, did not find one (E. K. Johnson et al., 2011; Köster & Schiller, 1997; Xie & Myers, 2015a). Likewise, the observation that passive exposure to a language reduces the language-familiarity effect has been reported by some studies (E. K. Johnson et al., 2011; Orena et al., 2015), but other studies have shown that the language-familiarity effect can be equally large whether listeners have prior experience with the foreign language or not (Perrachione & Wong, 2007; Xie & Myers, 2015a).

23.7.2 A Linguistic Processing Model

The second descriptive model inherits all the connections of the phonetic-familiarity model, but adds an important connection between speech processing (including especially word recognition and comprehension) and talker identification. There are a number of observations which do not seem to be well accounted for by the phonetic-familiarity model and which seem to suggest that processing the higher-level linguistic content of speech further facilitates native-language talker identification. First, even explicit and extended training on foreign-language talker identification does not reduce the magnitude of the language-familiarity effect for listeners with no linguistic competence in the foreign language, but such training does improve foreign-language talker identification for emerging bilinguals (Perrachione & Wong, 2007). Additionally, talker identification improves for meaningful speech compared to meaningless but phonologically-balanced nonsense speech (Goggin et al., 1991; Perrachione et al., 2015; Xie & Myers, 2015b), further indicating that meaningful and familiar linguistic units, like words, facilitate talker identification. Finally, listeners are more accurate identifying voices when they can compare and remember how different talkers say words, an effect that obtains only in a native language, not a foreign one (McLaughlin et al., 2015), which also suggests that part of the representation in memory for voices is memory for how they sound saying particular words. Together, these results suggest that accurate memory for voices takes advantage of high-level linguistic processes and representations that come with linguistic competence, not just passive familiarity with sound structure.

There are limitations on these data as well that nonetheless underscore a core importance for familiarity with phonological structure. In particular, the decrement in talker-identification performance between meaningful speech and meaningless but phonologically well-formed speech is much smaller than the corresponding decrement between meaningful and foreign-language speech (Goggin et al., 1991; Perrachione et al., 2015; Xie & Myers, 2015b), an observation that provides some insight into the relative importance of these features to accurate native-language talker identification.

Additionally, there is also some evidence that listeners cannot fully take advantage of familiar words in the absence of familiar phonetics. There are the numerous studies demonstrating a decrement in talker-identification accuracy when listening to one's native language, but in an unfamiliar regional or social accent (Doty, 1998; Goggin et al., 1991; Kerstholt et al., 2006; Perrachione et al., 2010; Stevenage et al., 2012). Goldstein and colleagues (1981) even found that English-speaking listeners were just as accurate recognizing voices in a voice line-up when they spoke Spanish as when the same voices spoke heavily Spanish-accented English, although most other studies have found smaller magnitude effects in an unfamiliar accent than an unfamiliar language (Goggin et al., 1991; Perrachione et al., 2010).

Why the availability of a higher-level speech-processing route might depend on the familiarity of the underlying phonetics is also an interesting question. Perhaps the contributions of phonetics and higher-order linguistic representations are indeed hierarchical. Alternatively, perhaps cognitive resources that would otherwise be available for talker identification are being usurped in the service of speech perception, mediating any performance gain from familiarity with the lexical content of speech. Future work is necessary to adjudicate whether and how the putative contribution of linguistic processing depends on the presence of familiar phonetics.

23.8 UNRESOLVED QUESTIONS ABOUT RECOGNIZING SPEAKERS ACROSS LANGUAGES

- Is improved talker-identification accuracy in a native language due to enhanced ability to *perceive* the relevant features that distinguish an individual talker, to *learn* those features, or to *remember* them when one encounters a voice again?
- Under the phonetic-familiarity hypothesis, is the information learned from passive exposure to foreign-language sounds (Orena et al., 2015) the same kind of information about these sounds that is gained through developing linguistic competence (Fleming et al., 2014; E. K. Johnson et al., 2011)?
- Can listeners develop passive phonological familiarity with a foreign language (Orena et al., 2015) without actually gaining some linguistic competence (particularly lexical representations) (E. K. Johnson et al., 2011; Perrachione & Wong, 2007)?
- Under the linguistic-processing hypothesis, can higher-level linguistic processing give rise to the language-familiarity effect even for phonologically unfamiliar (i.e. heavily accented) speech?
- How much do the typological or phonological similarities of the talker and listener's languages matter to the magnitude of the language-familiarity effect in talker identification (cf. Bent & Bradlow, 2003)?
- What role do familiar prosodic patterns in a native language play in talker identification?

23.9 SUMMARY AND CONCLUSION

One of the most reliable observations in voice-perception research is that listeners identify talkers more accurately when they can understand the language being spoken, compared to when they cannot. This language-familiarity effect arises from lifelong experiences listening to and recognizing talkers speaking in one's native language, and appears to depend primarily on familiarity with the phonological system of a language, but also takes advantage of higher-level linguistic representations, particularly memory for words. Superior native-language voice-processing skills emerge early and are refined throughout development. Although this voice-processing advantage is most prominent for one's native language, extensive and substantive experience with speech in a second language can improve talker-identification abilities in that language, as well. The language-familiarity effect in talker identification reveals the closely integrated psychological, and therefore neural, representations of talker identity and speech content, providing further insight into how the mind and brain extract core linguistic and social information from the single, convolved, communicative signal of speech.

ACKNOWLEDGEMENTS

This work was supported in part by NIH R03 DC014045.

REFERENCES

Bachorowski, J.-A. & Owren, M. J. (1999). Acoustic correlates of talker sex and individual talker identity are present in a short vowel segment produced in running speech. *The Journal of the Acoustical Society of America*, 106(2), 1054–1063. https://doi.org/10.1121/1.427115

Baumann, O. & Belin, P. (2008). Perceptual scaling of voice identity: common dimensions for different vowels and speakers. *Psychological Research PRPF*, 74(1), 110–120. https://doi.org/10.1007/s00426-008-0185-z

Belin, P., Bestelmeyer, P. E. G., Latinus, M., & Watson, R. (2011). Understanding voice perception. *British Journal of Psychology*, 102(4), 711–725. https://doi.org/10.1111/j.2044-8295.2011.02041.x

Belin, P., Zatorre, R. J., & Ahad, P. (2002). Human temporal-lobe response to vocal sounds. *Cognitive Brain Research*, 13(1), 17–26.

Belin, P., Zatorre, R. J., Lafaille, P., Ahad, P., & Pike, B. (2000). Voice-selective areas in human auditory cortex. *Nature*, 403(6767), 309–312.

Bent, T. & Bradlow, A. R. (2003). The interlanguage speech intelligibility benefit. *The Journal of the Acoustical Society of America*, 114(3), 1600–1610. https://doi.org/10.1121/1.1603234

Bergelson, E. & Swingley, D. (2012). At 6–9 months, human infants know the meanings of many common nouns. *Proceedings of the National Academy of Sciences*, 109(9), 3253–3258.

Blasi, A., Mercure, E., Lloyd-Fox, S., Thomson, A., Brammer, M., Sauter, D., … Murphy, D. G. M. (2011). Early specialization for voice and emotion processing in the infant brain. *Current Biology*, 21(14), 1220–1224. https://doi.org/10.1016/j.cub.2011.06.009

Bradlow, A. R., Nygaard, L. C., & Pisoni, D. B. (1999). Effects of talker, rate, and amplitude variation on recognition memory for spoken words. *Perception & Psychophysics*, 61(2), 206–219.

Bregman, M. R. & Creel, S. C. (2014). Gradient language dominance affects talker learning. *Cognition*, 130(1), 85–95.

Carrell, T. D. (1984). *Contributions of Fundamental Frequency, Formant Spacing, and Glottal Waveform to Talker Identification*. Doctoral dissertation, Department of Psychology, Indiana University, Bloomington, USA.

Chandrasekaran, B., Chan, A. H. D., & Wong, P. C. M. (2011). Neural processing of 'what' and 'who' information in speech. *Journal of Cognitive Neuroscience*, 23(10), 2690–2700. https://doi.org/10.1162/jocn.2011.21631

Creel, S. C., Aslin, R. N., & Tanenhaus, M. K. (2008). Heeding the voice of experience: the role of talker variation in lexical access. *Cognition*, 106(2), 633–664. https://doi.org/10.1016/j.cognition.2007.03.013

Doty, N. D. (1998). The influence of nationality on the accuracy of face and voice recognition. *The American Journal of Psychology*, 111(2), 191–214.

Dougherty, S. C. & Perrachione, T. K. (2016). *The Language-familiarity Effect in Talker Identification by Highly Proficient Bilinguals Depends on Second-language Immersion*. Presented at the 171st Meeting of the Acoustical Society of America, Salt Lake City, UT.

Fleming, D., Giordano, B. L., Caldara, R., & Belin, P. (2014). A language-familiarity effect for speaker discrimination without comprehension. *Proceedings of the National Academy of Sciences*, 111(38), 13795–13798.

Formisano, E., De Martino, F., Bonte, M., & Goebel, R. (2008). 'Who' is saying 'what'? Brain-based decoding of human voice and speech. *Science*, 322(5903), 970–973. https://doi.org/10.1126/science.1164318

Francis, A. L. & Driscoll, C. (2006). Training to use voice onset time as a cue to talker identification induces a left-ear/right-hemisphere processing advantage. *Brain and Language*, 98(3), 310–318. https://doi.org/10.1016/j.bandl.2006.06.002

Fristen, K. J. (1997). Imaging cognitive anatomy. *Trends in Cognitive Sciences*, 1(1), 21–27. https://doi.org/10.1016/S1364-6613(97)01001-2

Goggin, J. P., Thompson, C. P., Strube, G., & Simental, L. R. (1991). The role of language familiarity in voice identification. *Memory & Cognition*, 19(5), 448–458.

Goldstein, A. G., Knight, P., Bailis, K., & Conover, J. (1981). Recognition memory for accented and unaccented voices. *Bulletin of the Psychonomic Society*, 17(5), 217–220. https://doi.org/10.3758/BF03333718

Green, K. P., Tomiak, G. R., & Kuhl, P. K. (1997). The encoding of rate and talker information during phonetic perception. *Perception & Psychophysics*, 59(5), 675–692.

Grossmann, T., Oberecker, R., Koch, S. P., & Friederici, A. D. (2010). The developmental origins of voice processing in the human brain. *Neuron*, 65(6), 852–858. https://doi.org/10.1016/j.neuron.2010.03.001

Hillenbrand, J., Getty, L. A., Clark, M. J., & Wheeler, K. (1995). Acoustic characteristics of American English vowels. *The Journal of the Acoustical Society of America*, 97(5 Pt 1), 3099–3111.

Hollien, H., Majewski, W., & Doherty, E. T. (1982). Perceptual identification of voices under normal, stress and disguise speaking conditions. *Journal of Phonetics*, 10(2), 139–148.

Hollien, H., Majewski, W., & Hollien, P. A. (1974). Perceptual identification of voices under normal, stress, and disguised speaking conditions. *The Journal of the Acoustical Society of America*, 56(S1), S53–S53. https://doi.org/10.1121/1.1914230

Johnson, E. K., Westrek, E., Nazzi, T., & Cutler, A. (2011). Infant ability to tell voices apart rests on language experience. *Developmental Science*, 14(5), 1002–1011.

Johnson, K. (1990). The role of perceived speaker identity in Fo normalization of vowels. *The Journal of the Acoustical Society of America*, 88(2), 642–654.

Johnsrude, I. S., Mackey, A., Hakyemez, H., Alexander, E., Trang, H. P., & Carlyon, R. P. (2013). Swinging at a cocktail party: voice familiarity aids speech perception in the presence of a competing voice. *Psychological Science*, 24(10), 1995–2004. https://doi.org/10.1177/0956797613482467

Kadam, M. A., Orena, A. J., Theodore, R. M., & Polka, L. (2016). Reading ability influences native and non-native voice recognition, even for unimpaired readers. *The Journal of the Acoustical Society of America*, 139(1), EL6–EL12. https://doi.org/10.1121/1.4937488

Kaganovich, N., Francis, A. L., & Melara, R. D. (2006). Electrophysiological evidence for early interaction between talker and linguistic information during speech perception. *Brain Research*, 1114(1), 161–172. https://doi.org/10.1016/j.brainres.2006.07.049

Kamide, Y. (2012). Learning individual talkers' structural preferences. *Cognition*, 124(1), 66–71. https://doi.org/10.1016/j.cognition.2012.03.001

Kerstholt, J. H., Jansen, N. J. M., Van Amelsvoort, A. G., & Broeders, A. P. A. (2006). Earwitnesses: effects of accent, retention and telephone. *Applied Cognitive Psychology*, 20(2), 187–197. https://doi.org/10.1002/acp.1175

Kisilevsky, B. S., Hains, S. M., Lee, K., Xie, X., Huang, H., Ye, H. H., … Wang, Z. (2003). Effects of experience on fetal voice recognition. *Psychological Science*, 14(3), 220–224.

Kleinschmidt, D. F. & Jaeger, T. F. (2015). Robust speech perception: recognize the familiar, generalize to the similar, and adapt to the novel. *Psychological Review*, 122(2), 148–203. https://doi.org/10.1037/a0038695

Köster, O. & Schiller, N. O. (1997). Different influences of the native language of a listener on speaker recognition. *International Journal of Speech Language and the Law*, 4(1), 18–28.

Kreitewolf, J., Gaudrain, E., & von Kriegstein, K. (2014). A neural mechanism for recognizing speech spoken by different speakers. *NeuroImage*, 91, 375–385. https://doi.org/10.1016/j.neuroimage.2014.01.005

Kuhl, P. K. (2004). Early language acquisition: cracking the speech code. *Nature Reviews Neuroscience*, 5(11), 831–843. https://doi.org/10.1038/nrn1533

Kuhl, P. K. (2011). Who's talking? *Science*, 333(6042), 529–530. https://doi.org/10.1126/science.1210277

Kuhl, P. K., Tsao, F.-M., & Liu, H. M. (2003). Foreign-language experience in infancy: effects of short-term exposure and social interaction on phonetic learning. *Proceedings of the National Academy of Sciences of the United States of America*, 100(15), 9096–9101. https://doi.org/10.1073/pnas.1532872100

Kuhl, P. K., Williams, K. A., Lacerda, F., Stevens, K. N., & Lindblom, B. (1992). Linguistic experience alters phonetic perception in infants by 6 months of age. *Science*, 255(5044), 606–608.

Latinus, M. & Belin, P. (2011a). Anti-voice adaptation suggests prototype-based coding of voice identity. *Frontiers in Psychology*, 2. https://doi.org/10.3389/fpsyg.2011.00175

Latinus, M. & Belin, P. (2011b). Human voice perception. *Current Biology*, 21(4), R143–R145. https://doi.org/10.1016/j.cub.2010.12.033

Latinus, M., McAleer, P., Bestelmeyer, P. E. G., & Belin, P. (2013). Norm-based coding of voice identity in human auditory cortex. *Current Biology*, 23(12), 1075–1080. https://doi.org/10.1016/j.cub.2013.04.055

Lavner, Y., Rosenhouse, J., & Gath, I. (2001). The prototype model in speaker identification by human listeners. *International Journal of Speech Technology*, 4(1), 63–74. https://doi.org/10.1023/A:1009656816383

Levi, S. V. & Schwartz, R. G. (2013). The development of language-specific and language-independent talker processing. *Journal of Speech, Language, and Hearing Research*, 56(3), 913–920. https://doi.org/10.1044/1092-4388(2012/12-0095)

Magnuson, J. S. & Nusbaum, H. C. (2007). Acoustic differences, listener expectations, and the perceptual accommodation of talker variability. *Journal of Experimental Psychology. Human Perception and Performance*, 33(2), 391–409. https://doi.org/10.1037/0096-1523.33.2.391

McLaughlin, D. E., Dougherty, S. C., Lember, R. A., & Perrachione, T. K. (2015). *Episodic Memory for Words Enhances the Language Familiarity Effect in Talker Identification*. Presented at the Proceedings of the International Congress of Phonetic Sciences XVIII, Glasgow, Scotland.

Mehler, J., Bertoncini, J., Barrière, M., & Jassik-Gerschenfeld, D. (1978). Infant recognition of mother's voice. *Perception*, 7(5), 491–497. https://doi.org/10.1068/p070491

Mullennix, J. W. & Pisoni, D. B. (1990). Stimulus variability and processing dependencies in speech perception. *Perception & Psychophysics*, 47(4), 379–390.

Newman, R. S. & Evers, S. (2007). The effect of talker familiarity on stream segregation. *Journal of Phonetics*, 35(1), 85–103.

Nygaard, L. C. & Pisoni, D. B. (1998). Talker-specific learning in speech perception. *Perception & Psychophysics*, 60(3), 355–376.

Nygaard, L. C., Sommers, M. S., & Pisoni, D. B. (1994). Speech perception as a talker-contingent process. *Psychological Science*, 5(1), 42–46.

Open Science Collaboration (2015). PSYCHOLOGY. Estimating the reproducibility of psychological science. *Science*, 349(6251), aac4716. https://doi.org/10.1126/science.aac4716

Orena, A. J., Theodore, R. M., & Polka, L. (2015). Language exposure facilitates talker learning prior to language comprehension, even in adults. *Cognition*, 143, 36–40.

Palmeri, T. J., Goldinger, S. D., & Pisoni, D. B. (1993). Episodic encoding of voice attributes and recognition memory for spoken words. *Journal of Experimental Psychology: Learning, Memory, and Cognition*, 19(2), 309.

Pernet, C. R., McAleer, P., Latinus, M., Gorgolewski, K. J., Charest, I., Bestelmeyer, P. E. G., ... Belin, P. (2015). The human voice areas: spatial organization and inter-individual variability in temporal and extra-temporal cortices. *NeuroImage*, 119, 164–174. https://doi.org/10.1016/j.neuroimage.2015.06.050

Perrachione, T. K., Chiao, J. Y., & Wong, P. C. (2010). Asymmetric cultural effects on perceptual expertise underlie an own-race bias for voices. *Cognition*, 114(1), 42–55.

Perrachione, T. K., Del Tufo, S. N., & Gabrieli, J. D. E. (2011). Human voice recognition depends on language ability. *Science*, 333(6042), 595–595. https://doi.org/10.1126/science.1207327

Perrachione, T. K., Del Tufo, S. N., Winter, R., Murtagh, J., Cyr, A., Chang, P., ... Gabrieli, J. D. E. (2016). Dysfunction of rapid neural adaptation in dyslexia. *Neuron*, 92(6), 1383–1397. https://doi.org/10.1016/j.neuron.2016.11.020

Perrachione, T. K., Dougherty, S. C., McLaughlin, D. E., & Lember, R. A. (2015). *The Effects of Speech Perception and Speech Comprehension on Talker Identification*. Presented at the Proceedings of the International Congress of Phonetic Sciences XVIII, Glasgow, Scotland.

Perrachione, T. K., Pierrehumbert, J. B., & Wong, P. (2009). Differential neural contributions to native-and foreign-language talker identification. *Journal of Experimental Psychology: Human Perception and Performance*, 35(6), 1950.

Perrachione, T. K., Stepp, C. E., Hillman, R. E., & Wong, P. C. (2014). Talker identification across source mechanisms: experiments with laryngeal and electrolarynx speech. *Journal of Speech, Language, and Hearing Research*, 57(5), 1651–1665.

Perrachione, T. K. & Wong, P. C. (2007). Learning to recognize speakers of a non-native language: implications for the functional organization of human auditory cortex. *Neuropsychologia*, 45(8), 1899–1910.

Philippon, A. C., Cherryman, J., Bull, R., & Vrij, A. (2007). Earwitness identification performance: the effect of language, target, deliberate strategies and indirect measures. *Applied Cognitive Psychology*, 21(4), 539–550.

Remez, R. E., Fellowes, J. M., & Nagel, D. S. (2007). On the perception of similarity among talkers. *The Journal of the Acoustical Society of America*, 122(6), 3688–3696. https://doi.org/10.1121/1.2799903

Remez, R. E., Fellowes, J. M., & Rubin, P. E. (1997). Talker identification based on phonetic information. *Journal of Experimental Psychology: Human Perception and Performance*, 23(3), 651.

Schweinberger, S. R., Kawahara, H., Simpson, A. P., Skuk, V. G., & Zäske, R. (2014). Speaker perception. *Wiley Interdisciplinary Reviews: Cognitive Science*, 5(1), 15–25. https://doi.org/10.1002/wcs.1261

Sjerps, M. J., Mitterer, H., & McQueen, J. M. (2011). Listening to different speakers: on the time-course of perceptual compensation for vocal-tract characteristics. *Neuropsychologia*, 49(14), 3831–3846. https://doi.org/10.1016/j.neuropsychologia.2011.09.044

Stager, C. L. & Werker, J. F. (1997). Infants listen for more phonetic detail in speech perception than in word-learning tasks. *Nature*, 388(6640), 381–382. https://doi.org/10.1038/41102

Stevenage, S. V., Clarke, G., & McNeill, A. (2012). The 'other-accent' effect in voice recognition. *Journal of Cognitive Psychology*, 24(6), 647–653. https://doi.org/10.1080/20445911.2012.675321

Sullivan, K. P. H. & Kügler, F. (2001). Was the knowledge of the second language or the age difference the determining factor? *Forensic Linguistics*, 8(2), 1–8. https://doi.org/10.1558/sll.2001.8.2.1

Sullivan, K. P. H. & Schlichting, F. (2000). Speaker discrimination in a foreign language: first language environment, second language learners. *Forensic Linguistics*, 7(1), 95–111.

Theodore, R. M. & Miller, J. L. (2010). Characteristics of listener sensitivity to talker-specific phonetic detail. *The Journal of the Acoustical Society of America*, 128(4), 2090–2099. https://doi.org/10.1121/1.3467771

Theodore, R. M., Miller, J. L., & DeSteno, D. (2009). Individual talker differences in voice-onset-time: contextual influences. *The Journal of the Acoustical Society of America*, 125(6), 3974–3982. https://doi.org/10.1121/1.3106131

Thompson, C. P. (1987). A language effect in voice identification. *Applied Cognitive Psychology*, 1(2), 121–131.

Van Lancker, D. & Kreiman, J. (1987). Voice discrimination and recognition are separate abilities. *Neuropsychologia*, 25(5), 829–834.

von Kriegstein, K., Eger, E., Kleinschmidt, A., & Giraud, A. L. (2003). Modulation of neural responses to speech by directing attention to voices or verbal content. *Cognitive Brain Research*, 17(1), 48–55.

von Kriegstein, K. & Giraud, A.-L. (2004). Distinct functional substrates along the right superior temporal sulcus for the processing of voices. *NeuroImage*, 22(2), 948–955. https://doi.org/10.1016/j.neuroimage.2004.02.020

von Kriegstein, K., Smith, D. R. R., Patterson, R. D., Kiebel, S. J., & Griffiths, T. D. (2010). How the human brain recognizes speech in the context of changing speakers. *The Journal of Neuroscience*, 30(2), 629–638. https://doi.org/10.1523/JNEUROSCI.2742-09.2010

Wester, M. (2012). Talker discrimination across languages. *Speech Communication*, 54(6), 781–790.

Winters, S. J., Levi, S. V., & Pisoni, D. B. (2008). Identification and discrimination of bilingual talkers across languages. *The Journal of the Acoustical Society of America*, 123(6), 4524–4538.

Wong, P. C. M., Nusbaum, H. C., & Small, S. L. (2004). Neural bases of talker normalization. *Journal of Cognitive Neuroscience*, 16(7), 1173–1184. https://doi.org/10.1162/0898929041920522

Xie, X. & Myers, E. (2015a). The impact of musical training and tone language experience on talker identification. *The Journal of the Acoustical Society of America*, 137(1), 419–432.

Xie, X. & Myers, E. B. (2015b). *General Language Ability Predicts Talker Identification*. Presented at the Proceedings of the 37th Annual Meeting of the Cognitive Science Society, Austin, TX.

Zarate, J. M., Tian, X., Woods, K. J. P., & Poeppel, D. (2015). Multiple levels of linguistic and paralinguistic features contribute to voice recognition. *Scientific Reports*, 5, 11475. https://doi.org/10.1038/srep11475

Zhang, C., Pugh, K. R., Mencl, W. E., Molfese, P. J., Frost, S. J., Magnuson, J. S., … Wang, W. S.-Y. (2016). Functionally integrated neural processing of linguistic and talker information: an event-related fMRI and ERP study. *NeuroImage*, 124(Pt A), 536–549. https://doi.org/10.1016/j.neuroimage.2015.08.064

CHAPTER 24

....

PERCEIVING SPEAKER IDENTITY FROM THE VOICE

....

STEFAN R. SCHWEINBERGER AND ROMI ZÄSKE

24.1 INTRODUCTION AND HISTORY

....

THE biological importance of abilities to recognize an individual's identity from the voice may be exemplified by the fact that many animal species have developed such abilities. Early research on human voice recognition (before roughly the mid-1980s) was largely devoid of psychological theories, and tended to be driven mainly by three strands of research: (i) applied and forensic research into speaker identification (Saslove & Yarmey, 1980); (ii) intriguing developmental research showing that even newborn babies recognized and preferred their mothers' voices (DeCasper & Fifer, 1980); and, as discussed in the next section, (iii) substantial efforts from acoustic analyses to determine the signal parameters that are important for successful voice recognition (e.g. Bricker & Pruzansky, 1966; Pollack et al., 1954).

In the 1980s, Diana van Lancker and her colleagues were the first to describe brain-injured patients who had marked deficits in voice recognition, and coined the term *phonagnosia* as a selective deficit in recognizing speaker identity from the voices of familiar individuals. While these studies did not always include systematic tests for other forms of auditory agnosia, one of the important findings from these experiments was that the ability to recognize familiar or famous voices can be dissociated from the ability to discriminate between speaker identities for unfamiliar voices (Van Lancker & Canter, 1982; Van Lancker & Kreiman, 1987; Van Lancker et al., 1989). This finding not only was relevant to psychological theories of voice recognition but also almost coincided in time with the publication of the first influential cognitive model of face perception and face recognition (Bruce & Young, 1986). Remarkably, Bruce and Young also emphasized the need to distinguish between the processes that allow observers to identify faces of familiar persons from those that mediate the processing of identity in unfamiliar faces (e.g. in matching tasks or episodic memory tasks). While van Lancker's findings in brain-injured patients were later confirmed and extended in larger studies including more extensive sets of tests (Neuner & Schweinberger, 2000), cognitive models of voice perception (Belin et al., 2011, 2004) were proposed which essentially borrowed the functional architecture suggested by Bruce and Young (1986) for face perception.

24.2 THE ROLE OF THE SIGNAL

It is probably fair to say that the efforts to identify the acoustic parameters that allow perception of a speaker's identity (for an early review, see Hecker, 1971) were remarkably unsuccessful (Kuwabara & Sagisak, 1995), when compared with research into the acoustic profiles for other social signals such as emotion or gender in the voice. To give a few examples, voices signalling fear or panic are consistently characterized by high fundamental frequencies (F0) and fast speech rates, and sad voices exhibit low mean overall energy (Banse & Scherer, 1996). In the perception of voice gender, the importance of both F0 and formant frequencies is well established (e.g. Skuk & Schweinberger, 2014). By contrast, and despite considerable efforts, it seems that no acoustic parameters could be identified that signal speaker identity consistently.

In retrospect, this failure may simply indicate that whereas many communicative social signals are characterized by very systematic acoustic correlates, in order to recognize a speaker's identity, the perceptual system uses whatever acoustic cue is particularly salient or characteristic for that particular voice. This point is well illustrated by one of the first studies that investigated the identification of a large set of famous voices from brief samples of 2–4 seconds in duration (Van Lancker et al., 1985). Voices were presented either conventionally or temporally reversed (backward). The remarkable observation was that backward presentation (which essentially distorts phonetic information and temporal structures of segments and words, but preserves frequency and frequency ranges) had very different effects for different voices. For some famous voices, backward presentation resulted in virtually identical identification performance compared to forward presentation, whereas other voices were almost unrecognizable with backward presentation. This suggests that for some voices, acoustic cues that are preserved by temporal reversal are sufficient for identification, whereas other voices can only be identified by acoustic cues that are hampered by temporal reversal.

While the diagnosticity of acoustic parameters thus appears to depend heavily on the individual speaker, other aspects of the signal or task generated more consistent patterns of results. Unsurprisingly, voice-recognition performance was found to be inversely related to the number of speakers in a test set (e.g. Legge et al., 1984). Accordingly, comparing recognition performance in terms of percentage correct across different studies is rather meaningless unless speaker set size is taken into account. This needs to be kept in mind given that many studies—both older and more recent—worked with very small sets of speakers (often ten or even less) (see Andics et al., 2010; Bricker & Pruzansky, 1966; Compton, 1963; Latinus et al., 2011; Zäske et al., 2010).

As the voice signal unfolds over time, it is also hardly surprising that recognition performance increases with increasing duration and complexity of voice samples used in experiments. A study by Schweinberger, Herholz, and Sommer (1997) serves as an example for effects of sample duration on recognition performance for a relatively large set of familiar voices presented among unfamiliar voices (see Figure 24.1). There has been some debate

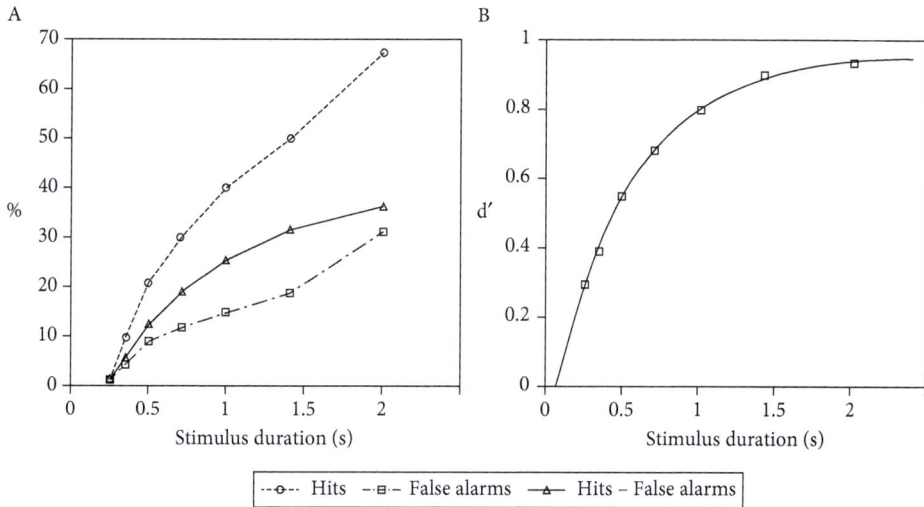

FIGURE 24.1 (A) Role of stimulus duration for the recognition of famous voices (N = 40) which were presented randomly among unfamiliar distractor voices (N = 20). Performance is expressed as the percentage of hits, false alarms, and hits minus false alarms as cumulated across stimulus duration, which was manipulated using a gating paradigm. Performance exceeded chance levels already at between 250 and 350 ms duration. (B) The same data as expressed by the sensitivity parameter (d') following signal detection analysis. The best-fitting negative exponential growth function relative to observed data (squares) is also shown. Gains were substantial within the first 1000–1500 ms, and reached asymptotic levels thereafter.

Republished with permission of American Speech-Language-Hearing Association, from *Journal of Speech, Language, and Hearing Research*, Schweinberger S.R., Herholz A, & Sommer W., 'Recognizing Famous Voices: Influence of Stimulus Duration and Different Types of Retrieval Cues', Volume 40, Copyright © 1997, American Speech-Language-Hearing Association.

about whether the benefit of longer samples originates from increased phonetic variability or from increased exposure duration per se. This is not an easy question, as both variables are typically confounded in natural speech. Although some researchers have argued for the importance of phonetic variety rather than duration for recognizing once-heard unfamiliar voices (Roebuck & Wilding, 1993), it is likely that both variability and exposure duration contribute to familiar voice recognition (Cook & Wilding, 1997).

Voice recognition and speech comprehension are often conceived as separate and independent abilities. There can be little doubt that this conceptual separation has its merits, and it indeed receives support from experimental, clinical, and neurophysiological data. At the same time, it has to be acknowledged that there is good evidence for systematic interactions between speech and voice perception. For instance, familiarity with a speaker's voice has been shown to facilitate speech comprehension (Nygaard et al., 1994). Conversely, voice recognition tends to be easier for speech in a listener's native language (Perrachione & Wong, 2007).

Overall then, this research suggests a number of practical recommendations for researchers who wish to investigate the identification of known speakers from the voice under relatively naturalistic conditions. First, a large (e.g. more than twenty) number of speakers should be used to counteract the danger that performance results from a discrimination of acoustic properties rather than genuine voice identification. Second, voice samples should be of both sufficient duration (e.g. more than 1500 ms) and phonetic variability to promote identification (e.g. Zäske et al., 2014). Third, while interference from speech content can be minimized by using relatively 'neutral' content which is devoid of semantic cues to speaker identity, voice identification should be tested with speech in a listener's native language.

24.3 SPEAKER FAMILIARITY, MENTAL REPRESENTATIONS, AND VOICE LEARNING

24.3.1 Identity Processing for Famous, Personally Familiar, and Unfamiliar Voices

Processing speaker identity from the voice has many facets: depending on the situation, we may identify a personally familiar speaker's voice over the telephone, a celebrity's voice on the radio or from a movie, or compare two unfamiliar voice samples to determine whether or not they were spoken by the same person. More generally, voice *identification* is exclusive to famous or familiar voices, and successful identification is characterized by two stages. First, a listener has to compare a heard voice with representations of known voices stored in long-term memory. Successful voice *recognition* can be said to have occurred if this comparison process results in the decision that the heard voice is indeed familiar. Note however, that 'familiar-only experiences' appear to be rather frequent in voice recognition (Hanley et al., 1998; Hanley & Turner, 2000). True identification requires a second step, during which the correspondence of the voice with a specific person is verified. This can be achieved via the production of the person's name or unique semantic information. By contrast, *discrimination* or *matching* tasks typically involve the comparison of two sequentially presented voice samples with one another, to determine whether or not they were spoken by the same (unfamiliar) speaker.

Striking dissociations between the recognition and identification of familiar voices on the one hand, and the discrimination of unfamiliar voices on the other hand (Neuner & Schweinberger, 2000; Van Lancker & Kreiman, 1987) suggest that it is important to consider familiar voice recognition and unfamiliar voice discrimination as separate abilities (Kreiman & Sidtis, 2011).

Two questions immediately arising from this insight are: what exactly characterizes the differences in mental representations of familiar and unfamiliar voices, and how exactly do voices become familiar? Regarding the first question, it has been suggested that familiar voices are recognized holistically, whereas unfamiliar voices tend to be processed in a featural manner that is strongly dependent on the individual voice sample (Kreiman & Sidtis, 2011). Beyond that general notion (which we certainly tend to agree with), the field currently lacks concrete models of how acoustic information could be represented to compute voice identity (but see Yamagishi et al., 2010, for an impressive system for personalized voice synthesis based on hidden Markov models). Although this is unfortunate, we may expect that the current and rapid advances in voice-morphing technology (see Kawahara & Skuk, this volume) will eventually promote conceptual progress. Morphing generally depends on computer algorithms that permit the creation of convincing and naturalistic stimulus continua between two sets of complex stimuli from the same perceptual category (e.g. between two voices, or between two faces). See Audio 24.1 for audio examples, including descriptions, of morphed voices used in Skuk et al. (2015).

At this point, we wish to direct the reader to several parallels with face-recognition research which may serve to justify our optimism. While the dissociation between familiar face recognition and unfamiliar face matching (e.g. Hancock et al., 2000; Malone et al., 1982; Megreya & Burton, 2006) precisely parallels the findings for voices, the foundations for image morphing (Benson & Perrett, 1991) were invented about ten years earlier than auditory morphing. Today, while the nature of mental representations of familiar faces is not yet fully understood, researchers have successfully implemented algorithms that computationally encode facial variability, for instance via principal components' analysis of images (e.g. Hancock et al., 1996). Dimensions of statistical variation both between different faces (Jenkins & Burton, 2008) and between images within individual known faces (Burton et al., 2011) have been successfully identified. This research has enhanced our understanding of how humans could mentally represent familiar faces in order to identify an individual from a novel image.

We eagerly anticipate novel methods to define, and experimentally manipulate, dimensions of statistical variation between voices of different known speakers. In parallel, it would be important to know how such representations are implemented in the brain via neuronal coding. Recent demonstrations that brain activity in auditory cortex can be reliably used to discriminate between three different speakers' voices (Formisano et al., 2008), however impressive, are only a first step in this direction.

24.3.2 Norm-Based Coding of Voice Identity

An influential account of voice memory proposes that voices are stored relative to an average prototypical voice which is located in the centre of a multidimensional space (Andics et al., 2010; Bruckert et al., 2010; Latinus et al., 2013; Lavner et al., 2001; Papcun et al., 1989; also cf. Latinus & Zäske, this volume). Accordingly, and in analogy to Valentine's (1991) multidimensional face-space framework, voices may be encoded along acoustic dimensions which are optimally suited to discriminate among all known voices. Research with unfamiliar voices suggests that such dimensions might include fundamental frequency, formant dispersion, and harmonics-to-noise ratio (Baumann & Belin, 2010; Latinus et al., 2013), but relevant research on familiar voices remains to be done. While the putative internal norm is often believed to represent the acoustic mean of all voices previously encountered, the precise determinants of the internal norm are debated. Extreme positions range from the assumption of some innate and stable template to the idea of a very transient template that only reflects the most recently heard voices.

We argue here that voice space is shaped by both long-term and more recent perceptual experience in a relatively flexible manner. Although recent perceptions will likely exert a disproportionately stronger influence in many instances, this flexibility may account both for differences between listeners and changes over time within a listener (e.g. Skuk et al., 2015).

Within the voice space, perceptually similar voices are thought to be stored in close neighbourhood, while dissimilar voices would be represented further apart. The more a given voice deviates from the prototype in terms of its acoustic parameters, the more distinctive it should be on a perceptual level, and the stronger its activation of voice-sensitive brain areas (Latinus et al., 2013).

The notion of a multidimensional voice space is compatible with data from auditory adaptation research showing that repeated exposure to an individual voice causes contrastive after-effects in voice-identity perception (Latinus & Belin, 2011a), similar to contrastive after-effects in the perception of voice categories (Schweinberger et al., 2008). Specifically, using auditory morphing (Kawahara et al., 1999), Latinus and Belin (2011a) created a voice space by averaging voices from sixteen male speakers uttering vowels. Voices of three further speakers (A, B, and C) were morphed with the average voice to create three continua of voice stimuli which systematically varied in identity strength between the original voices and their respective anti-voices. Anti-voices were extrapolated on this trajectory beyond the average voice. Thus, relative to the average, each anti-voice had the exact opposite acoustic characteristics of its original counterpart. Following adaptation to an anti-voice (e.g. anti-A speaker), participants were more likely to perceive the identity-ambiguous average voice as belonging to the respective original speaker (speaker A) compared to the other speakers (B or C). These contrastive after-effects of identity adaptation provide initial support for the notion that voices may be coded in a prototype-based fashion, similar to faces (Leopold et al., 2001). Since Latinus and Belin (2011a) used simple vowel stimuli and only a very small set of three voices, it is unclear, as yet, whether these results would transfer to more complex speech samples of familiar voices or to larger speaker sets.

Contrastive after-effects of adaptation have also been shown for other social signals in voices including voice gender, prosody, and age (Bestelmeyer et al., 2010; Skuk & Schweinberger, 2013a; Skuk et al., 2015; Zäske & Schweinberger, 2011; Zäske et al., 2010). Although these findings have occasionally been taken as evidence for opponent-coding neuronal mechanisms, there is relatively little research addressing specific models of neuronal coding of these various social signals in voices (compared to the visual modality; e.g. see Calder et al., 2008).

With respect to the voice-space framework, after-effects of adaptation may be explained in terms of a selective activation decrease in neurons coding individual voices or clusters of voices that belong to the same perceptual category (e.g. young voices, female voices). Many open questions remain. For instance, while it has been suggested that there may be separate norms for male and female voices (Latinus et al., 2013), it remains to be determined which (and how many) different norms exist for other classes of voices.

24.3.3 Voice Learning

Voice-recognition abilities are widely distributed in the animal kingdom (Kriengwatana et al., 2015) and likely have evolved in humans before speech (Belin, 2006). However, while humans can be experts for familiar voice recognition to the extent that they outperform modern voice-recognition technology (Latinus & Belin, 2011b), human perceivers can be extremely fallible when it comes to unfamiliar voice identification. Although these observations suggest that single or brief exposures are insufficient to acquire robust representations that permit reliable subsequent voice identification, it remains largely unclear how exactly unfamiliar voices become familiar during learning. Worse still, people often are hardly aware of their voice-recognition abilities. It has been shown that confidence in recognition accuracy is only weakly (or not at all) related to actual performance for unfamiliar speakers (Armstrong & McKelvie, 1996; Saslove & Yarmey, 1980). Accordingly, the predictive value of recognition confidence for the accuracy of earwitness testimony is highly questionable.

Because of its practical significance, human voice recognition has been subject to extensive forensic research following McGehee's (1937) seminal study. Since then, forensic researchers have investigated recognition of speakers whom listeners typically encountered for the first time during an experiment and who, thus, remained relatively unfamiliar. Voice recognition in these early stages of learning were found to be affected by various conditions including the nature, length, and quality of voice samples, retention intervals, number of voices learned, specific task and attentional demands, as well as characteristics of the speaker and listener (for reviews, see Clifford, 1980; Deffenbacher et al., 1989; Kreiman & Sidtis, 2011). For instance, recognition is improved when voices have been encoded intentionally rather than incidentally (Armstrong & McKelvie, 1996). Short delays between study and test may also increase recognition performance (Deffenbacher et al., 1989).

As voice learning often takes place while observing the speaker's face, researchers have asked if audiovisual face-voice learning facilitates subsequent voice recognition, compared to voice-only learning. This research produced mixed results (Armstrong & McKelvie, 1996; Cook & Wilding, 1997; Legge et al., 1984; McAllister et al., 1993; Sheffert & Olson, 2004; Stevenage et al., 2011), possibly because the beneficial effect of faces only emerges over time, and following initial costs that may be attributed to attentional capture of faces (Zäske et al., 2015). Redundant speaker information contained in voices and facial movements may help to establish and access multisensory speaker representations. Face-voice integration may therefore be particularly efficient when faces are presented as dynamic articulating faces along with the voices during learning (Sheffert & Olson, 2004) or recognition (Schweinberger et al., 2007).

Due to the focus on behavioural measures in most studies, little is known at present about the brain mechanisms underlying the transition from unfamiliar to familiar voices during learning (Schweinberger et al., 2014). One central mechanism that needs yet to be explored is how the perceptual system extracts, stores, and accesses *invariant* identity information across acoustically varying utterances within a given speaker, as opposed to between-speaker variability.

The relative robustness of familiar voice recognition against random stimulus variability and presentation conditions has been demonstrated by studies using personally familiar voices or trained-to-familiar voices in the laboratory. Although performance is affected by these following manipulations, familiar voices can often be recognized across various utterances (Skuk & Schweinberger, 2013b) including previously unheard or distorted utterances (Sheffert et al., 2002; Zäske et al., 2014), foreign languages (Zarate et al., 2015), very short excerpts of speech (Pollack et al., 1954; Schweinberger, Herholz, & Sommer, 1997), or even non-speech sounds such as when clearing one's throat (Skuk & Schweinberger, 2013b). At the same time, voices are consistently recognized more accurately from the initial study material than from novel utterances (Schweinberger, Herholz, & Stief, 1997; Zäske et al., 2014). See Audio 24.2 for audio examples, including descriptions, of voices used in the learning study by Zäske et al. (2014).

Together, these findings suggest that voice learning leads to the formation of both speech-invariant and speech-dependent voice representations. The notion of partial overlap in speaker and speech processing converges with studies showing that both abilities can dissociate on the one hand (Roswandowitz et al., 2014; Van Lancker & Canter, 1982) and are intertwined on the other hand (Nygaard et al., 1994; von Kriegstein et al., 2010).

24.4 INDIVIDUAL DIFFERENCES AND GROUP DIFFERENCES IN VOICE RECOGNITION

Interindividual variability in voice-recognition abilities is impressively exemplified by phonagnosia, the inability to recognize familiar voices. While first described as an acquired condition following right-hemispheric brain injury (Van Lancker & Canter, 1982), cases of developmental phonagnosia without known neurological cause have recently been reported (Garrido et al., 2009; Roswandowitz et al., 2014). Importantly, the impairment can selectively affect voice-identity processing, such that auditory processing of speech, music, and environmental sounds is preserved. Even the ability to discern affective information, gender, or age from voices can be preserved in selective cases (see Figure 24.2). The possibility remains that, similar to face-recognition abilities (Russell et al., 2009), voice-recognition abilities are normally distributed. Accordingly, individuals with developmental phonagnosia and super-recognizers (not yet identified in comprehensive case studies with extensive testing) may simply represent opposing ends of this spectrum. Preliminary evidence from large samples suggests that this may be the case, although the field suffers from a lack of sensitive and standardized tests to assess voice-recognition abilities (but see Aglieri et al., 2017; Mühl et al., 2017).

Could it be that voice-recognition ability is related to professional training? A reasonable presumption would be that trained listeners, such as phoneticians or speech pathologists, may have superior voice-recognition abilities. Although there is some evidence suggesting that this might be the case (Elaad et al., 1998; Schiller & Köster, 1998), more systematic research is needed to confirm these findings. Musical training has been related to improved discrimination of unfamiliar voices and recognition of newly-learned voices (Chartrand & Belin, 2006; Xie & Myers, 2015), although the directionality of these effects remains elusive. If musical training indeed enhances voice recognition, it remains to be determined whether musicians generalize their expertise in timbre and pitch processing from instruments to voices, or whether they use different cognitive strategies for voice-perception tasks.

Can clinical conditions affect voice-recognition ability? A group that has been discussed as having superior voice-recognition abilities are blind listeners. Several studies found small but significant effects to support this notion (Elaad et al., 1998; Föcker et al., 2012), although others reported similar identification rates for blind and sighted listeners (Winograd et al., 1984). In contrast to listener groups with superior voice-recognition abilities, there is initial evidence for impaired voice recognition in autistic individuals. Specifically, autism has been related to impaired familiar-voice recognition in children (Boucher et al., 1998) and voice-learning difficulties in adults (Schelinski et al., 2014). It is unclear at present whether

A. Famous - not famous

B. Identified/exposed

C. Summary of KH's performance

A - voice recognition
B - voice discrimination
C - vocal emotion
D - speech perception
E - environmental sounds
F - music processing

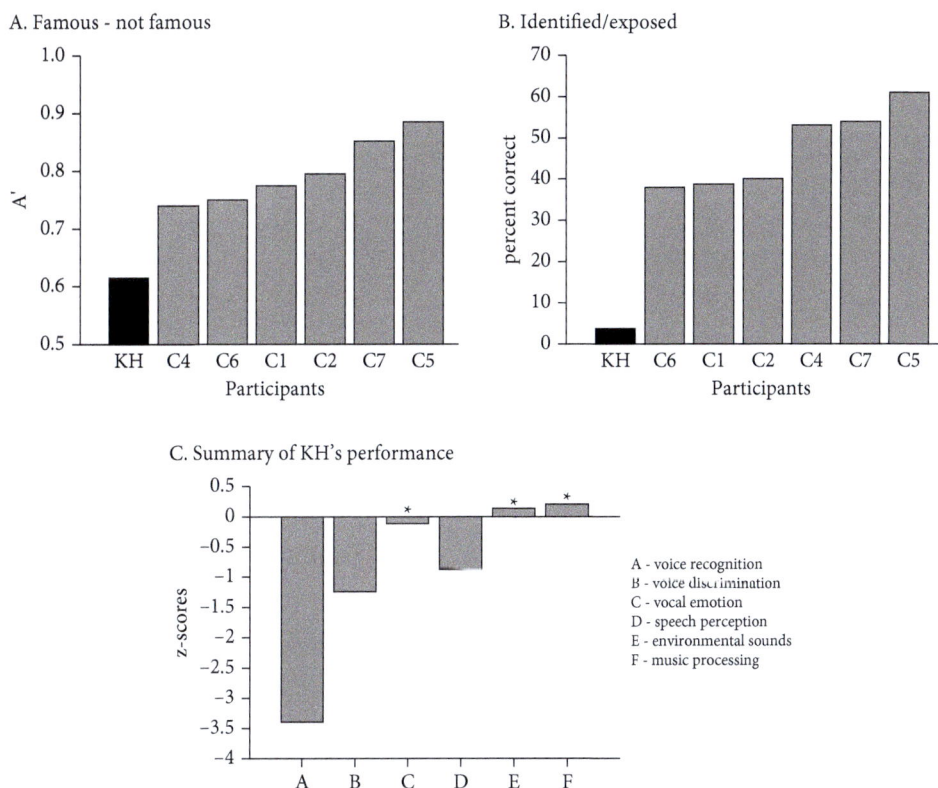

FIGURE 24.2 (A) Performance of phonagnosic participant KH in a test on the recognition of famous voices among unfamiliar distractor voices, compared with control participants' performance. A' reflects a signal detection parameter of performance in the famous/unfamiliar discrimination, and can vary from 0.5 (chance) to 1 (perfect). (B) Percentage of voices correctly identified, relative to the voices to which each participant was exposed. (C) Summary of KH's test performance (z-standardized) for each of several groups of tasks. Note the specificity of the impairment to voice recognition, with relatively preserved performance for unfamiliar voice discrimination, and completely preserved performance in tests on the perception of vocal emotion, environmental sounds, and music.

Reprinted from *Neuropsychologia*, Volume 47, Issue 1, Garrido L. et al., 'Developmental phonagnosia: A selective deficit of vocal identity recognition', pp. 123-31, Copyright © 2008 Elsevier Ltd, with permission from Elsevier, http://www.sciencedirect.com/science/article/pii/S0028393208003357

these deficits are due to reduced attention to social stimuli and/or impaired perceptual processing in autism. However, a new study on a non-clinical sample of young adults suggests that familiar voice-recognition abilities are negatively correlated with autistic traits—particularly those related to social communication, but not those related to attention to detail (Skuk et al., 2017). Furthermore, adults with dyslexia exhibit impaired voice learning relative to controls without reading disabilities (Perrachione et al., 2011). It has been argued that both reading abilities and voice learning rely on phonological processing which is impaired in dyslexia and may therefore also hamper voice learning.

Is there evidence for different voice-recognition abilities in women and men, or in listeners of different age groups? Although human voice-recognition abilities develop remarkably early in life (DeCasper & Fifer, 1980), such that even fetuses recognize their mother's voice (Kisilevsky et al., 2003), it is not until the age of 10 years that children reach adult levels of performance for unfamiliar voice recognition (Mann et al., 1979). Preliminary results could indicate a decline in voice-recognition abilities after 40 years of age (Clifford, 1980; Yonan & Sommers, 2000), as well as a specific age-related decline in a multi-talker environment (Rossi-Katz & Arehart, 2009), although more systematic research is needed to back up these findings.

It is not entirely clear whether male and female recognition abilities differ, as the few existing studies produced heterogeneous results. While one study did find better voice recognition in female listeners overall (Skuk & Schweinberger, 2013b), gender differences are often complicated by symmetrical (Roebuck & Wilding, 1993) or asymmetrical own-gender biases (OGBs) (Skuk & Schweinberger, 2013b; Wilding & Cook, 2000). In the study by Skuk and Schweinberger, forty pupils (aged 17–18 years) identified (named) twenty out of seventy classmates from the voice, using several utterance types. Both male and female listener groups exhibited considerable interindividual differences. Importantly, while female listeners identified male and female speakers with similar accuracy, male listeners exhibited an OGB such that they better identified male than female speakers. Interestingly, individual OGBs were related to differential pre-experimental contact with the speakers.

The notion that contact, and hence perceptual experience, with a certain group of speakers improves voice recognition may also explain other recently reported memory biases for voices. For instance, listeners find it easier to recognize voices from speakers who share their sociocultural background, compared to voices indicating a different origin based on sociocultural dialects (related to 'Black' and 'White' speakers; Perrachione et al., 2010), regional accents (Stevenage et al., 2012), or languages (Goggin et al., 1991; Perrachione & Wong, 2007; Zarate et al., 2015).

24.5 BRAIN CORRELATES OF SPEAKER-IDENTITY PROCESSING

One important step towards understanding how the brain processes speaker information is to identify the underlying brain areas. A major hallmark in this line of research was the discovery of voice-selective areas along the middle and anterior parts of the superior temporal sulcus (STS) bilaterally (Belin et al., 2000) by means of functional magnetic resonance imaging (fMRI). These 'temporal voice areas' (TVAs) show larger activity during passive listening to vocal sounds than to non-vocal control sounds, and are often regarded as the auditory equivalent of the fusiform face area (Kanwisher et al., 1997). The right TVA in particular is also activated by vocal sounds devoid of speech (Belin et al., 2002), indicating that this area is involved in non-linguistic processing of voice information.

Largely stimulated by those findings, current voice research is aimed at further segregating voice-sensitive areas within and outside TVAs onto which discrete voice-processing stages can be mapped (Blank et al., 2014). It is perhaps not surprising that areas in STS and superior temporal gyrus (STG) are not exclusively sensitive to voice identity, but are also sensitive to vocal expressions (for a meta-analysis, see Frühholz & Grandjean, 2013). Moreover, although the exact location of voice-sensitive regions varies between listeners (Ahrens et al., 2014; Pernet et al., 2015), voice-identity processing seems to recruit mainly right middle and anterior portions of the STS/STG, as well as the inferior frontal cortex (IFC).

In line with hierarchical models of voice processing (Belin et al., 2011, 2004; Campanella & Belin, 2007), neuroimaging research suggests that low-level voice information is analysed in primary auditory cortices before voices are structurally encoded and compared to long-term voice representations in (predominantly right) TVAs. Processing in TVAs is thought to be dependent on *acoustic* signal properties (Charest et al., 2013; Latinus et al., 2013), irrespective of speech content (Belin & Zatorre, 2003; Formisano et al., 2008; von Kriegstein et al., 2003), voice familiarity (Latinus et al., 2011; von Kriegstein & Giraud, 2004; von Kriegstein et al., 2003), and perceived identity (Andics et al., 2013). The right IFC, by contrast, has been linked to the *perception* of voice identity regardless of acoustic variability, following learning of initially unfamiliar voices (Andics et al., 2013; Latinus et al., 2011; Zäske, Hasan, & Belin, 2017). Importantly, and in line with behavioural findings (Bruckert et al., 2010; Mullennix et al., 2011; Papcun et al., 1989), fMRI research indicates that voices are coded relative to an acoustic and perceptual mean in right TVAs and IFC, respectively (Andics et al., 2013, 2011; Latinus et al., 2011, 2013; see also Section 24.3.2).

The network for processing voice identity may be more widely distributed depending on the level of voice familiarity and tasks (Blank et al., 2014). Voice-recognition tasks often entail prior knowledge of the speaker's face or name. In fact, listening to familiar voices can activate the fusiform face area (FFA) in the fusiform gyrus both for personally familiar speakers (von Kriegstein et al., 2005) and trained-to-familiar speakers (von Kriegstein & Giraud, 2006), in line with findings that the TVA and FFA are anatomically linked (Blank et al., 2011).

While the temporal resolution of neuroimaging techniques is too limited to investigate the neural correlates of voice perception in real time, electroencephalography (EEG) can provide information on the exact time course of voice-identity processing. The few studies that exist have been taken to suggest a similar timing of face and voice perception. For instance, voices are discriminated from other auditory object categories within the first 200 ms (Charest et al., 2009). A similar timing has been suggested for the assessment of voice familiarity in repetition paradigms (Beauchemin et al., 2006; Schweinberger, 2001). Other studies suggested that voice-identity processing begins around 250–300 ms for unfamiliar voices (Spreckelmeyer et al., 2009), personally familiar voices (Schweinberger, Kloth, & Robertson, 2011; Schweinberger, Walther, et al., 2011), and newly-learned voices (Zäske et al., 2014). For instance, Zäske et al. showed that compared to novel voices, previously learned voices induced a suppression of beta-band activity (16–17 Hz) between 290–370 ms after voice onset, with maximal effects at right-temporal and central sites. During learning, but at a similar latency (from ~250 ms), event-related potentials elicited by study voices were predictive of subsequent voice recognition. Importantly, both effects were independent of study-to-test changes in speech content (see Figure 24.3), and thus appear to reflect the acquisition of, and access to, speech-invariant voice representations, respectively.

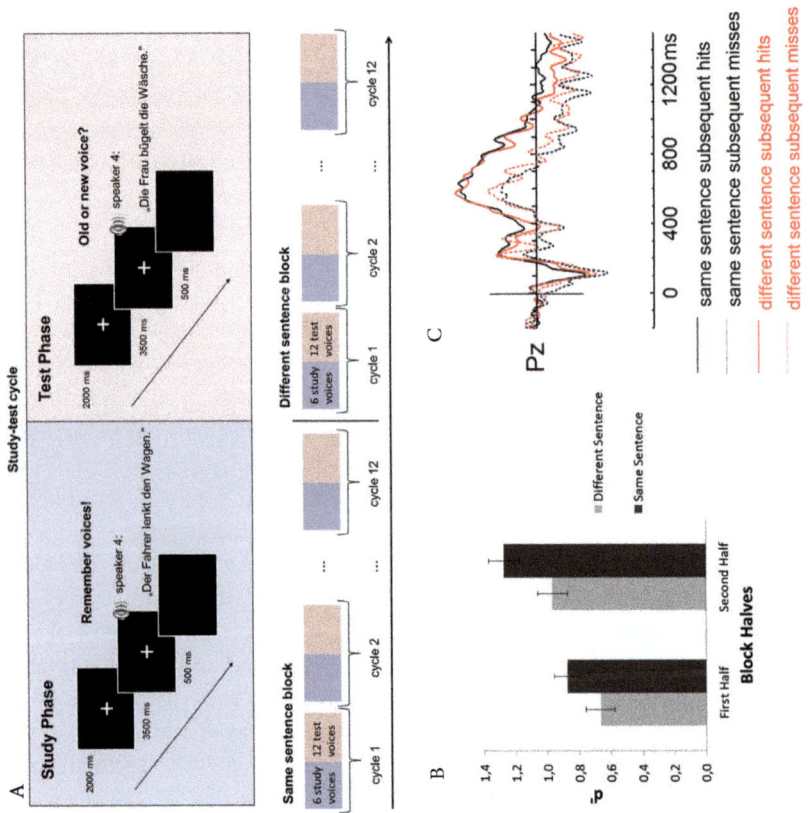

FIGURE 24.3 (A) Design of the learning study by Zäske et al. (2014), testing for voice recognition of voices from either same or different sentences than those heard during learning. (B) Performance scores (d′) show both moderate advantages for recognition from the same sentences and substantial performance in speaker recognition from different unheard sentences. (C) The 'Dm' effect for voices shows ERPs during the

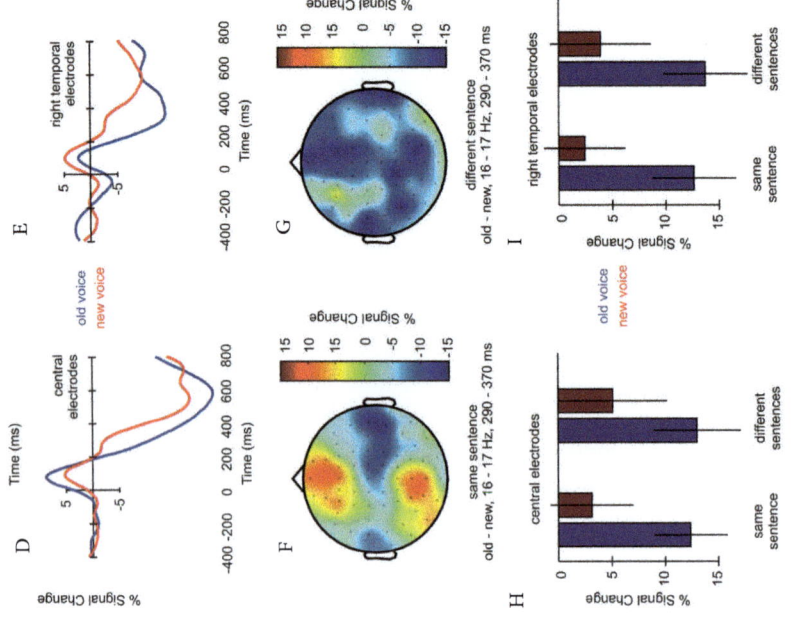

learning phase. Voices that were subsequently remembered elicited larger positivity than voices that were subsequently forgotten. Effects started already around 250 ms, and are shown for electrode Pz. (D–I) Between 290 and 370 ms after test voice onset, beta-band oscillations were systematically suppressed for learned compared to novel voices. This effect was independent of sentence condition, and was maximal at central and right temporal electrodes. (D) Waveforms showing the mean signal change (16–17 Hz) for old and new voices at a central electrode group. (E) Same as C but for a right temporal electrode group. (F) Scalp topography of the mean signal change, old versus new voices, for the 'same sentence' condition. (G) Same as F but for the 'different sentence' condition. (H) Mean signal change in each condition at the central electrode group. (I) Same as in (H) but at right temporal electrodes.

Reproduced with permission from Zäske R., Volberg G., Kovács G. & Schweinberger S.R., 'Electrophysiological Correlates of Voice Learning and Recognition,' *Journal of Neuroscience*, Volume 34, Issue 33, pp. 10821–31, Copyright © 2014 Society for Neuroscience, doi: 10.1523/JNEUROSCI.0581-14.2014

24.6 Audiovisual Face–Voice Integration in Speaker-Identity Perception

The recognition and identification of people is an important everyday ability, along with speech perception or the recognition of other people's emotional state. That said, a traditional assumption by scientists was that identity perception tends to be dominated by visual information from the face, with only a minor contribution from the voice (Bruce & Young, 1986; Walker et al., 1995). In parallel, speech perception had been typically considered a purely auditory process, at least before McGurk and Macdonald (1976) published their findings on a surprising and, now famous, perceptual illusion that demonstrates the automatic contribution of visual information from articulating faces to speech perception. Audiovisual integration (AVI) of high-level social information from speakers has received much scientific attention ever since (Calvert et al., 1998), although the major focus of that research was on the mechanisms of AVI relevant for speech perception (e.g. van Wassenhove et al., 2005), the perception of the spatial location of origin of a dynamic event (e.g. the ventriloquist illusion; see Calvert et al., 1998), or the perception of emotions from speakers (e.g. Hagan et al., 2009).

By comparison, research on AVI in the perception of speaker identity had been relatively neglected until recently. This may have been because identity is a temporally 'stable' social signal compared to rapidly changeable signals of speech or emotion. This is perhaps exemplified by a statement by Young and Bruce (2011) in a recent review on person perception: 'Our opinion at present is that although there is evidence of multimodality for a wide range of social signals, for the ecological reasons we outlined earlier this intermodal coupling will be tighter for speech than for emotion, and tighter for emotion than identity' (Young & Bruce, 2011, p. 969).

However, it also seems possible that the brain uses audiovisual correspondences whenever they are potentially useful for appropriately processing an event or episode. In fact, Welch and Warren (1980) proposed that in multisensory situations, perceivers tend to form what they call a 'unity assumption'—the assumption that two or more sensory signals are caused by the same underlying event. The unity assumption can be boosted by factors of the stimulation, such as the temporal correspondence of signals in different modalities. In that sense, the perception of a complex but familiar pattern of multisensory correspondence, like when a voice is perceived along with a dynamic face articulating in synchrony, may be a model case promoting audiovisual integration.

A number of more recent experiments indeed have demonstrated a role of face–voice integration in the perception of speaker identity from the voice (e.g. Schweinberger et al., 2007). They also showed that face–voice integration is reduced or absent when static faces are combined with voices (Schweinberger et al., 2007; but see also, Joassin et al., 2011), and that optimal face–voice integration occurs only in a relatively narrow window of audiovisual temporal synchrony (Robertson & Schweinberger, 2010). Moreover, electrophysiological studies suggest that face–voice AVI for the recognition of speaker identity begins approximately after 250 ms (Schweinberger, Kloth, & Robertson, 2011), and may be mediated by right anterior temporal brain activity. See Video 24.1 for audiovisual examples, including descriptions, used by Schweinberger, Kloth, and Robertson (2011).

An unsolved question in this research is whether audiovisual person recognition depends on the activation of a multisensory convergence zone, similar to the amodal 'person identity nodes' in Bruce-and-Young-type models of person recognition (Perrodin et al., 2015; Shah et al., 2001), or whether it reflects direct interactions between brain areas specialized for face and voice processing respectively (Blank et al., 2011; Schweinberger, Kloth, & Robertson, 2011). While a collection of papers in an edited volume (Belin et al., 2013) gives a good overview of studies on face–voice integration in person perception, an exciting development of the recent past is reflected in reports on brain mechanisms for voice recognition in other species (Perrodin et al., 2015). Voice cells (responding strongly to conspecific voices, and also differentially to individual voices) were reported in the monkey anterior temporal lobe (Perrodin et al., 2011).

Overall, there can be little doubt that a concerted effort to collect and link evidence from a variety of sources (human fMRI and scalp EEG data, animal single-cell recordings, and human intracranial recordings) will deliver an increasingly detailed picture of the brain mechanisms that mediate audiovisual speaker-identity perception (Abel et al., 2015; Perrodin et al., 2015).

24.7 CONCLUSIONS

The recognition and identification of people is an important everyday ability, but compared to face research, voice recognition has only more recently moved into the focus of researchers. Evidence from impairments (phonagnosia) shows that recognition and identification of voices of well-known speakers on the one hand, and the discrimination of speaker identity for unfamiliar voices on the other hand, represent separate abilities.

To adequately investigate voice identification, naturalistic speech samples with substantial phonetic variability are required. This is because—unlike for other social signals such as vocal emotion or gender—no consistent set of acoustic dimensions has been found to be crucial for voice-identity recognition; rather, different types of acoustic cues may be salient for different speakers.

We expect that foreseeable technological progress will promote better understanding of dimensions of statistical variation between familiar voices, as well as the nature of their mental representation. We also expect that the emerging large individual differences in voice-recognition abilities in the general population will become a focus for future research. It will be particularly important to see how these differences are reflected in neuronal responses measured by neuroscientists, who have established voice-sensitive areas in temporal cortex, and who are beginning to delineate the processes by which humans become familiar with previously unfamiliar voices.

Finally, we have discussed evidence for audiovisual face–voice integration in the perception of speaker identity, and have emphasized that the voice is typically perceived in the context of a person in real-life human interaction.

ACKNOWLEDGEMENT

The author's research has been supported by the Deutsche Forschungsgemeinschaft (DFG grant FOR1097).

References

Abel, T. J., Rhone, A. E., Nourski, K. V., Kawasaki, H., Oya, H., Griffiths, T. D., … Tranel, D. (2015). Direct physiologic evidence of a heteromodal convergence region for proper naming in human left anterior temporal lobe. *Journal of Neuroscience, 35*(4), 1513–1520. doi: 10.1523/jneurosci.3387-14.2015

Aglieri, V., Watson, R., Pernet, C. R., Latinus, M., Garrido, L., & Belin, P. (2017). The Glasgow Voice Memory Test: assessing the ability to memorize and recognize unfamiliar voices. *Behavior Research Methods, 49*(1), 97–110.

Ahrens, M.-M., Hasan, B. A. S., Giordano, B. L., & Belin, P. (2014). Gender differences in the temporal voice areas. *Frontiers in Neuroscience, 8*. doi: 10.3389/fnins.2014.00228

Andics, A., McQueen, J. M., & Petersson, K. M. (2013). Mean-based neural coding of voices. *NeuroImage, 79*, 351–360. doi: 10.1016/j.neuroimage.2013.05.002

Andics, A., McQueen, J. M., Petersson, K. M., Gal, V., Rudas, G., & Vidnyanszky, Z. (2010). Neural mechanisms for voice recognition. *NeuroImage, 52*(4), 1528–1540.

Armstrong, H. A. & McKelvie, S. J. (1996). Effect of face context on recognition memory for voices. *Journal of General Psychology, 123*(3), 259–270.

Banse, R. & Scherer, K. R. (1996). Acoustic profiles in vocal emotion expression. *Journal of Personality and Social Psychology, 70*(3), 614–636.

Baumann, O. & Belin, P. (2010). Perceptual scaling of voice identity: common dimensions for different vowels and speakers. *Psychological Research—Psychologische Forschung, 74*(1), 110–120.

Beauchemin, M., De Beaumont, L., Vannasing, P., Turcotte, A., Arcand, C., Belin, P., & Lassonde, M. (2006). Electrophysiological markers of voice familiarity. *European Journal of Neuroscience, 23*(11), 3081–3086.

Belin, P. (2006). Voice processing in human and non-human primates. *Philosophical Transactions of the Royal Society B: Biological Sciences, 361*(1476), 2091–2107.

Belin, P., Bestelmeyer, P. E., Latinus, M., & Watson, R. (2011). Understanding voice perception. *British Journal of Psychology, 102*, 711–725.

Belin, P., Campanella, S., & Ethofer, T. (2013). *Integrating Face and Voice in Person Perception.* New York, Heidelberg: Springer.

Belin, P., Fecteau, S., & Bedard, C. (2004). Thinking the voice: neural correlates of voice perception. *Trends in Cognitive Sciences, 8*(3), 129–135.

Belin, P. & Zatorre, R. J. (2003). Adaptation to speaker's voice in right anterior temporal lobe. *NeuroReport, 14*(16), 2105–2109.

Belin, P., Zatorre, R. J., & Ahad, P. (2002). Human temporal-lobe response to vocal sounds. *Cognitive Brain Research, 13*(1), 17–26.

Belin, P., Zatorre, R. J., Lafaille, P., Ahad, P., & Pike, B. (2000). Voice-selective areas in human auditory cortex. *Nature, 403*, 309–312.

Benson, P. J. & Perrett, D. I. (1991). Perception and recognition of photographic quality facial caricatures: implications for the recognition of natural images. *European Journal of Cognitive Psychology, 3*, 105–135.

Bestelmeyer, P. E. G., Rouger, J., DeBruine, L. M., & Belin, P. (2010). Auditory adaptation in vocal affect perception. *Cognition, 117*, 217–223.

Blank, H., Anwander, A., & von Kriegstein, K. (2011). Direct structural connections between voice- and face-recognition areas. *Journal of Neuroscience, 31*(36), 12906–12915.

Blank, H., Wieland, N., & von Kriegstein, K. (2014). Person recognition and the brain: merging evidence from patients and healthy individuals. *Neuroscience and Biobehavioral Reviews, 47,* 717–734. doi: 10.1016/j.neubiorev.2014.10.022

Boucher, J., Lewis, V., & Collis, G. (1998). Familiar face and voice matching and recognition in children with autism. *Journal of Child Psychology and Psychiatry and Allied Disciplines, 39*(2), 171–181. doi: 10.1017/s0021963097001820

Bricker, P. D. & Pruzansky, S. (1966). Effects of stimulus content and duration on talker identification. *Journal of the Acoustical Society of America, 40,* 1441–1449.

Bruce, V. & Young, A. (1986). Understanding face recognition. *British Journal of Psychology, 77,* 305–327.

Bruckert, L., Bestelmeyer, P., Latinus, M., Rouger, J., Charest, I., Rousselet, G. A., ... Belin, P. (2010). Vocal attractiveness increases by averaging. *Current Biology, 20*(2), 116–120.

Burton, A. M., Jenkins, R., & Schweinberger, S. R. (2011). Mental representations of familiar faces. *British Journal of Psychology, 102,* 943–958.

Calder, A. J., Jenkins, R., Cassel, A., & Clifford, C. W. G. (2008). Visual representation of eye gaze is coded by a nonopponent multichannel system. *Journal of Experimental Psychology—General, 137*(2), 244–261. doi: 10.1037/0096-3445.137.2.244

Calvert, G. A., Brammer, M. J., & Iversen, S. D. (1998). Crossmodal identification. *Trends in Cognitive Sciences, 2*(7), 247–253.

Campanella, S. & Belin, P. (2007). Integrating face and voice in person perception. *Trends in Cognitive Sciences, 11*(12), 535–543.

Charest, I., Pernet, C. R., Latinus, M., Crabbe, F., & Belin, P. (2013). Cerebral processing of voice gender studied using a continuous carryover fMRI design. *Cerebral Cortex, 23*(4), 958–966. doi: 10.1093/cercor/bhs090

Charest, I., Pernet, C. R., Rousselet, G. A., Quinones, I., Latinus, M., Fillion-Bilodeau, S., ... Belin, P. (2009). Electrophysiological evidence for an early processing of human voices. *BMC Neuroscience, 10*(127), 1–11.

Chartrand, J. P. & Belin, P. (2006). Superior voice timbre processing in musicians. *Neuroscience Letters, 405*(3), 164–167.

Clifford, B. R. (1980). Voice identification by human listeners: on earwitness reliability. *Law and Human Behavior, 4,* 373–394.

Compton, A. J. (1963). Effects of filtering and vocal duration upon identification of speakers, aurally. *Journal of the Acoustical Society of America, 35*(11), 1748. doi: 10.1121/1.1918810

Cook, S. & Wilding, J. (1997). Earwitness testimony: never mind the variety, hear the length. *Applied Cognitive Psychology, 11,* 95–111.

DeCasper, A. J. & Fifer, W. P. (1980). Of human bonding: newborns prefer their mothers' voices. *Science, 208,* 1174–1176.

Deffenbacher, K. A., Cross, J. F., Handkins, R. E., Chance, J. E., Goldstein, A. G., Hammersley, R., & Read, J. D. (1989). Relevance of voice identification research to criteria for evaluating reliability of an identification. *Journal of Psychology, 123*(2), 109–119.

Elaad, E., Segev, S., & Tobin, Y. (1998). Long-term working memory in voice identification. *Psychology, Crime & Law, 4*(2), 73–88.

Föcker, J., Best, A., Holig, C., & Röder, B. (2012). The superiority in voice processing of the blind arises from neural plasticity at sensory processing stages. *Neuropsychologia, 50*(8), 2056–2067.

Formisano, E., De Martino, F., Bonte, M., & Goebel, R. (2008). 'Who' is saying 'what'? Brain-based decoding of human voice and speech. *Science, 322*(5903), 970–973.

Frühholz, S. & Grandjean, D. (2013). Multiple subregions in superior temporal cortex are differentially sensitive to vocal expressions: a quantitative meta-analysis. *Neuroscience and Biobehavioral Reviews*, 37(1), 24–35. doi: 10.1016/j.neubiorev.2012.11.002

Garrido, L., Eisner, F., McGettigan, C., Stewart, L., Sauter, D., Hanley, J. R., … Duchaine, B. (2009). Developmental phonagnosia: a selective deficit of vocal identity recognition. *Neuropsychologia*, 47(1), 123–131.

Goggin, J. P., Thompson, C. P., Strube, G., & Simental, L. R. (1991). The role of language familiarity in voice identification. *Memory & Cognition*, 19(5), 448–458. doi: 10.3758/bf03199567

Hagan, C. C., Woods, W., Johnson, S., Calder, A. J., Green, G. G. R., & Young, A. W. (2009). MEG demonstrates a supra-additive response to facial and vocal emotion in the right superior temporal sulcus. *Proceedings of the National Academy of Sciences of the United States of America*, 106(47), 20010–20015.

Hancock, P. J. B., Bruce, V., & Burton, A. M. (2000). Recognition of unfamiliar faces. *Trends in Cognitive Sciences*, 4(9), 330–337.

Hancock, P. J. B., Burton, A. M., & Bruce, V. (1996). Face processing: human perception and principal components analysis. *Memory & Cognition*, 24, 26–40.

Hanley, J. R., Smith, S. T., & Hadfield, J. (1998). I recognise you but I can't place you: an investigation of familiar-only experiences during tests of voice and face recognition. *Quarterly Journal of Experimental Psychology*, 51A(1), 179–195.

Hanley, J. R. & Turner, J. M. (2000). Why are familiar-only experiences more frequent for voices than for faces? *Quarterly Journal of Experimental Psychology*, 53A(4), 1105–1116.

Hecker, M. H. L. (1971). Speaker Recognition: An Interpretive Survey of the Literature. *American Speech and Hearing Association Monographs, No. 16*. Washington, DC: American Speech and Hearing Association.

Jenkins, R. & Burton, A. M. (2008). 100% accuracy in automatic face recognition. *Science*, 319(5862), 435–435.

Joassin, F., Pesenti, M., Maurage, P., Verreckt, E., Bruyer, R., & Campanella, S. (2011). Cross-modal interactions between human faces and voices involved in person recognition. *Cortex*, 47(3), 367–376.

Kanwisher, N., McDermott, J., & Chun, M. M. (1997). The fusiform face area: a module in human extrastriate cortex specialized for face perception. *The Journal of Neuroscience*, 17(11), 4302–4311.

Kawahara, H., Masuda-Katsuse, I., & de Cheveigne, A. (1999). Restructuring speech representations using a pitch-adaptive time-frequency smoothing and an instantaneous-frequency-based Fo extraction: possible role of a repetitive structure in sounds. *Speech Communication*, 27(3–4), 187–207.

Kisilevsky, B. S., Hains, S. M. J., Lee, K., Xie, X., Huang, H. F., Ye, H. H., … Wang, Z. P. (2003). Effects of experience on fetal voice recognition. *Psychological Science*, 14(3), 220–224.

Kreiman, J. & Sidtis, D. (2011). *Foundations of Voice Studies: An Interdisciplinary Approach to Voice Production and Perception*. Chichester: Wiley-Blackwell.

Kriengwatana, B., Escudero, P., & ten Cate, C. (2015). Revisiting vocal perception in non-human animals: a review of vowel discrimination, speaker voice recognition, and speaker normalization. *Frontiers in Psychology*, 5. doi: 10.3389/fpsyg.2014.01543

Kuwabara, H. & Sagisak, Y. (1995). Acoustic characteristics of speaker individuality—control and conversion. *Speech Communication*, 16(2), 165–173. doi: 10.1016/0167-6393(94)00053-d

Latinus, M. & Belin, P. (2011a). Anti-voice adaptation suggests prototype-based coding of voice identity. *Frontiers in Psychology*, 2, Article 175.

Latinus, M. & Belin, P. (2011b). Human voice perception. *Current Biology*, 21(4), R143–R145. doi: 10.1016/j.cub.2010.12.033

Latinus, M., Crabbe, F., & Belin, P. (2011). Learning-induced changes in the cerebral processing of voice identity. *Cerebral Cortex*, 21(12), 2820–2828.

Latinus, M., McAleer, P., Bestelmeyer, P. E. G., & Belin, P. (2013). Norm-based coding of voice identity in human auditory cortex. *Current Biology*, 23(12), 1075–1080.

Lavner, Y., Rosenhouse, J., & Gath, I. (2001). The prototype model in speaker identification by human listeners. *International Journal of Speech and Technology*, 4, 63–74.

Legge, G. E., Grossmann, C., & Pieper, C. M. (1984). Learning unfamiliar voices. *Journal of Experimental Psychology: Learning, Memory, and Cognition*, 10, 298–303.

Leopold, D. A., O'Toole, A. J., Vetter, T., & Blanz, V. (2001). Prototype-referenced shape encoding revealed by high-level aftereffects. *Nature Neuroscience*, 4(1), 89–94.

Malone, D. R., Morris, H. H., Kay, M. C., & Levin, H. S. (1982). Prosopagnosia: a double dissociation between the recognition of familiar and unfamiliar faces. *Journal of Neurology, Neurosurgery, and Psychiatry*, 45, 820–822.

Mann, V. A., Diamond, R., & Carey, S. (1979). Development of voice recognition—parallels with face recognition. *Journal of Experimental Child Psychology*, 27(1), 153–165.

McAllister, H. A., Dale, R. H. I., Bregman, N. J., McCabe, A., & Cotton, C. R. (1993). When eyewitnesses are also earwitnesses—effects on visual and voice identifications. *Basic and Applied Social Psychology*, 14(2), 161–170. doi: 10.1207/s15324834basp1402_3

McGehee, F. (1937). The reliability of the identification of the human voice. *Journal of General Psychology*, 31, 53–65.

McGurk, H. & MacDonald, J. (1976). Hearing lips and seeing voices. *Nature*, 264, 746–748.

Megreya, A. M. & Burton, A. M. (2006). Unfamiliar faces are not faces: evidence from a matching task. *Memory & Cognition*, 34(4), 865–876.

Mühl, C., Sheil, O., Jarutyte, L., & Bestelmeyer, P. E. G. (2017). The Bangor Voice Matching Test: A standardized test for the assessment of voice perception ability. *Behavior Research Methods*. doi: 10.3758/s13428-017-0985-4.

Mullennix, J. W., Ross, A., Smith, C., Kuykendall, K., Conard, J., & Barb, S. (2011). Typicality effects on memory for voice: implications for earwitness testimony. *Applied Cognitive Psychology*, 25(1), 29–34. doi: 10.1002/acp.1635

Neuner, F. & Schweinberger, S. R. (2000). Neuropsychological impairments in the recognition of faces, voices, and personal names. *Brain and Cognition*, 44(3), 342–366.

Nygaard, L. C., Sommers, M. S., & Pisoni, D. B. (1994). Speech perception as a talker-contingent process. *Psychological Science*, 5, 42–46.

Papcun, G., Kreiman, J., & Davis, A. (1989). Long-term memory for unfamiliar voices. *Journal of the Acoustical Society of America*, 85, 913–925.

Pernet, C. R., McAleer, P., Latinus, M., Gorgolewski, K. J., Charest, I., Bestelmeyer, P. E. G., ... Belin, P. (2015). The human voice areas: spatial organization and inter-individual variability in temporal and extra-temporal cortices. *NeuroImage*, 119, 164–174. doi: 10.1016/j.neuroimage.2015.06.050

Perrachione, T. K., Chiao, J. Y., & Wong, P. C. M. (2010). Asymmetric cultural effects on perceptual expertise underlie an own-race bias for voices. *Cognition*, 114(1), 42–55. doi: 10.1016/j.cognition.2009.08.012

Perrachione, T. K., Del Tufo, S. N., & Gabrieli, J. D. E. (2011). Human voice recognition depends on language ability. *Science*, 333(6042), 595–595. doi: 10.1126/science.1207327

Perrachione, T. K. & Wong, P. C. M. (2007). Learning to recognize speakers of a non-native language: implications for the functional organization of human auditory cortex. *Neuropsychologia*, 45(8), 1899–1910.

Perrodin, C., Kayser, C., Abel, T. J., Logothetis, N. K., & Petkov, C. I. (2015). Who is that? Brain networks and mechanisms for identifying individuals. *Trends in Cognitive Sciences*, 19(12), 783–796. doi: 10.1016/j.tics.2015.09.002

Perrodin, C., Kayser, C., Logothetis, N. K., & Petkov, C. I. (2011). Voice cells in the primate temporal lobe. *Current Biology*, 21(16), 1408–1415. doi: 10.1016/j.cub.2011.07.028

Perrodin, C., Kayser, C., Logothetis, N. K., & Petkov, C. I. (2015). Natural asynchronies in audiovisual communication signals regulate neuronal multisensory interactions in voice-sensitive cortex. *Proceedings of the National Academy of Sciences of the United States of America*, 112(1), 273–278. doi: 10.1073/pnas.1412817112

Pollack, I., Pickett, J. M., & Sumby, W. H. (1954). On the identification of speakers by voice. *Journal of the Acoustical Society of America*, 26, 403–406.

Robertson, D. M. C. & Schweinberger, S. R. (2010). The role of audiovisual asynchrony in person recognition. *Quarterly Journal of Experimental Psychology*, 63(1), 23–30.

Roebuck, R. & Wilding, J. (1993). Effects of vowel variety and sample length on identification of a speaker in a line-up. *Applied Cognitive Psychology*, 7(6), 475–481. doi: 10.1002/acp.2350070603

Rossi-Katz, J. & Arehart, K. H. (2009). Message and talker identification in older adults: effects of task, distinctiveness of the talkers' voices, and meaningfulness of the competing message. *Journal of Speech, Language, and Hearing Research*, 52(2), 435–453. doi: 10.1044/1092-4388(2008/07-0243)

Roswandowitz, C., Mathias, S. R., Hintz, F., Kreitewolf, J., Schelinski, S., & von Kriegstein, K. (2014). Two cases of selective developmental voice-recognition impairments. *Current Biology*, 24(19), 2348–2353. doi: 10.1016/j.cub.2014.08.048

Russell, R., Duchaine, B., & Nakayama, K. (2009). Super-recognizers: people with extraordinary face recognition ability. *Psychonomic Bulletin & Review*, 16(2), 252–257.

Saslove, H. & Yarmey, A. D. (1980). Long-term auditory memory: speaker identification. *Journal of Applied Psychology*, 65, 111–116.

Schelinski, S., Riedel, P., & von Kriegstein, K. (2014). Visual abilities are important for auditory-only speech recognition: evidence from autism spectrum disorder. *Neuropsychologia*, 65, 1–11. doi: 10.1016/j.neuropsychologia.2014.09.031

Schiller, N. O. & Köster, O. (1998). The ability of expert witnesses to identify voices: a comparison between trained and untrained listeners. *Forensic Linguistics*, 5, 1–9.

Schweinberger, S. R. (2001). Human brain potential correlates of voice priming and voice recognition. *Neuropsychologia*, 39, 921–936.

Schweinberger, S. R., Casper, C., Hauthal, N., Kaufmann, J. M., Kawahara, H., Kloth, N., ... Zaske, R. (2008). Auditory adaptation in voice perception. *Current Biology*, 18(9), 684–688.

Schweinberger, S. R., Herholz, A., & Sommer, W. (1997). Recognizing famous voices: influence of stimulus duration and different types of retrieval cues. *Journal of Speech, Language, and Hearing Research*, 40, 453–463.

Schweinberger, S. R., Herholz, A., & Stief, V. (1997). Auditory long-term memory: repetition priming of voice recognition. *Quarterly Journal of Experimental Psychology*, 50A, 498–517.

Schweinberger, S. R., Kawahara, H., Simpson, A. P., Skuk, V. G., & Zäske, R. (2014). Speaker perception. *Wiley Interdisciplinary Reviews—Cognitive Science*, 5(1), 15–25.

Schweinberger, S. R., Kloth, N., & Robertson, D. M. C. (2011). Hearing facial identities: brain correlates of face-voice integration in person identification. *Cortex*, 47, 1026–1037.

Schweinberger, S. R., Robertson, D., & Kaufmann, J. M. (2007). Hearing facial identities. *Quarterly Journal of Experimental Psychology*, 60, 1446–1456.

Schweinberger, S. R., Walther, C., Zäske, R., & Kovács, G. (2011). Neural correlates of adaptation to voice identity. *British Journal of Psychology*, 102, 748–764.

Shah, N. J., Marshall, J. C., Zafiris, O., Schwab, A., Zilles, K., Markowitsch, H. J., & Fink, G. R. (2001). The neural correlates of person familiarity. A functional magnetic resonance imaging study with clinical implications. *Brain*, 124, 804–815.

Sheffert, S. M. & Olson, E. (2004). Audiovisual speech facilitates voice learning. *Perception & Psychophysics*, 66(2), 352–362.

Sheffert, S. M., Pisoni, D. B., Fellowes, J. M., & Remez, R. E. (2002). Learning to recognize talkers from natural, sinewave, and reversed speech samples. *Journal of Experimental Psychology: Human Perception and Performance*, 28(6), 1447–1469.

Skuk, V. G., Dammann, L. M., & Schweinberger, S. R. (2015). Role of timbre and fundamental frequency in voice gender adaptation. *Journal of the Acoustical Society of America*, 138(2), 1180–1193.

Skuk, V. G., Palermo, R., Broemer, L., & Schweinberger, S. R. (2017). Autistic traits are linked to individual differences in familiar voice identification. *Journal of Autism and Developmental Disorders*, 1–21. doi: 10.1007/s10803-017-3039-y

Skuk, V. G. & Schweinberger, S. R. (2013a). Adaptation aftereffects in vocal emotion perception elicited by expressive faces and voices. *PLoS One*, 8(11).

Skuk, V. G. & Schweinberger, S. R. (2013b). Gender differences in familiar voice identification. *Hearing Research*, 296, 131–140.

Skuk, V. G. & Schweinberger, S. R. (2014). Influences of fundamental frequency, formant frequencies, aperiodicity and spectrum level on the perception of voice gender. *Journal of Speech, Language, and Hearing Research*, 57, 285–296.

Spreckelmeyer, K. N., Kutas, M., Urbach, T., Altenmüller, E., & Müller, T. F. (2009). Neural processing of vocal emotion and identity. *Brain and Cognition*, 69(1), 121–126.

Stevenage, S. V., Clarke, G., & McNeill, A. (2012). The 'other-accent' effect in voice recognition. *Journal of Cognitive Psychology*, 24(6), 647–653. doi: 10.1080/20445911.2012.675321

Stevenage, S. V., Howland, A., & Tippelt, A. (2011). Interference in eyewitness and earwitness recognition. *Applied Cognitive Psychology*, 25(1), 112–118. doi: 10.1002/acp.1649

Valentine, T. (1991). A unified account of the effects of distinctiveness, inversion, and race in face recognition. *Quarterly Journal of Experimental Psychology*, 43A, 161–204.

Van Lancker, D. R. & Canter, G. J. (1982). Impairment of voice and face recognition in patients with hemispheric damage. *Brain & Cognition*, 1, 185–195.

Van Lancker, D. R. & Kreiman, J. (1987). Voice discrimination and recognition are separate abilities. *Neuropsychologia*, 25, 829–834.

Van Lancker, D. R., Kreiman, J., & Cummings, J. (1989). Voice perception deficits: neuroanatomical correlates of phonagnosia. *Journal of Clinical and Experimental Neuropsychology*, 11, 665–674.

Van Lancker, D. R., Kreiman, J., & Emmorey, K. (1985). Familiar voice recognition: patterns and parameters. Part I: recognition of backward voices. *Journal of Phonetics*, 13, 19–38.

van Wassenhove, V., Grant, K. W., & Poeppel, D. (2005). Visual speech speeds up the neural processing of auditory speech. *Proceedings of the National Academy of Sciences*, 102(4), 1181–1186.

von Kriegstein, K., Eger, E., Kleinschmidt, A., & Giraud, A. L. (2003). Modulation of neural responses to speech by directing attention to voices or verbal content. *Cognitive Brain Research*, 17(1), 48–55.

von Kriegstein, K. & Giraud, A. L. (2004). Distinct functional substrates along the right superior temporal sulcus for the processing of voices. *NeuroImage*, 22(2), 948–955.

von Kriegstein, K. & Giraud, A. L. (2006). Implicit multisensory associations influence voice recognition. *PLoS Biology*, 4(10), 1809–1820.

von Kriegstein, K., Kleinschmidt, A., Sterzer, P., & Giraud, A. L. (2005). Interaction of face and voice areas during speaker recognition. *Journal of Cognitive Neuroscience*, 17(3), 367–376.

von Kriegstein, K., Smith, D. R. R., Patterson, R. D., Kiebel, S. J., & Griffiths, T. D. (2010). How the human brain recognizes speech in the context of changing speakers. *Journal of Neuroscience*, 30(2), 629–638.

Walker, S., Bruce, V., & O'Malley, C. (1995). Facial identity and facial speech processing: familiar faces and voices in the McGurk effect. *Perception & Psychophysics*, 57, 1124–1133.

Welch, R. B. & Warren, D. H. (1980). Immediate perceptual response to intersensory discrepancy. *Psychological Bulletin*, 88, 638–667.

Wilding, J. & Cook, S. (2000). Sex differences and individual consistency in voice identification. *Perceptual and Motor Skills*, 91(2), 535–538. doi: 10.2466/pms.91.6.535-538

Winograd, E., Spence, M. J., & Kerr, N. H. (1984). Voice recognition—effects of orienting task, and a test of blind versus sighted listeners. *American Journal of Psychology*, 97(1), 57–70. doi: 10.2307/1422547

Xie, X. & Myers, E. (2015). The impact of musical training and tone language experience on talker identification. *Journal of the Acoustical Society of America*, 137(1), 419–432. doi: 10.1121/1.4904699

Yamagishi, J., Usabaev, B., King, S., Watts, O., Dines, J., Tian, J. L., … Kurimo, M. (2010). Thousands of voices for HMM-based speech synthesis-analysis and application of TTS systems built on various ASR corpora. *IEEE Transactions on Audio Speech and Language Processing*, 18(5), 984–1004.

Yonan, C. A. & Sommers, M. S. (2000). The effects of talker familiarity on spoken word identification in younger and older listeners. *Psychology and Aging*, 15(1), 88–99. doi: 10.1037//0882-7974.15.1.88

Young, A. W. & Bruce, V. (2011). Understanding person perception. *British Journal of Psychology*, 102, 959–974.

Zarate, J. M., Tian, X., Woods, K. J. P., & Poeppel, D. (2015). Multiple levels of linguistic and paralinguistic features contribute to voice recognition. *Scientific Reports*, 5. doi: 10.1038/srep11475

Zäske, R., Hasan, B. A. S., & Belin, P. (2017). It doesn't matter what you say: FMRI correlates of voice learning and recognition independent of speech content. *Cortex*, 94, 100–112. doi: 10.1016/j.cortex.2017.06.005

Zäske, R., Muehl, C., & Schweinberger, S. R. (2015). Benefits for voice learning caused by concurrent faces develop over time. *PLoS One*, 10(11). doi: 10.1371/journal.pone.0143151

Zäske, R. & Schweinberger, S. R. (2011). You are only as old as you sound: auditory aftereffects in vocal age perception. *Hearing Research*, 282(1–2), 283–288.

Zäske, R., Schweinberger, S. R., & Kawahara, H. (2010). Voice aftereffects of adaptation to speaker identity. *Hearing Research*, 268(1–2), 38–45.

Zäske, R., Volberg, G., Kovács, G., & Schweinberger, S. R. (2014). Electrophysiological correlates of voice learning and recognition. *Journal of Neuroscience*, 34(33), 10821–10831.

CHAPTER 25

PERCEPTUAL CORRELATES AND CEREBRAL REPRESENTATION OF VOICES—IDENTITY, GENDER, AND AGE

MARIANNE LATINUS AND ROMI ZÄSKE

25.1 INTRODUCTION

VOICES form a special class of auditory objects, the processing of which is supported by dedicated neural networks (Belin et al., 2000, 2004). Voices are not only the carriers of speech-related information, they also transmit a wealth of information about individuals such as their identity, gender, age, and affective state. Several neuropsychological models have described the functional organization of voice perception and concurred that it is a three-step process (Belin et al., 2004, 2011; Schirmer & Kotz, 2006). While Belin's (2004) model considers both paralinguisitic (e.g. emotion and identity) and linguistic information, Schirmer and Kotz's model (2006) only applies to emotion perception.

According to both models, voice perception starts with the processing of low-level acoustic information in subcortical nuclei and primary auditory cortex. After sensory processing, the models diverge slightly on what constitutes the second step. On the one hand, Belin's model describes a voice structural encoding stage that is both voice-specific and allows voice detection (Belin et al., 2011). This structural encoding is common to the processing of identity, affective information, and speech. On the other hand, Schirmer and Kotz (2006) describe the second stage as an integrative stage, during which affective information is combined into a 'gestalt'. Thereafter, voice identity, affect, and speech are further processed in independent but interacting pathways (Belin et al., 2004, 2011). Gender and age perception are often neglected in neuropsychological models of face

(Bruce & Young, 1986) and voice perception (Belin et al., 2004, 2011); yet, gender and age are crucial social information which can be discerned from voices with relatively high accuracy (e.g. for voice gender and age: Linville, 1996; Mullennix et al., 1995), and whose processing interacts with that of other social signals (e.g. identity and gender: Burton & Bonner, 2004).

Research on the perception of social signals in voices has addressed a range of issues. While some studies aim at assessing listeners' ability to perceive speaker characteristics, others are concerned with identifying the acoustic parameters that differentiate voices, and those used by listeners to extract identity, gender, and age. Finally, neuroscientists are interested in the cerebral mechanisms underlying these abilities. Since this strand of research has emerged relatively recently, our current understanding of the cerebral representation of voices is rather limited, particularly with respect to vocal age. This chapter describes the putative representation of voices by looking at perceptual, acoustical, and cerebral representation of voices.

25.2 ACOUSTIC AND PERCEPTUAL CORRELATES

25.2.1 Voice Identity

Voice production involves the whole body; as such, the voice reflects the physical characteristics of a speaker, and is therefore specific to each individual (Kreiman & Sidtis, 2011). Recognition of familiar voices is a widespread ability that has evolved in response to different environmental and behavioural demands (Sidtis & Kreiman, 2012). Over a lifetime, human listeners encounter hundreds of voices, some of which are stored in long-term memory. Voice-identity perception refers to the recognition of both unfamiliar and familiar voices (Van Lancker & Kreiman, 1987; Van Lancker et al., 1989). Familiar voice recognition refers to the act of recognizing a known voice, from a feeling of familiarity to speaker identification (i.e. the recollection of the speaker's name or associated semantic information). Familiar voice recognition encompasses several levels of familiarity (Blank et al., 2014; Kreiman & Sidtis, 2011) including personally-familiar and famous voices which a listener has known for a long time, heard in different contexts, and associated with multiple pieces of semantic information and feelings.

To control for spurious effects of different learning conditions for familiar voices, researchers often rely on voices learned during the course of an experiment (e.g. Andics et al., 2010; Latinus & Belin, 2011; Latinus et al., 2011; von Kriegstein & Giraud, 2006; Winters et al., 2008). 'Trained-to-familiar voices' (Kreiman & Sidtis, 2011) thus form a third level of familiarity, for which familiarity is acquired through extensive training over a relatively short period of time, and is associated with little semantic information.

Unfamiliar voice recognition refers either to the act of deciding whether a previously heard unknown voice is presented again or the act of discriminating between two voices. Increasing evidence suggests that the processing of familiar and unfamiliar voices are separate, but related (Cook & Wilding, 1997) abilities that partly rely on different cerebral mechanisms (Blank et al., 2014; Van Lancker & Kreiman, 1987; Van Lancker et al., 1989).

25.2.1.1 *Accuracy of Voice-Identity Perception*

Despite high intra-speaker variability, listeners perform fairly well at recognizing voices even across large variations in sound quality and content (Belin et al., 2011; Kreiman & Sidtis, 2011; Nakamura et al., 2001; Schweinberger, Herholz, & Sommer, 1997; Van Lancker et al., 1985; see also Schweinberge & Zäske, this volume). Although performance is in general well above chance, voice identification is not infallible (Sherrin, 2015). A large variability in identification performance has been reported across studies, speakers, and listeners (Lavner et al., 2001; Papcun et al., 1989; Sherrin, 2015; Skuk & Schweinberger, 2013b). For instance, Lavner and collaborators (2000) reported an accuracy rate of about 49% (chance level ~ 3%) in familiar speaker recognition from vowel samples lasting 500 ms. However, recognition accuracy varied greatly between both speakers (15–79%) and listeners (12–93%) (Lavner et al., 2001). Recognition accuracy of about 82% (range: 46.7–100%; chance level: 25%) was reported with 4-s speech samples (Van Lancker & Kreiman, 1987).

Listeners' performance on familiar voice recognition strongly depends on voice-sample duration, with longer samples yielding higher accuracy (Kreiman & Sidtis, 2011; Schweinberger, Herholz, & Sommer, 1997; Skuk & Schweinberger, 2013b), with a peak of performance observed for durations between 500 and 1000 ms (Schweinberger, Herholz, & Sommer, 1997; Van Lancker et al., 1985). Importantly, the increase in performance with increasing sample duration may not be related to sample duration per se, but rather to increasing linguistic variety in the voice samples (Bricker & Pruzansky, 1966; Hammersley & Read, 1996; Pollack et al., 1954).

Performance for unfamiliar voice discrimination also varies enormously across studies (Sell et al., 2015; Spreckelmeyer et al., 2009; Van Lancker & Kreiman, 1987). For voice-matching tasks using short (< 500 ms: Spreckelmeyer et al., 2009) and longer voice samples (Van Lancker et al., 1987), accuracies of 68% and ~87% were reported, respectively. In addition, listeners perform well on voice pairs with different phonetic content (Sell et al., 2015). As reported for familiar voices, voice sample duration also influences unfamiliar voice recognition, for which duration appears more crucial than linguistic variety (Cook & Wilding, 1997). In a large cohort of healthy participants, important individual differences were reported in an old/new voice judgement task with unfamiliar voices (Aglieri et al., 2016); mean accuracy was around 78% (set of six voices; range: 37.5–100%). It should be noted that in that study voice memory was assessed using the same tokens at study and test phases, and was lower than memory for non-vocal bell sounds. Lower performance in voice than bell recognition could arise from the overall higher homogeneity of the vocal sounds (same vowel) used in that study.

In summary, multiple studies have investigated the perception of identity from voices. These studies, relying on different tasks, paradigms, and methods, report a high variability in performance for both voice recognition and discrimination. While some authors argue that human listeners are good at identifying voices (Belin et al., 2004; Van Lancker et al., 1985), performance in voice-recognition tasks is relatively low compared with face recognition. Yet, the poor performance reported in experimental settings may not perfectly reflect people's ability to recognize voices in everyday life, which is in general far better, likely due to the presence of contextual information (Hammersley & Read, 1996). While there is evidence to suggest that some identity-related speaker information is available in voices, which of this listeners use to recognize speakers remains elusive.

25.2.1.2 *Acoustic Cues for Identity Perception*

Several studies have sought and failed to identify one cue, or a fixed set of acoustic cues, used to recognize all voices (Murry & Singh, 1980; e.g. Lavner et al., 2000; Schweinberger, 2001; reviewed in Kreiman & Sidtis, 2011). So far, a large number of acoustic features have been implicated in voice recognition, although the relative importance of these cues for speaker identification may vary between speakers (Van Lancker et al., 1985) and listeners (Lavner et al., 2001).

A study using professional impersonators demonstrated that voice identity was mainly associated with acoustic features reflecting the anatomy of the vocal tract, such as the difference between the fourth and fifth formants (Lopez et al., 2013). Yet, although shifting individual formant frequencies (F3 and F4 in particular; see Figure 25.1) disrupted familiar speaker recognition, the contribution of formants to identity perception was largely speaker-dependent (Lavner et al., 2000). More than individual formants, a manipulation of the voice spectral envelope induced large disruptions, with the lowest identification rates obtained when speaker-specific formants were replaced by the average of all speakers, suggesting a specific role for vocal tract information in voice-identity perception.

In a follow-up study, identification rate was significantly correlated with a combination of two or more acoustic features, in particular a combination of the fundamental frequency (F0) and the third formant (Lavner et al., 2001). Consistent with this finding, identity aftereffects with trained-to-familiar voices were found only when the original configuration of the voices was preserved, that is, by combining appropriate formant and fundamental frequencies (Latinus & Belin, 2012). This suggests that voice identity is encoded in a complex pattern of multiple acoustic cues among which formant frequencies, representing vocal-tract characteristics, and F0, as a means to glottal source information, appear to be crucial.

To study the acoustic cues involved in unfamiliar voice-identity perception, researchers often resort to correlational analysis between similarity judgements and acoustical measures of voices. This research has shown that voices are represented in a multidimensional voice space (Figure 25.1E), whose dimensions are well approximated by measures of pitch and spectral-shape information (e.g. F0 and formant frequencies/formant dispersion; Baumann & Belin, 2010; Sell et al., 2015). This suggests that these acoustic features are equally important for the encoding of unfamiliar voices. As a confirmation, a modification of both pitch and spectral-shape information impairs unfamiliar voice discrimination (Gaudrain et al., 2009; Sell et al., 2015), although the respective influence of each parameter varied between studies.

Listeners prove to be efficient in extracting invariant features in the vocal signal to recognize a person from novel utterances (Belin et al., 2011; Papcun et al., 1989; Schweinberger, Herholz, & Stief, 1997; Zäske et al., 2014); yet, to date, no universal set of acoustic parameters has been identified that reliably allows the identification of a human voice, suggesting that familiar voices are rather encoded as a 'gestalt-like' complex pattern (Belin et al., 2011; Kreiman & Sidtis, 2011; Kuwabara & Sagisak, 1995; Schweinberger et al., 2014; Sidtis & Kreiman, 2012). This gestalt-like pattern combines different acoustic cues about a voice, in particular information related to the anatomy of the glottal source and the vocal tract, represented by F0 and spectral-shape parameters such as formant frequencies and formant dispersion (see Figure 25.1).

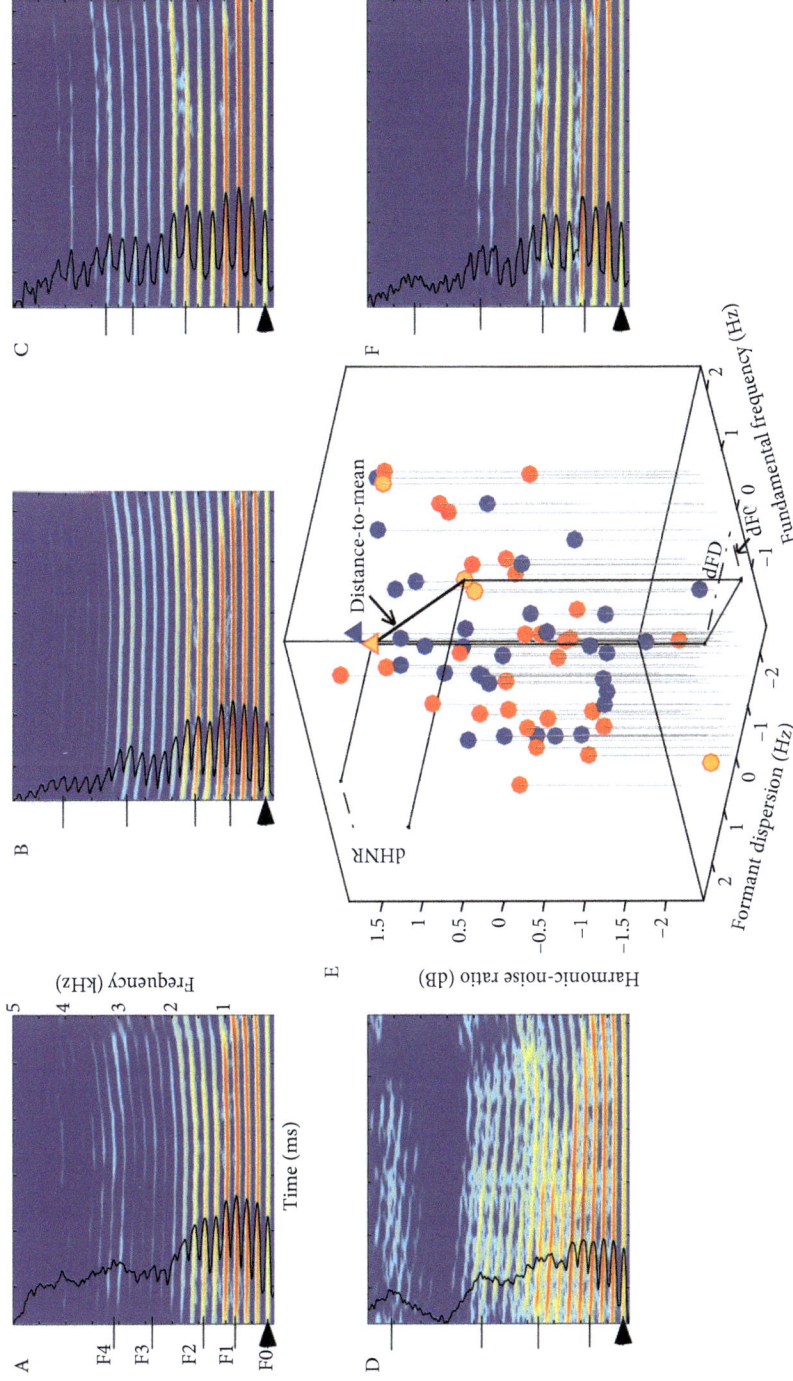

FIGURE 25.1 Acoustic cues for identity perception. (A, C, D, and F) Spectrograms of four different natural female voices, uttering the same syllable (see also Audio 25.1). Arrowheads indicate F0, lines indicate the first four formants (F1 to F4). Formant dispersion corresponds to the difference between formants: voices D and F have larger formant dispersion than voices C and F: (B) Spectrogram of the female voice prototype, corresponding to the average of thirty-two female voices (see also Audio 25.1). All five spectrograms are organized on a left–right axis depending on their fundamental frequencies (lower F0 on the left) and on a top–down axis based on their harmonic-to-noise ratio (HNR). HNR corresponds to the quantity of energy in the harmonics relative to outside the formants. It is particularly low for voice D. (E) A multidimensional voice space: voices are represented as individual points in the 3D space defined by their average log(F0), log(FD), and HNR, Z-scored by gender. (Red discs: female voices; blue discs: male voices; orange discs: voices illustrated by their spectrograms, following a similar spatial organization.) The prototypical voices (triangles) generated by averaging together all same-gender stimuli are located on top of the stimulus cloud owing to their high HNR value.

25.2.2 Voice Gender and Age

25.2.2.1 *Accuracy of Gender and Age Perception*

25.2.2.1.1 *Voice Gender*

Voice gender is among the most intensively studied speaker attributes and can be extracted from voices with high accuracy across various utterances or distortions. Accuracy usually increases with increasing phonemic variability and/or sample duration (reviewed in Kreiman & Sidtis, 2011). For instance, Lass et al. (1976) observed classification accuracies of 96%, 91%, and 75% for phonated, low-pass filtered and whispered vowels, respectively. Gender classification accuracies of ~80–90% have even been reported for voice samples as short as two phonation cycles (Owren et al., 2007). For sentences played backwards, listeners achieved 99% correct responses (Lass et al., 1978).

While listeners may be highly accurate and consistent in perceiving voice gender for gender-typical voices, substantial inter-individual differences emerge for the perception of gender-ambiguous voices (Pernet & Belin, 2012; Schweinberger et al., 2008; Skuk et al., 2015). Specifically, these studies created gender continua of voice samples by interpolating voice recordings between male and female speakers using auditory morphing (e.g. Kawahara & Matsui, 2003). When asked to classify the gender of voices drawn from these continua, listeners differed considerably with respect to the amount of 'femaleness' needed for voices to be perceived as male or female.

Recent voice experience has been identified as another important factor in gender perception (Mullennix et al., 1995; Schweinberger et al., 2008; Skuk et al., 2015; Zäske et al., 2013). Schweinberger and colleagues (2008) showed that prolonged listening to female voices causes subsequent gender-ambiguous voices to be perceived as more male, and vice versa (see Figure 25.2A). Similar aftereffects of adaptation have been demonstrated for vocal age (Schweinberger et al., 2011; Zäske et al., 2013), affective prosody (Bestelmeyer et al., 2010; Skuk & Schweinberger, 2013a), and speaker identity (Latinus & Belin, 2011, 2012; Zäske et al., 2010), revealing an enormous flexibility in the cerebral representation of non-linguistic social signals in voices.

Few studies have investigated the roles of speaker and listener characteristics on voice gender perception. With respect to speaker age, while higher accuracies have been observed for the perception of voice gender in adolescents' compared to children's voices (Amir et al., 2012), accuracy for children's voices is still well above chance (Amir et al., 2012; Ingrisano et al., 1980; Perry et al., 2001; Weinberg & Bennett, 1971). This may be due to both physiological differences and learned speaking patterns (Bennett, 1981; Cartei et al., 2014). However, it is less clear how gender is perceived in adult voices. One study found higher gender-classification accuracies for young (~20 years) compared to old (~70 years) voices, mainly because old female speakers were confused with men (Zäske et al., 2013), in line with earlier studies reporting higher classification accuracies for male compared to female voices (e.g. Amir et al., 2012; Bennett & Monterodiaz, 1982; Lass et al., 1976; Owren et al., 2007).

With respect to listener age, two studies reported no age-related differences in gender-classification accuracy, while comparing adults and children (6–9 year olds) (Bennett & Monterodiaz, 1982), and young and old adults (Schvartz & Chatterjee, 2012). Regarding listeners' gender, one study found an own-gender advantage for gender classifications such that listeners categorized same-gender voices faster than opposite gender voices, with no

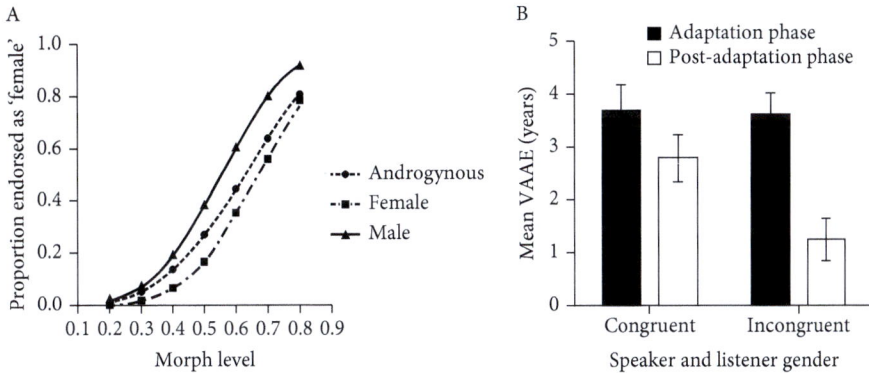

FIGURE 25.2 (**A**) Voice-gender aftereffects (VGAE; Schweinberger et al., 2008) reflected in higher proportions of 'female' responses to gender-morphed test voices (morph level reflects 'femaleness' of test voices) following adaptation to male and female voices. (**B**) Vocal- age aftereffects (VAAE; Zäske & Schweinberger, 2011) in age ratings of test voices depicted as difference values (young–old adaptation conditions) and depending on gender congruency of adaptor and test speakers in adaptation and post-adaptation phases. Note that the reduction of VAAEs in the post-adaptation phase relative to adaptation phase is significant only for incongruent speaker and listener gender (male speaker and female listener/female speaker and male listener). Error bars are standard errors of the mean (SEM).

(A) Reprinted from *Current Biology*, Volume 18, Issue 9, Schweinberger S.R. et al., 'Auditory Adaptation in Voice Perception', pp. 684–8, Copyright © 2008 Elsevier Ltd., with permission from Elsevier, http://www.sciencedirect.com/science/article/pii/S0960982208004545.

(B) Reprinted from *Hearing Research*, Volume 282, Issues 1–2, Zäske R. & Schweinberger S.R., 'You are only as old as you sound: Auditory aftereffects in vocal age perception', pp. 283–8, Copyright © 2008 Elsevier B.V., with permission from Elsevier, http://www.sciencedirect.com/science/article/pii/S0378595511001833

differences in accuracy (Latinus & Taylor, 2012). Another study reported that men and women can discriminate between male and female voices equally well overall, but that men exhibit better performance for female than for male voices (Junger et al., 2013). This was interpreted in terms of stronger attention to potential mates in men compared to women.

25.2.2.1.2 *Vocal Age*

The perception of vocal age is still poorly understood and research has been biased towards male adult voices judged by adult listeners. Overall, studies concur that vocal age can be discerned from voices with reasonable accuracy (Linville, 1996) and that chronological age and perceived age are positively correlated (e.g. Bruckert et al., 2006; Harnsberger et al., 2010; Neiman & Applegate, 1990; Shipp & Hollien, 1969). For sentence stimuli, an absolute error of ~10 years has recently been reported (Moyse, 2014) which parallels similar reports of ~6 years for static faces (Voelkle & Ebner, 2012). However, accuracy varies enormously between studies (for review, see Kreiman & Sidtis, 2011) depending on differences in tasks, stimulus materials, and speaker and listener characteristics.

With respect to task, listeners can be asked to sort voices into two or more categories or estimate age directly. For instance, when asked to assign adult voices to coarse categories of 'young' (< 35 years) and 'old' (> 65 years), listeners can be highly accurate for words (99%) and fairly accurate for sustained vowels (78%; Ptacek & Sander, 1966). Even whispered vowels provide sufficient cues for above-chance age recognition (Linville & Fisher, 1985) in categorization tasks with up to three categories. With more fine-grained age categories, or direct estimates, accuracy usually drops (e.g. Braun, 1996; Shipp & Hollien, 1969). As can be expected from statistical regression to the mean, young voices tend to be judged as older and old voices tend to be judged as younger. Across studies, a wide range of stimuli has been used including vowels, words, sentences, or phrases, which may or may not have been further manipulated. Not surprisingly, this research shows that with increasing availability of acoustic information, age estimates become more precise (Jacques & Rastatter, 1990; Linville & Fisher, 1985; Ptacek & Sander, 1966).

The accuracy of vocal-age ratings also varies with characteristics of speakers and listeners. Regarding speaker age, adult listeners find it easier to estimate young compared to older voices (Jacques & Rastatter, 1990; Moyse, 2014), particularly when children's voices are part of the sample (Hughes & Rhodes, 2010). As the physiological changes that determine voice quality may occur faster during childhood and adolescence than during adulthood (Moyse, 2014), listeners may be less likely to misjudge the age of children. With respect to listener age, Huntley et al. (1987) studied the ability of 120 male listeners to estimate the ages of 105 men aged 20–90 years from one sentence. Listeners were adolescents (9–15 years) and adults belonging to young (20–30 years), middle-aged (40–50 years), or older (60–84 years) groups. Effects of listener age emerged for young adult voices (20–30 years) which were overestimated, particularly by older listeners and adolescents. The authors reasoned that this might result from an underdeveloped concept of age in adolescents and a lack of contact to younger speakers for older listeners. Similarly, it has been speculated that asymmetrical contact may explain why older listeners estimated vocal age of their own age group more accurately than that of a young group (Moyse et al., 2014). Others found a general inferiority of the elderly in their ability to estimate vocal age, irrespective of speaker age (Linville & Fisher, 1985; Linville & Korabic, 1986; Moyse, 2014).

Due to these partly conflicting results, it is still unclear exactly how the age of speakers and listeners affects vocal-age perception. Owing to the lack of direct tests, it is further unknown if these effects are related to differential familiarity with particular groups of speakers (Moyse et al., 2014; Shipp & Hollien, 1969), or different perceptual abilities or strategies (Linville & Korabic, 1986).

Little is known on the roles of speaker and listener gender in age perception. Most studies have either focused on male *or* female speakers. There is some evidence that female listeners can judge age more accurately from female than from male voices (Neiman & Applegate, 1990). Since that study did not include male listeners, it cannot be established if this own-gender bias is confined to female listeners. A study using gender-balanced samples of speakers and listeners indicated that women judged male voices as older than female voices across a speaker-age continuum of ~20 to ~70 years (Zäske et al., 2013). There was no such effect for men, whose age estimations were similar for both speaker genders and also similar to those of women judging female voices. Overall, the highest accuracy was achieved by female listeners judging old male voices, in line with previous research (Hartman, 1979).

Further evidence of interactive effects of speaker and listener gender on vocal-age perception were reported for auditory aftereffects following vocal-age adaptation (Zäske & Schweinberger, 2011). Similar to voice gender, the perception of vocal age is subject to temporary distortions such that prolonged listening to young compared to old voices makes subsequent voices sound ~4 years older. While this contrastive aftereffect is independent of listener gender, it dissipates in a gender-specific fashion: faster recalibration of vocal-age perception was observed for opposite-gender speakers compared to same-gender speakers (cf. Figure 25.2B). This gender-specific recovery from age aftereffects may serve the need to accurately assess age in potential opposite-gender mates.

Overall, while researchers have begun to unravel important factors in the perception of voice gender and age, more systematic research is needed to understand the underlying mechanisms and their relation to the respective acoustic markers.

25.2.2.2 *Acoustic Correlates*

Due to physiological changes of respiratory and articulatory systems throughout the lifespan, human voices change in a systematic and partly gender-specific way (reviewed in Lee et al., 1999; Linville, 1996; Kreiman & Sidtis, 2011; Vorperian et al., 2009). Compared to young and middle-aged adults, children have higher Fo and formant frequencies, and relatively poor control over phonation and loudness, with hoarse voice quality. Furthermore, while initially slow, speaking rate increases as children grow older (Kreiman & Sidtis, 2011). Before puberty, the vocal tract and respiratory system develop similarly in boys and girls, with acoustic gender differences being subtle in children's voices, although acoustic differences emerge for formant frequencies by the age of 4 years (Perry et al., 2001; Vorperian & Kent, 2007).

During puberty, hormonal changes contribute to the sexual dimorphism found in adults, reflected in the anatomy of the vocal folds and vocal-tract cavities (Titze, 1989). In boys, adolescent voices start changing between 12.5 and 14.5 years of age (Hollien et al., 1994). With a marked growth and thickening of the vocal folds, mean Fo decreases more in boys than girls (Abitbol et al., 1999), resulting in lower perceived pitch for men (100–120 Hz) than women (200–220 Hz) (Simpson, 2009). Due to a lowering of the larynx during puberty, the male vocal tract is about 15% longer than that of females (Fant, 1966). Combined with larger laryngeal cavities (Chiba & Kajiyama, 1941) and differences in the articulatory system (Hillenbrand et al., 1995; Peterson & Barney, 1952), this leads to lower formant frequencies in males and characteristic gender differences in voice timbre. Furthermore, female voices are breathier than male voices due to larger glottal opening (e.g. Klatt & Klatt, 1990; Titze, 1989).

During young and middle age, Fo and formant frequencies continue to decrease for men and women, while speaking rate is fast, with stable phonation and good volume control (Kreiman & Sidtis, 2011). After the age of ~50 years, speaking rates decrease (Brown et al., 1989; Harnsberger et al., 2008; Ramig & Ringel, 1983; Shipp et al., 1992) and Fo becomes more variable (Gorham-Rowan & Laures-Gore, 2006; Linville, 1996; Ramig et al., 2001; Torre & Barlow, 2009), with further lowering of formant frequencies (Kreiman & Sidtis, 2011).

Gender-specific patterns of vocal ageing have been reported for various parameters (e.g. Fo, HNR, intensity). Specifically, while Fo tends to rise in older men due to atrophy of muscle tissue and increased stiffness of vocal-fold tissue, Fo falls in women after menopause due to hormonal changes causing vocal-fold oedema (Brown et al., 1989; Linville, 1996; Torre & Barlow, 2009). Moreover, while the amount of additive noise in female voices is lowest during childhood and old age, additive noise in male voices may decrease with increasing age (Stathopoulos et al., 2011). Regarding intensity, while older men (>60 years) speak louder than young men (Ryan, 1972), no change in average vocal intensity has been reported for women (Morris & Brown, 1994).

It needs to be noted that data on age-related changes of voice acoustic parameters originate primarily from cross-sectional studies and may therefore partly reflect sociocultural norms. Similarly, sexual dimorphism in voices may not only be the result of the anatomical make-up of male and female articulatory systems, but may also be shaped by learned speaking patterns (Simpson, 2009).

25.2.2.3 *Perceptually-Relevant Cues to Gender and Age*

Voices clearly contain a wide range of gender- and age-specific acoustic cues. However, which of these cues do listeners use to recognize a speaker's gender or age? Research on voice-gender stereotypes found that young listeners characterized male speech as deep, demanding, loud, and forceful, while female speech was described as high, fast, clear, gentle, emotional, and with a wide range in rate and pitch (Kramer, 1977). Psychophysical research has shown that Fo and formant frequencies may be the most salient cues to gender perception (e.g. Coleman, 1976; Lass et al., 1976; Pernet & Belin, 2012; Perry et al., 2001; Skuk & Schweinberger, 2014; Skuk et al., 2015). For instance, gender-classification accuracy for adult voices is higher for phonated compared to whispered vowels (Lass et al., 1976), although recognition accuracy is usually still above chance when pitch is unavailable (Ingemann, 1968; Lass et al., 1976; Schwartz & Rine, 1968), rendered atypical (Smith & Patterson, 2005), or ambiguous (Pernet & Belin, 2012; Skuk & Schweinberger, 2014). However, pitch information in otherwise gender-ambiguous voices may suffice for above-chance gender classification (Pernet & Belin, 2012; Skuk & Schweinberger, 2014).

Which acoustic cues of chronological age do listeners use to estimate age? Hartman and Danhauer (1976) had expert listeners characterize male adult voices that had been sorted into four adult-age categories by novices. The experts described the voices sounding oldest (50–60 years) as low-pitched, hoarse, and breathy, with a slow speaking rate and imprecise articulation, in line with a similar study by Ryan and Burk (1974). By contrast, young-sounding voices (< 30 years) were characterized as high-pitched, clear, and as speaking rapidly and precisely.

While vocal-age judgements and characterizations may in part reflect stereotypes of vocal ageing (Hummert et al., 1999), studies relating vocal-age ratings to acoustic measures overall confirm the previous observations, suggesting a role for temporal aspects such as speaking rate, Fo (instability), as well as vocal-tract resonances for vocal-age perceptions in both male (Harnsberger et al., 2008; Harnsberger et al., 2010; Jacques & Rastatter, 1990; Ptacek & Sander, 1966; Shipp et al., 1992; Smith & Patterson, 2005) and female voices (Linville & Fisher, 1985; Linville & Korabic, 1986).

25.3 CEREBRAL REPRESENTATION
OF VOICE IDENTITY

Influential models of face perception have proposed that faces are encoded in a multidimensional space as either points (exemplar-based model) or vectors relative to a facial norm (norm-based model) located at the centre of the space (Valentine, 1991). Both models make similar predictions for multiple behavioural measures, and differ mainly on whether stimulus encoding relies on a prototype. In contrast to the exemplar-based model, the norm-based model suggests that individual faces are represented in terms of their distance from a population prototype. Numerous studies have provided evidence for similarities in the processing and cerebral representation of facial and vocal information (reviewed in Yovel & Belin, 2013). Accordingly, accumulating evidence converges in demonstrating that voices, like faces, are encoded in a multidimensional space as deviations from an internal prototype which corresponds to the average of multiple voices of the same gender (see Figure 25.1; Andics et al., 2010, 2013; Latinus & Belin, 2011; Latinus et al., 2013; Lattner et al., 2003; Papcun et al., 1989).

25.3.1 Behavioural Evidence

Norm-based models assume that the prototype corresponds to the central tendency of a given category (Rosch et al., 1976). As such, its physical characteristics correspond to the average features observed in the population. In the case of voice perception, the prototype may therefore be characterized by average acoustical characteristics. A speaker with 'atypical' acoustic features (e.g. highly deviant features), will be located farther away from the prototype (see Figures 25.1E and 25.3A). Because voice density in the space decreases with increasing distance from the prototype, voices with highly-deviant features are less likely to be confused with neighbouring voices, and should be recognized more easily than voices with average acoustic characteristics.

Papcun and collaborators (1989) were the first to put forward a prototype-based model for voice perception. They asked participants to remember an unfamiliar target voice, and subsequently recognize it among nine new voices, after study-test delays of 1 to 4 weeks. They showed similar identification accuracies for voices previously rated as easy- versus hard-to-remember by independent listeners. Yet, easy-to-remember voices, that are farther away from the prototype, produced more false identifications than hard-to-remember voices, although the former were less likely to induce an erroneous response when used as foils. Accordingly, speaker recognition is linked to the deviance of vocal features from the average of all voices and to perceived voice distinctiveness, with higher recognition performance for more deviant and distinctive voices (Lavner et al., 2001; Skuk & Schweinberger, 2013b). These results were interpreted as evidence for a norm-based representation of voices.

Easy-to-remember voices, which have more distinctive acoustic features and are overall more deviant from the population's average, are encoded based on the features that distinguish them from other voices; these distinguishable features are more readily lost over time. By contrast, hard-to-remember voices, which are closer to the prototype and have more average features, are encoded as more robust representations, less sensitive to decay. It should be noted, however, that similar results would have been expected with an exemplar-based representation of voices (Valentine, 1991).

Similarity judgements between pairs of unfamiliar voices suggest that voices are represented in a two-dimensional space, the dimensions of which correlate with measures of Fo and formant frequencies (Baumann & Belin, 2010). This voice-identity space is largely independent of the linguistic content of the vocal stimuli, even though slight variations have

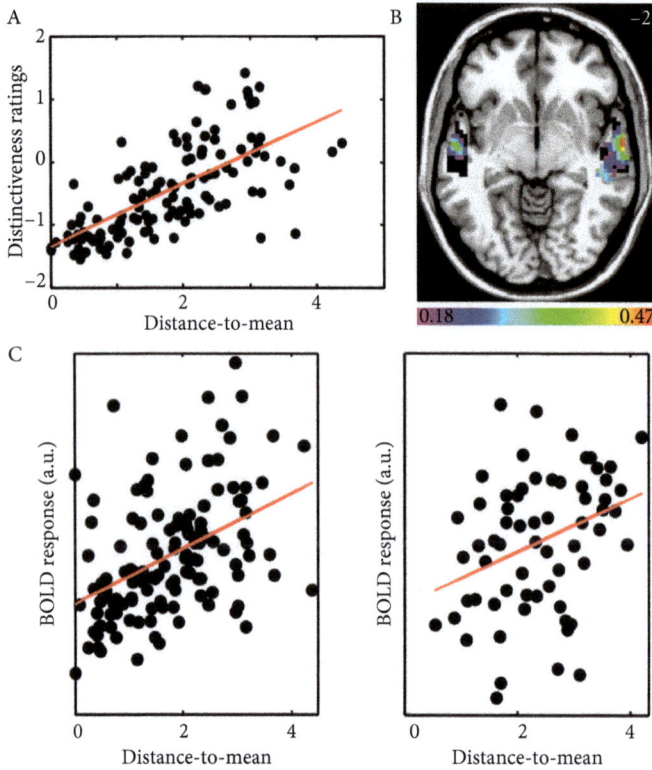

FIGURE 25.3 Cerebral representation of voice identity. (A) Correlation between distance-to-mean and distinctiveness ratings. (B) Cerebral activity in voice-sensitive cortex correlates with distance-to-mean. Colour scale indicates significant Spearman ρ values. (C) Illustration of the correlation between brain activity (BOLD response) and distance-to-mean in two independent experiments using different voice materials and participants.

been reported for different words (Sell et al., 2015). A representation of voices in a multidimensional space is also compatible with evidence of an own-language bias (Fleming et al., 2014; Hammersley & Read, 1996) where listeners are better at recognizing native- compared to foreign-language speakers. Accordingly, foreign-language speakers are more likely to be confused with one another as their representations are densely clustered in the periphery of the multidimensional space whose dimensions are optimal for discriminating between speakers of one's native language.

Studying attractiveness ratings of unfamiliar voices is also a means to understand the representation of voices (Bruckert et al., 2010; Yovel & Belin, 2013). Although evolutionary theory proposes that more typical stimuli are more attractive because they are good fitness indicators, a more cognitive-based account of this effect holds that typical stimuli, due to their similarity to an internal prototype, are easier to process and therefore more pleasant

(Winkielman et al., 2006). Accordingly, using morphing to generate voice composites, researchers demonstrated that increasing averageness was associated with increased perceived attractiveness (Bruckert et al., 2010). The increase in attractiveness ratings was explained by changes of two main acoustical parameters: (1) the distance-to-mean parameter (Figures 25.1E and 25.3A), that is, the Euclidean distance to the population average, created with auditory morphing (Kawahara & Matsui, 2003), in a two-dimensional space (whose dimensions were F0 and F1); and (2) the amount of spectro-temporal irregularities, approximated by measures of harmonic-to-noise ratio (HNR).

A principal component analysis on fifteen acoustical parameters further confirmed the role of these acoustic parameters in explaining the acoustic variability in a set of thirty-two male and thirty-two female voices. This analysis revealed that voices can be represented as points in a three-dimensional voice space whose dimensions can be approximated by F0, formant dispersion, and HNR (Figure 25.1; Latinus et al., 2013). Consistent with previous research, the Euclidean distance between individual voices and the population prototype in the three-dimensional voice space correlates with distinctiveness ratings of voices (Figure 25.1A; Latinus et al., 2013). The studies reviewed here provide correlational evidence that voices are represented in reference to an internal prototype; more causal evidence has been gathered through adaptation paradigms.

Adaptation paradigms rest on the principle that adaptation, induced by exposure to a stimulus over relatively long duration, alters the perception of subsequent stimuli. Perceptual aftereffects, which were traditionally used to study low-level perception, have recently allowed important new insights on the representation of social stimuli, such as faces and voices (Bestelmeyer et al., 2010; Leopold et al., 2001; Rhodes & Jeffery, 2006; Skinner & Benton, 2010; Webster & MacLin, 1999; Zäske et al., 2010). Importantly, perceptual aftereffects have provided compelling evidence that both faces (Leopold et al., 2001; Skinner & Benton, 2010) and voices (Latinus & Belin, 2011; Schweinberger et al., 2008; Zäske et al., 2010) are represented in reference to an internal prototype, favouring the prototype-based model over the exemplar-based model.

Latinus and Belin (2011) created anti-voice stimuli by extrapolating the features of the population prototype (created by averaging sixteen voices of the same gender) with respect to three natural voices. Anti-voice stimuli were used as adaptors in an adaptation paradigm in which probe stimuli were extracted from identity continua between the population prototype and each original voice. Following adaptation, the average voice, which had initially been perceived as neutral in terms of identity, was perceived more often as the voice opposite to the anti-voice adaptor, despite the anti-voice being perceived of as an unrelated identity (Latinus & Belin, 2011). Anti-voice stimuli yielded aftereffects not merely explained by adaptation to low-level information or perceptual distances between adaptors and probes. This study constituted the first direct evidence of a prototype-based coding of voice identity by demonstrating that adaptation was stronger for identity trajectories that passed through the average voice, highlighting its special role in the representation of voice identity.

25.3.2 Neurophysiological Evidence

Further evidence of a norm-based representation of voices comes from neurophysiological studies. In functional magnetic resonance imaging (fMRI), vocal sounds induce larger activity than non-vocal sounds in the upper bank of the superior temporal sulcus (STS), a region referred to as the temporal voice area (TVA; Figure 25.3B; Belin et al., 2000; Pernet et al., 2015). Similarly, voice sensitivity has also been reported within the latency range of the auditory P2 in electro/magnetoencephalography (E/MEG) studies: the occurring fronto-temporal positivity to voices (FTPV; Capilla et al., 2013; Rogier et al., 2010) is larger for vocal than non-vocal sounds (Capilla et al., 2013; Charest et al., 2009; De Lucia et al., 2010).

Adult participants showed sensitivity to voice prototypicality within the latency range of the FTPVm (~200 ms), with a cerebral source in bilateral temporal lobes (Lattner et al., 2003). Using a passive oddball design in MEG, Lattner and collaborators compared the mismatch response (MMR) evoked by a prototypical voice deviant (e.g. a female voice) and non-prototypical voice deviant (e.g. the same female voice in which Fo was modified so as to match it with the standard stimuli) presented in a stream of a standard male voice. Although acoustic differences between the standard male voice and the female voice deviants were greater for the prototypical than the non-prototypical voice deviant, a larger MMR was observed for the non-prototypical voice deviant. This enhanced response to non-prototypical vocal sounds was attributed to the existence of prototypes stored in long-term memory. This conclusion may be limited by the fact that stimuli were derived from only one speaker of each gender, such that it is unclear to which extent these effects would transfer to other speakers.

Alongside its sensitivity to vocal sounds relative to non-vocal sounds, the TVA is sensitive to acoustical cues that are characteristic of individual human voices (Andics et al., 2010; Belin & Zatorre, 2003; Formisano et al., 2008; Latinus et al., 2013). In particular, activity in the TVA is related to the acoustic dissimilarity between voices, suggesting its involvement in an acoustic-based representation of individual voices (Andics et al., 2010, 2013; Bestelmeyer et al., 2012, 2014; Charest et al., 2013; Latinus et al., 2011, 2013). Repetition-suppression paradigms, in which acoustic and perceptual distances between consecutive stimuli are modelled independently, allowed disentangling acoustical from perceptual processing of voices (Andics et al., 2010, 2013; Bestelmeyer et al., 2014; Charest et al., 2013; Latinus et al., 2011). Each of these studies reported an adaptation effect in the TVA linked to acoustic similarity.

The notion that voices are encoded relative to prototypes (see Section 25.1) has received support from correlational data linking acoustic measures of distance-to-mean with attractiveness ratings. Along those lines, neuroimaging studies showed an inverse relation between pleasantness/attractiveness ratings of voices and activity within the STS (MMR—Lattner et al., 2003; TVA—Bestelmeyer et al., 2012). An fMRI study further confirmed this finding by showing both correlational and causal evidence of norm-based coding of voices in the TVA (Figures 25.1C and 25.1D; Latinus et al., 2013). Participants passively listened to unfamiliar vocal sounds while their brain activity was recorded. In two experiments with different participants and stimuli, a strong correlation between TVA activity and distance-to-mean was observed. In a third experiment, the authors manipulated a subset of voices so as to bring some voices closer to and others farther away from the population prototype; as expected, activity was lower for voices moved toward the population prototype.

25.4 Cerebral Representation
of Voice Gender and Age

Perceptual aftereffects following voice adaptation suggest that voice gender is represented in a contrastive manner (e.g. Mullennix et al., 1995; Schweinberger et al., 2008) such that opponent neuron populations code male and female voices, respectively. It has been argued that voice gender aftereffects arise at a high perceptual level, and do not result from low-level adaptation to Fo or post-perceptual adaptation to gender concepts (Schweinberger et al., 2008).

Electrophysiological studies suggest that contrastive coding of voice gender is achieved within ~200 ms following voice onset: for instance, following voice adaptation, early auditory evoked potentials (N1 and P2) were reduced when test voices were congruent rather than incongruent with the gender of adaptor voices (Zäske et al., 2009). Consistently, Latinus and Taylor (2012) showed that voice gender is computed at ~200 ms following the processing of voice pitch (~50 ms), without prior adaptation.

fMRI research revealed several potential brain areas involved in the processing of voice gender. One group presented listeners with two-word sentences uttered by a male and a female speaker. Sentences were either natural or manipulated in pitch such that atypical voice qualities (i.e. a low-pitched female voice versus a high-pitched male voice) were created (Lattner et al., 2005). Results suggested that speaker gender is predominantly processed in the right hemisphere, with generally stronger responses to female compared to male voices. This was attributed to the greater biological or social relevance of female/high-pitched voices compared to male voices. Importantly, different voice characteristics were processed in functionally segregated areas: voice pitch was processed close and anterior to primary auditory cortex, voice-spectral information-modulated activity in the posterior superior temporal gyrus (STG) and areas surrounding the planum parietale bilaterally, and perceived 'voice naturalness' was processed in the right anterior STG. In line with Lattner and colleagues, Sokhi and others (2005) reported that the right anterior temporal gyrus near the STS responded more to female than to male voices. Conversely, male voices compared to female voices elicited stronger activity in the mesio-parietal precuneus area. Since only male listeners were tested, this finding has been interpreted as episodic-memory retrieval of the male listeners' own voices.

In contrast to the notion that different areas predominantly process one gender, fMRI research with gender-morphed voices suggests that overlapping neuron populations along the auditory ventral stream are involved in the processing of male and female voices (Charest et al., 2013; Junger et al., 2013). Specifically, while right anterior TVAs may be involved in a more general processing of acoustic properties (Charest et al., 2013), bilateral inferior prefrontal cortex, the cingulate cortex, and insula are sensitive to perceived gender ambiguity (Charest et al., 2013; Junger et al., 2013). However, it is unclear at present if these regions are the loci of categorical long-term representations for voice gender, or rather reflect attentional processes or general cognitive load during decision making. Along those lines, Junger et al. (2013) reported greater activation in fronto-temporal areas for voices with opposite gender to that of the listeners, possibly reflecting increased attention to potential mates.

Taken together, research on the neural basis of voice-gender processing is still in its infancy and future research is needed to further elucidate its underlying mechanisms. This is even more the case for vocal-age perception for which neurophysiological studies are virtually absent from the literature. However, behavioural evidence of aftereffects of adaptation suggests that vocal age may be coded by contrastive neuron populations (Zäske & Schweinberger, 2011; Zäske et al., 2013), analogous to voice gender (Schweinberger et al., 2008). Alternatively, it could be speculated that more than two types of neurons are involved in the representation of vocal age, especially when considering that children's voices may form a separate perceptual category.

Based on the overlap of age-related and gender-related acoustic cues, as well as the interaction of speaker age and gender at a perceptual level (cf. Section 25.2.2), one can assume that the cerebral representations of vocal age and gender are also intertwined. Behavioural evidence for this notion has been found in cross-categorical transfer effects of adaptation (Zäske et al., 2013). Specifically, vocal-age aftereffects were reduced but remained significant when voice gender was changed between adaptation and test, suggesting that vocal-age perception relies on both gender-dependent and gender-invariant representations. By contrast, voice-gender aftereffects in that study were not modulated by age congruence between adaptor and test voices, suggesting that gender in adult voices is represented independently of vocal age.

25.5 OUTSTANDING QUESTIONS

The research reviewed here clearly demonstrated that voices are encoded in a multidimensional voice space in terms of their deviation from an internal prototype. These studies raised new questions on the representation of voices. How does the prototype emerge during typical development? How are familiar voices encoded? On the one hand, it could be argued that the representation of voices in the multidimensional voice space is a mandatory process of voice perception. In this case, all voices, whether familiar or not, would first be encoded with respect to the population prototype. On the other hand, familiar voices may be processed through different mechanisms. Support for the latter hypothesis arises from different studies showing that the perception of familiar and unfamiliar voices involves different neural networks (Van Lancker & Kreiman, 1987; Van Lancker et al., 1989). Preliminary evidence showing only a weak relationship between distinctiveness ratings made by listeners who were either familiar or unfamiliar with the same set of voices, suggests an influence of familiarity on the position of the voice in the voice space (Skuk & Schweinberger, 2013b).

Latinus and collaborators (2013) raised questions on the nature of the space and the prototype. They proposed a three-dimensional space, whose dimensions correspond to fundamental frequency, formant dispersion, and HNR. The population prototypes were characterized by average spectral characteristics (Fo and formant dispersion), but a very smooth texture (e.g. a large HNR). A larger HNR for the prototype is a by-product of the averaging procedure used in their study. Yet, analysis of brain data demonstrated that this was a crucial aspect of the prototype, as the distance to the mathematical average of all voices (androgynous mathematical average) used in the experiment yielded no correlation with brain activity in the TVA. The same observation holds when using gender-specific mathematical averages (unpublished data from Latinus et al., 2013). This study further suggested that there were at least two population prototypes, one per gender, as distance-to-mean calculated to an androgynous prototype did not correlate with activity in the TVA.

Finally, is the prototype a single point at the centre of the space, or does it reflect a statistical distribution around the mean? Preliminary evidence suggests that the prototype is not a single point in the space, as similar correlations were observed for distance-to-mean calculated from the average of sixteen or thirty-two same-sex voices (unpublished data). This suggests that the 'prototype' corresponds to the statistical average around the mean, although it is characterized by highly-evident features (e.g. a large HNR). Future studies are needed to further explore these questions.

Thus far, it appears that there is at least one multidimensional space with two sex-specific prototypes. The possibility of another space for the encoding of familiar voices has been previously discussed, and raises questions regarding the existence of other prototypes, and potentially other voice spaces for representing voices depending on languages, emotional expression, or age. While there is some behavioural evidence for an interaction between the processing of vocal age and gender, it remains to be further explored how the perception of voice gender, age, and identity interact both at the perceptual and neural level.

References

Abitbol, J., Abitbol, P., & Abitbol, B. (1999). Sex hormones and the female voice. *Journal of Voice*, 13(3), 424–446.

Aglieri, V., Watson, R., Pernet, C., Latinus, M., Garrido, L., & Belin, P. (2016). The Glasgow Voice Memory Test: assessing the ability to memorize and recognize unfamiliar voices. *Behavior Research Methods*, 49(1), 97–110.

Amir, O., Engel, M., Shabtai, E., & Amir, N. (2012). Identification of children's gender and age by listeners. *Journal of Voice*, 26(3), 313–321.

Andics, A., McQueen, J. M., & Petersson, K. M. (2013). Mean-based neural coding of voices. *NeuroImage*, 79, 351–360.

Andics, A., McQueen, J. M., Petersson, K. M., Gal, V., Rudas, G., & Vidnyanszky, Z. (2010). Neural mechanisms for voice recognition. *NeuroImage*, 52(4), 1528–1540.

Baumann, O. & Belin, P. (2010). Perceptual scaling of voice identity: common dimensions for different vowels and speakers. *Psychological Research*, 74(1), 110–120.

Belin, P., Bestelmeyer, P. E. G., Latinus, M., & Watson, R. (2011). Understanding voice perception. *British Journal of Psychology*, 102(4), 711–725.

Belin, P., Fecteau, S., & Bedard, C. (2004). Thinking the voice: neural correlates of voice perception. *Trends in Cognitive Sciences*, 8(3), 129–135.

Belin, P. & Zatorre, R. J. (2003). Adaptation to speaker's voice in right anterior temporal lobe. *NeuroReport*, 14(16), 2105–2109.

Belin, P., Zatorre, R. J., Lafaille, P., Ahad, P., & Pike, B. (2000). Voice-selective areas in human auditory cortex. *Nature*, 403(6767), 309–312.

Bennett, S. (1981). Vowel formant frequency—characteristics of pre-adolescent males and females. *Journal of the Acoustical Society of America*, 69(1), 231–238.

Bennett, S. & Monterodiaz, L. (1982). Children's perception of speaker sex. *Journal of Phonetics*, 10(1), 113–121.

Bestelmeyer, P. E. G., Latinus, M., Bruckert, L., Rouger, J., Crabbe, F., & Belin, P. (2012). Implicitly perceived vocal attractiveness modulates prefrontal cortex activity. *Cerebral Cortex*, 22(6), 1263–1270.

Bestelmeyer, P. E. G., Maurage, P., Rouger, J., Latinus, M., & Belin, P. (2014). Adaptation to vocal expressions reveals multi-step perception of auditory emotion. *Journal of Neuroscience*, 34(24), 8098–8105.

Bestelmeyer, P. E. G., Rouger, J., DeBruine, L. M., & Belin, P. (2010). Auditory adaptation in vocal affect perception. *Cognition*, 117(2), 217–223.

Blank, H., Wieland, N., & von Kriegstein, K. (2014). Person recognition and the brain: merging evidence from patients and healthy individuals. *Neuroscience & Biobehavorial Reviews*, 47, 717–734.

Braun, A. (1996). Age estimation by different listener groups. *Forensic Linguistics*, 3, 65–73.

Bricker, P. D. & Pruzansky, S. (1966). Effects of stimulus content and duration on talker identification. *Journal of the Acoustical Society of America*, 40(6), 1441–1449.

Brown, W. S., Morris, R. J., & Michel, J. F. (1989). Vocal jitter in young adult and aged female voices. *Journal of Voice*, 3(2), 113–119.

Bruce, V. & Young, A. (1986). Understanding face recognition. *British Journal of Psychology*, 77 (Pt 3), 305–327.

Bruckert, L., Bestelmeyer, P. E. G., Latinus, M., Rouger, J., Charest, I., Rousselet, G. A., Kawahara, H., & Belin, P. (2010). Vocal attractiveness increases by averaging. *Current Biology*, 20(2), 116–120.

Bruckert, L., Lienard, J. S., Lacroix, A., Kreutzer, M. & Leboucher, G. (2006). Women use voice parameters to assess men's characteristics. *Proceedings of the Royal Society B: Biological Science*, 273(1582), 83–89.

Burton, A. M. & Bonner, L. (2004). Familiarity influences judgments of sex: the case of voice recognition. *Perception*, 33(6), 747–752.

Capilla, A., Belin, P., & Gross, J. (2013). The early spatio-temporal correlates and task independence of cerebral voice processing studied with MEG. *Cerebral Cortex*, 23(6), 1388–1395.

Cartei, V., Cowles, W., Banerjee, R., & Reby, D. (2014). Control of voice gender in pre-pubertal children. *British Journal of Developmental Psychology*, 32(1), 100–106.

Charest, I., Pernet, C., Latinus, M., Crabbe, F., & Belin, P. (2013). Cerebral processing of voice gender studied using a continuous carryover FMRI design. *Cerebral Cortex*, 23(4), 958–966.

Charest, I., Pernet, C. R., Rousselet, G. A., Quinones, I., Latinus, M., Fillion-Bilodeau, S., Chartrand, J. P., & Belin, P. (2009). Electrophysiological evidence for an early processing of human voices. *BMC Neuroscience*, 10, 127.

Chiba, T. & Kajiyama, M. (1941). *The Vowel: Its Nature and Structure*. Tokyo, Japan: Kaiseikan.

Coleman, R. O. (1976). Comparison of contributions of two voice quality characteristics to perception of maleness and femaleness in voice. *Journal of Speech and Hearing Research*, 19(1), 168–180.

Cook, S. & Wilding, J. (1997). Earwitness testimony: never mind the variety, hear the length. *Applied Cognitive Psychology*, 11(2), 95–111.

De Lucia, M., Clarke, S., & Murray, M. M. (2010). A temporal hierarchy for conspecific vocalization discrimination in humans. *Journal of Neuroscience*, 30(33), 11210–11221.

Fant, G. (1966). A note on vocal tract size factors and non-uniform F-pattern scalings. *Progress and Status Report—Computational Linguistics*, 29(1), 22–30.

Fleming, D., Giordano, B. L., Caldara, R., & Belin, P. (2014). A language-familiarity effect for speaker discrimination without comprehension. *Proceedings of the National Academy of Sciences of the USA*, 111(38), 13795–13798.

Formisano, E., De Martino, F., Bonte, M., & Goebel, R. (2008). 'Who' is saying 'what'? Brain-based decoding of human voice and speech. *Science*, 322(5903), 970–973.

Gaudrain, E., Li, S., Ban, V. S., & Patterson, R. D. (2009). The role of glottal pulse rate and vocal tract length in the perception of speaker identity. INTERSPEECH 2009, 10th Annual Conference of the International Speech Communication Association, September 6–10, 2009, Brighton, UK.

Gorham-Rowan, M. M. & Laures-Gore, J. (2006). Acoustic-perceptual correlates of voice quality in elderly men and women. *Journal of Communication Disorders*, 39(3), 171–184.

Hammersley, R. & Read, J. D. (1996). Voice identification by humans and computers. In: S. L. Sporer, R. S. Malpass, & G. Koehnken (eds) *Psychological Issues in Eyewitness Identification*. Psychology Press.

Harnsberger, J. D., Brown, W. S., Shrivastav, R., & Rothman, H. (2010). Noise and tremor in the perception of vocal aging in males. *Journal of Voice*, 24(5), 523–530.

Harnsberger, J. D., Shrivastav, R., Brown, W. S., Rothman, H., & Hollien, H. (2008). Speaking rate and fundamental frequency as speech cues to perceived age. *Journal of Voice*, 22(1), 58–69.

Hartman, D. E. (1979). Perceptual identity and characteristics of aging in normal male adult speakers. *Journal of Communication Disorders*, 12(1), 53–61.

Hartman, D. E. & Danhauer, J. L. (1976). Perceptual features of speech for males in four perceived age decades. *Journal of the Acoustical Society of America*, 59(3), 713–715.

Hillenbrand, J., Getty, L. A., Clark, M. J., & Wheeler, K. (1995). Acoustic characteristics of American English vowels. *Journal of the Acoustical Society of America*, 97(5 Pt 1), 3099–3111.

Hollien, H., Green, R., & Massey, K. (1994). Longitudinal research on adolescent voice change in males. *Journal of the Acoustical Society of America*, 96(5), 2646–2654.

Hughes, S. & Rhodes, B. C. (2010). Making age assessments based on voice: the impact of the reproductive viability of the speaker. *Journal of Social, Evolutionary, and Cultural Psychology*, 4(4), 290–304.

Hummert, M. L., Mazloff, D., & Henry, C. (1999). Vocal characteristics of older adults and stereotyping. *Journal of Nonverbal Behavior*, 23(2), 111–132.

Huntley, R., Hollien, H., & Shipp, T. (1987). Influences of listener characteristics on perceived age estimations. *Journal of Voice*, 1(1), 49–52.

Ingemann, F. (1968). Identification of speaker's sex from voiceless fricatives. *Journal of the Acoustical Society of America*, 44(4), 1142.

Ingrisano, D., Weismer, G., & Schuckers, G. H. (1980). Sex identification of preschool children's voices. *Folia Phoniatrica*, 32(1), 61–69.

Jacques, R. D. & Rastatter, M. P. (1990). Recognition of speaker age from selected acoustic features as perceived by normal young and older listeners. *Folia Phoniatrica*, 42(3), 118–124.

Junger, J., Pauly, K., Brohr, S., Birkholz, P., Neuschaefer-Rube, C., Kohler, C., ... Habel, U. (2013). Sex matters: neural correlates of voice gender perception. *NeuroImage*, 79, 275–287.

Kawahara, H. & Matsui, H. (2003). *Auditory Morphing Based on an Elastic Perceptual Distance Metric in an Interference-Free Time-Frequency Representation*. IEEE International Conference on Acoustics, Speech, and Signal Processing, 6–10 April 2003, Hong Kong, China.

Klatt, D. H. & Klatt, L. C. (1990). Analysis, synthesis, and perception of voice quality variations among female and male talkers. *Journal of the Acoustical Society of America*, 87(2), 820–857.

Kramer, C. (1977). Perceptions of female and male speech. *Language and Speech*, 20, 151–161.

Kreiman, J. & Sidtis, D. (2011). *Foundations of Voice Studies: An Interdisciplinary Approach to Voice Production and Perception.* Malden, MA: Wiley-Blackwell.

Kuwabara, H. & Sagisak, Y. (1995). Acoustic characteristics of speaker individuality: control and conversion. *Speech and Communication*, 16, 165–173. doi: 10.1016/0167-6393(94)00053-D

Lass, N. J., Hughes, K. R., Bowyer, M. D., Waters, L. T., & Bourne, V. T. (1976). Speaker sex identification from voiced, whispered, and filtered isolated vowels. *Journal of the Acoustical Society of America*, 59(3), 675–678.

Lass, N. J., Mertz, P. J., & Kimmel, K. L. (1978). The effect of temporal speech alterations on speaker race and sex identifications. *Language and Speech*, 21, 279–290.

Latinus, M. & Belin, P. (2011). Anti-voice adaptation suggests prototype-based coding of voice identity. *Frontiers in Psychology*, 2, article 175.

Latinus, M. & Belin, P. (2012). Perceptual auditory aftereffects on voice identity using brief vowel stimuli. *PLoS One*, 7(7), e41384.

Latinus, M., Crabbe, F., & Belin, P. (2011). Learning-induced changes in the cerebral processing of voice identity. *Cerebral Cortex*, 21(12), 2820–2828.

Latinus, M., McAleer, P., Bestelmeyer, P. E., & Belin, P. (2013). Norm-based coding of voice identity in human auditory cortex. *Current Biology*, 23(12), 1075–1080.

Latinus, M. & Taylor, M. J. (2012). Discriminating male and female voices: differentiating pitch and gender. *Brain Topography*, 25(2), 194–204.

Lattner, S., Maess, B., Wang, Y., Schauer, M., Alter, K., & Friederici, A. D. (2003). Dissociation of human and computer voices in the brain: evidence for a preattentive gestalt-like perception. *Human Brain Mapping*, 20(1), 13–21.

Lattner, S., Meyer, M. E., & Friederici, A. D. (2005). Voice perception: sex, pitch, and the right hemisphere. *Human Brain Mapping*, 24(1), 11–20.

Lavner, Y., Gath, I., & Rosenhouse, J. (2000). The effects of acoustic modifications on the identification of familiar voices speaking isolated vowels. *Speech Communication*, 30, 9–26.

Lavner, Y., Rosenhouse, J., & Gath, I. (2001). The prototype model in speaker identification by human listeners. *International Journal of Speech Technology*, 4(1), 63–74.

Lee, S., Potamianos, A., & Narayanan, S. (1999). Acoustics of children's speech: developmental changes of temporal and spectral parameters. *Journal of the Acoustical Society of America*, 105(3), 1455–1468.

Leopold, D. A., O'Toole, A. J., Vetter, T., & Blanz, V. (2001). Prototype-referenced shape encoding revealed by high-level aftereffects. *Nature Neuroscience*, 4(1), 89–94.

Linville, S. E. (1996). The sound of senescence. *Journal of Voice*, 10(2), 190–200.

Linville, S. E. & Fisher, H. B. (1985). Acoustic characteristics of perceived versus actual vocal age in controlled phonation by adult females. *Journal of the Acoustical Society of America*, 78(1), 40–48.

Linville, S. E. & Korabic, E. W. (1986). Elderly listeners estimates of vocal age in adult females. *Journal of the Acoustical Society of America*, 80(2), 692–694.

Lopez, S., Riera, P., Assaneo, M. F., Eguia, M., Sigman, M., & Trevisan, M. A. (2013). Vocal caricatures reveal signatures of speaker identity. *Scientific Reports*, 3, 3407.

Morris, R. J. & Brown, W. S. (1994). Age-related differences in speech intensity among adult females. *Folia Phoniatrica et Logopaedica*, 46(2), 64–69.

Moyse, E. (2014). Age estimation from faces and voices: a review. *Psychologica Belgica*, 54(3), 255–265.

Moyse, E., Beaufort, A., & Brédart, S. (2014). Evidence for an own-age bias in age estimation from voices in older persons. *European Journal of Ageing*, 11(3), 241–247.

Mullennix, J. W., Johnson, K. A., TopcuDurgun, M., & Farnsworth, L. M. (1995). The perceptual representation of voice gender. *Journal of the Acoustical Society of America*, 98(6), 3080–3095.

Murry, T. & Singh, S. (1980). Multidimensional analysis of male and female voices. *Journal of the Acoustical Society of America*, 68(5), 1294–1300.

Nakamura, K., Kawashima, R., Sugiura, M., Kato, T., Nakamura, A., Hatano, K., ... Kojima, S. (2001). Neural substrates for recognition of familiar voices: a PET study. *Neuropsychologia*, 39(10), 1047–1054.

Neiman, G. S. & Applegate, J. A. (1990). Accuracy of listener judgments of perceived age relative to chronological age in adults. *Folia Phoniatrica*, 42(6), 327–330.

Owren, M. J., Berkowitz, M., & Bachorowski, J. A. (2007). Listeners judge talker sex more efficiently from male than from female vowels. *Perception & Psychophysics*, 69(6), 930–941.

Papcun, G., Kreiman, J., & Davis, A. (1989). Long-term memory for unfamiliar voices. *Journal of the Acoustical Society of America*, 85(2), 913–925.

Pernet, C. R. & Belin, P. (2012). The role of pitch and timbre in voice gender categorization. *Frontiers in Psychology*, 3, 23–23.

Pernet, C. R., McAleer, P., Latinus, M., Gorgolewski, K. J., Charest, I., Bestelmeyer, P. E., ... Belin, P. (2015). The human voice areas: spatial organization and inter-individual variability in temporal and extra-temporal cortices. *NeuroImage*, 119, 164–174.

Perry, T. L., Ohde, R. N., & Ashmead, D. H. (2001). The acoustic bases for gender identification from children's voices. *Journal of the Acoustical Society of America*, 109(6), 2988–2998.

Peterson, G. E. & Barney, H. L. (1952). Control methods used in a study of the vowels. *Journal of the Acoustical Society of America*, 24(2), 175–184.

Pollack, I., Pickett, J. M., & Sumby, W. H. (1954). On the identification of speakers by voice. *Journal of the Acoustical Society of America*, 26(3), 403–406.

Ptacek, P. H. & Sander, E. K. (1966). Age recognition from voice. *Journal of Speech and Hearing Research*, 9, 273–277.

Ramig, L. A. & Ringel, R. L. (1983). Effects of physiological aging on selected acoustic characteristics of voice. *Journal of Speech and Hearing Research*, 26(1), 22–30.

Ramig, L. O., Gray, S., Baker, K., Corbin-Lewis, K., Buder, E., Luschei, E., Coon, H., & Smith, M. (2001). The aging voice: a review, treatment data and familial and genetic perspectives. *Folia Phoniatrica et Logopaedica*, 53(5), 252–265.

Rhodes, G. & Jeffery, L. (2006). Adaptive norm-based coding of facial identity. *Vision Research*, 46(18), 2977–2987.

Rogier, O., Roux, S., Belin, P., Bonnet-Brilhault, F. & Bruneau, N. (2010). An electrophysiological correlate of voice processing in 4- to 5-year-old children. *International Journal of Psychophysiology*, 75(1), 44–47.

Rosch, E., Mervis, C. B., Gray, W., Johnson, D., & Boyes-Braem, P. (1976). Basic objects in natural categories. *Cognitive Psychology*, 8, 382–439.

Ryan, W. J. (1972). Acoustic aspects of aging voice. *Journal of Gerontology*, 27(2), 265.

Ryan, W. J. & Burk, K. W. (1974). Perceptual and acoustic correlates of aging in speech of males. *Journal of Communication Disorders*, 7(2), 181–192.

Schirmer, A. & Kotz, S. A. (2006). Beyond the right hemisphere: brain mechanisms mediating vocal emotional processing. *Trends in Cognitive Sciences*, 10(1), 24–30.

Schvartz, K. C. & Chatterjee, M. (2012). Gender identification in younger and older adults: use of spectral and temporal cues in noise-vocoded speech. *Ear and Hearing*, 33(3), 411–420.

Schwartz, M. F. & Rine, H. E. (1968). Identification of speaker sex from isolated whispered vowels. *Journal of the Acoustical Society of America*, 44(6), 1736.

Schweinberger, S. R. (2001). Human brain potential correlates of voice priming and voice recognition. *Neuropsychologia*, 39(9), 921–936.

Schweinberger, S. R., Casper, C., Hauthal, N., Kaufmann, J. M., Kawahara, H., Kloth, N., . . . Zäske, R. (2008). Auditory adaptation in voice perception. *Current Biology*, 18(9), 684–688.

Schweinberger, S. R., Herholz, A., & Sommer, W. (1997). Recognizing famous voices: influence of stimulus duration and different types of retrieval cues. *Journal of Speech, Language and Hearing Research*, 40(2), 453–463.

Schweinberger, S. R., Herholz, A., & Stief, V. (1997). Auditory long term memory: repetition priming of voice recognition. *The Quarterly Journal of Experimental Psychology: Section A*, 50(3), 498–517.

Schweinberger, S. R., Walther, C., Zäske, R., & Kovacs, G. (2011). Neural correlates of adaptation to voice identity. *British Journal of Psychology*, 102(4), 748–764.

Sell, G., Suied, C., Elhilali, M., & Shamma, S. (2015). Perceptual susceptibility to acoustic manipulations in speaker discrimination. *Journal of the Acoustical Society of America*, 137(2), 911–922.

Sherrin, C. (2015). Earwitness evidence: the reliability of voice identifications. *Osgoode Hall Law Journal*, 56(3).

Shipp, T. & Hollien, H. (1969). Perception of aging male voice. *Journal of Speech, Language and Hearing Research*, 12(4), 703.

Shipp, T., Qi, Y. Y., Huntley, R., & Hollien, H. (1992). Acoustic and temporal correlates of perceived age. *Journal of Voice*, 6(3), 211–216.

Sidtis, D. & Kreiman, J. (2012). In the beginning was the familiar voice: personally familiar voices in the evolutionary and contemporary biology of communication. *Integrative Psychological & Behavioral Science*, 46(2), 146–159.

Simpson, A. P. (2009). Phonetic differences between male and female speech. *Language & Linguistics Compass*, 3, 621–640.

Skinner, A. L. & Benton, C. P. (2010). Anti-expression aftereffects reveal prototype-referenced coding of facial expressions. *Psychological Science*, 21(9), 1248–1253.

Skuk, V. G., Dammann, L. M., & Schweinberger, S. R. (2015). Role of timbre and fundamental frequency in voice gender adaptation. *Journal of the Acoustical Society of America*, 138(2), 1180–1193.

Skuk, V. G. & Schweinberger, S. R. (2013a). Adaptation aftereffects in vocal emotion perception elicited by expressive faces and voices. *PLoS One*, 8(11).

Skuk, V. G. & Schweinberger, S. R. (2013b). Gender differences in familiar voice identification. *Hearing Research*, 296, 131–140.

Skuk, V. G. & Schweinberger, S. R. (2014). Influences of fundamental frequency, formant frequencies, aperiodicity, and spectrum level on the perception of voice gender. *Journal of Speech, Language, and Hearing Research*, 57, 285–296.

Smith, D. R. R. & Patterson, R. D. (2005). The interaction of glottal-pulse rate and vocal-tract length in judgements of speaker size, sex, and age. *Journal of the Acoustical Society of America*, 118(5), 3177–3186.

Sokhi, D. S., Hunter, M. D., Wilkinson, I. D., & Woodruff, P. W. (2005). Male and female voices activate distinct regions in the male brain. *NeuroImage*, 27, 572–578.

Spreckelmeyer, K. N., Kutas, M., Urbach, T., Altenmuller, E.. & Munte, T. F. (2009). Neural processing of vocal emotion and identity. *Brain Cognition*, 69(1), 121–126.

Stathopoulos, E. T., Huber, J. E., & Sussman, J. E. (2011). Changes in acoustic characteristics of the voice across the life span: measures from individuals 4–93 years of age. *Journal of Speech, Language, and Hearing Research*, 54, 1011–1021.

Titze, I. R. (1989). Physiologic and acoustic differences between male and female voices. *Journal of the Acoustical Society of America*, 85, 1699–1707.

Torre, P. & Barlow, J. A. (2009). Age-related changes in acoustic characteristics of adult speech. *Journal of Communication Disorders*, 42(5), 324–333.

Valentine, T. (1991). A unified account of the effects of distinctiveness, inversion, and race in face recognition. *Quarterly Journal of Experimental Psychology A*, 43(2), 161–204.

Van Lancker, D. & Kreiman, J. (1987). Voice discrimination and recognition are separate abilities. *Neuropsychologia*, 25(5), 829–834.

Van Lancker, D., Kreiman, J., & Emmorey, K. (1985). Familiar voice recognition: patterns and parameters. Part I: Recognition of backward voices. *Journal of Phonetics*, 13, 19–38.

Van Lancker, D. R., Kreiman, J., & Cummings, J. (1989). Voice perception deficits: neuroanatomical correlates of phonagnosia. *Journal of Clinical and Experimental Neuropsychology*, 11(5), 665–674.

Voelkle, M. C. & Ebner, N. C. (2012). Let me guess how old you are: effects of age, gender, and facial expression on perceptions of age. *Psychology and Aging*, 25(265–277).

von Kriegstein, K. & Giraud, A. L. (2006). Implicit multisensory associations influence voice recognition. *PLoS Biology*, 4(10), e326.

Vorperian, H. K. & Kent, R. D. (2007). Vowel acoustic space development in children: a synthesis of acoustic and anatomic data. *Journal of Speech, Language and Hearing Research*, 50(6), 1510–1545.

Vorperian, H. K., Wang, S. B., Chung, M. K., Schimek, E. M., Durtschi, R. B., Kent, R. D., Ziegert, A. J., & Gentry, L. R. (2009). Anatomic development of the oral and pharyngeal portions of the vocal tract: an imaging study. *Journal of the Acoustical Society of America*, 125(3), 1666–1678.

Webster, M. A. & MacLin, O. H. (1999). Figural aftereffects in the perception of faces. *Psychonomic Bulletin & Review*, 6(4), 647–653.

Weinberg, B. & Bennett, S. (1971). Speaker sex recognition of 5-year-old and 6-year-old children's voices. *Journal of the Acoustical Society of America*, 50(4), 1210.

Winkielman, P., Halberstadt, J., Fazendeiro, T., & Catty, S. (2006). Prototypes are attractive because they are easy on the mind. *Psychological Science*, 17(9), 799–806.

Winters, S. J., Levi, S. V., & Pisoni, D. B. (2008). Identification and discrimination of bilingual talkers across languages. *Journal of the Acoustical Society of America*, 123(6), 4524–4538.

Yovel, G. & Belin, P. (2013). A unified coding strategy for processing faces and voices. *Trends in Cognitive Sciences*, 17(6), 263–271.

Zäske, R. & Schweinberger, S. R. (2011). You are only as old as you sound: auditory aftereffects in vocal age perception. *Hearing Research*, 282(1–2), 283–288.

Zäske, R., Schweinberger, S. R., Kaufmann, J. M., & Kawahara, H. (2009). In the ear of the beholder: neural correlates of adaptation to voice gender. *European Journal of Neuroscience*, 30(3), 527–534.

Zäske, R., Schweinberger, S. R., & Kawahara, H. (2010). Voice aftereffects of adaptation to speaker identity. *Hearing Research*, 268(1–2), 38–45.

Zäske, R., Skuk, V. G., Kaufmann, J. M., & Schweinberger, S. R. (2013). Perceiving vocal age and gender: an adaptation approach. *Acta Psychologica*, 144(3), 583–593.

Zäske, R., Volberg, G., Kovacs, G., & Schweinberger, S. R. (2014). Electrophysiological correlates of voice learning and recognition. *Journal of Neuroscience*, 34(33), 10821–10831.

CHAPTER 26

··

THE PERCEPTION
OF PERSONALITY TRAITS
FROM VOICES

··

PHIL MCALEER AND PASCAL BELIN

26.1 PERSONALITY FROM VOICES

··

EARLY work on personality from voices focused on determining status (Allport & Cantril, 1934; Herzog, 1933; Pear, 1931). Both Herzog and Pear, using questionnaires about speakers (Herzog—6, Pear—9) and large participant samples (2,700 and 4,000 respectively), found participants readily attributed traits such as trustworthiness to speakers based on similarity to acquaintances or stereotypes. Furthermore, physical characteristics such as height, age, and weight were quickly and somewhat accurately estimated, though still readily debated today (Pisanski et al., 2014, 2016; Smith et al., 2016). From there, Allport and Cantril (1934) established ten experiments, in a radio scenario, investigating listeners' ability to match information such as dominance, submissiveness (ascendance–submission scale), and outgoingness (extraversion–introversion) to eighteen male speakers. They defined 'voice' as including elements of pitch, rhythm, inflection (nowadays intonation/glide), and volume, separating it from 'speech' defined as the content or accent/language and vocabulary used. Allport and Cantril found that voices did convey information about personality but accuracy was not as robust as with physical attributes. Importantly, however, certain voices created consistent impressions across listeners even when the perception was wrong (i.e. an extrovert voice was perceived as such by all listeners irrespective of accuracy).

Extraversion was a key focus of early studies due to measures such as the Eysenck Personality Inventory (EPI) (Eysenck & Eysenck, 1965), a self-reported questionnaire allowing researchers to compare 'self' with 'other' percepts. Related to accuracy and utilizing the EPI, Kramer and Aronovitch (1970) found no correlation between self ratings of twenty-two speakers by eighteen listeners, irrespective of whether a passage was read in a neutral or emotional tone. Indeed, two prominent reviews (Kramer, 1963; Starkweather, 1961) stated the pessimistic view that deriving accurate personality from voices was a fallacy. What was evident, however, was that certain voices showed consistent ratings, with Kramer (1964) suggesting that this 'stereotyping' of voices was an interesting scope of research in itself.

Following this, Aronovitch (1976) explored the vocal parameters conveying consistent personality ratings. Ten-second excerpts of guided spontaneous speech, recorded from fifty-seven participants (thirty-two female), were rated by one hundred listeners on ten personality traits, using polar adjective scales (e.g. sociable–unsociable; kind–cruel). Four acoustical parameters were measured: rate—number of syllables per second; intensity—subjective loudness; sound:silence ratio—vocalized time over non-speech time per excerpt; fundamental frequency—pitch. Aronovitch found that participants' judgements were systematic with voices consistently labelled with specific traits. Furthermore, labelling was irrespective of sex of listener; an unsociable male was recognized by both males and females. In regards to acoustics, male voices were judged based on the variability of pitch and loudness, whereas female voices were judged on the average values of pitch and loudness—an effect Aronovitch related to the 'of-the-day' cultural stereotypes of the stability/variability of men/women.

Subsequently, this study has been a springboard to a wealth of research looking to derive the information and decisions that have a basis in vocal acoustics, both physical (Fitch, 1997; Hughes et al., 2004, 2009; Hughes & Rhodes, 2010; Krauss et al., 2002; Pisanski et al., 2014, 2016; Rendall et al., 2007; Smith et al., 2016; Titze, 1989) and perceptual (Anderson & Klofstad, 2012; Apicella & Feinberg, 2009; Apicella et al., 2007; Feinberg et al., 2008b; Jones et al., 2008, 2010; Klofstad et al., 2015, 2012; McAleer et al., 2014; Puts et al., 2007; Rezlescu et al., 2015).

Recently, studies have focused on trait preferences and how they influence decisions such as the products we buy and who we find funny, vote for, or find attractive (Apicella & Feinberg, 2009; Apicella et al., 2007; Cowan et al., 2015; Klofstad et al., 2015, 2012; Nass & Lee, 2001). Generally, findings reveal that both sexes perceive lower-pitched voices as more attractive (Feinberg et al., 2008a; Jones et al., 2010) due to connotations with physical dominance in males (Puts, Apicella, & Cardenas, 2012; Puts et al., 2007; Puts, Jones, & DeBruine, 2012) and social dominance (e.g. assertiveness, leadership) in both sexes (Borkowska & Pawlowski, 2011; Ohala, 1983; Puts et al., 2007; Tsantani et al., 2016). However, female preferences for male voices can be influenced by whether they are seeking short- or long-term partners (Apicella & Feinberg, 2009; Vukovic et al., 2011) and whether they are breastfeeding (Apicella & Feinberg, 2009) or taking contraceptives. In short, low-pitched male voices appear preferred when there is opportunity for procreation, given the association with strength and reproductive success, whilst high-pitched male voices are preferred when paternal instincts, stability, and longevity are required (Apicella & Feinberg, 2009; Apicella et al., 2007; O'Connor et al., 2014). For female voices, higher pitch could symbolize youth and fertility, but findings are inconsistent.

Tsantani et al. (2016) went as far as to suggest that the low-pitch male voice preference is generally independent of context, but preferences for female voices are contingent on who is listening and why they are judging. Finally, these findings have a degree of ecological and cross-cultural validity (Apicella & Feinberg, 2009), with low-pitched men of the Hadzi tribe, Tanzania, having more off-spring, perhaps relating to Darwinian fitness (Apicella et al., 2007). However, any true relationship may be stronger in facial judgements (Feinberg et al., 2008b; Vukovic et al., 2011), with attractiveness ratings being more influenced by visual than auditory signals (Rezlescu et al., 2015).

A second area of interest is how the perceived personality of politicians influences voting behaviour. For example, politicians with dominant faces win elections, and the difference in experimental preference is correlated to actual voter counts (Ballew & Todorov, 2007; Olivola et al., 2012; Todorov et al., 2005). Low-pitched voices are found to indicate trustworthiness and competence (Klofstad et al., 2012), related to leadership and charisma (Borkowska & Pawlowski, 2011; Ohala, 1983; Tsantani et al., 2016). Tigue et al. (2012) created low- and high-pitch versions of nine politicians' speeches and, using a two-alternative forced-choice task (2AFC), found low-pitch voices were often chosen as the preferred candidate. The effect held when using non-political candidates reading a standard text ('the rainbow passage'), suggesting speech content had no influence. Further analysis showed results were mediated by situational contexts, with low-pitched powerful voices preferred at wartime and low-pitched trustworthy voices preferred in general elections.

Again, Klofstad and colleagues (2012) found participants voted for low-pitched voices, after standardizing speaker and content within a pairing and controlling for historical voting. They suggested that females with low-pitched voices are competent and trustworthy, with strong leadership qualities, whilst men with low-pitched voices are more attractive to female voters and appear more competent to male voters. Recently, despite the theoretical thinking that participants prefer to vote for middle-aged candidates, Klofstad et al. (2015) confirmed that perceived strength and competence were more influential than age.

In short, a general overall preference for low-pitch voices may lead to fewer elected female candidates given the natural sex differences in pitch, resulting in female candidates and celebrities deliberately lowering their voice pitch through training (Ko et al., 2015; Pemberton et al., 1998). However, potential task effects may mask more pronounced gender-specific norm preferences (McAleer et al., 2014; Tsantani et al., 2016).

Elaborating on this point, we must consider the influence of what is asked and how the judgement is made. Klofstad et al. (2012) addressed speech content and found similar preferences to Tigue et al. (2012) using different vocalizations. Likewise, studies using vowels, one word, or neutral sentences have shown a low-pitch preference linked to attractiveness (Apicella & Feinberg, 2009; Feinberg et al., 2008b; Jones et al., 2010). Thus, in terms of differing utterances, preferences appear consistent and in line with Tsantani et al. (2016) who found content to have little influence. However, differences are noted in task (e.g. 2AFC versus Likert), creating contrasting results. Klofstad and colleagues (2012), using the 2AFC, found low-pitched males were rated as trustworthy; McAleer et al. (2014b), using a Likert scale, found high-pitched males were perceived as trustworthy. Likewise, 2AFC-driven studies reveal low-pitched females as dominant and attractive (Feinberg et al., 2008b; Tigue et al., 2012), whilst McAleer and colleagues found attractiveness relates to trustworthiness through vocal glide and intonation, not relative pitch. As such, more work is needed to explore how the task influences experimental findings. Perhaps the 2AFC forces participants to compare the voices within a pairing, whereas a Likert task may result in a more global comparison within the group or to an internalized collective norm (Latinus et al., 2013; Tsantani et al., 2016).

We will illustrate this point via perceived attractiveness of voices. The average face is thought to be the most attractive due to signalling good health and desirable genes, either implicitly or explicitly (Bruckert et al., 2010; Jastrow, 1885; Langlois & Roggman, 1990; Zebrowitz & Rhodes, 2004). Bruckert and colleagues tested this theory in voices. Sixty-four voices (thirty-two female) were morphed into composites based on averaging of two, four, eight, sixteen, and thirty-two voices, and rated on attractiveness using a visual analogue slider (extremely unattractive to extremely attractive); original voices were also rated for comparison. The thirty-two-voice composite of both sex was one of the highest-rated voices, indicating that vocal averageness is attractive. Acoustical analysis indicated a positive relationship between attractiveness and smoothness of voice, consistent with healthy, younger voices perceived as attractive (Hughes et al., 2002; Langlois et al., 2000; McAleer et al., 2014; Zebrowitz & Montepare, 2008; Zebrowitz & Rhodes, 2004). Furthermore, analysis found a negative relationship between attractiveness and distance-to-mean (an Euclidean measure incorporating pitch, harmonic-to-noise ratio, and formant dispersion), reiterating that voices further from the conglomerate norm are unusual (Latinus et al., 2013; Said et al., 2009) and unattractive.

In contrast, Re et al. (2012) found that compared to averages, lower male pitches were attractive, down to a limit of 96 Hz, whilst higher female pitches were attractive. They averaged thirty-two male and thirty-two female voices into gender-specific composites before creating new versions using the Pitch-Synchronous Overlap Add (PSOLA) method. They then used a 2AFC and a measure of constant stimuli paradigm to establish how attractiveness varied with pitch. Thus, the two studies are only loosely comparable as whilst Bruckert et al. allowed free movement of all acoustics, Re et al. deliberately constrained certain acoustics whilst manipulating pitch. Thus, different findings are perhaps to be expected. Yet as a comparison, it highlights that procedural differences to one theoretical question (attractiveness in voices) results in contrasting findings and that researchers should consider who or what our listeners are actually comparing in relation to real-world significance.

One final consideration is that real-world decisions are often not made unimodally. Zuckerman and Driver (1989) suggested the roles of face and voice on judgements depends on what is being asked and why. Surprisingly, they showed unimodal ratings were higher than bimodal, though this may have been driven by the traits studied or methodological limitations of the time. Subsequent emotion research found face and voice to have a combined effect on accuracy, but with the face being most influential (Watson et al., 2013). Yet, few have explored the face–voice trade-off in regards to personality; one example being Rezlescu et al. (2015). Approximately 150 participants rated twelve males on attractiveness, trustworthiness, and dominance. Results found both cues contributed for trustworthiness judgements, attractiveness from the face, and dominance by the voice. Thus, we use signals individually or combined, depending on the importance of the cue in that judgement (Rezlescu et al., 2015; Watson et al., 2013). However, this work is limited to a small sample of male stimuli and must be expanded to look at the interaction of listener and speaker sex. With the influx of interest in audiovisual research and the wealth of applications, the understanding of how to combine modalities to establish appropriate personalities is paramount.

26.2 SUMMARY SPACES—WHICH TRAIT TO JUDGE?

An overlooked element of Aronovitch's (1976) study was the reduction of fifty-four potential traits to a more manageable ten, based on the scales participants felt confident about using. Likewise, contemporaries to Aronovitch showed that, linguistically, many traits were redundant and could be removed with semantic analysis (Rosenberg et al., 1968; Wiggins,

1979). Scherer (1972), however, took a more empirical approach whilst testing the attribution of personality traits in mock-jury deliberations. Twelve American and twelve German male speakers, whose speech had been randomized via tape-splicing techniques, were rated by American and German female participants on eight scales (reduced from thirty-five through factor analysis) including neuroticism, dominance, likeability, and aggressiveness. Consistency of listener ratings was high for American males, but low for German males, by participant groups. Scherer proposed this related to differences in the complexity of Germanic tone and intonation potentially modified during stimuli production. Further factor analyses showed traits clustered into two categories—one of dependability and stability, and one of dominance. Scherer referred to these summary traits as the 'nice guy' and the 'leader', concluding that only one or two traits can be derived from a voice and all other traits are associated in 'halo clusters'.

Zuckerman and Driver (1989) used job applications and paragraphs from novels to explore 'halo' traits and attractiveness—the 'What is beautiful is good' theory (Dion et al., 1972). Using principal component analysis (PCA), ten five-point adjective scales (e.g. forceful, competent, lazy) were reduced to three orthogonal scales relating to traits of dominance, likeability, and achievement. Voices high on likeability and achievement scored high on attractiveness—evidence of halo traits working together. A similar relationship was identified by Montepare and Zebrowitz-McArthur (1987) investigating how adults with childlike-voices are perceived in terms of warmth and dominance when reciting the alphabet. They found younger voices were perceived as less competent, less dominant, but with higher warmth. Thus, despite the numerous traits a voice can be judged on, most traits appear redundant if you establish the 'key' traits all other traits correlate to—be it individual traits such as trust, dominance, and warmth (McAleer et al., 2014; Scherer, 1972; Zuckerman & Driver, 1989), or global traits such as those of the 'Big Five Personality Model' (McCrae & Costa, 1987; Norman, 1963; Zuckerman et al., 1990).

One overriding question is what purpose these summary traits serve. They exist for voices (McAleer et al., 2014; Scherer, 1972; Zuckerman & Driver, 1989), faces (Oosterhof & Todorov, 2008; Sutherland et al., 2013), group cohesion (Fiske et al., 2007), and semantics (Rosenberg et al., 1968; Wiggins, 1979). In general, the research addresses first impressions of a novel person—also called 'zero acquaintance' or 'thin-slice judgements' (Kenny et al., 1992; Kramer & Ward, 2010; Ward & Kramer, 2010; Zebrowitz & Montepare, 2008)—to establish the person as a friend/foe, triggering appropriate approach or avoidance behaviours (McAleer et al., 2014; McArthur & Baron, 1983; Oosterhof & Todorov, 2008). The roots of this theory are in a quartet of hypotheses relating to age, attraction, emotion, and familiarity—the overgeneralization hypotheses (McArthur & Baron, 1983; Zebrowitz & Collins, 1997; Zebrowitz & Montepare, 2008).

Secord (1958) suggested the attribution of a permanent personality trait is an extrapolation from a momentary percept of a fleeting emotion; a smiling person is a trustworthy person, whereas an angry person shouting is dominant and aggressive. As such, combining overgeneralizations and summary traits helps form quick impressions of a novel person's intent, albeit approachable or best avoided (trustworthiness), whilst dominance establishes their ability to carry out the intent. Thus, our complicated world is simplified through rapid, perhaps stereotypical, judgements.

The issue McAleer et al. (2014) raised was that prior first impressions' research in voices had made use of long passages and sentences (Berry, 1990; Zuckerman & Driver, 1989;

Zuckerman et al., 1990) or non-socially relevant vocal bursts (Montepare & Zebrowitz-McArthur, 1987; Scherer, 1972). (Although brief, socially-relevant stimuli have been utilized to focus on attractiveness; e.g. Ferdenzi et al., 2013.) As such, limited research existed on summary traits using stimuli pertinent to social first impressions—an issue given the variety of acoustical measures available in discourse (Scherer, 1972; Tomlinson & Fox Tree, 2011; Tyler, 2015) and the veracity of 'first impressions' after prolonged exposure. In contrast, face research utilizes short exposures of faces looking directly at the participant (Oosterhof & Todorov, 2008; Todorov et al., 2009; Willis & Todorov, 2006)—brief and socially relevant. Thus, if a vocal burst is akin to brief exposure of a static face (Belin et al., 2011, 2000; Yovel & Belin, 2013; Zatorre et al., 2004), we argued, and showed, that a vocal summary space was achievable from the single, sociably-relevant word, 'hello'.

The 'social voice space' is a two-dimensional space with orthogonal dimensions of valence (akin to trustworthiness, likeability, and warmth) and dominance (McAleer et al., 2014) (see Figure 26.1). The space was established through PCA of judgements, on ten scales (including attractiveness, dominance, and trustworthiness), from over 300 participants listening to thirty-two male and thirty-two female voices. The space has striking similarity to previous spaces, in particular for faces (Oosterhof & Todorov, 2008), with strong agreement across sex of voice. One noticeable difference is that male attractiveness is associated with dominance and trustworthiness, whereas female attractiveness is associated with trustworthiness alone. Regression analysis found attractiveness to be accurately established from the components of the summary space, suggesting attractiveness is perhaps a combination of traits and not a stand-alone trait in itself.

In terms of acoustics, to sound trustworthy, male voices should have a slightly higher pitch than average (compare Audio 26.1a, trustworthy and Audio 26.1b, untrustworthy)—a finding in contrast with previous studies (Klofstad et al., 2012; Tigue et al., 2012; Vukovic et al., 2008). For females, trustworthiness relates to the glide of the voice and whether they speak with a rising intonation (Audio 26.1c, untrustworthy) or a dropping intonation (Audio 26.1d, trustworthy), aligning with perceptions of low certainty associated with 'uptalk' (Tomlinson & Fox Tree, 2011; Tyler, 2015).

Additional associations between trustworthiness and harmonic-to-noise ratio (HNR) reiterated that older voices are perceived as more trustworthy (Schotz, 2007; cf. Ferrand, 2002). Dominance, evident in both sex, was a strong influence of formant dispersion, with lower dispersion associated with higher dominance—a well-known association found in both humans and animals (Hughes et al., 2009; Pisanski et al., 2016; Puts et al., 2007; Rendall et al., 2007; Smith et al., 2016; Vannoni & McElligott, 2008) (compare Audio 26.2a (dominant) with Audio 26.2b (non-dominant), and Audio 26.2c (dominant) with Audio 26.2d (non-dominant)).

Overall, we suggest that valence is connected to temporally variable features of the voice (pitch, intonation, glide), whilst dominance judgements are connected to more structurally rigid features of the voice (e.g. formant dispersion—a function of the distance from larynx to mouth) (McAleer et al., 2014). Oosterhof and Todorov (2008) found similar relationships in faces, with trustworthiness derived from malleable features (e.g. eyes, mouth) and dominance derived from facial structure and size.

Thus, a speaker's personality can be judged on numerous traits, yet a representation of any trait, including attractiveness, can be derived from whether the person sounds trustworthy and/or dominant. Questions remain though, including: how traits such as confidence are built (Jiang & Pell, 2015); what the connection is between perception and subsequent

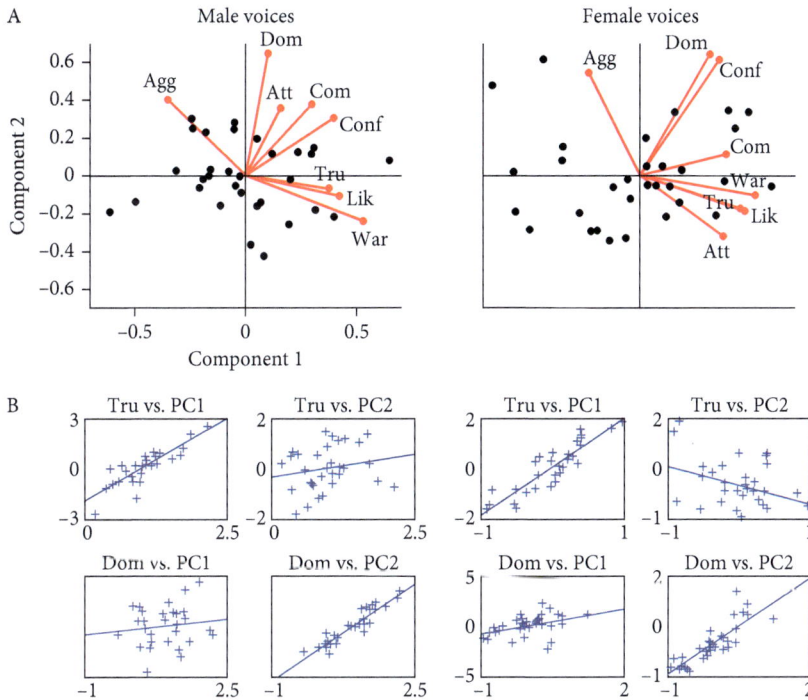

FIGURE 26.1 Principal component analysis solutions and main correlates of the social voice space. (**A**) The two-dimensional solution of the Principal Component Analysis for male (left) and female (right) voices (black dots). Labels equate to: Agg—aggressiveness; Att—attractiveness; Com—competence; Conf—confidence; Dom—dominance; Lik—likeability; Tru—trustworthiness; War—warmth. (**B**) Correlation plots between the ratings of trustworthiness (Tru—top row), dominance (Dom—bottom row), and the first (PC1) and second (PC2) principal components for male (left) and female (right) voices. Blue '+' represent individual voices. Trustworthiness was chosen arbitrarily over likeability due to the strong correlation between these two traits.

decision; what the influence is of the listener's own characteristics such as their personality, age, or social development; and how best to apply this understanding in technology using disembodied voices (e.g. sat navs and text-to-speech). In-depth consideration of future directions appears at the end of this chapter.

26.3 THE QUESTIONS OF CONSISTENCY AND ACCURACY

The two perennial questions surrounding personality judgements relate to consistency and accuracy. Here we address both, starting briefly with consistency across both listeners and time/duration, followed by detailed consideration of whether such judgements have any real-world validity.

26.3.1 Consistency

Aronovitch (1976) postulated that, despite weak correlations between listeners' judgements and speakers' self-rated judgements, the high internal agreement across listeners was no less informative. Indeed, listener agreement is a regular finding in the research. Be it through pairwise correlations (Rezlescu et al., 2015), Spearman-Brown reliability (Montepare & Zebrowitz-McArthur, 1987), or Cronbach Alphas (Hughes & Harrison, 2013; McAleer et al., 2014), findings all report listeners' agreement to be typically rather high. By illustration, Larrance and Zuckerman (1981) showed a Spearman-Brown inter-rater reliability for voice likeability of 0.77; Zuckerman and Driver (1989) found high inter-rater agreement for dominance, achievement, likeability, and attractiveness (0.92, 0.87, 0.81, and 0.85 respectively); likewise Montepare and Zebrowitz-McArthur (1987) for traits including warmth, vulnerability, and naïvety. More recently, Rezlescu et al. (2015) showed inter-rater agreement and reliability (all alphas > 0.88) for trustworthiness, dominance, and attractiveness, whilst McAleer et al. (2014) found high Cronbach Alphas across all traits (average = 0.92). Further, studies using the 2AFC regularly show preferences significantly different from chance (i.e. the point of no preference) (Feinberg et al., 2008b; Klofstad et al., 2015; Klofstad et al., 2012; Tsantani et al., 2016). In short, attributions to certain voices appear consistent across listeners. Yet how this agreement arises, perhaps via prototypical comparisons as for identity (Latinus et al., 2013), remains unanswered.

The second consideration regarding consistency is whether personality is attributed irrespective of duration of voicing. If such judgements are driven by acoustics, including pitch and intonation and their malleability (McAleer et al., 2014; Oosterhof & Todorov, 2008), then judgements may be expected to fluctuate with extended speech. Research is lacking; however, Rezlescu et al. (2015) in fact showed strong correlations between vowels from the same speaker for trustworthiness (r = 0.625), attractiveness (r = 0.729), and dominance (r = 0.632), whilst Tsantani et al. (2016) found no difference in pitch preferences for either forward or reversed 'hellos'. Whilst respective vocalization durations within both studies would be similar, they suggest stability across varying speech.

In faces, Bar et al. (2006) found a correlation between threat judgements after 39- and 1700-ms exposures (r = 0.546) but not for intelligence judgements, concluding that only survival-based first impressions are constant, and aligning with first impressions eliciting approach/avoidance behaviours (Oosterhof & Todorov, 2008). Likewise, Willis and Todorov (2006) showed that in judgements, only self-confidence, not correlation strength, increased with exposure duration suggesting a longevity for first impressions. Theoretically, a dual process has been proposed whereby rapid perceptual judgements become modulated and/or consolidated by later cognitive processes (Kahneman, 2011; Wood, 2014), consistent with Willis and Todorov (2006). Recent fMRI and event-related potential (ERP) studies confirmed this proposal for cognitive decision making (Fouragnan et al., 2015) and vocal confidence judgements (Jiang & Pell, 2015), though extensive research is required to elucidate how robust and lasting impressions are formed and updated.

26.3.2 Accuracy

In establishing what accuracy means, Funder (2012) states three potential measures. The first is self–other agreement whereby self ratings by the speaker (or close acquaintance) are compared to group ratings by naïve listeners. This was the approach of early work (Allport & Cantril, 1934; Pear, 1931) and is still used sporadically (Carney et al., 2007; Zebrowitz & Collins, 1997; Zebrowitz & Montepare, 2008), but is largely constrained to measures with a quantifiable ground-truth (Pisanski et al., 2016; Smith et al., 2016). General consensus suggests there is a moderate degree of self–other accuracy/agreement, but restricted to traits such as dominance, extraversion, and intelligence—arguably traits less variable across the lifespan (McAleer et al., 2014; Oosterhof & Todorov, 2008).

Funder's second measure is other–other agreement, looking for high inter-rater reliability across a large sample of participants. This measure is conceptually closer to consistency than accuracy, but if everyone perceives a voice as untrustworthy, then it is so, irrespective of ground-truth. Studies have regularly used this approach to infer traits such as attractiveness, dominance, and trustworthiness (Aronovitch, 1976; Borkowska & Pawlowski, 2011; Fruhen et al., 2015; Jones et al., 2010; Klofstad et al., 2015, 2012; McAleer et al., 2014; Rezlescu et al., 2015; Vukovic et al., 2011). This method, however, can be influenced by stereotyping voice patterns (e.g. a negative relationship between uptalk (ascending intonation) and certainty: Tomlinson & Fox Tree, 2011; Tyler, 2015). Likewise, self–other agreements may be erroneous due to the self-report nature or a speaker's self-serving bias (Alicke, 1985; Hughes & Harrison, 2013; Sedikides et al., 2014). Thus, the only true means of measuring accuracy according to Funder is behavioural prediction—when a judgement accurately predicts a speaker's actions. This however relies on the untested postulation of personality being context-independent (i.e. a trustworthy person is always trustworthy). As such, empirically quantifying the accuracy of personality judgements is a highly complex issue.

Theoretically, Scherer (1972) states that accuracy depends on a variety of factors including an actual relationship between voice and personality, a listener's ability to isolate appropriate cues to that personality, and a strong correspondence between actual and inferred traits. This bears striking resemblance to Funder's (1995) Realistic Accuracy Model (RAM), for personality in general. Caveating that the model merely proposes what must happen, Funder first proposes that the person being judged must behave in accordance with that trait, citing Zimbardo (1977) and that even shy people, judged aloof, often claim to be friendly. Secondly, he proposes that an appropriate action must be performed in front of the viewer/receiver and that they must be able to receive the relevant information (i.e. no point being friendly to a distracted person). Finally, the receiver must decode and utilize the cues appropriately (e.g. not mistaking friendliness for sarcasm).

Scherer (1972) and Funder (1995, 2012) clearly rely on the speaker's and listener's ability to project and receive cues appropriately, with failure resulting in an erroneous attribution. Where they differ is in the reliance of a true association between personality and vocal cues. Reiterating the overgeneralization hypothesis (Secord, 1958; Zebrowitz & Collins, 1997; Zebrowitz & Montepare, 2008), personality attribution occurs through extrapolating a momentary characteristic into an enduring trait, with an aim to elucidate approach/avoidance behaviours, irrespective of accuracy. If true, the link between vocal cues and personality may be weak at best, perhaps explaining previous low levels of 'accuracy' (e.g. Carney et al., 2007;

Olivola & Todorov, 2010; Zebrowitz & Montepare, 2008). However, we would argue that low accuracy is not concerning if the purpose of personality attribution is self-preservation. Akin to the smoke-detector principle (Nesse, 2005), or signal-detection theory, a degree of false alarms is expected if personality attribution is a remnant from a time when judgements resulted in life or death; for self-preservation, it is best to trigger with low levels of smoke than engulfing flames. Thus, it is perhaps not concerning that in regards to 'accuracy', personality attributions come up short.

Conversely, if first impressions are recurrently wrong or misleading, then we should question their relevance; an erroneous system is largely ineffective. However, as per Zebrowitz and Montepare (2008), we assume that the errors produced by an overgeneralization hypothesis are less maladaptive than alternative approaches. Indeed, according to Zebrowitz and Montepare, failure to integrate priors in our daily life makes it rather difficult to function as sociable humans. As such, research on personality attribution by populations with developmental problems may greatly advance our understanding. Ultimately, however, if our continued existence is the measure, then we are clearly capable of 'accurate' judgements despite the uncertainty of how best they are measured.

26.4 Future Directions

In this final section, we spotlight two key areas that would greatly enhance our understanding and application of personality judgements.

26.4.1 Neural Correlates of Personality Processing

Where and how personality is processed in the brain is a pertinent question. Jiang and Pell (2015), using ERPs, found that confidence is decoded in a two-step process, whereby an initial judgement determines the speaker as confident or not (~200 ms after speech onset) before a later judgement (~500 ms) categorizes the level of confidence (confident versus close-to-confident). Yet, despite insight into the time-locked process, such studies lack localization.

Using fMRI, Hensel et al. (2015) highlighted the inferior parietal cortex (IPC) and the dorsomedial prefrontal cortex (dmPFC) as activated in explicit judgements of trustworthiness and attractiveness. However, such judgements were explicit in nature, potentially resulting in elevated activation in cognitive areas. If first impressions are indeed beneficial for rapidly establishing personality, then they would be expected to function implicitly. In faces, an implicit negative relationship between trustworthiness and amygdala activation has indeed been shown (Todorov & Engell, 2008; Said et al., 2009), suggesting an alert system, and whilst the amygdala is involved in bimodal emotional judgements (Dolan et al., 2000; Vroomen & de Gelder, 2000), studies are needed on implicit attributions to unimodal voices. One focus would be on establishing the functional connectivity between the auditory cortex, the temporal voice areas, and amygdalae—a network proposed to create enriched speaker representations (Belin et al., 2011; Latinus & Belin, 2011; Pernet et al., 2015).

Beyond localization and connectivity, brain imaging could determine how differing personalities are represented across neurons. One proposition is that, as with identity (Latinus & Belin, 2011; Latinus et al., 2013; Lavner et al., 2001), personality is derived via norm-based coding (Bestelmeyer et al., 2012; McAleer et al., 2014). Morphing techniques have made it possible to merge voices, either by averaging different speakers into a conglomerate or by stepping from one speaker to another, highlighting the changes in the voices. Such morphing techniques have previously been used to explore attractiveness of averaging voices (Bruckert et al., 2010) and of manipulating changes in attractiveness (Bestelmeyer et al., 2012), as well as emotion and sex of speaker (Watson et al., 2013). Latinus et al. (2013), using vocal morphing, found identity to be a function of the distance-to-mean between an individual voice and a sex-specific prototype; for both natural and manipulated stimuli, voices distant from the prototype elicited increased activation in auditory regions of the temporal cortex. Regards personality, however, it is unknown whether a similar mechanism exists.

That said, consistent with Latinus et al.'s (2013) finding for distinct voices, Said et al. (2009) indicated increased activation for faces extremely untrustworthy/trustworthy or dominant/non-dominant (see also DeBruine et al., 2007). Thus we would hypothesize that personality is established via norm-based coding, testable through modern vocal-morphing techniques (Kawahara & Matsui, 2003; Latinus et al., 2013). For illustration, Figure 26.2 highlights a 'social voice space' based on prototypical 'hellos' along the two most salient dimensions issued from the PCA analysis—PC1, trustworthiness; PC2, dominance. The average, prototypical, and caricature 'hellos' for the two PCs, as generated through morphing, can be heard on Audio 26.3.

26.4.2 Changes with Ageing

Though few studies have addressed when concepts of personality become established, it is an area beginning to receive attention (Cogsdill et al., 2014; Ewing et al., 2015; Saxton et al., 2006, 2009). Cogsdill et al. (2014) found that 3- to 6-year-old children attributed trustworthiness, competence, and dominance to faces in a similar manner to adults. Likewise, Ewing et al. (2015) showed that 5- and 10-year-old children played trust games similarly to adults. However, Saxton et al. (2009) found attractiveness judgements only became consistent with adults when children reached puberty. Thus, we might suggest that survival-based judgements (e.g. trustworthiness) develop early in life, whereas other judgements (e.g. attractiveness) develop at relevant time points.

Beyond adolescence, and given the current ageing population, we should consider how personality judgements change as we age. The recognition of personality and emotion helps establish relationships, with failure to do so leading to isolation and mental health issues (Hawkley & Capitanio, 2015). A reason elderly people are taken advantage of may be due to their misattribution of personality. The limited work here shows more neutral stimuli being rated as trustworthy by older than by younger adults (Bailey et al., 2015; Li & Fung, 2014); likewise Ethier-Majcher et al. (2013) found older adults attributed trustworthiness to both happy and angry faces. Thus ageing, even healthily, alters how we perceive others. Two opposing theories suggest the cause is either a bottom–up change in the physical percept or, due to the socio-emotional selectivity theory (Carstensen, 2006), a top–down cognitive modulation/acceptance to avoid loneliness and exclusion. Combining vocal morphing with

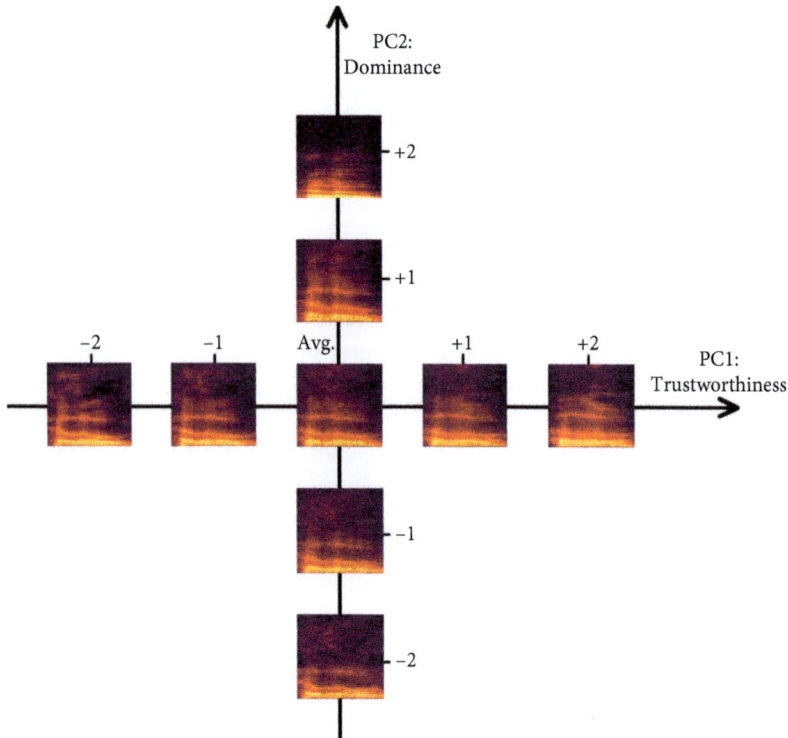

FIGURE 26.2 Prototypical and caricatured voices as extrapolated from the two principal components of the social voice space. Starting with an average voice at the centre of the social voice space (Avg.), it is possible to extrapolate voices, based on component weightings, to create the prototypical most (+1) trustworthy and dominant voices, as well as the prototypical least (−1) trustworthy and dominant voices. Further extrapolation leads to caricatured most (+2) trustworthy and dominant voices, as well as caricatured least (−2) trustworthy and dominant voices. The displayed traits are the two most salient dimensions issued from the PCA analysis of the social voice space. The average, prototypical, and caricature 'hellos' for the two PCs can be heard in Audio 26.3.

decision-making scenarios will enable us to parse both the perceptual and cognitive processes underlying how ageing affects our perception of voices.

26.5 APPLICATIONS IN THE REAL WORLD

Nowadays, disembodied voices are everywhere—our phone, the satnav; the check-out till—and inserting the correct voice improves user engagement (Nass & Lee, 2001); a satnav voice reportedly led to demands for a recall of BMWs (Nass & Brave, 2005; Takayama & Nass, 2008). Establishing how humans perceive and convey personality is fundamental in maximizing usable technology. Indeed, with a recent boom in social robotics, a key question is how to improve their acceptability (e.g. Destephe et al., 2015; Foster et al., 2012) through appropriate voices (Mitchell et al., 2011; Tinwell et al., 2015) and avoiding the uncanny valley (Mori, 1970). Furthering the understanding of the acoustics of personality, its 'vocal make-up', would rapidly advance our current technology.

Closer to home, the true malleability of the human voice is debatable, with some studies suggesting stability (e.g. DeGroot & Gooty, 2009) whilst others suggest flexibility depending on situation, either deliberately (Hughes et al., 2014) or subconsciously (Fraccaro et al., 2011, 2013), with some famous cases of vocal training (Ko et al., 2015). Clearly if the vocal make-up of a trait is known, then techniques could be developed to create a desired percept. An application of this would be in restoring socially-relevant and appropriate voicings to text-to-speech (TTS) aids for people with laryngeal deficits. Three million people in the USA and the UK use TTS, many using the same device with the same voice, creating a difficult communication environment for the speaker and listener (Mills et al., 2014). Through targeted research, improvement and personalization of TTS would greatly enhance the users' quality of life and communication ability. Similarly, with the increase of vocal databases including speech impairments (Grill & Tuckova, 2016), one could establish how traits are perceived across speaking abilities or by people who are blind (Kupers & Ptito, 2014) or have cochlear implants and hearing aids (Gilbers et al., 2015).

Advancing technology is a clear future impact of this work, but perhaps the simplest is improving people's awareness of the information contained in their voice. As we have seen, these percepts influence our decision making as well as whom we are attracted to, trust, vote for, and employ. Our simplest application may be in reducing snap impressions, in turn leading to more reasoned judgements about the embodied personalities behind the voices we hear.

26.6 Conclusions

Much has progressed in the eighty-five years since Pear (1931) first questioned the validity of personality attributions from voices. We have found halo traits and reduced them to their key dimensions. We have discovered people collectively assign the same trait to a voice irrespective of accuracy, and we have explored situations and decisions influenced simply by whether a voice is high-pitched or low, whether the intonation rises or falls. Yet, with the relatively recent development of modern imaging techniques, we are only at the grassroots of understanding the neuronal process involved in these percepts, these decisions. Clearly much is still to be realized as to how, when, and why we attribute personality traits so readily from voices. Nevertheless, with the abundance of technologies and medical developments using disembodied voices and everyday situations where the voice is our signal, it is an exciting area of research, full of application and impact.

References

Alicke, M. D. (1985). Global self-evaluation as determined by the desirability and controllability of trait adjectives. *Journal of Personality and Social Psychology*, 49(6), 1621–1630. doi: 10.1037/0022-3514.49.6.1621

Allport, G. W. & Cantril, H. (1934). Judging personality from voice. *Journal of Social Psychology,* 5(1), 37–54.

Anderson, R. C. & Klofstad, C. A. (2012). For love or money? The influence of personal resources and environmental resource pressures on human mate preferences. *Ethology,* 118(9), 841–849. doi: 10.1111/j.1439-0310.2012.02077.x

Apicella, C. L. & Feinberg, D. R. (2009). Voice pitch alters mate-choice-relevant perception in hunter-gatherers. *Proceedings of the Royal Society B: Biological Sciences,* 276(1659), 1077–1082. doi: 10.1098/rspb.2008.1542

Apicella, C. L., Feinberg, D. R., & Marlowe, F. W. (2007). Voice pitch predicts reproductive success in male hunter-gatherers. *Biology Letters,* 3(6), 682–684. doi: 10.1098/rsbl.2007.0410

Aronovitch, C. D. (1976). Voice of personality—stereotyped judgments and their relation to voice quality and sex of speaker. *Journal of Social Psychology,* 99(2), 207–220.

Bailey, P. E., Szczap, P., McLennan, S. N., Slessor, G., Ruffman, T., & Rendell, P. G. (2015). Age-related similarities and differences in first impressions of trustworthiness. *Cognition & Emotion,* 1–10. doi: 10.1080/02699931.2015.1039493

Ballew, C. C. & Todorov, A. (2007). Predicting political elections from rapid and unreflective face judgments. *Proceedings of the National Academy of Sciences of the United States of America,* 104(46), 17948–17953. doi: 10.1073/pnas.0705435104

Bar, M., Neta, M., & Linz, H. (2006). Very first impressions. *Emotion,* 6(2), 269–278. doi: 10.1037/1528-3542.6.2.269

Belin, P., Bestelmeyer, P. E. G., Latinus, M., & Watson, R. (2011). Understanding voice perception. *British Journal of Psychology,* 102, 711–725. doi: 10.1111/j.2044-8295.2011.02041.x

Belin, P., Zatorre, R. J., Lafaille, P., Ahad, P., & Pike, B. (2000). Voice-selective areas in human auditory cortex. *Nature,* 403(6767), 309–312. doi: 10.1038/35002078

Berry, D. S. (1990). Vocal attractiveness and vocal babyishness—effects on stranger, self, and friend impressions. *Journal of Nonverbal Behavior,* 14(3), 141–153. doi: 10.1007/Bf00996223

Bestelmeyer, P. E. G., Latinus, M., Bruckert, L., Rouger, J., Crabbe, F., & Belin, P. (2012). Implicitly perceived vocal attractiveness modulates prefrontal cortex activity. *Cerebral Cortex,* 22(6), 1263–1270. doi: 10.1093/cercor/bhr204

Borkowska, B. & Pawlowski, B. (2011). Female voice frequency in the context of dominance and attractiveness perception. *Animal Behaviour,* 82(1), 55–59. doi: 10.1016/j.anbehav.2011.03.024

Brown, B. L., Strong, W. J., & Rencher, A. C. (1973). Perceptions of personality from speech: effects of manipulations of acoustical parameters. *Journal of the Acoustical Society of America,* 54(1), 29–35.

Bruckert, L., Bestelmeyer, P., Latinus, M., Rouger, J., Charest, I., Rousselet, G. A., ... Belin, P. (2010). Vocal attractiveness increases by averaging. *Current Biology,* 20(2), 116–120. doi: 10.1016/j.cub.2009.11.034

Carney, D. R., Colvin, C. R., & Hall, J. A. (2007). A thin slice perspective on the accuracy of first impressions. *Journal of Research in Personality,* 41(5), 1054–1072. doi: 10.1016/j.jrp.2007.01.004

Carstensen, L. L. (2006). The influence of a sense of time on human development. *Science,* 312(5782), 1913–1915. doi: 10.1126/science.1127488

Cogsdill, E. J., Todorov, A. T., Spelke, E. S., & Banaji, M. R. (2014). Inferring character from faces: a developmental study. *Psychological Science,* 25(5), 1132–1139. doi: 10.1177/0956797614523297

Cordaro, D. T., Keltner, D., Tshering, S., Wangchuk, D., & Flynn, L. M. (2016). The voice conveys emotion in ten globalized cultures and one remote village in Bhutan. *Emotion,* 16(1), 117–128. doi: 10.1037/emo0000100

Cowan, M. L., Watkins, C. D., Fraccaro, P. J., Feinberg, D. R., & Little, A. C. (2015). It's the way he tells them (and who is listening): men's dominance is positively correlated with their preference for jokes told by dominant-sounding men. *Evolution and Human Behavior*, 37(2), 97–104.

DeBruine, L. M., Jones, B. C., Unger, L., Little, A. C., & Feinberg, D. R. (2007). Dissociating averageness and attractiveness: attractive faces are not always average. *Journal of Experimental Psychology: Human Perception & Performance*, 33(6), 1420–1430. doi: 10.1037/0096-1523.33.6.1420

DeGroot, T. & Gooty, J. (2009). Can nonverbal cues be used to make meaningful personality attributions in employment interviews? *Journal of Business and Psychology*, 24(2), 179–192. doi: 10.1007/s10869-009-9098-0

Destephe, M., Brandao, M., Kishi, T., Zecca, M., Hashimoto, K., & Takanishi, A. (2015). Walking in the uncanny valley: importance of the attractiveness on the acceptance of a robot as a working partner. *Frontiers in Psychology*, 6. doi: 10.3389/fpsyg.2015.00204

Dion, K., Berscheid, E., & Walster, E. (1972). What is beautiful is good. *Journal of Personality and Social Psychology*, 24(3), 285–290.

Dolan, R. J., Lane, R., Chua, P., & Fletcher, P. (2000). Dissociable temporal lobe activations during emotional episodic memory retrieval. *NeuroImage*, 11(3), 203–209. doi: 10.1006/nimg.2000.0538

Dunlap Jr, O. E. (1933). When Roosevelt goes on the air. *The New York Times, June 18th, 1933*.

Ethier-Majcher, C., Joubert, S., & Gosselin, F. (2013). Reverse correlating trustworthy faces in young and older adults. *Frontiers in Psychology*, 4, 592. doi: 10.3389/fpsyg.2013.00592

Ewing, L., Caulfield, F., Read, A., & Rhodes, G. (2015). Perceived trustworthiness of faces drives trust behaviour in children. *Developmental Science*, 18(2), 327–334. doi: 10.1111/desc.12218

Eysenck, H. J. & Eysenck, S. B. G. (1965). *Eysenck Manual of the Eysenck Personality Inventory*. London: University of London Press.

Feinberg, D. R., DeBruine, L. M., Jones, B. C., & Little, A. C. (2008a). Correlated preferences for men's facial and vocal masculinity. *Evolution and Human Behavior*, 29(4), 233–241. doi: 10.1016/j.evolhumbehav.2007.12.008

Feinberg, D. R., DeBruine, L. M., Jones, B. C., & Perrett, D. I. (2008b). The role of femininity and averageness of voice pitch in aesthetic judgments of women's voices. *Perception*, 37(4), 615–623. doi: 10.1068/p5514

Ferdenzi, C., Patel, S., Mehu-Blantar, I., Khidasheli, M., Sander, D., & Delplanque, S. (2013). Voice attractiveness: influence of stimulus duration and type. *Behavior Research Methods*, 45(2), 405–413. doi: 10.3758/s13428-012-0275-0

Ferrand, C. T. (2002). Harmonics-to-noise ratio: an index of vocal aging. *Journal of Voice*, 16(4), 480–487.

Fiske, S. T., Cuddy, A. J. C., & Glick, P. (2007). Universal dimensions of social cognition: warmth and competence. *Trends in Cognitive Sciences*, 11(2), 77–83. doi: 10.1016/j.tics.2006.11.005

Fitch, W. T. (1997). Vocal tract length and formant frequency dispersion correlate with body size in rhesus macaques. *Journal of the Acoustical Society of America*, 102(2), 1213–1222. doi: 10.1121/1.421048

Foster, M. E., Gaschler, A., Giuliani, M., Isard, A., Pateraki, M., & Petrick, R. P. A. (2012). *Two People Walk Into a Bar: Dynamic Multi-Party Social Interaction with a Robot Agent*. ICMI '12: Proceedings of the ACM International Conference on Multimodal Interaction, 3–10.

Fouragnan, E., Retzler, C., Mullinger, K., & Philiastides, M. G. (2015). Two spatiotemporally distinct value systems shape reward-based learning in the human brain. *Nature Communications*, 6, 8107.

Fraccaro, P. J., Jones, B. C., Vukovic, J., Smith, F. G., Watkins, C. D., Feinberg, D. R., ... DeBruine, L. M. (2011). Experimental evidence that women speak in a higher voice pitch to men they find attractive. *Journal of Evolutionary Psychology,* 9(1), 57–67. doi: 10.1556/JEP.9.2011.33.1

Fraccaro, P. J., O'Connor, J. J. M., Re, D. E., Jones, B. C., DeBruine, L. M., & Feinberg, D. R. (2013). Faking it: deliberately altered voice pitch and vocal attractiveness. *Animal Behaviour,* 85(1), 127–136.

Fruhen, L. S., Watkins, C. D., & Jones, B. C. (2015). Perceptions of facial dominance, trustworthiness and attractiveness predict managerial pay awards in experimental tasks. *Leadership Quarterly,* 26(6), 1005–1016. doi: 10.1016/j.leaqua.2015.07.001

Funder, D. C. (1995). On the accuracy of personality judgment: a realistic approach. *Psychological Review,* 102(4), 652–670.

Funder, D. C. (2012). Accurate personality judgment. *Current Directions in Psychological Science,* 21(3), 177–182. doi: 10.1177/0963721412445309

Gilbers, S., Fuller, C., Gilbers, D., Broersma, M., Goudbeek, M., Free, R., & Baskent, D. (2015). Normal-hearing listeners' and cochlear implant users' perception of pitch cues in emotional speech. *i-Perception,* 6(5). doi: 10.1177/0301006615599139

Grill, P. & Tuckova, J. (2016). Speech databases of typical children and children with SLI. *PLoS One,* 11(3). doi: 10.1371/journal.pone.0150365

Hawkley, L. C. & Capitanio, J. P. (2015). Perceived social isolation, evolutionary fitness and health outcomes: a lifespan approach. *Philosophical Transactions of the Royal Society B: Biological Sciences,* 370(1669). doi: 10.1098/rstb.2014.0114

Hensel, L., Bzdok, D., Muller, V. I., Zilles, K., & Eickhoff, S. B. (2015). Neural correlates of explicit social judgments on vocal stimuli. *Cerebral Cortex,* 25(5), 1152–1162. doi: 10.1093/cercor/bht307

Herzog, H. (1933). Stimme und personlichkeit/Voice and personality. *Zeitschrift für Psychologie und Physiologie der Sinnesorgane,* 130, 300–369.

Hughes, S. M., Dispenza, F., & Gallup, G. G. (2004). Ratings of voice attractiveness predict sexual behavior and body configuration. *Evolution and Human Behavior,* 25(5), 295–304. doi: 10.1016/j.evolhumbehav.2004.06.001

Hughes, S. M. & Harrison, M. A. (2013). I like my voice better: self-enhancement bias in perceptions of voice attractiveness. *Perception,* 42(9), 941–949.

Hughes, S. M., Harrison, M. A., & Gallup, G. G. (2002). The sound of symmetry—voice as a marker of developmental instability. *Evolution and Human Behavior,* 23(3), 173–180. doi: 10.1016/S1090-5138(01)00099-X

Hughes, S. M., Harrison, M. A., & Gallup, G. G. (2009). Sex-specific body configurations can be estimated from voice samples. *Journal of Social, Evolutionary, & Cultural Psychology,* 3, 343–355.

Hughes, S. M., Mogilski, J. K., & Harrison, M. A. (2014). The perception and parameters of intentional voice manipulation. *Journal of Nonverbal Behavior,* 38(1), 107–127. doi: 10.1007/s10919-013-0163-z

Hughes, S. M. & Rhodes, G. (2010). Making age assessments based on voice: the impact of the reproductive viability of the speaker. *Journal of Social, Evolutionary, & Cultural Psychology,* 4, 290–304.

Jastrow, J. (1885). Composite portraiture. *Science,* 6(134), 165–167. doi: 10.1126/science.ns-6.134.165

Jiang, X. M. & Pell, M. D. (2015). On how the brain decodes vocal cues about speaker confidence. *Cortex,* 66, 9–34. doi: 10.1016/j.cortex.2015.02.002

Jones, B. C., Feinberg, D. R., DeBruine, L. M., Little, A. C., & Vukovic, J. (2008). Integrating cues of social interest and voice pitch in men's preferences for women's voices. *Biology Letters, 4*(2), 192–194. doi: 10.1098/rsbl.2007.0626

Jones, B. C., Feinberg, D. R., DeBruine, L. M., Little, A. C., & Vukovic, J. (2010). A domain-specific opposite-sex bias in human preferences for manipulated voice pitch. *Animal Behaviour, 79*(1), 57–62. doi: 10.1016/j.anbehav.2009.10.003

Kahneman, D. (2011). *Thinking, Fast and Slow*. Canada: Doubleday.

Kawahara, H. & Matsui, H. (2003). Auditory morphing based on an elastic perceptual distance metric in an interference-free time-frequency representation. *2003 IEEE International Conference on Acoustics, Speech, and Signal Processing, Vol I, Proceedings* (pp. 256–259).

Kenny, D. A., Horner, C., Kashy, D. A., & Chu, L. C. (1992). Consensus at zero acquaintance—replication, behavioral cues, and stability. *Journal of Personality and Social Psychology, 62*(1), 88–97. doi: 10.1037//0022-3514.62.1.88

Klofstad, C. A., Anderson, R. C., & Nowicki, S. (2015). Perceptions of competence, strength, and age influence voters to select leaders with lower-pitched voices. *PLoS One, 10*(8). doi: e013377910.1371/journal.pone.0133779

Klofstad, C. A., Anderson, R. C., & Peters, S. (2012). Sounds like a winner: voice pitch influences perception of leadership capacity in both men and women. *Proceedings of the Royal Society B: Biological Sciences, 279*(1738), 2698–2704. doi: 10.1098/rspb.2012.0311

Ko, S. J., Sadler, M. S., & Galinsky, A. D. (2015). The sound of power: conveying and detecting hierarchical rank through voice. *Psychological Science, 26*(1), 3–14. doi: 10.1177/0956797614553009

Kramer, E. (1963). Judgment of personal characteristics and emotions from nonverbal properties of speech. *Psychological Bulletin, 60*(4), 408–420. doi: 10.1037/h0044890

Kramer, E. (1964). Personality stereotypes in voice—a reconsideration of the data. *Journal of Social Psychology, 62*(2), 247–251.

Kramer, E. & Aronovitch, C. D. (1970). Voice expression and rated etraversion. *Journal of Projective Techniques and Personality Assessment, 34*(5), 426–427. doi: 10.1080/0091651X.1970.10380278

Kramer, R. S. S. & Ward, R. (2010). Internal facial features are signals of personality and health. *Quarterly Journal of Experimental Psychology, 63*(11), 2273–2287. doi: 10.1080/17470211003770912

Krauss, R. M., Freyberg, R., & Morsella, E. (2002). Inferring speakers' physical attributes from their voices. *Journal of Experimental Social Psychology, 38*(6), 618–625. doi: 10.1016/S0022-1031(02)00510-3

Kupers, R. & Ptito, M. (2014). Compensatory plasticity and cross-modal reorganization following early visual deprivation. *Neuroscience and Biobehavioral Reviews, 41*, 36–52. doi: 10.1016/j.neubiorev.2013.08.001

Langlois, J. H., Kalakanis, L., Rubenstein, A. J., Larson, A., Hallam, M., & Smoot, M. (2000). Maxims or myths of beauty? A meta-analytic and theoretical review. *Psychological Bulletin, 126*(3), 390–423. doi: 10.1037/0033-2909.126.3.390

Langlois, J. H. & Roggman, L. A. (1990). Attractive faces are only average. *Psychological Science, 1*(2), 115–121. doi: 10.1111/j.1467-9280.1990.tb00079.x

Larrance, D. T. & Zuckerman, M. (1981). Facial attractiveness and vocal likability as determinants of nonverbal sending skills. *Journal of Personality, 49*(4), 349–362. doi: 10.1111/j.1467-6494.1981.tb00219.x

Latinus, M. & Belin, P. (2011). Anti-voice adaptation suggests prototype-based coding of voice identity. *Frontiers in Psychology, 2*. doi: 10.3389/fpsyg.2011.00175

Latinus, M., McAleer, P., Bestelmeyer, P. E. G., & Belin, P. (2013). Norm-based coding of voice identity in human auditory cortex. *Current Biology, 23*(12), 1075–1080. doi: 10.1016/j.cub.2013.04.055

Lavner, Y., Rosenhouse, J., & Gath, I. (2001). The prototype model in speaker identification by human listeners. *International Journal of Speech Technology, 4*, 63–74.

Li, T. & Fung, H. H. (2014). How avoidant attachment influences subjective well-being: an investigation about the age and gender differences. *Aging & Mental Health, 18*(1), 4–10. doi: 10.1080/13607863.2013.775639

McAleer, P., Todorov, A., & Belin, P. (2014). How do you say 'Hello'? Personality impressions from brief novel voices. *PLoS One, 9*(3). doi: e9077910.1371/journal.pone.0090779

McArthur, L. Z. & Baron, R. M. (1983). Toward an ecological theory of social-perception. *Psychological Review, 90*(3), 215–238.

McCrae, R. R. & Costa, P. T. (1987). Validation of the 5-factor model of personality across instruments and observers. *Journal of Personality and Social Psychology, 52*(1), 81–90. doi: 10.1037/0022-3514.52.1.81

Mills, T., Bunnell, H. T., & Patel, R. (2014). Towards personalized speech synthesis for augmentative and alternative communication. *Augmentative and Alternative Communication, 30*(3), 226–236. doi: 10.3109/07434618.2014.924026

Mitchell, W. J., Szerszen Sr, K. A., Lu, A. S., Schermerhorn, P. W., Scheutz, M., & Macdorman, K. F. (2011). A mismatch in the human realism of face and voice produces an uncanny valley. *i-perception, 2*(1), 10–12. doi: 10.1068/i0415

Montepare, J. M. & Zebrowitz-McArthur, L. (1987). Perceptions of adults with child-like voices in two cultures. *Journal of Experimental Social Psychology, 23*(4), 331–349. doi: 10.1016/0022-1031(87)90045-X

Mori, M. (1970). The uncanny valley. *Energy, 7*(4), 33–35.

Nass, C. & Brave, S. B. (2005). *Wired for Speech: How Voice Activates andEnhances the Human–Computer Relationship*. Cambridge, MA: MIT Press.

Nass, C. & Lee, K. M. (2001). Does computer-synthesized speech manifest personality? Experimental tests of recognition, similarity-attraction, and consistency-attraction. *Journal of Experimental Psychology—Applied, 7*(3), 171–181. doi: 10.1037//1076-898x.7.3.171

Nesse, R. M. (2005). Natural selection and the regulation of defenses—a signal detection analysis of the smoke detector principle. *Evolution and Human Behavior, 26*(1), 88–105. doi: 10.1016/j.evolhumbehav.2004.08.002

Norman, W. T. (1963). Toward an adequate taxonomy of personality attributes—replicated factor structure in peer nomination personality ratings. *Journal of Abnormal Psychology, 66*(6), 574. doi: 10.1037/h0040291

O'Connor, J. J. M., Pisanski, K., Tigue, C. C., Fraccaro, P. J., & Feinberg, D. R. (2014). Perceptions of infidelity risk predict women's preferences for low male voice pitch in short-term over long-term relationship contexts. *Personality and Individual Differences, 56*, 73–77. doi: 10.1016/j.paid.2013.08.029

Ohala, J. J. (1983). Cross-language use of pitch: an ethological view. *Phonetica, 40*(1), 1–18.

Olivola, C. Y., Sussman, A. B., Tsetsos, K., Kang, O. E., & Todorov, A. (2012). Republicans prefer Republican-looking leaders: political facial stereotypes predict candidate electoral success among right-leaning voters. *Social Psychological and Personality Science, 3*(5), 605–613. doi: 10.1177/1948550611432770

Olivola, C. Y. & Todorov, A. (2010). Fooled by first impressions? Reexamining the diagnostic value of appearance-based inferences. *Journal of Experimental Social Psychology, 46*(2), 315–324. doi: 10.1016/j.jesp.2009.12.002

Oosterhof, N. N. & Todorov, A. (2008). The functional basis of face evaluation. *Proceedings of the National Academy of Sciences of the United States of America,* 105(32), 11087–11092. doi: 10.1073/pnas.0805664105

Pear, T. H. (1931). *Voice and Personality.* London: Chapman and Hall Ltd.

Pemberton, C., McCormack, P., & Russell, A. (1998). Have women's voices lowered across time? A cross sectional study of Australian women's voices. *Journal of Voice,* 12(2), 208–213.

Pernet, C. R., McAleer, P., Latinus, M., Gorgolewski, K. J., Charest, I., Bestelmeyer, P. E., … Belin, P. (2015). The human voice areas: spatial organization and inter-individual variability in temporal and extra-temporal cortices. *NeuroImage,* 119, 164–174. doi: 10.1016/j.neuroimage.2015.06.050

Pisanski, K., Fraccaro, P. J., Tigue, C. C., O'Connor, J. J. M., Roder, S., Andrews, P. W., … Feinberg, D. R. (2014). Vocal indicators of body size in men and women: a meta-analysis. *Animal Behaviour,* 95, 89–99. doi: 10.1016/j.anbehav.2014.06.011

Pisanski, K., Jones, B. C., Fink, B., O'Connor, J. J. M., DeBruine, L. M., Roder, S., & Feinberg, D. R. (2016). Voice parameters predict sex-specific body morphology in men and women. *Animal Behaviour,* 112, 13–22. doi: 10.1016/j.anbehav.2015.11.008

Puts, D. A., Apicella, C. L., & Cardenas, R. A. (2012). Masculine voices signal men's threat potential in forager and industrial societies. *Proceedings of the Royal Society B: Biological Sciences,* 279(1728), 601–609. doi: 10.1098/rspb.2011.0829

Puts, D. A., Hodges, C. R., Cardenas, R. A., & Gaulin, S. J. C. (2007). Men's voices as dominance signals: vocal fundamental and formant frequencies influence dominance attributions among men. *Evolution and Human Behavior,* 28(5), 340–344. doi: 10.1016/j.evolhumbehav.2007.05.002

Puts, D. A., Jones, B. C., & DeBruine, L. M. (2012). Sexual selection on human faces and voices. *Journal of Sex Research,* 49(2–3), 227–243. doi: 10.1080/00224499.2012.658924

Re, D. E., O'Connor, J. J. M., Bennett, P. J., & Feinberg, D. R. (2012). Preferences for very low and very high voice pitch in humans. *PLoS One,* 7(3). doi: 10.1371/journal.pone.0032719

Rendall, D., Vokey, J. R., & Nemeth, C. (2007). Lifting the curtain on the Wizard of Oz: biased voice-based impressions of speaker size. *Journal of Experimental Psychology: Human Perception and Performance,* 33(5), 1208–1219. doi: 10.1037/0096-1523.33.5.1208

Rezlescu, C., Penton, T., Walsh, V., Tsujimura, H., Scott, S. K., & Banissy, M. J. (2015). Dominant voices and attractive faces: the contribution of visual and auditory information to integrated person impressions. *Journal of Nonverbal Behavior,* 39(4), 355–370. doi: 10.1007/s10919-015-0214-8

Rosenberg, S., Nelson, C., & Vivekanathan, P. S. (1968). A multidimensional approach to structure of personality impressions. *Journal of Personality and Social Psychology,* 9(4), 283. doi: 10.1037/h0026086

Said, C. P., Baron, S. G., & Todorov, A. (2009). Nonlinear amygdala response to face trustworthiness: contributions of high and low spatial frequency information. *Journal of Cognitive Neuroscience,* 21(3), 519–528. doi: 10.1162/jocn.2009.21041

Saxton, T. K., Caryl, P. G., & Roberts, S. C. (2006). Vocal and facial attractiveness judgments of children, adolescents and adults: the ontogeny of mate choice. *Ethology,* 112(12), 1179–1185. doi: 10.1111/j.1439-0310.2006.01278.x

Saxton, T. K., Debruine, L. M., Jones, B. C., Little, A. C., & Roberts, S. C. (2009). Face and voice attractiveness judgments change during adolescence. *Evolution and Human Behavior,* 30(6), 398–408. doi: 10.1016/j.evolhumbehav.2009.06.004

Scherer, K. R. (1972). Judging personality from voice—cross-cultural approach to an old issue in interpersonal perception. *Journal of Personality,* 40(2), 191. doi: 10.1111/j.1467-6494.1972.tb00998.x

Schotz, S. (2007). Acoustic analysis of adult speaker age. In: C. Müller (ed.) *Speaker Classification I, Lecture Notes in Computer Science, Vol. 1* (pp. 88–107). Berlin, Heidelberg: Springer.

Secord, P. F. (1958). The social stereotype and the concept of implicit personality theory. *American Psychologist*, 13(7), 329–329.

Sedikides, C., Meek, R., Alicke, M. D., & Taylor, S. (2014). Behind bars but above the bar: prisoners consider themselves more prosocial than non-prisoners. *British Journal of Social Psychology*, 53(2), 396–403. doi: 10.1111/bjso.12060

Smith, H. M., Dunn, A. K., Baguley, T., & Stacey, P. C. (2016). Matching novel face and voice identity using static and dynamic facial images. *Attention, Perception & Psychophysics*, 78(3), 868–879. doi: 10.3758/s13414-015-1045-8

Starkweather, J. A. (1961). Vocal communication of personality and human feelings. *Journal of Communication*, 11(2), 63–72. doi: 10.1111/j.1460-2466.1961.tb00330.x

Sutherland, C. A., Oldmeadow, J. A., Santos, I. M., Towler, J., Michael Burt, D., & Young, A. W. (2013). Social inferences from faces: ambient images generate a three-dimensional model. *Cognition*, 127(1), 105–118. doi: 10.1016/j.cognition.2012.12.001

Takayama, L. & Nass, C. (2008). Driver safety and information from afar: an experimental driving simulator study of wireless vs. in-car information services. *International Journal of Human-Computer Studies*, 66(3), 173–184.

Tigue, C. C., Borak, D. J., O'Connor, J. J. M., Schandl, C., & Feinberg, D. R. (2012). Voice pitch influences voting behavior. *Evolution and Human Behavior*, 33(3), 210–216. doi: 10.1016/j.evolhumbehav.2011.09.004

Tinwell, A., Grimshaw, G., & Nabi, D. A. (2015). The effect of onset asynchrony in audio-visual speech and the uncanny valley in virtual characters. *International Journal of Mechanisms and Robotic Systems*, 2(2), 97–110.

Titze, I. R. (1989). Physiologic and acoustic differences between male and female voices. *Journal of the Acoustical Society of America*, 85(4), 1699–1707. doi: 10.1121/1.397959

Todorov, A. & Engell, A. D. (2008). The role of the amygdala in implicit evaluation of emotionally neutral faces. *Social, Cognitive, and Affective Neuroscience*, 3(4), 303–312. doi: 10.1093/scan/nsn033

Todorov, A., Mandisodza, A. N., Goren, A., & Hall, C. C. (2005). Inferences of competence from faces predict election outcomes. *Science*, 308(5728), 1623–1626. doi: 10.1126/science.1110589

Todorov, A., Pakrashi, M., & Oosterhof, N. N. (2009). Evaluating faces on trustworthiness after minimal time exposure. *Social Cognition*, 27(6), 813–833.

Tomlinson Jr, J. M. & Fox Tree, J. E. (2011). Listeners' comprehension of uptalk in spontaneous speech. *Cognition*, 119(1), 58–69. doi: 10.1016/j.cognition.2010.12.005

Tsantani, M. S., Belin, P., Paterson, H. M., & McAleer, P. (2016). Low vocal pitch preference drives first impressions irrespective of context in male voices but not in female voices. *Perception*, 45(8), 946–963. doi: 10.1177/0301006616643675

Tyler, J. C. (2015). Expanding and mapping the indexical field: rising pitch, the uptalk stereotype, and perceptual variation. *Journal of English Linguistics*, 43(4), 284–310. doi: 10.1177/0075424215607061

Vannoni, E. & McElligott, A. G. (2008). Low frequency groans indicate larger and more dominant fallow deer (*Dama dama*) males. *PLoS One*, 3(9), e3113. doi: 10.1371/journal.pone.0003113

Vroomen, J. & de Gelder, B. (2000). Sound enhances visual perception: cross-modal effects of auditory organization on vision. *Journal of Experimental Psychology: Human Perception and Performance*, 26(5), 1583–1590.

Vukovic, J., Feinberg, D. R., Jones, B. C., DeBruine, L. M., Welling, L. L. M., Little, A. C., & Smith, F. G. (2008). Self-rated attractiveness predicts individual differences in women's preferences for masculine men's voices. *Personality and Individual Differences*, 45(6), 451–456. doi: 10.1016/j.paid.2008.05.013

Vukovic, J., Jones, B. C., Feinberg, D. R., Debruine, L. M., Smith, F. G., Welling, L. L., & Little, A. C. (2011). Variation in perceptions of physical dominance and trustworthiness predicts individual differences in the effect of relationship context on women's preferences for masculine pitch in men's voices. *British Journal of Psychology*, 102(1), 37–48. doi: 10.1348/000712610X498750

Ward, R. & Kramer, R. S. S. (2010). Accurate perceptions of personality from the static face. *Perception*, 39, 127–127.

Watson, R., Latinus, M., Noguchi, T., Garrod, O., Crabbe, F., & Belin, P. (2013). Dissociating task difficulty from incongruence in face-voice emotion integration. *Frontiers in Human Neuroscience*, 7, 744. doi: 10.3389/fnhum.2013.00744

Wiggins, J. S. (1979). Psychological taxonomy of trait-descriptive terms—interpersonal domain. *Journal of Personality and Social Psychology*, 37(3), 395–412. doi: 10.1037//0022-3514.37.3.395

Willis, J. & Todorov, A. (2006). First impressions: making up your mind after a 100-ms exposure to a face. *Psychological Science*, 17(7), 592–598. doi: 10.1111/j.1467-9280.2006.01750.x

Wood, T. J. (2014). Exploring the role of first impressions in rater-based assessments. *Advances in Health Science Education*, 19, 409–427. doi: 10.1007/s10459-013-9453-9

Yovel, G. & Belin, P. (2013). A unified coding strategy for processing faces and voices. *Trends in Cognitive Sciences*, 17(6), 263–271. doi: 10.1016/j.tics.2013.04.004

Zatorre, R. J., Bouffard, M., & Belin, P. (2004). Sensitivity to auditory object features in human temporal neocortex. *Journal of Neuroscience*, 24(21), 5078–5078.

Zebrowitz, L. A. & Collins, M. A. (1997). Accurate social perception at zero acquaintance: the affordances of a Gibsonian approach. *Personality and Social Psychology Review*, 1(3), 204–223. doi: 10.1207/s15327957pspr0103_2

Zebrowitz, L. A. & Montepare, J. M. (2008). Social psychological face perception: why appearance matters. *Social and Personality Psychology Compass*, 2(3), 1497. doi: 10.1111/j.1751-9004.2008.00109.x

Zebrowitz, L. A. & Rhodes, G. (2004). Sensitivity to 'bad genes' and the anomalous face overgeneralization effect: cue validity, cue utilization, and accuracy in judging intelligence and health. *Journal of Nonverbal Behavior*, 28(3), 167–185. doi: 10.1023/B:JONB.0000039648.30935.1b

Zimbardo, P. G. (1977). *Shyness*. New York, NY: Harcourt Brace/Jove.

Zuckerman, M. & Driver, R. E. (1989). What sounds beautiful is good—the vocal attractiveness stereotype. *Journal of Nonverbal Behavior*, 13(2), 67–82.

Zuckerman, M., Hodgins, H., & Miyake, K. (1990). The vocal attractiveness stereotype—replication and elaboration. *Journal of Nonverbal Behavior*, 14(2), 97–112. doi: 10.1007/Bf01670437

CHAPTER 27

VOCAL ATTRACTIVENESS

KATARZYNA PISANSKI AND DAVID R. FEINBERG

27.1 THE INTERDISCIPLINARY NATURE OF VOICE ATTRACTIVENESS RESEARCH

RESEARCH on voice attractiveness is highly interdisciplinary, incorporating findings from, but not limited to, psychology, neuroscience, animal behaviour, evolutionary theory, linguistics, and acoustic phonetics. Elements of each of these fields intertwine to paint a picture of why certain voices are more attractive than others. Attractiveness is important from an evolutionary perspective because it is a driving force behind our sexual urges, which in turn result in the passing on of our genes, the mechanism of evolutionary change. From a social perspective, we rely on voice attractiveness to find friends, fend off foes, network, and to climb social ladders or into bed sheets. From the perspective of cognitive neuroscience, the brain has evolved specific regions to process voices as opposed to other similar sounds (Belin et al., 2000). Indeed, voices are special in human perception. Attractive voices provide neural reward value (Bestelmeyer et al., 2012), and prototype-based voice perception drives the attractiveness of average voices (Bruckert et al., 2010). The mechanisms by which we perceive voices therefore shape which voices we ultimately prefer.

In this chapter, we examine voice attractiveness from evolutionary, social, and cognitive neuroscience perspectives. While each perspective is equally important, the majority of recent research on voice attractiveness has been in the evolutionary domain, thus the majority of this chapter focuses on the evolutionary perspective. However, it is our hope that although these approaches are presented in different sections, it is understood that these approaches are not at odds with one other, but rather explore the same problem through different lenses. We strongly encourage the cross-pollination of ideas across disciplines.

27.2 Evolution and Voice Attractiveness

Researchers studying voice attractiveness from an evolutionary perspective posit that non-verbal voice features, such as voice pitch, provide ecologically relevant information about the speaker that listeners are in turn sensitive to. Indeed, various parameters of the voice are linked to underlying biological, physiological, or psychological characteristics that can indicate a speaker's health, reproductive potential, social status, and emotional or motivational state. Voice parameters that indicate high mate quality are often perceived as attractive, arguably because sexual selection has operated on listeners to prefer such traits and on speakers to exploit listeners' perceptual biases, and/or because listeners have learned these preferences through experience. While several general patterns emerge, including consistent preferences for sex-typicality in sexually dimorphic acoustic parameters, voice preferences can also depend on individual differences, context, and culture, as reviewed in Sections 27.3.1 and 27.3.2 on vocal masculinity and vocal femininity, respectively.

27.3 Preferences for Sex-Typical Vocal Parameters

The key frequency components of the human voice are sexually dimorphic. Men's fundamental frequency (perceived as voice pitch) is on average 75% lower, and formant spacing (ΔF, affecting our perception of voice timbre) 18% lower relative to women's (based on weighted population averages; Pisanski, Fraccaro, et al., 2014). Sex differences in fundamental frequency and formants are related to a number of factors. For instance, pubertal surges in testosterone cause men's vocal folds to grow 60% longer (Kahane, 1978) and their larynges to descend a full vertebrate lower than women's, resulting in a vocal tract that is 10–15% longer in men (Lieberman et al., 2001)[1]. Men's fundamental frequency and formants remain inversely related to circulating levels of testosterone into adulthood (Bruckert et al., 2006; Cartei et al., 2014; Dabbs & Mallinger, 1999; Evans et al., 2008). Preferences for sex-typicality in these voice parameters (i.e. lower frequencies among men or 'vocal masculinity', and higher frequencies among women or 'vocal femininity') represent the most consistently reported preferences in the voice-attractiveness literature, and hence, constitute the bulk of this chapter.

27.3.1 Vocal Masculinity

The sex-typical pattern of relatively lower fundamental and/or formant frequencies that differentiate men's voices from women's voices is often referred to as vocal masculinity. While

---

[1] Morphological sex differences do not entirely account for the sex differences observed in fundamental frequency and formants. This hints at the possibility that men may modulate their voice frequencies more than women, for instance to exaggerate their apparent body size (Fitch, 2000; Morton, 1977; Ohala, 1983; Rendall et al., 2005). Indeed, recent research supports this prediction (Pisanski, Mora, et al., 2016).

masculinity can also be a social construct, here we are referring to the physical characteristics that differentiate men and women. Studies consistently indicate that women prefer lower fundamental frequency and/or formants compared to higher frequencies in men's voices, whether these voice parameters vary naturally (Babel et al., 2014; Collins, 2000; Hodges-Simeon et al., 2010; Oguchi & Kikuchi, 1997; Pisanski & Rendall, 2011; Zuckerman & Miyake, 1993) or are experimentally raised or lowered using computer software (Feinberg et al., 2005, 2006, 2011, 2012; Feinberg, DeBruine, Jones, & Little, 2008; Hodges-Simeon et al., 2010; Jones, Boothroyd, et al., 2010; Jones, Feinberg, et al., 2010; Little et al., 2011; Pisanski, Hahn, et al., 2014; Pisanski et al., 2012; Pisanski & Rendall, 2011; Re et al., 2012; Riding et al., 2006; Saxton et al., 2015; Tigue et al., 2012; Vukovic et al., 2008; Vukovic, Jones, et al., 2010). Preferences for vocal masculinity in men's voices are often stronger among female than male listeners (Babel et al., 2014; Jones, Feinberg, et al., 2010; Pisanski & Rendall, 2011). Moreover, while fundamental frequency and formants independently influence vocal attractiveness when manipulated separately (Pisanski & Rendall, 2011), fundamental and formant frequencies can interact such that low formants enhance the attractiveness of low pitch in men's voices and vice versa (Feinberg et al., 2011).

Men's vocal masculinity predicts mating and reproductive success (Apicella et al., 2007; Puts, 2005), body size and strength (Cartei et al., 2014; Pisanski, Fraccaro, et al., 2014; Sell et al., 2010), and may also indicate health (Pisanski et al., 2015; Vukovic, Feinberg, DeBruine, Smith, & Jones, 2010). Men with masculine voices may therefore be physically and/or genetically more fit and healthy than relatively feminine men. At the perceptual level, vocal masculinity is associated with a number of positive traits such as leadership, competence, physical prowess, social dominance, honesty, trustworthiness, and integrity (Klofstad et al., 2015; Puts et al., 2006; Tigue et al., 2012), but also with potentially threatening traits such as physical dominance, strength, and aggressiveness (Klofstad et al., 2012; Ohala, 1983; Puts et al., 2012). Women also perceive men with relatively lower fundamental frequency as more likely to cheat (O'Connor et al., 2011, 2014) and less likely to invest resources into the relationship and into potential offspring (O'Connor et al., 2012). These negative attributions may help to explain why women do not prefer very low fundamental frequencies below a threshold of 96 Hz (Re et al., 2012; Saxton et al., 2015).

Crucially, the perceived costs and benefits associated with vocal masculinity also present a trade-off for women. As a consequence, even though women show a general preference for vocal masculinity, the magnitude of this preference varies as a function of relevant factors as described in the remainder of this section. This systematic variation in vocal masculinity preferences is likely adaptive, as it may influence a woman to choose a masculine mate in specific contexts that ultimately maximize her reproductive success.

Preferences for relatively lower fundamental frequency in men's voices develop around the time of puberty (Saxton et al., 2006, 2010; Saxton, Debruine, et al., 2009) and are stronger among women having experienced relatively early puberty (Jones, Boothroyd, et al., 2010), those not taking hormonal contraception (Feinberg, DeBruine, Jones, & Little, 2008), those who perceive themselves as attractive or are perceived as attractive by others, and those with high fundamental frequency (Feinberg et al., 2012; Vukovic et al., 2008; Vukovic, Feinberg, et al., 2010). Together this suggests that women's vocal masculinity preferences are tuned to their current reproductive status or potential. Additional evidence for this hypothesis stems from studies indicating that women's preferences for low fundamental and/or formant frequencies peak during the most fertile, ovulatory phase of their menstrual cycles

(Feinberg et al., 2006; Hodges-Simeon et al., 2010; Puts, 2005) and increase with their oestra-diol levels (Pisanski, Hahn, et al., 2014)[2]. These within-woman shifts in masculinity prefer-ences, likely triggered by hormonal fluctuations, may function to increase the likelihood that women mate with masculine men when conception risk is highest (for example, see Penton-Voak et al., 1999; Roney & Simmons, 2008).

Women generally show stronger preferences for masculinity in men's voices (Feinberg et al., 2012; O'Connor, Pisanski, et al., 2014; Puts, 2005), as well as in men's faces, bodies, and odours (Little et al., 2011), when assessing potential short-term rather than long-term partners. This appears to be at least partly due to the perceived negative traits of mascu-line men, such as infidelity, low investment (O'Connor et al., 2012, 2011), or anti-sociality (Vukovic et al., 2011), that would be particularly costly in a long-term relationship. However, the influence of mating context on vocal masculinity preferences also depends on indi-vidual differences affecting the ratio of costs to benefits. For instance, women show rela-tively stronger vocal masculinity preferences for the short-term when they are ovulating (Puts, 2005). Feinberg et al. (2012) further showed that women's self-rated attractiveness predicted relatively higher vocal masculinity preferences for a long-term partner, whereas self-rated health predicted higher vocal masculinity preferences for a short-term partner. In fact, several studies have linked elevated health risks (for review, see Pisanski & Feinberg, 2013) and pathogen disgust (Jones et al., 2013) to relatively stronger masculinity preferences, suggesting that the benefits of choosing a masculine and thus potentially healthy mate are greater in cultures and among women for whom risk of infection is most probable.

There is a great need for cross-cultural studies in the biological and psychological sciences (Henrich et al., 2010). This includes research on voice attractiveness. We know that cultural factors such as pathogen prevalence and food availability affect women's facial and body masculinity preferences (for review, see Pisanski & Feinberg, 2013), but far less is known about the cultural factors affecting voice attractiveness. Studies examining voice preferences among the Tanzanian Hadza tribe indicate that Hadza men's vocal masculinity positively predicts their reproductive success (Apicella et al., 2007), body size, and strength (Puts, Apicella, Cardenas, 2012). Apicella & Feinberg (2009) further showed that Hadza women from Tanzania assessed men with lower fundamental frequency as better hunters; however, only Hadza women who were not breast-feeding indicated a preference to marry such men.

We encourage researchers to further test evolutionary and social hypotheses of human behaviour, including voice preferences, in diverse social and economic environments, to en-sure their generalizability and ecological validity, as well as to determine the influences of cultural, social, and economic factors on the expression of, preference for, and development of social attributions towards voices and voice preferences.

27.3.2 Vocal Femininity

The sex-typical pattern of relatively higher fundamental frequency and/or formants in women's than men's voices is often referred to as vocal femininity. In line with women's

---

[2] Similar cyclic shifts in women's preferences for masculine faces, bodies, and odours, in addition to voices, have recently become a popular topic of debate among researchers (see Gildersleeve et al., 2014; Wood et al., 2014).

preferences for sex-typicality in men's voices, studies indicate that men generally (although not always) prefer higher fundamental frequency and/or formants compared to lower frequencies in women's voices (Apicella & Feinberg, 2009; Babel et al., 2014; Borkowska & Pawlowski, 2011; Collins & Missing, 2003; Feinberg, DeBruine, Jones, & Perrett, 2008; Jones et al., 2008; Jones, Feinberg, et al., 2010; Little et al., 2011; Oguchi & Kikuchi, 1997; Pisanski et al., 2012; Pisanski & Rendall, 2011; Puts et al., 2011; Re et al., 2012). Higher fundamental frequency is preferred to the female population average (Feinberg, DeBruine, Jones, & Perrett, 2008), although digitally averaging voices together produces stimuli that both men and women consider attractive (Bruckert et al., 2010) (see also Section 27.8 on voice averageness). Studies testing for a potential upper limit to the attractiveness of high fundamental frequency in women's voices have produced mixed results (Borkowska & Pawlowski, 2011; Feinberg, DeBruine, Jones, & Perrett, 2008; Re et al., 2012). Interestingly, women are attuned to indices of vocal femininity in other women's voices (Borkowska & Pawlowski, 2011; Jones et al., 2008; Puts et al., 2013, 2011), particularly when assessing dominance (Jones, Feinberg, et al., 2010). Although this may reflect the monitoring of intrasexual competitors, few researchers have directly studied the role of voice in female–female competition.

Vocal femininity may be attractive because it communicates a woman's reproductive receptivity (Haselton & Gildersleeve, 2011). Indeed, fluctuations in sex hormones across the menstrual cycle and lifespan affect the female voice in various ways (for reviews, see Abitbol et al., 1999; Amir & Biron-Shental, 2004). For instance, the fundamental frequency of naturally-cycling women increases cyclically in the days immediately preceding ovulation (Bryant & Haselton, 2009; Fischer et al., 2011), decreases temporarily following childbirth (Pisanski et al., 2018), and decreases 8% on average following menopause (Lindholm et al., 1997). Men's assessments of vocal attractiveness are highest for women's voices recorded near ovulation (Fischer et al., 2011; Pipitone & Gallup, 2008; Puts et al., 2013) and lowest for voices recorded at menstruation (Pipitone & Gallup, 2012; but see Fischer et al., 2011). While cyclic changes in hormone levels may not predict cyclic changes in women's acoustic parameters (Fischer et al., 2011), higher oestrogen and progesterone levels (Puts et al., 2013), and to a lesser extent lower testosterone levels (Wheatley et al., 2014), predict men's assessments of women's vocal attractiveness. Men also prefer the voices of women near prime reproductive age (between 19 and 30 years) compared to those of circum-menopausal women (Röder et al., 2013; Wheatley et al., 2014). In addition to indicating fecundity, women's fundamental frequency correlates with various measures of body size and shape known to indicate health (Pisanski et al., 2015; Vukovic, Feinberg, et al., 2010).

Feminine voices systematically elicit in listeners a range of social stereotypes. Similar to men, whose attractively low fundamental frequency is associated with both positive and negative traits, high fundamental frequency among women is perceptually associated with femininity, fertility, youthfulness, and warmth, but also immaturity, babyishness, weakness, and lower levels of competence, intelligence, and dominance (Berry, 1992; Borkowska & Pawlowski, 2011; Collins & Missing, 2003; Feinberg, DeBruine, Jones, & Perrett, 2008; Jones et al., 2008; Klofstad et al., 2015, 2012; Montepare & Zebrowitz-Mcarthur, 1987; Robinson & McArthur, 1982). As a result, women often face the unfortunate conflict of sounding feminine *or* powerful.

Individual and environmental factors potentially contributing to variation in men's vocal femininity preferences remain largely understudied. Little et al. (2011) found that men preferred femininity in women's voices and faces relatively more in the context of short-term than long-term relationships, and that men's preferences for masculinity in potential long-term partners were consistent across modalities. The authors suggest that men may prefer relatively more masculine (i.e. stereotypically less attractive) women as long-term partners to minimize the probability of desertion or cuckoldry by an attractive mate. It is also possible that traits associated with vocal masculinity, such as assertiveness and competence, are desirable in long-term but not short-term female partners. Finally, a relatively stronger preference for lower women's voices may reflect a preference for an older, more mature partner (Berry, 1992; Collins & Missing, 2003; Feinberg, DeBruine, Jones, & Perrett, 2008; Zuckerman & Driver, 1989).

Only a handful of studies have examined vocal femininity preferences outside of Europe and North America. Montepare and Zebrowitz-McArthur (1987) showed that childlike voice qualities were associated with childlike attributions (e.g. weakness, ineptitude) in two samples of adult listeners from the United States and Korea, but did not measure voice attractiveness. Apicella & Feinberg (2009) found that Hadza men preferred women's voices with higher than lower fundamental frequency in the context of a potential wife; however, Hadza women's fundamental frequencies did not predict their reproductive success (Apicella et al., 2007). Wheatley et al. (2014) further found that vocal and facial attractiveness were positively correlated among both American and Hadza women. Men preferred the voices of women of reproductive age, but only among the Hadza, and those of physically smaller women, but only among Americans. These cross-cultural differences appear at least partially tied to differences in the age and body-size ranges of women from either culture (Wheatley et al., 2014).

27.4 BEYOND FUNDAMENTAL FREQUENCY AND FORMANTS

Fundamental and formant frequencies have been at the centre of voice attractiveness research. However, other sexually dimorphic parameters and/or those conveying socially-relevant information about speakers influence voice attractiveness. Like mean fundamental frequency, the standard deviation of fundamental frequency is sexually dimorphic; women's voices are characterized by more variable fundamental frequencies and are therefore perceived as less monotonous than are men's (Puts, Apicella, & Cardenas, 2012). The standard deviation of fundamental frequency also correlates negatively with men's reproductive success, testosterone levels, arm strength, self-reported dominance, and physical aggression (Hodges-Simeon et al., 2010; Hodges-Simeon et al., 2011; Puts, Apicella, & Cardenas, 2012), predicts variation in body shape in both sexes (Pisanski et al., 2015), increases near ovulation among women (Fischer et al., 2011), and decreases temporarily after pregnancy (Pisanski et al., 2018). Yet further experiments are needed to determine whether sex-typicality in fundamental-frequency variation is attractive, as current evidence is mixed (Hodges-Simeon et al., 2010; Ray et al., 1991; Riding et al., 2006).

Babel et al. (2014) found that breathiness was attractive in women's voices, whereas relatively shorter bouts of speech were attractive among men. Speech rate, speech duration, and breathiness are typically higher among women than men (Bradlow et al., 1996; Hughes et al., 2008; Klatt & Klatt, 1989; Simpson, 2009). Hence these findings may reflect preferences for sex-typicality in the voice. Vocal breathiness and hoarseness are also tied to vocal perturbation and noise parameters (Kreiman & Sidtis, 2011) that predict sex-specific variation in men's and women's body shapes (Pisanski et al., 2015), and vary across women's menstrual cycles (Fischer et al., 2011), and may therefore also indicate masculinity/femininity and fecundity. Some researchers have suggested that 'sexy' women's voices are characterized by breathiness and relatively lower fundamental frequency (Henton & Bladon, 1985; Riding et al., 2006; Tuomi & Fisher, 1979) because these qualities may communicate intimacy and arousal. Other studies show that a high harmonic-to-noise ratio, producing low perceptual hoarseness, is attractive in both men's and women's voices (Bruckert et al., 2010), whereas a creaky quality of voice referred to as 'vocal fry' is, in contrast, generally perceived as unattractive (Anderson et al., 2014; but see Yuasa, 2010).

Few studies have examined the attractiveness of loudness. Hodges-Simeon et al. (2010) found that men's voices with higher intensity were perceived as relatively more attractive by women for both short- and long-term mating contexts, regardless of women's menstrual-cycle phases. The authors suggest that voice intensity may indicate vigour and dominance; however, the underlying mechanism linking intensity to these traits is unclear.

27.5 Multimodality and Interactions

Non-verbal voice parameters combine with information gauged from other modalities—such as vision and olfaction—to affect judgements of attractiveness, suggesting that sexual selection may have operated on multiple modalities to communicate redundant or additive information about a person's mate value (Feinberg, 2008; Groyecka et al., 2017). In particular, numerous studies now report a positive relationship between judgements of voice and face attractiveness in both sexes (Collins & Missing, 2003; Hughes & Miller, 2015; Little et al., 2011; Saxton, Burriss, et al., 2009; Saxton et al., 2006; Skrinda et al., 2014; Wheatley et al., 2014). Voice attractiveness also correlates with body attractiveness (Hughes et al., 2004, 2008; Little et al., 2011; Saxton, Burriss, et al., 2009). Even within the acoustic modality, non-verbal voice parameters can interact with one another (Feinberg et al., 2011; Hughes et al., 2008) or with *verbal* aspects of speech (e.g. verbal indicators of social interest or socioeconomic status: Hodges-Simeon et al., 2010; Jones et al., 2008; O'Connor, Fraccaro, et al., 2014), to affect voice attractiveness. Objective and subjective measures of voice attractiveness can also differ between short speech sounds, such as vowels, and longer trains of read or free speech (e.g. indices of fertility in women's voices: Bryant & Haselton, 2009; Fischer et al., 2011; Lindholm et al., 1997). Taken together, these findings point to a need for more cross-modal research on voice attractiveness and for more ecologically valid studies that use longer, free speech stimuli produced in natural social contexts.

27.6 Social Approach to Voice Attractiveness

The studies reviewed here demonstrate that men and women with attractive voices are typically preferred as potential mates and succeed more often in contests with same-sex rivals (for reviews, see Feinberg, DeBruine, Jones, & Perrett, 2008; Puts, Jones, & DeBruine, 2012). It is perhaps unsurprising then that recent studies have shown that speakers manipulate the fundamental frequency, formants, and other features of their voices in socially-relevant ways, for example to sound more masculine (Cartei et al., 2012), dominant (Puts et al., 2006; Yuasa, 2010), physically larger (Pisanski, Mora, et al., 2016), or attractive and sexy (Fraccaro et al., 2013; Hughes et al., 2014; Tuomi & Fisher, 1979). In fact, studies suggest that men and women spontaneously alter their voices in response to attractive conversational partners (Anolli & Ciceri, 2002; Fraccaro et al., 2011; Hughes et al., 2010; Leongómez et al., 2014), but the specific acoustic properties of modulated speech and their effectiveness on listeners' perceptions of vocal attractiveness remain unclear (Pisanski, Cartei, et al., 2016).

Voice attractiveness can greatly influence social success beyond increasing mating opportunities. It has long been known that people associate attractiveness with goodness, commonly referred to as the 'what is beautiful is good' stereotype (Dion et al., 1972) or the 'halo effect' (Nisbett & Wilson, 1977). This phenomenon applies not only to physical attractiveness, but also voice attractiveness, wherein men and women with attractive voices are attributed with various positive attributes such as competence, kindness, and trustworthiness (Hughes & Miller, 2015; Zuckerman & Driver, 1989; Zuckerman & Miyake, 1993; Zuckerman et al., 1990). Recent studies suggest that these stereotypes can have serious implications in the real world. For example, people prefer to vote for hypothetical male and female leaders with more masculine than feminine voices (Klofstad et al., 2015, 2012; Tigue et al., 2012) and to hire potential female job candidates with lower, more attractive levels of vocal fry (Anderson et al., 2014). The recent influx of research in this field is revealing the great extent to which voice attractiveness can affect our everyday lives.

27.7 Cognitive Neuroscience and Voice Attractiveness

Researchers applying an evolutionary approach to voice attractiveness typically examine specific vocal parameters, such as fundamental and formant frequencies, because of the theoretical predictions stemming from the physiological and psychological correlates of these parameters. In cognitive neuroscience, the focus shifts from function to mechanism (Tinbergen, 1963), and hence produces a different set of predictions about voice attractiveness. Rather than focusing on *why* certain voices are attractive, cognitive neuroscience helps us to understand *how* the ways in which we produce and perceive voices influences their attractiveness. While tonotopy in the primary auditory cortex (Pantev et al., 1995; Romani et al., 1982) certainly aids in the frequency discrimination necessary to judge voice attractiveness, these auditory areas are general auditory processors and bear no special fruits to digest the way we represent voice attractiveness in the brain. Rather, voices appear to be individuated with reference to a mental prototype (Latinus & Belin, 2011; Latinus et al., 2013), and voice-selective areas in the brain (Belin et al., 2000) play an important role in this voice-prototype formation (Belin & Zatorre, 2003).

27.8 Voice Averageness

Many of the studies reviewed in Sections 27.3.1 and 27.3.2 suggest that relatively low- or high-frequency (i.e. masculine or feminine) voices are attractive because they provide clues to various ecologically relevant traits of the speaker. Yet, recent studies show that average voices—those that most closely fit our mental prototype of a voice—are also attractive (Bestelmeyer et al., 2012; Bruckert et al., 2010). In fact, they are more attractive than average.

Early experiments examining vocal averageness focused on single-voice parameters such as fundamental frequency (Feinberg, DeBruine, Jones, & Perrett, 2008; Re et al., 2012). In these studies, average fundamental frequency was judged attractive, but exaggerated sex-typical fundamental frequency was more attractive than the average. A more recent line of research, acoustically blending voices together using morphing technology, has demonstrated that increasing the number of voices in a prototype increases its attractiveness, and that the distance of a voice from the average in a multidimensional voice space predicts its relative attractiveness (Bestelmeyer et al., 2012; Bruckert et al., 2010). Voice averageness is not only attractive when manipulated using computer software; experiments using real, unmanipuated voices also show that average voices are attractive (Feinberg, DeBruine, Jones, & Perrett, 2008; McAleer et al., 2014). Whether the phenomenon that average voices are attractive is a by-product of the neural mechanisms underlying voice perception or a product of sexual selection need not be mutually exclusive. In the following section, we outline theories aimed at answering the question of why average voices are attractive.

27.9 Why Are Average Voices Attractive?

27.9.1 Averageness Indicates Health

Evolutionary explanations[3] for the attractiveness of voice averageness have focused on the sender rather than the perceiver. That is, being an average individual conveys certain messages to the perceiver about one's (the sender's) underlying quality as a potential mate. Health is one of the most important qualities people look for in a mate cross-culturally (Buss, 1989), so it is perhaps not surprising that researchers examining the attractiveness of averageness have linked it to health. People with average faces, and likely average voices, demonstrate a lower prevalence of disease and abnormalities than do less average people. Average individuals have relatively more heterozygous major histocompatibility complexes (MHCs)—referred to in humans as human leukocyte antigens (HLAs) (Lie et al., 2008; Roberts et al., 2005)—that code for the detection of differences between self and non-self in our immune systems. Thus, more average individuals, those with more heterozygous HLA profiles, will

---

[3] Although the term 'evolutionary explanations' may be a misnomer, because the evolution of brain structures and cognitive mechanisms need not parallel evolutionary explanations of behaviour, we use it here to refer to functionalist explanations.

have a higher probability of passing on genes to resist a higher number of pathogens than those with homozygous HLA profiles.

Aside from HLA and complex immune system genes, there are more parsimonious explanations as to why people associate averageness with healthiness. A group of average individuals excludes those who are extremely healthy and extremely unhealthy. The net effect is that a group of average people is, on average, not unhealthy. To take this further, most genetic abnormalities are quite rare. Conditions like Down syndrome and Turner syndrome, that result from genetic abnormalities, occur in less than one per cent of the population. Thus, a group of average individuals (i.e. within one standard deviation of the population average on a given trait) will not include people with these conditions. The group of average people will also exclude those with rare genetic abnormalities such as immunity to HIV, as on the whole, most mutations are deleterious rather than advantageous. Therefore, judging average individuals as attractive is a safe bet, because they have a low risk of genetic abnormality and a relatively stronger immune system.

A separate explanation as to why averageness is attractive, from a mechanistic viewpoint, is perceiver-based rather than sender-based. Here, there are two key lines of reasoning—the fluency of processing argument and the effects of mere exposure.

27.9.2 Fluency of Processing

Like faces, voices are processed using a prototype-based representation (Latinus & Belin, 2011; Latinus et al., 2013). We code new voices with reference to our internal representation of what the average voice sounds like. Experiments have shown that we may have different prototypes for male and female voices (Little et al., 2013) as adapting to male voice stimuli only affects subsequent perception of other male, but not female, voices and vice versa. Regardless of how separable these prototypes are or how many exist, voices closer to our internal prototype are processed more fluently than are those further from the prototype (Babel & McGuire, 2015). What this means for attractiveness is that we may prefer average voices not because they are relatively healthier, but because it is easy for our brains to process such voices (Winkielman et al., 2006). Of course, these explanations need not be mutually exclusive.

27.9.3 Mere Exposure

As long known in the advertising world, mere exposure to a stimulus increases our preference for it (Gordon & Holyoak, 1983; Rhodes et al., 2001; Zajonc, 1968). For instance, repeated exposure to music increases the speed at which we recognize it and makes it more attractive (Green et al., 2012; Peretz et al., 1998). Similarly, researchers have theorized that repeated exposure to a voice will increase its attractiveness (Feinberg, 2008). Our mental prototypes of voices are updated by repeated exposure (Belin & Zatorre, 2003; Latinus & Belin, 2011; Little et al., 2013), and hence, it stands to reason that average voices may be attractive because of the effects of mere exposure.

Mere exposure may be a self-reinforcing mechanism that helps maintain voice attractiveness, as we also have attentional biases towards familiar voices (Johnsrude et al., 2013). Yet, research on faces has shown that while adapting to highly unattractive faces increases their attractiveness, adapting to highly attractive faces decreases their attractiveness (DeBruine et al., 2007). People use similar cognitive mechanisms to process and evaluate the attractiveness of faces and voices (Campanella & Belin, 2007; Feinberg, 2008; Pisanski & Feinberg, 2013), suggesting that like faces, mere exposure or adaptation may have different effects on different types of voices.

27.10 Voice and Face Attractiveness

In all three perspectives on voice attractiveness discussed in this chapter, one apparent pattern emerges: voice and face attractiveness are related. From a functional perspective, both the voice and face can inform perceivers about mate quality. Behavioural studies indicate that people with attractive faces are typically judged as also having attractive voices and vice versa (Collins & Missing, 2003; Hughes & Miller, 2015; Little et al., 2011; Saxton, Burriss, et al., 2009; Saxton et al., 2006; Skrinda et al., 2014; Wheatley et al., 2014), regardless of whether audiovisual stimuli used in experiments are still images and voice recordings (Feinberg, DeBruine, Jones, & Perrett, 2008; Fraccaro et al., 2010), or videos (O'Connor et al., 2012, 2013). At the neural level, voice and face perception are integrated in the superior temporal sulcus (Campanella & Belin, 2007) and similar brain areas are active when attending either to an attractive voice (Bestelmeyer et al., 2012) or an attractive face (Aharon et al., 2001; O'Doherty et al., 2003), indicating that both modalities are processed similarly. Finally, from a social perspective, vocal-attractiveness stereotypes appear consistent across voice and face preferences (Hughes & Miller, 2015). Taken together, these studies are consistent with the idea that voice and face preferences reflect common features and mechanisms.

27.11 Conclusion

What makes a voice attractive? This remains an open question. Although we know that various acoustical features such as fundamental frequency and voice averageness are important, there is probably no single answer to the question of what makes a voice attractive. This is because voice attractiveness hinges on an interplay between the vocalizer and the listener, and different vocal qualities will be more or less attractive to different listeners at different times and in different social or cultural contexts. The work presented here represents our first foray into understanding voice attractiveness. We have only just begun to understand the dynamics of vocal modulation, how our brains process voices, the hormonal mechanisms underlying voice change and voice preferences, and even the social implications of voice attractiveness. Many of the recent advances in the study of voice attractiveness are the result of technological advances such as the ability to morph and manipulate voice features (Kawahara, 2006; Valbret et al., 1992). As better tools continue to be developed, we will acquire increasingly sophisticated ways to test previously untestable hypotheses about voice attractiveness.

REFERENCES

Abitbol, J., Abitbol, P., & Abitbol, B. (1999). Sex hormones and the female voice. *Journal of Voice*, 13(3), 424–446. http://doi.org/10.1016/S0892-1997(99)80048-4

Aharon, I., Etcoff, N., Ariely, D., Chabris, C. F., O'Connor, E., & Breiter, H. C. (2001). Beautiful faces have variable reward value: fMRI and behavioral evidence. *Neuron*, 32(3), 537–551.

Amir, O. & Biron-Shental, T. (2004). The impact of hormonal fluctuations on female vocal folds. *Current Opinion in Otolaryngology & Head and Neck Surgery*, 12(3), 180–184.

Anderson, R. C., Klofstad, C. A., Mayew, W. J., & Venkatachalam, M. (2014). Vocal fry may undermine the success of young women in the labor market. *PLoS One*, 9(5), e97506.

Anolli, L. & Ciceri, R. (2002). Analysis of the vocal profiles of male seduction: from exhibition to self-disclosure. *The Journal of General Psychology*, 129(2), 149–169. http://doi.org/10.1080/00221300209603135

Apicella, C. L. & Feinberg, D. R. (2009). Voice pitch alters mate-choice-relevant perception in hunter-gatherers. *Proceedings of the Royal Society B: Biological Sciences*, 276(1659), 1077–1082. http://doi.org/10.1098/rspb.2008.1542

Apicella, C. L., Feinberg, D. R., & Marlowe, F. W. (2007). Voice pitch predicts reproductive success in male hunter-gatherers. *Biology Letters*, 3(6), 682–684. http://doi.org/10.1098/rsbl.2007.0410

Babel, M. & McGuire, G. (2015). Perceptual fluency and judgments of vocal aesthetics and stereotypicality. *Cognitive Science*, 39(4), 766–787.

Babel, M., McGuire, G., & King, J. (2014). Towards a more nuanced view of vocal attractiveness. *PLoS One*, 9(2), e88616. http://doi.org/10.1371/journal.pone.0088616

Belin, P. & Zatorre, R. J. (2003). Adaptation to speaker's voice in right anterior temporal lobe. *NeuroReport*, 14(16), 2105–2109.

Belin, P., Zatorre, R. J., Lafaille, P., Ahad, P., & Pike, B. (2000). Voice-selective areas in human auditory cortex. *Nature*, 403(6767), 309–312.

Berry, D. S. (1992). Vocal types and stereotypes: joint effects of vocal attractiveness and vocal maturity on person perception. *Journal of Nonverbal Behavior*, 16(1), 41–54.

Bestelmeyer, P. E., Latinus, M., Bruckert, L., Rouger, J., Crabbe, F., & Belin, P. (2012). Implicitly perceived vocal attractiveness modulates prefrontal cortex activity. *Cerebral Cortex*, 22(6), 1263–1270.

Borkowska, B. & Pawlowski, B. (2011). Female voice frequency in the context of dominance and attractiveness perception. *Animal Behaviour*, 82(1), 55–59. http://doi.org/10.1016/j.anbehav.2011.03.024

Bradlow, A. R., Torretta, G., & Pisoni, D. B. (1996). Intelligibility of normal speech I: global and fine-grained acoustic-phonetic talker characteristics. *Speech Communication*, 20, 255–272.

Bruckert, L., Bestelmeyer, P., Latinus, M., Rouger, J., Charest, I., Rousselet, G. A., ... Belin, P. (2010). Vocal attractiveness increases by averaging. *Current Biology*, 20(2), 116–120. http://doi.org/10.1016/j.cub.2009.11.034

Bruckert, L., Lienard, J.-S., Lacroix, A., Kreutzer, M., & Leboucher, G. (2006). Women use voice parameters to assess men's characteristics. *Proceedings of the Royal Society B: Biological Sciences*, 273(1582), 83–89. http://doi.org/10.1098/rspb.2005.3265

Bryant, G. A. & Haselton, M. G. (2009). Vocal cues of ovulation in human females. *Biology Letters*, 5(1), 12–15. http://doi.org/10.1098/rsbl.2008.0507

Buss, D. M. (1989). Sex differences in human mate preferences: evolutionary hypotheses tested in 37 cultures. *Behavioral and Brain Sciences*, 12(01), 1–14.

Campanella, S. & Belin, P. (2007). Integrating face and voice in person perception. *Trends in Cognitive Sciences*, 11(12), 535–543.

Cartei, V., Bond, R., & Reby, D. (2014). What makes a voice masculine: physiological and acoustical correlates of women's ratings of men's vocal masculinity. *Hormones and Behavior*, 66(4), 569–576. http://doi.org/10.1016/j.yhbeh.2014.08.006

Cartei, V., Cowles, H. W., & Reby, D. (2012). Spontaneous voice gender imitation abilities in adult speakers. *PLoS One*, 7(2), e31353. http://doi.org/10.1371/journal.pone.0031353

Collins, S. A. (2000). Men's voices and women's choices. *Animal Behaviour*, 60(6), 773–780. http://doi.org/10.1006/anbe.2000.1523

Collins, S. A. & Missing, C. (2003). Vocal and visual attractiveness are related in women. *Animal Behaviour*, 65(5), 997–1004. http://doi.org/10.1006/anbe.2003.2123

Dabbs, J. M. & Mallinger, A. (1999). High testosterone levels predict low voice pitch among men. *Personality and Individual Differences*, 27(4), 801–804. http://doi.org/10.1016/S0191-8869(98)00272-4

DeBruine, L. M., Jones, B. C., Unger, L., Little, A. C., & Feinberg, D. R. (2007). Dissociating averageness and attractiveness: attractive faces are not always average. *Journal of Experimental Psychology: Human Perception and Performance*, 33(6), 1420.

Dion, K., Berscheid, E., & Walster, E. (1972). What is beautiful is good. *Journal of Personality and Social Psychology*, 24, 285–290.

Evans, S., Neave, N., Wakelin, D., & Hamilton, C. (2008). The relationship between testosterone and vocal frequencies in human males. *Physiology & Behavior*, 93(4-5), 783–788. http://doi.org/10.1016/j.physbeh.2007.11.033

Feinberg, D. R. (2008). Are human faces and voices ornaments signaling common underlying cues to mate value? *Evolutionary Anthropology: Issues, News, and Reviews*, 17(2), 112–118. http://doi.org/10.1002/evan.20166

Feinberg, D. R., DeBruine, L. M., Jones, B. C., & Little, A. C. (2008). Correlated preferences for men's facial and vocal masculinity. *Evolution and Human Behavior*, 29(4), 233–241. http://doi.org/10.1016/j.evolhumbehav.2007.12.008

Feinberg, D. R., DeBruine, L. M., Jones, B. C., Little, A. C., O'Connor, J. J. M., & Tigue, C. C. (2012). Women's self-perceived health and attractiveness predict their male vocal masculinity preferences in different directions across short- and long-term relationship contexts. *Behavioral Ecology and Sociobiology*, 66(3), 413–418. http://doi.org/10.1007/s00265-011-1287-y

Feinberg, D. R., DeBruine, L. M., Jones, B. C., & Perrett, D. I. (2008). The role of femininity and averageness of voice pitch in aesthetic judgments of women's voices. *Perception*, 37(4), 615–623. http://doi.org/10.1068/p5514

Feinberg, D. R., Jones, B. C., DeBruine, L. M., O'Connor, J. J. M., Tigue, C. C., & Borak, D. J. (2011). Integrating fundamental and formant frequencies in women's preferences for men's voices. *Behavioral Ecology*, 22(6), 1320–1325. http://doi.org/10.1093/beheco/arr134

Feinberg, D. R., Jones, B. C., Law Smith, M. J., Moore, F. R., DeBruine, L. M., Cornwell, R. E., ... Perrett, D. I. (2006). Menstrual cycle, trait estrogen level, and masculinity preferences in the human voice. *Hormones and Behavior*, 49(2), 215–222. http://doi.org/10.1016/j.yhbeh.2005.07.004

Feinberg, D. R., Jones, B. C., Little, A. C., Burt, D. M., & Perrett, D. I. (2005). Manipulations of fundamental and formant frequencies influence the attractiveness of human male voices. *Animal Behaviour*, 69(3), 561–568. http://doi.org/10.1016/j.anbehav.2004.06.012

Fischer, J., Semple, S., Fickenscher, G., Jürgens, R., Kruse, E., Heistermann, M., & Amir, O. (2011). Do women's voices provide cues of the likelihood of ovulation? The importance of sampling regime. *PLoS One*, 6(9), e24490. http://doi.org/10.1371/journal.pone.0024490

Fitch, W. T. (2000). The evolution of speech: a comparative review. *Trends in Cognitive Sciences*, 4(7), 258–267. http://doi.org/10.1016/S1364-6613(00)01494-7

Fraccaro, P. J., Feinberg, D. R., DeBruine, L. M., Little, A., Watkins, C. D., & Jones, B. C. (2010). Correlated male preferences for femininity in female faces and voices. *Evolutionary Psychology: An International Journal of Evolutionary Approaches to Psychology and Behavior*, 8(3), 447–461.

Fraccaro, P. J., Jones, B. C., Vukovic, J., Smith, F. G., Watkins, C. D., Feinberg, D. R., ... Debruine, L. M. (2011). Experimental evidence that women speak in a higher voice pitch to men they find attractive. *Journal of Evolutionary Psychology*, 9(1), 57–67. http://doi.org/10.1556/JEP.9.2011.33.1

Fraccaro, P. J., O'Connor, J. J., Re, D. E., Jones, B. C., DeBruine, L. M., & Feinberg, D. R. (2013). Faking it: deliberately altered voice pitch and vocal attractiveness. *Animal Behaviour*, 85(1), 127–136.

Gildersleeve, K., Haselton, M. G., & Fales, M. R. (2014). Do women's mate preferences change across the ovulatory cycle? A meta-analytic review. *Psychological Bulletin*, 140(5), 1205–1259. http://doi.org/10.1037/a0035438

Gordon, P. C. & Holyoak, K. J. (1983). Implicit learning and generalization of the 'mere exposure' effect. *Journal of Personality and Social Psychology*, 45(3), 492.

Green, A. C., Bærentsen, K. B., Stødkilde-Jørgensen, H., Roepstorff, A., & Vuust, P. (2012). Listen, learn, like! Dorsolateral prefrontal cortex involved in the mere exposure effect in music. *Neurology Research International*, 2012.

Groyeck, A., Pisanski, K., Sorokowska, A., Havlicek, J., Karwowski, M., Puts, D., Roberts, C., & Sorokowski, C. (2017). Attractiveness is multimodal: Beauty is also in the nose and ear of the beholder. *Frontiers in Psychology*, 8, 778. doi: 10.3389/fpsyg.2017.00778

Haselton, M. G. & Gildersleeve, K. (2011). Can men detect ovulation? *Current Directions in Psychological Science*, 20(2), 87–92. http://doi.org/10.1177/0963721411402668

Henrich, J., Heine, S. J., & Norenzayan, A. (2010). The weirdest people in the world? *Behavioral and Brain Sciences*, 33(2–3), 61–83. http://doi.org/10.1017/S0140525X0999152X

Henton, C. J. & Bladon, R. A. W. (1985). Breathiness in normal female speech. *Language and Communication*, 5(3), 221–227.

Hodges-Simeon, C. R., Gaulin, S. J. C., & Puts, D. A. (2010). Different vocal parameters predict perceptions of dominance and attractiveness. *Human Nature*, 21(4), 406–427. http://doi.org/10.1007/s12110-010-9101-5

Hodges-Simeon, C. R., Gaulin, S. J. C., & Puts, D. A. (2011). Voice correlates of mating success in men: examining 'contests' versus 'mate choice' modes of sexual selection. *Archives of Sexual Behavior*, 40(3), 551–557. http://doi.org/10.1007/s10508-010-9625-0

Hughes, S. M., Dispenza, F., & Gallup Jr, G. G. (2004). Ratings of voice attractiveness predict sexual behavior and body configuration. *Evolution and Human Behavior*, 25(5), 295–304. http://doi.org/10.1016/j.evolhumbehav.2004.06.001

Hughes, S. M., Farley, S. D., & Rhodes, B. C. (2010). Vocal and physiological changes in response to the physical attractiveness of conversational partners. *Journal of Nonverbal Behavior*, 34(3), 155–167.

Hughes, S. M. & Miller, N. E. (2015). What sounds beautiful looks beautiful stereotype: the matching of attractiveness of voices and faces. *Journal of Social and Personal Relationships*, 33(7), 1–14.

Hughes, S. M., Mogilski, J. K., & Harrison, M. A. (2014). The perception and parameters of intentional voice manipulation. *Journal of Nonverbal Behavior*, 38(1), 107–127. http://doi.org/10.1007/s10919-013-0163-z

Hughes, S. M., Pastizzo, M. J., & Gallup Jr., G. G. (2008). The sound of symmetry revisited: subjective and objective analyses of voice. *Journal of Nonverbal Behavior*, 32(2), 93–108. http://doi.org/10.1007/s10919-007-0042-6

Johnsrude, I. S., Mackey, A., Hakyemez, H., Alexander, E., Trang, H. P., & Carlyon, R. P. (2013). Swinging at a cocktail party: voice familiarity aids speech perception in the presence of a competing voice. *Psychological Science*, 24(10), 1995–2004.

Jones, B. C., Boothroyd, L., Feinberg, D. R., & DeBruine, L. M. (2010). Age at menarche predicts individual differences in women's preferences for masculinized male voices in adulthood. *Personality and Individual Differences*, 48(7), 860–863. http://doi.org/10.1016/j.paid.2010.02.007

Jones, B. C., Feinberg, D. R., DeBruine, L. M., Little, A. C., & Vukovic, J. (2008). Integrating cues of social interest and voice pitch in men's preferences for women's voices. *Biology Letters*, 4(2), 192–194. http://doi.org/10.1098/rsbl.2007.0626

Jones, B. C., Feinberg, D. R., DeBruine, L. M., Little, A. C., & Vukovic, J. (2010). A domain-specific opposite-sex bias in human preferences for manipulated voice pitch. *Animal Behaviour*, 79(1), 57–62. http://doi.org/10.1016/j.anbehav.2009.10.003

Jones, B. C., Feinberg, D. R., Watkins, C. D., Fincher, C. L., Little, A. C., & DeBruine, L. M. (2013). Pathogen disgust predicts women's preferences for masculinity in men's voices, faces, and bodies. *Behavioral Ecology*, 24(2), 373–379. http://doi.org/10.1093/beheco/ars173

Kahane, J. C. (1978). A morphological study of the human prepubertal and pubertal larynx. *American Journal of Anatomy*, 151(1), 11–19. http://doi.org/10.1002/aja.1001510103

Kawahara, H. (2006). STRAIGHT, exploitation of the other aspect of vocoder: perceptually isomorphic decomposition of speech sounds. *Acoustical Science and Technology*, 27, 349–353.

Klatt, D. H. & Klatt, L. C. (1989). Analysis, synthesis, and perception of voice quality variations among female and male talkers. *Journal of the Acoustical Society of America*, 87(2), 820–857.

Klofstad, C. A., Anderson, R. C., & Nowicki, S. (2015). Perceptions of competence, strength, and age influence voters to select leaders with lower-pitched voices. *PLoS One*, 10(8), e0133779. http://doi.org/10.1371/journal.pone.0133779

Klofstad, C. A., Anderson, R. C., & Peters, S. (2012). Sounds like a winner: voice pitch influences perception of leadership capacity in both men and women. *Proceedings of the Royal Society of London B: Biological Sciences*, 279(1738), 2698–2704. http://doi.org/10.1098/rspb.2012.0311

Kreiman, J. & Sidtis, D. (2011). *Foundations of Voice Studies: An Interdisciplinary Approach to Voice Production and Perception*. Wiley-Blackwell. Retrieved from: http://eu.wiley.com/WileyCDA/WileyTitle/productCd-0631222979.html

Latinus, M. & Belin, P. (2011). Anti-voice adaptation suggests prototype-based coding of voice identity. *Frontiers in Psychology*, 2, 175.

Latinus, M., McAleer, P., Bestelmeyer, P. E., & Belin, P. (2013). Norm-based coding of voice identity in human auditory cortex. *Current Biology*, 23(12), 1075–1080.

Leongómez, J. D., Binter, J., Kubicová, L., Stolařová, P., Klapilová, K., Havlíček, J., & Roberts, S. C. (2014). Vocal modulation during courtship increases proceptivity even in naive listeners. *Evolution and Human Behavior*, 35(6), 489–496. http://doi.org/10.1016/j.evolhumbehav.2014.06.008

Lie, H. C., Rhodes, G., & Simmons, L. W. (2008). Genetic diversity revealed in human faces. *Evolution*, 62(10), 2473–2486.

Lieberman, D. E., McCarthy, R. C., Hiiemae, K. M., & Palmer, J. B. (2001). Ontogeny of postnatal hyoid and larynx descent in humans. *Archives of Oral Biology*, 46(2), 117–128. http://doi.org/10.1016/S0003-9969(00)00108-4

Lindholm, P., Vilkman, E., Raudaskoski, T., Suvanto-Luukkonen, E., & Kauppila, A. (1997). The effect of postmenopause and postmenopausal HRT on measured voice values and vocal symptoms. *Maturitas*, 28(1), 47–53.

Little, A. C., Connely, J., Feinberg, D. R., Jones, B. C., & Roberts, S. C. (2011). Human preference for masculinity differs according to context in faces, bodies, voices, and smell. *Behavioral Ecology*, 22(4), 862–868. http://doi.org/10.1093/beheco/arr061

Little, A. C., Feinberg, D. R., DeBruine, L. M., & Jones, B. C. (2013). Adaptation to faces and voices: unimodal, cross-modal, and sex-specific effects. *Psychological Science*, 24(11), 2297–2305.

McAleer, P., Todorov, A., Belin, P., & Larson, C. R. (2014). How do you say 'Hello'? Personality impressions from brief novel voices. *PloS One*, 9(3), e90779.

Montepare, J. M. & Zebrowitz-Mcarthur, L. (1987). Perceptions of adults with childlike voices in two cultures. *Journal of Experimental Social Psychology*, 23(4), 331–349.

Morton, E. S. (1977). On the occurrence and significance of motivation-structural rules in some bird and mammal sounds. *The American Naturalist*, 111(981), 855–869.

Nisbett, R. E. & Wilson, T. D. (1977). The halo effect: evidence for unconscious alteration of judgment. *Journal of Personality and Social Psychology*, 34, 250–256.

O'Connor, J. J., Fraccaro, P. J., & Feinberg, D. R. (2012). The influence of male voice pitch on women's perceptions of relationship investment. *Journal of Evolutionary Psychology*, 10(1), 1–13. http://doi.org/10.1556/JEP.10.2012.1.1

O'Connor, J. J., Fraccaro, P. J., Pisanski, K., Tigue, C. C., & Feinberg, D. R. (2013). Men's preferences for women's femininity in dynamic cross-modal stimuli. *PloS One*, 8(7), e69531.

O'Connor, J. J., Fraccaro, P. J., Pisanski, K., Tigue, C. C., O'Donnell, T. J., & Feinberg, D. R. (2014). Social dialect and men's voice pitch influence women's mate preferences. *Evolution and Human Behavior*, 35(5), 368–375. http://doi.org/10.1016/j.evolhumbehav.2014.05.001

O'Connor, J. J., Pisanski, K., Tigue, C. C., Fraccaro, P. J., & Feinberg, D. R. (2014). Perceptions of infidelity risk predict women's preferences for low male voice pitch in short-term over long-term relationship contexts. *Personality and Individual Differences*, 56, 73–77. http://doi.org/10.1016/j.paid.2013.08.029

O'Connor, J. J., Re, D. E., & Feinberg, D. R. (2011). Voice pitch influences perceptions of sexual infidelity. *Evolutionary Psychology*, 9(1), 64–78.

O'Doherty, J., Winston, J., Critchley, H., Perrett, D., Burt, D. M., & Dolan, R. J. (2003). Beauty in a smile: the role of medial orbitofrontal cortex in facial attractiveness. *Neuropsychologia*, 41(2), 147–155.

Oguchi, T. & Kikuchi, H. (1997). Voice and interpersonal attraction. *Japanese Psychological Research*, 39(1), 56–61. http://doi.org/10.1111/1468-5884.00037

Ohala, J. J. (1983). An ethological perspective on common cross-language utilization of Fo of voice. *Phonetica*, 41(1), 1–16.

Pantev, C., Bertrand, O., Eulitz, C., Verkindt, C., Hampson, S., Schuierer, G., & Elbert, T. (1995). Specific tonotopic organizations of different areas of the human auditory cortex revealed by simultaneous magnetic and electric recordings. *Electroencephalography and Clinical Neurophysiology*, 94(1), 26–40.

Penton-Voak, I. S., Perrett, D. I., Castles, D. L., Kobayashi, T., Burt, D. M., Murray, L. K., & Minamisawa, R. (1999). Menstrual cycle alters face preference. *Nature*, 399(6738), 741–742.

Peretz, I., Gaudreau, D., & Bonnel, A.-M. (1998). Exposure effects on music preference and recognition. *Memory & Cognition*, 26(5), 884–902.

Pipitone, N. & Gallup, G. G. (2008). Women's voice attractiveness varies across the menstrual cycle. *Evolution and Human Behavior*, 29(4), 268–274. http://doi.org/10.1016/j.evolhumbehav.2008.02.001

Pipitone, N. & Gallup, G. G. (2012). The unique impact of menstruation on the female voice: implications for the evolution of menstrual cycle cues: menstruation and voice. *Ethology*, 118(3), 281–291. http://doi.org/10.1111/j.1439-0310.2011.02010.x

Pisanski, K., Bhardwaj, K., & Reby, D. (2018). Women's voice pitch lowers after pregnancy. *Evolution & Human Behavior*. https://doi.org/10.1016/j.evolhumbehav.2018.04.002.

Pisanski, K., Cartei, V., McGettigan, C., Raine, J., & Reby, D. (2016). Voice modulation: A window into the origins of human vocal control? *Trends in Cognitive Science*, 20(4), 304–318.

Pisanski, K. & Feinberg, D. (2013). Cross-cultural variation in mate preferences for averageness, symmetry, body size, and masculinity. *Cross-Cultural Research*, 47(2), 162–197. http://doi.org/10.1177/1069397112471806

Pisanski, K., Fraccaro, P. J., Tigue, C. C., O'Connor, J. J. M., Röder, S., Andrews, P. W., … Feinberg, D. R. (2014). Vocal indicators of body size in men and women: a meta-analysis. *Animal Behaviour*, 95, 89–99. http://doi.org/10.1016/j.anbehav.2014.06.011

Pisanski, K., Hahn, A. C., Fisher, C. I., DeBruine, L. M., Feinberg, D. R., & Jones, B. C. (2014). Changes in salivary estradiol predict changes in women's preferences for vocal masculinity. *Hormones and Behavior*, 66(3), 493–497. http://doi.org/10.1016/j.yhbeh.2014.07.006

Pisanski, K., Jones, B. C., Fink, B., O'Connor, J. J. M., DeBruine, L., Roder, S., & Feinberg, D. R. (2015). Voice parameters predict sex-specific body morphology in men and women. *Animal Behaviour*, 112, 13–22. http://doi.org/10.1016/j.anbehav.2015.11.008

Pisanski, K., Mishra, S., & Rendall, D. (2012). The evolved psychology of voice: evaluating interrelationships in listeners' assessments of the size, masculinity, and attractiveness of unseen speakers. *Evolution and Human Behavior*, 33(5), 509–519. http://doi.org/10.1016/j.evolhumbehav.2012.01.004

Pisanski, K., Mora, E., Pisanski, A., Reby, D., Sorokowski, P., Franckowiak, T., & Feinberg, D. (2016). Volitional exaggeration of body size through fundamental and formant frequency modulation in humans. *Scientific Reports*, 6, 34389. doi: 10.1038/srep34389

Pisanski, K. & Rendall, D. (2011). The prioritization of voice fundamental frequency or formants in listeners' assessments of speaker size, masculinity, and attractiveness. *Journal of the Acoustical Society of America*, 129(4), 2201. http://doi.org/10.1121/1.3552866

Puts, D. (2005). Mating context and menstrual phase affect women's preferences for male voice pitch. *Evolution and Human Behavior*, 26(5), 388–397. http://doi.org/10.1016/j.evolhumbehav.2005.03.001

Puts, D., Apicella, C. L., & Cardenas, R. A. (2012). Masculine voices signal men's threat potential in forager and industrial societies. *Proceedings of the Royal Society B: Biological Sciences*, 279(1728), 601–609. http://doi.org/10.1098/rspb.2011.0829

Puts, D., Bailey, D. H., Cárdenas, R. A., Burriss, R. P., Welling, L. L. M., Wheatley, J. R., & Dawood, K. (2013). Women's attractiveness changes with estradiol and progesterone across the ovulatory cycle. *Hormones and Behavior*, 63(1), 13–19. http://doi.org/10.1016/j.yhbeh.2012.11.007

Puts, D., Barndt, J. L., Welling, L. L. M., Dawood, K., & Burriss, R. P. (2011). Intrasexual competition among women: vocal femininity affects perceptions of attractiveness and flirtatiousness. *Personality and Individual Differences*, 50(1), 111–115. http://doi.org/10.1016/j.paid.2010.09.011

Puts, D., Gaulin, S. J. C., & Verdolini, K. (2006). Dominance and the evolution of sexual dimorphism in human voice pitch. *Evolution and Human Behavior*, 27(4), 283–296. http://doi.org/10.1016/j.evolhumbehav.2005.11.003

Puts, D., Jones, B. C., & DeBruine, L. M. (2012). Sexual selection on human faces and voices. *The Journal of Sex Research*, 49(2–3), 227–243. http://doi.org/10.1080/00224499.2012.658924

Ray, G. B., Ray, E. B., & Zahn, C. J. (1991). Speech behaviour and social evaluation: an examination of medical messages. *Communication Quarterly*, 39(2), 119–129.

Re, D. E., O'Connor, J. J. M., Bennett, P. J., & Feinberg, D. R. (2012). Preferences for very low and very high voice pitch in humans. *PLoS One*, 7(3), e32719. http://doi.org/10.1371/journal.pone.0032719

Rendall, D., Kollias, S., Ney, C., & Lloyd, P. (2005). Pitch (F0) and formant profiles of human vowels and vowel-like baboon grunts: the role of vocalizer body size and voice-acoustic allometry. *The Journal of the Acoustical Society of America*, 117(2), 944. http://doi.org/10.1121/1.1848011

Rhodes, G., Halberstadt, J., & Brajkovich, G. (2001). Generalization of mere exposure effects to averaged composite faces. *Social Cognition*, 19(1), 57–70.

Riding, D., Lonsdale, D., & Brown, B. (2006). The effects of average fundamental frequency and variance of fundamental frequency on male vocal attractiveness to women. *Journal of Nonverbal Behavior*, 30(2), 55–61. http://doi.org/10.1007/s10919-006-0005-3

Roberts, S. C., Little, A. C., Gosling, L. M., Perrett, D. I., Carter, V., Jones, B. C., … Petrie, M. (2005). MHC-heterozygosity and human facial attractiveness. *Evolution and Human Behavior*, 26(3), 213–226.

Robinson, J. & McArthur, L. Z. (1982). Impact of salient vocal qualities on causal attribution for a speaker's behavior. *Journal of Personality and Social Psychology*, 43(2), 236.

Röder, S., Fink, B., & Jones, B. (2013). Facial, olfactory, and vocal cues to female reproductive value. *Evolutionary Psychology*, 11(2), 392–404. Retrieved from http://www.epjournal.net/wp-content/uploads/EP11392404.pdf

Romani, G. L., Williamson, S. J., & Kaufman, L. (1982). Tonotopic organization of the human auditory cortex. *Science*, 216(4552), 1339–1340.

Roney, J. R. & Simmons, Z. L. (2008). Women's estradiol predicts preference for facial cues of men's testosterone. *Hormones and Behavior*, 53(1), 14–19. http://doi.org/10.1016/j.yhbeh.2007.09.008

Saxton, T. K., Burriss, R. P., Murray, L. K., Rowland, H. M., & Roberts, S. C. (2009). Face, body, and speech cues independently predict judgments of attractiveness. *Journal of Evolutionary Psychology*, 7, 23–35.

Saxton, T. K., Caryl, P. G., & Craig Roberts, S. (2006). Vocal and facial attractiveness judgments of children, adolescents and adults: the ontogeny of mate choice. *Ethology*, 112(12), 1179–1185. http://doi.org/10.1111/j.1439-0310.2006.01278.x

Saxton, T. K., Debruine, L. M., Jones, B. C., Little, A. C., & Roberts, S. C. (2009). Face and voice attractiveness judgments change during adolescence. *Evolution and Human Behavior*, 30(6), 398–408. http://doi.org/10.1016/j.evolhumbehav.2009.06.004

Saxton, T. K., Kohoutova, D., Craig Roberts, S., Jones, B. C., DeBruine, L. M., & Havlicek, J. (2010). Age, puberty and attractiveness judgments in adolescents. *Personality and Individual Differences*, 49(8), 857–862. http://doi.org/10.1016/j.paid.2010.07.016

Saxton, T. K., Mackey, L. L., McCarty, K., & Neave, N. (2015). A lover or a fighter? Opposing sexual selection pressures on men's vocal pitch and facial hair. *Behavioral Ecology*, 27(2), 512–519. http://doi.org/10.1093/beheco/arv178

Sell, A., Bryant, G. A., Cosmides, L., Tooby, J., Sznycer, D., von Rueden, C., … Gurven, M. (2010). Adaptations in humans for assessing physical strength from the voice. *Proceedings of the Royal Society B: Biological Sciences*, 277(1699), 3509–3518. http://doi.org/10.1098/rspb.2010.0769

Simpson, A. P. (2009). Phonetic differences between male and female speech. *Language and Linguistics Compass*, 3(2), 621–640. http://doi.org/10.1111/j.1749-818x.2009.00125.x

Skrinda, I., Krama, T., Kecko, S., Moore, F. R., Kaasik, A., Meija, L., … Krams, I. (2014). Body height, immunity, facial and vocal attractiveness in young men. *Naturwissenschaften*, 101(12), 1017–1025. http://doi.org/10.1007/s00114-014-1241-8

Tigue, C. C., Borak, D. J., O'Connor, J. J. M., Schandl, C., & Feinberg, D. R. (2012). Voice pitch influences voting behavior. *Evolution and Human Behavior*, 33(3), 210–216. http://doi.org/10.1016/j.evolhumbehav.2011.09.004

Tinbergen, N. (1963). On aims and methods of ethology. *Zeitschrift Für Tierpsychologie*, 20(4), 410–433.

Tuomi, S. K. & Fisher, J. E. (1979). Characteristics of simulated sexy voice. *Folia Phoniat*, 31, 242–249.

Valbert, H., Mouline, E., & Tubach, J. (1992). Voice transformation using PSOLA technique. *Speech and Communication*, 11, 175–187.

Vukovic, J., Feinberg, D., DeBruine, L., Smith, F., & Jones, B. (2010). Women's voice pitch is negatively correlated with health risk factors. *Journal of Evolutionary Psychology*, 8(3), 217–225. http://doi.org/10.1556/JEP.8.2010.3.2

Vukovic, J., Feinberg, D. R., Jones, B. C., DeBruine, L. M., Welling, L. L. M., Little, A. C., & Smith, F. G. (2008). Self-rated attractiveness predicts individual differences in women's preferences for masculine men's voices. *Personality and Individual Differences*, 45(6), 451–456. http://doi.org/10.1016/j.paid.2008.05.013

Vukovic, J., Jones, B. C., DeBruine, L., Feinberg, D. R., Smith, F. G., Little, A. C., ... Main, J. (2010). Women's own voice pitch predicts their preferences for masculinity in men's voices. *Behavioral Ecology*, 21(4), 767–772. http://doi.org/10.1093/beheco/arq051

Vukovic, J., Jones, B. C., Feinberg, D. R., DeBruine, L. M., Smith, F. G., Welling, L. L. M., & Little, A. C. (2011). Variation in perceptions of physical dominance and trustworthiness predicts individual differences in the effect of relationship context on women's preferences for masculine pitch in men's voices: vocal attractiveness, trust and dominance. *British Journal of Psychology*, 102(1), 37–48. http://doi.org/10.1348/000712610X498750

Wheatley, J. R., Apicella, C. A., Burriss, R. P., Cárdenas, R. A., Bailey, D. H., Welling, L. L. M., & Puts, D. A. (2014). Women's faces and voices are cues to reproductive potential in industrial and forager societies. *Evolution and Human Behavior*, 35(4), 264–271. http://doi.org/10.1016/j.evolhumbehav.2014.02.006

Winkielman, P., Halberstadt, J., Fazendeiro, T., & Catty, S. (2006). Prototypes are attractive because they are easy on the mind. *Psychological Science*, 17(9), 799–806.

Wood, W., Kressel, L., Joshi, P. D., & Louie, B. (2014). Meta-analysis of menstrual cycle effects on women's mate preferences. *Emotion Review*, 6(3), 229–249. http://doi.org/10.1177/1754073914523073

Yuasa, I. P. (2010). Creaky voice: a new feminine voice quality for young urban-oriented upwardly mobile American women? *American Speech*, 85, 315–337. http://doi.org/10.1215/00031283-2010-018

Zajonc, R. B. (1968). Attitudinal effects of mere exposure. *Journal of Personality and Social Psychology*, 9(2p2), 1.

Zuckerman, M. & Driver, R. (1989). What sounds beautiful is good: the vocal attractiveness stereotype. *Journal of Nonverbal Behavior*, 13, 67–82.

Zuckerman, M., Hodgins, H., & Miyake, K. (1990). The vocal attractiveness stereotype: replication and elaboration. *Journal of Nonverbal Behavior*, 14, 97–112.

Zuckerman, M. & Miyake, K. (1993). The attractive voice: what makes it so? *Journal of Nonverbal Behavior*, 17(2), 119–135.

CHAPTER 28

VOICE PROCESSING
Implications for Earwitness Testimony

SARAH STEVENAGE

28.1 INTRODUCTION

WHILST voice processing is undoubtedly important in our everyday social encounters, it assumes particular importance in a forensic context, when the nature of the crime sometimes makes the voice the only cue from which to determine identity. Such a situation may arise when crimes are committed under cover of darkness or poor light, when the perpetrator is hidden from full view or wears a mask or disguise, or when the perpetrator is not seen at all through direction or desire to 'look away'. In these situations, our reliance on the face as a primary cue to identity is compromised, and the voice assumes greater importance. This is even clearer when the perpetrator is not actually physically present, such as when making a bomb threat, a ransom demand, or a threatening phone call. In each of these instances, the voice becomes paramount in helping to identify the perpetrator, and in helping to clear any innocent suspects of the crime. Early literature suggested the importance of voice pitch, together with the changes in intonation and the rhythm of a speech pattern (Brown, 1981; Van Dommelen, 1990). Indeed, voice researchers held the view that a spectral analysis or 'voiceprint' may be unique, and thus as valuable as the fingerprint in telling one person apart from another (Kersta, 1962). Taken together, these early views were sufficient for judges to deem voice recognition admissible within court proceedings as a way of determining identity.

Two legal cases are particularly notable in this regard. The first describes the case of Bruno Hauptmann who was tried, convicted, and later executed for the kidnap and murder of the son of Charles Lindbergh in 1941. Hauptmann was convicted partly on the basis of voice recognition testimony by Lindbergh himself. He claimed that he recognized Hauptmann's voice from the ransom drop two years earlier during which Hauptmann was heard to utter the words 'Hey doc, here doc, over here ...' The case highlights that the jury was sufficiently convinced by this testimony to make a conviction despite the facts that Hauptmann's voice was unfamiliar, the initial phrase consisted only of six words, and the delay between initial hearing and eventual identification was substantial. Nevertheless, a conviction was made and a sentence was carried out.

The second legal case of relevance is that against Guy Paul Morin. In 1992, in the state of Ontario, Canada, Morin was tried and convicted of the rape and murder of Christine Jessop, a 9-year-old neighbour. Again, voice-recognition evidence contributed to the conviction. In this case, the evidence was provided by the victim's mother, Janet, who claimed to recognize Morin's voice saying 'Help me, help me. Oh God, help me' on the eve of her daughter's funeral. Janet identified this voice as belonging to her neighbour, Morin. Moreover, she testified that this voice matched the voice she had heard on the day of the murder itself. The testimony was deemed admissible because of the familiarity that the witness had with the defendant. However, the influence of a time delay between the two speech samples, and the time delay between the eve of the funeral and the eventual identification, were overlooked. In fact, DNA evidence eventually cleared Guy Morin of all charges and he was released from custody having served three years of a sentence he did not deserve. The voice testimony in this case was false.

These two cases suggest a clear need for caution when evaluating earwitness testimony in the absence of a full understanding of the factors that influence it. Particularly pertinent in this regard is the finding of Yarmey et al. (2001). In the only study of its type, they showed that the *prediction* of someone's voice-recognition ability far exceeded their actual ability. In other words, we believe that people are better as earwitnesses than they actually are. Given that juries are comprised of lay people with no particular expertise in the area of voice recognition, the same overestimation of earwitness performance may be likely in their minds too. The present chapter will provide an overview of the essential capabilities of the earwitness in an attempt to understand what they *are* able to report on, and what may be too much of a challenge. First, however, a consideration is provided of the place of voice-recognition evidence in court.

28.2 VOICES IN COURT

Voice recognition has been used in court as a means to establish guilt from as early as the sixteenth century. Initially, judges were quite willing to accept voice-recognition evidence in court. However, more recently, and with cases such as those in the 'Introduction' in mind, research has urged for caution in accepting earwitness testimony in court. The concern is twofold. First, the voice-recognition literature lacks the same extensive research base that exists with face recognition regarding reliability and error rates. Second, the legal and court procedures are yet to be fully and satisfactorily defined regarding voice recognition. Indeed, voice recognition is conducted through adjusting those processes defined for face recognition, and questions of admissibility are determined on a case-by-case basis. Ormerod (2001, p. 596) describes this situation as a significant concern, suggesting that 'adapting rules evolved for eyewitnesses could be more dangerous than having no rules at all if it engenders a false sense of security against mis-identification'. Moreover, without a clearly-defined set of rules and procedures regarding voice-recognition evidence, there exist no clear grounds for appeal against mistakes.

With this in mind, the decision regarding admissibility of voice-recognition evidence sits with the trial judge. S(he) has the responsibility of determining whether the evidence is of sufficient quality to be relied on in court, and this decision principally rests on the familiarity of the speaker to the witness, and the conditions under which the voice was heard. If these are not satisfied, a judge may deem evidence in a particular case to be inadmissible.

A related but potentially even more problematic issue may exist with the process of voice recognition by a jury following the presentation of a recording of the perpetrator, and the oral evidence of the defendant in court (*R* v *O'Doherty* [2002]). Whilst the jury has the right to listen to recorded evidence, and to make a comparison to the defendant's voice, several factors make this risky. Indeed, their unfamiliarity with the speaker, their lack of qualified expertise in voice recognition, and the stress of making an identification in the courtroom setting (with all the biases that this may bring), point to considerable concern over such a practice.

With these concerns in mind, and on the basis of an appeal in the case of *R* v *Hersey* [1998], there is now a requirement that the judge warn the jury of the special need for caution when considering voice-recognition evidence, with reference to the specifics of the particular case. This so-called 'Turnbull direction' (*R* v *Turnbull* [1977]) requires that the judge spell out for the jury the risks of mistaken identification, and the reasons why a witness may be mistaken in this particular case, whilst also stressing that an honest witness may be convincing but incorrect.

The 'Turnbull direction' provides some guidance to jurors who ultimately have the responsibility of weighing the evidence. However, it remains the case that whilst judges may know of some of the factors that render voice recognition unreliable for court purposes (such as a lack of familiarity, a short voice clip, a time delay, or intentional disguise), they may be unaware of other less obvious factors. Consequently, expert testimony is often requested in order to advise the court regarding the reliability of an earwitness identification. Given all these factors, one plausibly may ask 'what can we tell from a voice?'

28.3 WHAT CAN WE TELL FROM A VOICE?

The literature suggests that there are a number of characteristics that can be determined about a speaker. For example, whilst our estimates of height and weight of a speaker tend not to be reliable (Gonzalez, 2003), we can generally tell the biological sex of a speaker. The primary cue for sex judgements in adult speakers is fundamental frequency (F0) or vocal pitch, with females generally having higher-pitched voices than males. On this basis, the accuracy of sex identification for 18-year-old speakers was high (but not perfect) at 87% (Amir et al., 2011). However, Amir et al. noted that it was possible to determine speaker sex at above-chance levels of 69%, even when the targets were young (pre-pubertal) speakers who did not differ in pitch. (See also Weinberg and Bennett (1971) who report a 74% accuracy in sex identification of 5–6-year-old boys and girls.) Successful sex judgements of these young speakers was based on the listeners' sensitivity to other characteristics of the vocal tract such as vowel formant differences. Consequently, in all but the most extreme instances, one may consider that the earwitness is sufficiently able to detect sex-related vocal cues, making sex classification reliable.

Earwitnesses may also be able to provide an age judgement of an individual based on their voice. Whilst fundamental frequency is important to age estimates of younger speakers, it does not vary greatly after the vocal changes triggered by puberty (Hughes & Rhodes, 2010). Nevertheless, age variations do still exist in linguistic factors such as speech complexity and fluency (Kemper et al., 2003). Similarly, age variations exist in vocal characteristics, with older speakers showing more 'shimmer' (through less control of the airways) and a slower speech rate than younger speakers. Indeed, if a voice is artificially sped up by 10% it is estimated to be younger, and if artificially slowed down by 10% it is estimated to be older, than it really is (Skoog-Waller et al., 2015).

Our sensitivity to these cues underpins good age perception. Nevertheless, biases do exist in vocal-age judgements, with younger speakers tending to be judged as older, and older speakers tending to be judged as younger, than their chronological age (Moyse, 2014). In addition, there is some evidence for an own-age bias in which older listeners are better able to judge the age of speakers from their own age group compared to speakers who are younger than themselves (Moyse et al., 2014).

It is also worth noting the way in which the age estimates are collected. The first method is to obtain absolute estimates of age which can then be correlated with actual chronological age. In a review of such studies, Moyse (2014) notes correlations between 0.68 and 0.88, and an absolute error of about 10 years. This compares with an absolute error of about 5 years when judging age from the face. The weakness of this approach, however, is that a systematic error in age estimates could nevertheless produce a high correlation whilst providing values that are quite far from the truth. Consequently, the second method of obtaining age estimates is to ask participants for categorical decisions in which a speaker is assigned to an age bracket. When this method is used, performance is much better. Indeed, Ptacek and Sander (1966) report 99% accuracy when sorting speech into two categories (under 35 years; over 65 years), and this compares with an accuracy of 83.1% when sorting faces into three age categories (18–25 years; 35–45 years; 55–75 years) (Anastasi & Rhodes, 2006). With these factors taken into account, speaker-age judgements may be considered to have broad accuracy when provided by adult earwitnesses with good hearing, and when using categorical decisions.

In addition to these broad speaker characteristics, earwitnesses are also able to discern aspects of emotional state from a speaker's voice. In this regard, several studies show a capacity to identify the basic emotions of anger, disgust, fear, sadness, and joy from the voice compared to a neutral state. Within the parallel field of face processing, these basic emotions are well understood in terms of their identification from facial expressions both across cultures and across literate and pre-literate groups. As a consequence, the common view amongst face researchers is that the perception of emotion from faces is universal (Ekman & Friesen, 1971). More recent work on voice processing suggests that the perception of these emotions from the voice is also universal (see Scherer et al., 2001). Indeed, Pell et al. (2009) showed 64% accuracy when labelling native-language sentences with one of six expression labels. Moreover, this fell only marginally to 56% accuracy when labelling non-native sentences. Both levels of performance are significantly above chance given the six alternatives available to the listeners, suggesting that vocal expression can be recognized regardless of language. Moreover, this is demonstrated even though individual speakers may vary in how they display vocal emotions.

More impressive, however, are the results of a time-course analysis which revealed that vocal emotions can be identified with accuracy as quickly as half a second after voice onset (Pell & Kotz, 2011). Predictably, fear was identified with greatest speed (517 ms), followed by sadness (576 ms) and anger (710 ms), with happiness (977 ms) and disgust (1486 ms) showing recognition over a longer time frame. This pattern makes evolutionary sense in a context in which immediate threat is important to detect. Indeed, the voice seems to be particularly important, compared to the face, when quickly communicating negative emotional states. Having said this, emotional identification is superior when a witness is presented with both the face and the voice as dual sources of input, compared to when they have either the face or the voice in isolation (Barkhuysen et al., 2010).

The literature also suggests that a listener can detect a host of other temporary speaker states through their voice. For instance, they can detect increased anxiety in a speaker's voice through characteristics including raised mean pitch, raised maximum pitch, and increased pauses (Laukka et al., 2008). Moreover, they can detect speaker certainty using language-specific intonation patterns to determine whether someone believes what they are saying, or is asking for clarification or reassurance (del Mar Vanrell et al., 2012). Similarly, vocal characteristics can signal levels of intoxication in a speaker (Klingholz et al., 1988). However, background noise or hiss, together with voice strain, illness, or simple individual differences, may mimic the intoxicated voice, making it possible to draw a false conclusion of intoxication in a sober individual. As such, whilst several speaker states, and especially emotional states, can be determined with reliability by the earwitness, other speaker states may be misattributed given the broad range of speaker variability that we experience.

28.4 Speaker Identification

Arguably, the most important decision that an earwitness can make surrounds the identity of the speaker. Certainly, the ability to know who one is talking to serves us well in any social encounter. However, the capacity to identify and name an individual from their voice is of immeasurable value within a forensic context. In this regard, the literature suggests that whilst our voice-recognition performance is above chance, it does not approach the level of performance associated with face recognition and may not always be reliable.

This level of difficulty is surprising given our obvious need as social animals to be able to tell one person apart from another. It is also surprising given that we start life as newborns with a notable sensitivity to the voice. Innovative work using a variety of methods has shown that infants at just 1 month old prefer their mother's voice over an unfamiliar female voice (see Panneton Cooper et al., 1997). This early preference is believed to reflect exposure to the mother's voice whilst still in the womb. Indeed, measurement of the fetal heart rate through the mother's abdomen during gestation shows selective responding to the mother's voice relative to an unfamiliar female's voice in the last months before birth (Kisilevsky et al., 2009). By 6 months old, the infant is capable of combining faces and voices together in a multimodal manner (Trehub et al., 2009). Moreover, by 7 months old, the infant is able to tell speakers apart when they are speaking in the infant's native tongue, despite the infant not being able to speak or necessarily understand all that is said (Johnson et al., 2011). These findings, taken together, indicate that an infant comes into the world primed to attend to voices, yet by adulthood, this ability may have been overtaken by an attention to faces.

Against this backdrop, it would be unwise, however, to consider that *all* adult earwitnesses will be unreliable and *all* voices will be poorly recognized. Indeed, there are several factors that will encourage good performance. For instance, when recognizing the voices of familiar classmates, performance was better in female listeners than in male listeners overall, with males showing an own-sex bias by identifying male speakers better than female speakers (Skuk & Schweinberger, 2013). Moreover, voice recognition tends to be better in listeners who have conversed with the target speaker, as opposed to those who have merely engaged in passive listening (Hammersley & Read, 1985).

A considerable literature also notes an advantage when recognizing voices that are speaking in the listener's mother tongue. In this regard, speaking in a foreign language significantly affects the accuracy of voice recognition. Goggin et al. (1991) showed that monolingual listeners identified bilingual speakers with significantly higher accuracy and confidence when they spoke in a familiar language rather than in an unfamiliar language. This was replicated by Phillipon et al. (2007) using a line-up task in which monolingual English listeners were asked to pick out the English- or French-speaking target from a line-up of English- or French-speaking foils. As in the previous study, Phillipon et al. noted significantly better performance when the language was familiar. However, they also noted that whilst there was poorer recognition of speakers when the language was unfamiliar, this circumstance also gave rise to a worrying level of mistaken identifications. In fact, 46.7% of listeners inappropriately chose the wrong speaker from a line-up when the target was present, and 93.3% of listeners inappropriately chose the wrong speaker from a line-up when the target was absent. Each of these selections is a mistaken identification and, in a legal context, represents the identification of an innocent party.

More recently, the literature would suggest that the basis for the own-language effect discussed here may be much more fine-grained than we might think. Indeed, recent research suggests that it is a familiarity with the *sound structure* of a language that is important, rather than the ability to comprehend what is said. In this regard, Fleming et al. (2014) showed an advantage when English-speaking listeners were asked to discriminate between different speakers speaking in English and in Mandarin. Intriguingly, however, the sound clips in this study had been temporally reversed so as to remove comprehension. Despite this, discrimination was still better for English speakers than for Mandarin speakers, suggesting a basic importance of familiarity with the phonological structure of the language being spoken.

Alongside these findings, the literature also suggests that voice recognition is better when the voice is relatively unchanged (in terms of wording or emotional tone) between initial hearing and later test (Read & Craik, 1995). Performance is also better when longer speech clips are provided (Cook & Wilding, 1997; Yarmey & Matthys, 1991) and when the delay between study and test is relatively short (Clifford et al., 1981; McGehee, 1937; Papcun et al., 1989; Saslove & Yarmey, 1980; Yarmey & Matthys, 1991). Indeed, delays of up to 24 hours have rather little effect on performance compared to delays of weeks or months. Finally, tests of voice recognition also suggest that performance is better when the target voice sounds distinctive. Indeed, Yarmey (1991) showed that descriptions of voices were remembered better over a week when the voice was distinctive rather than typical. Similarly, distinctive-sounding voices elicited better recognition, and fewer false identifications, than did typical-sounding voices (Mullenix et al., 2011; Orchard & Yarmey, 1995; cf. Papcun et al., 1989).

28.5 THE INFLUENCE OF SPEAKER FAMILIARITY

Dwarfing all these influences on voice recognition, however, the major factor that appears to benefit voice recognition is speaker familiarity (for an overview, see Yarmey, 1995). Indeed, given our capacity to recognize familiar speakers, be they family, friends, or known celebrities from radio or television, it is tempting to conclude that all voice recognition is good. In fact, several researchers now consider that the processes involved in recognizing a familiar speaker are quite different to those used when recognizing an unfamiliar or once-heard speaker (Clifford, 1980; Papcun et al., 1989; van Lancker et al., 1985). More specifically, they suggest that familiar-speaker recognition relies on a comparison to a stored prototype, whilst unfamiliar-speaker recognition relies on a perceptual pattern-matching process.

An early demonstration of the benefit of familiarity is provided by Hollien et al. (1982). They explored the capacity to recognize ten English speakers who were asked to speak in a normal, stressed, or disguised style. When the speakers spoke normally, recognition performance was near-perfect amongst listeners who knew the speakers. Moreover, it only fell to 79% when those speakers tried to disguise their voices. In contrast, those who did not know the speakers recognized only half of them when speaking normally, and were substantially affected by disguise.

Such a level of performance when recognizing familiar speakers is noteworthy. However, it may be wise to apply a degree of caution in assuming all familiar speakers to be this easily recognized. Indeed, Goldstein and Chance (1985) revealed a somewhat different picture. They asked twenty fraternity 'brothers' to identify twenty voices. Nine were drawn from their own fraternity and were thus familiar, whilst the remaining eleven were unfamiliar. Results showed that 60% of the participants could recognize all nine familiar voices. Moreover, six of the eleven unfamiliar voices were inappropriately recognized as members of the fraternity (see also Ladefoged, 1978; Rose & Duncan, 1995). On the one hand, one may view these results as being indicative of encouraging levels of performance, and indeed 60% of listeners showing perfect performance is impressive. However, these results also suggested that familiarity with a speaker is not a guarantee of good voice recognition.

Two further studies also serve to illustrate this point. First, Hughes and Nicholson (2010) showed a surprising level of performance in a test of own-voice recognition. In this study, participants listened to voices counting from one to ten so that content was constant and neutral. One of the voices was their own, and participants were asked to indicate whether each voice in the test set was theirs or not. Overall, performance again looks impressive with accuracy levels exceeding 90%. However, what was surprising in this study was that participants' recognition of their own voice was significantly worse (91%) than recognition of a voice as unfamiliar (98%). This occurred despite the assumption that their own voice would be of maximal familiarity and would thus elicit maximal accuracy in the recognition task. The authors note that the sound of one's own voice is usually perceived both through reverberation in the bones as well as through the airwaves (see Maurer & Landis, 1990). As such, one's own voice may sound different when played through speakers rather than when heard live, and a disruptive reaction ('that's not me!') may underlie the poor self-recognition results.

The second study of note avoids this issue and is provided by Ladefoged and Ladefoged (1980). They conducted a unique study in which one of the authors attempted to recognize twenty-nine familiar voices from speech clips of increasing length. The results showed improvement in the ability to recognize these voices as the clips got longer, with 31% accuracy from the single word 'hello', 66% accuracy from a single sentence, and 83% accuracy when presented with a full 30 seconds of continuous speech. Strikingly though, the participant was unable to recognize his own mother from 'hello' or from the single sentence, and was only able to signal her 'possible familiarity' from the longest clip available.

The results highlighted in this section, taken together, indicate that familiarity with a voice is an important factor in voice recognition—hence its use by the trial judge when determining admissibility. However, the present results also indicate that familiarity is not a guarantee of accurate recognition.

28.6 Why Are We Poor at Recognizing Voices—A Question of Priorities?

The example of Ladefoged (Ladefoged & Ladefoged, 1980) may indicate the importance of expectation when recognizing voices. Indeed, it is possible that Ladefoged did not expect his mother's voice to be in the corpus of voices to be recognized. In a similar vein, Fenn et al. (2011) showed blindness to a change of speaker during a telephone conversation—a finding that they attributed to an expectation that the speaker would not change mid-call. These findings serve as a reminder that voice recognition occurs in a social context, and that that context is important in determining performance levels.

In this regard, several explanations now exist to account for our relatively poor voice-recognition skills. First, and perhaps most influential, is the view of Belin and colleagues (2004, 2011). They described the voice as an 'auditory face' from which we are capable of extracting several strands of information: *speech* (what is said), *affect* (how it is said), and *identity* (who said it). This view is supported by the identification of anatomically distinct regions in the brain responsible for each processing strand. Moreover, clinical dissociations may be implied through the fact that aphasic patients have an inability to process speech content but can process vocal identity and affect, whereas phonagnosic patients have an inability to process vocal identity but can still process speech and affect (see Hailstone et al., 2010).

Belin's framework allows the conjecture that vocal identification is a difficult task because it may not be a priority. After all, the identification task can easily be achieved by looking at the face which, most of the time, accompanies the voice (Stevenage & Neil, 2014). Consequently, rather than processing the identity of a speaker from their voice, the priority may be to determine what they are saying (see Goggin et al., 1991) or how they are feeling (Scherer, 2003). This is a tempting conclusion; however, more and more research is emerging to suggest that the three processing strands of *speech, affect,* and *identity* may interact. Indeed, young adult listeners in particular appear to process voice segments simultaneously for both identity and speech (Naveh-Benjamin, 1996). In this vein, a body of evidence exists which confirms the interaction between speech strands. For instance, Nygaard and Kalish (1994) and Lander and Davies (2008) showed that, despite identity-related cues being irrelevant for the task at hand, familiarity with a speaker facilitates speech reading in hard-to-hear conditions. Similarly, several authors have shown that a change in speaker identity significantly impairs word memory (see Church & Schacter, 1994; Palmeri et al., 1993; Pollack et al., 1954; Sheffert & Fowler, 1995). In a more applied context, familiarity also helps in the tracking of a target speaker's message, and in dismissing a non-target speaker's message, amidst other voices (Johnsrude et al., 2013). These findings indicate that identity can affect speech processing, suggesting that vocal identity is not completely ignored when processing these other aspects of a voice.

Perhaps the most intriguing demonstration of this interaction is provided by Aruffo and Shore (2012). They revealed that identity can also affect perception of the well-known 'McGurk effect' (McGurk & MacDonald, 1976)—a speech-processing illusion in which the face is seen to say one thing ('ba') while the voice is heard to say another thing ('ga'). Traditionally, the observer resolves the incongruence by hearing either a blend 'da' or a combination 'bga' of the two percepts, and the illusion is so robust that the perceiver cannot override it even when they know its basis. However, Aruffo and Shore (2012) were interested in whether a participant would still be susceptible to the illusion when their own face and voice were used as stimuli. Their results indicated that the illusion was still exhibited when the participant's own face was paired with another voice. This was explained by the fact that participants do not often see their own faces speaking, and this lack of familiarity with the lip movements of their own face meant that the illusion persisted. In contrast, however, the strength of the illusion was significantly reduced when the participant's own voice was paired with another face, suggesting that the familiarity of the participant's own voice was able to influence speech processing even in this powerful illusory context. This provides a compelling indication that the identity and speech channels are not independent.

Given the literature reviewed, the identity of a voice appears to be processed alongside speech and affect, even when the processing of identity per se is not the priority. Accordingly, identity-related information is likely to be available to the listener. In this regard, in order to account for mistakes in a voice-recognition task one would have to assume that these identity cues receive *less* conscious attention compared to speech or affective cues.

28.7 REDUNDANCY OF VOCAL-IDENTITY INFORMATION?

The notion of relative importance in Belin's 'auditory faces' framework fits well alongside a second account of voice recognition. According to this second account, voice recognition is weak relative to face recognition because the identification of a target individual is so easily and so usually achieved from the accompanying face. Indeed, four lines of evidence now exist to suggest that recognition is consistently weaker from the voice than from the face. First, voices of familiar individuals elicit more 'familiar only' experiences in which the listener knows that they know the individual but cannot recall any further details (Ellis et al., 1997; Hanley et al., 1998). Second, voices elicit more tip-of-the-tongue states in which a listener knows exactly who the individual is but is unable to retrieve their name (Ellis et al., 1997). Third, voices prove to be weaker as a trigger for semantic information about an individual

(Barsics & Brédart, 2011, 2012; Brédart et al., 2009; Hanley & Damjanovic, 2009; Hanley et al., 1998), and when trying to remember episodic information about when that individual was last seen (Barsics & Brédart, 2011, 2012; Damjanovic & Hanley, 2007). Finally, even when voices are optimally presented, research shows them to be more vulnerable to distraction between study and test compared to faces (Stevenage et al., 2013). In fact, voice recognition and face recognition can only be equated when a substantial level of blurring is applied to reduce the quality of the face (Damjanovic & Hanley, 2007; Hanley & Damjanovic, 2009).

Two mechanisms have been offered to account for this weakness of voices compared to faces and, whilst not mutually exclusive, they have different characterizations (for a discussion, see Stevenage et al., 2012). First, relative to faces, our *ability* to discriminate between voices may be reduced (differential confusability). Second, relative to faces, our *need* to process identity from voices may be reduced (differential utilization).

Several literatures may lend support for the latter ideas, and each stem from the interaction that occurs when faces and voices are co-presented. Take, for instance, the results of a study by Stevenage et al. (2014) in which celebrity faces and voices were combined to form either congruous pairs (face and voice belonged to the same individual) or incongruous pairs (face and voice belonged to different individuals). When participants were asked to recognize the faces, the presence of an incongruous voice did not affect performance relative to the congruous condition. However, when asked to recognize the voices, performance was significantly and negatively affected by the co-presentation of an incongruous face, suggesting that the face dominated over the voice in the incongruous percept. This was taken by the authors to demonstrate the relative weakness of voices compared to faces for identification.

In a similar design, several studies now demonstrate what has come to be known as the 'facial overshadowing effect'. This reflects the fact that voice recognition is worse at test when the face accompanied the voice at study than when the voice was presented alone at study. Cook and Wilding (1997) demonstrated this effect by asking participants to study two voices (one male, one female) uttering a single sentence at study. One week later, the participants were asked to identify each speaker from a six-person target-present line-up. Study and test conditions varied in a complex design, but the important conditions for the purposes of this discussion included (i) study via audiovisual presentation followed by a voice test; and (ii) study via audio-only presentation followed by a voice test. The results indicated a measurable drop in performance when the face was present at study. This result is notable given its demonstration in a forensically realistic line-up test after a one-week delay, and a similar result is reported by Joassin et al. (2004). Interestingly, this effect was minimized when familiarity with the voice was increased (Cook & Wilding, 2001). However, it was not affected by an instruction to attend to the voice only.

Together, these results suggested that initial orientation to the face may be an unconscious and unstoppable action. Consequently, Cook and Wilding (2001) reasoned that if attention could be directed to the face *before* the voice was presented, then this may reduce or remove the facial overshadowing effect. The results completely supported this conjecture, suggesting that the overshadowing may arise from an automatic direction of attention to the face. By extension, this automatic orientation to the face may underpin its dominance in the more usual situation where face and voice are co-presented.

More recently, Tomlin (2015) has queried whether the facial overshadowing effect is truly the result of facial distraction at study, or whether overshadowing may be observed from *any* visual stimulus. In a well-controlled series of studies, participants were either asked to study a voice or a voice–face combination, prior to a same/different voice test. However, half the participants saw the faces presented upright (the standard facial overshadowing condition) and half the participants saw the faces presented inverted. Inversion provided a natural opportunity to test whether overshadowing was attributable to the face-ness or the visual-ness of the accompanying stimulus. The inverted faces were identical in complexity, luminance, and contrast to the upright faces, and yet were more difficult to perceive as meaningful faces when compared to upright faces (for a review of inversion effects, see Valentine, 1991). The results confirmed that the overshadowing effect only emerged in the standard face overshadowing condition; indeed, it was removed entirely when the accompanying faces were inverted. This suggested that the facial overshadowing effect arose because of the psychosocial significance of faces per se, rather than due to their visual nature. Equally, it suggested that the facial overshadowing effect could not be attributable to a simple dual-task cost when presented with both a face and a voice to study.

Consequently, whilst vocal identification may be a lower priority than speech and affect processing when listening to the voice, vocal identification may also be a less skilled, or overshadowed, task when the voice is presented alongside the face. These two explanations taken together may provide a useful account of the difficulties associated with voice recognition.

28.8 Voice Variability

The chapter so far has centred on the capacity of an earwitness to determine useful information about an individual from their voice. Whilst we have considered listener characteristics, voice-clip characteristics, and testing characteristics, there is one more source of variation that may be important to our understanding of voice recognition capability. In short, voice recognition may be relatively weak (compared to face recognition) because an individual can change their voice quite considerably at will. Given this, the current chapter ends with a consideration of vocal variation and disguise.

Useful in this regard is a paper that tests the influence of ten different vocal disguises on the capacity of an automated speaker recognition system (Zhang & Tan, 2008). These disguises include raising or lowering of the vocal pitch, and increasing or decreasing of speech rate, together with disguise by whispering, pinching the nose, applying masking tape to the mouth, holding a pencil between the teeth, speaking with chewing gum in the mouth, or speaking in an affected accent. The results suggested that whilst there was individual variation in the success with which a disguise may be achieved across different speakers, the performance of the automated system was most significantly impaired by disguise that substantially distorted either articulation or pitch cues. In this regard, the application of masking tape to the mouth and the use of whispers affected the automated system to the greatest extent, followed by raising the pitch, speaking with chewing gum, lowering the pitch, or speaking with a pinched nose or a pencil between the teeth. Alteration of speaking rate had a minimal effect perhaps because speaking rate has such high inter- and intra-speaker variability anyway. Similarly, within this study, alteration of accent had a minimal effect, as the system had been trained to have a world view of voices across language and accent.

These results are intriguing and raise the question of whether the human listener will be similarly affected by vocal variation or disguise compared to the automated system. In this regard, the empirical literature is surprisingly sparse, and much more attention is encouraged to this area of human voice processing. The available literature does, however, mirror the overall findings from the field of computer science. Indeed, Clifford (1980) notes recognition accuracy levels of 65% for a normal voice, versus 26% for a disguised voice (type of disguise left to the speaker), in a test where chance level performance was around 15%.

In some sense, this may be considered surprising, as intra-speaker variation is commonplace within our realm of human experience. Indeed, a single speaker may sound very different due to changes in health or emotional state. As such, one might consider that our voice-processing system should demonstrate greater tolerance if we are to recognize familiar speakers across these natural changes. Contrary to this assumption, empirical studies by Clifford and Denot (unpublished) and by Saslove and Yarmey (1980) both show impaired voice-recognition performance when the speaker's emotional state changed between study and test (angry–calm) relative to a no-change baseline (calm–calm). As such, the literature suggests that listeners are easily fooled by a change to an individual's voice even when that change arises through natural variation.

In a similar vein, evidence suggests that voice recognition may also be affected by the unconscious way in which our voices vary depending on who we are speaking with. The adoption of 'motherese' when speaking to an infant provides a case in point. Motherese is characterized by both a raised vocal pitch and an increase in intonation, creating a sing-song quality that infants preferentially orientate towards. In this particular example, infants at just one month of age can differentiate between an unfamiliar female when speaking in motherese and when speaking in an adult-directed manner (Panneton Cooper et al., 1997). These results suggest that we are sensitive to changes in vocal pitch and timing as they arise within a voice, and we differentiate between voices that vary on these dimensions. As a consequence, variation of a single speaker's voice along these dimensions may naturally and readily lead a listener to the mistaken conclusion that there are instead, two different speakers.

Finally within this section, it is important to consider the effect of non-malicious but intentional changes to the voice. Accordingly, a small set of studies has explored the effect of an intentional whisper on voice recognition. Whispering appears to be a particularly successful mode of disguise in that it can be performed by most speakers and effectively reduces the variation in pitch both between speakers and within a single speaker's utterance. It also is associated with a significant reduction in the ability to recognize a speaker (Orchard & Yarmey, 1995; Pollack et al., 1954; Yarmey et al., 2001). To put it into context, Pollack et al. (1954) reported that participants required a clip of three times the length if they were to identify a speaker from a whisper compared to a normal voice.

Taking this body of work together, it is clear that vocal variation, both between speakers and within speakers, can be considerable. If we assume that vocal identification is achieved through comparing an instance with some stored representation, the full tolerance required to enable us to identify an individual despite this variation may render our recognition system inefficient. Far more likely is a scenario in which reasonable tolerance bands are set for voice recognition, with the result that we are unlikely to be able to identify an individual speaker under all possible perturbations of their voice. Much more research is required to document and determine the extent of our human ability when recognizing disguised voices. Moreover, there would be clear value in extending that research to consider the recognition of intentionally and maliciously disguised voices as they may emerge in a forensic context.

28.9 Conclusion

In reviewing the body of research available to us, it is highly likely that our capacity when processing the voice is shaped by at least three factors. We have considered here the impact of the voice as a source of *identity*-related information, alongside *speech* and *affect*. We have considered also the relative value of the voice as a source of identity-related information compared to the face. Last but not least, we have considered the extent of variability, both intentional and unintentional, that makes the voice hard to identify. It is suggested here that all factors are important and combine to make vocal identification a task of some difficulty. So, should we trust the earwitness?

The answer to this question is necessarily conditional. We can trust the earwitness for some decisions such as those about the age, sex, and emotional state of the speaker. However, the extent to which we can trust them for other decisions linked to identity appears to depend on a host of factors to do with the speaker, the listener, and the precise listening and testing conditions. In light of the weight of evidence, some earwitness judgements will be more reliable than others. However, earwitness identification is likely to be problematic unless the most optimal of conditions have been available. The 'Turnbull direction' (see Section 28.2) to jurors reminds them of the need for caution in evaluating earwitness identifications in a court setting. However, it is prudent also to remember that earwitness evidence, if available, is just one line of evidence within an investigation. Indeed, in line with the UK Police and Criminal Evidence (PACE) guidelines (1984), no conviction can be made on the basis of witness evidence alone—additional forensic evidence is always required.

It is worthwhile, however, to reflect on an article by Hollien (2012) which offers thoughts as to the optimal methods for eliciting an earwitness identification. Based on his analysis, witness training is unlikely to make a substantial difference to witness reliability. However, the way in which an identification is conducted can be influential. Key in this regard is the importance of remembering that voices are not like faces. Thus, voice line-ups should not blindly mimic face line-ups. An optimal process will utilize a comprehensive review approach in which all line-up voices may be listened to and replayed before a decision is required. As with face line-ups, clear and unbiased instructions should allow witnesses to report that a voice is not in the line-up. However, most important in the line-up process is the construction of the line-up itself, taking due account of both the need for foils with a range of similarities to the target and of the conditions under which that target was initially experienced. Unclear at this stage is the response to factors such as the number and selection of foil speakers, the consideration of what the speakers say, and the response required when a suspect has a strong regional or national accent. These factors emerge as questions for future research if we are to work towards a complete understanding of vocal processing by the earwitness.

References

Amir, O., Engel, M., Shabtai, E., & Amir, N. (2011). Identification of children's gender and age by listeners. *Journal of Voice,* 26(3), 313–321. doi: 10.1016.j.jvoice.2011.06.001

Anastasi, J. S. & Rhodes, J. G. (2006). Evidence for an own-age bias in face recognition. *North American Journal of Psychology*, 8, 237–252.

Aruffo, C. & Shore, D. I. (2012). Can you McGurk yourself? Self-face and self-voice in audiovisual speech. *Psychonomic Bulletin and Review,* 19, 66–72. doi: 10.3758/s13423-011-0176-8

Barkhuysen, P., Krahmer, E., & Swerts, M. (2010). Crossmodal and incremental perception of audiovisual cues to emotional speech. *Language and Speech,* 53(1), 3–30. doi: 10.1177/0023830909348993

Barsics, C. & Brédart, S. (2011). Recalling episodic information about personally known faces and voices. *Consciousness and Cognition,* 20, 303–308. doi: 10.1016/j.concog.2010.03.008

Barsics, C. & Brédart, S. (2012). Recalling semantic information about newly learned faces and voices. *Memory,* 20(5), 527–534. doi: 10.1080/09658211.2012.683012

Belin, P., Bestelmeyer, P. E. G., Latinus, M., & Watson, R. (2011). Understanding voice perception. *British Journal of Psychology,* 102, 711–725. doi: 10.1111/j.2044-8295.2011.02041.x

Belin, P., Fecteau, S., & Bédard, C. (2004). Thinking the voice: neural correlates of voice perception. *Trends in Cognitive Sciences,* 8(3), 129–135.

Brédart, S. & Barsics, C. (2012). Recalling semantic and episodic information from faces and voices: a face advantage. *Current Directions in Psychological Science,* 21(6), 378–381.

Brédart, S., Barsics, C., & Hanley, R. (2009). Recalling semantic information about personally known faces and voices. *European Journal of Cognitive Psychology,* 21(7), 1013–1021. doi: 10.1080/09541440802591821

Brown, R. (1981). An experimental study of the relative importance of acoustic parameters for auditory speaker recognition. *Language and Speech,* 24(4), 295–310.

Church, B. A. & Schacter, D. L. (1994). Perceptual specificity of auditory priming: implicit memory for voice intonation and fundamental frequency. *Journal of Experimental Psychology: Learning, Memory and Cognition,* 20, 521–533.

Clifford, B. R. (1980). Voice identification by human listeners. *Law and Human Behavior,* 4(4), 373–394.

Clifford, B. R. & Denot, H. (unpublished). *Visual and Verbal Testimony and Identification under Conditions of Stress.*

Clifford, B. R., Rathborn, H., & Bull, R. (1981). The effects of delay on voice recognition accuracy. *Law and Human Behavior,* 5(2–3), 201–208.

Cook, S. & Wilding, J. (1997). Earwitness testimony 2: voices, faces and context. *Applied Cognitive Psychology,* 11, 527–541.

Cook, S. & Wilding, J. (2001). Earwitness testimony: effects of exposure and attention on the face overshadowing effect. *British Journal of Psychology,* 92, 617–629.

Damjanovic, L. & Hanley, J. R. (2007). Recalling episodic and semantic information about famous faces and voices. *Memory and Cognition,* 35(6), 1205–1210. doi: 10.3758/BF03193594

Del Mar Vanrell, M., Mascaró, I., Torres-Tamarit, F., & Prieto, P. (2012). Intonation as an encoder of speaker-certainty: information and confirmation yes-no questions in Catalan. *Language and Speech,* 56(2), 163–190. doi: 10.1177/0023830912443942

Ekman, P. & Friesen, W. (1971). Constants across cultures in the face and emotion. *Journal of Personality and Social Psychology,* 17(2), 124–129.

Ellis, H. D., Jones, D. M., & Mosdell, N. (1997). Intra- and inter-modal repetition priming of familiar faces and voices. *British Journal of Psychology,* 88, 143–156.

Fenn, K. M., Shintel, H., Atkins, A. S., Skipper, J. I., Bond, V. C., & Nusbaum, H. C. (2011). When less is heard than meets the ear: change deafness in a telephone conversation. *Quarterly Journal of Experimental Psychology,* 64(7), 1442–1456.

Fleming, D., Giordano, B. L., Caldara, R., & Belin, P. (2014). A language-familiarity effect for speaker discrimination without comprehension. *PNAS,* 111(38), 13795–13798. doi: 10.1073/pnas.14013853111

Goggin, J. P., Thompson, C. P., Strube, G., & Simental, L. R. (1991). The role of language familiarity in voice identification. *Memory and Cognition,* 19, 448–458.

Goldstein, A. G. & Chance, J. E. (1985). *Voice Recognition: The Effects of Faces, Temporal Distribution of 'Practice' and Social Distance.* Paper presented at the Annual Meeting of the Midwestern Psychology Association, Chicago, IL.

Gonzalez, J. (2003). Estimation of speakers' weight and height from speech: a re-analysis of data from multiple studies by Lass and colleagues. *Perceptual Motor Skills,* 96, 297–304.

Hailstone, J. C., Crutch, S. J., Bestergaard, M. D., Patterson, R. D., & Warren, J. D. (2010). Progressive associative phonagnosia: a neuropsychological analysis. *Neuropsychologia,* 48, 1104–1114.

Hammersley, R. & Read, J. D. (1985). The effect of participation in a conversation on recognition and identification of the speakers' voices. *Law and Human Behavior,* 9(1), 71–81.

Hanley, J. R. & Damjanovic, L. (2009). It is more difficult to retrieve a familiar person's name and occupation from their voice than from their blurred face. *Memory,* 17, 830–839.

Hanley, J. R., Smith S. T., & Hadfield, J. (1998). I recognize you but can't place you. An investigation of familiar-only experiences during tests of voice and face recognition. *Quarterly Journal of Experimental Psychology,* 51A(1), 179–195.

Hollien, H. (2012). On earwitness line-ups. *Investigative Sciences Journal,* 4(1), 1–17.

Hollien, H., Majewski, W., & Doherty, E. T. (1982). Perceptual identification of voices under normal, stress and disguise speaking conditions. *Journal of Phonetics,* 10(2), 139–148.

Hughes, S. M. & Nicholson, S. E. (2010). The processing of auditory and visual recognition of self-stimuli. *Consciousness and Cognition,* 19, 1124–1134. doi: 10.1016/jconcog.2010.03.001

Hughes, S. & Rhodes, B. C. (2010). Making age assessments based on voice: the impact of the reproductive viability of the speaker. *Journal of Social, Evolutionary and Cultural Psychology,* 4, 290–304. doi: 10.1037/h0099282

Joassin, F., Maurage, P., Bruyer, R., Crommelinck, M., & Campanella, S. (2004). When audition alters vision: an event-related potential study of the cross-modal interactions between faces and voices. *Neuroscience Letters,* 369, 132–137.

Johnson, E. K., Westrek, E., Nazzi, T., & Cutler, A. (2011). Infant ability to tell voices apart rests on language experience. *Developmental Science,* 14(5), 1002–1011. doi: 10.1111/j.1467-7687.2001.01052x

Johnsrude, I. S., Mackey, A., Hakyemez., H., Alexander, E., Trang, H. P., & Carlyon, R. P. (2013). Swinging at a cocktail party: voice familiarity aids speech perception in the presence of a competing voice. *Psychological Science,* 24(10), 1995–2004. doi: 10.1177/0956797613482467

Kemper, S., Herman, R. E., & Lian, C. H. T. (2003). The cost of doing two things at once for young and older adults: talking while walking, finger tapping and ignoring speech of noise. *Psychology and Aging,* 18, 181–192. doi: 10.1037/0882-7974.18.2.181

Kersta, L. G. (1962). Voiceprint identification. *Nature,* 196, 1253–1257.

Kisilevsky, B. S., Hains, S. M. J., Brown, C. A., Lee, C. T., Cowperthwaite, B., Stutzman, S. S., … Wang, Z. (2009). Fetal sensitivity to properties of maternal speech and language. *Infant Behavior and Development,* 32, 59–71. doi: 10.1016/jinfbeh.2008.10.002

Klingholz, F., Penning, R., & Liebhardt, E. (1988). Recognition of low-level alcohol intoxication from speech signal. *Journal of Acoustical Society of America,* 84(3), 929–935. doi: 0001-4966/88/090929-07

Ladefoged, P. (1978). Expectation affects identification by listening. *UCLA Working Papers in Phonetics,* 41, 41–42.

Ladefoged, P. & Ladefoged, J. (1980). The ability of listeners to identify voices. *UCLA Working Papers in Phonetics,* 49, 43–51.

Lander, K. & Davies, R. (2008). Does face familiarity influence speech readability? *Quarterly Journal of Experimental Psychology*, 61(7), 961–967. doi: 10.1080.17470210801908476

Laukka, P., Linnman, C., Åhs, F., Pissiota, A., Frans, Ö., Faria, V., ... Furmark, T. (2008). In a nervous voice: acoustic analysis and perception of anxiety in social phobics' speech. *Journal of Nonverbal Behaviour*, 32, 195–214. doi: 10.1007/s10919-008-005-9

McGehee, F. (1937). The reliability of identification of the human voice. *Journal of General Psychology*, 27, 249–271.

McGurk, H. & MacDonald, J. (1976). Hearing lips and seeing voices. *Nature*, 264, 746–748.

Maurer, D. & Landis, T. (1990). Role of bone conduction in the self-perception of speech. *Folia Phoniatrica*, 42, 226–229.

Moyse, E. (2014). Age estimation from faces and voices: a review. *Psychologica Belgica*, 54(3), 255–265. doi: http://dx.doi.org/10.5332/pb.aq

Moyse, E., Beaufort, A., & Brédart, S. (2014). Evidence for an own-age bias in age estimation from voices in older persons. *European Journal of Ageing*, 11(3), 241–247. doi: 10.1007/s10433-014-0305-0

Mullenix, J. W., Ross, A., Smith, C., Kuykendall, D., Conard, J., & Barb, S. (2011). Typicality effects on memory for voice: implications for earwitness testimony. *Applied Cognitive Psychology*, 25(1), 29–34. doi: 10.1002/acp.1635

Naveh-Benjamin, M. (1996). Effects of perceptual and conceptual processing on memory for words and voice: different patterns for young and old. *Quarterly Journal of Experimental Psychology, A*, 49(3), 780–796. doi: 10.1080/713755640

Nygaard, L. C. & Kalish, M. L. (1994). Modelling the effect of learning voices on the perception of speech. *Journal of the Acoustical Society of America*, 95, 2873.

Orchard, T. & Yarmey, A. D. (1995). The effects of whispers, voice sample duration, and voice distinctiveness on criminal speaker identification. *Applied Cognitive Psychology*, 9(3), 249–260.

Ormerod, D. (2001). Sounds familiar? Voice identification evidence. *Criminal Law Review*, August, 595–622.

Palmeri, T. J., Goldinger, S. D., & Pisoni, D. B. (1993). Episodic encoding of voice attributes and recognition memory for spoken words. *Journal of Experimental Psychology: Learning, Memory and Cognition*, 19(2), 309–328.

Panneton Cooper, R., Abraham, J., Berman, S., & Staska, M. (1997). The development of infants' preference for motherese. *Infant Behavior and Development*, 20(4), 477–488.

Papcun, G., Kreiman, J., & Davis, A. (1989). Long-term memory for unfamiliar voices. *Journal of the Acoustical Society of America*, 85(2), 913–925.

Pell, M. C. & Kotz, S. A. (2011). On the time course of vocal emotion recognition. *PLoS One*, 6(11), e27256. doi: 10.1371/journal.pone.0027256

Pell, M. C., Monetta, L., Paulmann, S., & Kotz, S. A. (2009). Recognizing emotions in a foreign language. *Journal of Nonverbal Behaviour*, 33, 107–120. doi: 10.1007/s10919-008-0065-7

Phillipon, A. C., Cherryman, J., Bull, R., & Vrij, A. (2007). Earwitness identification performance: the effect of language, threat, deliberate strategies and indirect measures. *Applied Cognitive Psychology*, 21, 539–550. doi: 10.1002/acp.1296

Police and Criminal Evidence Act (1984). https://www.gov.uk/guidance/police-and-criminal-evidence-act-1984-pace-codes-of-practice [Accessed: 27th November, 2015]

Pollack, L., Pickett, J. M., & Sumby, W. H. (1954). On the identification of speakers by voice. *Journal of the Acoustical Society of America*, 26, 403–406.

Ptacek, P. H. & Sander, E. K. (1966). Age recognition from voice. *Journal of Speech and Hearing Research*, 9, 273–277.

R v *Hersey* [1998]. Crim LR 281.

R v *O'Doherty* [2002]. NI 263.

R v *Turnbull* [1977]. QB 224.

Read, D. & Craik, F. I. M. (1995). Earwitness identification: some influences on voice recognition. *Journal of Experimental Psychology: Applied*, 1(1), 6–18.

Rose, P. & Duncan, S. (1995). Naïve auditory identification and discrimination of similar voices by familiar listeners. *Forensic Linguistics*, 10, 1–17.

Saslove, H. & Yarmey, A. D. (1980). Long-term auditory memory: speaker identification. *Journal of Applied Psychology*, 65(1), 111–116.

Scherer, K. R. (2003). Vocal communication of emotion: a review of research paradigms. *Speech Communication*, 40, 227–256.

Scherer, K. R., Banse, R., & Wallbott, H. (2001). Emotion inferences from vocal expression correlate across languages and cultures. *Journal of Cross-Cultural Psychology*, 32, 76–92.

Sheffert, S. M. & Fowler, C. A. (1995). The effects of voice and visible speaker change on memory for spoken words. *Journal of Memory and Language*, 34, 665–685.

Skoog Waller, S., Eriksson, M., & Sörqvist, P. (2015). Can you hear my age? Influences of speech rate and speech spontaneity on estimation of speaker age. *Frontiers in Psychology*, 6, 978. doi: 10.3389/fpsyg.2015.00978

Skuk, V. G. & Schweinberger, S. R. (2013). Gender differences in familiar voice identification. *Hearing Research*, 296, 131–140. doi: 10.1016/j.heares.2012.11.004

Stevenage, S. V., Hugill, A. R., & Lewis, H. (2012). Integrating voice recognition into models of person perception. *Journal of Cognitive Psychology*, 24(4), 409–419. doi: http://dx.doi.org/10.1080/20445911.2011.642859

Stevenage, S. V. & Neil, G. J. (2014). Hearing faces and seeing voices: the integration and interaction of face and voice processing. *Psychologica Belgica*, 54(3), 266–281. doi: http://dx.doi.org/10.5334/pb.ar

Stevenage., S. V., Neil, G. J., Barlow, J., Dyson, A., Eaton-Brown, C., & Parsons, B. (2013). The effect of distraction on face and voice recognition. *Psychological Research*, 77(2), 167–175. doi: http://dx.doi.org/10.1007.s00425-012-0450-z

Stevenage. S. V., Neil, G. J., & Hamlin, I. (2014). When the face fits: recognition of celebrities from matching and mismatching faces and voices. *Memory*, 22(3), 284–294. doi: http://dx.doi.org/10.1080/09658211.2013.781654

Tomlin, R., Stevenage, S. V., & Hammond, S. (2016). Putting the pieces together: Revealing face-voice integration through the facial overshadowing effect. *Visual Cognition*. doi: http://dx.doi.org/10.1080/13506285.2016.1245230

Trehub, S. E., Plantinga, J., & Brcic, J. (2009). Infants detect cross-modal cues to identity in speech and singing. *The Neurosciences and Music III: Disorders and Plasticity*, 1169, 508–511. doi: 10.1111/j.1749-6632.2009.04851.x

Valentine, T. (1991). A unified account of the effects of distinctiveness, inversion and race in face recognition. *Quarterly Journal of Experimental Psychology*, 43A, 161–204. doi: http://dx.doi.org/10.1080/14640849108400966

Van Dommelen, W. A. (1990). Acoustic parameters in human speaker recognition. *Language and Speech*, 33(3), 259–272.

van Lancker, D., Kreiman, J., & Emmorey, K. (1985). Familiar voice recognition: patterns and parameters. Part I: recognition of backwards voices. *Journal of Phonetics*, 13, 19–38.

Weinberg, B. & Bennett, S. (1971). Speaker sex recognition of 5- and 6-year-old children's voices. *Journal of the Acoustical Society of America*, 50(4 part 2), 1210–1213.

Yarmey, A. D. (1991). Descriptions of distinctive and non-distinctive voices over time. *Journal of the Forensic Sciences Society,* 31(4), 421–428.

Yarmey, A. D. (1995). Earwitness speaker identification. *Psychology, Public Policy and Law,* 1(4), 792–816.

Yarmey, A. D. & Matthys, E. (1991). Voice identification of an abductor. *Applied Cognitive Psychology,* 6(5), 367–377.

Yarmey, A. D., Yarmey, A. L., Yarmey, M. J., & Parliament, L. (2001). Commonsense beliefs and the identification of familiar voices. *Applied Cognitive Psychology,* 15, 283–299. doi: 10.1002/acp.702

Zhang, C. & Tan, T. (2008). Voice disguise and automatic speaker recognition. *Forensic Science International,* 175, 118–122. doi: 10.1061/j.forsciint.2007.05.019.

CHAPTER 29

....

VOICES IN THE CONTEXT OF HUMAN FACES AND BODIES

....

BENJAMIN KREIFELTS AND THOMAS ETHOFER

29.1 INTRODUCTION

IN everyday life, perception is driven by more than one sensory channel, and thus integration of information across sensory modalities is rather the rule than the exception. In this chapter, we review recent studies regarding the neural correlates of multimodal integration of emotional information derived from faces, voices, and bodies.

Integration of information obtained via different sensory channels usually improves accuracy and shortens response latencies (Schroger & Widmann, 1998). This is of particular importance for emotional signals as they can indicate information which is crucial for the survival of the individual or for successful interaction within social groups.

29.2 VOICES AND FACES—BEHAVIOURAL EFFECTS

At the behavioural level, audiovisual emotions are classified faster and with higher accuracy than emotional signals which are exclusively presented via the auditory or visual modality (Collignon et al., 2008; Kreifelts et al., 2007; see Video 29.1 for example stimuli). Such integration effects remain intact over a long lifespan (Lambrecht et al., 2012) and are more pronounced in women than in men (Collignon et al., 2010). Several studies have documented facilitated processing of emotional signals for stimuli carrying congruent versus incongruent information across facial expressions and speech melody (de Gelder & Vroomen, 2000; Dolan et al., 2001; Massaro & Egan, 1996). Furthermore, emotions perceived via one modality have the potential to influence perception of affective information in other sensory modalities (de Gelder & Vroomen, 2000; Ethofer, Anders, Erb, et al., 2006; Massaro & Egan,

1996). Such crossmodal biases occur mostly in an automatic manner (Collignon et al., 2008; de Gelder & Vroomen, 2000; Ethofer, Anders, Erb, et al., 2006; Focker et al., 2011; Vroomen et al., 2001) and irrespective of the social context (Piwek et al., 2015), but can be modulated at least to some extent by attentional resources (Takagi et al., 2015).

29.3 Voices and Faces—Electrophysiological Studies

Several studies investigating event-related potentials (ERPs) (i.e. recording of electric brain responses over the human scalp) by means of electroencephalography (EEG) and magnetencephalography (MEG) have been conducted and have compared time courses of stimuli, with congruent to incongruent stimuli (i.e. same versus different emotions expressed in voice and face), to determine the exact onset of interactions. Incongruent non-verbal emotional information from voice and face yielded a mismatch negativity response about 180 ms after stimulation onset, indicating an early modulation of auditory processing by conflicting visual information (de Gelder et al., 1999). Further support for such early effects has been described in a subsequent study which demonstrated that the auditory N1 component at around 110 ms after onset of an emotional voice is enhanced by an emotionally congruent facial expression. This effect, however, only occurred for upright faces and was abolished by inversion (Pourtois et al., 2000), a manipulation which effectively hinders recognition of emotional facial expressions (White, 1999). Thus, the authors of this study concluded that the N1 enhancement is driven by perceived facial emotion and not by low-level visual features of the stimuli. Results obtained in cortical blind patients demonstrated a modulation of the N1 component by congruent faces, but not pictures (de Gelder et al., 2002), which indicates binding of emotions in face–voice combinations independent of an intact striate cortex.

Comparison of ERPs to face–voice combinations versus voice stimuli resulted in a strong reduction of the N100 amplitude, lending further support to early crossmodal interactions (Jessen & Kotz, 2011; Kokinous et al., 2015; see also Figure 29.1). Emotionally-congruent stimuli also yielded a shorter latency of the positive deflection following the N1-P1 component about 220 ms post stimulus onset (Pourtois et al., 2002) and might constitute an electrophysiological correlate of faster responses to emotionally-congruent as compared to emotionally-incongruent audiovisual information (de Gelder & Vroomen, 2000; Dolan et al., 2001; Massaro & Egan, 1996). Modulations of early ERP components by congruity of non-verbal emotional information across the auditory and visual modalities can be already demonstrated in 7-month-old infants (Grossmann et al., 2006). This indicates that integration and recognition of audiovisual emotional signals is already possible at early developmental stages. Modulations of ERP responses to emotional prosody occur even during unconscious presentation of emotional faces, arguing for a mandatory process (Doi & Shinohara, 2015).

In summary, results from ERP studies argue for an early and automatic multisensory crosstalk of about 110–220 ms for congruency effects, while differentiation between emotional and neutral stimuli appears to occur at later stages including P200, P300, and N250

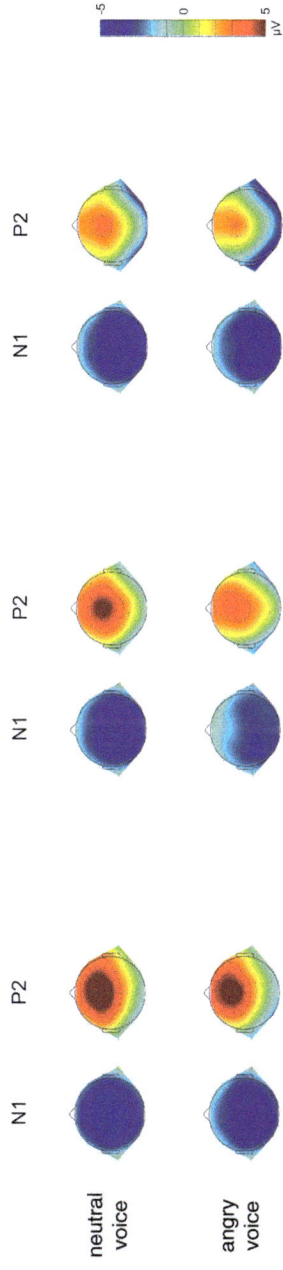

FIGURE 29.1 Modulation of auditory N1 and P2 suppression by audiovisual congruency. N1–P2 complex of the auditory evoked potential (AEP) to voice onset (top) and corresponding voltage distributions (bottom) for the two emotion categories (neutral voice, solid line; angry voice, dotted line) in the different visual context conditions (left: auditory-only; middle: audiovisual-congruent; right: audiovisual-incongruent). N1 topographies are plotted in time windows centred on the individual condition peaks ± 20 ms; P2 topographies are plotted from 177–217 ms for neutral and from 205–245 ms for angry conditions.

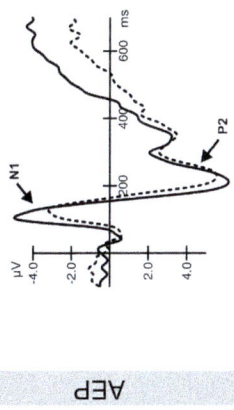

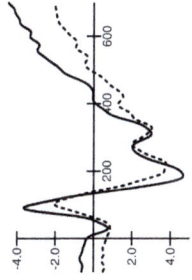

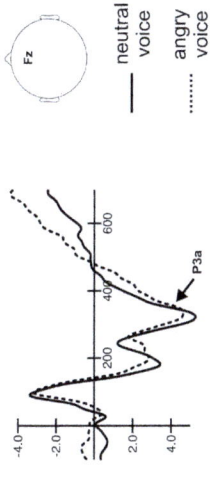

Adapted from Kokinous J., Kotz S.A., Tavano A., & Schröger E., 'The role of emotion in dynamic audiovisual integration of faces and voices', Social Cognitive and Affective Neuroscience, Volume 10, Issue 5, pp. 713–20, doi: 10.1093/scan/nsu105, by permission of Oxford University Press.

(Ho et al., 2015; Liu et al., 2012). MEG studies, including source localization, revealed the right posterior temporal sulcus (pSTS) as a possible neural substrate for audiovisual integration processes concerning facial and vocal emotions (Hagan et al., 2009), while no crossmodal effects were observed within unisensory areas (Chen et al., 2010).

29.4 Voices and Faces—
Neuroimaging Studies

29.4.1 Face-Voice Integration in the Right Posterior Temporal Sulcus

There is a large body of neuroimaging evidence implicating the cortex adjacent to the pSTS as the central module of audiovisual integration processes. This has been demonstrated for a large variety of stimuli including animals (Beauchamp, Lee, et al., 2004), tools (Beauchamp, Argall, et al., 2004), speech (Wright et al., 2003), letters (van Atteveldt et al., 2004), and emotional information in face–voice combinations (Ethofer, Pourtois, & Wildgruber, 2006; Kreifelts et al., 2007; Pourtois et al., 2005; Robins et al., 2009) which is in line with data from animal studies indicating converging projections to the pSTS from visual and auditory areas (Jones & Powell, 1970; Seltzer & Pandya, 1978). Inhibitory stimulation of this area by transcranial direct current stimulation (tDCS) can disrupt speech recognition of auditory as well as visual stimuli (Riedel et al., 2015). It has to be acknowledged, however, that the superior temporal sulcus (STS) is a structure with high inter-individual variability (Ochiai et al., 2004), which is not fully accounted for in group studies relying on 3D-normalization techniques as implemented, for example, in Statistical Parametric Mapping (SPM) software (Ashburner & Friston, 2005).

A functional magnetic resonance imaging (fMRI) study, aiming at a precise localization of the audiovisual integration area within the pSTS and specifically addressing this inter-individual variance, revealed that the audiovisual integration area within the pSTS can be pinpointed at the bifurcation of the STS in its two posterior-ascending branches and arises exactly at a spatial overlap of the voice-sensitive region in the mid portion (or posterior trunk section) of the STS and the face-sensitive region in the posterior-ascending branch of the STS in its posterior section (Kreifelts et al., 2009; see also Figure 29.2).

There has been much debate in the past concerning the correct statistical criteria for localizing multisensory areas (Beauchamp, 2005; Ethofer, Pourtois, & Wildgruber, 2006) with fMRI. Electrophysiological results obtained by magnetencephalography revealed supra-additive responses (Hagan et al., 2009) to audiovisual stimuli. The supra-additivity criterion demands that the response to audiovisual stimuli (AV) is larger than the sum of responses to visual (V) and auditory (A) stimuli: AV > A + V. Haemodynamic responses of the pSTS measured by fMRI, however, typically revealed much lower signal amplitudes to AV stimuli. Thus, most studies on audiovisual integration in fMRI studies rely on the so-called maximum criterion which demands that the response to AV stimuli be larger than the maximum of A and V responses: AV > max (A, V). Within the framework of neuroimaging studies, this is typically investigated by conjunction contrasts (Nichols et al., 2005): AV—A ∩ AV—V.

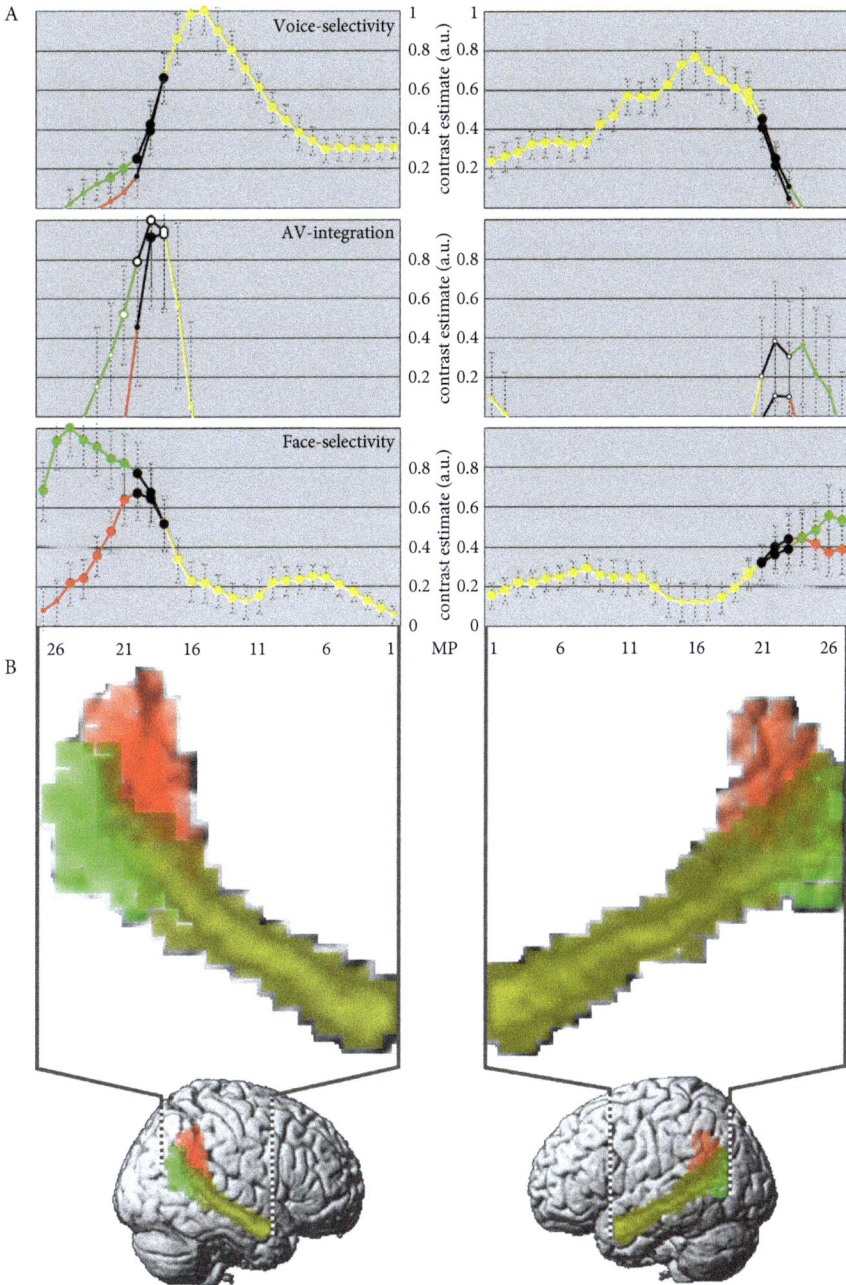

FIGURE 29.2 Cerebral correlates of voice selectivity, audiovisual integration of non-verbal emotional information, and face selectivity along the superior temporal sulcus. (A) Peak-normalized beta estimates (a.u.) for voice selectivity, audiovisual integration, and face selectivity for twenty-seven measuring points along the superior temporal sulcus. Error bars represent the SEM. Large dots stand for significant results with p < 0.05 in a one-sample t-test across subjects, while small dots denote non-significant results. Additional central white dots represent a significant positive correlation (p < 0.05) between the individual

One possible explanation for smaller enhancement of fMRI responses to AV stimuli is the non-linearity regarding the neurovascular coupling of the blood-oxygen-level dependent (BOLD) effects, and it has been demonstrated that the BOLD response to two stimuli in temporal proximity is strongly overpredicted by summing the responses to the two stimuli presented in isolation (Friston et al., 1998; Mechelli et al., 2001). Other explanations include the fact that less than 25% of the neurons in multisensory regions are responsive to stimuli from more than one sensory modality (Wallace et al., 1992), and that these neurons are distributed in an intertwined and overlapping fashion (Romanski, 2012) resulting in a patchy distribution of fMRI responses in the pSTS (Beauchamp, Argall, et al., 2004).

The participation of the pSTS audiovisual integration area, located at the bifurcation of the STS, in processing affective information has been established on several levels. First, it responds stronger to AV stimuli that express emotional information, and this has been demonstrated for a broad variety of emotional categories (Jansma et al., 2014; Kreifelts et al., 2007). Second, activation in pSTS to AV stimuli is correlated with the gain in behavioural accuracy for correct classification of the expressed emotions through audiovisual integration (Kreifelts et al., 2007). Third, the right pSTS is the only region that shows a correlation between emotional intelligence, as obtained by the self-report emotional intelligence test (Schutte et al., 1998), and haemodynamic responses of the audiovisual integration effect (Kreifelts et al., 2010). Fourth, the right pSTS shows specific adaptation effects in a continuous carry-over design. That is, fMRI amplitude in this area was diminished in response to stimuli in which the emotion in facial expressions was similar to the vocal emotion of the preceding stimulus (Watson et al., 2014).

29.4.2 Connectivity of the Right Posterior Temporal Sulcus

While these studies provide compelling evidence for the involvement of pSTS cortices in various aspects of audiovisual integration and also for specific contributions to judgement of emotional signals, it is less clear how the pSTS interacts with other brain areas during these processes. According to a model on integration of face and voice in person perception (Campanella & Belin, 2007), integration of vocal and facial affective cues is accomplished by heteromodal areas in the pSTS which exert a top–down control on unimodal areas for

---

integration effect, AV—max (A, V) and trait emotional intelligence, as estimated by the self-report emotional intelligence test. (B) Representation of the inter-individual variability of the superior temporal sulcus as a probability map (n = 24) superimposed on a standard brain. Yellow = trunk section of the STS, red = anterior terminal ascending branch of the STS, green = posterior terminal ascending branch of the STS. Stronger colours denote higher probabilities, indicating an increasing spatial variability in the course of the STS from the trunk section to the branches. Same colour code as in (A).

Adapted from *Neuropsychologia*, Volume 47, Issue 14, Kreifelts B., Ethofer T., Shiozawa T., Grodd W., & Wildgruber D., 'Cerebral representation of non-verbal emotional perception: fMRI reveals audiovisual integration area between voice- and face-sensitive regions in the superior temporal sulcus', pp. 3059–66, Copyright © 2009 Elsevier Ltd, with permission from Elsevier, http://www.sciencedirect.com/science/article/pii/S0028393209002930

processing of emotional signals, such as extrastriate fusiform gyrus (FG) (Surguladze et al., 2003; Vuilleumier et al., 2001), as well as associative auditory cortex in the middle part of the superior temporal sulcus (mSTS) (Ethofer, Anders, Wiethoff, et al., 2006; Ethofer et al., 2007; Grandjean et al., 2005; Wiethoff et al., 2008). In line with this hypothesis, psycho-physiological interaction (PPI) analyses (Friston et al., 1997) revealed enhanced connectivity between the pSTS to FG and mSTS areas during perception of audiovisual emotional information (Kreifelts et al., 2007).

A diffusion tensor imaging (DTI) study (Ethofer et al., 2013; see also Figure 29.3) specifically addressing the structural connectivity profile of areas for unimodal voice and face perception, as well as audiovisual integration of facial and vocal affective cues, revealed a strong connectivity of pSTS areas with associative auditory cortices in the mSTS, but not the FG. These findings converge with the view of separable pathways for processing of invariant facial features in the FG and changeable aspects, such as emotional expressions, in the STS (Haxby et al., 2000), while functional interactions between FG and STS areas are probably mediated by back-projections to earlier visual areas, such as the occipital face area. As a possible output projection of the audiovisual integration area in the pSTS, consistent fibre projections along the ventral part of the superior longitudinal fasciculus (SLF) towards inferior frontal cortex areas were identified (Ethofer et al., 2013)—a structural connection which was also implicated in processing social cues in gaze movements (Ethofer et al., 2011). The inferior frontal cortex (IFC) showed a consistent repetition-suppression effect for AV trials (Ethofer et al., 2013), replicating previous results on specific adaptation effects during perception of emotional prosody (Ethofer, Kreifelts, et al., 2009), which is in line with animal data proposing convergent visual and auditory projections to this area (Chavis & Pandya, 1976; Jones & Powell, 1970).

These combined structural and functional data point to a key role of the IFG for judgement and integration of emotional signals in prosody and facial expressions, as a module within the extended system for face and voice perception. Further evidence for such distributed systems comes from a recent study using multivoxel pattern analysis (Li et al., 2015)—a technique that can be used to identify the perceived emotion based on the spatial activation profile across voxels in voices (Ethofer, Van de Ville, et al., 2009) and faces (Said et al., 2010). This study revealed that the decoding accuracy is enhanced for audiovisual trials, and that the informative voxels are not restricted to STS areas but are also found in right FG as well as bilateral frontal areas.

29.4.3 The Amygdala

Another area which has been repeatedly demonstrated to participate in multimodal integration processes is the amygdala, which also receives converging visual and auditory projections (McDonald, 1998; Murray & Mishkin, 1985; Pitkänen, 2000). Neuroimaging studies in humans demonstrated enhanced responses to emotional faces (Breiter et al., 1996; Morris et al., 1996) and voices (Wiethoff et al., 2009). A pioneering study relying on comparison of emotionally-congruent versus incongruent signals in voice and face (pairings of fear and happiness expressed by facial expression and prosody) revealed increased activation to congruent stimuli, which was particularly pronounced if fear was expressed in both sensory modalities (Dolan et al., 2001).

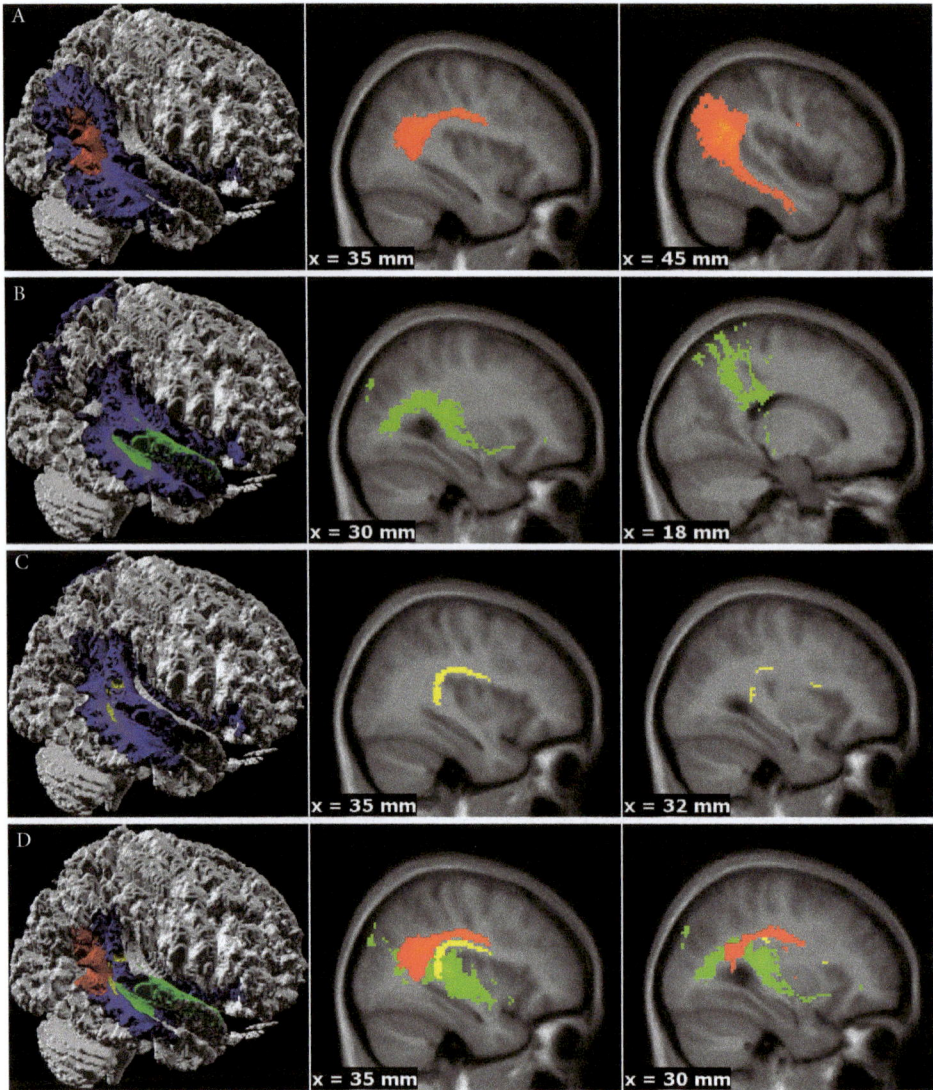

FIGURE 29.3 Structural connection profile of the face-sensitive (A), voice-sensitive (B), and audiovisual integration areas (C) along the right STS and conjunction of projections from these three brain areas (D) displayed on the border between grey and white matter of the 3D mean-normalized T1-weighted image. Brain regions showing consistent fibre connections in more than half of the participants are shown in blue (left panels). Statistical comparison of fibre pathways revealed predominant projections along the dorsal superior longitudinal fasciculus for the face-selective areas (red), external capsule for voice-selective areas (green), and ventral superior longitudinal fasciculus for audiovisual integration areas (yellow).

Reprinted from *NeuroImage*, Volume 76, Ethofer T. et al., 'Functional responses and structural connections of cortical areas for processing faces and voices in the superior temporal sulcus', pp. 45–56, Copyright © 2013 Elsevier Inc., with permission from Elsevier, http://www.sciencedirect.com/science/article/pii/S105381191300219X

A particular role for binding emotional information in voice and face for fear has been further established by demonstrating that the response amplitude in the left amygdala correlates with a more negative evaluation of neural and fearful facial expressions in the presence of fearful (but not happy) prosody (Ethofer, Anders, Erb, et al., 2006). The right FG also showed a modulation of its responses to faces in the presence of fearful prosody, and a PPI analysis confirmed increased connectivity between left amygdala and right FG during perception of fearful voices (Ethofer, Pourtois, & Wildgruber, 2006).

A recent study, using Granger causality mapping (Roebroeck et al., 2005) to investigate flow of information processing across different brain areas using the amygdala as seed regions, replicated this finding, demonstrating that the amygdala receive input from the right FG, but also other areas including STS, IFG, putamen, thalamus, anterior and posterior cingulate cortex, as well as temporal pole areas (Jansma et al., 2014). A similar set of brain areas has been found in a study addressing responses to congruent emotional face–voice combinations (Klasen et al., 2011), while incongruent stimuli yielded enhanced activation in a cingulate-fronto-parietal network involved in conflict monitoring and resolution (Müller et al., 2011). A recent study also suggested that anterior cingulate cortex and anterior insula provide feedback during detection of mismatch between auditory and visual speech signals, with triggering of responses during perception of incongruent information (Moris Fernandez et al., 2015).

In summary, pSTS and amygdala have been consistently demonstrated to be key nodes for integration of audiovisual emotional information. However, recent findings substantiate the importance of network analyses and inclusion of brain areas beyond these well-established integration modules to improve our understanding on the neural substrates of audiovisual integration and to elucidate how they interact with other brain networks.

29.5 VOICES AND BODIES

While the perception of emotions in voices in the context of faces and the underlying integrative mechanisms has been studied for several decades now, research on the combined perception of voices and bodies is still in its infancy. This area of research mainly builds on studies from three neighbouring areas—emotional voice perception; integration of emotional faces and voices; and perception of emotional body movements, gestures, and postures, often termed 'emotional body language'. Studies on emotional body language have been used to develop an influential model of the neural structures subserving its processing (de Gelder, 2006), which posits three interconnected systems. The first system, including amygdala, superior colliculus, thalamus, and striatum, is supposed to sustain the fast and automatic perception of emotional body signals and the reflex-like expression of responsive emotional motor patterns. Activity in the second system, consisting of the insula, somatosensory cortex, anterior cingulate cortex, and ventromedial prefrontal cortex, reflects body awareness of emotional body language. The third system is thought to consist of a cortical network which includes the lateral occipital cortex, fusiform gyrus, superior temporal sulcus, the intraparietal lobule, the premotor cortex, and the amygdala. The de Gelder model of emotional body language processing (2006) assumes that in this cortical network, with its subcortical connections, emotional information from body expressions is decoded into a detailed conscious perception of emotional body expressions, a representation of their behavioural consequences, and adequate responses to the perceived emotional information.

Interestingly, there appear to be strong neuroanatomical analogies between emotional body processing and emotional face processing. Similar to the fusiform face area (Kanwisher et al., 1997), there exist specialized cortical modules in the fusiform gyrus (Peelen & Downing, 2005; Schwarzlose et al., 2005) and the lateral occipito-temporal cortex close to the middle occipital gyrus (i.e. extrastriate body area) (Downing et al., 2001) which selectively respond to human bodies and are sensitive to emotional body movements (Peelen et al., 2007; van de Riet et al., 2009). In addition, similar to dynamic representations of emotional facial expressions (e.g. Kreifelts et al., 2007), the pSTS exhibits stronger responses to dynamic body expressions of emotion than to neutral expressions (Kret et al., 2011).

29.6 VOICES AND BODIES— BEHAVIOURAL EFFECTS

In a first set of experiments on the integration of vocal and bodily expressions of emotion, van den Stock and colleagues demonstrated that congruent task-irrelevant body expressions of emotions facilitate the perception of emotional information in speech prosody (Van den Stock et al., 2007), and vice versa (Van den Stock et al., 2008). Notably, the methodology progressed from static representations of body expressions to dynamic representations between the two studies. Taken together, these results bear a striking resemblance to the facilitation effects between facial and vocal emotion expressions observed earlier by the same group using similar experimental designs (de Gelder & Vroomen, 2000). A follow-up study with masked emotional body expressions indicated that these facilitation effects occur irrespective of the visual awareness of the body expressions and of whether the emotional voice or body expression is task-relevant (Stienen et al., 2011). Very recently, these findings were extended to more complex social situations (i.e. dyadic interactions) with impoverished visual stimulation in the form of point light displays. Piwek and colleagues (2015) observed audiovisual integration effects with facilitated classification of the emotion present in the interaction for bimodal stimulation as compared to unimodal visual or auditory stimulation.

29.7 VOICES AND BODIES—ELECTROPHYSIOLOGICAL AND NEUROIMAGING STUDIES

At the level of ERPs, the combined processing of emotional prosody and body language led to a reduction of the N100, which was interpreted as an early influence of visual information on voice processing (Jessen & Kotz, 2011). Moreover, audiovisual stimulation was associated with an increase in the P200. While the use of video sequences without blurred faces argues for a particularly high ecological validity of the stimulation conditions, it remains difficult to say which of the visual components (i.e. emotional body language, facial expressions, or both) led to the observed audiovisual integration effects.

Another ERP study (Jessen et al., 2012) reports increased perceptual sensitivity to emotional information, under both low and high auditory noise conditions, during audiovisual presentation of emotional whole-body movements and emotional prosody at the behavioural level. Beyond the replication of a reduction of the N100 amplitude under audiovisual stimulation, a decreased latency of the N100 under audiovisual stimulation solely under high auditory noise conditions argues that this reduced latency represents a neural correlate of the increased behavioural facilitation effects under the high-noise condition. Moreover, earlier peaking of the N100 for emotional than for neutral expressions, under the audiovisual as compared to the unimodal auditory condition, points to emotion-specific audiovisual integration effects at the neural level.

Frequency analyses in the same study finally revealed an emotion-modulated suppression of beta-band oscillations, thought to reflect biological motion perception around 200–400 ms after voice onset. Greater decreases in beta power between audiovisual and auditory stimuli that occurred in high-noise as compared to low-noise conditions were for emotional stimuli only, while no difference was observed for neutral stimuli. This observation is in accordance with the so-called 'inverse effectiveness principle' derived from the response patterns of multisensory neurons. Here, the less effective unimodal stimuli are in generating a neural response, the more powerful are the relative effects of supra-additivity observed after bimodal stimulation.

This suggests a modulation of audiovisual integration of voice and body movements by their emotional content. A source localization analysis pointed to the right superior parietal cortex as generator of this beta-power suppression pattern, highlighting this area as a potential neural emotion-specific integration module for bimodal voice–body signals. A recent fMRI neuroimaging study on emotion effects during cerebral multisensory body–voice perception (Jessen & Kotz, 2015) yielded somewhat counterintuitive results. While audiovisual emotional stimuli (i.e. interjections combined with whole-body movements) led to stronger activation of the fusiform gyrus than neutral stimuli, the reverse contrast yielded activations most prominently around the pSTS. Additionally, the activation difference for neutral versus emotional stimuli was greater for audiovisual stimuli than for either monomodal visual or auditory stimuli. The authors explain this obvious contrast of their results with the literature on audiovisual emotion perception with differences in experimental design and stimulus material. Based on an average delay of around 600 ms between the onset of the body expression and the vocal stimulus, they offer priming effects rather than audiovisual sensory integration effects as a source of the results.

Taken together, these behavioural, electrophysiological, and neuroimaging studies demonstrate some striking similarities between the integration of emotions expressed in voice and whole-body movements and the results obtained in studies on voice–face emotion integration, with a clear trend towards dynamic depictions of body movements and therefore higher ecological validity. Regarding the localization of the neuronal sources of behavioural and electrophysiological correlates of audiovisual integration of vocal and whole-body expressions of emotions, especially in comparison to observed voice–face integration effects, more fMRI and MEG studies, preferentially applying comparable experimental designs, are needed.

29.8 The Integration of Emotional Cues from Voice, Face, and Body Expressions in Psychiatric Disorders

Alterations and parial impairments with regard to the evaluation and correct recognition of emotional signals are characteristics of many, if not most, psychiatric disorders (e.g. schizophrenia, anxiety disorders, autism spectrum disorders (ASD), affective disorders, personality disorders, addiction). Some of these disorders are thought to be linked with genuine alterations in sensory crossmodal integration processes (e.g. schizophrenia, ASD), while some are more likely associated with alterations in attentional and evaluative processes during the perception of audiovisual cues (e.g. anxiety disorders, affective disorders, personality disorders). Some disorders, finally, appear to be associated with alterations in both areas (i.e. schizophrenia, ASD).

The number of studies investigating crossmodal processes during the perception of vocal emotional signal in the context of facial or bodily cues in psychiatric disorders has grown very fast in past years. In the following, we will review the findings from recent studies performed to elucidate potential deficits in the audiovisual perception of such cues in several psychiatric disorders.

29.8.1 Schizophrenia

Studies demonstrate that deficits in vocal and facial emotion recognition in schizophrenic patients (e.g. Addington et al., 2012; Corcoran et al., 2015; Kucharska-Pietura et al., 2005; Weisgerber et al., 2015), which are already present in still-healthy high-risk-for-psychosis individuals (Addington et al., 2012), progress during the course of the disorder (Kucharska-Pietura et al., 2005) and may even predict the transition of at-risk individuals to clinical psychosis (Corcoran et al., 2015). First studies on crossmodal processing of audiovisual emotional cues in schizophrenia have been performed.

De Gelder et al. (2005) first reported a decreased effect of emotional prosody on the categorization of emotional faces and an increased impact of emotional facial expressions on the categorization of emotional prosody. The latter finding was then challenged by a later, and considerably larger, study by the same research group which indicated a decreased impact of visual emotion on the evaluation of vocal emotion, applying a a 2×2 congruence/incongruence design (de Jong et al., 2009). Additionally, this effect was found to be specific for schizophrenia when compared to a control group of non-schizophrenic psychotic patients included in the same study. A follow-up study, including neutral visual and auditory distractor stimuli as attention modulators, demonstrated that the influence of emotional facial expressions on the evaluation of emotional voices is reduced by visual distractors to a greater degree than by auditory distractors in healthy individuals, while crossmodal interactions in the schizophrenic group remained intact, which was interpreted as an indicator of a deficiency in regulatory effects of modality-specific attention in schizophrenia (de Jong et al., 2010).

With regard to symptoms and cognitive impairments, it could be shown that deficiencies in emotional face–voice integration are correlated with negative symptoms and reduced executive functions (Castagna et al., 2013). First evidence for the neural underpinnings of altered integration of emotional voices and faces in schizophrenia comes from an ERP study. Müller and colleagues found not only reduced amplitudes of P1 and P2 to faces, irrespective of the presence or the emotional quality of the voice, but observed that the P1 amplitude reduction for emotionally incongruent voice–face pairs was rendered non-significant for congruent voice–face pairs. This not only corroborates deficits in neural face processing in schizophrenia but also suggests alterations in early audiovisual face–voice integration processes and, more importantly, that alterations in face processing can be restored through congruent emotional voices. As a caveat, it needs to be mentioned though that the electrophysiological effects were not met by corresponding behavioural effects in this study.

Notably, the assumption of deficient audiovisual emotion integration in schizophrenia is also challenged by a smaller study in schizophrenic and schizo-affective patients, with the finding of an intact audiovisual facilitation effect in an emotion-labelling paradigm where decreased labelling accuracy of emotional voices and faces in the monomodal condition were not observable in the bimodal condition (Simpson et al., 2013). Eye-tracking data from the same study offer a potential partial explanation for the normalization of emotion recognition under bimodal stimulation: while fixation time on the mouth as an emotionally salient feature, in contrast to fixation time on the eye region, was decreased during the visual monomodal condition in the psychosis group, fixation times for the most salient facial regions (i.e. eyes and mouth) normalized under bimodal stimulation.

In the only presently available study on the integration of emotional voices and emotional body language in schizophrenia, van den Stock and colleagues reported reduced signs of audiovisual integration with a decreased influence of voice cues on the categorization of body expressions (Van den Stock et al., 2011).

Data on the neuronal sources of reported behavioural and electrophysiological alterations in audiovisual integration of non-verbal emotional cues from voice and face in patients with schizophrenia (e.g. using fMRI or MEG) is still lacking. However, there is data on audiovisual speech integration (Szycik et al., 2009) demonstrating altered activation in several fronto-temporal brain areas when contrasting audiovisual congruence versus incongruence conditions in schizophrenia patients. A follow-up analysis (Szycik et al., 2010) on the previously mentioned study additionally shows divergent connectivity patterns of Broca's area and the right pSTS for congruent and incongruent audiovisual speech between individuals suffering from schizophrenia and healthy individuals, which the authors suggest implies less adaptive processing of audiovisually congruent and incongruent speech.

29.8.2 Autism Spectrum Disorder

Beyond the well-known deficits in emotion recognition from monomodal cues, it could be recently demonstrated that individuals with autism spectrum disorder (ASD) show decreased behavioural correlates of audiovisual integration with regard to emotion recognition accuracy and response times using dynamic audiovisual cues (Charbonneau et al., 2013). In addition, it has been suggested that this alteration might be due to altered multisensory temporal binding in ASD (Wallace & Stevenson, 2014). At the level of automatic facial responses to emotional information from faces and voices, it was observed, in a facial MEG study, that patients with pervasive developmental disorder (PDD) had a heightened response to happy and fearful faces, but an intact response to audiovisual affective information, arguing against an impairment in multimodal emotion processing at this level of perception (Magnee et al., 2007).

The first electrophysiological study in a patient group from the autism spectrum (i.e. pervasive developmental disorder) evidenced a diminished N2 response for emotionally congruent face–voice combinations which were most strongly driven by face–voice pairs, including fearful rather than happy voices (Magnee et al., 2008). The same research group later showed that, additionally, alterations of ERP multisensory integration correlates in ASD are dependent on concurrent attentional demands (Magnee et al., 2011).

First evidence for alterations in the processing of multimodal non-verbal information from face–voice combinations, at the neuroimaging level, came from a study by Hall and colleagues (2003). In a small PET study, they demonstrated reduced activation of the inferior frontal cortex and fusiform gyrus, and also a potentially compensatorily increased activation in the anterior cingulate cortex, the thalamus, and the temporal pole. However, in this specific study, no behavioural differences were observed. These results were largely corroborated by a very small fMRI study in which decreased activation for congruent emotional faces and voices was observed not only in the orbitofrontal cortex and occipital region but also in the superior temporal, parahippocampal, and posterior cingulate gyri (Loveland et al., 2008). Recently, an increased activation in several parieto-frontal brain areas, during audiovisual emotion matching in teenagers with ASD as compared to typically developed individuals, was proposed as the cerebral correlate of a compensatory mechanism during multimodal emotion processing (Doyle-Thomas et al., 2014).

29.8.3 Other Disorders

With regard to anxiety disorders, to date, little evidence on potential alterations of multimodal emotional integration has been accumulated, but it has recently been emphatically called for (Peschard et al., 2014). However, existing evidence (Koizumi et al., 2011) already makes it very clear that attention and interpretation biases present in anxiety disorders will have to be factored into this kind of research, specifically with regard to any emotional information which might be perceived as threatening.

In the area of affective disorders, first studies (Doose-Grünefeld et al., 2015; Müller et al., 2014; Van Rheenen and Rossell, 2014) investigated crossmodal interaction effects of emotional voices on the evaluation of emotional faces in patients with major depressive disorder (Doose-Grünefeld et al., 2015; Müller et al., 2014) and bipolar disorder (Van Rheenen & Rossell, 2014). A first study in depression found altered cerebral emotional incongruence effects in depressed patients in the absence of behavioural alterations, with a lack of parietal and prefrontal deactivation specifically for the perception of fearful voices in the context of happy faces (Müller et al., 2013). Additionally, the same study demonstrated an alteration in the integration of emotional and neutral cues from voice and face in depressed patients, with increased responses to emotional-neutral face–voice combinations in the posterior STG and the middle cingulate cortex, which represents a reversal of the activation pattern observed in the control group. A behavioural follow-up study with a somewhat larger sample (Doose-Grünefeld et al., 2015) then revealed a negative (i.e. reversed) effect of happy voices on face valence ratings, and a lacking negative effect of fearful voices on the evaluation of happy faces, in depressed patients.

The only available audiovisual emotional integration study in (a mixed group of) bipolar patients detected the lack of increased response times to emotionally incongruent face-voice combinations, while no alterations were observed with regard to crossmodal effects on the accuracy of recognition of emotional facial expressions (Van Rheenen & Rossell, 2014). Here, further research will be needed not only to reconcile the partially divergent findings but also to clarify the source of observed alterations in audiovisual emotional integration in affective disorders (i.e. valence biases/ emotional blunting versus basic alterations in sensory integration).

Interestingly, a lacking audiovisual facilitation effect during the bimodal processing of emotional faces and voices (Maurage et al., 2007) was observed in alcohol-dependent individuals. Using ERPs, the same group described an anger-specific alteration in neural processing during audiovisual emotion perception (Maurage et al., 2008). These findings were later complemented by an fMRI study indicating a reduction or even lack of the cerebral correlates of audiovisual emotion integration (Maurage et al., 2013). Moreover, reduced connectivity between unimodal and bimodal brain regions was observed in alcohol dependence in this study. Nevertheless, it remains unresolved if these alterations will prove to be emotion- or even anger-specific, if they are cause or consequence of alcohol dependence, and if they represent domain-specific alterations or rather reflect one aspect of global damage of the brain.

Taken together, the studies reviewed in this section represent a fast-growing beachhead in the research exploring the cerebral and psychophysical underpinnings of altered multimodal perception of emotional cues in states of psychiatric disease. While, on the one hand, this type of research might certainly enhance our understanding of mechanisms of disease in the context of complex social-perception processes, on the other hand, thus refined models of psychiatric diseases might lead to the development of therapeutic approaches designed to alleviate difficulties in the perception and integration of non-verbal signals in such disorders.

As a final caveat, it does need to be added that, unfortunately, not all of the studies reviewed here employed analysis approaches which conform to the principles of audiovisual integration as demonstrated in the first part of this chapter—or rather, on the positive side, there is still plenty of room to perform analytically rigorous studies on audiovisual emotion integration in psychiatric disorders.

REFERENCES

Addington, J., Piskulic, D., Perkins, D., Woods, S. W., Liu, L., & Penn, D. L. (2012). Affect recognition in people at clinical high risk of psychosis. *Schizophrenia Research,* 140, 87–92.

Ashburner, J. & Friston, K. J. (2005). Unified segmentation. *NeuroImage,* 26, 839–51.

Beauchamp, M. S. (2005) Statistical criteria in fMRI studies of multisensory integration. *Neuroinformatics,* 3, 93–113.

Beauchamp, M. S., Argall, B. D., Bodurka, J., Duyn, J. H., & Martin, A. (2004a). Unraveling multisensory integration: patchy organization within human STS multisensory cortex. *Nature Neuroscience*, 7, 1190–1192.

Beauchamp, M. S., Lee, K. E., Argall, B. D., & Martin, A. (2004b). Integration of auditory and visual information about objects in superior temporal sulcus. *Neuron*, 41, 809–823.

Breiter, H. C., Etcoff, N. L., Whalen, P. J., Kennedy, W. A., Rauch, S. L., Buckner, R. L., ... Rosen, B. R. (1996). Response and habituation of the human amygdala during visual processing of facial expression. *Neuron*, 17, 875–887.

Campanella, S. & Belin, P. (2007). Integrating face and voice in person perception. *Trends in Cognitive Sciences*, 11, 535–543.

Castagna, F., Montemagni, C., Maria Milani, A., Rocca, G., Rocca, P., Casacchia, M., & Bogetto, F. (2013). Prosody recognition and audiovisual emotion matching in schizophrenia: the contribution of cognition and psychopathology. *Psychiatry Research*, 205, 192–198.

Charbonneau, G., Bertone, A., Lepore, F., Nassim, M., Lassonde, M., Mottron, L., & Collignon, O. (2013). Multilevel alterations in the processing of audio-visual emotion expressions in autism spectrum disorders. *Neuropsychologia*, 51, 1002–1010.

Chavis, D. A. & Pandya, D. N. (1976). Further observations on corticofrontal connections in the rhesus monkey. *Brain Research*, 117, 369–386.

Chen, Y. H., Edgar, J. C., Holroyd, T., Dammers, J., Thonnessen, H., Roberts, T. P., & Mathiak, K. (2010). Neuromagnetic oscillations to emotional faces and prosody. *European Journal of Neuroscience*, 31, 1818–1827.

Collignon, O., Girard, S., Gosselin, F., Roy, S., Saint-Amour, D., Lassonde, M., & Lepore, F. (2008). Audio-visual integration of emotion expression. *Brain Research*, 1242, 126–135.

Collignon, O., Girard, S., Gosselin, F., Saint-Amour, D., Lepore, F., & Lassonde, M. (2010). Women process multisensory emotion expressions more efficiently than men. *Neuropsychologia*, 48, 220–225.

Corcoran, C. M., Keilp, J. G., Kayser, J., Klim, C., Butler, P. D., Bruder, G. E., Gur, R. C., & Javitt, D. C. (2015). Emotion recognition deficits as predictors of transition in individuals at clinical high risk for schizophrenia: a neurodevelopmental perspective. *Psychological Medicine*, 45, 2959–2973.

De Gelder, B. (2006). Towards the neurobiology of emotional body language. *Nature Reviews Neuroscience*, 7, 242–249.

De Gelder, B., Bocker, K. B., Tuomainen, J., Hensen, M., & Vroomen, J. (1999). The combined perception of emotion from voice and face: early interaction revealed by human electric brain responses. *Neuroscience Letters*, 260, 133–136.

De Gelder, B., Pourtois, G., & Weiskrantz, L. (2002). Fear recognition in the voice is modulated by unconsciously recognized facial expressions but not by unconsciously recognized affective pictures. *Proceedings of the National Academy of Science of the United States of America*, 99, 4121–4126.

De Gelder, B. & Vroomen, J. (2000). The perception of emotions by ear and by eye. *Cognition & Emotion*, 14, 289–311.

De Gelder, B., Vroomen, J., De Jong, S. J., Masthoff, E. D., Trompenaars, F. J., & Hodiamont, P. (2005). Multisensory integration of emotional faces and voices in schizophrenics. *Schizophrenia Research*, 72, 195–203.

De Jong, J. J., Hodiamont, P. P., & De Gelder, B. (2010). Modality-specific attention and multisensory integration of emotions in schizophrenia: reduced regulatory effects. *Schizophrenia Research*, 122, 136–143.

De Jong, J. J., Hodiamont, P. P., Van Den Stock, J., & De Gelder, B. (2009). Audiovisual emotion recognition in schizophrenia: reduced integration of facial and vocal affect. *Schizophrenia Research*, 107, 286–293.

Doi, H. & Shinohara, K. (2015). Unconscious presentation of fearful face modulates electro-physiological responses to emotional prosody. *Cerebral Cortex*, 25, 817–832.

Dolan, R. J., Morris, J. S., & De Gelder, B. (2001). Crossmodal binding of fear in voice and face. *Proceedings of the National Academy of Sciences of the United States of America*, 98, 10006–10010.

Doose-Grünefeld, S., Eickhoff, S. B., & Muller, V. I. (2015). Audiovisual emotional pro-cessing and neurocognitive functioning in patients with depression. *Frontiers in Integrated Neuroscience*, 9, 3.

Downing, P. E., Jiang, Y., Shuman, M., & Kanwisher, N. (2001). A cortical area selective for visual processing of the human body. *Science*, 293, 2470–2473.

Doyle-Thomas, K. A., Goldberg, J., Szatmari, P., & Hall, G. B. (2014). Neurofunctional under-pinnings of audiovisual emotion processing in teens with autism spectrum disorders. *Frontiers in Psychiatry*, 4, 48.

Ethofer, T., Anders, S., Erb, M., Droll, C., Royen, L., Saur, R., ... Wildgruber, D. (2006). Impact of voice on emotional judgment of faces: an event-related fMRI study. *Human Brain Mapping*, 27, 707–714.

Ethofer, T., Anders, S., Wiethoff, S., Erb, M., Herbert, C., Saur, R., Grodd, W., & Wildgruber, D. (2006). Effects of prosodic emotional intensity on activation of associative auditory cortex. *NeuroReport*, 17, 249–253.

Ethofer, T., Bretscher, J., Wiethoff, S., Bisch, J., Schlipf, S., Wildgruber, D., & Kreifelts, B. (2013). Functional responses and structural connections of cortical areas for processing faces and voices in the superior temporal sulcus. *NeuroImage*, 76, 45–56.

Ethofer, T., Gschwind, M., & Vuilleumier, P. (2011). Processing social aspects of human gaze: a combined fMRI-DTI study. *NeuroImage*, 55, 411–419.

Ethofer, T., Kreifelts, B., Wiethoff, S., Wolf, J., Grodd, W., Vuilleumier, P., & Wildgruber, D. (2009). Differential influences of emotion, task, and novelty on brain regions underlying the processing of speech melody. *Journal of Cognitive Neuroscience*, 21, 1255–1268.

Ethofer, T., Pourtois, G., & Wildgruber, D. (2006). Investigating audiovisual integration of emotional signals in the human brain. *Progress in Brain Research*, 156, 345–361.

Ethofer, T., Van De Ville, D., Scherer, K., & Vuilleumier, P. (2009). Decoding of emotional in-formation in voice-sensitive cortices. *Current Biology*, 19, 1028–1033.

Ethofer, T., Wiethoff, S., Anders, S., Kreifelts, B., Grodd, W., & Wildgruber, D. (2007). The voices of seduction: cross-gender effects in processing of erotic prosody. *Social, Cognitive, and Affective Neuroscience*, 2, 334–337.

Focker, J., Gondan, M., & Roder, B. (2011). Preattentive processing of audio-visual emotional signals. *Acta Psychologica*, 137, 36–47.

Friston, K. J., Buechel, C., Fink, G. R., Morris, J., Rolls, E., & Dolan, R. J. (1997). Psychophysiological and modulatory interactions in neuroimaging. *NeuroImage*, 6, 218–229.

Friston, K. J., Josephs, O., Rees, G., & Turner, R. (1998). Nonlinear event-related responses in fMRI. *Magnetic Resonance in Medicine*, 39, 41–52.

Grandjean, D., Sander, D., Pourtois, G., Schwartz, S., Seghier, M. L., Scherer, K. R., & Vuilleumier, P. (2005). The voices of wrath: brain responses to angry prosody in meaningless speech. *Nature Neuroscience*, 8, 145–146.

Grossmann, T., Striano, T., & Friederici, A. D. (2006). Crossmodal integration of emotional in-formation from face and voice in the infant brain. *Developmental Science*, 9, 309–315.

Hagan, C. C., Woods, W., Johnson, S., Calder, A. J., Green, G. G., & Young, A. W. (2009). MEG demonstrates a supra-additive response to facial and vocal emotion in the right superior temporal sulcus. *Proceedings of the National Academy of Sciences of the United States of America*, 106, 20010–20015.

Hall, G. B., Szechtman, H., & Nahmias, C. (2003). Enhanced salience and emotion recognition in autism: a PET study. *American Journal of Psychiatry*, 160, 1439–1441.

Haxby, J. V., Hoffman, E. A., & Gobbini, M. I. (2000). The distributed human neural system for face perception. *Trends in Cognitive Sciences*, 4, 223–233.

Ho, H. T., Schroger, E., & Kotz, S. A. (2015). Selective attention modulates early human evoked potentials during emotional face-voice processing. *Journal of Cognitive Neuroscience*, 27, 798–818.

Jansma, H., Roebroeck, A., & Munte, T. F. (2014). A network analysis of audiovisual affective speech perception. *Neuroscience*, 256, 230–241.

Jessen, S. & Kotz, S. A. (2011). The temporal dynamics of processing emotions from vocal, facial, and bodily expressions. *NeuroImage*, 58, 665–674.

Jessen, S. & Kotz, S. A. (2015). Affect differentially modulates brain activation in uni- and multisensory body-voice perception. *Neuropsychologia*, 66, 134–143.

Jessen, S., Obleser, J., & Kotz, S. A. (2012). How bodies and voices interact in early emotion perception. *PLoS One*, 7, e36070.

Jones, E. G. & Powell, T. P. (1970). An anatomical study of converging sensory pathways within the cerebral cortex of the monkey. *Brain*, 93, 793–820.

Kanwisher, N., Mcdermott, J., & Chun, M. M. (1997). The fusiform face area: a module in human extrastriate cortex specialized for face perception. *Journal of Neuroscience*, 17, 4302–4311.

Klasen, M., Kenworthy, C. A., Mathiak, K. A., Kircher, T. T., & Mathiak, K. (2011). Supramodal representation of emotions. *Journal of Neuroscience*, 31, 13635–13643.

Koizumi, A., Tanaka, A., Imai, H., Hiramatsu, S., Hiramoto, E., Sato, T., & De Gelder, B. (2011). The effects of anxiety on the interpretation of emotion in the face-voice pairs. *Experimental Brain Research*, 213, 275–282.

Kokinous, J., Kotz, S. A., Tavano, A., & Schroger, E. (2015). The role of emotion in dynamic audiovisual integration of faces and voices. *Social, Cognitive, and Affective Neuroscience*, 10, 713–720.

Kreifelts, B., Ethofer, T., Grodd, W., Erb, M., & Wildgruber, D. (2007). Audiovisual integration of emotional signals in voice and face: an event-related fMRI study. *NeuroImage*, 37, 1445–1456.

Kreifelts, B., Ethofer, T., Huberle, E., Grodd, W., & Wildgruber, D. (2010). Association of trait emotional intelligence and individual fMRI- activation patterns during the perception of social signals from voice and face. *Human Brain Mapping*, 31, 979–991.

Kreifelts, B., Ethofer, T., Shiozawa, T., Grodd, W., & Wildgruber, D. (2009). Cerebral representation of non-verbal emotional perception: fMRI reveals audiovisual integration area between voice- and face-sensitive regions in the superior temporal sulcus. *Neuropsychologia*, 47, 3059–3066.

Kret, M. E., Pichon, S., Grezes, J., & De Gelder, B. (2011). Similarities and differences in perceiving threat from dynamic faces and bodies. An fMRI study. *NeuroImage*, 54, 1755–1762.

Kucharska-Pietura, K., David, A. S., Masiak, M., & Phillips, M. L. (2005). Perception of facial and vocal affect by people with schizophrenia in early and late stages of illness. *British Journal of Psychiatry*, 187, 523–528.

Lambrecht, L., Kreifelts, B., & Wildgruber, D. (2012). Age-related decrease in recognition of emotional facial and prosodic expressions. *Emotion*, 12, 529–539.

Li, Y., Long, J., Huang, B., Yu, T., Wu, W., Liu, Y., Liang, C., & Sun, P. (2015). Crossmodal integration enhances neural representation of task-relevant features in audiovisual face perception. *Cerebral Cortex*, 25, 384–395.

Liu, T., Pinheiro, A., Zhao, Z., Nestor, P. G., Mccarley, R. W., & Niznikiewicz, M. A. (2012). Emotional cues during simultaneous face and voice processing: electrophysiological insights. *PLoS One*, 7, e31001.

Loveland, K. A., Steinberg, J. L., Pearson, D. A., Mansour, R., & Reddoch, S. (2008). Judgments of auditory-visual affective congruence in adolescents with and without autism: a pilot study of a new task using fMRI. *Perceptual and Motor Skills*, 107, 557–575.

Magnee, C. M., De Gelder, B., Van Engeland, H., & Chantal, K. (2008). Atypical processing of fearful face-voice pairs in pervasive developmental disorder: an ERP study. *Clinical Neurophysiology*, 119, 2004–2010.

Magnee, M. J., De Gelder, B., Van Engeland, H., & Kemner, C. (2007). Facial electro-myographic responses to emotional information from faces and voices in individuals with pervasive developmental disorder. *Journal of Child Psychology & Psychiatry*, 48, 1122–1130.

Magnee, M. J., De Gelder, B., Van Engeland, H., & Kemner, C. (2011). Multisensory integration and attention in autism spectrum disorder: evidence from event-related potentials. *PLoS One*, 6, e24196.

Massaro, D. W. & Egan, P. B. (1996). Perceiving affect from the voice and the face. *Psychonomic Bulletin & Review*, 3, 215–221.

Maurage, P., Campanella, S., Philippot, P., Pham, T. H., & Joassin, F. (2007). The crossmodal facilitation effect is disrupted in alcoholism: a study with emotional stimuli. *Alcohol*, 42, 552–559.

Maurage, P., Joassin, F., Pesenti, M., Grandin, C., Heeren, A., Philippot, P., & De Timary, P. (2013). The neural network sustaining crossmodal integration is impaired in alcohol-dependence: an fMRI study. *Cortex*, 49, 1610–1626.

Maurage, P., Philippot, P., Joassin, F., Pauwels, L., Pham, T., Prieto, E. A., ... Campanella, S. (2008). The auditory-visual integration of anger is impaired in alcoholism: an event-related potentials study. *Journal of Psychiatry & Neuroscience*, 33, 111–122.

Mcdonald, A. J. (1998). Cortical pathways to the mammalian amygdala. *Progress in Neurobiology*, 55, 257–332.

Mechelli, A., Price, C. J., & Friston, K. J. (2001). Nonlinear coupling between evoked rCBF and BOLD signals: a simulation study of hemodynamic responses. *NeuroImage*, 14, 862–872.

Moris Fernandez, L., Visser, M., Ventura-Campos, N., Avila, C., & Soto- Faraco, S. (2015). Top-down attention regulates the neural expression of audiovisual integration. *NeuroImage*, 119, 272–285.

Morris, J. S., Frith, C. D., Perrett, D. I., Rowland, D., Young, A. W., Calder, A. J., & Dolan, R. J. (1996). A differential neural response in the human amygdala to fearful and happy facial expressions. *Nature*, 383, 812–815.

Müller, V. I., Cieslik, E. C., Kellermann, T. S., & Eickhoff, S. B. (2014). Crossmodal emotional integration in major depression. *Social, Cognitive, and Affective Neuroscience*, 9, 839–848.

Müller, V. I., Cieslik, E. C., Laird, A. R., Fox, P. T., & Eickhoff, S. B. (2013). Dysregulated left inferior parietal activity in schizophrenia and depression: functional connectivity and characterization. *Frontiers in Human Neuroscience*, 7, 268.

Müller, V. I., Habel, U., Derntl, B., Schneider, F., Zilles, K., Turetsky, B. I., & Eickhoff, S. B. (2011). Incongruence effects in crossmodal emotional integration. *NeuroImage*, 54(3), 2257–2266.

Murray, E. A. & Mishkin, M. (1985). Amygdalectomy impairs crossmodal association in monkeys. *Science*, 228, 604–606.

Nichols, T., Brett, M., Andersson, J., Wager, T., & Poline, J. B. (2005). Valid conjunction inference with the minimum statistic. *NeuroImage*, 25, 653–660.

Ochiai, T., Grimault, S., Scavarda, D., Roch, G., Hori, T., Riviere, D., Mangin, J. F., & Regis, J. (2004). Sulcal pattern and morphology of the superior temporal sulcus. *NeuroImage*, 22, 706–719.

Peelen, M. V., Atkinson, A. P., Andersson, F., & Vuilleumier, P. (2007). Emotional modulation of body- selective visual areas. *Social, Cognitive and Affective Neuroscience*, 2, 274–283.

Peelen, M. V. & Downing, P. E. (2005). Selectivity for the human body in the fusiform gyrus. *Journal of Neurophysiology*, 93, 603–608.

Peschard, V., Maurage, P., & Philippot, P. (2014). Towards a cross-modal perspective of emotional perception in social anxiety: review and future directions. *Frontiers in Human Neuroscience*, 8, 322.

Pitkänen, A. (2000). Connectivity of the rat amygdaloid complex. In: J. P. Aggleton (ed.) *The Amygdala. A Functional Analysis* (pp. 31–115). New York, Oxford University Press.

Piwek, L., Pollick, F., & Petrini, K. (2015). Audiovisual integration of emotional signals from others' social interactions. *Frontiers in Psychology*, 6, article 611.

Pourtois, G., De Gelder, B., Bol, A., & Crommelinck, M. (2005). Perception of facial expressions and voices and of their combination in the human brain. *Cortex*, 41, 49–59.

Pourtois, G., De Gelder, B., Vroomen, J., Rossion, B., & Crommelinck, M. (2000). The time-course of intermodal binding between seeing and hearing affective information. *NeuroReport*, 11, 1329–1333.

Pourtois, G., Debatisse, D., Despland, P. A., & De Gelder, B. (2002). Facial expressions modulate the time course of long latency auditory brain potentials. *Brain Research: Cognitive Brain Research*, 14, 99–105.

Riedel, P., Ragert, P., Schelinski, S., Kiebel, S. J., & Von Kriegstein, K. (2015). Visual face-movement sensitive cortex is relevant for auditory-only speech recognition. *Cortex*, 68, 86–99.

Robins, D. L., Hunyadi, E., & Schultz, R. T. (2009). Superior temporal activation in response to dynamic audio-visual emotional cues. *Brain and Cognition*, 69, 269–278.

Roebroeck, A., Formisano, E., & Goebel, R. (2005). Mapping directed influence over the brain using Granger causality and fMRI. *NeuroImage*, 25, 230–242.

Romanski, L. M. (2012). Integration of faces and vocalizations in ventral prefrontal cortex: implications for the evolution of audiovisual speech. *Proceedings of the National Academy of Sciences of the United States of America*, 109 (Suppl. 1), 10717–10724.

Said, C. P., Moore, C. D., Engell, A. D., Todorov, A., & Haxby, J. V. (2010). Distributed representations of dynamic facial expressions in the superior temporal sulcus. *Journal of Vision*, 10, 11.

Schroger, E. & Widmann, A. (1998). Speeded responses to audiovisual signal changes result from bimodal integration. *Psychophysiology*, 35, 755–759.

Schutte, N., Malouff, J., Hall, L., Haggerty, D., Cooper, J., Golden, C., & Dornheim, L. (1998). Development and validation of a measure of emotional intelligence. *Personality and Individual Differences*, 25, 167–177.

Schwarzlose, R. F., Baker, C. I., & Kanwisher, N. (2005). Separate face and body selectivity on the fusiform gyrus. *Journal of Neuroscience*, 25, 11055–11059.

Seltzer, B. & Pandya, D. N. (1978). Afferent cortical connections and architectonics of the superior temporal sulcus and surrounding cortex in the rhesus monkey. *Brain Research*, 149, 1–24.

Simpson, C., Pinkham, A. E., Kelsven, S., & Sasson, N. J. (2013). Emotion recognition abilities across stimulus modalities in schizophrenia and the role of visual attention. *Schizophrenia Research*, 151, 102–106.

Stienen, B. M., Tanaka, A., & De Gelder, B. (2011). Emotional voice and emotional body postures influence each other independently of visual awareness. *PLoS One*, 6, e25517.

Surguladze, S. A., Brammer, M. J., Young, A. W., Andrew, C., Travis, M. J., Williams, S. C., & Phillips, M. L. (2003). A preferential increase in the extrastriate response to signals of danger. *NeuroImage*, 19, 1317–1328.

Szycik, G. R., Munte, T. F., Dillo, W., Mohammadi, B., Samii, A., Emrich, H. M., & Dietrich, D. E. (2009). Audiovisual integration of speech is disturbed in schizophrenia: an fMRI study. *Schizophrenia Research*, 110, 111–118.

Szycik, G. R., Ye, Z., Mohammadi, B., Dillo, W., Te Wildt, B. T., Samii, A., … Munte, T. F. (2010). Maladaptive connectivity of Broca's area in schizophrenia during audiovisual speech perception: an fMRI study. *Neuroscience*, 253, 274–282.

Takagi, S., Hiramatsu, S., Tabei, K., & Tanaka, A. (2015). Multisensory perception of the six basic emotions is modulated by attentional instruction and unattended modality. *Frontiers in Integrated Neuroscience*, 9, 1.

Van Atteveldt, N., Formisano, E., Goebel, R., & Blomert, L. (2004). Integration of letters and speech sounds in the human brain. *Neuron*, 43, 271–282.

Van De Riet, W. A., Grezes, J., & De Gelder, B. (2009). Specific and common brain regions involved in the perception of faces and bodies and the representation of their emotional expressions. *Social Neuroscience*, 4, 101–120.

Van Den Stock, J., De Jong, S. J., Hodiamont, P. P., & De Gelder, B. (2011). Perceiving emotions from bodily expressions and multisensory integration of emotion cues in schizophrenia. *Social Neuroscience*, 6, 537–547.

Van Den Stock, J., Grezes, J., & De Gelder, B. (2008). Human and animal sounds influence recognition of body language. *Brain Research*, 1242, 185–190.

Van Den Stock, J., Righart, R., & De Gelder, B. (2007). Body expressions influence recognition of emotions in the face and voice. *Emotion*, 7, 487–494.

Van Rheenen, T. E. & Rossell, S. L. (2014). Multimodal emotion integration in bipolar disorder: an investigation of involuntary cross-modal influences between facial and prosodic channels. *Journal of the International Neuropsychology Society*, 20, 525–533.

Vroomen, J., Driver, J., & De Gelder, B. (2001). Is cross-modal integration of emotional expressions independent of attentional resources? *Cognitive, Affective, and Behavioral Neuroscience*, 1, 382–387.

Vuilleumier, P., Armony, J. L., Driver, J., & Dolan, R. J. (2001). Effects of attention and emotion on face processing in the human brain: an event-related fMRI study. *Neuron*, 30, 829–841.

Wallace, M. T., Meredith, M. A., & Stein, B. E. (1992). Integration of multiple sensory modalities in cat cortex. *Experimental Brain Research*, 91, 484–488.

Wallace, M. T. & Stevenson, R. A. (2014). The construct of the multisensory temporal binding window and its dysregulation in developmental disabilities. *Neuropsychologia*, 64C, 105–123.

Watson, R., Latinus, M., Noguchi, T., Garrod, O., Crabbe, F., & Belin, P. (2014). Crossmodal adaptation in right posterior superior temporal sulcus during face-voice emotional integration. *Journal of Neuroscience*, 34, 6813–6821.

Weisgerber, A., Vermeulen, N., Peretz, I., Samson, S., Philippot, P., Maurage, P., … Constant, E. (2015). Facial, vocal and musical emotion recognition is altered in paranoid schizophrenic patients. *Psychiatry Research*, 229, 188–193.

White, M. (1999). Representation of facial expressions of emotion. *American Journal of Psychology*, 112, 371–381.

Wiethoff, S., Wildgruber, D., Grodd, W., & Ethofer, T. (2009). Response and habituation of the amygdala during processing of emotional prosody. *NeuroReport*, 20, 1356–1360.

Wiethoff, S., Wildgruber, D., Kreifelts, B., Becker, H., Herbert, C., Grodd, W., & Ethofer, T. (2008). Cerebral processing of emotional prosody—influence of acoustic parameters and arousal. *NeuroImage*, 39, 885–893.

Wright, T. M., Pelphrey, K. A., Allison, T., Mckeown, M. J., & Mccarthy, G. (2003). Polysensory interactions along lateral temporal regions evoked by audiovisual speech. *Cerebral Cortex*, 13, 1034–1043.

....

CHAPTER 30

LINGUISTIC 'FIRST IMPRESSIONS'
Accents as a Cue to Person Perception

....

PATRICIA E.G. BESTELMEYER

30.1 INTRODUCTION

....

SPEECH conveys meaning via words and sentences. This semantic meaning and the grammatical structure of language has been the traditional object of study by linguists and psychologists for many decades. However, spoken language can also provide meaning beyond the semantic content of words and can offer much social information about the speaker and the speech situation. For example, individuals from different regions sound and talk differently even when the spoken language is the same. Accent refers to this variation in pronunciation of the same language spoken by different communities (Wardhaugh, 1992).

While the grammar between accents of the same language is largely or completely the same, the differences between accents are due to phonetic, phonological, and prosodic variations. Native speakers can perceive accent differences and categorize accented speakers (e.g. Clopper & Pisoni, 2007; Clopper et al., 2012) as well as identify which region of the country the speaker is from (Clopper & Pisoni, 2004). Studies have also shown that listeners make reliable social judgements about the friendliness and intelligence of the speaker (e.g. Clopper & Pisoni, 2007; Giles, 1970; Luhman, 1990). Hence, a speaker's accent is an important source of social information to the listener.

Accents are generally associated with certain group memberships and can *index* a particular geographical origin, ethnic background, or social class such as level and type of education (Labov, 2006). One of the most widely-cited examples of the significant social (and potentially lethal) impact of accents is the biblical story of 'Shibboleth'. In this story, two Semitic tribes, the Ephraimites and the Gileadites, are at war. After the Gileadites win the battle, they set up a barrier across the River Jordan to kill any fugitives of Ephraim who try to return to their territory. This barrier can only be crossed alive with the correct 'password', that is, the pronunciation of the word *shibboleth* with a Gileadite accent. The Ephraimites who had no *sh* sound in their language pronounced the word with an *s* (rather than *sh*) and were therefore revealed as the enemy and slaughtered. More modern versions of 'Shibboleth' still exist and there are several historic examples in which linguistic change and nationalist movements co-occurred, underlining the role of language change in ethnic group relations (e.g. repression of the official language of the Ottoman Empire in favour of a more modern version of Turkish to underline its identification with central Asia; Khleif, 1979).

30.2 STUDYING ATTITUDES TOWARDS DIFFERENT ACCENTS

Social scientists, predominantly sociolinguists, have studied the social influences of accents on listeners, for many different varieties, using two main methodologies—direct and indirect approaches (Garrett et al., 2003). Direct methods involve overt questioning of listeners about certain accents using interviews, questionnaires, or rating scales. This approach has been criticized because the listeners' verbal or written responses of their attitudes may not be the same as their actual reactions towards a particular accent (Knops & van Hout, 1988). In other words, the participant may not feel comfortable disclosing their opinions about a particular accent to the researcher. There are related issues with this method such as a tendency to give socially appropriate responses, experimenter bias (a subject responding in a way to please the experimenter), acquiescence bias (where respondents agree to any question, independent of content), as well as other issues related to hypothetical questions that may be difficult to understand, or leading questions (Garrett et al., 2003). In addition, sociolinguists who wanted to observe everyday speech were creating a situation during these interviews that was unusual and affected the formality of the speech (Labov called this situation the 'observer's paradox'; see Labov, 1972, p. 209). Despite these drawbacks, this qualitative method is probably the most commonly used approach in sociolinguistic studies.

The indirect approach is synonymous with the 'matched guise technique' (Lambert et al., 1960). Lambert developed this technique because he doubted that overt responses matched privately held beliefs about accents. This procedure uses speech recordings of actors reading the same neutral passage while imitating the different accents of interest. These recordings are then validated by independent judges and rated for authenticity (i.e. typicality of the accent for a given region). Once the stimulus material has been created, a new group of participants rates each speaker, one after the other, on a range of personality characteristics (e.g. social desirability) using bipolar rating scales. This technique allows further quantitative analyses, such as factor analysis, to determine the evaluative dimensions used to judge accents. The most frequently observed dimensions of accent judgements and their speakers are prestige (e.g. educated), social attractiveness (e.g. nice), and dynamism (e.g. energetic) (Zahn & Hopper, 1985). Analyses of variance then allow to differentiate accent groups (e.g. 'Brummie' is more or less attractive than Glaswegian). This technique has the advantage of controlling potential acoustic confounds, such as pitch or harmonics-to-noise ratio ('smoothness') of the voice, which we know affect vocal attractiveness ratings (Bestelmeyer et al., 2012; Bruckert et al, 2010).

Sceptics have criticized the indirect method because repeated presentations of the same passage with repeated instructions of rating the speaker may lead to unreliable responses by an unengaged participant. It is also possible, particularly if the speakers had to imitate a large number of different accents, that the accent was not authentic enough or was even misperceived by the judge (for a detailed description of the pros and cons of each technique, see Garrett et al., 2003). Nevertheless, this elegant method, if well prepared and counterbalanced, is more likely to tap into listener's actual opinions about different varieties of speech. It has led to a range of international studies that are comparable and has allowed for the isolating of the dimensions typically used to describe accents (prestige, social attractiveness, and dynamism; Garrett et al., 2003).

30.3 THE EFFECTS OF ACCENT ON SOCIAL EVALUATION

Empirical research on 'linguistic first impressions' arguably began with Pear (1931), Professor of Psychology at Manchester University. He asked 200 listeners to provide personality profiles of a variety of voices heard during a recording of a radio drama (including likeability of the 'Cockney' accent). He noticed that a speaker's voice and accent could dramatically affect person perception. In a later study, he had nine different speakers (including children and individuals from different social classes) read a short text about a skating incident. The BBC broadcast the same text nine times over three days, and the *Radio Times* published a personality questionnaire to be completed and sent back to the BBC. Several thousand listeners responded to questions about voice gender, age, profession of the speaker, and the 'locality affecting speech'. Age and gender were accurately judged, as well as estimates with respect to the geographical background of the speaker and their professions, suggesting that speech variations provide detailed hints to a speaker's age, gender, geographical background, and social class.

The domain of sociolinguistics began as a quest to understand language variation and its social implications. William Labov is one of the pioneers who studied the unique accent of people on Martha's Vineyard, an island community off the east coast of the United States with a population of around 6,000. Labov (1966) studied the variation of diphthongs [aw] and [ay] by interviewing a number of speakers from different social backgrounds and ages. He found that the younger generation moved away from the norms of the New England accent to an accent unique to inhabitants of the island. Speakers who particularly identified themselves as 'Vineyarders' and rejected the values of the mainland had particularly strong accents (e.g. the Chilmark fishermen). Later, Trudgill (1974) was interested in the effects of social class and gender on accent variation. He investigated his questions by looking at the final consonant in words like 'walking' or 'talking' pronounced in Standard English versus 'walkin' or 'talkin' as the non-standard version of many accents. Trudgill discovered that non-standard versions of pronunciation were more common in lower social classes. He also learned that men are more likely to use non-standard forms. Trudgill confirmed Pear's observation that both gender and social class affect accent production.

Typically, a language will have a standard form which prescribes the grammar, spelling, and pronunciation, for example, BBC English in the UK (also known as Queen's English or Received Pronunciation/RP), General American in the USA, and Castilian Spanish in Spain. This should not be confused with being 'accent-free' (i.e. RP is still a type of accent). Standard accents generally receive positive evaluations, for example, they favourably affect listeners' perceptions of the speaker's education, status, personality, similarity with the rater, and even attractiveness (e.g. Ball, 1983; Giles, 1970; Stewart et al., 1985). Information conveyed by standard accented speech is also more easily understood and recalled (Ryan & Sebastian, 1980).

Regional and non-native varieties usually fall under the definition of non-standard accents. In contrast to standard accents, many studies have highlighted the usually negative social perceptions of non-standard speech and even stigmatization of non-native accented speakers (Gluszek & Dovidio, 2010a,b). For instance, foreign-accented speakers have been shown to be less credible than native speakers (Lev-Ari & Keysar, 2010), with an obvious negative impact on foreign job seekers or sales representatives. A foreign accent is also a signal of not being native-born (Derwing & Munro, 2009; Moyer, 2004) and therefore possibly not being able to speak the language fluently, irrespective of the speaker's actual language competence (Lindemann, 2002). In addition to these negative perceptions of listeners, foreign- but not regional-accented speakers in the USA have reported lower feelings of social belonging mediated by perceived problems in communicating (Gluszek & Dovidio, 2010a). The reason why foreign accents are generally rated negatively may be due to increased cognitive load when trying to understand heavily accented messages (e.g. Adank et al., 2009).

While speakers of non-standard speech have often been found to be at a disadvantage compared to speakers of standard varieties (particularly when the accent is broad; Gluszek et al., 2011), regional accents can occasionally be upgraded depending on the context of the situation. For example, craftsmen with a non-standard accent have been rated as more masculine and more skilled at their job (Giles et al., 1992). Another prominent example of non-standard accent preference is when group membership is salient. One large online survey, conducted in association with the BBC, asked participants about their own accent as well as to rate thirty-four accents, which included most major regional British and global (e.g. Australian) varieties, on social attractiveness and prestige (e.g. 'how much prestige do you think is associated with this accent?'). The survey confirmed earlier research in that standard varieties were favoured on dimensions of prestige and attractiveness, while many regional varieties were downgraded (e.g. the urban accent of Birmingham, 'Brummie'). Interestingly, the informant's own regional variety had robust effects on the ratings of non-standard varieties in that their own accent, and those similar to it, were favoured. The accent identical to the respondent's own accent was rated similarly to Standard English in terms of social attractiveness and was next in line to standard varieties on prestige (Coupland & Bishop, 2007; but see also Edwards, 1982; Hurt & Weaver, 1972; Mulac et al., 1974; Ryan & Sebastian, 1980). This study is one of the first that clearly illustrates the importance of an additional variable in the social evaluation of speech—the speaker's *own accent*.

Applied research supports the impact of this own-accent bias. In higher education, for example, North American students rated North American teachers more favourably and recalled more information from their lessons than from teachers who spoke British or

Malaysian-accented English (Gill, 1994). Similarly, a recent study on 'earwitness' memory reported an interaction between witness accent and offender's accent in that Scottish and English earwitnesses were less confident in their judgement and more prone to confuse offenders who spoke in a different accent to their own (Stevenage et al., 2012; for a similar result with familiar versus unfamiliar accented speech, see also Philippon et al., 2007). Individuals with out-group accents may sound more alike and may therefore be more easily confused (Williams et al., 1999).

30.4 SOCIAL IDENTITY THEORY AS AN EXPLANATION FOR THE OWN-ACCENT BIAS

One possible explanation for the positive bias towards own-accented speakers comes from social psychology. Humans perceive their surroundings in terms of categories in which they compare the sensory information to several stored representations of objects, individuals, or social situations. Social categorization involves classifying individuals in terms of the groups they belong to (in-group) or do not belong to (out-group) and is a fundamental process in person perception (Bartlett, 1932; Bruner, 1957). Social theorists have argued that, in addition to our personal identities, these social categories are so important to us that our identity is partially based on these group memberships (e.g. Tajfel & Turner, 1979; Turner et al., 1987). Tajfel (1979) proposed that the groups (e.g. social class) individuals belonged to were an important source of pride and self-esteem. Thus the groups we belong to shape our attitudes, determine the language we speak, and which accent we have.

The purpose of the formation of these categories is thought to simplify the overwhelming environment that the perceiver is confronted with (Brewer, 1988; Fiske & Neuberg, 1990), but this computational reductionism comes with costs. Social identity theory (SIT) predicts that group membership causes an enhancement and favouritism of the in-group at the expense of the out-group. In other words, group members of an in-group may discriminate against the out-group to boost their self-image. SIT has found support in numerous experimental studies, which have reported that the mere perception of belonging, or even just the awareness of the presence of two distinct groups, is sufficient for a bias towards or favouring of the in-group (Billig & Tajfel, 1973; Doise et al, 1972; Tajfel & Billig, 1974; Tajfel et al., 1971; Turner, 1975). Later studies have suggested that this bias occurs without conscious awareness and involves positive affect towards the in-group (Dovidio & Gaertner, 1993), even when the in-group is novel or based on arbitrary categorization (Otten & Moskowitz, 2000). Ethnolinguistic identity theory (based on SIT; Giles & Johnson, 1981) highlights the connection between language and social identity, as well as language, as a marker for group membership.

According to these theories, language can enhance a speaker's social identity and pride for one's own group. Social or ethnolinguistic identity theory provides cognitive psychologists and neuroscientists with a testable framework. In other words, we should be able to detect neural correlates of this bias in the listener's brain.

SIT also provides a framework for explaining the well-researched phenomenon of speech imitation and accommodation. Speakers often converge their speech pattern to the speech of their conversational partner. For example, imitation of speech patterns has been found for speech rate (Giles et al., 1991), prosody (Goldinger, 1998), style (Kappes et al., 2009), and also regional accent (Delvaux & Soquet, 2007). Imitative behaviour during social interaction is generally linked with increased likeability and closeness (e.g. Chartrand & Bargh, 1999). A more specific example comes from Pardo et al. (2012) who showed that room-mates' self-reported closeness correlated with phonetic convergence. Conversely, speech divergence, such as a more pronounced accent, may help speakers to make themselves more distinct and favourably different from an out-group (Bourhis, 1979; Giles, 1977, 1978, 1979; Giles et al., 1977; Giles & Johnson, 1981; Hogg & Abrams, 1988).

30.5 THE EVOLUTION OF ACCENTS

The connection between social-group inferences and spoken language has been known and explored (for an interesting review, see Giles & Johnson, 1981). However, even *non-speech* vocalizations can index social-group relations (Lewis, 1975). With regards to non-human animals, it has typically been claimed that vocal production is hard-wired (i.e. genetically determined and independent of environmental influences) (e.g. Simmons et al., 2003). However, more recent evidence actually suggests that call production in non-human animals also exists and may reflect a 'group-distinctive identifier', with very alike vocalizations consolidating social bonds (Tyack, 2008). Hence, speculatively put, other non-human animals may also have a form of accent or at least a 'precursor' to accents.

For example, Seyfarth and Cheney (2014) have noted that in a number of social primate species, individuals can identify members of their social group by their voice alone. Gibbons are small apes and close-living relatives of humans. This species has received much scientific attention due to their characteristic song structure that varies between individuals and gibbon subspecies. A recent study has analysed the acoustic structure of several hundred gibbon duets. It found a strong positive correlation between the similarity of song structure, the gibbons' genetic relatedness, and geographic distance. In other words, the more similar the song between pairs of gibbons, the more likely the gibbons belonged to the same species and lived more closely together (Van Ngoc et al., 2011; for increased geographic distance and dissimilarity in birdsong of the same species, see also Lachlan et al., 2013). Not only are these vocalizations useful to unravel genetic relatedness and geographic origins, but they also highlight their social usefulness in strengthening groups.

Gibbons are not the only example amongst non-human animals to have group-dependent vocalizations. A study which received lots of media attention, by the BBC and others, investigated whether the social environment affected the vocalizations of young goats, another highly social and vocal species (Briefer & McElligott, 2012). The researchers examined the acoustic structure of vocalizations by full and half siblings raised in the same group or different social groups. Goat calls of full siblings were more alike than those of half siblings, and vocalizations of half siblings were more alike if they were raised by the same rather than different social groups. Interestingly, the similarity of calls between siblings converged with time if they were raised together. This vocal convergence has been shown in other mammals such as bats, dolphins, harbour seals, and elephants (e.g. Tyack, 2008). This vocal plasticity affected by the animal's social environment may be an early prerequisite to vocal learning and language evolution.

30.6 THE DEVELOPMENT OF ACCENTS

The ability to discriminate vocal acoustic structure in humans begins before birth. Term fetuses are able to discriminate their mother's voice from that of a stranger, as demonstrated by increased fetal heartbeat to the mother's voice (Kisilevsky et al., 2003). Only a few months later, neonates are able to discriminate and recognize the voices of their parents (Ockleford et al., 1988) and can discriminate languages of different rhythmic classes (Nazzi et al., 1998). At five months of age, before any significant speech-production ability, North American children can differentiate between American and British English accents at the sentence level. Similarly, Butler et al. (2011) have shown that five and seven month olds can differentiate their own regional accent from another regional accent but are unable to distinguish two unfamiliar regional accents. Thus at this age, children seem to have already developed an acoustic prototype or acoustic reference system for their native language and accent. At roughly the same age, infants were also found to show a looking preference to speakers who speak with their native accent compared to a foreign accent (Kinzler et al., 2007).

By five years of age, accents play a significant role in children's social appraisals whereby they tend to choose other children as friends who speak with their native accent compared to a comprehensible foreign accent (Kinzler et al., 2007; Kinzler et al., 2011). Typically, all else being equal, children will favour same-race children over other-race children. However, if accent and race are pitted against each other, five year olds will prefer children with the same, native accent as theirs, independently of the child's race (Kinzler et al., 2009). While we know about the ubiquitous stereotypes, prejudices, and tragedies that can result from unacceptance of individuals of other races in almost any country, it is a new development in the literature to think of accents as a potentially powerful marker of out-groups.

Regional-accent recognition is less well studied than foreign-accent recognition and seems to appear a little later in development. For example, children as old as six years are able to differentiate between foreign and native accents but not between different, unfamiliar regional accents (Floccia et al., 2009; Girard et al., 2008). However, by seven to ten years of age, children are able to differentiate various regional Dutch accents (van Bezooijen, 1994). While children at this age can tell the difference between regional accents, the literature on regional-accent *preferences* is unclear.

Labov (1965) claimed that children do not realize the social significance of accents until they reach their early teens. However, there is now evidence to suggest that Labov's initial estimate was perhaps conservative. For example, five- and six-year-old children can already successfully differentiate their home accent from a foreign accent and reliably associate cultural items with the home and foreign accent but not another non-home regional accent (Wagner et al., 2014). Given the importance of accents to adult's social judgements, it does make sense that children develop a rudimentary understanding of the social significance of accents relatively quickly.

A complication of research on social attitudes is that much has been investigated in terms of the development of *language* attitudes in bilingual children but not necessarily attitudes towards the characteristic regional *accent*. For example, bilingual children of Welsh and English will have different attitudes towards Welsh and English depending on the type of school (e.g. Welsh immersion versus predominantly English) and their age. Children in Welsh-medium schools prefer Welsh to English during adolescence, while the attitude of children in mixed schools or English schools changes from Welsh towards English as the children get older (Lewis, 1975). Similarly, Schneiderman (1976) found that young bilingual Franco-Ontarian children will favour French, the language of their in-group.

Regarding the relatively neglected research topic of accent preference, most of the work has focused on the preference for regional (but not necessarily home accents) versus standard accents. For example, seven-year-old Welsh children seem to prefer their own accent and react negatively towards Standard English, although by the age of ten, the children show similar reactions to the standard variety as the adults, with a preference for the Standard English accent (Giles et al., 1983; Price et al., 1983). Often the attitude towards the actual *accent* is not as such assessed. However, Lambert et al. (1975) have shown that Franco-American high-school and college students expressed increasingly more positive attitudes as they got older towards their local variety of French, even though it is a minority language. However, several studies have found that children will develop a tendency to prefer the standard variety rather than their own accent (e.g. Cremona & Bates, 1977). While the exact developmental pattern of social preference for own or standard accents is still to be determined, these findings in developmental sociolinguistics are in support of the conclusion that young children and adolescents already use accents as a symbol of group membership or social desirability.

One of the ways children may learn how to discriminate between accents and attribute certain traits to them is via television productions. A now classic study by Lippi-Green (1997) analysed all animated Disney films between 1938 and 1994. All characters who uttered more than just single words were included in the analysis, resulting in a sample size of 371 characters. Systematic patterns emerged on how accents were used across the different roles. She found that most characters spoke with a native English accent, particularly mainstream American English. Only 9% of characters spoke with a foreign accent. Lippi-Green then divided her characters into four groups based on their motivation and actions (i.e. positive, negative, mixed, and unclear). She found that twice as many foreign as compared with native-accented speakers were portrayed as negative characters. While the number of speakers was very low, all characters with African-American vernacular English accents appeared as non-human animals. The author concludes that 'what children learn from the entertainment industry is to be comfortable with *same* and to be wary about *other*, and that language is a prime and ready diagnostic for this division between what is approachable and what is best left alone' (Lippi-Green, 1997, p. 103).

Accent production appears early in development because it is so closely associated with speech acquisition. The acoustic contour of newborn babies' cries is already similar to that of the language they were exposed to prenatally. Thus, French newborns tend to produce rising melody contours, while German newborns produce falling contours (Mampe et al., 2009). By the age of ten months, there are distinct differences in the babbling of babies raised in different countries (de Boysson-Bardies, 1993). At approximately five years of age, children often shift their accents to be more similar to that of their peers (Labov, 1964). This shift can be striking in the case of children who have moved to another country with the same language. For example, an analysis of Canadian children's speech demonstrated how their vowels shifted over time to approximate those of their new British peers (Chambers, 1992). This process may not be perfect and depends on the age at which the children are exposed to the new accent (Deser, 1989; Kerswill & Williams, 2000; Payne, 1980). Interestingly, how well children can approximate the new regional (or national) variety is dependent on how socially integrated they are with their new peer group. Thus children who are more integrated and have a rich social network of friends are more likely to adjust their accent than children with smaller social networks (Berthele, 2002), although it is not clear whether similar amounts of non-social exposure to the new accent would do the same trick.

30.7 THE NEUROSCIENCE OF ACCENTS

The neuropsychology of accent production has received much media attention due to curious reports of patients who, as a result of a brain injury, suddenly speak with a 'foreign' accent. This phenomenon is a rare speech disorder and was coined 'foreign accent syndrome'. It was first reported in 1907 by French neurologist, Pierre Marie. Phonetic errors on consonants and vowels, as well as prosodic errors (including stress and rhythm), characterize the syndrome, and in listeners, these errors are perceived as a foreign accent. To date, there are only approximately seventy recorded cases worldwide, most commonly following a stroke (Liu et al., 2015). The exact cause of foreign accent syndrome has been debated (e.g. Blumstein & Kurowski, 2006; Moen, 2000) with more recent evidence suggesting that there may be a disconnection between the planning of articulation and motor control (Scott et al., 2006). The lesion site can be tiny and go unnoticed in anatomical scans but frequently affect subcortical structures (e.g. basal ganglia) or white matter in ventral to primary motor cortex (Liu et al., 2015).

Due to the strangeness of the phenomenon, but also the severity with which it affects the patient's quality of life, some of these patients have been interviewed on television chat shows and for tabloid articles. One well-known sufferer in the UK is Kath Lockett, who has survived a severe brain condition relatively unscathed except for her speech impediment which sounds like the British national speaks with an Italian accent. Speaking to Phillip Schofield and Amanda Holden on ITV's 'This Morning' in October 2014, Kath Lockett said: 'I feel like I've been robbed—now I'm either Italian, Lithuanian, Russian, Polish. I have no homeland now—I want to go home.' Due to the rarity and heterogeneity of the condition, it probably only tells us little about the neuropsychology of accent production but it does again underline the importance of accents to social identity.

The neuroscience of accent perception has only recently gained momentum with a study that investigated the neural substrates of accent processing of standard Dutch and an artificial, novel variation of Dutch (Adank et al., 2012). It revealed that bilateral mid and superior temporal gyri, planum temporale, as well as left inferior frontal gyrus are involved in processing accents. Some of the reported activations overlapped with regions that also respond preferentially to vocal compared to non-vocal sounds, known as the temporal voice areas (Belin & Zatorre, 2000; Bestelmeyer et al., 2011; Grandjean et al., 2005; Lewis et al., 2009).

There is only one study to date that has investigated the neural underpinnings of the social effects of accents on listeners (Bestelmeyer et al., 2015), in particular, the neural basis for the preference of own versus other accents. Participants from Scotland or Southern England

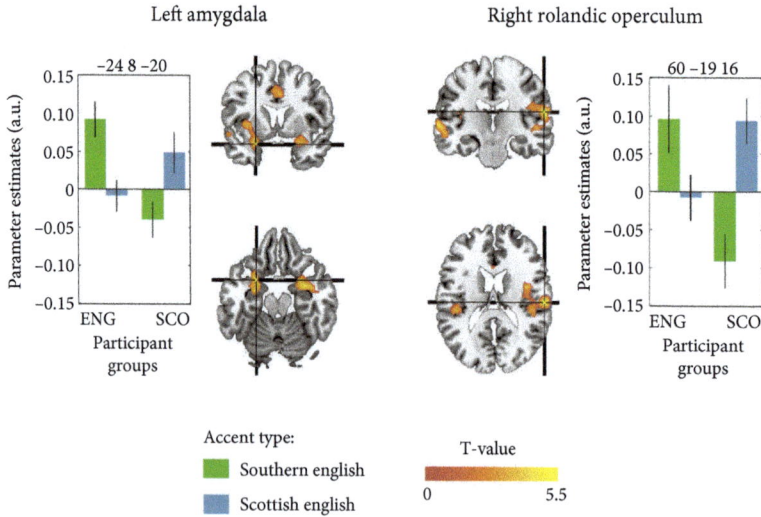

FIGURE 30.1 Overlay of brain activation in response to the interaction between participant group (from Scotland and Southern England) and accent type of the speakers in bilateral amygdalae and bilateral auditory association cortices. The bar graphs represent the BOLD signal in the areas that show the cross hair with stronger activations after repetitions of the listener's own accent compared to the accent of the out-group.

listened to women pronouncing four-digit numbers in three types of accents (Scottish, Southern English, and General American; listen to Audio 30.1 for samples). Cerebral activity in several regions, including bilateral amygdalae, revealed a significant interaction between the participants' own accent and the accent they listened to: while repetition of their own accents elicited an enhanced neural response, repetition of the other group's accent resulted in reduced responses classically associated with adaptation (see Figure 30.1). Our findings suggest that increased social relevance of, or greater emotional sensitivity to, in-group accents may underlie the own-accent bias. Our results provide a neural marker for the bias associated with accents, and show that the neural response to speech is partly shaped by the geographical background of the listener. These results are the first report of a neural signature for group membership based on phonetic variations of the same language.

30.8 CONCLUSION

This chapter reviewed the multidisciplinary literature on the social perception and behaviour towards accents, as well as their development and evolution. A neglected but potentially important finding is the general preference for speakers who 'sound like us'. Recently, neuroscientific evidence supports the notion that we process our own accents differently from accents of another region despite familiarity with, and comprehension of, the out-group's accent (e.g. via media). Hence, the way for stereotypes, and even prejudice, based on accents is paved. Awareness of this issue is limited because most stereotypic features discussed in the literature are visible (e.g. race or sex). What remains to be seen is what drives this bias towards individuals who sound like us. Is our brain's reaction related to greater attentional capture of speakers of our own accent or is it related to a greater, possibly emotional, affiliation with speakers who sound like us? As society becomes increasingly more geographically mobile and interconnected, the understanding and alleviating of social bias based not only on sex, race, and religion but also on accents, is essential.

REFERENCES

Adank, P., Davis, M. H., & Hagoort, P. (2012). Neural dissociation in processing noise and accent in spoken language comprehension. *Neuropsychologia*, 50(1), 77–84. doi: 10.1016/j.neuropsychologia.2011.10.024

Adank, P., Evans, B. G., Stuart-Smith, J., & Scott, S. K. (2009). Comprehension of familiar and unfamiliar native accents under adverse listening conditions. *Journal of Experimental Psychology: Human Perception and Performance*, 35(2), 520–529. doi: 10.1037/a0013552

Ball, P. (1983). Stereotypes of Anglo-Saxon and non-Anglo-Saxon accents: some exploratory Australian studies with the Matched Guise Technique. *Language Sciences*, 5, 163–183.

Bartlett, F. C. (1932). *Remembering: A Study in Experimental and Social Psychology*. New York: Cambridge University Press.

Belin, P. & Zatorre, R. J. (2000). Auditory perception and functional magnetic resonance imaging— fMRI. *Revue De Neuropsychologie*, 10(4), 603–621.

Berthele, R. (2002). Learning a second dialect: a model of idiolectal dissonance. *Multilingua*, 21, 327–344.

Bestelmeyer, P. E. G., Belin, P., & Grosbras, M.-H. (2011). Right temporal TMS impairs voice detection. *Current Biology*, 21, R838–839.

Bestelmeyer, P. E. G., Belin, P., & Ladd, D. R. (2015). A neural marker for social bias toward in-group accents. *Cerebral Cortex*, 25, 3953–3961.

Bestelmeyer, P. E. G., Latinus, M., Bruckert, L., Crabbe, F., & Belin, P. (2012). Implicitly perceived vocal attractiveness modulates prefrontal cortex activity. *Cerebral Cortex*, 22, 1263–1270.

Billig, M. & Tajfel, H. (1973). Social categorization and similarity in intergroup behaviour. *European Journal of Social Psychology*, 3(1), 27–52. doi: 10.1002/ejsp.2420030103

Blumstein, S. E. & Kurowski, K. (2006). The foreign accent syndrome: a perspective. *Journal of Neurolinguistics*, 19(5), 346–355. doi: 10.1016/j.jneuroling.2006.03.003

Bourhis, R. Y. (1979). Language in ethnic interaction. In: H. Giles & R. Saint-Jacques (eds) *Language and Ethnic Relations*. Elmsford, NY: Pergamon.

Brewer, M. B. (ed.) (1988). *A Dual Process Model of Impression Formation* (Vol. 1). Hillsdale, NJ: Lawrence Erlbaum.

Briefer, E. F. & McElligott, A. G. (2012). Social effects on vocal ontogeny in an ungulate, the goat, *Capra hircus. Animal Behaviour*, 83(4), 991–1000. doi: 10.1016/j.anbehav.2012.01.020

Bruckert, L., Bestelmeyer, P., Latinus, M., Rouger, J., Charest, I., Rousselet, G. A., Kawahara, H., & Belin, P. (2010). Vocal attractiveness increases by averaging. *Current Biology*, 20(2), 116–120. doi: 10.1016/j.cub.2009.11.034

Bruner, J. S. (1957). On perceptual readiness. *Psychological Review*, 64, 123–152.

Butler, J., Floccia, C., Goslin, J., & Panneton, R. (2011). Infants' discrimination of familiar and unfamiliar accents in speech. *Infancy*, 16(4), 392–417. doi: 10.1111/j.1532-7078.2010.00050.x

Chambers, J. K. (1992). Dialect acquisition. *Language*, 68(4), 673–705. doi: 10.2307/416850

Chartrand, T. L. & Bargh, J. A. (1999). The chameleon effect: the perception-behavior link and social interaction. *Journal of Personality and Social Psychology*, 76(6), 893–910. doi: 10.1037//0022-3514.76.6.893

Clopper, C. G. & Pisoni, D. B. (2004). Some acoustic cues for the perceptual categorization of American English regional dialects. *Journal of Phonetics*, 32(1), 111–140. doi: 10.1016/s0095-4470(03)00009-3

Clopper, C. G. & Pisoni, D. B. (2007). Free classification of regional dialects of American English. *Journal of Phonetics*, 35(3), 421–438. doi: 10.1016/j.wocn.2006.06.001

Clopper, C. G., Rohrbeck, K. L., & Wagner, L. (2012). Perception of dialect variation by young adults with high-functioning autism. *Journal of Autism and Developmental Disorders*, 42(5), 740–754. doi: 10.1007/s10803-011-1305-y

Coupland, N. & Bishop, H. (2007). Ideologised values for British accents. *Journal of Sociolinguistics*, 11(1), 74–93.

Cremona, C. & Bates, E. (1977). The development of attitudes toward dialect in Italian children. *Journal of Psycholinguistic Research*, 6, 223–232.

de Boysson- Bardies, B. (1993). Ontogeny of language-specific syllabic production. In: B. de Boysson-Bardies, S. de Schoen, P. Jusczyk, P. F. MacNeilage, & J. Morton (eds) *Developmental Neurocognition: Speech and Face Processing in the First Year of Life*. Dordrecht: Kluwer Academic Publishers.

Delvaux, V. & Soquet, A. (2007). The influence of ambient speech on adult speech productions through unintentional imitation. *Phonetica*, 64(2–3), 145–173. doi: 10.1159/000107914

Derwing, T. M. & Munro, M. J. (2009). Putting accent in its place: rethinking obstacles to communication. *Language Teaching*, 42, 476–490. doi: 10.1017/s026144480800551x

Deser, T. (1989). Dialect transmission and variation: an acoustic analysis of vowels in six urban Detroit families'. *York Papers in Linguistics*, 13, 115–128.

Doise, W., Csepeli, G., Dann, H. D., Gouge, C., Larsen, K., & Ostell, A. (1972). Experimental investigation into formation of intergroup representations. *European Journal of Social Psychology*, 2(2), 202–204.

Dovidio, J. F. & Gaertner, S. L. (1993). Stereotypes and evaluative intergroup bias. In: D. M. Mackie & D. L. Hamilton (eds) *Affect, Cognition, and Stereotyping* (pp. 167–193). San Diego: Academic Press.

Edwards, J. R. (1982). Language attitudes and their implications among English speakers. In: E. B. Ryan & H. Giles (eds) *Attitudes Towards Language Variation* (pp. 20–33). London: Edward Arnold.

Fiske, S. T. & Neuberg, S. L. (1990). *A Continuum of Impression Formation, from Category Based to Individuating Processes: Influence of Information and Motivation on Attention and Interpretation*. San Diego, CA: Academic Press.

Floccia, C., Butler, J., Goslin, J., & Ellis, L. (2009). Regional and foreign accent processing in English: can listeners adapt? *Journal of Psycholinguistic Research*, 38(4), 379–412. doi: 10.1007/s10936-008-9097-8

Garrett, P., Coupland, N., & Williams, A. (2003). *Investigating Language Attitudes: Social Meanings of Dialect, Ethnicity and Performance*. Cardiff, UK: University of Wales Press.

Giles, H. (1970). Evaluative reactions to accents. *Educational Review*, 22, 211–227.

Giles, H. (1977). Social psychology and applied linguistics: towards an integrative approach. *ITL Review of Applied Linguistics*, 35, 27–42.

Giles, H. (1978). Linguistic differentiation between ethnic groups. In: H. Tajfel (ed.) *Differentiation Between Social Groups*. London: Academic Press.

Giles, H. (1979). Ethnicity markers in speech. I. In: K. Scherer & H. Giles (eds) *Social Markers in Speech*. Cambridge: Cambridge University Press.

Giles, H., Bourhis, R. Y., & Taylor, D. M. (1977). Towards a theory of language in ethnic group relations. In: H. Giles (ed.) *Language, Ethnicity and Intergroup Relations* (pp. 307–348). London: Academic Press.

Giles, H., Coupland, J., & Coupland, N. (1991). *Contexts of Accommodation: Developments in Applied Sociolinguistics*. Cambridge: Cambridge University Press.

Giles, H., Harrison, C., Creber, C., Smith, P., & Freeman, N. (1983). Developmental and contextual aspects of British children's language attitudes. *Language and Communication*, 3, 1–6.

Giles, H., Henwood, K., Coupland, N., Harriman, J., & Coupland, J. (1992). Language attitudes and cognitive mediation. *Human Communication Research*, 18(4), 500–527. doi: 10.1111/j.1468-2958.1992.tb00570.x

Giles, H. & Johnson, P. (1981). The role of language in ethnic group relations. I. In: J. C. Turner & H. Giles (eds) *Intergroup Behavior*. Oxford, UK: Blackwell.

Gill, M. M. (1994). Accent and stereotypes: their effect on perceptions of teachers and lecture comprehension. *Journal of Applied Communication Research*, 22, 348–361.

Girard, F., Floccia, C., & Goslin, J. (2008). Perception and awareness of accents in young children. *British Journal of Developmental Psychology*, 26, 409–433. doi: 10.1348/026151007X251712

Gluszek, A. & Dovidio, J. F. (2010a). Speaking with a nonnative accent: perceptions of bias, communication difficulties, and belonging in the United States. *Journal of Language and Social Psychology*, 29(2), 224–234. doi: 10.1177/0261927X09359590

Gluszek, A. & Dovidio, J. F. (2010b). The way they speak: a social psychological perspective on the stigma of nonnative accents in communication. *Personality and Social Psychology Review*, 14(2), 214–237. doi: 10.1177/1088868309359288

Gluszek, A., Newheiser, A.-K., & Dovidio, J. F. (2011). Social psychological orientations and accent strength. *Journal of Language and Social Psychology*, 30(1), 28–45. doi: 10.1177/0261927X10387100

Goldinger, S. D. (1998). Echoes of echoes? An episodic theory of lexical access. *Psychological Review*, 105(2), 251–279. doi: 10.1037//0033-295X.105.2.251

Grandjean, D., Sander, D., Pourtois, G., Schwartz, S., Seghier, M. L., Scherer, K. R., & Vuilleumier, P. (2005). The voices of wrath: brain responses to angry prosody in meaningless speech. *Nature Neuroscience*, 8(2), 145–146. doi: 10.1038/nn1392

Hogg, M. A. & Abrams, D. (1988). *Social Identifications: A Social Psychology of Intergroup Relations and Group Processes*. London, UK: Routledge.

Hurt, H. T. & Weaver, C. H. (1972). Negro dialect, ethno-centricism, and the distortion of information in the communicative process. *Central States Speech Journal*, 23, 118–125.

Kappes, J., Baumgaertner, A., Peschke, C., & Ziegler, W. (2009). Unintended imitation in nonword repetition. *Brain and Language*, 111(3), 140–151. doi: 10.1016/j.bandl.2009.08.008

Kerswill, P. & Williams, A. (2000). Creating a new town koine: children and language change in Milton Keynes. *Language in Society*, 29(1), 65–115.

Khleif, B. B. (1979). Language as identity—toward an ethnography of Welsh nationalism. *Ethnicity*, 6(4), 346–357.

Kinzler, K. D., Corriveau, K. H., & Harris, P. L. (2011). Children's selective trust in native-accented speakers. *Developmental Science*, 14(1), 106–111. doi: 10.1111/j.1467-7687.2010.00965.x

Kinzler, K. D., Dupoux, E., & Spelke, E. S. (2007). The native language of social cognition. *Proceedings of the National Academy of Sciences of the United States of America*, 104, 12577–12580.

Kinzler, K. D., Shutts, K., DeJesus, J., & Spelke, E. S. (2009). Accent trumps race in guiding children's social preferences. *Social Cognition*, 27, 623–634.

Kisilevsky, B. S., Hains, S. M. J., Lee, K., Xie, X., Huang, H. F., Ye, H. H., Zhang, K., & Wang, Z. P. (2003). Effects of experience on fetal voice recognition. *Psychological Science*, 14(3), 220–224. doi: 10.1111/1467-9280.02435

Knops, U. & van Hout, R. (1988). *Language Attitudes in the Dutch Language Area.* Dordrecht: Foris.

Labov, W. (1964). Stages in the acquisition of standard English. In: R. Shuy, A. Davis, & R. Hogan (eds) *Social Dialects and Language Learning* (pp. 77–104). Champaign, IL: National Council of Teachers of English.

Labov, W. (1965). *Stages in the Acquisition of Standard English.* Champaign, IL: National Council of Teachers of English.

Labov, W. (1972). *Sociolinguistic Patterns.* Philadelphia: University of Pennyslvania.

Labov, W. (2006). *The Social Stratification of English in New York City* (2nd edn). New York: Cambridge University Press.

Lachlan, R. F., Verzijden, M. N., Bernard, C. S., Jonker, P.-P., Koese, B., Jaarsma, S., ... ten Cate, C. (2013). The progressive loss of syntactical structure in bird song along an island colonization chain. *Current Biology*, 23(19), 1896–1901. doi: 10.1016/j.cub.2013.07.057

Lambert, W. E., Giles, H., & Picard, O. (1975). Language attitudes in a French-American community. *International Journal of the Sociology of Language*, 4, 127–152.

Lambert, W. E., Hodgson, R. C., Gardner, R. C., & Fillenbaum, S. (1960). Evaluational reactions to spoken language. *Journal of Abnormal and Social Psychology*, 60, 44–51.

Lev-Ari, S. & Keysar, B. (2010). Why don't we believe non-native speakers? The influence of accent on credibility. *Journal of Experimental Social Psychology*, 46(6), 1093–1096. doi: 10.1016/j.jesp.2010.05.025

Lewis, G. (1975). Attitudes to language among bilingual children and adults in Wales. *International Journal of the Sociology of Language*, 4, 103–121.

Lewis, J. W., Talkington, W. J., Walker, N. A., Spirou, G. A., Jajosky, A., Frum, C., & Brefczynski-Lewis, J. A. (2009). Human cortical organization for processing vocalizations indicates representation of harmonic structure as a signal attribute. *Journal of Neuroscience*, 29, 2283–2296.

Lindemann, S. (2002). Listening with an attitude: a model of native-speaker comprehension of nonnative speakers in the United States. *Language in Society*, 31, 419–441.

Lippi-Green, R. (1997). *English with an Accent: Language, Ideology, and Discrimination in the United States.* London and New York: Routledge.

Liu, H. E., Qi, P., Liu, Y. L., Liu, H. X., & Li, G. (2015). Foreign accent syndrome: two case reports and literature review. *European Review for Medical and Pharmacological Sciences*, 19(1), 81–85.

Luhman, R. (1990). Appalachian English stereotypes: language attitudes in Kentucky. *Language in Society*, 19, 331–348.

Mampe, B., Friederici, A. D., Christophe, A., & Wermke, K. (2009). Newborns' cry melody is shaped by their native language. *Current Biology*, 19(23), 1994–1997. doi: 10.1016/j.cub.2009.09.064

Moen, I. (2000). Foreign accent syndrome: a review of contemporary explanations. *Aphasiology*, 14(1), 5–15. doi: 10.1080/026870300401577

Moyer, A. (2004). *Age, Accents, and Experience in Second Language Acquisition: An Integrated Approach to Critical Period Inquiry*. Clevedon, UK: Multilingual Matters.

Mulac, A., Hanley, T. D., & Prigge, D. Y. (1974). Effects of phonological speech foreignness upon three dimensions of attitude of selected American listeners. *Quarterly Journal of Speech*, 60(4), 411–420.

Nazzi, T., Bertoncini, J., & Mehler, J. (1998). Language discrimination by newborns: toward an understanding of the role of rhythm. *Journal of Experimental Psychology: Human Perception and Performance*, 24(3), 756–766. doi: 10.1037//0096-1523.24.3.756

Ockleford, E. M., Vince, M. A., Layton, C., & Reader, M. R. (1988). Responses of neonates to parents and others voices. *Early Human Development*, 18(1), 27–36. doi: 10.1016/0378-3782(88)90040-0

Otten, S. & Moskowitz, G. B. (2000). Evidence for implicit evaluative in-group bias: affect-biased spontaneous trait inference in a minimal group paradigm. *Journal of Experimental Social Psychology*, 36, 77–89.

Pardo, J. S., Gibbons, R., Suppes, A., & Krauss, R. M. (2012). Phonetic convergence in college roommates. *Journal of Phonetics*, 40(1), 190–197. doi: 10.1016/j.wocn.2011.10.001

Payne, A. (1980). Factors controlling the acquisition of the Philadelphia dialect by out-of-state children. In: W. Labov (ed.) *Locating Language in Time and Space* (pp. 143–178). New York: Academic Press.

Pear, T. H. (1931). *Voice and Personality*. London: Chapman and Hall.

Philippon, A. C., Cherryman, J., Bull, R., & Vrij, A. (2007). Earwitness identification performance: the effect of language, target, deliberate strategies and indirect measures. *Applied Cognitive Psychology*, 21(4), 539–550. doi: 10.1002/acp.1296

Price, S., Fluck, M., & Giles, H. (1983). The effects of language of testing on bilingual pre-adolescents' attitudes towards Welsh and varieties of English. *Journal of Multilingual and Multicultural Development*, 4, 149–161.

Ryan, E. B. & Sebastian, R. J. (1980). The effects of speech style and social class background on social judgements of speakers. *British Journal of Social and Clinical Psychology*, 19, 229–233.

Schneiderman, E. (1976). An examination of the ethnic and linguistic attitudes of bilingual children. *ITL Review of Applied Linguistics*, 33, 59–72.

Scott, S. K., Clegg, F., Rudge, P., & Burgess, P. (2006). Foreign accent syndrome, speech rhythm and the functional neuroanatomy of speech production. *Journal of Neurolinguistics*, 19(5), 370–384. doi: 10.1016/j.jneuroling.2006.03.008

Seyfarth, R. M. & Cheney, D. L. (2014). The evolution of language from social cognition. *Current Opinion in Neurobiology*, 28, 5–9. doi: 10.1016/j.conb.2014.04.003

Simmons, A. M., Popper, A. N., & Fay, R. R. (2003). *Acoustic Communication*. New York: Springer.

Stevenage, S. V., Clarke, G., & McNeill, A. (2012). The effect of regional accent on voice recognition. *Journal of Cognitive Psychology*, 24(6), 647–653.

Stewart, M. A., Ryan, E. B., & Giles, H. (1985). Accent and social-class effects on status and solidarity evaluations. *Personality and Social Psychology Bulletin*, 11(1), 98–105. doi: 10.1177/0146167285111009

Tajfel, H. & Billig, M. (1974). Familiarity and categorization in intergroup behavior. *Journal of Experimental Social Psychology*, 10(2), 159–170. doi: 10.1016/0022–1031(74)90064-x

Tajfel, H., Billig, M. G., Bundy, R. P., & Flament, C. (1971). Social categorization and intergroup behavior. *European Journal of Social Psychology*, 1(2), 149–177. doi: 10.1002/ejsp.2420010202

Tajfel, H. & Turner, J. C. (1979). An integrative theory of inter-group conflict. In: W. G. Austin & S. Wrochel (eds) *The Social Psychology of Inter-Group Relations*. Monterey, CA: Brooks/ Cole.

Trudgill, P. (1974). Sex, covert prestige and linguistic change in the urban British English of Norwich. *Language and Society*, 1, 179–195.

Turner, J. C. (1975). Social comparison and social identity—some prospects for intergroup behavior. *European Journal of Social Psychology*, 5(1), 5–34.

Turner, J. C., Hogg, M. A., Oakes, P. J., Reicher, S. D., & Wetherell, M. S. (1987). *Rediscovering the Social Group: A Self-Categorization Theory*. Oxford: Blackwell.

Tyack, P. L. (2008). Convergence of calls as animals form social bonds, active compensation for noisy communication channels, and the evolution of vocal learning in mammals. *Journal of Comparative Psychology*, 122(3), 319–331. doi: 10.1037/a0013087

van Bezooijen, R. (1994). Aesthetic evaluation of Dutch language varieties. *Language and Communication*, 14, 253–263.

Van Ngoc, T., Hallam, C., Roos, C., & Hammerschmidt, K. (2011). Concordance between vocal and genetic diversity in crested gibbons. *BMC Evolutionary Biology*, 11, 36. doi: 10.1186/1471-2148-11-36

Wagner, L., Clopper, C. G., & Pate, J. K. (2014). Children's perception of dialect variation. *Journal of Child Language*, 41(5), 1062–1084. doi: 10.1017/s0305000913000330

Wardhaugh, R. (1992). *An Introduction to Linguistics* (2nd edn). Oxford: Blackwell.

Williams, A., Garrett, P., & Coupland, N. (1999). Dialect recognition. In: D. R. Preston (ed.) *Handbook of Perceptual Dialectology*. Philadelphia: John Benjamins.

Zahn, C. & Hopper, R. (1985). Measuring language attitudes: the speech evaluation instrument. *Journal of Language and Social Psychology and Aging*, 4, 113–123.

PART VI

MACHINE-BASED GENERATION AND DECODING OF VOICES

CHAPTER 31

···

VOICE MORPHING

···

HIDEKI KAWAHARA AND VERENA G. SKUK

31.1 INTRODUCTION

VOICE perception is a result of evolution and ontogenetic development. It is a collection of many non-linear subsystems. The ideal stimulus for testing such a non-linear system is the natural voice, as our auditory system evolved to perceive it optimally. However, it is difficult to directly control attributes of natural speech sounds while assuring quantitative reproducibility. It is also difficult to manipulate the natural speech sounds to the desired direction for testing a perceptual attribute of interest. Voice morphing provides a means to solve these difficulties.

31.2 WHAT IS VOICE MORPHING?

31.2.1 Definition

In the broadest definition, voice morphing is a procedure to make a given voice sound like a different voice. Voice morphing provides the means to quantify perceptual effects of physical sound attribute modifications. This strategy requires an accurate analysis method to derive a parametric representation of a speech sample and a high-quality voice synthesis procedure to generate natural sounding synthesized voices from the (modified) parametric representation. This chapter introduces three types of voice morphing, with their underlying technical backgrounds, and discusses their application in voice-perception research.

31.2.2 Three Types of Morphing

The first morphing type uses one example voice to generate a new modified voice. In this chapter, we refer to this morphing as 'voice morphing with one reference'. When only one example is available, the analysed parameter values of the reference voice are modified to synthesize a new voice. This type of morphing is a close relation to voice conversion, which is discussed in Hirose (this volume).

The second morphing type uses two examples to generate a new modified voice. We refer to this morphing as 'voice morphing with two references' and it is an auditory counterpart of commonly known visual face morphing (Steyvers, 1999; Sutherland et al., 2017; Wolberg, 1998). This chapter mainly discusses voice morphing with two references. Potential applications of this morphing for auditory perception research were suggested by Slaney et al. (1996).

The third morphing type, which we will introduce, is called 'generalized morphing'. It enables extrapolation as well as interpolation of arbitrarily many numbers of voices. It also enables selective manipulation of specific combinations of fundamental parameters. Voice morphing with two references is a special case of this generalized morphing, which was recently introduced by Kawahara et al. (2013) to solve difficulties encountered using the second type of morphing in previous voice-perception research to generate averaged voices (Bruckert et al., 2010). Although no significant application is published yet, this chapter introduces this generalized morphing because it provides a flexible framework to implement a morphing procedure using new parametric representations and is conceptually clear and straightforward.

31.2.3 Morphing as a Research Tool

An important feature, which makes morphing a useful tool for voice-perception research, is the stimulus continuum generation between given voice examples. By adjusting the mixing weight of parameters, related for example to the voice pitch and vocal tract length, arbitrary intermediate voices can be generated, including a replica of the voices provided at each end. This generation capability is essential because it enables the creation of a stimulus continuum spanning two different typical examples of a perceptual attribute of interest, without requiring detailed prior knowledge of physical correlates of the attribute.

31.3 Technology Behind Morphing

31.3.1 Requirement

A voice-morphing method which is appropriate for voice-perception research should satisfy the following criteria. First, the generated voice should be perceptually identical to the original reference voice, when no modifications on parametric representations are introduced. Second, a generated voice from a set of modified parametric representations of voice should sound like an instance of a natural voice. Third, the element of the parametric representations to be changed should be adjustable independently without introducing degradations in the synthesized voice. Fourth, a small modification of parameter values should result in a minor perceptual difference of the generated sound. A number of voice-morphing procedures have been proposed based on various types of representations, focusing on different requirements. However, no existing method satisfies all these criteria simultaneously and strictly.

For small modifications, waveform-based processing methods provide high-quality modified voices while discarding flexibility and continuity. Concatenative synthesis (Hunt & Black, 1996) and PSOLA (Pitch Synchronous Overlap and Add; Moulines & Charpentier, 1990) are representative examples. However, since flexibility and continuity are of primary importance for voice morphing, the analysis and synthesis-based methods are preferable. While advances in recent decades have made analysis and synthesis-based methods applicable to voice morphing, there remain limitations in modified voice quality, especially when modifications are extreme. The following section briefly reviews parametric representations of speech sounds by focusing on their application to voice morphing.

31.3.2 Parametric Representation of Speech Sounds

31.3.2.1 *VOCODER*

Speech analysis and synthesis methods decompose speech into a set of parameters. The first VOCODER decomposed speech sounds into an excitation signal followed by a set of resonators. The excitation-signal generator consists of a pulse generator and a noise generator. The excitation parameters are fundamental frequency (Fo) and an indicator of voicing (voiced or unvoiced). The characterizing parameters of the resonators are their resonance frequencies (Dudley, 1939). Dudley's classic paper already discussed the application of VOCODER for investigating perceptual effects of excitation and resonator parameters. The structural similarity of VOCODER to the human speech production process made VOCODER-type systems appropriate tools for studying speech communication. The underlying idea was formulated later as the source filter model (Fant, 1970). The repetitive valving of airflow by vocal-fold vibration generates the excitation source. The vocal tract shape determines resonance frequencies of the filter, in other words, formant frequencies. The relation of these parameters to the voice-production process and perceived attributes have been studied extensively. However, obtaining reliable estimates of these parameters is still a challenging problem. Also, synthesizing a signal that sounds perceptually close to the original natural voice, based only on Fo and formant frequencies, is rarely successful.

Using more comprehensive source and filter representations, generation of a signal that sounds close to the original natural voice is possible. A review paper on statistical parametric speech synthesis provides a summary of such representations (Zen et al., 2009). There are three successful groups of filter implementations: (1) linear prediction coefficients (LPC), (2) cepstrum, and (3) Fo-adaptive spectrum envelope. Each filter representation provides a model, which is necessary to interpolate when used in morphing.

31.3.2.2 *Linear Prediction Coefficients Family*

Linear prediction coefficients (LPC) provide a statistical estimate of the model parameters, which is equivalent to the one-dimensional acoustic tube model of the vocal tract (Makhoul, 1975). Formant frequencies and bandwidths have a one-to-one correspondence to the roots of the polynomial equation made from LPC analysis. Sagayama and Itakura (1986,

2002) theoretically clarified all one-to-one correspondence between LPC family parameters as autocorrelation coefficients, LPC, partial correlation (PARCOR), and so on. The most useful parameter representation which uniquely corresponds to LPC is line spectrum frequencies (LSF; Itakura, 1975), which is the parameter widely used in mobile communications. Even though LPC family parameters provide the best statistical estimate of the all-pole spectral model (Itakura & Saito, 1970; Makhoul, 1975), the actual speech spectrum deviates from the calculated all-pole spectrum. The harmonic structure of the power spectrum of voiced sounds, the difference between the glottal source waveform and a pulse, and resonance and anti-resonance caused by the three-dimensional vocal tract shape are major contributing factors of this deviation.

31.3.2.3 *Cepstrum*

A power spectrum of voiced sound is a product of the power spectrum of the source signal and the squared absolute value of the vocal tract transfer function. Logarithmic conversion of the power spectrum is the sum of logarithmic conversion of each one. The cepstrum is the inverse Fourier transform of the logarithmic transformation of the power spectrum. Since the inverse Fourier transform is a linear operation, the cepstrum of a voiced sound is a sum of cepstrum of the source and the transfer function (Oppenheim, 1969). A power spectrum is in the frequency domain, and its corresponding cepstrum is in the quefrency domain (quefrency is the anagram of frequency). The periodic repetition of the glottal source signal corresponds to periodic peaks in higher quefrency region. The spectrum envelope information mainly corresponds to the cepstrum components in the lower quefrency region. These correspondences make separation of periodic structure and spectrum envelope using cepstrum easy. The separated spectrum envelope can be used to design the filter for synthesizing speech and the Fo value derived from the quefrency peak can be used to generate the excitation source signal. The spectrum envelope based on cepstrum can alleviate difficulties pointed out for LPC-based spectrum envelope.

Current statistical speech-synthesis systems (Zen et al., 2009) widely use Mel cepstrum (Imai, 1983), which takes advantage of human auditory characteristics. The human auditory system uses a non-linear frequency axis. Frequency resolution is roughly proportional to frequency. Mel cepstrum is defined using this non-linear frequency axis instead of using the linear frequency axis (Imai, 1983). However, the quefrency region of the periodicity peak and the spectrum envelope are overlapping, and it causes smearing and periodic interference of the estimated spectrum envelope.

31.3.2.4 *STRAIGHT*

STRAIGHT (Kawahara et al., 1999) and TANDEM-STRAIGHT (Kawahara et al., 2008) are the modern versions of VOCODER, which provide flexible and high-quality speech-manipulation procedures, using the following Fo-adaptive spectrum analysis. The harmonic structure of the power spectrum of voiced sounds is understood to be a sampling operation of underlying spectrum envelope values at harmonic frequencies. Then, spectrum-envelope estimation is a discrete-to-analogue conversion problem. Since spectrum envelope of speech sounds consists of rapidly changing components which do not satisfy the condition required by Shannon's sampling theory, the consistent sampling theory (Unser, 2000) is used to derive the spectrum envelope in STRAIGHT. Finally, the spectrum-envelope estimation of STRAIGHT is implemented as a localized smoothing operation of the logarithmic power spectrum with Fo-adaptive preprocessing in the time domain (Kawahara & Morise, 2011). These Fo-adaptive localized procedures allow STRAIGHT to alleviate difficulties found in LPC- and cepstrum-based spectrum-envelope estimation.

LPC-, cepstrum-, and STRAIGHT-based representations are not exclusive. A STRAIGHT spectrum envelope can generate a Mel cepstrum via a logarithmic spectrum. It also can generate LPC-family parameters via autocorrelation, which is derived using inverse Fourier transform of power-spectrum representation of the STRAIGHT spectrum. However, fine details in the STRAIGHT spectrum deteriorate by these conversions.

31.3.2.5 *Sinusoidal Model*

The sinusoidal model (McAuley & Quatieri, 1986) represents speech sounds using a sum of weighted sinusoids. The recent extension of the model provides close to the original high-quality reproduction (Degottex & Stylianou, 2013). Sinusoidal models are also applicable to implement morphing procedures by introducing relevant parameter interpolation models.

31.3.3 Voice Morphing with One Reference

Figure 31.1 shows a schematic diagram of voice morphing with one reference. The analysis method decomposes input speech into a set of parametric representations and coordinates of parameters. For example, time and frequency are the parameter coordinates for STRAIGHT, and the parameters on the coordinates are Fo, aperiodicity, and the spectrum envelope. Similarly, time and quefrency are the parameter coordinates for the cepstrum parameter. Time and the formant index (first, second, and so on) are the parameter coordinates for formant VOCODERs. Time and distance from the lip are the parameter coordinates for the vocal tract area function. The modification procedure modifies each parameter and coordinate. The synthesis process generates the voice signal from the modified set of parameters and coordinates. If the modification procedure does not change the parameter values, the synthesized results should sound perceptually identical to the reference voice.

Permissible manipulations depend on the nature of the parameters and coordinates. For example, manipulated Fo should be positive and mapping from the original to manipulated time coordinate should be monotonic. Manipulated spectral levels represented using dB can have any value.

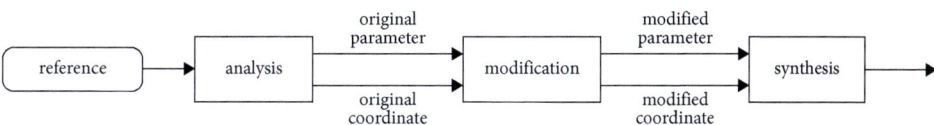

FIGURE 31.1 Schematic diagram of voice morphing with one reference.

31.3.4 Voice Morphing with Two References

Figure 31.2 shows a schematic diagram of voice morphing with two references. Analysed parameters and coordinates of two references are interpolated or extrapolated to generate the modified parameters and coordinates. The modified parameters and coordinates are inputs to the synthesis procedure, which produces the morphed voice.

The combination of relevant conversion and inverse conversion assures morphed parameters and coordinates to be permissible. For Fo modification, appropriate conversion is linear interpolation or extrapolation of logarithmic Fo frequencies, and the inverse conversion is exponential of the resulting logarithmic Fo value. This combination of conversion and inverse conversion assures the resulting Fo has a positive value. Similarly, using linear interpolation or extrapolation of logarithmic derivatives of the mapping of time coordinates for conversion, and using integration of the exponential of the resulting value as the inverse conversion, assures that the produced mapping of time coordinates is monotonic. For modification of the mapping of frequency coordinates, the similar set of conversion and inverse conversion is relevant. For modification of unconstrained values, such as dB-represented levels, linear interpolation itself is appropriate. In Figure 31.2, by changing the contribution weight for the reference-1 from 1 to 0 and that for the reference-2 from 0 to 1, in steps, while keeping their sum to one, a stimulus continuum spanning from reference-1 to reference-2 is generated. Setting different weights to each parameter and coordinate enables parameter-selective morphing.

31.3.5 Generalized Voice Morphing

Figure 31.3 shows a schematic diagram of generalized morphing (Kawahara et al., 2013). This morphing enables mixing of arbitrarily many numbers of voices to generate a morphed voice. Using constraints to keep the sum of contribution weights for each physical parameter or coordinate to 1, allows the morphed voice to traverse the high-dimensional space spanned by given references. In addition to this generalization of the number of voices, generalized morphing enables analysis frame-dependent setting of contribution weights. In other words, the contribution weight has three indices—the reference voice identifier index, the frame position identifier index, and the parameter and coordinate identifier index. When the number of reference voices is two, it is morphing with two references; for arbitrary numbers of reference voices, it is called 'morphing with N references'.

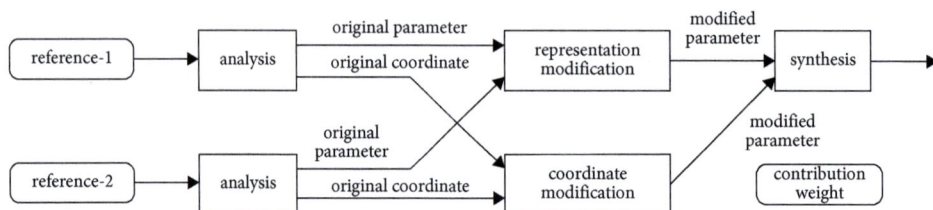

FIGURE 31.2 Schematic diagram of voice morphing with two references.

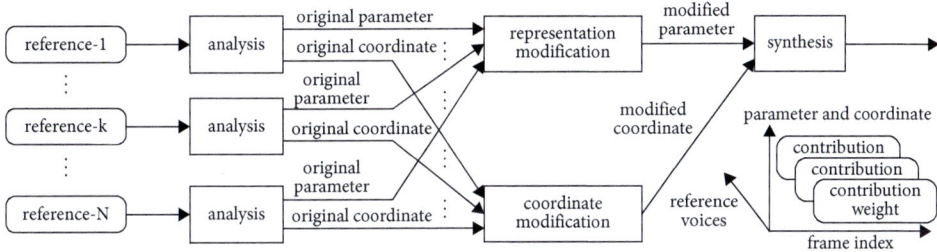

FIGURE 31.3 Schematic diagram of generalized morphing.

© 2013 IEEE. Reprinted, with permission, from Kawahara H. et al., 'Temporally variable multi-aspect N-way morphing based on interference-free speech representations', *IEEE Proceedings,* doi:10.1109/APSIPA.2013.6694355.

31.3.6 Future Directions of Voice Morphing

Generalized morphing can be implemented using different parametric representations. Using parameters closely correlated with physical parameters of voice production and articulation systems may alleviate degradations caused by extreme manipulation of attributes, such as exaggeration or caricaturing. Morphing using a vocal tract area function, which is a set of relative cross-sectional areas of a one-dimensional vocal tract model defined as a function of distance from the mouth opening, instead of using vocal tract transfer function, is an example of such directions (Arakawa et al., 2010). Studies on estimation of articulatory parameters (e.g. vocal tract area function, tongue shape, jaw opening) and voice excitation source parameters (e.g. glottal source waveform, Liljencrants-Fant (LF) model parameters; Fant et al., 1985) are also useful for further extensions. See Vinciarelli (this volume) and Schmitt and Schuller (this volume) for estimation and use of these parameters.

In image morphing, several types of morphing algorithms are available (Wolberg, 1998). The generalized morphing introduced in this chapter corresponds to an extension of mesh morphing of images. The other image morphing algorithms may have counterparts in the morphing of voices. For example, the multi-level free-form deformation can be applied by defining an appropriate hierarchical structure in speech sounds for automating the morphing process. Taking concepts found in the image-morphing field is an exciting future direction. It is important to note though the difference that the time and frequency axes of voice morphing are not exchangeable, while the vertical and horizontal axes of image morphing can be rotated and exchanged. In 2017, an audio-morphing paradigm based on deep learning was introduced (Engel, 2017). Application of this revolutionary morphing in voice-communication research will open new and prospective opportunities.

31.4 Morphing Procedure and Tools

31.4.1 An Example of STRAIGHT-Based Morphing

To provide a specific example, this section briefly introduces a voice-morphing framework based on TANDEM-STRAIGHT. This introduction includes descriptions of both a set of tools for preparing the morphing source materials and a set of supporting tools for generating morphed voice samples. It further includes notes on interactive tools for exploitation and demonstrations.

The generalized morphing framework can be implemented using different voice representations. The tools introduced here provide a guideline or template for developing morphing procedures based on other available systems (e.g. Praat: Boersma & Weenink, 2016; COVAREP: Degottex et al., 2014) and different parametric representations mentioned in the previous sections. The STRAIGHT-based morphing tools introduced in this section are available for academic use (Kawahara, 2002).

31.4.2 Preparation of Morphing Materials

Coordinates of all given voice parameters have to be aligned properly to prevent quality degradation in generated morphed sounds. For example, if the first formant of one reference voice is aligned to the second formant of another reference voice, the morphed voices sound unnatural and degraded. Similarly, if a temporal location of one reference voice, where formants are in transition, is aligned to a stable location of another reference voice, the morphed voices sound degraded.

Tools for preparing materials consist of a reference marker and a target marker. In our example used here, we select one of the N reference voices as 'reference' and we name the other reference voices as 'target'. The reference marker is to assign anchors to the selected example. The target marker is used to assign corresponding anchors by comparing the target anchors assigned on the reference representation. We designed the tools introduced here for voice-perception studies. Manual assignment of anchors is intended to provide full control of the morphing procedure to researchers. For other applications, such as special sound effects in post-production, automatic morphing methods might be preferable.

Figure 31.4 shows a graphical user interface (GUI) of the reference marker. One of the reference voices is selected to assign reference anchors. (The sentence 'I love you', spoken with 'pleasant' emotion, is used in this example.) The upper image shows a spectrographic representation of the filter characteristics of the given voice example. The filter characteristics are envelope spectra by STRAIGHT analysis. The lower panel shows the waveform and magnitude of the spectral difference between adjacent frames. Vertical white lines in the image indicate temporal anchors. Green circles on the white lines indicate frequency anchors. The toolbar of this GUI provides the means to add, delete, and adjust these anchors and zoom in, zoom out, and panning functions of the image. The GUI saves the completed anchor information and the speech parameter as a set of files of the reference voice.

Figure 31.5 shows a GUI for the target anchor assignment voices. The GUI shows the reference and the target voice representations side by side. The toolbar of this GUI provides similar functions for adjusting anchors of the target. The GUI highlights the corresponding time or frequency anchor in the reference representation (right-side image in Figure 31.5) when an anchor in the target representation is interactively adjusted. The GUI provides sound playback of each original voice and the morphed voice to verify the relevance of the current anchor assignment.

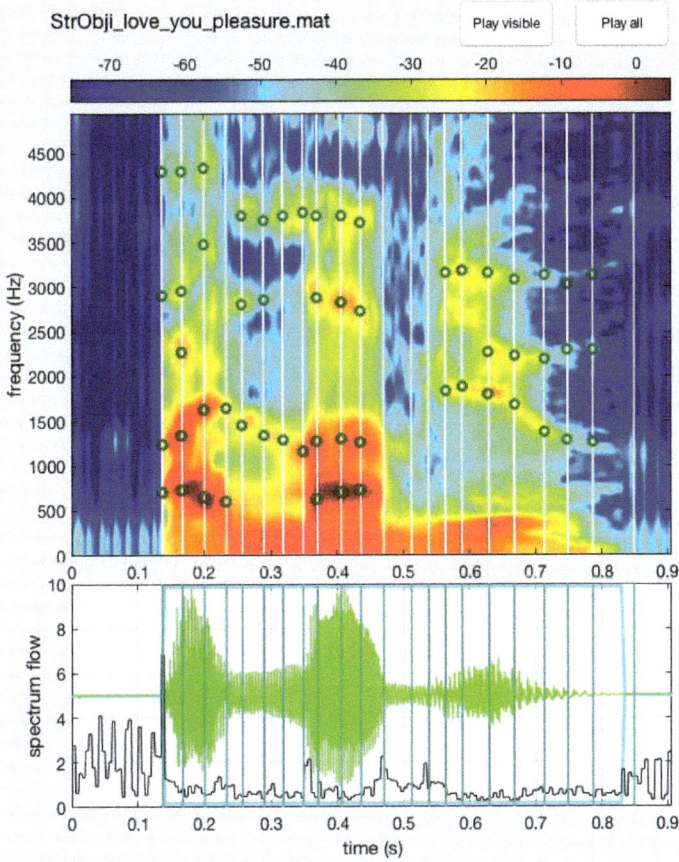

FIGURE 31.4   A graphical user interface (GUI) of the reference marker.

31.4.3 Supporting Tools for Generating Morphed Voices

31.4.3.1 *Stimulus Generation*

The primary use of morphing is to generate a stimulus continuum spanning from one example to the other example. A command interpreter for generating the morphed voice—which reads indexed contribution weights, speech parameter files (consisting of STRAIGHT analysis results), and associated time and frequency anchor files—is prepared. Any stimulus continuum is generated by properly designing indexed contribution weights and using this interpreter.

The other commonly used stimuli are the averaged voice and caricatured voice. The averaged voice is generated by assigning equal value, namely reciprocal of the number of reference voices, to each contribution weight and using this interpreter. Extrapolation morphing exaggerates the deviation of the target from the averaged voice. In other words, this procedure caricatures the target.

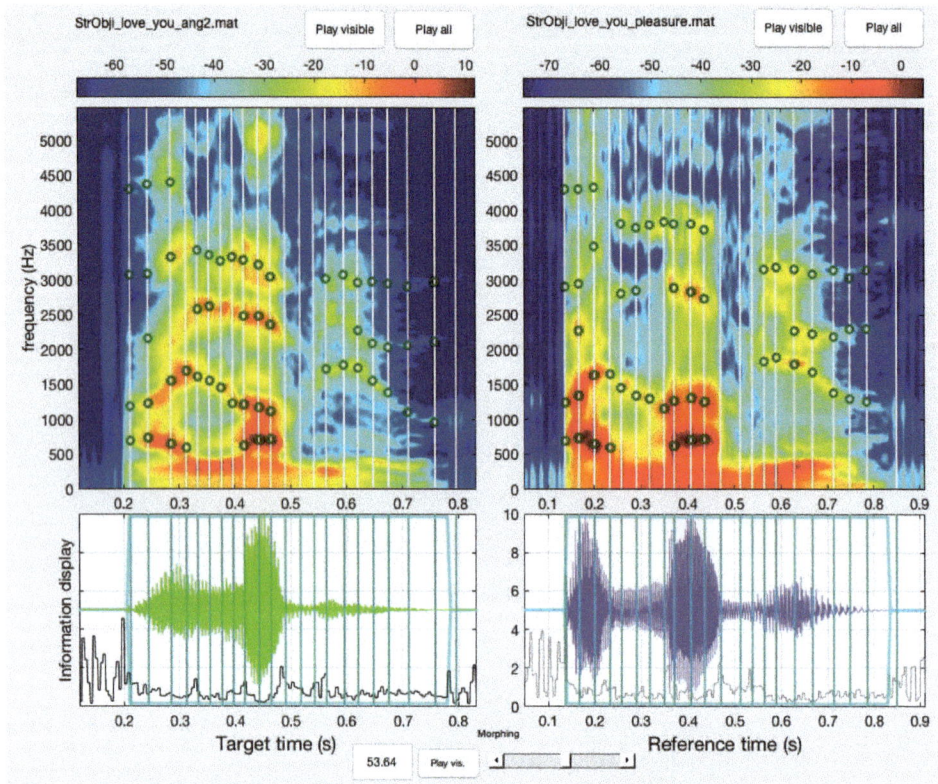

FIGURE 31.5   A graphical user interface (GUI) of the target anchor preparation.

31.4.4   Interactive Tool

The command interpreter introduced in the previous paragraph is for generation of systematic test stimuli. It is relevant for designing full-scale subjective tests. GUI-based interactive tools are useful for the earlier stage of investigations, where flexibility and quick turn-around of tests are essential.

Figure 31.6 shows four example snapshots of an interactive three-way morphing GUI, which allows the user to adjust the contribution weights of three voices. This example shows interaction using the sentence 'I love you', spoken with three different emotions—pleasure, anger, and sadness. The grey sphere is the controller for interactive manipulation. When release action after dragging takes place, the morphed sound is synthesized and played back. The ratios of the three triangular areas formed by the grey and coloured spheres define the contribution weights of the three voices. For example, in the top right image, voices assigned to green and blue balls have positive weights. The voice assigned to the red colour has a negative weight. This setting generates an anti-pleasant morphed voice.

In each image, the bottom left coloured bars represent contribution weights. The bottom right image shows the morphed filter information and the top right plot shows Fo trajectories of the original voices and the morphed voice. The original Fo trajectories are represented using lines similar in colour to the spheres. The black line represents

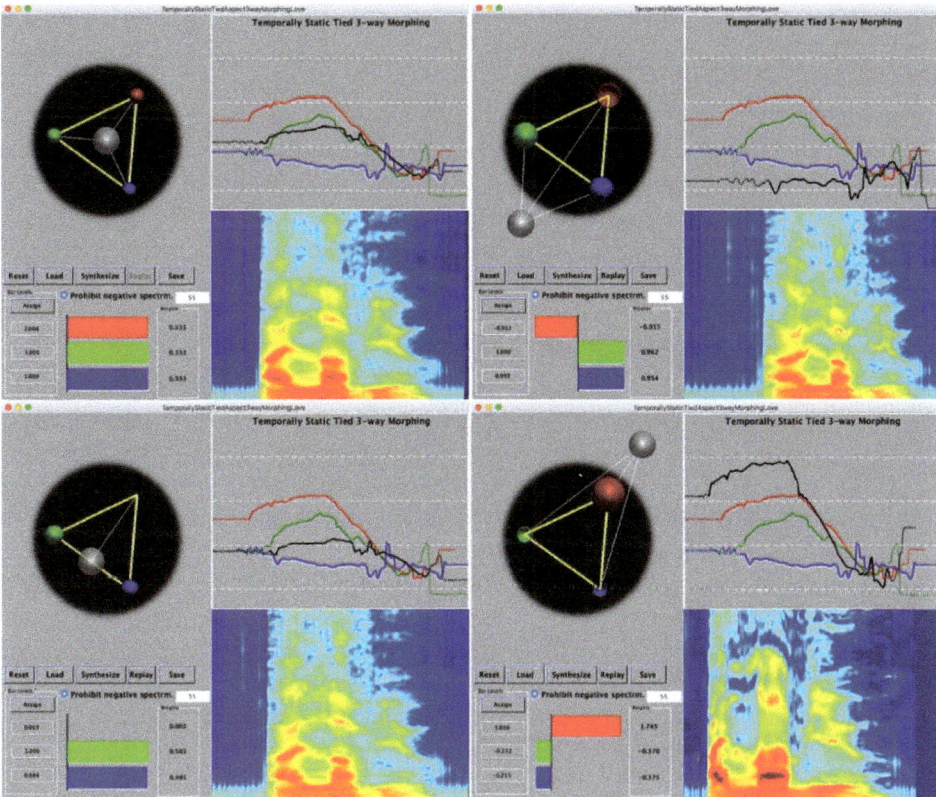

FIGURE 31.6 Interactive three-way morphing GUI snapshots. Red, green, and blue spheres represent locations of 'pleasure', 'anger', and 'sadness', respectively. Anticlockwise, from top left to top right, images represent 'average', 'between pleasure and anger', 'exaggerated pleasure', and 'anti-pleasure' morphed expressions.

the Fo trajectory of the morphed voice. Using three-dimensional haptic interfaces enables interactive tool design for up to four-way morphing. Creating interactive interfaces for general N-way morphing of more than four voices needs application-specific modifications.

31.5 APPLICATION TO
VOICE-PERCEPTION RESEARCH

Dramatic advances in the understanding of face perception within the last thirty years have been achieved by making intense use of computer graphics (Bruce & Young, 2012, p. 96) and image-morphing technology (Sutherland et al., 2017), which together have allowed extensive and widespread use of face morphing. In contrast, voice morphing is still in its infancy, but the improvement of algorithms and development of new tools and applications offer new possibilities for voice researchers from various disciplines. In the last decade, voice morphing has become a powerful tool for the investigation of linguistic, paralinguistic, and extralinguistic cues in voices (Schweinberger et al., 2014). The separation of source and filter characteristics, and the ability to manipulate the synthesized voice quality by mutually independent parameters, give researchers precise physical control over stimulus qualities and 'provides a quantitative evaluation of perceptual effects of manipulated parameters' (Schweinberger et al., 2014).

In this section, we review studies that used the three aforementioned concepts of voice morphing with one, two, or n references, to investigate mainly voice (indexical) identity and to discuss possible implications and future research approaches.

31.5.1 Voice Morphing with One Reference

Voice morphing with one reference relates to the transformation of a single-source speaker's voice into many different voice qualities, depending on the precise transformation applied. It has, for instance, been used to change adult male or female voices into voices of the opposite sex or children's voices by incremental upward and downward shifting of Fo, formants, or both Fo and formants. Listeners then rated the perceived gender or naturalness of voice quality based on the resulting synthesized voices. From these ratings, researchers could infer the relative importance of Fo and vocal-tract resonances for the categorization of voice gender. The results tended to show an advantage of Fo over formant frequencies (Gelfer & Mikos, 2005; Hillenbrand & Clark, 2009), although some studies found a more comparable contribution of Fo and vocal-tract resonances (Assmann et al., 2006; Smith et al., 2007). Discrepancies between studies could depend on the stimuli and speakers used (Skuk & Schweinberger, 2014).

Unsurprisingly, voice transformations become more difficult if the desired changes require complex modifications in multiple acoustical dimensions simultaneously (e.g. Fo, formants, amplitude levels, jitter, shimmer, timing), and especially since these parameters are also likely to vary over time. For instance, the transformation of young into elderly-sounding voices requires expert knowledge about both the underlying acoustical parameters that have to be changed as well as the handling of the software to apply such modifications. Morphing between two references may require less specialist knowledge about the acoustic parameters to be changed.

31.5.2 Voice Morphing with Two References

Voice morphing with two references may be used to produce voice samples that vary systematically along a continuum spanned by the two references. It can be used, for instance, to generate perceptually 'middle-aged' voices, which may only require morphing between representative young and old speech samples (Figure 31.7). While basic phonetic knowledge is useful to find corresponding key features in the utterances, there is no need to address in detail the acoustical changes involved (Zäske & Schweinberger, 2011). To create perceptually efficient morphs, it may not be necessary to morph all parameters along a continuum, since parameters that are perceptually irrelevant with respect to a specific social signal may be fixed at a specific morph level. Selective morphing of individual parameters (e.g. Fo, timbre, timing; Figure 31.8) is in fact a powerful method to evaluate the relative

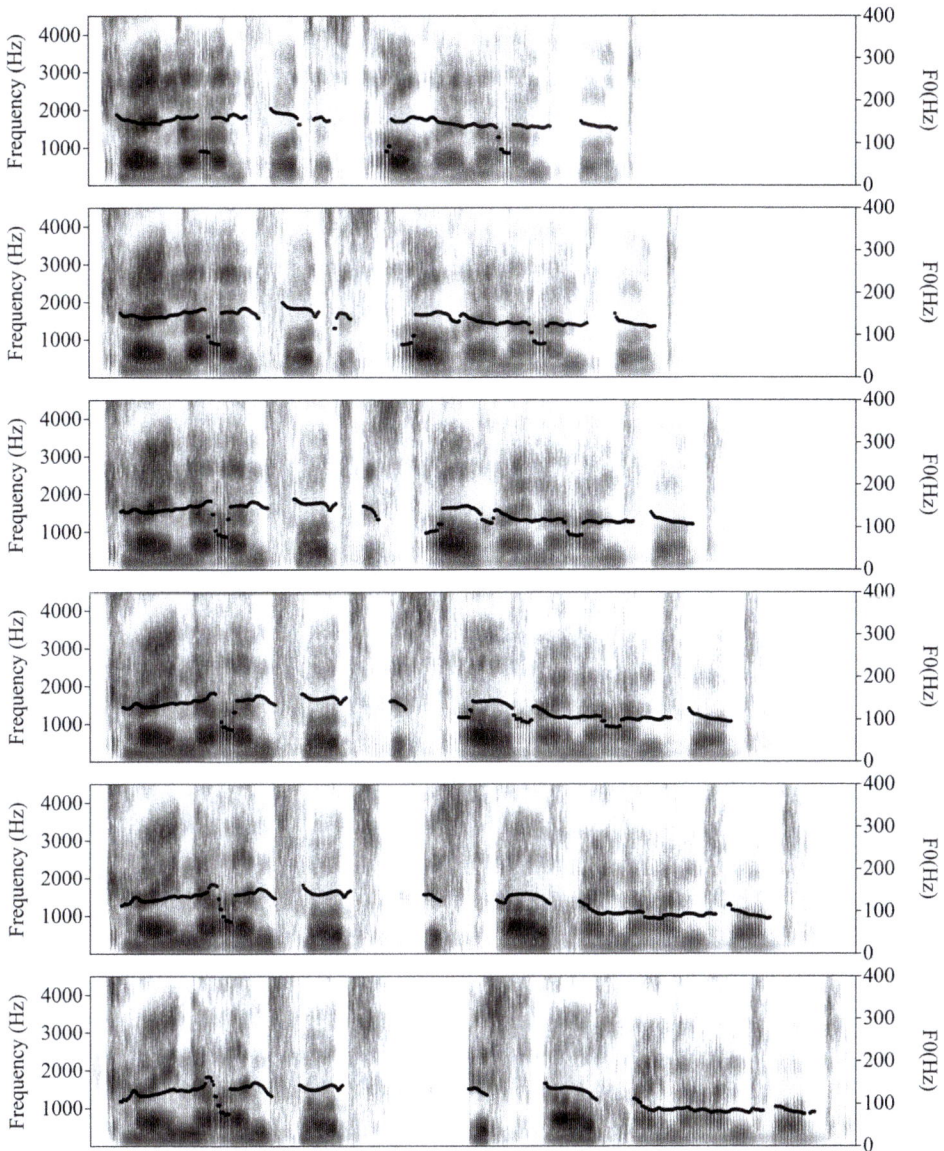

FIGURE 31.7 Spectrograms and Fo contour of morphed voices of a German sentence 'Keine antwort ist auch eine antwort' ['No answer is an answer as well'] resulting from the interpolation of a 22-year-old male speaker (top) with a 71-year-old male speaker (bottom). Audio 31.1 provides corresponding audio samples.

impact of these cues on perception (e.g. Bruckert et al., 2010, for attractiveness; Skuk & Schweinberger, 2014, for voice gender). This approach is particularly useful if little is known about the acoustic correlates of the perceptual attribute (cf. Schweinberger et al., 2014).

However, voice morphing offers more than a method to control acoustical changes in stimuli and measure their percepts. In combination with perceptual adaptation paradigms,

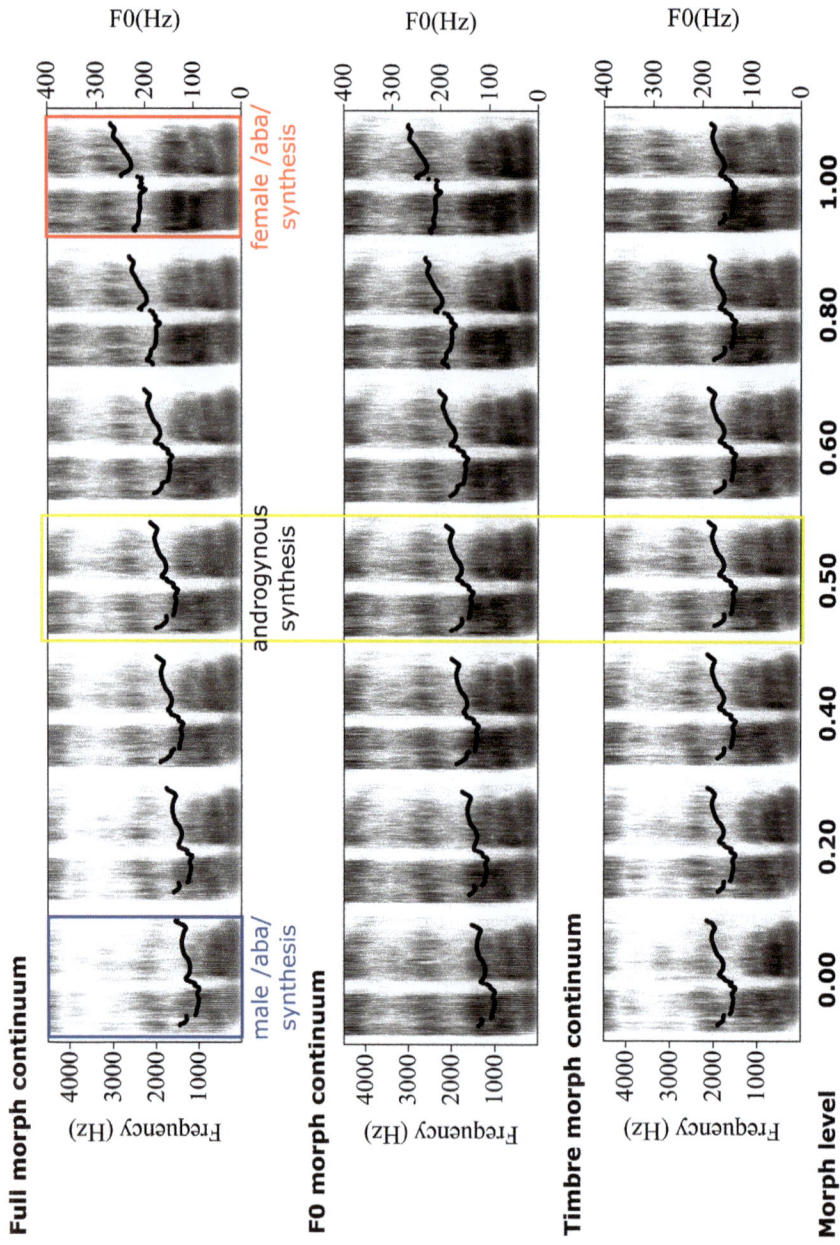

FIGURE 31.8 Spectrograms and Fo contours of three parameter morph continua between a male and a female /aba/, in which different TANDEM-STRAIGHT parameters are morphed from male to female in steps of 0.20, with an additional intermediate (0.5) 'androgynous' morph level. The morph level refers to the proportion of 'femaleness' contained in the voice morph. Shown are: a full morph continuum (top row), in which all parameters but time axis are morphed from a male voice (blue frame) to a female voice (red frame); a Fo morph continuum (middle row), in which the TANDEM-STRAIGHT parameter Fo is morphed from male to female, while all other parameters are kept constant at the 'androgynous' morph level; and a timbre morph continuum (bottom row), in which the Fo and time parameter are kept constant at the 'androgynous' level, while the residual parameters vary from male to female. The intermediate 0.5 morph level is perceptually the same in all three morph continua (yellow frame). Audio 31.2 provides corresponding audio samples.

it provides a powerful tool to investigate the neuronal representation of socially-relevant stimulus qualities. Perceptual adaptation is a phenomenon according to which the exposure (or adaptation) to a certain stimulus quality subsequently causes the presented stimuli to be perceived in a contrastive manner (Grill-Spector et al., 2006). Contrastive after-effects are well investigated for various low-level stimulus qualities like motion, colour, or temperature, and are also shown for the perception of speech sounds (e.g. McQueen, 2010) and complex stimulus properties in both faces (for review, see Webster & MacLeod, 2011) and voices.

The perceptual representation of voice gender was first investigated in an adaptation design by Mullennix et al. (1995) using natural and synthesized voices. They found some evidence for adaptation, but their results were inconsistent and not reliable across experiments, most likely due to the use of synthesized and not natural-sounding test and adaptor voices. More than ten years later, and using natural-sounding morphed voices as test and adaptor stimuli, Schweinberger et al. (2008) were the first to report consistent contrastive after-effects in voice-gender perception. Specifically, morphed gender-ambiguous test voices were perceived as more female after adaptation to male voices and vice versa. The adaptation effects were present in individual listeners, strongest for the most ambiguous stimuli, and still measurable after minutes. Most importantly, the effects cannot be explained by a simple contrastive response bias or a low-level adaptation to pitch, as indicated by three control experiments.

Following these promising initial findings, a number of studies used morphed voices to investigate the processing of other socially-relevant cues in voices. High-level contrastive after-effects were also found for vocal affect (Bestelmeyer et al., 2010; Skuk & Schweinberger, 2013), vocal age (Zäske & Schweinberger, 2011; Zäske et al., 2013), and voice identity (Zäske et al., 2010), suggesting the existence of specialized neuron populations coding these stimulus qualities (see Latinus & Zäske, this volume). However, the precise nature of these representations is still a matter of debate and currently under investigation.

To disentangle the relative importance of individual acoustical cues involved in these higher-level processes, follow-up studies used modified voice adaptors in which some of the relevant acoustic information was either removed (Hubbard & Assmann, 2013), rendered uninformative (Skuk et al., 2015), or exaggerated by caricaturing (Bestelmeyer et al., 2010). The results from these studies generally show that after-effects cannot be solely explained by low-level adaptation to acoustical stimulus characteristics, but are likely based on a recalibration of higher-level representations. However, there are also some discrepancies with respect to the importance of Fo and timbre for the processing of voice gender. Some studies suggest a major role of timbre (Pernet & Belin, 2012; Skuk et al., 2015), whereas others advocate an exclusive dependency on Fo (Hubbard & Assmann, 2013). One possible explanation for these discrepancies is that adaptation fails when the adaptors do not contain a fully-preserved natural spectrum, i.e. both Fo and timbre (Hubbard & Assmann, 2013; Mullennix et al., 1995; Schweinberger et al., 2008). If this is true, it emphasizes the importance of using naturalistic stimuli— and, by the very same argument, the important methodological advance provided by voice morphing compared with other voice-manipulation techniques such as voice conversion methods (for review, see Ling et al., 2015).

Further, studies used morphed stimuli in combination with ERP (event-related potentials), fMRI (functional magnetic resonance imaging), or TMS (transcranial magnetic stimulation) to investigate in more detail the timing of social-signal processing, or to find or confirm brain regions related to higher-level voice processing (e.g. Bestelmeyer et al., 2012,

2014; Charest et al., 2013; Donhauser et al., 2014; Latinus et al., 2011; Latinus & Taylor, 2012; Schweinberger et al., 2011; Watson et al., 2014; Zäske et al., 2009). Latinus et al. (2011), for instance, used an fMRI-adaptation design to distinguish acoustic- from identity-based representation of voices. They found that the processing of voice identity appears to be subserved by a large network of brain areas ranging from the superior temporal pole, involved in an acoustic-based representation of unfamiliar voices, to areas along the convexity of the inferior frontal cortex for identity-related processing of familiar voices.

31.5.3 Voice Morphing with N References

Researchers are highly interested in mechanisms involved in memorizing and recognizing speaker identity. As many attempts to identify a unitary set of acoustic features that underlie voice identification have failed, it has been suggested that listeners use whatever cue is characteristic (distinctive) to recognize a speaker (for a recent review, see Schweinberger et al., 2014). One theory based on this idea suggests that voices, like faces, are represented in memory relative to a perceptual norm (Papcun et al., 1989). The norm is the centre of a higher-dimensional space (see Latinus & Zäske, this volume). While the exact dimensions of the voice space are still a matter of debate (but see Latinus et al., 2013), it is further suggested that the more distant a voice is located from the norm, the more distinctive it sounds.

Morphing with n references now provides a means to creating average voices (also referred to as prototypes or norms) that are devoid of identity-specific distinctive features. An average voice comprises the average acoustical properties across all voices contained in the morph (e.g. average pitch contour, average formant frequencies, average timing). For instance, when morphing only voices of one speaker sex, one obtains a gender-specific prototype (e.g. Pernet & Belin, 2012), while the morphing of similar numbers of both male and female voices would yield an androgynous-sounding average voice.

The first study that created average voices was conducted by Bruckert et al. (2010). They used recursively applied pair-wise morphing to generate averages of /had/ utterances: thirty-two original voice samples were randomly paired and morphed with one another to result in sixteen two-voice averages. This process was repeated to yield averages of four, eight, sixteen, and thirty-two voices. Bruckert et al. (2010) showed that averaging across increasing numbers of voices increased perceived attractiveness of the resulting voices, which could partly be explained by the spectrotemporal smoothing (i.e. the reduction of aperiodic noise) and higher similarity to the gender-specific prototypes.

Subsequently, Latinus and Belin (2012) provided initial evidence for a norm-based coding of voice identity by implementing an adaptation experiment in a virtual voice space. Participants first learned to discriminate three different male-voice identities, and then performed a three-alternative forced-choice identification task on identity-reduced test voices. These were generated by morphing the individual voice identities with an average voice (i.e. a morphing of sixteen male speaker utterances). The test voices were presented either in isolation (baseline) or following adaptation to matching anti-voices or non-matching anti-voices (see Figure 31.9; see also Latinus & Zäske, this volume). Results revealed slightly stronger after-effects for test voices preceded by matching anti-voices, compared with other adaptors. These results are similar to adaptation after-effects observed for facial identity (Leopold et al., 2001) and support the norm-based coding hypothesis of voice identity.

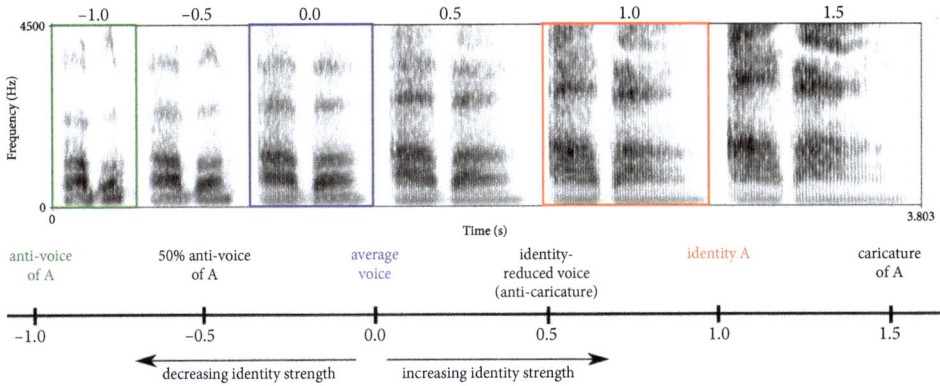

FIGURE 31.9 Spectrograms of /aba/ morphs resulting from interpolations and extrapolations of a 25-year-old male speaker (identity A) with an average voice made from thirty-two speakers. The morph continuum ranges from the anti-voice with an identity strength (IS) of −1 to a caricature of 1.5 IS. The numbers indicate the identity strength (i.e. the proportion of identity A). The anti-voice is a type of caricature of the average in that its properties are extrapolated from those of voice A. Voice A has higher Fo and formants and a longer duration than the average voice, so the anti-voice yields lower Fo, lower formants, and shorter duration than the average voice. The caricature uses the same principles to extend beyond voice A as we used to morph between voice A and the average (i.e. the caricature is more different from the average than voice A is). Audio 31.3 provides a corresponding audio sample.

As a limitation, it is unclear to what extent these results from short voice-identity learning sessions with brief vowel stimuli would generalize to recognition of familiar voices from natural speech samples (i.e. from speech that involves stable long-term identity representations). It thus remains an open question of whether the existence of prototype-based coding can be confirmed for larger sets of familiar speakers and more ecologically-valid stimuli, such as (minimal) sentences (Schweinberger et al., 2014).

31.5.4 Limitations and Future of Research Using Voice Morphing

At present, most studies that use 2- or N-way morphing use rather short utterances (e.g. vowels, vowel–consonant–vowel sequences, words like 'had') as stimuli, which has several advantages. Shorter stimuli are mostly devoid of meaning or regionalism and can be used cross-culturally if the sounds occur in the languages or cultures of question. Further, they can be used to show that valid social information can be efficiently processed based on short excerpts of voices. Moreover, the processing of these stimuli can easily be compared with the processing of other auditory stimulus classes, like environmental sounds or animal vocalizations.

However, our understanding of voice perception would also profit from the use of longer and more phonetically-rich stimuli. It is, for instance, well established that longer speech samples allow more accurate and reliable perception of speaker identity (Schweinberger et al., 1997) or age (Linville, 1996). Moreover, since some indexical cues are simply absent in brief stimuli, the relevance of acoustical cues in relation to social-signal perception in natural speech may necessitate the use of longer stimuli. At the same time, morphing of more ecologically-valid stimuli like sentences (Zäske et al., 2010), and especially the creation of average voices, is still technically challenging. It requires phonetic expertise to determine correct placement of anchors, and even with experience it can sometimes be hard to find corresponding key features across all utterances, as not all speakers produce the same utterances in a similar way (Smith & Hawkins, 2012).

While prior editing of voices and the deleting of some artefacts (e.g. clicks, smacks) might be useful and recommended, any editing should be done with care in order not to eliminate valuable information about a speaker. The misalignment of time or frequency anchors may cause perceivable artefacts or smearing of (formant) frequencies. The averaging of many voices may lead to a flattening of the Fo contour and a highly periodic and regular signal, which may sound robotic and synthesized, and it is, for instance, unclear whether the finding of Bruckert et al. (2010)—that averaging increases attractiveness—is true for sentence stimuli. However, voice averaging may further be a promising method to investigate the perception of other highly-relevant social signals, such as first impressions or personality, as has recently been investigated for faces, using facial averages

Furthermore, extrapolation of acoustic parameters may cause caricatures as well as anti-voices sounding fairly unnatural or 'weird'. Extrapolation of the time parameter may cause, for instance, phoneme durations or voice-onset times to be unnaturally shortened or lengthened. Extrapolation of Fo may result in unnatural frequency ranges, too wide or narrow harmonics, and unnaturally variable pitch contours, and therefore changes in intonation. Similarly, extreme shifts of formants may result in unnatural formant transitions and formant positions, possibly leading to changes in perceived phoneme category.

However, these or other consequences should not keep researchers from using potentially unnatural-sounding stimuli, and for mainly two reasons. First, our ability to recognize voices and speech can be remarkably robust in the face of many acoustic modifications, including severe degradation and exaggerations. Second, 'weird' but controlled stimuli have been shown to be highly valuable in the visual domain. Researchers presented, for instance, average and anti-faces (e.g. Leopold et al., 2001), expanded and contracted faces (e.g. Webster & MacLin, 1999), faces with unnatural positioning of eyes or mouth (e.g. Cooper & Wojan, 2000), or extreme forms of facial caricatures (e.g. Benson & Perrett, 1991) to investigate perception. Moreover, selective interpolation or extrapolation of individual acoustic parameters may be used to investigate individual differences in voice processing, similar to recent work showing that good and bad face recognizers differ with respect to usage of shape but not texture information in faces (Kaufmann et al., 2013).

In conclusion, and despite some apparent limitations, the possibilities of voice morphing are manifold. The technique provides unique potential to address open questions related to acoustical and neuronal correlates of voice perception, and can be used to broaden our understanding of (vocal) person perception and social interaction.

References

Arakawa, A. et al. (2010). *High quality voice manipulation method based on the vocal tract area function obtained from sub-band LSP of STRAIGHT spectum*. IEEE International Conference on Acoustics, Speech, and Signal Processing, Dallas, Texas, pp. 4834–4837.

Assmann, P. F., Dembling, S., & Nearey, T. M. (2006). *Effects of frequency shifts on perceived naturalness and gender information.* Interspeech 2006, Pittsburg, PA, pp. 889–892.

Benson, P. J. & Perrett, D. I. (1991). Synthesizing continuous-tone caricatures. *Image and Vision Computing,* 9(2), 123–129.

Bestelmeyer, P. E. G. et al. (2012). Implicitly perceived vocal attractiveness modulates prefrontal cortex activity. *Cerebral Cortex,* 22(6), 1263–1270.

Bestelmeyer, P. E. G. et al. (2014). Adaptation to vocal expressions reveals multistep perception of auditory emotion. *The Journal of Neuroscience,* 34(24), 8098–8105.

Bestelmeyer, P. E. G., Rouger, J., DeBruine, L. M., & Belin, P. (2010). Auditory adaptation in vocal affect perception. *Cognition,* 117(2), 217–223.

Boersma, P. & Weenink, D. (2016). *Praat: doing phonetics by computer* [computer program]. Available online at: http://www.praat.org/ [Accessed: 24th December 2016]

Bruce, V. & Young, A. W. (2012). *Face Perception* (1st edn). New York: Psychology Press.

Bruckert, L. et al. (2010). Vocal attractiveness increases by averaging. *Current Biology,* 20(2), 116–120.

Charest, I. et al. (2013). Cerebral processing of voice gender studied using a continuous carryover fMRI design. *Cerebral Cortex,* 23(4), 958–966.

Cooper, E. E. & Wojan, T. J. (2000). Differences in the coding of spatial relations in face identification and basic-level object recognition. *Journal of Experimental Psychology—Learning Memory and Cognition,* 26(2), 470–488.

Degottex, G. et al. (2014). *COVAREP: a cooperative voice analysis repository for speech technologies.* Available online at: http://covarep.github.io/covarep [Accessed: 24th December 2016]

Degottex, G. & Stylianou, Y. (2013). Analysis and synthesis of speech using an adaptive fullband harmonic model. *IEEE Transactions on Audio, Speech, and Language Processing,* 21(10), 2085–2095.

Donhauser, P. W., Belin, P., & Grosbras, M.-H. (2014). Biasing the perception of ambiguous vocal affect: a TMS study on frontal asymmetry. *Social, Cognitive, and Affective Neuroscience,* 9(7), 1046–1051.

Dudley, H. (1939). Remaking speech. *Journal of the Acoustical Society of America,* 11(2), 169–177.

Engel, J., Resnick, C., Roberts, A. et al. (2017). *Neural audio synthesis of musical notes with WaveNet autoencoders.* ArXiv e-prints, Cornell University Library. arXiv:1704.01279[cs.LG]

Fant, G. (1970). *Acoustic Theory of Speech Production.* Hauge: Mouton.

Fant, G., Liljencrants, J., & Lin, Q. (1985). A four parameter model of glottal flow. *STL-QPSR,* 26(4), 1–13.

Gelfer, M. P. & Mikos, V. A. (2005). The relative contributions of speaking fundamental frequency and formant frequencies to gender identification based on isolated vowels. *Journal of Voice,* 19(4), 544–554.

Grill-Spector, K., Henson, R., & Martin, A. (2006). Repetition and the brain: neural models of stimulus-specific effects. *Trends in Cognitive Sciences,* 10(1), 14–23.

Hillenbrand, J. M. & Clark, M. J. (2009). The role of f0 and formant frequencies in distinguishing the voices of men and women. *Attention, Perception, & Psychophysics,* 71(5), 1150–1166.

Hubbard, D. J. & Assmann, P. F. (2013). Perceptual adaptation to gender and expressive properties in speech: the role of fundamental frequency. *Journal of the Acoustical Society of America,* 133(4), 2367–2376.

Hunt, A. J. & Black, A. W. (1996). *Unit selection in a concatenative speech synthesis system using a large speech database.* IEEE International Conference on Acoustics, Speech, and Signal Processing, Atlanta, GA, pp. 373–376.

Imai, S. (1983). *Cepstral analysis synthesis on the mel frequency scale*. IEEE International Conference on Acoustics, Speech, and Signal Processing, Boston, pp. 93–96.

Itakura, F. (1975). Line spectrum representation of linear predictor coefficients of speech signals. *Journal of the Acoustical Society of America*, 57(S1), S35–S35.

Itakura, F. & Saito, S. (1970). A statistical method for estimation of speech spectral density and formant frequencies. *IEICE Transactions on Fundamentals of Electronics, Communications and Computer Science*, 53–A(1), 35–42.

Kaufmann, J. M., Schulz, C., & Schweinberger, S. R. (2013). High and low performers differ in the use of shape information for face recognition. *Neuropsychologia*, 51(7), 1310–1319.

Kawahara, H. (2002). *STRAIGHT information page*. Available online at: http://www. wakayama-u.ac.jp/~kawahara/STRAIGHTadv/ [Accessed: 15th May 2017]

Kawahara, H., Masuda-Katsuse, I., & de Cheveigné, A. (1999). Restructuring speech representations using a pitch-adaptive time-frequency smoothing and an instantaneous frequency-based F0 extraction: possible role of a repetitive structure in sounds. *Speech Communication*, 27(3–4), 187–207.

Kawahara, H. & Morise, M. (2011). Technical foundations of TANDEM-STRAIGHT, a speech analysis, modification and synthesis framework. *Sadhana*, 36(5), 713–727.

Kawahara, H., Morise, M., Banno, H., & Skuk, V. G. (2013). *Temporally variable multi-aspect N-way morphing based on interference-free speech representations*. Asia-Pacific Signal and Information Processing Association Annual Summit and Conference, Kaohsiung, 2013, pp. 1–10.

Kawahara, H. et al. (2008). *TANDEM-STRAIGHT: a temporally stable power spectral representation for periodic signals and applications to interference-free spectrum, F0, and aperiodicity estimation*. IEEE International Conference on Acoustics, Speech and Signal Processing, Las Vegas, USA, pp. 3933–3936.

Latinus, M. & Belin, P. (2011). Anti-voice adaptation suggests prototype-based coding of voice identity. *Frontiers in Psychology*, 2(175), 1–12.

Latinus, M. & Belin, P. (2011). Human voice perception. *Current Biology*, 21(4), R143-R145.

Latinus, M. & Belin, P. (2012). Perceptual auditory aftereffects on voice identity using brief vowel stimuli. *PLoS One*, 7(7), e41384.

Latinus, M., Crabbe, F., & Belin, P. (2011). Learning-induced changes in the cerebral processing of voice identity. *Cerebral Cortex*, 21(12), 2820–2828.

Latinus, M., McAleer, P., Bestelmeyer, P. E., & Belin, P. (2013). Norm-based coding of voice identity in human auditory cortex. *Current Biology*, 23(12), 1075–1080.

Latinus, M. & Taylor, M. J. (2012). Discriminating male and female voices: differentiating pitch and gender. *Brain Topography*, 25(2), 194–204.

Leopold, D. A., O'Toole, A. J., Vetter, T., & Blanz, V. (2001). Prototype-referenced shape encoding revealed by high-level aftereffects. *Nature Neuroscience*, 4(1), 89–94.

Ling, Z.-H. et al. (2015). Deep learning for acoustic modeling in parametric speech generation: a systematic review of existing techniques and future trends. *IEEE Signal Processing Magazine*, 32(3), 35–52.

Linville, S. E. (1996). The sound of senescence. *Journal of Voice*, 10(2), 190–200.

Makhoul, J. (1975). Linear prediction: a tutorial review. *Proceedings of IEEE*, 63(4), 561–580.

McAuley, R. & Quatieri, T. (1986). Speech analysis/synthesis based on a sinusoidal representation. *IEEE Transactions on Acoustics, Speech, and Signal Processing*, 34(4), 744–754.

McQueen, J. (2010). Phonetic categorisation. *Language and Cognitive Processes*, 11(6), 655–664.

Moulines, E. & Charpentier, F. (1990). Pitch-synchronous waveform processing techniques for text-to-speech synthesis using diphones. *Speech Communication*, 9(5–6), 453–467.

Mullennix, J. W., Johnson, K. A., Topcu-Durgun, M., & Farnsworth, L. M. (1995). The perceptual representation of voice gender. *Journal of the Acoustical Society of America*, 98(6), 3080–3095.

Oppenheim, A. V. (1969). Speech analysis-synthesis system based on homomorphic filtering. *Journal of the Acoustical Society of America*, 45(2), 458–465.

Papcun, G., Kreiman, J., & Davis, A. (1989). Long-term memory for unfamiliar voices. *Journal of the Acoustical Society of America*, 85(2), 913–925.

Pernet, C. R. & Belin, P. (2012). The role of pitch and timbre in voice gender categorization. *Frontiers in Psychology*, 3(23), 1–11.

Sagayama, S. & Itakura, F. (1986). *Duality theory of composite sinusoidal modeling and linear prediction.* IEEE International Conference on Acoustics, Speech, and Signal Processing, Tokyo, pp. 1261–1264.

Sagayama, S. & Itakura, F. (2002). Symmetry between linear predictive coding and composite sinusoidal modeling. *Electronics and Communications in Japan (Part III: Fundamental Electronic Science)*, 85(6), 42–54.

Schweinberger, S. R. et al. (2008). Auditory adaptation in voice perception. *Current Biology*, 18(9), 684–688.

Schweinberger, S. R. et al. (2014). Speaker perception. *Wiley Interdisciplinary Reviews: Cognitive Science*, 5(1), 15–25.

Schweinberger, S. R., Herholz, A., & Sommer, W. (1997). Recognizing famous voices: influence of stimulus duration and different types of retrieval cues. *Journal of Speech, Language, and Hearing Research*, 40(2), 453–463.

Schweinberger, S. R., Walther, C., Zäske, R., & Kovacs, G. (2011). Neural correlates of adaptation to voice identity. *British Journal of Psychology*, 102(4), 748–764.

Skuk, V. G., Dammann, L. M., & Schweinberger, S. R. (2015). Role of timbre and fundamental frequency in voice gender adaptation. *Journal of the Acoustical Society of America*, 138(2), 1180–1193.

Skuk, V. G. & Schweinberger, S. R. (2013). Adaptation aftereffects in vocal emotion perception elicited by expressive faces and voices. *PLoS One*, 8(11), e81691.

Skuk, V. G. & Schweinberger, S. R. (2014). Influences of fundamental frequency, formant frequencies, aperiodicity, and spectrum level on the perception of voice gender. *Journal of Speech, Language, and Hearing Research*, 57(1), 285–296.

Slaney, M., Covell, M., & Lassiter, B. (1996). *Automatic audio morphing.* IEEE International Conference on Acoustics, Speech, and Signal Processing, Atlanta, USA, pp. 1001–1004.

Smith, D. R. R., Walters, T. C., & Patterson, R. D. (2007). Discrimination of speaker sex and size when glottal-pulse rate and vocal-tract length are controlled. *Journal of the Acoustical Society of America*, 122(6), 3628–3639.

Smith, R. & Hawkins, S. (2012). Production and perception of speaker-specific phonetic detail at word boundaries. *Journal of Phonetics*, 40(2), 213–233.

Steyvers, M. (1999). Morphing techniques for manipulating face images. *Behavior Research Methods, Instruments, & Computers*, 31(2), 359–369.

Sutherland, C. A. M., Rhodes, G., & Young, A. W. (2017). Facial image manipulation: A tool for investigating social perception. *Social, Psychological, and Personality Science*, 8(5), 538–551. doi: 10.177/1948550617697176

Unser, M. (2000). Sampling—50 years after Shannon. *Proceedings of the IEEE*, 88(4), 569–587.

Watson, R. et al. (2014). Crossmodal adaptation in right posterior superior temporal sulcus during face–voice emotional integration. *Journal of Neuroscience*, 34(20), 6813–6821.

Webster, M. A. & MacLeod, D. I. A. (2011). Visual adaptation and face perception. *Philosophical Transactions of the Royal Society of London B: Biological Sciences,* 366(1571), 1702–1725.

Webster, M. A. & MacLin, O. H. (1999). Figural aftereffects in the perception of faces. *Psychonomic Bulletin & Review,* 6(4), 647–653.

Wolberg, G. (1998). Image morphing: a survey. *The Visual Computer,* 14(8), 360–372.

Zäske, R. & Schweinberger, S. R. (2011). You are only as old as you sound: auditory aftereffects in vocal age perception. *Hearing Research,* 282(1), 283–288.

Zäske, R., Schweinberger, S. R., Kaufmann, J. M., & Kawahara, H. (2009). In the ear of the beholder: neural correlates of adaptation to voice gender. *European Journal of Neuroscience,* 30(3), 527–534.

Zäske, R., Schweinberger, S. R., & Kawahara, H. (2010). Voice aftereffects of adaptation to speaker identity. *Hearing Research,* 268(1), 38–45.

Zäske, R., Skuk, V. G., Kaufmann, J. M., & Schweinberger, S. R. (2013). Perceiving vocal age and gender: an adaptation approach. *Acta Psychologica,* 144(3), 583–593.

Zen, H., Tokuda, K., & Black, A. W. (2009). Statistical parametric speech synthesis. *Speech Communication,* 51(11), 1039–1064.

....

CHAPTER 32

MACHINE-BASED DECODING OF VOICES AND HUMAN SPEECH

....

ALESSANDRO VINCIARELLI

32.1 INTRODUCTION

....

FIGURE 32.1 shows the *threshold of hearing*— the minimum intensity required for a sound to be heard—as a function of frequency. The lowest part of the curve corresponds to the frequencies typical of human speech (roughly between 20 and 400 Hz). Thus, human ears are most sensitive to human voices than to any other sound in the environment. From an evolutionary point of view, the most likely explanation is that speech has been a key advantage for our species (Dunbar et al., 2005). Therefore, it is not surprising to observe that technology has made major efforts aimed at dealing automatically with speech signals (Pieraccini, 2012).

The earliest technological approaches revolving around speech signals date back to the first half of the twentieth century. It is in this period that the diffusion of telecommunications fostered the development of coding systems (i.e. automatic methodologies capable of representing a signal in as compact a form as possible). The main goal of these efforts was to improve the efficiency of transmissions (i.e. to convey as much information as possible using as little data as possible). In parallel, research laboratories started to work on automatic speech recognition (ASR)—the task of automatically transcribing speech signals (Pieraccini, 2012). After a pioneering stage, it was during the seventies that ASR technologies made the most important progress. The reason is twofold. On the one hand, it was in this period that computers became powerful enough to deal with the ASR problem. On the other hand, it was in the seventies that the statistical methodologies that still today underlie most ASR approaches made their first appearance in the speech-technology community.

The initial ASR attempts targeted relatively simple tasks like the automatic transcription of phone numbers. In this case, the predefined list of words that a speech-recognition system can actually transcribe is limited ('zero', 'one', 'two', …, 'nine'). Furthermore, the utterances are not connected (i.e. they are separated by silences long enough to easily segment

Absolute threshold of hearing

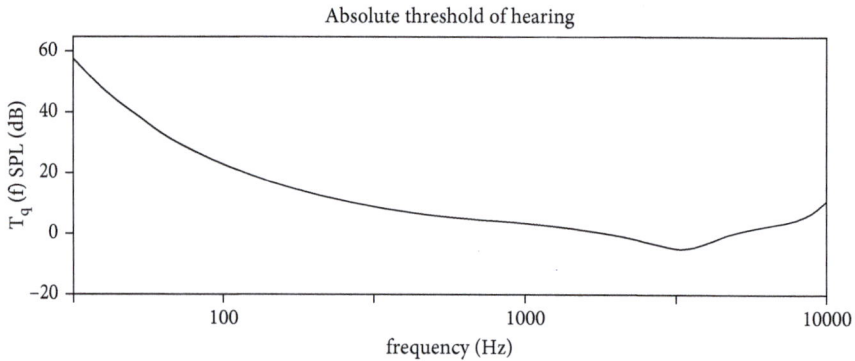

FIGURE 32.1 Absolute threshold of hearing (TOH). The TOH is plotted on a logarithmic scale and shows how the energy necessary to hear frequencies between 50 and 4000 kHz is significantly lower than the energy needed for other frequencies.

the speech stream into individual words). Over the years, the efforts have addressed increasingly more challenging recognition tasks—first, the automatic transcription of people reading written texts (the data does not include noise, there are no disfluencies or grammatical errors, language models can constrain effectively the space of the transcription hypotheses to be searched); then, the recognition of spontaneous speech in naturalistic settings (the data includes noise, there are disfluencies and grammatical errors, the language models constrain, to a limited extent, the space of possible transcription hypotheses). Applications like Siri and Cortana®, capable of effectively interacting with their users via speech, come at the end of this long process and rely on unprecedented large volumes of data available through the development of internet-based services and the diffusion of mobile platforms.

Typically, ASR approaches include a normalization step aimed at eliminating, or at least attenuating, variability in the speech signal that is not relevant to the automatic transcription problem. Normalization methodologies target the suppression of variability due to sources like, for example, echoes or environmental noise. Furthermore, they target non-verbal and paralinguistic aspects of speech such as prosody (loudness, pitch, speaking rate, etc.), vocalizations (laughter, crying, etc.), use of silence and pauses, overlapping speech, turn-taking, and so on. The reason is that these elements do not change the transcription (*what* people say) even if they contribute to its sense (*how* people say it). However, the last 10–15 years have witnessed increasingly more efforts aimed at analysis and understanding of non-verbal components of speech, especially in fields like computational paralinguistics (Schuller & Batliner, 2013) and social signal processing (SSP) (Vinciarelli et al., 2009, 2012). This has led to approaches for the automatic analysis of a wide spectrum of social and psychological phenomena that speech conveys, including emotions, personality, dominance, roles, effectiveness of delivery. The efforts in this direction have made it clear that it is not possible to correctly transcribe speech without taking into account communicative aspects that paralanguage and non-verbal communication convey. However, a full integration between ASR and SSP has still to be achieved.

The goal of this chapter is to provide a short introduction to the aforementioned technologies, and in particular the main technological and methodological issues and components. The rest of the chapter is organized as follows: Section 32.2 introduces automatic speech recognition and its state of the art; Section 32.3 shows how the computing community deals with non-verbal aspects of speech; and Section 32.4 draws some conclusions.

32.2 AUTOMATIC SPEECH RECOGNITION

ASR is the task of automatically transcribing speech data. In mathematical terms, this corresponds to mapping a signal $S = (s_0, s_1, \ldots, s_N)$ into a sequence of words $W = (w_1, w_2, \ldots, w_T)$, where s_k is the kth sample of the signal and N is the total number of samples in S. Sample s_k is a physical measurement, typically air pressure, made at time $k\Delta t$, where Δt is the length in seconds of the time interval between two consecutive measurements. When using a microphone, the physical measurement that accounts for air pressure is the displacement of an elastic membrane, positioned inside the microphone, with respect to its position of equilibrium. The value of Δt is constant during a recording and it is called *sampling period*. Its inverse is the *sampling frequency F* in Hertz (i.e. the number of times per second that a measurement has been done during the recording). In the case of speech, the typical sampling frequency is 44 kHz when high quality is required (e.g. broadcast material or commercial audio products) and 8 kHz when low quality is sufficient (e.g. phone and radio communications).

Figure 32.2 shows the main components of an ASR system. The *front-end* is the step that takes the signal S as input and gives, as output, a representation of it suitable for further processing. In current state-of-the-art ASR technologies, the representation is a sequence $X = (\vec{x}_1, \vec{x}_2, \ldots, \vec{x}_M)$ of observation vectors, where M is the total number of vectors in sequence X. The observation vector $\vec{x}_k$ is extracted from a short analysis window—the typical length is 30 ms—that starts at time kB, where B is the interval of time between the start of two consecutive analysis windows (in the most frequent case, $B = 10$ ms). Typically, two consecutive windows are partially overlapping (with the parameters mentioned earlier in this section, the overlap is 20 ms).

The rationale behind such a representation is that spoken sentences are sequences of *phonemes*, the atomic sounds that compose every word in a given language. Ideally, there

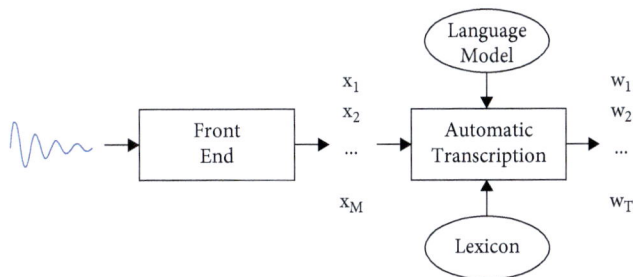

FIGURE 32.2 The main technological components of an automatic speech recognition system. The front-end takes, as input, the speech signals and gives, as output, a sequence of observation vectors. Automatic transcription maps the sequence of vectors into a sequence of words.

should be one observation vector per phoneme, but it is not possible to know, a priori, where the phonemes are. Windows positioned at regular time steps do not correspond exactly to phonemes. However, they are expected to entirely include one phoneme at least in some cases. This is the reason why the windows must be long enough to frequently enclose one phoneme, but short enough to rarely include two consecutive phonemes. The use of statistical approaches for the transcription step (see next paragraph) allows one to deal with the uncertainty in the position of the windows with respect to the actual phonemes.

The second stage, the actual transcription step, takes X as input and gives, as output, the sequence of words $W = (w_1, \ldots, w_T)$ that is the final output of the ASR system. In general, the transcription relies not only on X but also on two linguistic resources, namely the *lexicon* and the *language model*. The lexicon L is the list of words that the system can actually give as output. In other words, every $w_i \in W$ must be one of the entries of the lexicon L. If the signal contains a word that is not in the lexicon, the system will still give, as output, one of the words of the lexicon, typically the one that is closest from a phonetic point of view. The language model is a probability distribution $p(W)$ that estimates how probable a given transcription W is. Language models are typically obtained by counting the occurrences of individual words and N-grams (sequences of N consecutive words) in large corpora of text. The main role of the lexicon and language model is to constrain the space of the hypotheses to search (i.e. to eliminate those transcriptions that are too unlikely to be considered).

State-of-the-art ASR systems find the transcription $\hat{W}$ that satisfies the following equation:

$$\hat{W} = \arg\max_{W \in W_L} p(X, W) p(W) \tag{1}$$

where $p(X, W)$ is a probability distribution defined over the joint space of observation and word sequences, and W_L is the set of all possible sequences of words belonging to the lexicon L. In other words, an ASR system takes into account all possible transcriptions for a given observation sequence X and, for each transcription, estimates the probability $p(X, W)p(W)$. Then, the transcription that corresponds to the largest probability is retained as the actual transcription of the input speech data. Given that the number of transcriptions is prohibitively large, the lexicon and language model are used to eliminate all transcriptions that are unlikely to match the observation sequence X.

The description in the previous paragraph shows that, from a technical point of view, the most distinctive aspects of an ASR system are the type of information that X conveys and the approach adopted to estimate $p(W, X)p(W)$. Furthermore, the lexicon L typically characterizes the application domain for which the ASR system has been designed, from the simple transcription of phone numbers (only ten items in the lexicon corresponding to the digits from zero to nine) to the transcription of unconstrained conversations (up to 100,000 items in the lexicon expected to cover 90–95% of all words used in a generic conversation). The rest of this section focuses on front-end and automatic transcription.

32.2.1 Front-End Transcription

The extraction of the observation vectors from the speech signal is typically referred to as *feature extraction* because the components of the observation vectors are called *features*.

These latter are physical measurements expected to convey information relevant to the recognition of the words being uttered. In particular, the features are expected to be different and stable for different phonemes. The assumption of stability over time intervals comparable to the duration of a phoneme is known as *piecewise quasi-stationarity assumption* and it underlies virtually every ASR approach proposed in the literature.

The features most commonly extracted from the speech signals are the *mel-frequency cepstral coefficients* (MFCC) (Zheng et al., 2001) and the *perceptual linear prediction* (PLP) coefficients (PLP) (Hermansky, 1990). In both cases, the goal is to obtain a smooth version of the *spectral envelope* (i.e. the curve of the frequency-amplitude plan that describes the way the energy of a sound is distributed across different frequencies). The main difference between the actual distribution and the envelope is that the latter is designed to be steady (no jumps of the first derivative) and smooth (no major oscillations) while following as closely as possible the actual distribution. In intuitive terms, the spectral envelope can be thought of as the curve that connects the maxima of a spectrum, hence the use of the term 'envelope'.

MFCC and PLP coefficients are the most commonly adopted features, but the literature provides a large number of other methodologies. However, the overall attempt is always to account for the spectral properties in the most compact possible way while conveying all the information necessary to correctly transcribe the signals.

32.2.2 Automatic Transcription

The transcription step aims at finding the sequence of lexicon words $\hat{W}$ that satisfies Equation (1). In intuitive terms, $\hat{W}$ is the sequence of lexicon entries that maximizes the joint probability of W and X multiplied by the probability of W. The main approaches adopted in the literature to estimate $p(X, W)$ and $p(W)$ are the *Hidden Markov Models* (Rabiner, 1989) and the *N-gram models* (Manning & Schütze, 1999).

The main assumption underlying Hidden Markov Models (HMM) is that there is a sequence of non-observable (hidden) states fundamental to the sequence of observations X. In the case of ASR, the sequence of the states corresponds to a sequence of phonemes that compose the words in W. Typically, there are three states for every phoneme, namely *onset*, *apex*, and *offset*. From a technical point of view, the sequence of states corresponding to a word is obtained by concatenating multiple HMMs, each corresponding to a phoneme. Overall, the expression of $p(X, W)$ in the case of a HMM is as follows:

$$p(X, W) = \pi_{s1} b_{s1}(\vec{x}_1) \prod_{k=2}^{M} a_{s_k s_{k-1}} b_{sk}(\vec{x}_k) \qquad (2)$$

where s_j is the jth state in the sequence of states that underlies W, π_{s1} is the probability of starting with state$_1$ (i.e. the probability of starting the sequence with a certain phoneme), $a_{sk\ sk-1}$ is the probability of a transition between state s_{k-1} and s_k, and $b_{sk}(\vec{x})$ is the probability of observing $\vec{x}$ when the underlying state is s_k (the *emission probability function*). Since self-transitions are possible, the HMMs can accommodate variations in length of the same phoneme (multiple observations can be attributed to the same underlying state).

The values of π_{sk} are typically obtained by counting the number of times in a given collection of spoken data that an utterance starts with a certain phoneme and, hence, the underlying HMM starts with a certain state. Similarly, the transition probabilities are estimated by counting how frequently, in a collection of spoken data, a given state s_i is followed by another state s_j. In the case of the emission probability functions, the most common approach to get the explicit expression of $b_s(\vec{x})$ is the application of the expectation-maximization (Bilmes, 1998). In general, the emission probability functions correspond to mixtures of Gaussians:

$$b_s(\vec{x}) = \sum_{k=1}^{G} \alpha_k \, N(\vec{x} \,|\, \Sigma_{ks}, \vec{\mu}_{ks})\tag{3}$$

where the *mixing coefficients* α_k sum up to 1, $N(.)$ is a multivariate Gaussian, Σ_{ks} and $\vec{\mu}_{ks}$ are covariance matrix and mean of Gaussian k in the mixture of state s. Figure 32.3 shows how the HMMs work in practice.

The transcription step actually consists of finding the sequence of states (hence of phonemes and words) that better accounts for the observation sequence X. Such a task is performed with the *Viterbi algorithm* (Forney, 1973) that is capable of finding the sequence of states that maximizes the probability $p(W, X)$. However, the search through all possible sequences W can be constrained with a language model $p(W)$ so that the computational effort is reduced. The most common approach to estimate $p(W)$ is the N-gram model. The reason is not only that this model appears to be the most effective, but also that it naturallys fit the Viterbi algorithm. The expression of $p(W)$ with an N-gram model is as follows:

$$p(W) = \prod_{k=N}^{T} p(w_k \,|\, w_{k-1}, w_{k-2}, \& , w_{k-N+1})\tag{4}$$

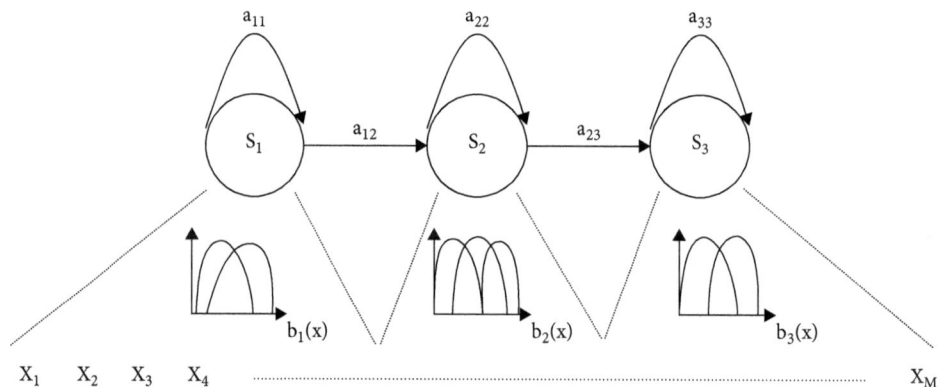

FIGURE 32.3 Schematic showing how a left–right hidden Markov model (HMM) works. The emission probability density functions associated to the states allow one to estimate the probabilities of an observation vector *xx* belonging to one of the states. The transition probabilities allow one to estimate the probability of passing from one state to the other.

where N is the *order* of the model, w_k is the kth word of W, and T is the total number of words in W. While being simple, the N-gram model has been shown to be more effective than models trying to take into account the meaning of the words or the grammar of a language.

The main role of $p(W)$ in the transcription is to lower the probability of transcriptions that, while making sense from an acoustic point of view, are not necessarily observable in a given language. This applies in particular to short sequences that include only *function words* (i.e. terms that are content-independent but allow one to build grammatically correct sentences—articles, prepositions, etc.). Such short sequences include expressions such as '*there is a*' and '*it is on*', that, while being frequent, can often be confused with longer words. In general, content words are less frequent than function words (roughly one third of all the words appearing in a corpus occur only once), but the acoustic evidence is sufficiently strong to counterbalance the low value of $p(W)$.

32.3 Non-Verbal Vocal Behaviour

Besides extracting features from the speech signal, the front-end of an ASR system typically tries to eliminate any source of variablity that is not relevant to the automatic transcription of what is being said, a step typically referred to as *normalization*. This applies to variability resulting from gender, age, emotional state, accent, speaking style, and any other factor that, while influencing the way something is said, does not influence the transcription of an utterance. The reason is that the ASR performances increase when there is a consistent relationship between the phonemes being uttered and the features being extracted. However, these sources of variability have recently become the focus of domains like computational paralinguistics (Schuller & Batliner, 2013) and SSP (Vinciarelli et al., 2012). The reason is that non-verbal components of speech prosody, voice quality, vocalizations, disfluencies, intonation, and so on, convey socially and psychologically relevant information about speakers and their interaction.

Figure 32.4 shows the main technological components of systems that analyse non-verbal communication in speech. Like in the case of ASR, speech data is first segmented into short analysis windows (typically 20–30 ms) that overlap each other and start at regular

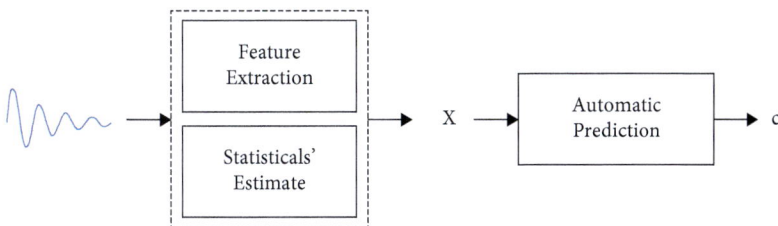

FIGURE 32.4 The main technological components of a system aimed at computational paralinguistics or speech-based social signal processing. The first step is the extraction of the features (short-term initially and then statistics), while the second step is the inference of the social or psychological phenomena of interest.

time-steps (typically 10 ms). In this way, it is possible to extract short-term properties from the speech signals (i.e. properties that can be expected to be relatively stable for no more than a few tens of milliseconds or the time that someone can hold a stable configuration of the articulators). The result is that, for a given short-term property, it is possible to obtain as many measurements as there are analysis windows that fit in the data (e.g. in the case of 30-ms windows that start at regular time-steps of 10 ms, one second of speech yields 970 measurements). These measurements are then summarized with statistics like average, variance, entropy, minimum, and maximum. In this way, while not taking into account every single value of a measurement, it is still possible to have an idea of its distribution over a speech sample.

The ultimate goal of the process previously discussed is to represent a speech sample as a vector of physical properties that account for how a person speaks. Once such a vector is available, it is then possible to apply statistical approaches that can be used to infer the traits attributed by people. The short-term properties adopted in the different works presented in the literature cover the most important speech properties. The measurements most commonly adopted target pitch (the fundamental frequency), energy, and speaking rate (i.e. the *big three* of prosody). Intuitively, these measurements account for the sound of the voice, how loud a person speaks, and how fast he or she does it, respectively. The statistics account for the distribution of the measurements, in particular, the average accounts for the values that occur most frequently, the variance for how wide is the range of the measurement, the entropy for its variability, minimum and maximum (used only rarely because they can be outliers) for the dynamic range, etc. Other short-term properties account for voice spectral properties such as MFCC (Zheng et al., 2001), harmonic-to-noise ratio (de Krom, 1993), spectral tilt (Jackson et al., 1985), etc.

The prediction step is performed using a wide spectrum of classification and regression approaches. The former are adopted when non-verbal behaviour is used to infer categorical information like, for example, which of the six basic emotions a speaker is displaying (Scherer, 2003) or which role someone is playing in a meeting (Garg et al., 2008). The latter are adopted when non-verbal behaviour is used to infer dimensional information like, for example, emotions represented in the valence-arousal space or personality assessed along the 'Big Five' traits (five major dimensions that have been shown to capture most individual differences—openness, conscientiousness, extraversion, agreeableness, neuroticism). From a mathematical point of view, a classifier is a function $f(\vec{x})$ that maps a vector $\vec{x}$ into c, where this latter is a class that belongs to a predefined set $C = \{c_1, c_2, ..., c_N\}$ (N is the total number of classes). In contrast, a regressor is a function $f(\vec{x})$ that maps a vector $\vec{x}$ into a real number y. The choice between classifiers and regressors depends on the particular problem being targeted. The literature proposes a large number of classifiers and regressors, but some of the most popular and effective are support vector machines (Hearst et al., 1998), deep neural networks (Bengio, 2009), LASSO (Tibshirani, 1996), logistic regression (Hosmer Jr & Lemeshow, 2004), and Gaussian processes (Rasmussen, 2006).

While in the case of ASR, all systems address the same problem—the automatic transcription of speech recordings—in the case of SSP and computational paralinguistics, the technologies presented in the literature address a large number of different issues. The earliest approaches focused on emotion (for an extensive survey, see Scherer, 2003), but the latest technologies have applied methodologies like those described in this section to infer from speech information such as role, conflict, dominance, synchrony, interest, personality, developmental disease in children, and depression. The rest of this section provides a short state-of-the-art review of the main problems addressed in the literature.

32.3.1 Analysis of Social Signals and Paralanguage

The computing literature proposes a large number of approaches aimed at inferring socially and psychologically relevant phenomena from speech recordings (Schuller & Batliner, 2013; Vinciarelli et al., 2009, 2012). One of the problems that has been addressed most extensively is that of emotion recognition (i.e. the automatic identification of the emotions that speakers experience based on the physical characteristics of their speech). The problem has been the subject not only of many articles (for an extensive survey, see Scherer, 2003) but also of several international benchmarking campaigns in which a large number of different approaches have been adopted and compared (Schuller et al., 2011, 2009). As a result, it has been possible to perform a meta-analysis showing that there is a set of features—called the *Geneva minimalistic acoustic parameter set* (GeMAPS)—that appears to be more reliable than others in conveying information about the emotional state of a speaker (Eyben et al., 2016).

In recent years, the attention has shifted towards other problems that can be addressed using the approach depicted in Figure 32.4. In particular, a large number of works and an international benchmarking campaign (Schuller et al., 2012) have been dedicated to the inference of personality traits—both self-assessed and attributed—from non-verbal aspects of speech (Vinciarelli & Mohammadi, 2014). Unlike in the case of the emotions, no feature set has been shown to be more reliable than others. However, a few indications emerge from the literature. The first is that all works addressing the problem of the relationship between speech and personality from a computing point of view adopt trait-based personality models (i.e. models that represent personality as a D-dimensional vector where every component accounts for a behavioural dimension). In most cases, the traits correspond to the 'Big Five' (Digman, 1996). The second is that the only task that can be performed with satisfactory performance is the prediction of whether a person is above or below median with respect to every trait. Finally, the third is that not all traits can be inferred equally well from speech. In particular, the performances tend to be satisfactory only for extraversion and conscientiousness.

Another domain where there has been a significant effort has been the recognition of the roles that people play in a particular social setting (Dong et al., 2007; Garg et al., 2008; Zancanaro et al., 2006). The main difference with respect to the problems already mentioned in this section is that, in this case, it is necessary to analyse recordings that include multiple voices. However, the proposed approaches remain similar to those depicted in Figure 32.4. The only difference is that there is a preliminary speaker diarisation step (i.e. a segmentation of the audio recordings into intervals in which only one person is expected to speak) (Anguera et al., 2012; Tranter & Reynolds, 2006). This allows one to use not only the features that have been adopted for the inference of emotions and personality, but also features that account for turn-taking, including speaking-time distribution across speakers, adjacency matrices, amount of overlapping speech, etc. (Vinciarelli et al., 2009, 2012). The main limitation of this area is that the roles tend to be specific for a given setting and, unlike the case of constructs like personality or phenomena like the emotions, it is not possible to identify a general set of roles that applies to all possible contexts.

In the case of other social and psychological phenomena, the number of works was not sufficiently large to give rise to a research community, but the approaches stem directly from those adopted for the other problems mentioned in this section and, overall, replicate the scheme of Figure 32.4. Such phenomena include, for example, dominance (Jayagopi et al., 2009), conflict (Kim et al., 2014), mimicry (Michelet et al., 2012), depression (Scibelli et al., 2016), and interest (Yeasin et al., 2006).

32.4 Conclusions

This chapter has provided a general introduction to the problem of machine-based decoding of speech and human voice. Such a definition encompasses all technologies that automatically infer information from speech signals, whether this means to automatically transcribe what a speaker is saying (the domain is, in this case, automatic speech recognition) or to predict information about social and psychological aspects of speakers and their interactions with others (the domains are, in this case, social signal processing and computational paralinguistics).

One of the main messages of the chapter is that the approaches adopted to infer information from speech can be described in terms of two general schemes. The first, underlying most automatic speech recognition systems, has been depicted in Figure 32.2. The second, underlying most systems aimed at SSP and computational paralinguistics, has been depicted in Figure 32.4. A crucial problem in both cases is the extraction of features (i.e. automatic measurements that account for the physical properties of speech). In the case of the problems that have been addressed most extensively in the literature (ASR and emotion recognition), it has been possible to identify feature sets that are more reliable than the others or, at least, lead to satisfactory performances in the majority of the experimental settings. In the case of those problems that have been addressed more recently and less extensively, the identification of reliable features is still an open issue.

With regards the aspect of machine intelligence (i.e. the computational approach aimed at mapping the features into information of interest—transcriptions or social and psychological phenomena), the state of the art in ASR is the adoption of hidden Markov models, statistical sequential models that can take into account temporal aspects of the data they take as input. In the case of SSP and computational paralinguistics, the variety of approaches is wider because the data is typically represented with a single vector and, then, any type of classifier or regressor can be applied. However, deep neural networks have started to be used more and more frequently both in ASR and in the other domains, and they are likely to become one of the most common approaches, if not the dominant approach, in years to come.

The main application field of the technologies described in this chapter is likely to be human–computer interaction in all its multiple aspects, from speech-based personal assistants like Siri and Cortana®, to social robots expected to understand the inner state of their users. The main challenges concern the possibility of working in naturalistic environments where noise and lack of constraints make it difficult to extract proper features and to limit the space of possible outcomes, respectively. Furthermore, speech technologies are used increasingly more frequently in non-technological fields such as social psychology and cognitive neuropsychology. This will hopefully result in new insights about human speech and its crucial role in our life.

References

Anguera, X., Bozonnet, S., Evans, N., Fredouille, C., Friedland, G., & Vinyals, O. (2012). Speaker diarization: a review of recent research. *IEEE Transactions on Audio, Speech, and Language Processing*, 20(2), 356–370.

Bengio, Y. (2009). Learning deep architectures for AI. *Foundations and Trends in Machine Learning*, 2(1), 1–127.

Bilmes, J. (1998). *A gentle tutorial of the EM algorithm and its application to parameter estimation for Gaussian mixture and hidden Markov models*. Technical Report 510, International Computer Science Institute, 1998.

de Krom, G. (1993). A cepstrum-based technique for determining a harmonics-to-noise ratio in speech signals. *Journal of Speech, Language, and Hearing Research*, 36(2), 254–266.

Digman, J. M. (1996). The curious history of the Five-Factor Model. In: J. S. Wiggins (ed.) *The Five-Factor Model of Personality* (pp. 1–20). New York: Guilford Press.

Dong, W., Lepri, B., Cappelletti, A., Pentland, A., Pianesi, F., & Zancanaro, M. (2007). *Using the influence model to recognize functional roles in meetings*. Proceedings of the Ninth International Conference on Multimodal Interfaces, Nov 12–15, 2007, Nagoya, Japan (pp. 271–278).

Dunbar, R., Barrett, L., & Lycett, J. (2005). *Evolutionary Psychology: A Beginner's Guide*. Oneworld Publications.

Eyben, F., Scherer, K. R., Schuller, B. W., Sundberg, J., André, E., Busso, C., ... Narayanan, S. S. (2016). The Geneva minimalistic acoustic parameter set (GeMAPS) for voice research and affective computing. *IEEE Transactions on Affective Computing*, 7(2), 190–202.

Forney, G. D. (1973). The Viterbi algorithm. *Proceedings of the IEEE*, 61(3), 268–278.

Garg, N. P., Favre, S., Salamin, H., Hakkani Tür, D., & Vinciarelli, A. (2008). *Role recognition for meeting participants: an approach based on lexical information and social network analysis*. Proceedings of the ACM International Conference on Multimedia (pp. 693–696).

Hearst, M. A., Dumais, S. T., Osman, E., Platt, J., & Scholkopf, B. (1998). Support vector machines. *IEEE Intelligent Systems and their Applications*, 13(4), 18–28.

Hermansky, H. (1990). Perceptual linear predictive (PLP) analysis of speech. *Journal of the Acoustical Society of America*, 87(4), 1738–1752.

Hosmer Jr, D. W. & Lemeshow, S. (2004). *Applied Logistic Regression*. John Wiley & Sons.

Jackson, P., Ladefoged, M., Huffman, M., & Antonãnzas Barroso, N. (1985). Measures of spectral tilt. *Journal of the Acoustical Society of America*, 77(S1), S86–S86.

Jayagopi, D. B., Hung, H., Yeo, C., & Gatica-Perez, D. (2009). Modeling dominance in group conversations using nonverbal activity cues. *IEEE Transactions on Audio, Speech, and Language Processing*, 17(3), 501–513.

Kim, S., Valente, F., Filippone, M., & Vinciarelli, A. (2014). Predicting continuous conflict perception with Bayesian Gaussian processes. *IEEE Transactions on Affective Computing*, 5(2), 187–200.

Manning, C. D. & Schütze, H. (1999). *Foundations of Statistical Natural Language Processing*. MIT Press.

Michelet, S., Karp, K., Delaherche, E., Achard, C., & Chetouani, M. (2012). *Automatic imitation assessment in interaction.* International Workshop on Human Behavior Understanding, 7 October 2012, Vilamoura, Portugal (pp. 161–173).

Pieraccini, R. (2012). *The Voice in the Machine.* MIT Press.

Rabiner, L. R. (1989). A tutorial on hidden Markov models and selected applications in speech recognition. *Proceedings of the IEEE, 77*(2), 257–286.

Rasmussen, C. E. (2006). *Gaussian Processes for Machine Learning.* MIT Press.

Scherer, K. R. (2003). Vocal communication of emotion: a review of research paradigms. *Speech Communication, 40*(1), 227–256.

Schuller, B. & Batliner, A. (2013). *Computational Paralinguistics: Emotion, Affect and Personality in Speech and Language Processing.* John Wiley & Sons.

Schuller, B., Batliner, A., Steidl, S., & Seppi, D. (2011). Recognising realistic emotions and affect in speech: state of the art and lessons learnt from the first challenge. *Speech Communication, 53*(9), 1062–1087.

Schuller, B., Steidl, S., & Batliner, A. (2009). *The Interspeech 2009 emotion challenge.* Proceedings of Interspeech 2009 (pp. 312–315).

Schuller, B., Steidl, S., Batliner, A., Nöth, E., Vinciarelli, A., Burkhardt, F., Van Son, R., Weninger, F., Eyben, F., & Bocklet, T. (2012). *The Interspeech 2012 speaker trait challenge.* Proceedings of Interspeech 2012 (pp. 254–257).

Scibelli, F., Troncone, A., Likforman-Sulem, L., Vinciarelli, A., & Esposito, A. (2016). How major depressive disorder affects the ability to decode multimodal dynamic emotional stimuli. *Frontiers in ICT, 3,* 16.

Tibshirani, R. (1996). Regression shrinkage and selection via the lasso. *Journal of the Royal Statistical Society B, 58*(1), 267–288.

Tranter, S. E. & Reynolds, D. A. (2006). An overview of automatic speaker diarization systems. *IEEE Transactions on Audio, Speech, and Language Processing, 14*(5), 1557–1565.

Vinciarelli, A. & Mohammadi, G. (2014). A survey of personality computing. *IEEE Transactions on Affective Computing, 5*(3), 273–291.

Vinciarelli, A., Pantic, M., & Bourlard, H. (2009). Social signal processing: survey of an emerging domain. *Image and Vision Computing Journal, 27*(12), 1743–1759.

Vinciarelli, A., Pantic, M., Heylen, D., Pelachaud, C., Poggi, I., D'Errico, F., & Schroeder, M. (2012). Bridging the gap between social animal and unsocial machine: a survey of social signal processing. *IEEE Transactions on Affective Computing, 3*(1), 69–87.

Yeasin, M., Bullot, B., & Sharma, R. (2006). Recognition of facial expressions and measurement of levels of interest from video. *IEEE Transactions on Multimedia, 8*(3), 500–508.

Zancanaro, M., Lepri, B., & Pianesi, F. (2006). *Automatic detection of group functional roles in face to face interactions.* Proceedings of the Eighth International Conference on Multimodal Interfaces, Nov 2–4, 2006, Alberta, Canada (pp. 28–34).

Zheng, F., Zhang, G., & Song, Z. (2001). Comparison of different implementations of MFCC. *Journal of Computer Science and Technology, 16*(6), 582–589.

CHAPTER 33

MACHINE-BASED DECODING OF PARALINGUISTIC VOCAL FEATURES

MAXIMILIAN SCHMITT AND BJÖRN SCHULLER

33.1 INTRODUCTION

MACHINE *learning* is a major discipline in computer science, dealing with the question of how to imitate biological learning for technical purposes. Within the audio domain, a field of growing interest is *computational paralinguistics* (i.e. the machine analysis of 'how' *and* 'what' a speaker says aiming at the automatic recognition of speaker *states* and *traits*). This has numerous possible applications, such as, for example, automated market research or a more natural human–computer interaction through a virtual agent. Speaker states such as emotion evolve quickly over time. Speaker traits, in contrast, are describing permanent characteristics of a person such as gender, personality, or mother tongue, and alter—if at all—only in the long run. Somewhere in between are longer-term speaker states such as being intoxicated, having flu, or age.

The task of the machine is to find the optimum mapping between a speech signal and, for example, the current emotional state of the speaker. One of the first questions when building an intelligent machine is how the different possible states, the so-called *targets*, are modelled. There are two generally different approaches: speaker states and traits can be expressed either by a finite set of categories or as a value on a continuous scale. One example for categories is the 'Big Six' emotions by Ekman (Ekman, 1999)—*anger, disgust, fear, happiness, sadness*, and *surprise*. For the continuously-valued representation, the most common way is to use the two dimensions *arousal* and *valence* when dealing with emotion. As not all emotions can be described on this two-dimensional plane, further dimensions, such as *dominance* (Burkhardt et al., 2005), are sometimes added. As another example, one typical approach to model speaker personality-related traits is the Big-Five ('OCEAN') model of personality (Wiggins, 1996), consisting of five dimensions—*openness, conscientiousness, extraversion, agreeableness*, and *neuroticism*.

When the targets are defined, a classifier or, in the case of continuous targets, a regressor must usually be learned. In machine learning or, to be precise, in *supervised learning*, this is accomplished by giving the machine a large number of examples of speech signals, together with the corresponding targets. These examples are the so-called *training data*; their number and selection has a crucial influence on the performance of the final system. If the training database is too small, the examples are not (sufficiently) representative, or, if the target labels are not reliable, the classifier (or regressor) will not generalize well enough, meaning that the accuracy of its predictions is insufficient for the application.

For supervised learning, many different approaches exist, and some of them are introduced in Section 33.3. Most of those methods, however, do not work on the raw audio signal but on *features*, which are extracted from the signal in a first step. A typical chain for the analysis of human affect (or other states and traits) is displayed in Figure 33.1. As described, the first step is usually the extraction of acoustic low-level descriptors (LLDs) on *frame level* (i.e. the computation of feature vectors that describe short-term properties of the speech signal) (Schuller, 2012). As the frame-level audio features (i.e. the LLDs) do not contain enough information to recognize the state of the speaker, several successive frames must be observed and summarized. The duration of those *segments* depends on several aspects (e.g. the target labels and the employed machine-learning scheme). Very often, the speech is segmented on *utterance level* (i.e. a spoken sentence or statement of the speaker). In a fully automatic approach, this segmentation can be the result of *voice-activity detection* (Eyben, Weninger, Squartini, & Schuller, 2013).

There are different ways to summarize the information of the frame-level features from one segment. Two common approaches to get such *suprasegmental* features are described in Section 33.2—*functionals* and the *bag-of-words method*.

As an alternative to or complement for the acoustic feature space, *linguistic* features can be considered. For the recognition of emotion and further states and traits in speech, the exploitation of emotional keywords or phrases can be of benefit, especially for the prediction of valence. To obtain a textual representation of the spoken words (i.e. the transcription of what is said in written language), *automatic speech recognition* (ASR) (Schuller et al., 2009; Wöllmer, Weninger, et al., 2013) is usually applied. The resulting text document is then further processed using techniques from *natural language processing* (NLP), such as a *bag-of-words* representation (Schuller, Mousa, & Vasileios, 2015).

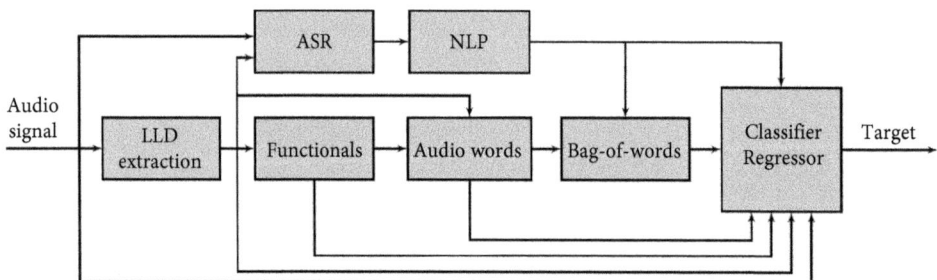

FIGURE 33.1 Exemplary speech-processing chain for the analysis of human affect and further states and traits.

The features are finally fed into a machine-learning scheme. As described in Section 33.3, methods may work on different representations, on segment level, frame level, or even on the raw audio signal.

33.2 Vocal Features

In this section, the most common acoustic low-level descriptors are first introduced; then, two techniques are explained that can be used to obtain a feature-space representation of the whole audio segment—functionals and bags-of- words.

33.2.1 Low-Level Descriptors

LLDs are extracted from the audio waveform in order to obtain the short-term acoustic properties of the human voice signal. The computation is based on frames of approximately 25–60 ms in length. During these short periods of time, the audio signal is assumed to be quasi-stationary (i.e. its properties are not supposed to vary during these time intervals). Successive frames usually have an overlap of between 50 % and 75 % (i.e. the distance between the centres of adjacent frames, the so-called *hopsize*, is between 6 ms and 30 ms).

Most LLDs are based on the *magnitude spectrum* of the signal frames, which is mostly obtained by the *discrete Fourier transform* (DFT) (Schuller, 2013). For the computation of the DFT, a fast algorithm exists with the *fast Fourier transform* (FFT). In general, the Fourier transform is based on the fact that a signal can be represented by the sum of a limited number of weighted sinusoids. Prior to the DFT, the samples within each frame are weighted with a window function, such as the *Hamming*, the *von Hann*, or a *Gaussian* window. Each window has specific properties which make it more or less suitable with regard to the application (Schuller, 2013).

A commonly used group of features are the prosodic features, which are related to:

- *Intensity*: can be approximated by the signal energy of the frame. The more sophisticated approach of (perceived) *loudness* modelling also takes into account psycho-acoustic effects, such as *masking* or frequency dependencies (Zwicker & Fastl, 2013).
- *Intonation*: is usually derived from the *fundamental frequency* of the human voice ('Fo'). Fo or (perceived) 'pitch' tracking is a quite challenging task, where many different approaches have been proposed (Schuller, 2013).
- *Speed*: describes the rhythm of the speaker. One simple method to obtain a rhythmic feature is to exploit the rate of changes between *voiced* and *unvoiced* frames and the duration of pauses.

Note that in voiced frames, a fundamental frequency can be detected, whereas this is not the case for unvoiced frames.

Another relevant group are the voice-quality features. Very well-known voice-quality features are the *harmonic-to-noise ratio* and the *microprosodic* features, *jitter* and *shimmer*.

Jitter is a measurement of the slight variations in successive period lengths of the fundamental frequency; shimmer describes the variations of the loudness of the voice between
those periods.

Further feature types comprise the spectral and cepstral features. The spectral features
are computed directly from the spectrum. Typical examples are the *spectral centroid, spectral flux,* or *spectral roll-off.* Cepstral features, on the other hand, are computed from the so-
called *cepstrum,* which can be computed by the inverse Fourier transform of the logarithm
of the spectrum. This procedure is motivated by the concept of the *source-filter model,* in
which a voice or similar signal is modelled in the frequency domain as the product (multiplication) of a harmonic source signal (usually an 'excitation' pulse train in the time domain) and the frequency response of a filter that shapes the (excited) sound. The filter
represents the transmission path of the source signal, which is, in the case of a speech signal,
predominantly the vocal tract. Taking the logarithm in the frequency domain converts the
product of the source and filter spectra into a sum. This sum is preserved during the inverse
Fourier transform due to its linear property. As a result, harmonic content with low amplitudes can be recognized and separated easily from the filter part. The probably most-spread
feature in speech analysis is derived from cepstral analysis—the Mel-frequency cepstral coefficients (MFCCs). Compared to the coefficients of the cepstrum, two modifications are
applied to the algorithm in order to obtain MFCCs. First, the bands of the power spectrum are summarized according to the *Mel scale* (i.e. a non-linear frequency scale aiming to
model the human auditory perception of frequencies). The Mel scale can be approximated
by (O'Shaughnessy, 1987)

$$f_{\text{mel}} = 2595 \cdot \log_{10}\left(1 + \frac{f}{700}\right) \tag{1}$$

The filters have a triangular shape in the frequency domain where their centre frequencies are distributed according to the Mel scale. With this mapping step, a dimensionality reduction is performed. After taking the logarithm, an inverse transform is
applied in order to decorrelate the Mel-spectrum coefficients. Instead of the inverse
discrete Fourier transform (IDFT), the *discrete cosine transform* (DCT) is applied
more often, and further alternatives are used. The whole processing chain is shown in
Figure 33.2. From the resulting coefficients, those with the indexes 0 to 12 are mostly
used in speech analysis. In ASR (speech-to-text), Mel-frequency cepstral coefficients
are the most widely spread feature; pitch, which is mainly a speaker-dependent feature
in non-tonal languages, is attenuated during the computation process, whereas the filter
responses of the vocal tract, which contain the information on the articulated vowels,
are preserved.

An overview of further relevant acoustic features can be found in Schuller (2013). From all
described LLDs, their differences in evolution over time—the so-called *delta coefficients*—
can also be computed, to augment the feature space, since, after all, the speech signal is represented as a contour of acoustic frame-level features over time. In order to reduce the impact
of noise on the speech-analysis process, *smoothing* can be applied (e.g. using a *moving
average filter*).

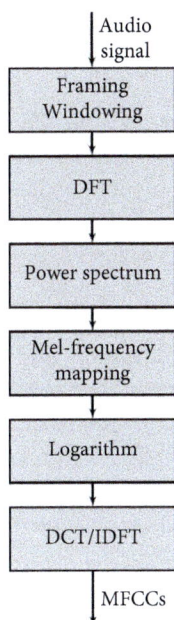

FIGURE 33.2 Computation of Mel-frequency cepstral coefficients.

33.2.2 Functionals

Once the contour of all LLDs over time has been extracted, the typical (yet optional) next step is to derive some statistics of them over a longer segment, to reach a *suprasegmental* feature vector representation. The most popular functionals used are the *mean value* and the *standard deviation* of the LLDs over each segment. Other commonly used functionals comprise *higher-order moments* (e.g. variance, skewness, kurtosis), *extrema* (maximum and minimum), *quartiles, percentiles*, and *regression coefficients*, as well as spectral LLD analysis. Note that hierarchical processing can be chosen, just as in the case of LLDs, where derived LLDs are frequently found. Examples include means of extrema or spectral coefficients of the number of segments, etc.

Naturally, the optimum choice of LLDs and corresponding functionals highly depends on the task at hand, just like the employed machine-learning model does. Nevertheless, some standardized feature sets have broadly established themselves in the community of computational paralinguistics. A recent dominant example is the *ComParE* feature set, which was introduced with the INTERSPEECH 2013 Computational Paralinguistics Challenge (Schuller et al., 2013) and has been used since in follow-up challenges. This set is a large-scale 'brute-forced' feature set, which consists of functionals from sixty-five LLDs and their delta coefficients—in total, 6,373 features per segment. It has been the result of steady refinement, and proven to be suitable for a variety of speech-recognition tasks including personality (Schuller et al., 2012), pathology (Schuller et al., 2013), cognitive and physical load (Schuller et al., 2014), and eating condition (Schuller et al., 2015). One drawback of such large-scale feature sets is, however, that there is a risk of *over-fitting* (i.e. the model adapts too much to the given training examples and does not generalize in a way that provides the same performance on unknown data).

In contrast to the ComParE feature set, the Geneva Minimalistic Acoustic Parameter Set (GeMAPS) is a small, expert-knowledge-based feature set recommendation made by a larger group of experts. It comprises only eighteen LLDs with selected functionals, resulting in a feature vector of size 62 (Eyben et al., 2016). An extended version of this set (eGeMAPS) has been introduced, comprising eighty-eight features in total. GeMAPS has proven to be suitable for the prediction of short-term speaker states (Ringeval et al., 2014, 2015). The criteria for the selection of the acoustic features were mainly their potential capabilities to model the physiological changes in voice production related to emotion and affect.

Compared to this expert-based, handcrafted selection of features, methods of *automatic feature selection* exist (Eyben et al., 2013). Applied to large-scale acoustic feature sets, such as ComParE, an improvement in performance can possibly be achieved.

Various tools have been introduced to extract acoustic LLDs and corresponding functionals from audio data. One popular example is *openSMILE* (Eyben, Weninger, Groß, & Schuller, 2013), which provides a large number of features relevant for the analysis of human speech, general sound, and also music. It provides the aforementioned standard feature sets and several further feature sets used in challenges in the field.

33.2.3 Audio Words

Instead of using functionals, LLD contours can be further processed in other ways. The LLDs of one frame can be considered as a vector of 'continuous numbers', which may then be subject to *vector quantization*. This means that the whole vector is assigned to a template vector from a *codebook* of audio words, sometimes also referred to as a *dictionary*. It is usually learned from the LLDs computed from training data by applying a clustering algorithm, such as *k-means* (Pancoast & Akbacak, 2012) or *expectation maximization* (EM) (Grzeszick et al., 2015) clustering. An even simpler way to generate a codebook is to select the required number of feature vectors randomly or distributed equidistantly from the training data (Rawat et al., 2013).

The assignment step is based on the distance between the LLD vector and the audio words from the codebook. Typically, the audio word w with the smallest *Euclidean distance* or further-suited distance measure is then assigned to each LLD vector F:

$$w = \arg\min_{w'} \sqrt{\sum_{m=1}^{M}\left(F_m - C_{w',m}\right)^2}, \tag{2}$$

with the w'-th audio word $C_{w'}$, the index of the LLD m, and the number of LLDs M. In Figure 33.3, the process of vector quantization is exemplified by a short segment of audio consisting of fifteen frames of Mel-frequency cepstral coefficients with indexes 1–12 and logarithmized energy as LLDs. A codebook of five audio words has been learned beforehand. For each LLD vector, the index of the audio word which is closest in terms of the Euclidean distance is specified.

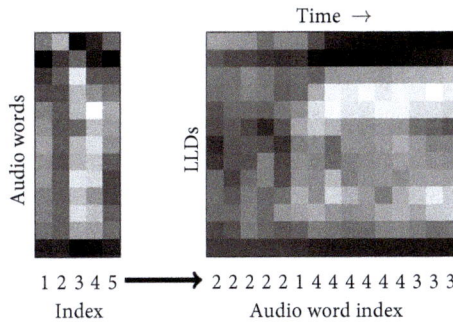

FIGURE 33.3 Example for vector quantization. The codebook consists of five audio words.

The motivation behind vector quantization is to obtain a compact representation of each frame in the audio signal. Given the fact that a whole segment can now be described by a sequence of integers (specifying the audio word indexes in the codebook), this results in a very compressed representation of the speech signal. This can be compared to the most frequent type of linguistic features (i.e. the transcription of the spoken words in a speech segment). Thus, the 'audio words' are suitable for further processing with methods inspired by *natural language processing*. The first of these methods is the bag-of-words method, which is then called *bag-of-audio-words* and will be described in Section 33.2.4. Other potential ideas would include stemming or retagging, which is similar to part-of-speech tagging (i.e. assigning broader word classes such as noun, verb, and adjective), by, for example, a hierarchical clustering of audio words. Obviously, also 'stopping' by selection of audio words is feasible. Additionally, more refined versions of audio words could be reached (e.g. with variable length) by means of, for example, dynamic warping-enabled clustering. Finally, audio words can be built from functional-based vectors rather than LLDs.

33.2.4 Bag-of-Words

In the bag-of-words (BoW) method, the words (or other linguistic cues, such as syllables or characters) within a document are represented as a *histogram* of their frequencies of occurrence. This means that, for each term in a dictionary, it is counted how often it is present in the text at hand. The histogram vector of *term frequencies*, which is of the same size as the dictionary, is then the feature vector to be fed into the classifier (Schuller, Mousa, & Vasileios, 2015).

In the audio domain, once the frame-level features have been assigned to audio words, the same procedure can be performed as for linguistic units. This bag-of-audio-words (BoAW) method has received increasing attention in various audio-recognition tasks, but mostly in *acoustic event detection* (Grzeszick et al., 2015; Lim et al., 2015; Plinge et al., 2014) and *multimedia event detection* (Liu et al., 2010; Pancoast & Akbacak, 2012; Rawat et al., 2013), although also in *music information retrieval* (Riley et al., 2008), *speech-based emotion recognition* (Pokorny et al., 2015; Schmitt, Ringeval, et al., 2016), and healthcare (Schmitt, Janott, et al., 2016). Also, in the field of image and video content analysis, the corresponding *bag-of-visual-words* is now a well-established approach (Fei-Fei & Perona, 2005; Sivic et al., 2005).

Moreover, in recognition tasks where different modalities are available, the bags from different domains can be easily fused in an *early fusion* approach, where the bags are simply concatenated to form a single, larger-feature vector (Joshi et al., 2013). This applies especially for speech-recognition tasks as both the acoustic and linguistic domains are always available.

The open-source toolkit, termed *openXBOW*, has recently been published (Schmitt & Schuller, 2016), providing bag-of-words-based 'crossmodal' representations of arbitrary numerical (acoustic and video) and symbolic (textual) features.

In the basic bag-of-words approach, the order of each word, and hence its context, is not taken into account, even though it might imply some important information. To overcome this problem, *n-grams* can be exploited (Schuller, Mousa, & Vasileios, 2015). Using n-grams, the dictionary does not only consist of single words, but also of sequences of up to *n* words. The grams that are present in the dictionary are again learned from the training data, so that only relevant sequences are considered. The approach can easily be adopted for bag-of-audio-words, by adding sequences of audio words to the framework (Pancoast & Akbacak, 2013).

The resulting bags (i.e. frequency histograms) can further be processed in order to make them more robust, with the ultimate goal to improve the recognition performance on unseen data samples. The necessity to apply the methods introduced in the following depends on both the data and the used machine-learning scheme, as different methods are able to cope, more or less, with differing histogram-based feature representations.

In order to compress the range of the (words') term frequency (TF) i, the logarithm is very often applied, as expressed in the equation

$$TF_{\log,i} = \log(TF_i + c), \tag{3}$$

where c is a constant, mostly chosen as 1 in order to avoid negative values. Another very common modification is to choose the *term frequency inverse document frequency* (TF-IDF), in which the TF is multiplied with the *inverse document frequency* (IDF) measure. The IDF for each term i is computed as

$$IDF_i = \log\left(\frac{N}{DF_i}\right), \tag{4}$$

where N is the number of instances in the training data, and DF_i (document frequency) is the number of instances therein where the term (e.g. word) i is present. Instance here refers to one sample in the available data (i.e. one speech segment in the case of voice analysis). The motivation behind IDF is to increase the weight of rare words in the histogram, which are assumed to be more meaningful than words occurring very often.

In a further step, the bag-of-word histograms can be *normalized*. This might be beneficial if the given segments vary in length, as the ranges of the TFs are then larger for segments of longer duration. Normalization can be considered by, for example, dividing each TF by the *absolute* or the *Euclidean length* of the histogram, or even by the number of frames in the segment.

Finally, it must be stated that the described extensions of bag-of-words are not always beneficial and that their usefulness depends on many parameters (Schmitt, Janott, et al.,

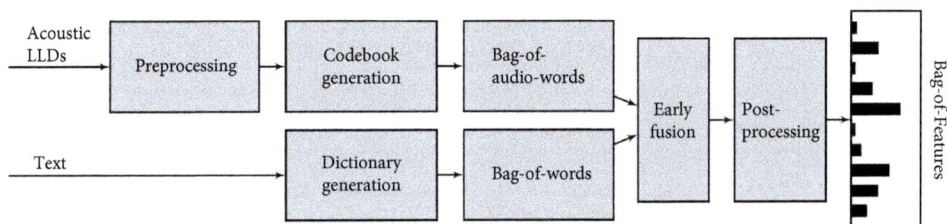

FIGURE 33.4 Bag-of-features processing chain for multimodal input.

2016). Thus, the optimum configuration is ideally evaluated each time a term frequency histogram-based representation is used. The whole process of multimodal bag-of-words' generation with early fusion of acoustic and linguistic (and potentially further) features is displayed in Figure 33.4. In general, one can also speak of *bag-of-features* implicating linguistic, acoustic, and/or visual words. As an initial step, a *preprocessing* of the LLDs (in case of linguistics, these are usually strings) might be necessary if the ranges of their values differ. If we consider, for instance, Mel-frequency cepstral coefficients and pitch, the variance of the pitch contour is usually larger, so that pitch would have a higher impact on the Euclidean distance in the word-assignment step. Thus, either a *standardization, unity-based normalization*, or further suited representation of the LLDs is mostly beneficial. The difference between both techniques is that in unity-based normalization (also known as *feature scaling*), all values are mapped onto a scale of, for example, −1 to +1 (by normalization to the minimum/maximum occurring value), whereas in standardization, after subtraction of the mean value, each LLD is divided by its standard deviation. Therefore, standardization is less prone to outliers in the LLDs; however, the resulting range of standardized values is not fixed. Both techniques can be conducted in an *online approach*, in which the required parameters (e.g. in the case of standardization, mean and standard deviation for each LLD) are computed from all LLDs in the training data and then stored in the system to be used with all sample instances that need to be classified. *Postprocessing* in Figure 33.4 refers to the aforementioned term frequency weighting and histogram normalization methods.

33.3 DECODING

Once a suitable representation of all acoustic and/or linguistic information in a speech segment has been found, the representation needs to be *decoded* in order to reach a prediction for the respective target (e.g. the emotion). The most critical aspect is typically the availability and the proper selection of the training data. As shown in the following sections, each machine-learning model needs a large number of examples in each category (in case of a classification task) or in different ranges (in case of a regression task). If the training data has not been chosen carefully, the resulting model will usually not generalize well enough. This could be the case if, for instance, training data has been recorded only in silent environments but the system is supposed to work also in noisy or more generally speaking 'mismatched' environments. Another problem can arise if the subjects have not been well selected. Speakers should be balanced in both age and gender, and ideally represent all ages and types of the general population, if expected to work for these. However, the low amount of available training data is usually the most problematic bottleneck.

Decoding can be done on different levels: (1) on *frame level*; (2) on *segment level*; and (3) even on the plain signal, usually referred to as *end-to-end learning*. This section gives a brief review of machine-learning methods that can be employed on the aforementioned levels.

33.3.1 Frame-Level Decoding

In frame-level decoding, the sequence of LLDs—or the sequence of audio words—is directly fed into a machine-learning algorithm. In this section, two types of models that can be used with sequential data are introduced—*hidden Markov models* and (recurrent) *neural networks*.

33.3.1.1 *Hidden Markov Models*

Hidden Markov models (HMMs) (Rabiner, 1989) are one of the most used learning algorithms in many speech-processing tasks. They are based on *Markov chains*, a statistical process given by a number of states and transition probabilities between all states. The main characteristic of Markov chains is that the subsequent state depends only on a finite number of previous states (in a first-order Markov chain, only the current state). In HMMs, the current state cannot be observed directly, but only estimated through its *emission* (also called *observation*) based on a second probabilistic process in addition to the probabilistic state transitions. HMMs are especially suitable for ASR, where the spoken words are modelled on different levels: on the first level, there is often an HMM for each phoneme where the emissions are the measured LLDs (e.g. Mel-frequency cepstral coefficients) (Gales & Young, 2008); on the second level, an HMM can, for example, model a linguistic word with the phonemes as their emissions.

Formally, an HMM is given by a set of states (S) and a set of possible emissions (X). The transition probabilities between all states are described by a matrix (A), and the probability, that a state emits a certain element of X is defined by another matrix (B). For each HMM, the two Markov properties apply: (1) the probability of the following state depends only on the current state, and (2) the probability of the current emission depends only on the current state.

Different models of HMMs have been introduced so far, differing in the number of states and in the positivity of their state transition probabilities. In Figure 33.5, a three-state *linear left–right model* is shown. A linear left–right model ('stay or move') is commonly used in ASR as linguistic information in speech is encoded in an ordered sequence of phonemes. By having self-transitions (loops) in the model, different durations of, for example, spoken sounds, or simply different speech rates, can be captured. Thus, an HMM is able to *warp* the signal in time. The 'start' and 'end' state in the model shown in Figure 33.5 have been introduced to simplify the further calculations.

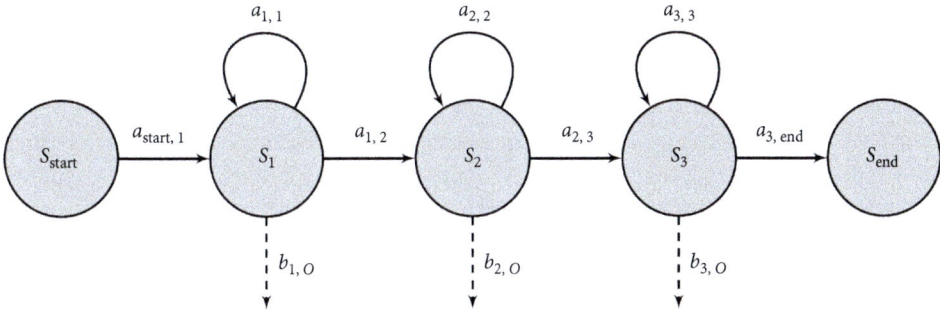

FIGURE 33.5 Linear left–right hidden Markov model with three hidden states.

In general, each HMM represents the conditional probability $p(\mathbf{x}|c)$, which denotes the probability of observing the sequence $\mathbf{x}$ under the hypothesis that it belongs to class c. Given a sequence of T observations in an audio segment, this probability can be computed as

$$p(\mathbf{x}|c) = \sum_{\text{seq}} a_{S_{\text{start}},S_1} \prod_{t=1}^{T} b_{st,xt} a_{st,st+1},\tag{5}$$

where the summation is executed over all possible sequences of states. Alternatively, exploiting the *Viterbi algorithm*, a speed-up is achieved while still obtaining good results (Jelinek, 1997). In this case, the conditional probability turns into the following equation, taking only the most probable state sequence into account:

$$\hat{p}(\mathbf{x}|c) = \left\{ a_{S_{\text{start}},S_1} \prod_{t=1}^{T} b_{st,xt} a_{st,st+1} \right\}.\tag{6}$$

So far, the assumption has been made that there is a finite number of observations (e.g. audio words) and, therefore, the probabilities in matrix B are discrete. In audio-recognition tasks, however, the emission probabilities in B are usually modelled continuously by *Gaussian mixture models* (GMMs) (Jelinek, 1997) as, for example, the LLDs are continuously valued. The emission probability density functions (PDFs) for each state s are determined by

$$b_s(x_t) = \sum_{m=1}^{M} c_{s,m} \mathcal{N}(x_t; \mu_{s,m}, \Sigma_{s,m}),\tag{7}$$

for a GMM consisting of M mixtures, mixture weights $c_{s,m}$, and the PDF of the multivariate Gaussian distribution $\mathcal{N}(\cdot; \mu, \Sigma)$ with mean vector μ and covariance matrix Σ.

In order to train the model, its parameters (i.e. the elements of matrices A and B) need to be learned based on a given training data set of audio sequences and corresponding labels. In the case of ASR, the labels are the transcriptions of the speech segments (one HMM is then usually trained per phoneme or word); in the case of emotion recognition, the emotion labels (one HMM is then usually trained per emotion class). For parameter estimation in HMMs, the *Baum-Welch* algorithm is usually employed, which is an instance of the previously mentioned expectation maximization algorithm. For further details, we refer to the corresponding literature (Baum et al., 1970; Schuller, 2013).

In the recognition phase, all HMMs are evaluated applying, for example, the Viterbi algorithm. Consequently, the HMM with the highest posterior probability is supposed to be the correct model for the respective target (e.g. a word, an emotion, further speaker state or trait). Classification can be realized by the *maximum a posteriori* (MAP) estimate,

$$\hat{c} = \arg\max_{c} \; p(c|\mathbf{x}), \quad c = 1, \ldots, C, \tag{8}$$

where $\hat{c}$ is the most likely out of C classes, and $\mathbf{x}$ is the sequence of observations. Exploiting Bayes' theorem,

$$p(c|\mathbf{x}) = \frac{p(\mathbf{x}|c) \cdot p(c)}{p(\mathbf{x})} \tag{9}$$

and as the prior probability $p(\mathbf{x})$ is the same for all classes, Equation 8 can be transformed into

$$\hat{c} = \arg\max_{c} p(\mathbf{x}|c) \cdot p(c), \quad c = 1, \ldots, C \tag{10}$$

If all classes are presumed to have the same probability, the MAP is identical to the *maximum likelihood* (ML) estimate.

In the case of ASR, the term in Equation 10 splits up into an HMM, denoted by $p(x|c)$ and defining the *acoustic model* (AM), and a prior probability $p(c)$, defining the *language model* (LM). In fact, the acoustic model usually consists of several HMMs. Also, the language model can be refined by using the aforementioned n-grams with linguistic words. Then, a whole sequence of words W is modelled as

$$p(W) = \prod_{i=1}^{n} p(w_i \mid w_{i-(n-1)}, \ldots, w_{i-1}). \tag{11}$$

This is especially advantageous for homophones (e.g. 'piece' and 'peace') or words with similar pronunciations (e.g. 'affect' and 'effect'). As an example, the language model would favour 'I read a book' over 'I red a book'.

Though HMMs are most popular in ASR, they can be used for arbitrary classification problems (e.g. emotion recognition in speech) (Schuller et al., 2003). As mentioned, each emotional state is then represented by an HMM, where the one with maximum likelihood is chosen based on the given speech signal. The language model can then model the probability of emotion transitions, such as whether it is more likely to change from angry to neutral to happy, or to change from angry to happy to angry, etc. Several open-source toolkits have been published providing training and decoding of HMMs, such as *Sphinx* (Walker et al., 2004), *HTK* (Young et al., 2006), and *Kaldi* (Povey et al., 2011).

33.3.1.2 *Artificial Neural Networks*

In recent years, however, research on computational paralinguistics (and ASR) has mostly abandoned HMMs due to their susceptibility to background noise and other factors such as the fact that discriminative learning is harder to realize. The prevailing research is now re-focusing on another fundamental approach in machine learning—*artificial neural networks* (ANNs). The basic idea is to create a model which is inspired by the information processing in the human brain, or more generally, in the human nervous system.

First research in this domain was published in the 1940s by McCulloch and Pitts, who were proposing a model of *neurons* as simple cells providing the processing of binary signals (McCulloch & Pitts, 1943). A common neuron model is displayed in Figure 33.6. The elements of an M-dimensional input vector x are weighted individually and summed up, and a bias w_0 is added. Then, a *non-linear activation function* is applied to the result, which can be realized by, for example, a *step function* or a *sigmoid function* $f(u) = \dfrac{1}{1 + \exp(-\alpha u)}$ with the steepness parameter α. The optimum activation function depends on the task at hand. The whole (multilayer) ANN is then a network consisting of several neurons, where the output of each neuron ($\hat{y}$) is an input to another neuron:

$$\hat{y} = f\left(\sum_{m=0}^{M} w_m x_m \right); \quad x_0 = 1. \tag{12}$$

As displayed in Figure 33.7, the cells are arranged in different layers, where all outputs of one layer are propagated to all inputs to the next layer in the case of a *feed forward* neural network. In a *recurrent* neural network (RNN), the outputs are also propagated to the same or even previous layers. The step of one propagation is then synchronized with a clock where, in each clock cycle, a new input feature vector is given to the input layer of the recurrent neural network. Altogether, the ANN involves a sequence of non-linear transformations of the input data, providing the final predictions in the output layer. The input layer usually simply

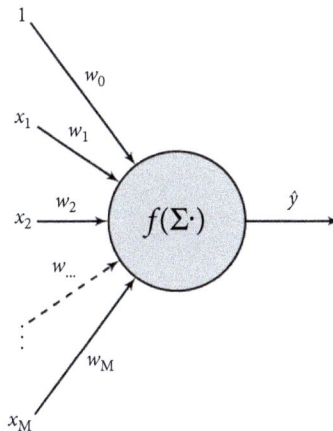

FIGURE 33.6 Neuron—the basic component of artificial neural networks.

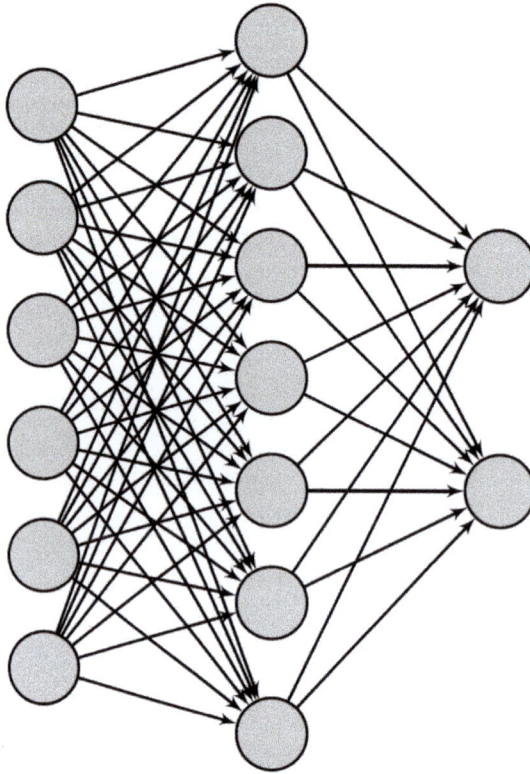

FIGURE 33.7 A feedforward neural network with one hidden layer. Each circle represents a neuron.

propagates the input values to the second layer and involves no weighting, summation, or non-linearity. The layers, which are neither input nor output, are called *hidden layers*. The output layer usually has a dimensionality according to the number of possible targets. Thus, if it handles a binary decision task (two classes), there are two neurons in the output layer, each one providing a likelihood for the corresponding class. Suited functions such as the *softmax* function can be used to normalize the output to the range of 0 to 1, and thus reflect posterior probabilities per class. In the case of a (single-task) regression problem, there is usually one neuron per predicted variable.

The process of learning the weights of all neurons is time-consuming and computationally intensive. The common practice is the *back propagation* method with *stochastic gradient descent* (Rumelhart et al., 1986).

Whilst research on ANN was on the fringes from the 1970s onwards, it has experienced a powerful revival since the first decade of the twenty-first century. This has been driven mainly by two factors: (1) the increasing performance of computers, especially parallel architectures such as graphics processing units (GPUs), that are a fundamental requirement to the time-consuming training of ANNs; and (2) the proposal of new architectures, particularly *long short-term memory recurrent neural networks* (LSTM-RNNs) (Hochreiter & Schmidhuber, 1997). In this context, new methods of (pre-)training 'deep' networks (i.e. up to hundreds of hidden layers) such as layer-wise unsupervised learning and 'drop-out' learning (randomly omitting neurons during iterations), or suited activation functions such as 'rectified linear units', are to be mentioned.

Nowadays, ANNs are mostly *deep neural networks*, which have at least two hidden layers. *Deep learning* has evolved as a new research field of machine learning in computer science and is applied to a large variety of tasks, such as handwriting recognition, ASR, medical image analysis, and music synthesis, to mention only a few. Popular modern architectures of deep learning (LeCun et al., 2015) comprise *restricted Boltzmann machines* (RBMs) (Hinton & Salakhutdinov, 2006), *convolutional neural networks* (CNN) (Simard et al., 2003), and the aforementioned LSTM-RNN. CNNs are mostly used in the context of spatially distributed data (e.g. images). In this approach, local regions in the signal are iteratively processed in a convolutional layer of neurons with globally equal weights. By a successive *pooling* layer, the outputs of the convolutional layers are downsampled. The final layers of a CNN are then fully connected, so that the compressed information from all regions can be combined.

In contrast, recurrent neural networks are preferably used with sequential data, such as speech signals, as they can model both the long-term and short-term evolution of the signal, based on the sequence of LLDs. The core of LSTM-RNNs are the *long short-term memory cells*. They are able to store activations from an earlier time instant in the signal for an arbitrary time. For this reason, they overcome the *vanishing gradient problem*, which was one of the major drawbacks of recurrent neural networks in audio recognition. The fundamental principle of an LSTM cell is displayed in Figure 33.8. A common neuron (shown at the top of the cell) is complemented by a memory and three *gate neurons*, controlling the flow of the activation by scaling it with their outputs at different stages of the cell. The *input gate* scales the input to the memory. The incoming activation is then stored in the so-called *error carousel*, where it can remain for an arbitrary number of time steps. This is accomplished by a loop which is controlled by the *forget gate,* scaling the recurring activation of the cell memory. The actual output of the LSTM cell is controlled by the third gate, the *output gate*. Besides the activations from outside the cell, the stored activation itself is also passed to all

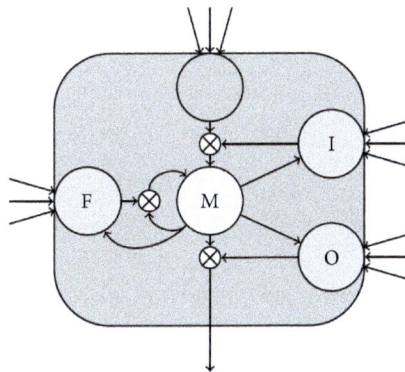

FIGURE 33.8 Long short-term memory cell. I: input gate, F: forget gate, O: output gate, M: memory.

gates as an input. The behaviour of the gate neurons has to be learned in addition to the original neuron. However, the same set of three gates can control several neurons to reduce the number of free parameters to be learned from data.

LSTM-RNNs have successfully been used for a great variety of audio-recognition tasks, such as voice-activity detection (Eyben, Weninger, Squartini, & Schuller, 2013), social-signal detection (Brückner & Schuller, 2014), acoustic-novelty detection (Marchi et al., 2015), emotion recognition (Wöllmer, Kaiser, et al., 2013), and feature enhancement (Zhang et al., 2016) in paralinguistics. It seems noteworthy that dynamic-sequence learning is possible with recurrent neural networks, similar to the warping abilities in HMMs.

In LSTM-RNNs, all weights in each cell of the network must be learned, based on the given training data. Several open-source tools that are able to train LSTM-RNNs and other neural architectures have been published, including *CURRENNT* (Weninger et al., 2015) and *TensorFlow* (Abadi et al., 2016). This simplifies the application tremendously as efficient implementation is a challenge.

33.3.2 Segment-Level Decoding

In segment-level decoding, the feature vector representing the segment (e.g. the vector of functionals and/or the bag-of-words derived per spoken unit, such as words or phrases) is fed into the machine-learning model to predict either a discrete class or a continuous label. Formally spoken, in the case of classification, the class $\hat{c}$ with the highest posterior probability given the feature vector x is chosen according to a MAP estimation (see Equation 8).

Many different learning methods have emerged (e.g. *Bayes classifier, k-nearest neighbour, decision trees, random forests*) and each one has its pros and cons. However, probably the most commonly used method in the field of speaker-state and trait analysis, including emotion recognition from speech, is the *support vector machine* (SVM) for classification tasks and its counterpart *support vector regression* (SVR) for regression tasks (Cortes & Vapnik, 1995). In the following, only SVM will be further discussed, but most of the theory can easily be adapted to derive SVR (Schuller, 2013).

The principle of SVMs is to find an optimum separating hyperplane between two classes in the feature space. The feature space is constructed from the feature vectors x in the training data. The goal of an SVM is now to find the hyperplane in the feature space which separates the classes with the widest 'channel' between the instances of both classes. Likewise as in ANNs, training is discriminative, as in general, an ideal separation is not feasible due to outliers in the training data; *slack variables* have been introduced, through which a certain number of outliers are allowed. The amount of error can be controlled by the so-called *complexity* parameter of an SVM. The basic principle is exemplified in Figure 33.9. The margins on both sides of the hyperplane are represented as dashed lines and the area in between should ideally be free of instances. The instances on the margins on both sides are named *support vectors* and define the equation of the hyperplane in the feature space. With the binary labels $y_l \in \{-1, +1\}$, the feature vectors x_l where $a_l > 0$ for the support vectors, a scalar bias b, and the size of the training set L, the prediction for a sample instance x_i is based on the following decision function:

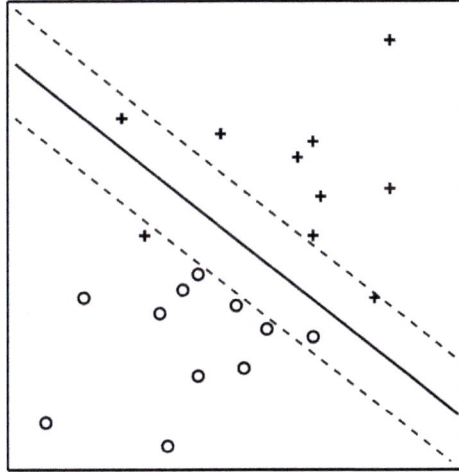

FIGURE 33.9 Support vector machine classifier in a binary classification task based on a two-dimensional feature space. Outliers are present in the training data.

$$\hat{y}(x_t) = \text{sign}\left(\sum_{l=1}^{L} y_l a_l x_l \cdot x_t + b\right),$$ (13)

where

$$\text{sign(u)} = \begin{cases} +1 & \text{if } u > 0, \\ 0 & \text{if } u = 0, \\ -1 & \text{if } u < 0. \end{cases}$$ (14)

As shown in the example, it is usually better to tolerate some training samples within the margin in order to get a wider channel. The result is consequently called a *soft margin*. If no outliers were allowed between the margins on both sides, the result would be a *hard margin* and a narrower channel. Such a model normally does not generalize well and is subject to overfitting. That is why the complexity parameter must always be tuned in order to be sure to obtain a good model. This process is referred to as *hyperparameter optimization*, in which several SVMs are trained with different complexities, typically in a certain range of values ≤ 1. Each SVM is then evaluated on independent validation data and the SVM with the best performance (the lowest error) is finally selected as the optimum model.

So far, we were making the assumption that, disregarding the outliers, the feature space was somehow linearly separable into two parts. This might not always be the case though, especially if the space is low-dimensional. In order to tackle this problem, the feature vectors can be transformed into a space of higher dimension, using a non-linear transformation. In an SVM, (suited) transformations do not need to be computed explicitly as in the final decision function; only the dot product between the training instances and a sample instance is present (see Equation 13). Such suited functions describing the dot product between the transformed feature vectors are named *kernels* and the way of using them is called *kernel trick*. A multitude of kernel functions have so far been introduced, and the most established ones are the *linear*, the *polynomial*, and the *Gaussian* (RBF) kernel. Selection of the most suitable one is normally subject to trial and error (Hsu et al., 2003). Empirically, we can say that the linear kernel normally works well with large-feature vectors (e.g. with the aforementioned ComParE feature set). However, combinations of multiple kernels can also be used.

Finally, one might need to build a classifier for more than two classes. As SVMs can, in their usually preferred 'basic' version, only do binary decisions, multiple SVMs are trained and their outputs are combined. The two most popular schemes applied are referred to as *one-vs-one* and *one-vs-all* (Hsu & Lin, 2002), where each class is trained against each other or all remaining ones.

So far, many implementations of SVM have been published and are available to the research community. One popular example is the open-source library LIBSVM (Chang & Lin, 2011) which supports several kernels, optimization methods, multi-class classification, and regression.

Deep neural networks (e.g. LSTM-RNN) can also be employed for classification or regression on the segment level. In the special case of recurrent neural networks, the information from adjacent segments is usually also taken into account for the predictions at the present moment in time, similar to a language model.

33.3.3 End-to-End Learning

Besides exploiting the extracted acoustic features from the speech signal, a machine-learning model can also be learned directly on the raw audio signal, in a procedure called *end-to-end learning*. It has successfully been applied to speech-based emotion recognition (Trigeorgis et al., 2016) and is also of great interest in ASR (Graves & Jaitly, 2014), even though most approaches that have been proposed, so far, still use a handcrafted time-frequency transform in the first step. It has, however, already been shown that it is feasible to automatically learn meaningful representations from the speech signal by methods of deep learning (Jaitly & Hinton, 2011). This process is usually referred to as *feature learning*.

An architecture for end-to-end learning for emotion recognition, similar to that proposed by Trigeorgis et al. (2016), is shown in Figure 33.10. It learns a suitable representation of the

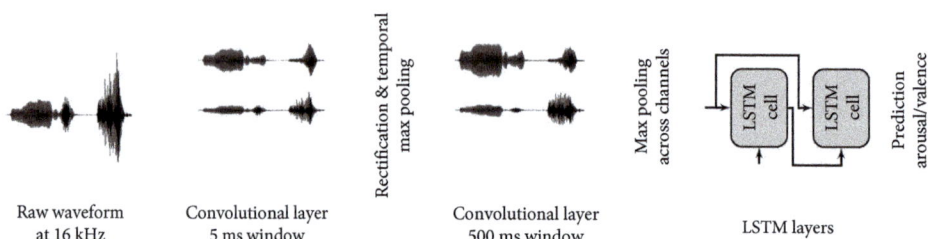

FIGURE 33.10 End-to-end learning architecture for speech-based emotion and further states and traits recognition.

signal incorporating all information relevant to the emotion. Hence, the first layers in the network replace the conventional handcrafted acoustic features in a certain way. The first step is a temporal convolutional layer consisting of forty parallel filters with a window size of 5 ms, extracting fine-scale spectral information. Then, a half-wave rectifier is applied, which means that all parts of the band signals that are below zero are set to zero. This step is motivated by the rectifying property of the cochlear transduction in the human ear. The rectified band signals are then pooled by a factor of two, resulting in a downsampled representation. Subsequently, there is another convolutional layer of forty parallel filters, this time with a window size of 500 ms, in order to capture characteristics of the speech signal on a longer scale. The output signals are then again maximum pooled, this time across the channels, which results in a huge dimensionality reduction. Finally, the remaining compressed representation is fed into a conventional LSTM-RNN, which provides the emotion predictions in terms of the two dimensions, arousal and valence. The number of LSTM cells found to be sufficient for this task was 128.

Interestingly, the outputs of some cells within a neural network trained for emotion recognition were observed as closely correlated with 'typical' prosodic features such as loudness and fundamental frequency (Trigeorgis et al., 2016). This accounts for the finding that affective states are encoded in prosody (Gunes et al., 2011). It has also been found that the filters learned by deep neural networks have a bandpass behaviour which is very similar to the filtering process in the human inner ear (Tüske et al., 2014).

33.4 CONCLUSION

Finally, it must be stated that there is an almost infinite number of methods with regard to both features describing the content of a speech signal and models to decode the audio information. The best-suited approach always depends on many parameters, such as the final application, the recording environment, and the amount of available training data, to mention only a few. This chapter is, by far, not exhaustive and accounts only for a reasonable selection of ways to proceed in machine recognition of human voice. More information about specific topics is found in the corresponding references.

In the future, one can assume a trend towards cross-lingually, cross-culturally, and environmentally robust speaker-state and trait analysers. These will likely target a whole range of speaker attributes simultaneously rather than assessing, for example, emotion in isolation, to exploit interdependencies of the states and traits such as between emotion and personality. Their high interdependence is obvious, as all different states and traits impact on the same one vocal-production mechanism and the cognitive process choosing the words to be said. Likely, these engines will be trained on huge amounts of data which will be increasingly labelled in weakly supervised ways such as by active, semi-supervised, and reinforcement learning. Likely, deep learning or similar approaches of 'holistic' end-to-end learning will play an increasing role, ultimately leading to the advent of such technology in a broad range of everyday applications, such as, for example, emotionally sensitive virtual agents, health monitoring, and personalized recommendation engines.

REFERENCES

Abadi, M., Agarwal, A., Barham, P., Brevdo, E., Chen, Z., Citro, C., … Zheng, X. (2016). TensorFlow: large-scale machine learning on heterogeneous distributed systems. *arXiv preprint*, arXiv:1603.04467

Baum, L. E., Petrie, T., Soules, G., & Weiss, N. (1970). A maximization technique occurring in the statistical analysis of probabilistic functions of Markov chains. *The Annals of Mathematical Statistics*, 41(1), 164–171.

Brückner, R. & Schuller, B. (2014). *Social Signal Classification Using Deep BLSTM Recurrent Neural Networks*. Proceedings of ICASSP, IEEE, Florence, Italy, pp. 4856–4860.

Burkhardt, F., Paeschke, A., Rolfes, M., Sendlmeier, W., & Weiss, B. (2005). *A Database of German Emotional Speech*. Proceedings of INTERSPEECH, ISCA, Lisbon, Portugal, pp. 1517–1520.

Chang, C.-C. & Lin, C.-J. (2011). LIBSVM: a library for support vector machines. *ACM Transactions on Intelligent Systems and Technology*, 2(3), 27.

Cortes, C. & Vapnik, V. (1995). Support-vector networks. *Machine Learning*, 20(3), 273–297.

Ekman, P. (1999). Basic emotions. In: T. Dalgleish & M. J. Power (eds) *Handbook of Cognition and Emotion* (pp. 301–320). New York: John Wiley & Sons.

Eyben, F., Scherer, K., Schuller, B., Sundberg, J., André., E., Busso, C., … Truong, K. (2016). The Geneva minimalistic acoustic parameter set (GeMAPS) for voice Research and Affective Computing. *IEEE Transactions on Affective Computing*, 7(2), 190–202.

Eyben, F., Weninger, F., Groß, F., & Schuller, B. (2013). *Recent Developments in openSMILE, the Munich Open-Source Multimedia Feature Extractor*. Proceedings of MM 2013, ACM, Barcelona, Spain, pp. 835–838.

Eyben, F., Weninger, F., & Schuller, B. (2013). *Affect Recognition in Real-life Acoustic Conditions—A New Perspective on Feature Selection*. Proceedings of INTERSPEECH, ISCA, Lyon, France, pp. 2044–2048.

Eyben, F., Weninger, F., Squartini, S., & Schuller, B. (2013). *Real-life Voice Activity Detection with LSTM Recurrent Neural Networks and an Application to Hollywood Movies*. Proceedings of ICASSP, IEEE, Vancouver, Canada, pp. 483–487.

Fei-Fei, L. & Perona, P. (2005). *A Bayesian Hierarchical Model for Learning Natural Scene Categories*. Proceedings of CVPR, Vol. 2, IEEE, San Diego, CA, USA, pp. 524–531.

Gales, M. & Young, S. (2008). The application of hidden Markov models in speech recognition. *Foundations and Trends in Signal Processing*, 1(3), 195–304.

Graves, A. & Jaitly, N. (2014). *Towards End-to-End Speech Recognition with Recurrent Neural Networks*. Proceedings of ICML, Vol. 14, Beijing, China, pp. 1764–1772.

Grzeszick, R., Plinge, A., & Fink, G. A. (2015). *Temporal Acoustic Words for Online Acoustic Event Detection*. Proceedings of GCPR, Aachen, Germany, pp. 142–153.

Gunes, H., Nicolaou, M. A., & Pantic, M. (2011). Continuous analysis of affect from voice and face. In: A. A. Salah & T. Gevers (eds) *Computer Analysis of Human Behavior* (pp. 255–291). Springer.

Hinton, G. E. & Salakhutdinov, R. R. (2006). Reducing the dimensionality of data with neural networks. *Science*, 313(5786), 504–507.

Hochreiter, S. & Schmidhuber, J. (1997). Long short-term memory. *Neural Computation*, 9(8), 1735–1780.

Hsu, C.-W., Chang, C.-C., & Lin, C.-J. (2003). *A Practical Guide to Support Vector Classification*. Technical report, Department of Computer Science, National Taiwan University, Taipei, Taiwan.

Hsu, C.-W. & Lin, C.-J. (2002). A comparison of methods for multiclass support vector machines. *IEEE Transactions on Neural Networks*, 13(2), 415–425.

Jaitly, N. & Hinton, G. (2011). *Learning a Better Representation of Speech Soundwaves Using Restricted Boltzmann Machines*. Proceedings of ICASSP, IEEE, Prague, Czech Republic, pp. 5884–5887.

Jelinek, F. (1997). *Statistical Methods for Speech Recognition*. MIT Press.

Joshi, J., Goecke, R., Alghowinem, S., Dhall, A., Wagner, M., Epps, J., Parker, G., & Breakspear, M. (2013). Multimodal assistive technologies for depression diagnosis and monitoring. *Journal on MultiModal User Interfaces*, 7(3), 217–228.

LeCun, Y., Bengio, Y., & Hinton, G. (2015). Deep learning. *Nature*, 521(7553), 436–444.

Lim, H., Kim, M. J., & Kim, H. (2015). *Robust Sound Event Classification Using LBP-HOG Based Bag-of-Audio-Words Feature Representation*. Proceedings of INTERSPEECH, ISCA, Dresden, Germany, pp. 3325–3329.

Liu, Y., Zhao, W.-L., Ngo, C.-W., Xu, C.-S., & Lu, H.-Q. (2010). *Coherent Bag-of Audio Words Model for Efficient Large-Scale Video Copy Detection*. Proceedings of CIVR, ACM, Xi'an, China, pp. 89–96.

Marchi, E., Vesperini, F., Weninger, F., Eyben, F., Squartini, S., & Schuller, B. (2015). *Non-Linear Prediction with LSTM Recurrent Neural Networks for Acoustic Novelty Detection*. Proceedings of IJCNN, IEEE, Killarney, Ireland.

McCulloch, W. S. & Pitts, W. (1943). A logical calculus of the ideas immanent in nervous activity. *The Bulletin of Mathematical Biophysics*, 5(4), 115–133.

O'Shaughnessy, D. (1987). *Speech Communication: Human and Machine*. Addison-Wesley Publishing Co.

Pancoast, S. & Akbacak, M. (2012). *Bag-of-Audio-Words Approach for Multimedia Event Classification*. Proceedings of INTERSPEECH, ISCA, Portland, USA, pp. 2105–2108.

Pancoast, S. & Akbacak, M. (2013). *N-Gram Extension for Bag-of-Audio-Words*. Proceedings of ICASSP, IEEE, Vancouver, Canada, pp. 778–782.

Plinge, A., Grzeszick, R., & Fink, G. A. (2014). *A Bag-of- Features Approach to Acoustic Event Detection*. Proceedings of ICASSP, IEEE, Florence, Italy, pp. 3732–3736.

Pokorny, F., Graf, F., Pernkopf, F., & Schuller, B. (2015). *Detection of Negative Emotions in Speech Signals Using Bags-of-Audio-Words*. Proceedings of ACII, AAAC, IEEE, Xi'an, China, pp. 879–884.

Povey, D., Ghoshal, A., Boulianne, G., Burget, L., Glembek, O., Goel, N., ... Vesely, K. (2011). *The Kaldi Speech Recognition Toolkit*. Proceedings of IEEE Workshop on Automatic Speech Recognition and Understanding, Big Island, HI, USA.

Rabiner, L. R. (1989). A tutorial on hidden Markov models and selected applications in speech recognition. *Proceedings of IEEE*, 77(2), 257–286.

Rawat, S., Schulam, P. F., Burger, S., Ding, D., Wang, Y., & Metze, F. (2013). *Robust Audio-Codebooks for Large-Scale Event Detection in Consumer Videos*. Proceedings of INTERSPEECH, ISCA, Lyon, France, pp. 2929–2933.

Riley, M., Heinen, E., & Ghosh, J. (2008). *A Text Retrieval Approach to Content-Based Audio Hashing*. Proceedings of ISMIR, Philadelphia, PA, USA, pp. 295–300.

Ringeval, F., Amiriparian, S., Eyben, F., Scherer, K., & Schuller, B. (2014). *Emotion Recognition in the Wild: Incorporating Voice and Lip Activity in Multimodal Decision Level Fusion*. Proceedings of ICMI, ACM, Istanbul, Turkey, pp. 473–480.

Ringeval, F., Marchi, E., Méhu, M., Scherer, K., & Schuller, B. (2015). *Face Reading from Speech—Predicting Facial Action Units from Audio Cues*. Proceedings of INTERSPEECH, ISCA, Dresden, Germany, pp. 1977–1981.

Rumelhart, D. E., Hinton, G. E., & Williams, R. J. (1986). Learning representations by back-propagating errors. *Nature*, 323, 533–536.

Schmitt, M., Janott, C., Pandit, V., Qian, K., Heiser, C., Hemmert, W., & Schuller, B. (2016). *A Bag-of-Audio-Words Approach for Snore Sounds' Excitation Localisation.* Proceedings of ITG Speech Communication, ITG/VDE, IEEE, Paderborn, Germany, pp. 230–234.

Schmitt, M., Ringeval, F., & Schuller, B. (2016). *At the Border of Acoustics and Linguistics: Bag-of-Audio-Words for the Recognition of Emotions in Speech.* Proceedings of INTERSPEECH, ISCA, San Francsico, CA, USA, pp. 495–499.

Schmitt, M. & Schuller, B. (2016). OpenXBOW—introducing the Passau open-source crossmodal bag-of-words toolkit. *arXiv preprint*, arXiv:1605.06778

Schuller, B. (2012). The computational paralinguistics challenge. *IEEE Signal Processing Magazine*, 29(4), 97–101.

Schuller, B. (2013). *Intelligent Audio Analysis, Signals and Communication Technology.* Springer.

Schuller, B., Batliner, A., Steidl, S., & Seppi, D. (2009). *Emotion Recognition from Speech: Putting ASR in the Loop.* Proceedings of ICASSP, IEEE, Taipei, Taiwan, pp. 4585–4588.

Schuller, B., Mousa, A. E.-D., & Vasileios, V. (2015). Sentiment analysis and opinion mining: on optimal parameters and performances. *WIREs Data Mining and Knowledge Discovery*, 5, 255–263.

Schuller, B., Rigoll, G., & Lang, M. (2003). *Hidden Markov Model-Based Speech Emotion Recognition.* Proceedings of ICASSP, Vol. II, IEEE, Hong Kong, China, pp. 1–4.

Schuller, B., Steidl, S., Batliner, A., Epps, J., Eyben, F., Ringeval, F., Marchi, E., & Zhang, Y. (2014). *The INTERSPEECH 2014 Computational Paralinguistics Challenge: Cognitive and Physical Load.* Proceedings of INTERSPEECH, ISCA, Singapore, pp. 427–431.

Schuller, B., Steidl, S., Batliner, A., Hantke, S., Hönig, F., Orozco-Arroyave, J. R., … Weninger, F. (2015). *The INTERSPEECH 2015 Computational Paralinguistics Challenge: Degree of Nativeness, Parkinson's and Eating Condition.* Proceedings of INTERSPEECH, ISCA, Dresden, Germany, pp. 478–482.

Schuller, B., Steidl, S., Batliner, A., Nöth, E., Vinciarelli, A., Burkhardt, F., … Weiss, B. (2012). *The INTERSPEECH 2012 Speaker Trait Challenge.* Proceedings of INTERSPEECH, ISCA, Portland, OR, USA, pp. 254–257.

Schuller, B., Steidl, S., Batliner, A., Vinciarelli, A., Scherer, K., Ringeval, F., … Kim, S. (2013). *The INTERSPEECH 2013 Computational Paralinguistics Challenge: Social Signals, Conflict, Emotion, Autism.* Proceedings of INTERSPEECH, ISCA, Lyon, France, pp. 148–152.

Simard, P. Y., Steinkraus, D., & Platt, J. C. (2003). *Best Practices for Convolutional Neural Networks Applied to Visual Document Analysis.* Proceedings of ICDAR, IEEE, Edinburgh, UK, pp. 958–962.

Sivic, J., Russell, B. C., Efros, A. A., Zisserman, A., & Freeman, W. T. (2005). *Discovering Object Categories in Image Collections.* Technical report, MIT CSAIL.

Trigeorgis, G., Ringeval, F., Brueckner, R., Marchi, E., Nicolaou, M. A., Schuller, B., & Zafeiriou, S. (2016). *Adieu Features? End-to-End Speech Emotion Recognition using a Deep Convolutional Recurrent Network.* Proceedings of ICASSP, IEEE, Shanghai, China, pp. 5200–5204.

Tüske, Z., Golik, P., Schlüter, R., & Ney, H. (2014). *Acoustic Modeling with Deep Neural Networks using Raw Time Signal for LVCSR.* Proceedings of INTERSPEECH, ISCA, Singapore, Singapore, pp. 890–894.

Walker, W., Lamere, P., Kwok, P., Raj, B., Singh, R., Gouvea, E., Wolf, P., & Woelfel, J. (2004). *Sphinx-4: A Flexible Open Source Framework for Speech Recognition.* Technical report, Sun Microsystems, Inc.

Weninger, F., Bergmann, J., & Schuller, B. (2015). Introducing CURRENNT: the Munich open-source CUDA RecurRent neural network toolkit. *Journal of Machine Learning Research*, 16, 547–551.

Wiggins, J. S. (ed.) (1996). *The Five-Factor Model of Personality: Theoretical Perspectives*. New York: Guilford.

Wöllmer, M., Kaiser, M., Eyben, F., Schuller, B., & Rigoll, G. (2013). LSTM-modeling of continuous emotions in an audiovisual affect recognition framework. *Image and Vision Computing*, 31(2), 153–163.

Wöllmer, M., Weninger, F., Geiger, J., Schuller, B., & Rigoll, G. (2013). Noise robust ASR in reverberated multisource environments applying convolutive NMF and long short-term memory. *Computer Speech and Language*, 27(3), 780–797.

Young, S., Evermann, G., Gales, M., Hain, T., Kershaw, D., Liu, X., ... Woodland, P. (2006). *The HTK Book (v3.4)*. Cambridge University.

Zhang, Z., Ringeval, F., Han, J., Deng, J., Marchi, E., & Schuller, B. (2016). *Facing Realism in Spontaneous Emotion Recognition from Speech: Feature Enhancement by Autoencoder with LSTM Neural Networks*. Proceedings of INTERSPEECH, ISCA, San Francsico, CA, USA, pp. 3593–3597.

Zwicker, E. & Fastl, H. (2013). *Psychoacoustics: Facts and Models, Vol. 22*. Springer Science & Business Media.

....

CHAPTER 34

NEUROCOMPUTATIONAL MODELS OF VOICE AND SPEECH PERCEPTION

....

BERND J. KRÖGER

34.1 MAPS AND STREAMS IN THE BRAIN: A COMPREHENSIVE FUNCTIONAL MODEL

....

EVEN a simple model of voice and speech perception comprises fourteen neural network modules, two neural hubs, and twenty bidirectional neural pathways or streams (see Figure 34.1) in order to be capable of reproducing basic behavioural features of voice and speech perception.

Auditory perception starts with *auditory input processing* (e.g. first spectral analysis at the cochlear level) and forwarding the neural signal, via the thalamus, towards the primary auditory cortex (Kandel et al., 2000). Here, speech and voice perception start with spectrotemporal analysis within the temporal lobe (Belin et al., 2000; Hickok & Poeppel, 2007; Zatorre et al., 2002), carried out in the *auditory feature network*. Subsequently, language-specific phonological feature and syllable neural representations become activated during speech perception within the *phonological network* (Hickok & Poeppel, 2007; Obleser et al., 2010). This network already uses top-down knowledge from the mental lexicon (*lexical network*; Hickok & Poeppel, 2007) and subsequently leads to an activation of lexical items within the lexical network together with concept activation via a *semantic hub* (Patterson et al., 2007). All these modules are located within the temporal lobe, while semantic information is represented in a widely-distributed cortical *conceptual network* (Hickok & Poeppel, 2007, p. 398). The lexical network is associated with a *combinatorial network*, also located within the temporal lobe. This network processes syntactic information of utterances (Hickok & Poeppel, 2007, p. 398) and thus— together with concept activations of a current utterance—performs speech comprehension and ends at the comprehension level (see top level of Figure 34.1). This stream from the auditory feature network, via the phonological and lexical networks towards the combinatorial network, is mainly located in

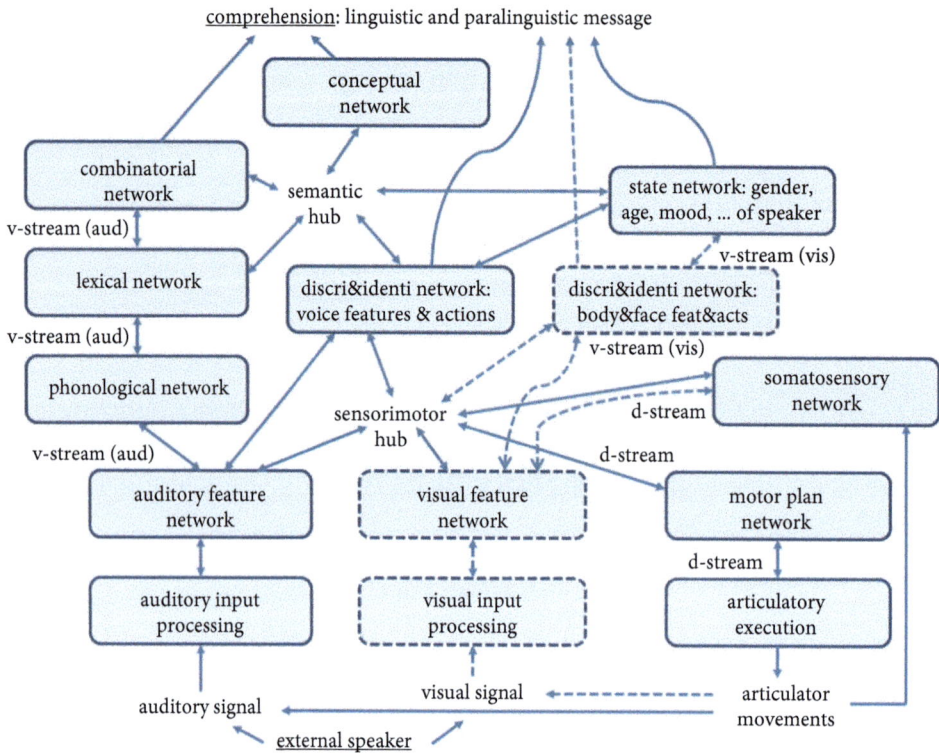

FIGURE 34.1 Network modules (boxes), hubs, and streams (arrows) in a functional model of voice and speech perception; v-stream = ventral stream, d-stream = dorsal stream for auditory (aud) and visual (vis) processing, respectively. Networks and streams for visual processing are labelled as dashed lines. Locations of network modules and hubs within the brain are listed in Table 34.1.

the temporal lobe and called the *ventral stream of speech perception* (Hickok & Poeppel, 2007, p. 394ff). (The neurophysiological locations of all network modules and hubs within our model are listed in detail in Table 34.1.)

For speech perception, a second neural stream exists and is called the *dorsal stream of speech perception* (Hickok & Poeppel, 2007, p. 399ff). This stream plays an important role in speech acquisition, because motor and sensory representations of syllables and words are acquired simultaneously (speech imitation; see e.g. Kröger et al., 2014). This stream is activated as well in perception of distorted speech (i.e. speech perceived in noisy environments; perception of unclear, slurred, or disordered speech). While the ventral stream of speech perception takes place within one cortical lobe (i.e. the temporal lobe), the dorsal stream involves motor-speech areas within the frontal lobe as well, and thus needs a neural association between the temporal and frontal lobe. This stream starts (or ends) at the sensorimotor interface (Hickock & Poeppel, 2007, p. 395ff), also called the *sensorimotor hub*. This hub links sensory and motor streams (Figure 34.1) and is located at the edge of the temporal, parietal, and occipital lobe. Within the frontal lobe, speech perception can activate the *motor plan network* (Figure 34.1), while *articulatory execution* via the primary motor areas is

Table 34.1 Neurophysiological location of network modules and hubs within the brain

Network module or hub	Location	Reference
Articulatory execution	Posterior frontal lobe (primary motor cortex); basal ganglia; thalamus; inferior cerebellum; bilateral	Hickok & Poeppel (2007), Riecker et al. (2005)
Auditory feature network	Supratemporal gyrus, STG (primary auditory cortex and unimodal association cortex); anterior-lateral superior cortex; bilateral	Obleser et al. (2010), Zatorre et al. (2002)
Auditory input processing	Cochlea; thalamus; primary auditory cortex; bilateral	e.g. Kandel et al. (2000)
Combinatorial network	Anterior middle temporal gyrus, aMTG; anterior inferior temporal sulcus, aITS; left dominant	Hickok & Poeppel (2007)
Conceptual network	Widely distributed: frontal, parietal, temporal, occipital lobe	Hickok & Poeppel (2007), Patterson et al. (2007)
Discrimination & selection network (body & face, features & actions)	Superior temporal gyrus; fusiform face area	Adolphs (2002a)
Discrimination & selection network (voice features & actions)	Upper bank of superior temporal sulcus, STS; bilateral ('voice selective areas')	Belin et al. (2010)
Lexical network (lexical interface)	Posterior middle temporal gyrus, pMTG; posterior inferior temporal sulcus, pITS; bilateral, weak left bias	Hickok & Poeppel (2007)
Motor plan network (preparatory network)	Supplementary motor area, SMA; dorsolateral frontal cortex; anterior insula; superior cerebellum; left dominant for speech	Golfinopoulos et al. (2010), Hickok & Poeppel (2007), Riecker et al. (2005)
Phonological network	Middle to posterior portions of superior temporal sulcus, STS, bilateral; weak left bias	Hickok & Poeppel (2007)
Semantic hub (semantic interface)	Anterior temporal lobe; bilateral	Patterson et al. (2007)
Sensorimotor hub (sensorimotor interface)	Area in sylvian fissure at pariotemporal boundary (area Spt); left dominant	Hickok & Poeppel (2007)
Somatosensory network	Anterior parietal lobe (ventral somatosensory cortex, vSC); anterior supramarginal gyrus, aSMG; bilateral	Golfinopoulos et al. (2010)
State network: gender, age, mood, etc. of speaker	Temporal lobe, hypermodal regions; integrated portions of auditory and visual 'what' pathways	Kriegstein et al. (2010), Frühholz et al. (2014), Bestelmeyer et al. (2014), Watson et al. (2014)
Visual feature network	Occipital lobe, unimodal regions	e.g. Kandel et al. (2000)
Visual input processing	Retina; thalamus; primary visual cortex; bilateral	e.g. Kandel et al. (2000)

inhibited. In this case, speech perception also involves a *somatosensory network* (Figure 34.1) by activating the somatosensory expectations for the (inhibited) motor execution of a perceived speech item (Kröger et al., 2014).

In many daily situations in our lives, voice and speech perception is an important element of social interaction or communication processes. Thus, beside the pure *linguistic information*, the listener or interlocutor is interested as well in gathering *paralinguistic information* about, for example, who is speaking (e.g. speaker's gender, age, health state, emotional or affective state) or what is the speaker's real intention, which is perhaps not directly given in the linguistic shape of an utterance (e.g. identification of irony or sarcasm). To answer these questions, information concerning co-speech facial and hand-arm gestures as well as the speaker's voice quality and its changes during an utterance or conversational turn is used by the listener (Kröger et al., 2011). Thus, communication as well needs non-linguistic voice perception together with visual perception of facial features and of bodily movements, in addition to pure speech perception, in order to get the information that is 'beside pure text'.

Like speech perception, non-linguistic voice perception starts with *auditory input processing* and a spectrotemporal analysis, executed within the *auditory feature network* (Figure 34.1). This primary auditory analysis is linked with a higher-level *discrimination and identification network for voice features and voice actions* (Figure 34.1), also called the voice-selective network (Belin et al., 2000). This network is capable of discriminating voice quality and intonation cues (Bänziger & Scherer 2005; Gobl & Chasaide, 2003) and thus helps to identify gender, age, and emotional or affective state of a speaker (see link towards speaker-state network in Figure 34.1). However, for processing emotional or affective states for identity perception, an additional close link is needed between auditory and visual processing (Collignon et al., 2008; Schweinberger et al., 2007; Watson et al., 2014). This link occurs in our model by introducing a visual processing network. The basic *visual input processing* and first visual feature analysis within the *visual feature network* is performed within the occipital lobe. This basic visual-processing stream is directly linked with a higher-level *visual discrimination and identification network for facial and bodily features and actions* (Figure 34.1), which can be assumed to be located within the superior temporal gyrus (Adolphs, 2002a). This higher-level part of the visual-processing stream is mainly integrated in the ventral stream of visual perception (Rauschecker & Scott, 2009; see also Figure 34.1).

As introduced in this chapter, it is important for the neural activation of features within the (hypermodal) *speaker-state network* that auditory speech and voice information, as well as visual information of bodily and facial actions (movements), is processed within one (hypermodal) network. In addition, the visual discrimination and identification network for facial and bodily features and actions (Figure 34.1) may profit from activations of the *motor plan network* as well as from activations within the *somatosensory network* (Figure 34.1), which is part of the *dorsal stream of visual perception* (Rauschecker & Scott, 2009). This motor-related dorsal stream helps to identify facial, as well as other bodily co-speech actions (movements), and also voice quality (Kröger et al., 2010). The resulting neural activation patterns for describing features of the speaker (gender, age, emotional and affective state; hypermodal association areas of the temporal lobe, combining information from auditory and visual 'what' streams; Kröger et al., 2010) and identification of voice features and features of co-speech hand-arm actions, as well as of co-speech facial actions, give a representation of paralinguistic information for comprehending the deep intention of a spoken utterance (see arrows to the comprehension level in Figure 34.1). Voice features can change from phrase to phrase (Kröger et al., 2011). Thus, a quotation of the motor plan network via the sensori-motor hub may also be helpful here in order to identify voice colour in terms of laryngeal vocal-fold adjustment actions (e.g. abduction or adduction actions for a more smooth or more harsh voice; Kröger et al., 2011).

Last but not least, it should be mentioned that the model proposed here separates a *ventral stream for visual and auditory perception* (Hickok & Poeppel, 2007; Rauschecker & Scott, 2009), while only one dorsal stream is lined out in our model for visual and auditory processing (e.g. for processing not only auditory vocal cues but also visual facial and bodily cues). Thus, the motor plan network (Figure 34.1) as well as the *articulatory execution network* (Figure 34.1) comprise the speech-production system, the facial system, as well as the whole-body system, as far as it is important in speech-communication processes.

34.2 Neurocomputational Modelling

Neurocomputational modelling aims for a detailed modelling of functional neurobiological processes. Because we are still not able to understand neural processes in depth, most researchers call their neural models 'neurologically plausible' or at least 'biologically inspired'. However, that is not necessarily a disadvantage because it is a goal of modelling to make generalizations in order to understand the overall functioning of the modelled system and to uncover basic functional principles of that neural system. These generalizations comprise the following points:

(i)   Different degrees of abstractions exist for functional neural network models. *Rate neuron models* (see the following) are more abstract than *spiking neuron models*.

(ii) Sensory, motor, or cognitive information is represented in *neural maps*, also called *neural populations* or *neuron ensembles*. Specific information (i.e. specific *neural states*) leads to specific *neural activation patterns* within a neural map.

(iii) Within a large-scale neural model (e.g. a model which comprises cognitive and sensorimotor components), we can separate *neural network modules* and *neural streams*. Neural network modules comprise neural maps connected by neural mappings for processing neural states. Neural streams mainly forward neural states.

(iv) Modelling allows a clear separation between *architecture of the neural model* and *acquired knowledge*. The knowledge is mainly stored within neural link weights within neural mappings. Before a neural large-scale model is capable of working properly (e.g. to recognize words or faces, or to produce words or gestures), a simulation of knowledge acquisition is required.

34.2.1 Model Neurons

The basic unit of each neural network module is the *model neuron*. Large-scale models typically comprise millions of model neurons in order to be capable of simulating perceptual or motor tasks (i.e. in order to simulate behaviour) (e.g. Eliasmith et al., 2012). Like a real biological neuron, a model neuron accumulates incoming neural spikes from upstream-connected model neurons via its input neural connections and continuously calculates its nucleus action potential. If the threshold activation of the model neuron is passed, the model neuron generates a new spike and propagates this electrical pulse towards downstream-connected model neurons. Neural spike pulse generation (e.g. Kandel et al., 2000) is modelled in spiking model neurons like *leaky-integrate-and-fire neurons* (Tal & Schwartz, 1997). This type of spiking neuron model is used in contemporary large-scale neural models (e.g. Eliasmith et al., 2012). A simpler model-neuron approach is the rate neuron model. Here, the *neuron activation rate* in spikes/s is the main model-neuron parameter, while spike pulse patterns are not simulated (e.g. Kohonen, 2001).

In both cases (i.e. spiking and rate-model neurons) a model neuron represents a bundle of neighbouring natural neurons, which fire more or less simultaneously. This representation of a model neuron by a bundle of natural neurons is important especially in the case of the rate neuron approach, because activation rates can only be calculated properly if a sufficient mean number of neural spikes is available per time interval. If we want to calculate activation rates for example for 20-ms to 50-ms time intervals—which is typical for auditory processing—one model neuron should sum up spike pulses from round about 1,000 natural neurons in order to get a still sufficient amount of spikes per time interval (round about twenty to fifty spikes in this example) in the case of a low-firing rate of one spike per natural neuron.

34.2.2 Neural Maps

A specific neural state, representing specific sensory, motor, or abstract cognitive information, appears as a specific neural activation pattern within a neural map. The model neurons within a map are of the same type and the groups of natural neurons, representing each model neuron, are located near together within the brain. Higher-level maps (i.e. mainly neural maps, representing hypermodal cognitive information) often use *local representations* of neural states (e.g. word map, syllable maps in lexical and phonological network modules; Figure 34.2). Here, only one model neuron is activated at a moment and each neuron within that neural map represents one specific state or piece of information. For example, in the case of the mental lexicon, one model neuron represents one word at the lemma level (e.g. Dell & O'Seaghdha, 1992; see word map in Figure 34.2). Neural connections (neural mappings) between different neural maps at cognitive levels are *sparse*. That is, each neuron of one map is connected with only a few (perhaps round about ten) other model neurons of other neural maps. For example, in the case of the mental lexicon, each lemma model neuron, representing a specific word, is only connected with a few neurons within the concept state map (also called *concept map*; Figure 34.2); (e.g. the lemma model neuron representing the word 'human' is connected with only a few concept neurons representing the concepts 'is living', 'has two legs', 'is intelligent', etc.).

Within sensory or motor neural networks, states are implemented by *distributed representations* (e.g. the mapping between the phonetic syllable map and feature maps within auditory feature, motor plan, and somatosensory network modules in Figure 34.2). Here, different activation patterns within a map represent different states, and all neurons within a neural feature map can potentially be activated for the representation of a specific sensory or motor state. Examples for motor plan states or for auditory states of syllables are given

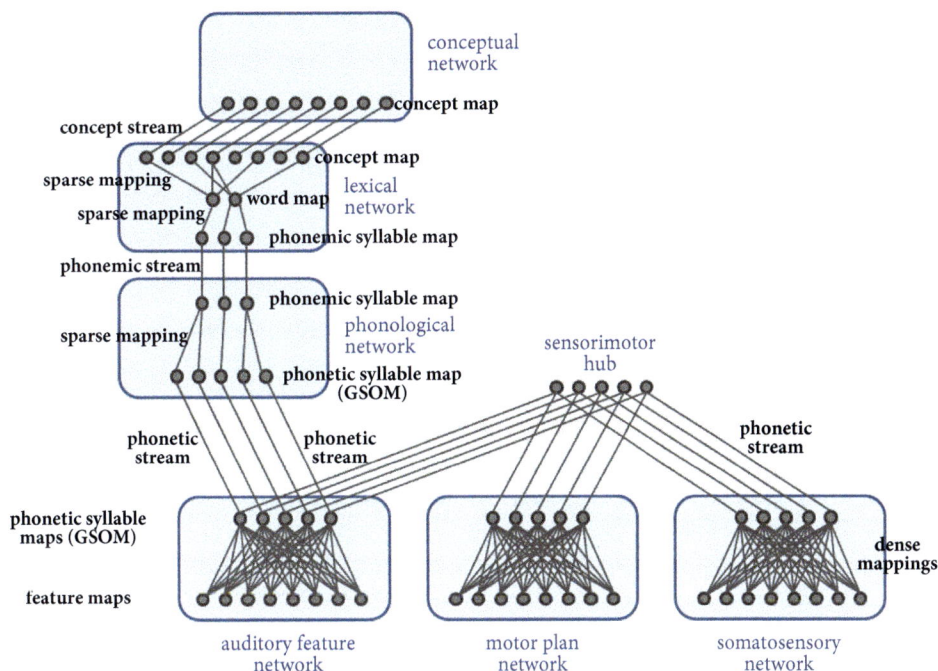

FIGURE 34.2 Exemplification of the detailed network structure for some network modules (boxes), hubs, and streams, defined in our functional model of voice and speech perception (see Figure 34.1). Here, neural maps are represented as arrays of model neurons (represented by dot arrays) and lines indicate bidirectional connections between model neurons. The phonetic syllable map is equivalent with the phonetic map and is implemented as a self-organizing map (SOM; see Kröger et al., 2009, 2014) or as a growing self-organizing map (GSOM; see Cao et al., 2014). In the lexical network, only two words are listed on the word map (lemma map, see text); one of these words is composed of two syllables, the other of only one syllable. The difference between the phonemic and phonetic syllable map is that a phonemic syllable may occur in different phonetic realizations (e.g. the phonemic syllable /ta/ as [ta] and as [tʰa]).

in Kröger et al. (2014). Here, auditory states are represented as 'mental spectrograms' and the neurons within the auditory state map together provide the spectrogram information (i.e. represent different points in time and different frequency intervals). The existence of these types of neural state maps is underpinned experimentally (e.g. by Pasley et al., 2012). In most cases, neural connections (neural mappings) between sensory or motor maps are dense, even if one of the connected maps (in Figure 34.2, the phonetic syllable map) uses a local representation. Thus, each neuron of one neural map is connected with each neuron of the other map. If we assume a map representing, for instance, 2,000 syllables within a language (local representation: one neuron represents one syllable), each neuron of this map is connected with each neuron of the auditory state map (i.e. 2,000 neurons as well). Thus, the dense neural mapping consists of 40,000 neural associations (cf. Kröger et al., 2014; connection of phonetic syllable state map with auditory state map), representing the knowledge concerning the mental auditory images of these (already trained) syllables.

34.2.3 Neural Network Module

While neural streams just forward neural information within a neural system without changing that information, it is the main task of a network module to process or transform neural information. A neural network module comprises at least two neural maps (m1 and m2) which are interconnected (i.e. associated) by neural mapping. The task of the mapping is to process a neural state (s1 in m1), in order to generate (activate) a new (transformed) state (s2 in m2). This is done, for example, in a lexical network, if s1 is a local activation pattern for a word within the lemma map m1 (Dell & O'Seaghdha, 1992; see word state map in Figure 34.2) and if m2 is the concept activation pattern for that specific word, represented by s2 within concept state map m2 (Figure 34.2). Or if s1 is the local activation of a neuron, representing a syllable within the phonetic syllable map m1 (see Kröger et al., 2014), s2 could represent the distributed activation pattern of the mental auditory image of that syllable within auditory feature map m2, and s3 could represent the motor plan of that syllable within motor plan map m3 (Figure 34.2).

Within our voice and speech perception network (Figure 34.1), the auditory feature network comprises an auditory feature map (also called auditory state map in Kröger et al., 2014), a self-organizing phonetic syllable state map, and a dense neural mapping connecting both maps (Cao et al., 2014; Kröger et al., 2009, 2014). The motor plan network comprises a copy of the same phonetic syllable representation, linked by the dorsal stream via the sensorimotor hub (Figure 34.2). This phonetic syllable state map is associated with a motor plan map via a dense mapping (Kröger et al., 2014). Both dense mappings from phonetic syllable state to auditory states as well as to motor states, as well as a third dense mapping between phonetic syllable states and the somatosensory state of the acquired syllable, are learned and stored during speech acquisition (Kröger et al., 2014). A lexical network—comprising a conceptual map, a lemma map, and a phonological map—is exemplified by Dell and O'Seaghdha (1992) (see also Figure 34.2).

Streams connect neural maps between different network modules. Streams differ from mappings in the way that they do not connect each neuron of one map with each neuron of the other map but, rather, only one neuron of one map with one neuron of the other map (see concept stream, phonemic stream, and phonetic streams in Figure 34.2). Thus, a neural stream can be realized as a stream of parallel-directed axons. This enables the copying of an activation pattern of an interface map (input or output map at the end of each network module; see Figure 34.2) of one neural network module to an interface map of another network module. In the case of a neural hub, all interface maps of the co-activated network modules should have available the same neural representation (same type of map). A neural hub, in addition, includes a central neural map in order to be capable of forwarding a current neural activation pattern to all network modules connected with that hub (see the neural map representing the sensorimotor hub in Figure 34.2). Input or output maps of a neural module connected with the hub, need to be connected to those parts of the central neural map of the hub which carry the information required by that module.

34.2.4 Knowledge Acquisition

While the coarse architecture of a functional neural network (e.g. as outlined in Figure 34.1) is already defined by evolution (i.e. locations of network modules and of streams, occurring in defined parts of the brain and connecting defined parts), most mappings within network modules (i.e. the link weights of all neural connections between all maps within a network module) need to be adjusted during speech acquisition, to take account of, for example, whether a connection is inhibitory or exhibitory, or how strong the effect of inhibition or exhibition is. Currently, learning is not easy to model in spiking neuron models. Thus, in the case of language-specific sensorimotor learning, we used self-organizing learning algorithms for rate models (e.g. for establishing the mappings between syllable state maps and auditory and motor state maps; Kröger et al., 2014). In the case of voice and emotion recognition, it may be possible that some information is already transferred by evolutionary processes and thus needs not to be learned. It has been shown that identification and recognition of basic emotions from auditory (voice) and visual (facial) cues is already existent directly after birth (Adolphs, 2002b).

Only parts of the model network introduced in Figure 34.1 are currently computer-implemented. Auditory, motor, and somatosensory networks are included in the implemented production model introduced by Guenther et al. (2006) and by Guenther and Vladusich (2012). A strict separation of motor planning and articulatory execution within neurocomputational modelling was introduced by Kröger et al. (2009, 2014). Neurocomputational models of visual processing, including modelling of cognitive processes, have already been developed (e.g. Eliasmith et al., 2012; Sun et al., 1999). Neurocomputational models of the mental lexicon (i.e. the interconnection of lexical, phonological, and conceptual networks) are described, for example, by Dell and O'Seaghdha (1992), Dell et al. (1999), and Roelofs (1997). The first steps towards a cognitive model for processing semantics and syntax of sentences (combinatorial network) has been introduced by Eliasmith (2013).

The network labelled in Figure 34.1 as the state network for representing different speakers and emotional or affective states or moods (state network in Figure 34.1) can be interpreted as a part of the concept network. It is separated here with respect to the fact that these concepts or states result from discrimination and identification processes carried out in both discrimination and identification networks (i.e. for voice as well as for body and face features and actions; see Figure 34.1). These networks need to be realized and implemented in the near future, because the voice can be seen as an important part of modelling communication processes. Currently, researchers are more concerned with the modelling of speech than of voice processing, but voice processing becomes more and more important as an integral part of neurocomputational models, especially in the case of modelling neural processes of (speech) communication in face-to-face situations, where emotional states as well as paralinguistic information are important (see Schmitt & Schuller, this volume).

34.3 GATHERING KNOWLEDGE FOR VOICE AND SPEECH PERCEPTION

While basic locations of network modules, as well as of streams and hubs (see Figure 34.1), were shaped during evolution, indicating comparable locations within brains of different human individuals and overlap with comparable functional brain regions in other primates (e.g. Rauschecker & Scott, 2009), this is only partially the case for the organization of states within neural maps and for the link weight values within most mappings. Because different individuals acquire different mother tongues, they have to learn different syllable structures and phoneme systems. Moreover, because language acquisition proceeds differently from child to child, even if the same mother tongue is acquired, language-specific networks within the lexical, phonological, as well as higher-level auditory feature, motor plan, and somatosensory networks exhibit the same functionality but develop differently during acquisition at the level of neural-state representation.

For voice perception, it is well known that the child always recognizes the voice of his or her primary caregiver, and automatically pays much attention to that voice and to the acts of the caregiver in comparison to the voice and acts of other persons within the child's environment. In the case of there being more than one caregiver or teacher, the child is capable of differentiating these individuals, and especially their voices, because the child always needs to adapt to different learning scenarios with respect to different caregivers or teachers. Thus, the development of the neural networks within the voice-processing units of our neural model of voice and speech perception up to the state network, which processes personal features of different individuals like age and gender (see Figure 34.1), needs to evolve very early in life so that we can identify our caregivers in order to make language and speech learning easier. Because voice perception is closely related with emotion recognition, it should be stated here as well that the neural representation and processing of emotions is not innate (see the current discussion on basic emotions in, for example, Mason & Capitanio, 2012). Thus, the perception or recognition of emotions—like voice perception and recognition of different individuals—may develop fast, but there are a lot of arguments that the associated networks are not completely developed by the time of birth (Mason & Capitanio, 2012).

From imaging studies it is possible to identify regions, for example, for voice processing or for speech processing, but it is not possible per se to find identical locations for different voices, words, or phonemes. That is not just because the local neuron groups (ensembles) representing a voice, word, or phoneme are so small that they cannot be resolved by functional imaging devices, but it is also because the (self-)organization of neural representations of voices with respect to other human features, of lexemes with respect to their concepts, and of phonemes with respect to words as well as with respect to motor and sensory (e.g. auditory) syllable states within a neural network, develop in different ways with respect to different learning scenarios (i.e. different interactions of learning individuals with the world). We already have shown in our modelling studies that the overall organization, for example of the phonetic map, is the same for different instances of the model (representing different individuals), but that the concrete location of different syllables within that map differs, at least by rotation or mirroring of the whole map from model instance to model instance with respect to different trainings (Kröger et al., 2009).

Neurocomputational modelling of knowledge acquisition has been carried out in the case of speech. For early phases of speech acquisition, a babbling and imitation phase can be separated (e.g. Guenther et al., 2006; Kröger et al., 2009). During babbling, the child activates random motor plans and executes these in order to establish first associations between motor plans on the one hand and auditory and somatosensory expectations on the other hand. During imitation, the child reproduces words and utterances of teachers (caregivers) and, in addition, may activate the already existing lexical entry and its associated concepts, and thus trains neural associations between auditory and motor representations and cognitive representations of a word or utterance. We can model these processes by using neurobiologically inspired approaches, at least for word production and word recognition (e.g. Cao et al., 2014; Li et al., 2004).

Natural learning is mainly reinforcement learning and, thus, guided learning. Natural learning is not a strict supervised learning because the child, for example, associates auditive states with words and their cognitive concepts, while it is unclear whether first associations during a longer learning period are correct or not. Correct associations can only be secured step by step, after many trials accompanied by rewards (or more importantly, no reward in the case of wrong associations) and thus by reinforcement, given by the caregiver. In the case of strict supervised learning, both neural representations of the objects or states have always to be associated correctly. This is the case during babbling, because motor plans and sensory results are activated nearly simultaneously (after articulation and phonation), but here, the problem is to choose an effective training set (training items are almost random). So, in the case of biological realistic training, the child often directs the caregiver to items she/he wants to hear and the child forms hypotheses concerning the word and its concepts, but the reproduction of the word and, thus, the auditory and motor affiliate of the word, as well as the cognitive association of the word with cognitive concepts, may be at least only partially correct during first learning trials. In current modelling approaches, these facts are only partially taken into consideration.

In many cases of neurocomputational modelling of speech acquisition, the training scenario is simplified by already feeding the model with just correct information, but modelling of real learning from face-to-face caregiver–child interactions is not tried yet. In order to do that, it would be necessary to train avatars which act in a realistic communicational environment. In these kinds of scenarios, more realistic knowledge concerning different individuals can be fed to the avatar as a result of face-to-face communication-training scenarios with different individuals. In addition, it should be mentioned that the opposite process of learning (i.e. forgetting) can also be modelled by introducing processes which lead to a slow decrease of the synaptic strength of excitatory as well as of inhibitory synaptic connections, established during learning (e.g. Li et al., 2002). Forgetting of knowledge occurs during ageing or, for example, as a result of neurological diseases. This aspect is interesting for voice and speech perception models in order to simulate performance losses in identity perception (e.g. during ageing).

Last but not least, the close interaction between learning, perception, and production should be emphasized. Speech learning is done by reproducing heard words and utterances, and by simultaneously activating cognitive states representing the meaning of the words or utterances. Thus, neural streams and neural networks for production and perceptions are shaped simultaneously, and it is well known that in specific perceptual situations, the motor networks (production networks) are activated as well (see dorsal stream of speech perception, as introduced earlier in this chapter). In the case of the voice, the production-perception link exists as well for different voice qualities. If we hear a hoarse voice, we immediately try to clear our own throat because we have activated the motor imagery of the hoarse voice of our communication partner within our own vocal apparatus. Thus, it can also be expected that the laryngeal adjustments for different phonation states—responsible, for example, for a breathy, normal, or pressed voice—are easily perceived because we are capable of activating a mental motor plan image for these different voice types of one speaker. However, the production–perception link may not hold or only partially hold for the identification of voices of different speakers, because an individual cannot mimic different laryngeal anatomies. Thus, in parallel to face identification, it can be assumed that voice identification is a passive process, but that visual cues are important in order to generate hypotheses concerning correlates of voice parameters with gender, age, body indices, etc.

34.4 FUTURE DIRECTIONS

Some parts of the voice and speech perception model introduced here (and in Figure 34.1) are still fictional. Especially, to my knowledge, there exists no neurocomputational model of voice perception yet. However, voice perception is a mandatory part of speech perception in a biologically plausible model, if modelling of natural communication processes (at least as part of speech-acquisition processes) is aimed for. Thus, we have outlined in this chapter a concept—how voice perception could be integrated in a neurocomputational model of speech processing. Voice perception though, besides speech perception, should also be seen as a 'stand alone' network, for example in scenarios where it is necessary to identify humans by voice features but without understanding the language they speak. Moreover, it is important to see voice perception as an important part of identification of the affective and emotional state of a person, which needs not necessarily be tightly coupled with speech perception. However, voice and speech perception should be seen as a compact unit if viewed as an integral part of uncovering the message that an interlocutor wants to communicate to us, for example in face-to-face communication scenarios.

In our opinion, a neurobiological model of voice perception should be closely related to facial perception as well as to speech perception. The analogy to visual perception of faces is twofold: (i) it holds for the identification of voices,which is very similar to the identification of different individuals with respect to different faces, and (ii) it holds for the identification of voice actions (i.e. changing voice qualities for signalling different emotional states), which is comparable to the perception of facial actions (cf. Kröger et al., 2010, 2011). The link to speech perception firstly results from the fact that the voice provides the basic carrier signal for speech (i.e. formants or vocal-tract resonances need to be excited by the glottal voice signal) and is part of signalling segmental information (e.g. voiced versus voiceless sounds), as well as suprasegmental or prosodic linguistic information, by the intonation contour. Thus, it is an aim of future neurocomputational modelling to initially develop approaches covering voice and speech production and perception.

REFERENCES

Adolphs, R. (2002a). Neural systems for recognizing emotion. *Current Opinion in Neurobiology*, 12, 169–177.
Adolphs, R. (2002b). Recognizing emotion from facial expressions: psychological and neurological mechanisms. *Behavioral and Cognitive Neuroscience Reviews*, 1, 21–62.
Bänziger, T. & Scherer, K. R. (2005). The role of intonation in emotional expressions. *Speech Communication*, 46, 252–267.

Belin, P., Zatorre, R. J., Lafaille, P., Ahad, P., & Pike, B. (2000). Voice-selective areas in human auditory cortex. *Nature*, 403, 309–312.

Bestelmeyer, P. E. G., Maurage, P., Rouger, J., Latinus, M., & Belin, P. (2014). Adaptation to vocal expressions reveals multistep perception of auditory emotion. *Journal of Neuroscience*, 34, 8098–8105.

Cao, M., Li, A., Fang, Q., Kaufmann, E., & Kröger, B. J. (2014). Interconnected growing self-organizing maps for auditory and semantic acquisition modeling. *Frontiers in Psychology*, 5, 236. doi: 10.3389/fpsyg.2014.00236

Collignon, O., Girard, S., Gosselin, F., Roy, S., Saint-Amour, D., Lassonde, M., & Lepore, F. (2008). Audio-visual integration of emotion expression. *Brain Research*, 1242, 126–135.

Dell, G. S., Chang, F., & Griffin, Z.M. (1999). Connectionist models of language production: lexical access and grammatical encoding. *Cognitive Science*, 23, 517–542.

Dell, G. S. & O'Seaghdha, P. G. (1992). Stages of lexical access in language production. *Cognition*, 42, 287–314.

Eliasmith, C. (2013). *How to Build a Brain*. Oxford: Oxford University Press.

Eliasmith, C., Stewart, T.C., Choo, X., Bekolay, T., DeWolf, T., & Tan, Y. (2012). A large-scale model of the functioning brain. *Science*, 338, 1202–1205.

Frühholz, S., Trost, W., & Grandjean, D. (2014). The role of the medial temporal limbic system in processing emotions in voice and music. *Progress in Neurobiology*, 123, 1–17.

Gobl, C. & Chasaide, A. N. (2003). The role of voice quality in communicating emotion, mood and attitude. *Speech Communication*, 40, 189–212.

Golfinopoulos, E., Tourville, J. A., Bohland, J. W., Ghosh, S. S., & Guenther, F. H. (2011). fMRI investigation of unexpected somatosensory feedback perturbation during speech. *NeuroImage*, 55, 1324–1338.

Guenther, F. H., Ghosh, S. S., & Tourville, J. A. (2006). Neural modeling and imaging of the cortical interactions underlying syllable production. *Brain and Language*, 96, 280–301.

Guenther, F. H. & Vladusich, T. (2012). A neural theory of speech acquisition and production. *Journal of Neurolinguistics*, 25, 408–422.

Hickok, G. & Poeppel, D. (2007). The cortical organization of speech processing. *Nature Reviews Neuroscience*, 8, 393–402.

Kandel, E. R., Schwartz, J. H., & Jessel, T. M. (2000). *Principles of Neural Science* (4th edn). New York: McGraw-Hill.

Kohonen, T. (2001). *Self-Organizing Maps* (3rd edn). Berlin: Springer.

Kröger, B. J., Birkholz, P., Kaufmann, E., & Neuschaefer-Rube, C. (2011). Beyond vocal tract actions: speech prosody and co-verbal gesturing in face-to-face communication. In: B. J. Kröger & P. Birkholz (eds) *Studientexte zur Sprachkommunikation: Elektronische Sprachsignalverarbeitung* (pp. 195–204). Dresden, Germany: TUD Press.

Kröger, B. J., Kannampuzha, J., & Neuschaefer-Rube, C. (2009). Towards a neuro-computational model of speech production and perception. *Speech Communication*, 51, 793–809.

Kröger, B. J., Kannampuzha, J., & Kaufmann, E. (2014). Associative learning and self-organization as basic principles for simulating speech acquisition, speech production, and speech perception. *EPJ Nonlinear Biomedical Physics*, 2, 2.

Kröger, B. J., Kopp, S., & Lowit, A. (2010). A model for production, perception, and acquisition of actions in face-to-face communication. *Cognitive Processing*, 11, 187–205.

Li, P., Farkas I., & MacWhinney, B. (2004). Early lexical development in a self-organizing neural network. *Neural Networks*, 17, 1345–1362.

Li, S. C. & Sikström, S. (2002). Integrative neurocomputational perspectives on cognitive aging, neuromodulation, and representation. *Neuroscience & Biobehavioral Reviews*, 26, 795–808.

Mason, W. A. & Capitanio, J. P. (2012). Basic emotions: a reconstruction. *Emotion Review*, 4, 238–244.

Obleser, J., Leaver, A. M., Van Meter, J., & Rauschecker, J. P. (2010). Segregation of vowels and consonants in human auditory cortex: evidence for distributed hierarchical organization. *Frontiers in Psychology*, 1, 232. doi: 10.3389/fpsyg.2010.00232

Pasley, B. N., David, S. V., Mesgarani, N., Flinker, A., Shamma, S. A., Crone, N. E., Knight, R. T., & Chang, E. F. (2012). Reconstructing speech from human auditory cortex. *PLoS Biology*, 10(1), e1001251. doi: 10.1371/journal.pbio.1001251

Patterson, K., Nestor, P. J., & Rogers, T. T. (2007). Where do you know what you know? The representation of semantic knowledge in the human brain. *Nature Reviews Neuroscience*, 8, 976–987.

Rauschecker, J. P. & Scott, S. K. (2009). Maps and streams in the auditory cortex: nonhuman primates illuminate human speech processing. *Nature Neuroscience*, 12, 718–724.

Riecker, A., Mathiak, K., Wildgruber, D., Erb, M., Hertrich, I., Grodd, W., & Ackermann, H. (2005). fMRI reveals two distinct cerebral networks subserving speech motor control. *Neurology*, 64, 700–706.

Roelofs, A. (1997). The WEAVER model of word-form encoding in speech production. *Cognition*, 64, 249–284.

Schweinberger, S. F., Robertson, D., & Kaufmann, J. M. (2007). Hearing facial identities. *The Quarterly Journal of Experimental Psychology*, 60, 1446–1456.

Sun, H., Liu, L., & Guo, A. (1999). A neurocomputational model of figure-ground discrimination and target tracking. *IEEE Transactions on Neural Networks*, 10, 860–884.

Tal, D. & Schwartz, E. L. (1997). Computing with the leaky integrate-and-fire neuron: logarithmic computation and multiplication. *Neural Computation*, 9, 305–318.

von Kriegstein, K., Smith, D. R. R., Patterson, R. D., Kiebel, S. J., & Griffiths, T. D. (2010). How the human brain recognizes speech in the context of changing speakers. *The Journal of Neuroscience*, 30, 629–638.

Watson, R., Latinus, M., Charest, I., Crabbe, F., & Belin, P. (2014). People-selectivity, audiovisual integration and heteromodality in the superior temporal sulcus. *Cortex*, 50, 125–136.

Zatorre, R. J., Belin, P., & Penhune, V. B. (2002). Structure and function of auditory cortex: music and speech. *Trends in Cognitive Sciences*, 6, 37–46.

CHAPTER 35

··

VOICE AND SPEECH
SYNTHESIS—HIGHLIGHTING
THE CONTROL OF PROSODY

··

KEIKICHI HIROSE

35.1 INTRODUCTION

ATTEMPTS to synthesize human voice/speech have a very long history. In 1779, Christian Kratzenstein constructed acoustic resonators for five vowels, and, in 1791, Wolfgang von Kempelen developed a speech machine which could also generate consonants (Flanagan, 1972). Although several attempts to mimic human speech sounds using mechanical devices followed, it was necessary to wait until the early 1900s for the start of the development of practical speech synthesizers. The famous speech synthesizer, Voder (Voice operating demonstrator), was developed by H. Dudley, and its speech sounds were demonstrated during New York's World Fair in 1939 (Dudley et al., 1939). In Voder, the human-speech generation process was simulated using electrical circuits, and short sentence speech could be generated through manual control of circuits, though it required a trained person. Voder consisted of voiced and unvoiced source waveform generators, and filters to mimic resonances of vocal tracts; Voder is the basis of source-filter model-based speech synthesis systems.

Vocal-tract resonances of vowels and some voiced consonants (such as nasals) are called formants. Formants (and anti-resonances for nasals, etc.) have been studied well and, by constructing rules to control them, the realization of speech in various voice qualities and utterance styles was expected. We can see several works on formant-based speech synthesis from 1953 (Klatt, 1987).

Obtaining correct formants is not always an easy task, and manual corrections are required to avoid low-quality sounds. Linear prediction (LP) is a technique to decompose speech sounds into sources (residuals) and resonances (LP coefficients), originally developed for low bit-rate speech coding. One of the good points of the method is that the analysis of speech sounds is straightforward and can be done automatically. In the mid 1960s, speech-synthesis experiments based on LP were conducted, and later were carried out using LP-related technologies—PARCOR (PARtial auto-CORrelation) and LSP (line spectrum pair).

It is possible to model articulatory organs and to calculate acoustic parameters (such as formants) of corresponding sounds. Such articulatory speech synthesis attracted researchers' attention, since it can mimic the whole process of speech sound generation by humans without constructing mechanical articulatory organs. An articulatory synthesizer was first reported in 1958, and several others followed (Klatt, 1987).

In order to generate speech sounds given a text, processes to analyse the text and to relate the analysis results with speech features are necessary besides the speech sound generation process. Such a text-to-speech (TTS) conversion system was first developed by Noriko Umeda and others in 1968. In 1979, the MITalk system was produced at MIT, and then the famous Klattalk system was developed in 1981 (Klatt, 1987). These were the basis of an epoch-making commercial speech synthesizer, DECtalk. Although these systems used formant synthesizers, we can also see a number of systems with LP-based speech synthesizers. Since then, many TTS conversion systems have been developed, targeting major languages around the world.

The source-filter model can well represent the process of human speech generation. The synthetic speech quality, however, shows a certain degradation—a problem that is difficult to solve in spite of a number of works devoted to it. This situation led to the method of directly handling speech waveforms without converting them into acoustic parameters. This waveform concatenation method was already common in applications such as announcing times of the day: embedding a speech phrase expressing time in a carrier sentence speech. However, in order to realize a wide variety of sentence speech, a scheme was necessary to concatenate speech waveforms in phonemes and/or syllables.

Time-domain pitch synchronous overlap add (TD-PSOLA), developed by E. Moulines and F. Charpentier in 1985, is a technique to change fundamental frequencies of speech waveforms without decomposing them into source and filter components (Moulines & Charpentier, 1990). In addition, the advance of computers made it possible to select the best match to the context from a huge number of speech segments in real time. Based on these backgrounds, TTS conversion systems with waveform concatenation were developed. Later, owing to increased sizes of speech corpora, concatenation-based speech synthesis was realized at the Advanced Telecommunications Research (ATR) Institute International without (basically) changing fundamental frequencies (Black & Taylor, 1994), and many commercial TTS systems with highly natural speech are now available.

Although the quality of synthetic speech was largely improved, speech synthesis by waveform concatenation requires a large speech corpus of the speaker and speaking style to be synthesized. In order to realize a new voice quality with a new style, it is necessary to prepare such a speech corpus, which is time-consuming and costly. A sophisticated speech synthesis method based on the source-filter model needs to be developed. By representing the acoustic feature space with a statistical framework (such as Gaussian distributions), the 'best' acoustic-feature trajectories for speech synthesis need not be in the speech corpus, and, therefore, the size of the speech corpus can be largely reduced.

The hidden Markov model (HMM) was first used to represent acoustic-feature trajectories for speech recognition, and then introduced to speech synthesis. Synthetic speech with a new voice quality and new styles can be realized from a very limited speech corpus through HMM-adaptation techniques (Tokuda et al., 2013). When generating continuous speech, speech segments need to be concatenated. This process results in degradation of synthetic speech quality. The problem is solved in HMM-based synthesis, since concatenation is done in a model basis under a maximum likelihood criterion. Because of these advantages, many research works have been dedicated to HMM-based speech synthesis, and synthetic speech of a high quality (although with slightly more degradation compared to top waveform concatenation systems) is now available. More recently, another statistical-based speech synthesis system—(deep) neural-network-based speech synthesis—has been gaining researchers' attention because of its flexibility in handling acoustic-feature statistics (Ling et al., 2015). Better, or at least comparable, speech quality is already available.

Statistical-based handling of acoustical parameters considerably improved voice-conversion technology. Voice conversion is a method for converting speech of a speaker to that of another (target) speaker, given a small set of utterances of the same sentences spoken by both speakers. The technique can also be used to change utterance styles (such as to generate emotional speech) from a reading style. Acoustic-feature spaces of both speakers are represented by Gaussian mixtures, and conversion is realized through soft mapping of Gaussian distributions between speakers (Stylianou et al., 1998). It is also possible to relate features of both speakers using neural networks without assuming Gaussian distributions.

In the following sections, after briefly introducing the necessary processes of generating speech from text, formant synthesis is first explained as a landmark speech-synthesis technology. It is currently not used, but is based on the human speech generation process, and may give us hints for future development of speech-synthesis technology. Then, concatenation-based synthesis and HMM-based synthesis are explained. In speech synthesis, segmental and prosodic features of speech need to be handled. The situation is different from speech recognition, where prosodic features are rather ignored. Speech-quality degradation in prosodic features is an important issue in speech synthesis. Prosodic features are spread over a long time span, and their frame-by-frame handling is not appropriate. In addition, when synthesizing speech that varies in terms of reading styles and contains various elements such as attitudes and emotions, the importance of prosody control becomes more evident. This chapter focuses on this topic, and introduces a model for fundamental frequency (Fo) contours, with an example of application in HMM-based speech synthesis.

Several websites such as http://www.festvox.org/history/klatt.html and http://piisami.net/dippa/appa.html have good sound demonstrations on synthetic speech, provided in historical order, starting from Vocoder speech. We can also generate HMM-based synthetic speech by accessing http://www.cstr.ed.ac.uk/projects/festival/.

35.2 TEXT-TO-SPEECH CONVERSION AND CONCEPT-TO-SPEECH CONVERSION

Speech synthesis with text input is called text-to-speech conversion. It is widely used as a way to read out various texts, including e-mails. It also plays an important role in providing aids for visually impaired persons. When a text is given, it needs to be analysed to find out how it is related to the speech to be synthesized. Although the process is highly language-independent, it includes morpheme, syntactic, and semantic analyses (text analyses) to segment the text into morphemes/words and to find out syntactic structures (mutual relations of morphemes/words). In order to conduct the process correctly, knowledge on the topic is necessary. For instance, in languages without apparent indication of word boundaries, like Japanese, morpheme analysis is prone to errors without proper knowledge. The Japanese phrase '東海上' can be decomposed in two ways—'東海 + 上 (on Tokai area)' or '東 + 海上 (on Eastern sea)'—with different phoneme sequences. Knowledge on whether Tokai is the topic or not is necessary for correct parsing.

Based on the results of analysis, the text-to-speech conversion system makes decisions regarding pronunciation including prosody (i.e. word accent, stress, intonation, rhythm, and tempo). Although the author will not go into details of the process, it is worth pointing out that it is difficult to conduct the process without errors for an arbitrary text. Since the relation between linguistic information and pronunciation is affected by the nature of human speech generation, the process is usually somewhat simplified. For instance, deeper syntactic boundaries may not always correspond to deeper prosodic boundaries, because of constraints of human respiratory systems. In many text-to-speech conversion systems, part-of-speech information is used instead of precise information of syntactic structures.

Another possible input to speech synthesis is the contents of information to be transmitted. When speech is generated as outputs of spoken dialogue systems or robots, written texts may not be given as inputs. In these cases, sentences need to be generated first from the contents; we need text generation instead of text analysis (Young & Fallside, 1979). This type of speech synthesis is often known as concept-to-speech conversion. Although text-to-speech conversion is used in many spoken dialogue systems and robots (because of a rather limited variety of speech outputs), it is problematic. When generating texts, precise information on morphemes/words and syntax is available. We can even obtain discourse information, such as key words conveying important information. These should be reflected in speech outputs, especially their prosodic features (Kiriyama et al., 2002; Takada et al., 2007). However, it is difficult to realize this in most text-to-speech conversion systems, since their text analyses are simplified.

35.3 METHODS OF SPEECH SOUND GENERATION

There are several ways to generate speech sounds from phoneme sequences with prosodic information: vocal tract analogue (articulatory synthesis), terminal analogue (formant synthesis), analysis-synthesis (parametric synthesis), and waveform concatenation methods. While vocal tract analogue consists in simulating movements of articulatory organs during phonations, terminal analogue is based on simulating movements of poles and zeros of speech spectra. In vocal-tract analogue, speech spectra are calculated from vocal-tract shapes before synthesizing speech. Source waveforms are simplified, such as (low-pass filtered) impulse trains for voiced speech and as white Gaussian noise for voiceless speech. Several models of voiced-source waveforms were later developed and used. In Klattalk, a model with breathiness noise is used for the female voice (Klatt, 1987). Both methods mimic human speech generation, and have the ability to generate various types of speech not relying on a huge speech corpus. In turn, since vocal tract shapes and poles/zeros cannot be obtained straightforwardly, they cannot benefit well from a large speech corpus. The quality of synthetic speech obtainable by these methods is rather limited, despite a large amount of research works.

Analysis-synthesis methods represent speech signals with parameters through speech-analysis techniques such as linear prediction and cepstral analysis. These methods are similar to terminal analogue in that they are based on source-filter modelling of speech, but the difference is that speech waveforms are parameterized analytically and can be reconstructed completely (not counting the effects of windowing and phases) from parameters. This enables handling of and thus benefiting from a large speech corpus. As for the source waveforms, starting from a single impulse for each pitch period, schemes were introduced to handle residual waveforms in linear prediction vocoder, which then evolved into speech-coding techniques such as code-excited linear prediction (Schroeder & Atal, 1985).

Waveform concatenation methods have been widely used for text-to-speech conversion since the development of TD-PSOLA (Moulines & Charpentier, 1990)—a technique to change fundamental frequency (and duration) in the time domain (Figure 35.1). Although TD-PSOLA can change fundamental frequencies up to around +/−20% without serious degradation of speech quality, it requires pitch marks for pitch-wise windowing, which may include errors. These errors may cause buzzing sounds. (Note: TD-PSOLA is a useful technique to generate speech stimuli where prosodic features vary systematically. These speech stimuli are used for listening experiments to find out categorical boundaries of human perception.) Owing to a larger size of speech corpus, waveform concatenation without pitch modification can generate highly natural speech, and is now widely used in commercial speech synthesizers.

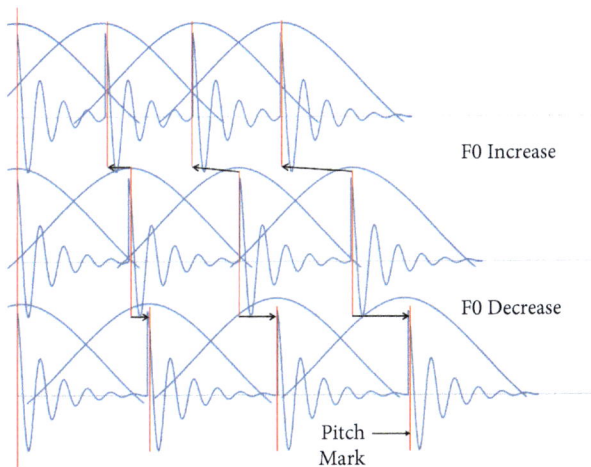

FIGURE 35.1 Scheme of changing fundamental frequencies by TD-PSOLA (Moulines & Charpentier, 1990).

Selection of speech segments for concatenation from a huge number of candidates in the speech corpus is crucial for the quality of corpus-based speech synthesis. In the case of waveform concatenation without pitch manipulation, the methods are often called selection-based speech synthesis. Selection is done taking two types of costs into consideration: selection cost and concatenation cost (Black & Campbell, 1995). Selection cost reflects how the segment matches the speech to be synthesized. For this, various parameters are considered, including one or two preceding and following phonemes, position (of segment) in the sentence, and so on. The importance of parameters related to fundamental frequency grows in selection-based speech synthesis, since fundamental frequency is basically not modified. It is possible to generate speech features using another speech-synthesis method (such as HMM-based speech synthesis), and to use them as references for selection costs (Donovan & Woodland, 1999). Segments selected as the best ones from the selection cost viewpoint are not always the best for the concatenation process; a larger mismatch at a concatenation point may degrade the speech quality. Therefore, spectral mismatch (concatenation cost) is also counted for selection. The selection cost and concatenation cost can be assumed as state-occupancy cost and state-transition cost of HMM-based recognition, respectively. Then, a Viterbi algorithm can be used for the unit selection process (Hunt & Black, 1995). Many research works have focused on efficient segment search and speech corpus size reduction.

Here, terminal analogue speech synthesis is viewed in more detail, though currently it is not used for text-to-speech synthesis systems. It is an epoch-making technology in speech-synthesis history, and the author thinks that researchers should revisit the technology when speech synthesis reaches its ultimate goal—to 'create' speech not relying on a (large) speech corpus. In the terminal analogue method, a speech spectrum is represented as the multiplication of a source spectrum and a vocal tract transfer function. In general, a transfer function as a real coefficient rational function is represented as follows, using poles and zeros:

$$H(s) = G \frac{(s - s_{01})(s - s_{02}) \cdots (s - s_{0n})}{(s - s_{p1})(s - s_{p2}) \cdots (s - s_{pm})} \tag{1}$$

where $s\,(= \sigma + j\omega)$ is complex frequency, and $s_{p1}, s_{p2}, \cdots s_{pm}$ are poles and $s_{01}, s_{02}, \cdots s_{0n}$ are zeros. A set of complex conjugate poles corresponds to a resonance, and a set of complex conjugate zeros corresponds to an anti-resonance. By representing poles and zeros as second-order IIR filters, and connecting then in cascade, a vocal transfer function is realized. Temporal movements of central frequencies and bandwidths of resonances/anti-resonances should be given for speech synthesis, but they are rather difficult to obtain precisely (especially frequencies of anti-resonances and bandwidths of resonances). In order to cope with the situation, methods with parallel concatenation of resonant filters were developed. It is possible to adjust spectral peaks directly. However, we should note that parallel concatenation of resonant filters is represented as a sum of all pole transfer functions, and pseudo zeros appear in transfer functions. Considering these situations, the famous Klattalk synthesizer adopts both type of concatenations—cascade concatenation for vowels and vowel-like sounds (semi-vowels and nasals), and parallel concatenation for other consonants (Klatt, 1980).

35.4 HIDDEN MARKOV MODEL-BASED SPEECH SYNTHESIS

As mentioned in the previous section, high-quality synthetic speech is obtainable by con-catenation-based methods. The waveform concatenation method can generate synthetic speech close to the human voice. However, these methods require a large speech corpus of the speaker and the style to be synthesized. The ultimate goal of speech synthesis should be to generate speech in any voice quality and speech style, as required by a user. This goal is difficult to realize by the waveform concatenation method only, since in order to implement a new voice quality with a new style, it is necessary to prepare such a speech corpus from the beginning. A scheme is necessary to control voice quality and speech style ideally without such a speech corpus, or at least from a small amount of data.

Analysis-synthesis methods have better flexibility than waveform concatenation methods, and work with a smaller speech corpus. Many research works focused on the unit and way of concatenation, but there were certain limitations on the speech quality. The major reason for this situation is that the methods included a great deal of heuristics, which made the best process unclear. There were numerous discussions on concatenation units, concatenation methods, and so on, without clear conclusions. (Note that, as for the concatenation units, several units were investigated regarding the size/design of the speech corpus and method of concatenation, including di-phone, C(consonant)–V(vowel), CVC, VCV, and non-uniform units; Sagisaka (1988).) Introduction of statistical technologies made it possible to conduct selection and concatenation processes using the maximum likelihood criterion. Currently, a good quality of speech is obtainable by statistical parametric speech synthesis methods such as hidden Markov model (HMM)-based speech synthesis (Tokuda et al., 2013) and, recently, deep neural network (DNN)-based speech synthesis (Ling et al., 2015). They are attracting considerable attention from researchers, since flexible control of voice quality and speech styles is possible through statistical adaptation techniques. Here, HMM-based speech synthesis is viewed briefly and especially in terms of how it differs from HMM-based speech recognition.

In speech recognition, recognition rates degrade considerably due to speaker-to-speaker variations of pronunciation. In order to cope with this situation, HMMs are trained using speech from a number of speakers. On the other hand, in speech synthesis, speech from one speaker is used to mimic his/her sounds. Thus, HMMs for speech synthesis should be trained for various contexts. In most cases, the units used in an HMM are phonemes for both speech recognition and speech synthesis. For speech recognition, a phoneme is divided into several cases, counting preceding and following phonemes as the context, and the resulting HMMs are called 'tri-phone models'. For speech synthesis, various contexts other than these are counted—part of speech/conjugation of current/preceding/following words, position of the phoneme in the word, etc. The contexts are language-dependent. So, for English, two preceding/following phonemes are counted, while in Japanese, one preceding and one following phoneme are counted, for instance. Prosodic features not (directly) counted in speech recognition should be included in the models for speech synthesis. There are many contexts related to prosody, such as lengths and accent types of preceding/current/following accent phrases. Combination of these contexts produces an enormous number of cases, and causes a data sparseness problem for HMM training. To cope with this, segmentation of training data is conducted using such methods as binary decision trees with leaf nodes being context labels. The segmentation is stopped based on an MDL (minimum description length) criterion or the like, so that each leaf node has a certain amount of training data.

As mentioned already, prosodic features are not handled explicitly in speech recognition. This is because inclusion of prosodic features in speech-feature vectors causes rather negative effects on recognition performance. The situation is different for speech synthesis; prosodic features need to be handled properly to generate high-quality synthetic speech. Furthermore, when synthesizing speech with various styles, such as emotional speech, the importance of prosodic features may increase even further. When including fundamental frequencies in the feature vector of an HMM, some consideration should be made: no fundamental frequencies are observable for unvoiced speech segments. In order to cope with this situation, a multi-space probability distribution (MSD) HMM was proposed, where fundamental frequencies at voiced frames and 'no pitch' at unvoiced frames were modelled as events in different spaces (Tokuda et al., 1999). In order to properly model phoneme durations, an HSMM (hidden semi-Markov model), where the number of self-transitions (transition to the same state) for each state of an HMM is assumed to follow a Gaussian (or Gamma) distribution, is used in speech synthesis (Zen et al., 2007).

The key issue of analysis-synthesis methods is how precisely they can obtain envelopes of spectra, which represent vocal transfer characteristics. Mel-frequency cepstrum coefficients (MFCCs) are commonly used for both speech recognition and synthesis, but they are obtained somewhat differently. While, in speech recognition, (mel-)cepstrum coefficients are calculated directly from spectra without knowing fundamental frequencies, a pitch synchronous speech analysis method, called STRAIGHT (Kawahara et al., 2008), is widely used in speech synthesis to obtain 'more precise' spectrum envelope shapes on the frequency–time plane. The current high quality of HMM-based synthetic speech is partly due to STRAIGHT analysis.

When modelling speech using an HMM, HMM state density is usually represented by (a mixture of) Gaussian distributions. Although it is a better representation than vector quantization of acoustic feature space, it has a certain limitation in representing actual acoustic-feature distributions. To overcome this limitation, deep learning schemes, such as deep belief networks, are used. It is also possible to map linguistic information of input text to output acoustic features of speech using DNNs (Ling et al., 2015).

35.5 VOICE CONVERSION

Voice conversion is a technology to convert speech into another speech with a different quality/style, keeping the (linguistic) content of an utterance, and is attracting researchers' attention as one of the key technologies for providing a wide variety of synthetic speech that does not rely on large speech corpora. Conversion is usually done without knowing the linguistic content of speech. Although HMM adaptation techniques developed for speaker adaptation in speech recognition can also be used for the purpose, given a parallel corpus of the original and target speech, better conversion can be done by the voice-conversion scheme. Here, a 'parallel' corpus is one containing the original and target speech of the same sentences. The feature space of the original speech is mapped to that of the target speech using linear conversion, which is represented by the following equation:

$$\hat{y}_t = Wx_t + b \tag{2}$$

where $\hat{y}_t$ and x_t are (estimated) feature vectors of the target and original speech, respectively. Conversion matrix W and vector b are obtainable through training using the parallel corpus, but we should note that they vary intricately in the feature spaces. To cope with this situation, feature spaces are represented by mixtures of Gaussian distributions (Gaussian mixture model, GMM), and correspondences between distributions of both feature spaces are trained using the parallel corpus (Stylianou et al., 1998). In order to keep correspondences between mixtures of both spaces, methods were developed, including those to obtain Gaussian distributions for connected vectors of original and target speeches (Kain & Macon, 2002; Toda et al., 2007). Several efforts were then conducted to realize conversion when the parallel corpus was not obtainable (Mouchtaris et al., 2006; Ohtani et al., 2009). Recently, DNN-based methods have been developed to directly relate feature vector spaces between original and target speeches, with good results obtained.

If single Gaussians are assumed for one-dimensional parameters of the original and target speech, equation 2 becomes

$$\hat{y}_t = \frac{\sigma^{(y)}}{\sigma^{(x)}}(x_t - \mu^{(x)}) + \mu^{(y)}. \tag{3}$$

where $\mu^{(y)}$, $\mu^{(x)}$ ($\sigma^{(y)}$, $\sigma^{(x)}$) are averages (and standard deviations) of the parameters after and before conversion. This simple conversion is often applied to fundamental frequencies. This conversion can only generate an expanded or shrunken figure (on the frequency axis) of the original Fo contour, and cannot handle conversions including speaking-style changes. One possible way to solve this situation is to assume an Fo contour model during conversion (see Section 35.6).

35.6 SYNTHESIS OF PROSODIC FEATURES

35.6.1 Modelling of Fo Contours

Speech features can be divided into two groups—segmental and prosodic features. Segmental features appear as envelopes in speech spectra, and play a major role in transmitting phoneme information. On the other hand, prosodic features are features of vocal fold vibrations, and realize speech prosody, such as intonation, rhythm, and tempo. Unlike segmental features, prosodic features have no direct correspondence with written text and are unique to spoken language. They play important roles in human communications. Although segmental features have major roles in the transmission of linguistic information, such as word meanings, the roles of prosodic features are more evident for higher-level information, such as at syntactic and discourse levels. They become dominant for paralinguistic and non-linguistic information, such as attitudes and emotions. Therefore, control of prosodic features is an important issue in speech synthesis. Improper control may cause serious degradation in speech quality. Although selection-based speech synthesis does not include a speech-generation process, prosodic features are often generated as targets for selecting speech units.

In order to generate prosodic features for speech synthesis, it is necessary to relate linguistic information (such as word accent, stress position, syntactic structure, and so on) of input text with prosodic features. For this purpose, many rule-based and statistical methods were developed with models to parameterize prosodic features. Although source power and phoneme duration are important features to be controlled in speech synthesis, fundamental frequency is mainly addressed here, since the relations with linguistic information are somewhat visible as Fo movements and many research works have been conducted.

Before going into details of Fo contour generation in speech synthesis, it should be pointed out that Fos should be handled as logarithmic values. Formerly, it was pointed out that the female voice was accompanied by larger Fo movements as compared to male voices, sometimes leading to the conclusion that the female voice is more expressive than the male voice. However, if we view Fo contours of male and female voices, they are similar, with differences only in the bias level. Moreover, an extension of the vocal tract causes an exponential increase of Fo. Now, it is widely recognized that Fos need to be handled in a logarithmic scale.

In the early days of speech synthesis, Fo contours were represented as piecewise straight lines connecting Fos at points representing syllables. Several rules were developed to generate sentence Fo contours under this framework. Concatenation of Fos in syllable units was also widely used, especially for Chinese speech, which is known as a typical tonal language. For English, a metrical grid modelling was developed, where Fo contours are represented as shifts between four tone-curves (Pierrehumbert, 1979). Motivated by this modelling, a well-known system for prosodic labelling was developed—Tone and Break Indices (ToBI) (Silverman et al., 1992). Versions for various languages were developed later. Although a rather good quality was realized with the controls based on the aforementioned models/ systems, using either rule-based or corpus-based methods, there were certain limitations because they only modelled Fo movements and were not based on the human process of Fo contour generation.

Fo contours of sentences appear as piecewise curves decoupled at unvoiced periods (and pauses). Although no Fo is observable at unvoiced periods, a sentence Fo contour is well interpreted as a fully continuous curve with unvoiced periods in between. It is generally recognized that an Fo contour consists of global and local movements, which may be related to phrasing and accentuation, respectively. Also, prosody has a hierarchical structure, from a shorter time span covering a syllable/word to a longer time span covering a phrase/sentence/ paragraph. Models should well relate the prosodic structure with Fo movements.

The ToBI system counts the hierarchical structure of prosody as ToBI tiers. However, it is a labelling scheme, and does not aim at parametric representations of Fo contours. Several models have been developed for this purpose, including Tilt (Taylor, 2000) and PENTA (Xu, 2005). However, most models only try to trace observed Fo movements and fail to decompose Fo contours into their constituents with clear physical meanings. PENTA includes the concept of tilted pitch target, which is useful for tonal languages. Phrase or longer time-span movements of Fo are not clear in the model. There are several attempts to model Fo contours as superposition of components representing gradual movements of longer time spans and sharp movements of shorter time spans (Bailly & Holm, 2005; Hirst & Espesser, 1993). However, in many cases, an Fo contour is decomposed simply as a smoothed Fo contour and residuals. For instance, MOMEL uses spline curves for smoothing, and phrase-level and word/syllable-level Fo movements are not well decomposed. Focusing on the multi-scale feature of wavelet transform, continuous wavelet transform is used to represent the hierarchical structure of prosody (Vainio et al., 2015). However, the relation between decomposed components and linguistic information of the utterance is still not clear enough.

Öhman (1967) introduced an important feature into Fo modelling—command response. While an Fo contour is (quasi-)continuous, linguistic information conveyed by prosody is discrete. A better view is supposed to be obtainable for prosody if discrete commands are introduced into the model. Unfortunately, model commands were multi-level step functions, which made relations with linguistic information unclear.

35.6.2 Generation Process Model of Fo Contours

The generation process model of Fo contours, often referred to as 'Fujisaki's model', has two important features related to Fo modelling—it is superpositional, and it is a command-response model (Hirose & Fujisaki, 1982). It describes Fo contours in a logarithmic scale as the superposition of phrase and accent components, represented as responses to impulse-like and step-wise commands, respectively. The model has a clear advantage in that both components are represented as responses to discrete commands, which have clear relations with linguistic information of the utterance. The response functions are responses of second-order linear systems, which are well-known physical constraints when a system is controlled by inertia and damping. A phrase component $G_p(t)$ is formulated as the following function of time t:

$$G_p(t) = \begin{cases} \alpha^2 t \exp(-\alpha t), & t \geq 0 \\ 0, & t \geq 0 \end{cases}, \tag{4}$$

while an accent component $G_a(t)$ is formulated as:

$$G_a(t) = \begin{cases} \min\left[1-(1+\beta t)\exp(-\beta t), \gamma\right], & t \geq 0 \\ 0, & t < 0 \end{cases}. \tag{5}$$

α and β are time constants for the phrase- and accent-control mechanisms, respectively. Since these parameters are tightly related to the mechanical system of the larynx, they are considered to be similar for all utterances, and can be fixed as approximately 3.0 s^{-1} for α and 20.0 s^{-1} for β, when analysing Fo contours. The ceiling parameter γ can be fixed as 0.9.

Then, an Fo contour is given by the sum of phrase and accent components as:

$$\log F0(t) = \ln F_b + \sum_{i=1}^{I} A_{pi} G_p(t - T_{0i}) + \sum_{j=1}^{J} A_{aj} \left\{ G_a(t - T_{1j}) - G_a(t - T_{2j}) \right\}. \tag{6}$$

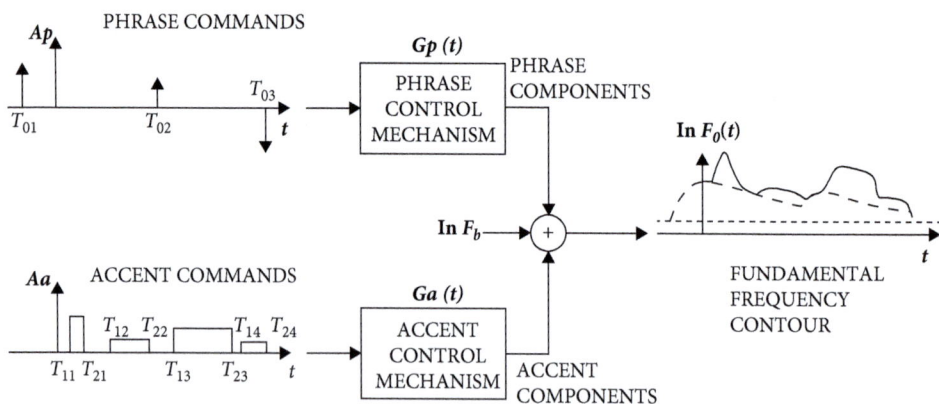

FIGURE 35.2 Generation process model for sentence Fo contours (Fujisaki & Hirose, 1984).

Reproduced from Fujisaki H. & Hirose K., 'Analysis of voice fundamental frequency contours for declarative sentences of Japanese', *The Journal of the Acoustical Society of Japan (E)*, Volume 5, No. 4, pp. 233–42, Copyright © 1984 Acoustical Society of Japan, reprinted with permission.

Here, F_b is the bias level, i is the number of phrase commands, j is the number of accent commands, A_{pi} is the magnitude of the ith phrase command, A_{aj} is the amplitude of the jth accent command, T_{0i} is the onset time of the ith phrase command, T_{1j} is the onset time of the jth accent command, and T_{2j} is the reset time of the jth accent command. A schematic view of the model is given in Figure 35.2.

With this model, Fo contours are generated by assigning command locations and amplitudes corresponding to input texts. Rule-based and corpus-based (binary decision tree, neural network) methods have been developed for Japanese and other languages (Hirose et al., 1986, 2005) (also Audios 35.1 and 35.2). By handling Fo contours in the framework of the model, 'flexible' control of prosodic features becomes possible. A corpus-based method has been developed to predict differences in the model commands between source and target utterances of the same linguistic content (Ochi et al., 2009). Applying the predicted differences to the Fo contours of the source speech, those of the target speech are realized. A large speech corpus is not necessary to train the model command differences. The validity of the method has been shown through experiments on prosodic emphasis (Hirose, 2015) and speaking-style/voice conversion (Hirose et al., 2011) (also Audios 35.3 and 35.4).

35.6.3 Fo Contour Generation in Hidden Markov Model-Based Speech Synthesis

By statistical parametric speech synthesis (HMM-based speech synthesis and DNN-based speech synthesis), Fo values can be related to linguistic information in a frame-by-frame manner. This is an advantage when training acoustic models using a large amount of speech corpus, since we can handle raw Fo data directly. However, we should also note that the frame-by-frame processing includes an inherent problem in handling prosodic features. Prosodic features are related to words, phrases, sentences, and even paragraphs, and should be viewed in wider time spans. Relations between frames are taken into account as time-derivative (Δ and Δ^2) features and/or by handling several frames in one process, but they are not enough. Generated speech often has oversmoothed Fo contours with occasional Fo undulations not observable in human speech. Moreover, the relation between generated Fo contours and linguistic (and para-/non-linguistic) information conveyed by them is unclear, making further processing, such as adding emphasis or changing speaking styles, not straightforward.

Several schemes were developed to represent the hierarchical structure of prosody in HMM-based speech synthesis. Fo contours were decomposed into several layers by arranging level-dependent questions for the context clustering in HMM-based speech synthesis (Lei et al., 2010; Zen & Braunschweiler, 2009). These works aimed at realizing better Fo control in HMM-based speech synthesis, but the relation between the resulting decomposition and linguistic information is still not clear enough.

Hsia et al. (2010) applied a hierarchical modelling of prosodic units to generate global Fo movements, and combined them with frame-by-frame Fos generated by HMM-based speech synthesis. They introduced a syllable-level Fo layer, which is considered to be suitable for Chinese. The modelling is based on approximating global Fo movements with Legendre polynomials, which cannot represent phrase components well. The method generates global Fo movements outside HMM-based speech synthesis processes.

One major issue of HMM-based speech synthesis is how to handle voiceless phoneme periods, where Fo values are unavailable. Although MSD-HMM is commonly used (Tokuda et al., 1999), it is pointed out that MSD-HMM has a limitation in representing Fo movements around voiced/voiceless boundaries. This is because derivative features such as Δ and Δ^2 are usually included in feature parameters of HMMs (to capture temporal movements of acoustical features), and they are not well represented around voiced/unvoiced boundaries. In order to cope with the problem, methods were developed to assume 'pseudo' Fo values for unvoiced periods and to handle Fos as a continuous curve (Yu & Young, 2011). This type of method requires an additional stream of voiced/unvoiced labels. When Fo contours are modelled by the generation process model, for instance, 'reasonable' (pseudo) Fo values are obtained.

35.6.4 Generation Process Model and Hidden Markov Model-Based Speech Synthesis

Because of the ability of interpreting prosody, introducing the generation process model constraint into HMM-based speech synthesis is attractive. However, the model commands are not amenable to being handled in a frame-by-frame manner. Although an effort was reported to represent the model in a statistical framework to cope with the problem, it was not combined with HMM-based speech synthesis (Kameoka et al., 2013). A simple way to approximate Fo contours of speech with the model, and to use these Fos for HMM training, was attempted with successful results (Hashimoto et al., 2012) (also Audio 35.5).

As mentioned already, a major advantage of the generation process model is that it can nicely decompose an observed Fo contour into phrase and accent components. Phrase components represent gradual Fo declination corresponding to phrasing, while accent

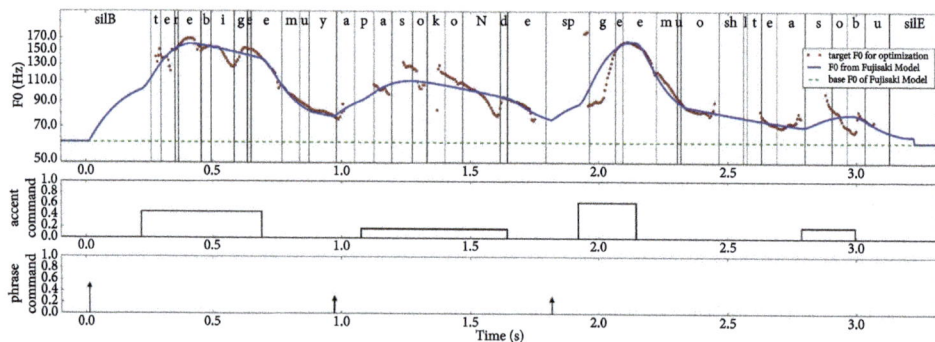

FIGURE 35.3 An example of observed Fos (in red dots) and their approximation by the generation process model (noted as Fo model, in blue solid line). The model parameters (accent and phrase commands) are also shown. ('terebigeemuya pasokoNde geemuoshite asobu': '(We) played games with TV gamers and/or personal computers'.)

Reproduced from Hirose K., Hashimoto H., Saito D., & Minematsu N., 'Superpositional modeling of fundamental frequency contours for HMM-based speech synthesis', *Proceedings of the 8th International Conference on Speech Prosody*, pp.771–5, Copyright © 2016.

components represent local Fo humps corresponding to word accents. Since they are differently related to linguistic information of the utterance, better control of prosody can be expected by handling them separately. This idea is realized in a scheme of predicting model commands—first, phrase commands, and then accent commands, taking the predicted phrase commands into consideration (Hirose et al., 2005). Huang et al. (2012) developed a similar method for Chinese.

Figure 35.3 shows an example of Fo contour approximation by this model. Although the approximated Fo contour is close to that of the utterance, some discrepancies are observable. The generation process model only takes phrase and accent components into account, and does not account for micro-prosodic Fo movements. Also, minor Fo undulations without clear correspondence to linguistic information are ignored. Furthermore, Fo contours may not strictly follow a (critically-damped) second-order linear system, causing minor deviations from the model. These discrepancies are called Fo residuals and are primarily related to phoneme identities.

From these considerations, a method was developed to decompose Fo contours into three layers—phrase component, accent component, and Fo residual—in the framework of the generation process model, and to handle each of them as a different stream in the training and synthesis processes of HMM-based speech synthesis (Hirose et al., 2016). Figure 35.4 shows a sentence Fo contour generated by the original HMM-based speech synthesis (MSD-HMM without Fo contour decomposition) and that generated by the method developed as just described (with Fo contour decomposition), together with that of natural utterance (target Fo contour). Fo contours closer to target utterances are obtainable with improved speech quality (Audio 35.6).

The benefit of handling Fo contours as three streams is clear from the result of context clustering (Figure 35.5). Questions regarding longer time spans such as breath group length and sentence length are selected for phrase component Fos, while questions regarding (accent

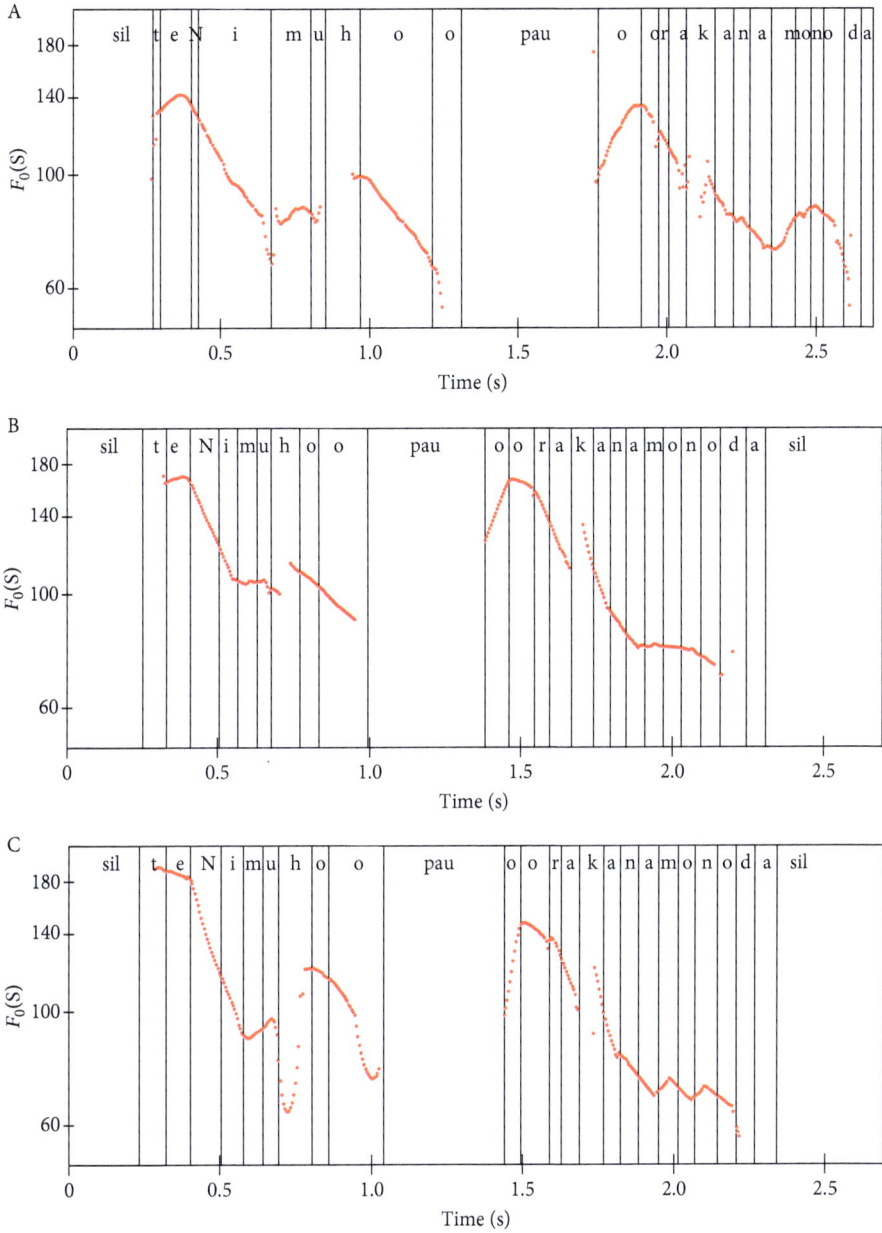

FIGURE 35.4 Fo contours generated by the two versions of HMM-based speech synthesis, as compared to Fo contour of the target utterance: (A) target, (B) original HMM-based, and (C) multi-stream. ('teNimuhoo oorakana monoda': '(He) is such a flawless, natural, and generous (person)'.)

(A)

(B)

(C)

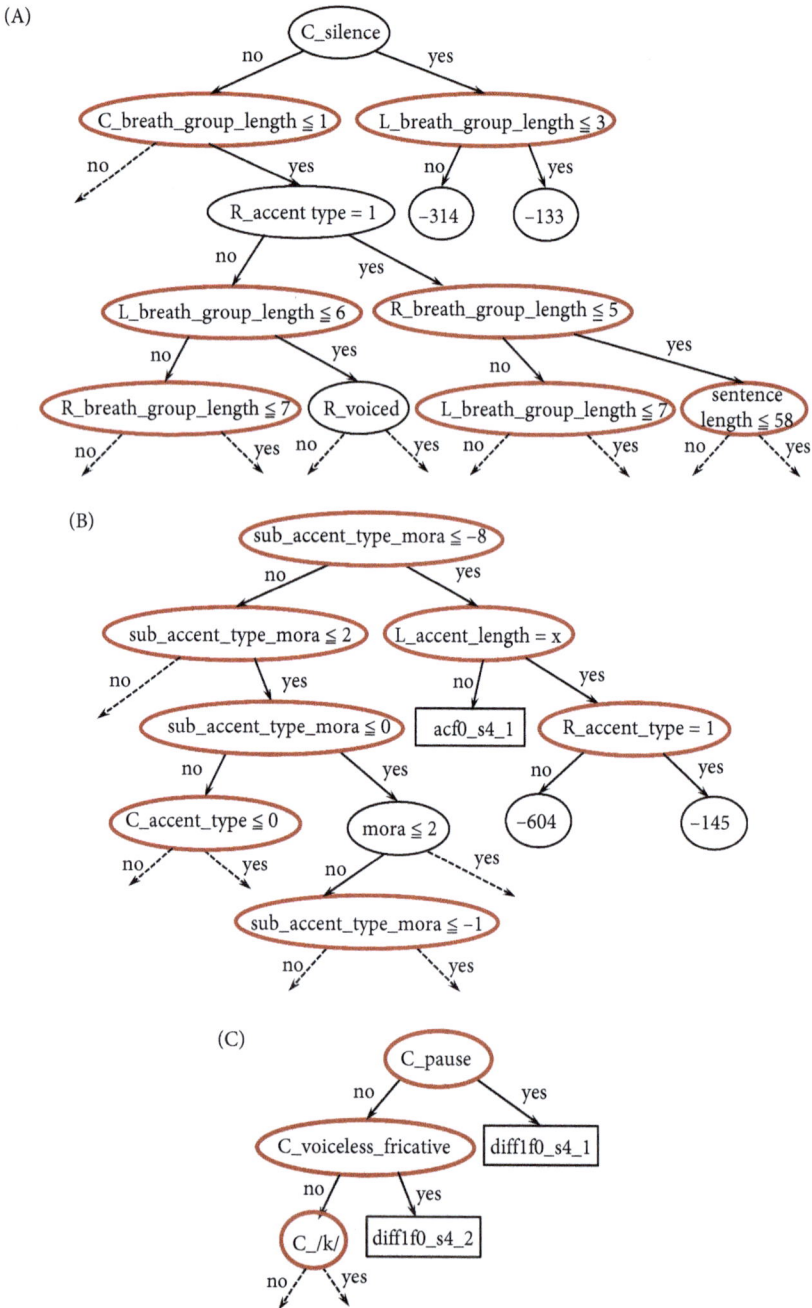

FIGURE 35.5 Parts of binary decision trees (near root nodes) obtained as the results of context clustering for (A) phrase component Fos, (B) accent component Fos, and (C) Fo residuals. Nodes highlighted with thick red circles are questions related to breath groups/sentences for (A), accent phrases for (B), and phonemes for (C).

types of) accent phrases are selected for accent component Fos. Questions on phoneme identities are selected for Fo residuals.

By the proposed method, generated Fo contours are represented as the sum of three contours—two contours generated from HMMs trained using phrase and accent components of the generation process model, and one contour generated from HMMs trained using Fo residuals. Extraction of model commands is considered to be easy for the former two contours, leading to flexible and systematic control of prosody as already mentioned.

35.7 CONCLUSION

Attempts to mimic human speech generation led to source-filter modelling with several vocoder techniques, including linear prediction, cepstrum, and, recently, STRAIGHT. Several speech-synthesis systems were developed based on these techniques. Systems based on articulatory and formant synthesis were also developed. However, despite researchers' efforts, the quality of synthetic speech remained rather low. This situation led to waveform concatenation without the process of dividing speech into source and vocal tract features. Although the quality was largely improved, owing to a huge amount of speech corpus used as material for speech synthesis, the lack of flexibility in speech qualities and utterance styles made it necessary to improve vocoder-based techniques. This was realized by statistical parametric synthesis, in the form of HMM-based and DNN-based schemes.

Now, a rather high quality is obtainable, and sophisticated voice-conversion techniques have also been developed. It has become possible even to convert one's speech to a different language, maintaining voice quality. However, with regard to the prosodic features of speech, research work is necessary for the handling of them in the speech-synthesis process, while keeping their relation with linguistic and para-/non-linguistic information. Frame-by-frame methods especially have certain limitations in handling prosodic features. In order to solve this situation, prosody models become important, and schemes need to be developed to handle them in statistical parametric speech synthesis. This has led to a technique to realize various utterance styles of speech that do not rely on a speech corpus.

In recent academic conferences on speech synthesis, many research works related to DNN-based speech synthesis have been reported. Although they are not introduced here, DNN-based speech synthesis is very attractive, since it can handle acoustic features in other than a frame-by-frame manner, making it easier to incorporate prosody modelling into the synthesis process.

Developing sophisticated speech-synthesis systems from the beginning may not be an easy task. Now, researchers can have the benefit of open software: several speech-synthesis systems are obtainable from http://www.cstr.ed.ac.uk/projects/festival/ and http://hts.sp.nitech.ac.jp/ (HMM-based speech synthesis).

REFERENCES

Bailly, G. & Holm, B. (2005). SFC: a trainable prosodic model. *Speech Communication*, 46(3–4), 348–364.

Black, A. & Campbell, N. (1995). *Optimizing selection of units from speech database for concatenative synthesis*. Proceedings of EUROSPEECH, Vol. 1, pp. 581–584.

Black, A. & Taylor, P. (1994). *CHATR: a generic speech synthesis system*. Proceedings of International Conference on Computational Linguistics, Vol. 2, pp. 983–986.

Donovan, R. & Woodland, P. (1999). A hidden Markov-model-based trainable speech synthesizer. *Computer Speech and Language*, 13, 223–241.

Dudley, H., Riesz, R. R., & Watkins, S. S. A. (1939). A synthetic speaker. *Journal of Franklin Institute*, 227(6), 739–882.

Flanagan, J. (1972). Voices of men and machines. *Journal of the Acoustical Society of America*, 51(5), 1375–1387.

Fujisaki, H. & Hirose, K. (1984). Analysis of voice fundamental frequency contours for declarative sentences of Japanese. *Journal of the Acoustical Society of Japan (E)*, 5(4), 233–242.

Hashimoto, H., Hirose, K., & Minematsu, N. (2012). *Improved automatic extraction of generation process model commands and its use for generating fundamental frequency contours for training HMM-based speech synthesis*. Proceedings of Interspeech 2012 meeting, Portland, USA.

Hirose, K. (2015). Use of generation process model for improved control of fundamental frequency contours in HMM-based speech synthesis. In: K. Hirose & J. Tao (eds) *Speech Prosody in Speech Synthesis: Modeling and Generation of Prosody for High Quality and Flexible Speech Synthesis* (pp. 145–159). Springer-Verlag.

Hirose, K. & Fujisaki, H. (1982). *Analysis and synthesis of voice fundamental frequency contours of spoken sentences*. Proceedings of IEEE International Conference on Acoustics, Speech and Signal Processing, Vol. 2, pp. 950–953.

Hirose, K., Fujisaki, H., & Kawai, H. (1986). *Generation of prosodic symbols for rule-synthesis of connected speech of Japanese*. Proceedings of IEEE International Conference on Acoustics, Speech and Signal Processing, Tokyo, Vol. 4, pp. 2415–2418.

Hirose, K., Hashimoto, H., Saito, D., & Minematsu, N. (2016). *Superpositional modeling of fundamental frequency contours for HMM-based speech synthesis*. Proceedings of International Conference on Speech Prosody, pp. 771–775.

Hirose, K., Ochi, K., Mihara, R., Hashimoto, H., Saito, D., & Minematsu, N. (2011). *Adaptation of prosody in speech synthesis by changing command values of the generation process model of fundamental frequency*. Proceedings of INTERSPEECH, pp. 2793–2796.

Hirose, K., Sato, K., Asano, Y., & Minematsu, N. (2005). Synthesis of F_0 contours using generation process model parameters predicted from unlabeled corpora: application to emotional speech synthesis. *Speech Communication*, 46(3–4), 385–404.

Hirst, D. & Espesser, R. (1993). Automatic modelling of fundamental frequency curves using a quadratic spline function. *Travaux de l'Institut de Phonétique d'Aix*, 15, 75–85.

Hsia, C. C., Wu, C. H., & Wu, J. Y. (2010). Exploiting prosody hierarchy and dynamic features for pitch modeling and generation in HMM-based synthesis. *IEEE Transactions in Audio, Speech, and Language Processing*, 18(8), 1994–2003.

Huang, Y. C., Wu, C. H., & Weng, S. T. (2012). *Hierarchical prosodic pattern selection based on Fujisaki model for natural Mandarin speech synthesis*. Proceedings of IEEE International Symposium on Chinese Spoken Language Processing, pp. 79–83.

Hunt, A. & Black, A. (1995). *Unit selection in a concatenative speech synthesis system using large speech database*. IEEE International Conference on Acoustics, Speech and Signal Processing, Vol. 1, pp. 373–376.

Kain, A. & Macon, M. W. (2002). *Spectral voice conversion for text-to-speech synthesis*. Proceedings of IEEE International Conference on Acoustics, Speech and Signal Processing, pp. 285–288.

Kameoka, H., Yoshizato, K., Ishihara, T., Ohishi, Y., Kashino, K., & Sagayama, S. (2013). *Generative modeling of speech F_0 contours*. Proceedings of INTERSPEECH, pp. 1826–1830.

Kawahara, H., Morise, M., Takahashi, T., Nishimura, R., Irino, T., & Banno, H. (2008). *Tandem-STRAIGHT: a temporally stable power spectral representation for periodic signals and applications to interference-free spectrum, F_0 and aperiodicity estimation*. Proceedings of IEEE International Conference on Acoustics, Speech and Signal Processing, pp. 3933–3936.

Kiriyama, S., Hirose, K., & Minematsu, N. (2002). *Control of prosodic focuses for reply speech generation in a spoken dialogue system of information retrieval on academic documents*. Proceedings of International Conference on Speech Prosody, pp. 431–434.

Klatt, D. (1987). Review of text-to-speech conversion. *Journal of the Acoustical Society of America*, 82(3), 737–793.

Klatt, D. (1980). Software for a cascade/parallel formant synthesizer. *Journal of the Acoustical Society of America*, 67(3), 971–995.

Lei, M., Wu, Y., Soong, F., Ling, Z., & Dai, L. (2010). *A hierarchical F_0 modeling method for HMM-based speech synthesis*. Proceedings of INTERSPEECH, pp. 2170–2173.

Ling, Z., Kang, S., Zen, H., Senior, A., Schuster, M., Qian, X., Meng, H., & Deng, L. (2015). Deep learning for acoustic modeling in parametric speech generation. *IEEE Signal Processing Magazine*, 35–52.

Mouchtaris, A., Spiegel, J., & Mueller, P. (2006). Nonparallel training for voice conversion based on a parameter adaptation approach. *IEEE Transactions on Audio, Speech, and Language Processing*, 14(3), 952–963.

Moulines, E. & Charpentier, F. (1990). Pitch synchronous waveform processing techniques for text-to-speech synthesis using diphones. *Speech Communication*, 9, 453–467.

Ochi, K., Hirose, K., & Minematsu, N. (2009). *Control of prosodic focus in corpus-based generation of fundamental frequency contours of Japanese based on the generation process model*. Proceedings of IEEE International Conference on Acoustics, Speech and Signal Processing, pp. 4485–4488.

Öhman, S. (1967). Word and sentence intonation: a quantitative model. *Speech Transmission Laboratory—Quarterly Progress and Status Report, Dept. of Speech Communication, Royal Institute of Technology*, 8(2–3), 20–54.

Ohtani, Y., Toda, T., Saruwatari, H., & Shikano, K. (2009). *Many-to-many eigenvoice conversion with reference voice*. Proceedings of INTERSPEECH, pp. 1623–1626.

Pierrehumbert, J. (1979). Intonation synthesis based on metrical grids. *Journal of the Acoustical Society of America*, 63(Suppl. 1), S131.

Sagisaka, Y. (1988). *Speech synthesis by rule using an optimal selection of non-uniform synthesis units*. Proceedings of IEEE International Conference on Acoustics, Speech and Signal Processing, pp. 679–632.

Schroeder, M. & Atal, B. (1985). *Code-excited linear prediction (CELP): high-quality speech at very low bit rates*. Proceedings of IEEE International Conference on Acoustics, Speech and Signal Processing, Vol. 10, pp. 937–940.

Silverman, K., Beckman, M., Pitrelli, J., Ostendorf, M., Wightman, C., Price, P., Pierrehumbert, J., & Hirschberg, J. (1992). ToBI: a standard for labelling English prosody. *Proceedings of International Conference on Spoken Language Processing*, Vol. 2, pp. 867–870.

Stylianou, Y., Cappe, O., & Moulines, E. (1998). Continuous probabilistic transform for voice conversion. *IEEE Transactions on Speech and Audio Processing*, 6(2), 131–142.

Takada, S., Yagi, Y., Hirose, K., & Minematsu, N. (2007). *A framework of reply speech generation for concept-to-speech conversion in spoken dialogue systems*. Proceedings of INTERSPEECH, pp. 1286–1289.

Taylor, P. (2000). Analysis and synthesis of intonation using the Tilt model. *Journal of the Acoustical Society of America*, 107(3), 1997–1714.

Toda, T., Black, A. W., & Tokuda, K. (2007). Voice conversion based on maximum-likelihood estimation of spectral parameter trajectory. *IEEE Transactions on Audio, Speech and Language Processing*, 15(8), 2222–2235.

Tokuda, K., Masuko, T., Miyazaki, N., & Kobayashi, T. (1999). *Hidden Markov models based on multispace probability distribution for pitch pattern modeling*. Proceedings of IEEE International Conference on Acoustics, Speech and Signal Processing, pp. 229–232.

Tokuda, K., Nankaku, Y., Toda, T., Zen, H., Yamagishi, J., & Oura, K. (2013). Speech synthesis based on hidden Markov models. *Proceedings of IEEE*, 101(5), 1234–1252.

Vainio, M., Suni, A., & Alto, D. (2015). Emphasis, word prominence, and continuous wavelet transform in the control of HMM-based synthesis. In: K. Hirose & J. Tao (eds) *Speech Prosody in Speech Synthesis: Modeling and Generation of Prosody for High Quality and Flexible Speech Synthesis* (pp. 173–188). Springer-Verlag.

Xu, Y. (2005). Speech melody as articulatorily implemented communicative functions. *Speech Communications*, 46, 220–251.

Young, S. & Fallside, F. (1979). Speech synthesis from concept: a method for speech output from information systems. *Journal of the Acoustical Society of America*, 66, 685–695.

Yu, K. & Young, S. (2011). Continuous F_0 modeling for HMM based statistical parametric speech synthesis. *IEEE Transactions on Audio, Speech, and Language Processing*, 19(5), 1071–1079.

Zen, H. & Braunschweiler, N. (2009). *Context-dependent additive log F_0 model for HMM-based speech synthesis*. Proceedings of INTERSPEECH, pp. 2091–2094.

Zen, H., Tokuda, K., Masuko, T., Kobayashi, T., & Kitamura, T. (2007). Hidden semi-Markov model based speech synthesis system. *IEICE Transactions on Information and Systems*, E90-D(5), 825–834.

CHAPTER 36

....

VOICE BIOMETRICS FOR FORENSIC SPEAKER RECOGNITION APPLICATIONS

....

VOLKER DELLWO, PETER FRENCH, AND LEI HE

36.1 INTRODUCTION

....

RECOGNIZING individuals is a crucial social procedure performed intuitively and usually unconsciously by humans and many animal species. Together with visual cues such as face, body shape, and motion, a person's voice plays an essential role in the recognition process. Indeed, voice in itself often carries sufficient information to allow recognition, in particular when visual cues are not available (e.g. on the telephone or over the radio) or impaired (e.g. in reduced light or darkness). When we listen to the television or the radio, the voices of many politicians, actors, public speakers, and others can typically be recognized without effort. Recognizing a person by voice is also essential in certain institutional contexts, such as when a telephone caller wishes to have access to information concerning his/her bank account or when the identity of a speaker recorded in connection with a crime is unknown or disputed. In such cases, the recognition process is more formal and based on so-called voice 'biometrics'.

The term 'biometrics' is often used ambiguously, as indicated by its definition in the *Oxford English Dictionary*:

> The use of unique physical characteristics (fingerprints, iris pattern, etc.) to identify individuals, typically for the purposes of security. Also (with pl.concord): the physical characteristics that can be so used. (Oxford University Press, 2017, entry: biometrics)

This means that biometrics can refer either to unique physical characteristics that may be input to a system used to recognize individuals, or it may refer to the processing of such data in performing the recognition process. This distinction may be particularly important in the case of voice recognition as the mere existence of a physical characteristic of identity does not automatically make it applicable for recognition. Also, different systems may use different types and constellations of characteristics in the process of recognizing an individual, and no system uses the full gamut of information available. With automatic systems, for example, the process of voice recognition is primarily based on amassed and 'smoothed' short-term spectral information, while idiosyncrasies in the temporal structure of the signal are for the most part disregarded, even though it is known that temporal variability between speakers exists (Dellwo et al., 2015; He & Dellwo, 2016, 2017; Leemann, Kolly, & Dellwo, 2014). In order to disambiguate the term 'biometric', then, we hereon refer to the voice features that vary between individuals as *biometric features* and the process of using biometric features for individual recognition purposes as *biometric recognition*.

In Section 36.2 of the chapter we discuss the concept of biometric voice features and in Section 36.3, the principles of biometric voice recognition. In Section 36.4 we present some ideas on future recognition technology that might become relevant when certain methodological obstacles can be overcome. While the chapter is predominantly concerned with voice recognition for forensic purposes, we also give consideration to commercially-orientated voice-recognition applications, as this contributes to a more thorough understanding of the concepts.

The terms *recognition* and *identification* are often used interchangeably, but sometimes their usage can be confounding. While in the automatic voice-recognition literature, the term *speaker identification* was applied for so-called closed-set recognition in which the most probable match of a limited number of voices is found for an unknown voice (Reynolds, 1995), the term is often used in the forensic literature for the question of whether two voice samples derived from the same or from different speakers (Hollien et al., 2016). However, because of the alleged implication that identification potentially suggests an unambiguous assignment of the same speaker, the terminology was changed to *speaker comparison* (French & Harrison, 2007; Morrison, 2010; Nolan, 1999) in forensic settings and is now typically used throughout the forensic speech community. In this chapter, we use *speaker recognition* to refer to any process of identity attribution based on voice. In the forensic context, we refer to these processes as *forensic speaker comparison*.

36.2 Biometric Features: Physiological and Behavioural

We define biometric features as the aspects of the voice that carry information concerning the speaker and we define voice as any acoustic output of a speaker that is produced by the organs of speech, typically, but not necessarily, with the aim of communication. Two types of biometric features are distinguished in the general literature. First, there are characteristics of the voice that may be attributed to the individual's anatomy and physiology. These are referred to as *physiological* biometric features (often also referred to as *fixed biometrics;* see Section 36.2.1). Second, there are those that are the result of acquired or learned behaviour. These are referred to as *behavioural* biometric features (see Section 36.2.2). As we shall see in Section 36.2.3, in respect to speech, the dichotomy is something of an over-simplification as with many voice biometric features, the relative contributions of physiology and learning are difficult to disentangle and they arise from a complex interaction between the two

(Nolan, 1999). For the purposes of exposition, however, it is helpful to bear with the distinction in the first instance.

36.2.1 Physiological Biometric Features

Physiological biometric features are all characteristics that enter the acoustic speech signal as a result of individual dimensions of the articulators (in particular, the vocal tract) and the movement behaviour of the articulators that results out of their particular design (size, weight, etc.). Examples of voice features that we place into this category also include neuromotor-based speech pathologies, such as stammering, aspects of the realization of alveolar and dental consonants arising from the configuration of the individual speaker's dentition, multiple release bursts in velar plosive consonants (i.e. sounds produced by placing the tongue against the soft palate or velum—[k] and [g]) caused by flaccidity of the velum, certain aspects of voice quality related to the configuration of the vocal tract and larynx, and general voice pitch as a function of vocal folds' mass, length, controlling musculature, and so on. In practice, the forensic scientist typically analyses vocal tract resonances (formants), voice quality, and fundamental frequency to gain knowledge about a speaker's vocal tract and larynx dimensions respectively.

For voice research, the idea of physiological biometric features has been adapted from other biometric domains such as fingerprints or DNA, where the character of physiological fixation is more apparent. Even though the recognition of fingerprints is also problembound and recognition errors can occur (Cole, 2005), those problems are typically related to the recognition techniques in that variable positions and pressures during the application of a fingerprint can lead to signal variability. With physiological voice biometric features the situation is different. Such biometrics are the result of the vocal apparatus and this apparatus—unlike DNA or fingerprints—is not fixed in time but changes as a result of short-term (e.g. influenza that causes swelling of the mucous membrane) and long-term development (e.g. ageing influences on vocal tract shape). When speaker recognition is carried out over the range of a few years, the influences of anatomical changes on biometric voice features can be severe. Such situations frequently occur in forensic speaker comparison as the time delay between a recording of a perpetrator's voice and of a suspect may easily be a few years. In Section 36.2.3 we therefore extensively discuss the variability of speech biometric features.

36.2.2 Behavioural Biometric Features

Behavioural biometric features of voice are, to a large extent, the product of a speaker's linguistic socialization and psychosocial orientations (i.e. speakers learn and adopt the social, regional, and ethnic norms of the speech communities in which they live, identify with, and aspire to). That this should apply to the vowel and consonant pronunciations that collectively characterize a language and accent is perhaps very obvious. However, it may not be so obvious that linguistic learning encompasses aspects of voice quality too.

'Voice quality' refers to effects produced within the larynx (harsh voice, creaky voice, breathy voice, etc.) and to effects resulting from adopting postures, or settings, of supralaryngeal organs, i.e. those situated higher up in the vocal tract (lip-rounding, open jaw, denasality, etc.). Phonatory effects and supralaryngeal settings are undoubtedly partly physiological biometric features, being related to the physical properties of an individual speaker's laryngeal and vocal tract dimensions and configuration. However, the fact that learning also plays a part has become increasingly clear from sociophonetic studies. In respect of British English, for example, Trudgill (1974) reported that working-class speakers in Norwich exhibited creaky phonation, tense vocal tracts, raised larynges, a high degree of nasality, and lowering of the body of the tongue. A study by Knowles (1978) indicated that the accent of Merseyside was characterized by raising and restriction of the tongue body, constriction of the pharynx, speaking with the jaw held relatively close, and denasality. Esling's (1978) research on Edinburgh accents found that working-class speakers spoke in harsh voice, raised their larynges, narrowed their pharyngeal cavities, and protruded their jaws. Also, Stuart-Smith (1999) reported that working-class Glasgow accents were characterized by whispery voice, lax vocal tracts, and raised and retracted tongue body. Middle-class Glasgow accents were distinguished from working-class speech by the absence of these effects. Stevens and French (2012) reported that the voices of male speakers of Standard Southern British English were characterized by fronted tongue body, advanced tongue tip, and sibilance (see also San Segundo et al., 2017).

Studies have also noted age, gender, and ethnic group related patterns (cf. Esling, 1978; Henton & Bladon, 1988; Szakay, 2012; Torgersen & Szakay, 2012; Wormald, 2016), thereby demonstrating that a speaker's voice quality in some measure derives not only from learning at the overall accent level but also from adopting the norms appertaining to subgroups of speakers within accent communities.

The learning a speaker undergoes with regard to voice quality may result in some reduction in the physiological biometric potential of this aspect of speech: 'at a group level, any individual's congenital "default" settings are likely to be varied through social and linguistic socialisation towards ethnic, social-class and regional norms' (French & Stevens, 2013, p. 190).

Further, behavioural biometric features of voice may be found in respect to prosody (i.e. rate of speaking, rhythm, and intonation). Speech is produced by a constant and careful coordination of about two hundred muscles (Marchal, 2009). It seems inevitably the case that not all muscles can be actively controlled by the speaker in the same way. Numerous articulatory movements are thus possibly much less contributing to perceptually salient acoustic information, in particular in their temporal organization (Dellwo et al., 2015). This includes the durational characteristics of phonetic units (e.g. voice onset time—VOT, segments, syllables, consonantal or vocalic intervals) and also dynamic changes of other acoustic domains, such as formant frequencies and intensity changes as a function of time (He & Dellwo, 2016, 2017; McDougall, 2004, 2006).

Two types of dynamic properties of the articulatory motor plant exist—controllable properties and intrinsic properties (Perrier, 2012). Controllable properties can be controlled by the speaker's central nervous system, such as muscle force, stiffness and direction of joints and other tissues. Intrinsic properties like friction, weight, and damping characteristics of the motor plant cannot be voluntarily controlled by the speaker. The controllable properties allow speakers of the same language or dialect to coordinate their articulators in such a way that the resultant phonetic units are similar enough across speakers to maximize mutual intelligibility. For example, while producing a voiceless stop, native English speakers usually produce longer VOT than native French speakers. The speakers in both groups voluntarily control the constriction time of the articulators to abide by the categorical perception cut-off in each language.

However, within the constraint of VOT duration, speakers also show a fair amount of individual difference (Allen et al., 2003) and VOT is highly correlated with speech rate. Speech rate is heavily influenced by a variety of situational factors (e.g. emotion) rather than being inborn. However, since speech rate is to a high degree dependent on up and down movements of the jaw, it seems plausible that the resonance characteristics of the jaw should stand in relationship to speaker individual rates (i.e. larger cavities mean larger articulators mean slower rates). Such individual differences come from speaker-specific biomechanical constraints of the articulators. In addition to VOT, individual differences were also observed in phonemic, voicing, and segmental durations (Johnson et al., 1984; Wretling & Eriksson, 1998).

Moreover, the individual biomechanics of the articulator also influence intensity variability of the signal. There is evidence that the degree of mouth aperture (largely determined by jaw and lip movement) is related to the intensity fluctuation of the signal (Chandrasekaran et al., 2009). Since jaw and lip articulation contains speaker-specific information, such idiosyncrasy can be captured by intensity-based rhythm measures (He & Dellwo, 2016). He and Dellwo (2017) tested whether acoustic features of the intensity curve related to opening or closing gestures of the mouth movements contain speaker-specific information. Measures based on the speed of intensity decrease (from an intensity peak to its neighbouring trough point) explained approximately 70% of the between-speaker variability, suggesting that the closing movements of the mouth contained more speaker-specific information.

Speaker-specific articulation is not only reflected in the dynamic change of intensity levels in an utterance, but is also reflected in the dynamic change of formant frequencies. The shape of the vocal tract is changing continuously as a function of articulation movements, resulting in speaker-specific formant dynamics (McDougall, 2004, 2006).

36.2.3 Variability of Biometric Features Within and Between Speakers

The reliability of voice biometric processes in legal and commercial contexts is not absolute. Problems may arise in particular from two sources—high levels of variability within individual voices (within-speaker variation), and low levels of variation across speakers (between-speaker variation).

Leaving aside deliberate voice disguise for the moment, which brings with it its own problems (Künzel, 2000), in the short term, within-speaker variation may arise from the use of alcohol (Künzel & Braun, 2003) or drugs (Papp, 2008; Papp et al., 2011), smoking (Schwab et al., 2017), illnesses (notably colds and flu), changes in affective states (happiness, sadness, anger) (Sobin & Alpert, 1999), accommodation of one's own speech habits to those of interlocutors (Kim et al., 2011), and changes in accent or formality of speaking style in accordance with one's perception of the communicative needs of the situation (French & Stevens, 2013). Long-term changes arise, inter alia, from the continuing development of the speech organs over the lifetime of a speaker. As the organs change, so does their acoustic 'output' (i.e.

the voice). When speaker recognition is carried out from recordings spanning a long time period, the influences of anatomical changes on biometric voice features can be substantial (Rhodes et al., 2017). Such situations frequently arise in forensic speaker comparison, where the time delay between a criminal recording and a comparison recording of a suspect may easily be several years.

For male speakers, an obvious and well-known example of a long-term, age-related alteration is the so-called 'voice change' that marks the transition from childhood to adulthood. This change results from the production of testosterone which causes rapid growth of the larynx thickening and lengthening of the vocal folds. Resonating cavities and sinuses also expand. The overall effect of these changes, which usually take place over no more than a few months and are completed by around 15 years of age, is that the voice becomes lower-pitched—usually around a full octave lower—and the resonance frequencies of vowels become lower too (Harries et al., 1998). Less obvious and more gradual, however, is the lowering of the lowest vowel resonance that continues into middle age (Rhodes et al., 2017). Men's voice pitch may also continue to decrease until around age 40 years. Then, following a period of relative stability, pitch will increase again into old age, this process usually beginning somewhere between 60 and 80 years of age. Albeit less dramatic than for males, there is also 'voice change' for women, again involving pitch and vowel resonance lowering, which occurs around the time of menarche. The picture between menarche and menopause is variable and rather complex. However, the time from menopause to old age is generally marked by a downdrift in pitch (Baken & Orlikoff, 2000). In addition to pitch and resonance changes, for both sexes the progression from mid life to old age normally sees an increase in 'harshness' or 'roughness' in phonation, as well as an increased breathiness and possible whisperiness resulting from leakage of air at the vocal folds as a function of ossification of the cartilage tissue of the larynx (Wilcox & Horii, 1980).

Between-speaker convergence has been noted as arising from relatively low levels of variability across speakers in respect of vocal tract dimensions (Xue & Hao, 2003, 2006), and through common linguistic socialization. Individual speakers converge in adopting the social, regional, and ethnic norms of the speech communities in which they live, identify with, and aspire to. Very obviously this is so in respect of their adopting the vowel and consonant pronunciations (Babel, 2012; Pardo et al., 2012) that collectively characterize their language and accent. Convergence is more conspicuous among people of the same dialectal variation (Kim et al., 2011). Further, it is becoming increasingly clear from sociophonetic studies that convergence also applies with regard to the prosody of speech (i.e. those features of talk that concern its temporal and rhythmic organization)—rate of delivery (Putman & Street, 1984), amplitude of syllables relative to one another, and intonation (i.e. the 'melodies' of speech resulting from the rise and fall of pitch over the course of utterances) (Leemann, Kolly, & Dellwo, 2014; Leemann, Mixdorft, et al., 2014). Further, between-speaker convergence within accent communities is known to entail voice quality too.

Speakers may also deliberately bring about temporary organic changes in an attempt to disguise their voice—a common phenomenon in forensic recordings. Some parts of the vocal tract are readily amenable to such manipulations. It is possible, for example, to shorten the tract by artificially raising the larynx or to distend the pharynx, which is a major resonating chamber. For this reason, there have been attempts to obtain physiological biometric measurements associated with resonance cavities that are more difficult to alter—the nasal cavity, for example (Amino & Arai, 2009; Amino et al., 2006). A further advantage of the nasal cavity is that, in the course of speaking, its shape remains comparatively unchanged, thereby making it a potential source of stable biometric data from non-disguised speech too.

Similarly, the anatomy of the hypopharynx (the lower part of the pharynx), while having an impact on acoustic characteristics of speech, in particular speaker-specific characteristics in higher-frequency bands, is not amenable to deliberate manipulation by someone wishing to disguise their voice, and again remains relatively fixed over long-term stretches of speech. Kitamura et al. (2005) measured the morphological structure of the hypopharynx (mid-sagittal and transverse sections) using MRI during sustained vowel production. The geometry remained similar across the production of different vowels for each speaker, while between-speaker anatomical differences were found to be large. The transfer functions of the hypopharynges of different speakers showed idiosyncratic effects in spectral characteristics above 2.5 kHz.

A further cavity not amenable to deliberate manipulation or natural short-term segment-related changes is the piriform recess or sinus (the small pear shaped cavity found between each lateral wall of the pharynx and the higher part of the larynx). A study by Dang and Honda (1997) indicated that the morphology of this sinus contributed to antiresonances (areas of low energy) in the spectral region of 4–5 kHz (also see Kitamura & Akagi, 1996). Effects arising from the individual architecture of this sinus have once more the potential as relatively stable physiological biometric voice data.

In addition to its contributing to long-term changes in the male voice, temporary changes to testosterone levels may affect male voices in the short term too (Dabbs & Mallinger, 1999). Level changes may be brought about by dietary factors, physical exercise level fluctuations, alteration to sleep patterns, sexual activity, and, in fact, change over the course of a day, being higher in the morning than the afternoon (Resko & Eik-Nes, 1966). Dabbs & Mallinger (1999) measured the salivary testosterone levels in males and females. They found that in males, but not in females, the level has a significant negative correlation with pitch. There are two possible reasons for this. First, as already stated, testosterone may increase the mass, length, and tension of the vocal folds. Second, it may bring about changes in vocal style, one of which is pitch lowering (Evans et al., 2008). This latter, behavioural explanation is not implausible, as it is known, for example, that males may lower their larynxes to sound attractive to females, thereby creating lowered resonance characteristics (Evans et al., 2006). This may have implications for forensic voice analysis when, for instance, dealing with anonymous sexual harassment calls. Potentially, the vocal tract resonances of the caller could be lower during such a call than those found in later recordings of the perpetrator used for comparison purposes.

The two tendencies then—intra-speaker variation and inter-speaker convergence—pose problems for the task of an expert attempting to uniquely identify an individual by his or her voice. Intra-speaker variation means that two or more recordings of the same speaker may vary in a range of ways that could give rise to a *missed* identification or *false elimination*, and inter-speaker convergence could give rise to the situation where different speakers appeared so similar as to bring about a *false identification*. We return to these problems later in the chapter.

36.3 BIOMETRIC SPEAKER RECOGNITION

Biometric speaker recognition is a process in which the identity of one or more speakers is recognized based on voice evidence. There are a wide variety of scenarios in speaker recognition of which the two main ones are referred to as *identification* and *verification* in the automatic speaker-recognition literature (Reynolds, 1995). Identification refers to the closed-set problem (see Section 36.1). In forensics it can at best be relevant in situations where a larger number of suspects might have produced the recording of a perpetrator, where it might help to narrow down the choice to the most probable match (Petr Motlicek, personal communication). A problem with closed-set speaker identification is that in any case the most probable match will be identified. In absurd cases, speaker identification will provide an answer to the question of which of ten female speakers is most likely to match the voice of a male speaker. This means that an a priori assumption needs to be present that excludes the occurrence of such cases.

In forensic scenarios, the question is often whether two voice samples (typically a sample of a perpetrator and that of a suspect) have derived from the same or different speakers. This speaker comparison process is also referred to as *speaker verification* or *authentication* in the automatic literature. Speaker verification is characterized by the fact that a claim is present about the speaker identity (e.g. two voice samples derived from the same speaker). This is true for automatic access systems and forensic speaker recognition scenarios alike. Here, a system can be both a phonetically naïve human listener, an expert analyst, or a computer system. The system is presented with two voice samples, one of which the identity of its source is non-disputed (known sample) and one of which the identity is unknown. The claim, then, is that the unknown sample was produced by the same speaker as the known sample. Subsequently, the system tests the hypothesis of whether the claim is correct (Ho; same-speaker hypothesis) or, alternatively, whether the claim is incorrect (H1; different-speaker hypothesis). Given this situation, a recognition system can make two possible mistakes. The voice samples presented could have been produced by two different speakers, but the system responds as though they were from one and the same speaker. This error is referred to as a *false acceptance* or *false positive*. In the second possible mistake, the voice samples could have been produced by one and the same speaker, but the system responds as though they were two different speakers. This error is referred to as a *false rejection* or *false negative*.

In automatic access systems, the claim is always that the speakers of known and unknown samples are identical. Automatic access systems can allow physical access to a building or computer system or virtual access to an internet bank account, for example, based on a speaker-recognition process. The known sample here is a recording of the speaker's voice in the system, which the speaker will recognize as his or her own, and the unknown sample is provided at the point when the person requires access. In this situation, speakers have an interest in being recognized (i.e. they are almost always cooperative). In forensic speaker comparison, the most typical scenario is that the known sample is provided by a suspect of a crime and the unknown sample derived from a recording produced by a perpetrator during the crime. In numerous cases, the speech act in the recording is actually the crime itself (e.g. sexual harassment calls, bomb threats, kidnap calls). In such situations, two claims exist in theory. The prosecution claims that the H0 is correct (i.e. perpetrator and suspect are identical), while the defence claims that H1 is correct.

The term 'speaker verification' is typically not applied in forensic speaker comparison scenarios as the automatic literature in the case of access systems, for example, only knows a binary output (yes or no), even though this decision is based on a threshold value in a continuous probability scale. In forensic environments, the output of a system is always a continuous estimation of the strength of evidence (Drygajlo et al., 2014). The underlying processes, however, are mostly identical. A more severe difference between access system verification and forensic speaker recognition probably lies in the way the evidence might be willingly manipulated by the speakers to produce a system error. In access systems, the most likely scenario is that an imposter claims the identity of another person to gain un-authorized access (e.g. to a bank account). The imposter's strategy is then to imitate the voice of the speaker of the known sample. In the case of the system falsely recognizing the voice and providing access, the imposter is successful. In forensic cases, this strategy is reversed. In almost all scenarios, the suspect has an interest in the system responding as though the known and unknown voice samples are from different speakers. In case the unknown and known samples are from the same speaker, the strategy of the suspect will be to disguise his/her voice to make the system produce a false rejection. For this reason, speakers in forensic speaker comparison scenarios are referred to as uncoopera-tive speakers. In both commercial and forensic speaker comparison, however, the false positives are the more dramatic mistakes. In access systems, it might mean that an im-poster gains access to a bank account; in forensic speaker comparison, it might mean that an innocent suspect is sentenced.

36.3.1 Naïve and Expert Human Speaker Recognition Systems

All humans are speaker recognition systems with more or less high performance. Speaker verification occurs in everyday situations. When a family member calls home (e.g. a husband phoning his wife) and asks for confidential information, then the caller makes a same-speaker claim by simply saying 'hi, it's me' (meaning: 'I am the speaker of the voice samples you have stored as your husband'). The wife subsequently carries out a verification process based on the voice sample perceived over the phone and either con-firms or rejects the same-speaker hypothesis. The example shows that speaker verifica-tion occurs constantly in daily life and humans, without degrees in voice analysis and the accompanying technical detail, can perform the process reliably in most cases. This natural speaker recognition ability of humans also plays a role in law enforcement actions in cases when no physical recording of a perpetrator's voice is present but there is a re-cording in the memory of an earwitness. In such situations, the reliability of a particular human to recognize speakers based on their voice is of most interest and can be acquired with the help of psychological tests (Blatchford & Foulkes, 2006; Foulkes & Barron, 2000; Hammersley & Read, 1996).

Forensic voice experts, who might be referred to as human expert speaker comparison systems, also make use of their natural speaker recognition abilities, but these abilities have been trained systematically. In practice, an initial auditory screening of voice is always ap-plied before any other action is taken. Further, the forensic expert typically makes use of acoustic measurements to judge the acoustic similarities or dissimilarities between voices. Such analysis can be the following, amongst others:

- *Fundamental frequency of oscillation* (Fo) is the result of the rate of vocal fold vibration. Lindh and Eriksson (2007) developed an Fo baseline measure (baseline = the average Fo of a person: the standard deviation of Fo of the same person × a constant) and tested this for different speaking styles, vocal efforts, and recording qualities. Within-speaker variability was low among these different conditions, which makes the measures appropriate for between-speaker comparisons. Fo is probably the variable that has been most studied in terms of within- and between-speaker variability. Künzel (2000) tested one hundred subjects with text-reading on five occasions during a period of six months, using their normal voices and two disguise conditions (raised Fo, lowered Fo, denasalization by pinching nose). Results revealed a relationship between the Fo of a speaker's natural speech behaviour and the kind of disguise he/she will use in an incriminating phone call (speakers with higher-than-average Fo tend to increase their Fo levels, those with lower-than-average Fo prefer to disguise their voices by lowering Fo). Fo is also the variable for which probably most population statistics are available to date (for German: Jessen et al., 2005; for Standard Southern British English: Hudson et al., 2007). Fo can have a varying significance depending on the language system. For example, speakers of tone languages differ from each other in the realization of particular linguistic tones (Chan, 2016).
- *Formant frequencies*, determined by the cross-sectional areas and the length of the vocal tract (Fant, 1960; Stevens, 1998), are typically applied in comparisons. Differences in vocal tract anatomy results in between-speaker formant differences which have been applied for forensic purposes (e.g. McDougall, 2006; Morrison, 2009; Pang & Rose, 2012; Rose & Simmons, 1996; Zhang et al., 2006). The advantage of the acoustic analysis over an auditory one is that some formant information cannot be picked up by the human voice (e.g. formant 3 cannot reliably be monitored auditorily and varies between 2 and 3 kHz). Formant frequencies can be speaker-specific in a number of different dimensions—centre formant frequencies of vowels (Rose, 2003), formant dynamics over time (McDougall, 2006), and long-term formant distribution (Nolan & Grigoras, 2005).
- *Voice quality variability* between speakers can be examined using auditory (Laver, 1980) and acoustic approaches (Nolan, 2005). Breathy voice has an increase in the open quotient of the vocal folds, which changes the amplitude of the first harmonic relative to the second harmonic (H1–H2) (Kreiman et al., 2012). Individual differences in H1–H2 have been observed by Jessen (1997) and Kreiman et al. (2012).
- *Prosodic features* of speech—like the articulation rate and the way speakers deviate from an average rate—may vary consistently between speakers (Cao & Wang, 2011; Dellwo et al., 2015; Jessen, 2009). Within-syllable temporal variability has also been shown to be a feature that can be used for recognition purposes (Shriberg et al., 2005). For higher-level temporal and amplitude variability on a phrase level, numerous recent studies have pointed out strong and robust variability between speakers (Dellwo et al., 2015; He & Dellwo, 2016, 2017; Leemann, Kolly, & Dellwo, 2014). To our knowledge, the findings have not yet been applied in case work.

The parameters for identification might vary for different voices, which is why the approaches to voice comparison must be flexible enough to be changed on a case by case basis. Finally, deciding which variables are important and how they should be interpreted is one of the most crucial decisions taken by experts.

36.3.2 Automatic Speaker Recognition Systems

Automatic speaker recognition systems follow the same fundamental principles as human recognition systems. In case of speaker verification, the system compares two voice samples against the same or different hypothesis. Whilst humans have lifelong experience with voices and voice variability, a machine needs to receive such information in a learning phase which is then followed by the test phase. Both phases contain the extraction of speech parameters and building speaker models. In the training phase, the models of enrolled speakers and a background model are built. In the test phase, the model of an unknown speaker (seeking to be verified) is built and compared with the enrolled speaker model and the background model to decide whether the unknown speaker should be accepted or rejected (cf. Drygajlo, 2012 and Hansen & Hasan, 2015, for a detailed description of automatic methods in forensics).

The comparison method between humans and machines is fundamentally different. The basic idea behind automatic systems is to collect frequency-domain characteristics of a speaker produced by static positions of the vocal tract. Such static positions are gained by studying frequency-domain characteristics during short intervals of the speech signal that are short enough to have little influence from dynamic articulatory processes but that are long enough to contain enough information to construct a full frequency spectrum. Given that a fundamental period in voice has a minimal duration of about 12 msec in low-pitched male speakers, the length of an analysis window needs to be at least that. Typically, a value of around 20 msec is used to ensure that at least one male pitch period is captured by the window. Since the articulatory process of speech can be viewed as a vocal pulse that is created by one excitation of the vocal folds that is then filtered in the resonance cavities of the vocal tract, an analysis window of 20 msec takes a snapshot of that process.

A subsequent analysis of speech intervals includes spectral features (e.g. Besacier & Bonastre, 2000; Damper & Higgins, 2003; Franco-Pedroso et al., 2012; Zilovic et al., 1998), glottal excitation features (e.g. Gudnason & Brookes, 2008; Plumpe et al., 1999), and amplitude/duration features (e.g. Reynolds et al., 2002). Although the choice of features differs between systems, based on specific needs, the most widely-used features which yield satisfactory results are the Mel-frequency cepstral coefficients (MFCCs). The general idea behind MFCCs is to segregate the information in the signal produced by the filter from the information produced by the signal. This information contains the closest approximation of the static vocal tract at a particular point.

MFCCs are produced for each windowed signal in the short time interval (frame). For each frame, a spectrum is received that contains lots of noise and discontinuities that is smoothed by a filter bank containing the most crucial frequency-domain information. For each filter band, the centre frequency in the linear scale (Hertz scale) is transformed into the Mel scale. The values in each Mel-frequency band are then averaged. Next, the discrete cosine transform (similar to the Fourier transform, but only real numbers are used in this process) is applied to the spectral vector in each frame, which yields the MFCCs. One MFCC provides a snapshot of the vocal tract at this particular configuration. Multiple MFCC snapshots hence provide information about the vocal tract in numerous positions. From about 30 seconds of speech signal, we can gain enough MFCC frames that contain snapshots of the vocal tract in different positions and allow to build statistical models about the assumed characteristics of this vocal tract.

After obtaining the speech parameters (or feature vectors) of the unknown speaker, the enrolled speakers, and the background speakers, it is possible to build the speaker models and to compare the likelihoods of the speech sample of the unknown speaker coming from the enrolled speakers as well as from the background speakers. With an increase in likelihood that the unknown speaker comes from the enrolled speakers as opposed to the background speakers, the strength of evidence for the same-speaker hypothesis increases (Morrison, 2010; Rose, 2002). A variety of statistical methods can underlie the calculation of likelihood ratios, such as Gaussian mixture models (e.g. Reynolds, 1995; Reynolds & Rose, 1995; Reynolds et al., 2000; Xiang & Berger, 2003), hidden Markov models (e.g. Tisby, 1991; Yu et al., 1995), or neural networks (e.g. Kenny et al., 2014; Xiang & Berger, 2003).

36.3.3 Automatic, Acoustic, Aural—Which Method is the Best?

The question of whether automatic, acoustic, and/or aural methods are the best has been a matter of longstanding debate. While in the very beginnings of forensic speech analysis, purely aural methods were applied, the advent of speech-processing techniques (in particular digital technology) has introduced many ways of analysing speaker-specific information based on objective acoustic measurements. While automatic systems were initially met with severe antagonism by the forensic community, they are increasingly becoming an integral part of the voice-comparison process. A recent survey of INTERPOL (Morrison et al., 2016) revealed that a human-supervised automatic method is, along with auditory spectrographic methods, the second most common technique worldwide.

Guidelines for the usage of fully and partly automatic techniques in forensic speaker comparison are set out in Drygajlo et al. (2015). The acceptance of automatic methods in court can vary widely from country to country, which has a major impact on their use. The application of different techniques is also influenced by the experience of the forensic investigator. As there is no one single perfect method, it seems reasonable to combine evidence from many different analysis methods and not to neglect methods based on human analytical listening (Hansen & Hasan, 2015; Hollien et al., 2016). Indeed, Hughes et al. (2017) showed concrete examples in which auditory voice analysis remedies errors produced by an automatic recognition device. This provides strong support for the view that automatic systems must be combined with human analysis methods.

36.4 FUTURE VISIONS

One of the major drawbacks of voice biometric recognition is probably the fact that the variability of voice biometric features is not yet well understood. With an increasing level of understanding, a number of other applications relevant to forensics can be conceived. Since there is a relationship between anatomical formations of the visible parts of the vocal tract (lips, size of the jaw, nasal shape, etc.), it seems plausible that such visible speaker-specific characteristics can be predicted from voice to some degree. Such applications would allow the drawing of visual images of the parts of the articulators of perpetrators for which only a voice sample is present. Such visual correlates might be present particularly in speech sounds that are produced at predominantly visible places of articulation (bilabial, labio-dental, nasals) or in suprasegmental information that stands in close relationship with the movement of articulators like the jaw (e.g. amplitude dynamics, timing characteristics).

There have been numerous behavioural results in the recent past pointing at the fact that relationships between voices and faces can be predicted, to some degree, by humans (Kamatchi et al., 2003; Lander et al., 2007; Sutter & Dellwo, 2013). There have also been studies allowing that closer descriptions of other anatomical properties of the body might be possible. Hansen et al. (2015) found that speaker height can be predicted from speech to some degree. Sell et al. (2010) found that listeners can estimate upper body strength from voices, especially in male listeners. They found that, in particular, formant dispersions (average distances between formant frequencies) showed a negative correlation with strength measures, while best correlation was obtained for height. Evans et al. (2006) found a significant negative relationship between formant dispersion and body shape and weight. Similar evidence was provided by Fitch (1997) for monkeys.

However, vocal tract characteristics and body size are not always closely related (Gonzalez, 2004) and such dissociations should be expected because of the evolutionary development of the human larynx which was relatively free from skeletal size constraints. Numerous studies reported null effects for voice–shape relationships (Collins, 2000; Bruckert et al., 2006; Künzel, 1989; Lass & Brown, 1978). Future research will show whether and, if yes, to what degree, facial cues can be predicted from voice and whether this can aid law enforcement.

36.5 Conclusions

In this chapter, we explained some key concepts concerning voice biometric features and how such features can be used in speaker recognition. We demonstrated that more knowledge needs to be gained, in particular about the variability of voice biometric features. Future research needs especially to disambiguate the interaction between physiological and acquired biometrics to make voice biometric information a more reliable option for person-recognition purposes.

In summary, our knowledge about voice biometric features is far from perfect and so are our methods to carry out forensic speaker comparisons. This, however, does not only apply to speech but probably to all areas of forensic investigation including fingerprinting and DNA (Saks & Koehler, 2008). With any prosecution, it is inevitably the case that false accusations are possible. Does it mean that we have to give up the task and stop carrying out forensic research? For speaker comparison, the question has been discussed for many decades (Braun & Künzel, 1998) and the answer seems quite obvious. Law enforcement agencies demand evidence from speaker comparisons in many cases. It is absolutely necessary that such evidence is provided by forensic phonetic experts who understand the complex nature of voice evidence as described in this chapter. Only the expert is able to advise the court appropriately about the strengths and limitations of forensic speaker comparison.

There is almost certainly a misconception in the public view about the capability of voice-biometric methods, created by a simplified picture of voice recognition in criminal movies and vastly overstating what can be done in practice. Such mental pictures are, on occasion, taken into the courtroom and lead to falsely high expectations. It is certainly one of the tasks of a forensic voice expert to remedy this by clarifying the true nature of voice evidence. Despite the many obstacles and limitations, there is an impressive and ever-growing number of cases in which such evidence has contributed significantly to solving crime, and this will continue into the future.

References

Allen, J. S., Miller, J. L., & DeSteno, D. (2003). Individual talker differences in voice-onset-time. *Journal of the Acoustical Society of America*, 113, 544–552.

Amino, K. & Arai, T. (2009). Speaker-dependent characteristics of the nasals. *Forensic Science International*, 185, 21–28.

Amino, K., Sugawara, T., & Arai, T. (2006). Idiosyncrasy of nasal sounds in human speaker identification and their acoustic properties. *Acoustical Science and Technology*, 27, 233–235.

Babel, M. (2012). Evidence for phonetic and social selectivity in spontaneous phonetic imitation. *Journal of Phonetics*, 40, 177–189.

Baken, R. J. & Orlikoff, R. F. (2000). *Clinical Measurement of Speech and Voice* (2nd edn). San Diego: Singular Publishing.

Besacier, L. & Bonastre, J. F. (2000). Subband architecture for automatic speaker recognition. *Signal Processing*, 80, 1245–1259.

Blatchford, H. & Foulkes, P. (2006). Identification of voices in shouting. *International Journal of Speech, Language and the Law*, 13, 241–254.

Braun, A. & Künzel, H. J. (1998). Is forensic speaker identification unethical—or can it be unethical not to do it? *Forensic Linguistics*, 5, 10–21.

Breitenstein, C., Lancker, D. V., & Daum, I. (2001). The contribution of speech rate and pitch variation to the perception of vocal emotions in a German and an American sample. *Cognition and Emotion*, 15, 57–79.

Bruckert, L., Liénard, J. S., Lacroix, A., Kreutzer, M., & Leboucher, G. (2006). Women use voice parameters to assess men's characteristics. *Proceedings of the Royal Society of London B: Biological Sciences*, 273, 83–89.

Cao, H. & Wang, Y. (2011). *A forensic aspect of articulation rate variation in Chinese*. Proceedings of the International Congress of Phonetic Sciences (ICPhS), Hong Kong, pp. 396–399.

Chan, R. K. (2016). Speaker variability in the realisation of lexical tones. *International Journal of Speech, Language and the Law*, 23, 195–214.

Chandrasekaran, C., Trubanova, A., Stillittano, S., Caplier, A., & Ghazanfar, A. A. (2009). The natural statistics of audiovisual speech. *PLoS Computational Biology*, 5(7), e1000436.

Cole, S. A. (2005). More than zero: accounting for error in latent fingerprint identification. *Journal of Criminal Law and Criminology*, 95, 985–1078.

Collins, S. A. (2000). Men's voices and women's choices. *Animal Behaviour*, 60, 773–780.

Dabbs Jr, M. & Mallinger, A. (1999). High testosterone levels predict low voice pitch among men. *Personality and Individual Differences*, 27, 801–804.

Damper, R. I. & Higgins, J. E. (2003). Improving speaker identification in noise by subband processing and decision fusion. *Pattern Recognition Letters*, 24, 2167–2173.

Dang, J. & Honda, K. (1997). Acoustic characteristics of the piriform sinus in models and humans. *Journal of the Acoustical Society of America*, 101, 456–465.

Dellwo, V., Leemann, A., & Kolly, M.-J. (2015). Rhythmic variability between speakers: articulatory, prosodic, and linguistic factors. *Journal of the Acoustical Society of America*, 137, 1513–1528.

Drygajlo, A. (2012). Automatic speaker recognition for forensic case assessment and interpretation. In: A. Neustein & H.A. Patil (eds) *Forensic Speaker Recognition* (pp. 21–39). Springer International Publishing.

Drygajlo, A. (2014). From speaker recognition to forensic speaker recognition. In: *International Workshop on Biometric Authentication* (pp. 93–104). Springer International Publishing.

Drygajlo, A., Jessen, M., Gfroerer, S, Wagner, I., Vermeulen, J., & Niemi, T. (2015). *Methodological Guidelines for Best Practice in Forensic Semiautomatic and Automatic Speaker Recognition*. Frankfurt: Verlag für Polizeiwissenschaft.

Esling, J. H. (1978). The identification of features of voice quality in social groups. *Journal of the International Phonetic Association*, 8, 18–23.

Evans, S., Neave, N., & Wakelin, D. (2006). Relationships between vocal characteristics and body size and shape in human males: an evolutionary explanation for a deep male voice. *Biological Psychology*, 72, 160–163.

Evans, S., Neave, N., Wakelin, D., & Hamilton, C. (2008). The relationship between testosterone and vocal frequencies in human males. *Physiology and Behavior*, 93, 783–788.

Fant, G. (1960). *Acoustic Theory of Speech Production*. The Hague: Mouton.

Foulkes, P. & Barron, A. (2000). Telephone speaker recognition amongst members of a close social network. *Forensic Linguistics*, 7, 180–198.

Fitch, W. T. (1997). Vocal tract length and formant frequency dispersion correlate with body size in rhesus macaques. *Journal of the Acoustical Society of America*, 102, 1213–1222.

Franco-Pedroso, J., Gonzalez-Rodriguez, J., Gonzalez-Dominguez, J., & Ramos, D. (2012). Fine-grained automatic speaker recognition using cepstral-trajectories in phone units. In: C. Donohue, S. Ishihara, & W. Steed (eds) *Quantitative Approaches to Problems in Linguistics: Studies in Honour of Phil Rose* (pp. 185–195). München: LINCOM.

French, J. P. & Harrison, P. (2007). Position statement concerning use of impressionistic likelihood terms in forensic speaker comparison cases. *International Journal of Speech, Language and the Law*, 14, 137–144.

French, P. & Stevens, L. (2013). Forensic speech science. In: M. J. Jones & R.-A. Knight (eds) *The Bloomsbury Companion to Phonetics* (pp. 183–197). London: Bloomsbury.

Gonzalez, J. (2004). Formant frequencies and body size of speaker: a weak relationship in adult humans. *Journal of Phonetics*, 32, 277–287.

Gudnason, J. & Brookes, M. (2008). *Voice source cepstrum coefficients for speaker identification*. IEEE International Conference on Acoustics, Speech and Signal Processing (ICASSP), Las Vegas, pp. 4821–4824.

Hammersley, R. & Read, J. D. (1996). Voice identification by humans and computers. In: S. L. Sporer, R. S. Malpass, & G. Koehnken (eds) *Psychological Issues in Eyewitness Identification* (pp. 117–152). Mahwah, NJ: Erlbaum.

Hansen, J. H. L. & Hasan, T. (2015). Speaker recognition by machines and humans. *IEEE Signal Processing Magazine*, 32(6), 74–99.

Hansen, J. H. L., Williams, K., & Boril, H. (2015). Speaker height estimation from speech: Fusing spectral regression and statistical acoustic models. *Journal of the Acoustical Society of America*, 138(2), 1052–1067.

Harries, M. L. I., Hawkins, S., Hacking, J., & Hughes, I. A. (1998). Changes in the male voice at puberty: vocal fold length and its relationship to the fundamental frequency of the voice. *Journal of Laryngology and Otology*, 112, 451–454.

He, L. & Dellwo, V. (2016). The role of syllable intensity in between-speaker rhythmic variability. *International Journal of Speech, Language and the Law*, 23, 243–273.

He, L. & Dellwo, V. (2017). Between-speaker variability in temporal organizations of intensity contours. *Journal of the Acoustical Society of America*, 141, EL488–EL494.

Henton, C. & Bladon, A. (1988). Creak as a sociophonetic marker. In: L. M. Hyman & C. N. Li (eds) *Language, Speech, and Mind: Studies in Honour of Victoria A. Fromkin* (pp. 3–29). London: Routledge.

Hollien, H., Didla, G., Harnsberger, J. D., & Hollien, K. A. (2016). The case for aural perceptual speaker identification. *Forensic Science International*, 269, 8–20.

Hudson, T., de Jong, G., McDougall, K., Harrison, P., & Nolan, F. (2007). *Fo statistics for 100 young male speakers of Standard Southern British English*. Proceedings of the International Congress of Phonetic Sciences (ICPhS), Saarbrücken, pp. 1809–1812.

Hughes, V. Harrison, P., Foulkes, P., French, P., Kavanagh, C., & San Segundo, E. (2017). *The complementarity of automatic, semi-automatic, and phonetic measures of vocal tract output in forensic voice comparison*. Presentation at the 26th International Association for Forensic Phonetics and Acoustics (IAFPA) Annual Conference, Split, July 2017.

Jessen, M. (1997). Speaker-specific information in voice quality parameters. *Forensic Linguistics*, 4, 84–103.

Jessen, M. (2009). Forensic phonetics and the influence of speaking style on global measures of fundamental frequency. In: G. Grewendorf & M. Rathert (eds) *Formal Linguistics and Law* (pp. 115–139). Bern: Mouton de Gruyter.

Jessen, M., Köster, O., & Gfroerer, S. (2005). Influence of vocal effort on average and variability of fundamental frequency. *International Journal of Speech, Language and the Law*, 12, 174–213.

Johnson, C. C., Hollien, H., & Hicks Jr, J.W. (1984). Speaker identification utilizing selected temporal speech features. *Journal of Phonetics*, 12, 319–326.

Kamachi, M., Hill, H., Lander, K., & Vatikiotis-Bateson, E. (2003). Putting the face to the voice: matching identity across modality. *Current Biology*, 13, 1709–1714.

Kenny, P., Gupta, V., Stafylakis, T., Ouellet, P., & Alam, J. (2014). *Deep neural networks for extracting Baum- Welch statistics for speaker recognition*. Proceedings of Odyssey, Joensuu, pp. 293–298.

Kim, M., Horton, W. S., & Bradlow, A. R. (2011). Phonetic convergence in spontaneous conversations as a function of interlocutor language distance. *Laboratory Phonology*, 2, 125–156.

Kitamura, T. & Akagi, M. (1996). Relationship between physical characteristics and speaker individualities in speech spectral envelopes. *Journal of the Acoustical Society of America*, 100, 2600.

Kitamura, T., Honda, K., & Takemoto, H. (2005). Individual variation of the hypopharyngeal cavities and its acoustic effects. *Acoustical Science and Technology*, 26, 16–26.

Knowles, G. (1978). *Scouse, the Urban Dialect of Liverpool*. Unpublished doctoral thesis, University of Leeds.

Kreiman, J., Shue, Y. L., Chen, G., Iseli, M., Gerratt, B. R., Neubauer, J., & Alwan, A. (2012). Variability in the relationships among voice quality, harmonic amplitudes, open quotient, and glottal area waveform shape in sustained phonation. *Journal of the Acoustical Society of America*, 132, 2625–2632.

Künzel, H. J. (1989). How well does average fundamental frequency correlate with speaker height and weight? *Phonetica*, 46, 117–125.

Künzel, H. J. (2000). Effects of voice disguise on speaking fundamental frequency. *Forensic Linguistics*, 7, 150–179.

Künzel, H. J. & Braun, A. (2003). The effect of alcohol on speech prosody. Proceedings of the 15th International Congress of Phonetic Sciences, Barcelona, Spain, pp. 2645–2648.

Lander, K., Hill, H., Kamachi, M., & Vatikiotis-Bateson, E. (2007). It's not what you say but the way you say it: matching faces and voices. *Journal of Experimental Psychology: Human Perception and Performance*, 33, 905–914.

Lass, N. J. & Brown, W. S. (1978). Correlational study of speakers' heights, weights, body surface areas, and speaking fundamental frequencies. *Journal of the Acoustical Society of America*, 63, 1218–1220.

Laver, J. (1980). *The Phonetic Description of Voice Quality*. Cambridge: Cambridge University Press.

Leemann, A., Kolly, M.-J., & Dellwo, V. (2014). Speech-individuality in suprasegmental temporal features: implications for forensic voice comparison. *Forensic Science International*, 238, 59–67.

Leemann, A., Mixdorff, H., O'Reilly, M., Kolly, M.-J., & Dellwo, V. (2014). Speaker individuality in Fujisaki model fo features: implications for forensic voice comparison. *International Journal of Speech, Language and the Law*, 21, 343–370.

Lindh, J. & Eriksson, A. (2007). Robustness of long time measures of fundamental frequency. *Proceedings of INTERSPEECH*, Antwerp, pp. 2025–2028.

Marchal, A. (2009). *From Speech Physiology to Linguistic Phonetics*. London: ISTE Ltd.

McDougall, K. (2004). Speaker-specific formant dynamics: an experiment on Australian English / aɪ/. *International Journal of Speech, Language and the Law*, 11, 103–130.

McDougall, K. (2006). Dynamic features of speech and the characterization of speakers: towards a new approach using formant frequencies. *International Journal of Speech, Language and the Law*, 13, 89–126.

Morrison, G. S. (2009). Likelihood-ratio-based forensic speaker comparison using parametric representations of the formant trajectories of diphthongs. *Journal of the Acoustical Society of America*, 125, 2387–2397.

Morrison, G. S. (2010). Forensic voice comparison. In: I. Freckelton & H. Selby (eds) *Expert Evidence*. Sydney: Thomson Reuters.

Morrison, G. S., Sahito, F. H., Jardine, G., Djokic, D., Clavet, S., Berghs, S., & Dorny, C. G. (2016). INTERPOL survey of the use of speaker identification by law enforcement agencies. *Forensic Science International*, 263, 92–100.

Nolan, F. (1999). Speaker recognition and forensic phonetics. In: W. J. Hardcastle & J. Laver (eds) *The Handbook of Phonetic Sciences*. Blackwell Publishing/Blackwell Reference Online. http://www.blackwellreference.com/subscriber/tocnode.html?id=g9780631214786_chunk_g978063121478625 [Last accessed on 1st August 2017]

Nolan, F. (2005). Forensic speaker identification and the phonetic description of voice quality. In: W. J. Hardcastle & J. Mackenzie Beck (eds) *A Figure of Speech: A Festschrift for John Laver* (pp. 385–411). Mahwah NJ: Erlbaum.

Nolan, F. & Grigoras, C. (2005). A case for formant analysis in forensic speaker identification. *International Journal of Speech, Language and the Law*, 12, 143–173.

Oxford University Press (2017). Entry: biometrics, Oxford English Dictionary. http://www.oed.com/view/Entry/273387?redirectedFrom=biometrics#eid [Last accessed on 29th July 2017]

Pang, J. & Rose, P. (2012). *Likelihood ratio-based forensic voice comparison with the Cantonese diphthong / ei/ F-pattern*. Proceedings of the 14th Australasian International Conference on Speech Science and Technology, Sydney, pp. 205–208.

Perrier, P. (2012). Gesture planning integrating knowledge of the motor plant's dynamics: a literature review from motor control and speech motor control. https://halshs.archives-ouvertes.fr/hal-00714458/ [Last accessed on 29th July 2017]

Papp V. (2008). *The Effects of Heroin on Speech and Voice Quality.* Unpublished MSc dissertation, University of York.

Papp, V., Schreuder, M., Theunissen, E., & Ramakerers, J. (2011). *Reference corpus of Dutch drug users I: MDMA/Ecstasy.* Presentation at the 20th International Association for Forensic Phonetics and Acoustics (IAFPA) Annual Conference, Vienna, July 2011.

Pardo, J. S., Gibbons, R., Suppes, A., & Krauss, R. M. (2012). Phonetic convergence in college roommates. *Journal of Phonetics,* 40, 190–197.

Plumpe, M. D., Quatieri, T. F., & Reynolds, D. A. (1999). Modeling of the glottal flow derivative waveform with application to speaker identification. *IEEE Transactions on Speech and Audio Processing,* 7, 569–586.

Putman, W. B. & Street, R. L. (1984). The conception and perception of noncontent speech performance: implications for speech-accommodation theory. *International Journal of the Sociology of Language,* 46, 97–114.

Resko, J. A. & Eik-Nes, K. B. (1966). Diurnal testosterone levels in peripheral plasma of human male subjects. *The Journal of Clinical Endocrinology and Metabolism,* 26, 573–576.

Reynolds, D., Andrews, W., Campbell, J., Navrátil, J., Peskin, B., Adami, A., ... Xiang, B. (2002). SuperSID project final report: exploiting high-level information for high-performance speaker recognition. http://www.clsp.jhu.edu/vfsrv/ws2002/groups/supersid/SuperSID_Final_Report_CLSP_WS02_2003_10_06.pdf [Last accessed on 5th January 2017]

Reynolds, D. A. (1995). Speaker identification and verification using Gaussian mixture speaker models. *Speech Communication,* 17, 91–108.

Reynolds, D. A. & Rose, R. C. (1995). Robust text-independent speaker identification using Gaussian mixture speaker models. *IEEE Transactions on Speech and Audio Processing,* 3, 72–83.

Reynolds, D. A., Quatieri, T. F., & Dunn, R. B. (2000). Speaker verification using adapted Gaussian mixture models. *Digital Signal Processing,* 10, 19–41.

Rhodes, R., French, P., Harrison, P., Kirchhübel, C., & Wormald, J. (2017). *Which questions, propositions and 'relevant populations' should a speaker comparison expert assess?* Presentation at the 26th International Association for Forensic Phonetics and Acoustics (IAFPA) Annual Conference, Split, July 2017.

Rose, P. (2002). *Forensic Speaker Identification.* London: Taylor & Francis.

Rose, P. Osanai. T., & Kinoshita, Y. (2002). *Strength of forensic speaker identification evidence: multispeaker formant and cepstrum-based segmental discrimination with a Bayesian likelihood ratio as threshold.* Proceedings of the 9th Australian International Conference on Speech Science and Technology, Melbourne, pp. 303–308.

Rose, P. & Simmons, A. (1996). *F-pattern variability in disguise and over the telephone-comparisons for forensic speaker identification.* Proceedings of the 6th Australian International Conference on Speech Science and Technology, Adelaide, pp. 121–126.

Saks, M. J. & Koehler, J. J. (2008). The individualization fallacy in forensic science evidence. *Vanderbilt Law Review,* 61, 199–219.

San Segundo, E., Foulkes, P., French, J. P., Harrison, P., Hughes, V., & Kavanagh, C. (2017). A simplified vocal profile analysis protocol for the assessment of voice quality and speaker similarity. *Journal of Voice,* 35(5), 644.e11–644.e27.

Schwab, S., Amato, M. S., Dellwo, V., & Fernández Trinidad, M. (2017). *Can we hear nicotine craving?* Presentation at the 26th International Association for Forensic Phonetics and Acoustics (IAFPA) Annual Conference, Split, July 2017.

Sell, A., Bryant, G. A., Cosmides, L., Tooby, J., Sznycer, D., Von Rueden, C., ... Gurven, M. (2010). Adaptations in humans for assessing physical strength from the voice. *Proceedings of the Royal Society of London B: Biological Sciences,* 277, 3509–3518.

Shriberg, E., Ferrer, L., Kajarekar, S., Venkataraman, A., & Stolcke, A. (2005). Modeling prosodic feature sequences for speaker recognition. *Speech Communication*, 46, 455–472.

Sobin, C. & Alpert, M. (1999). Emotion in speech: the acoustic attributes of fear, anger, sadness, and joy. *Journal of Psycholinguistic Research*, 28, 347–365.

Stevens, K. (1998). *Acoustic Phonetics*. Cambridge, MA: MIT Press.

Stevens, L. & French, P. (2012). *Voice quality in studio quality and telephone transmitted recordings*. Presentation at the British Association of Academic Phonetics Conference, Leeds, March 2012.

Stuart-Smith, J. (1999). Glasgow: accent and voice quality. In: P. Foulkes & G. Docherty (eds) *Urban Voices* (pp. 203–222). London: Arnold.

Sutter, S. & Dellwo, V. (2013). Audiovisuelle sprechererkennung durch linguistisch naive personen. *Revue Tranel (Travaux Neuchâtelois de Linguistique)*, 59, 167–181.

Szakay, A. (2012). Voice quality as a marker of ethnicity in New Zealand: from acoustics to perception. *Journal of Sociolinguistics*, 16, 382–397.

Tisby, N. Z. (1991). On the application of mixture AR hidden Markov models to text independent speaker recognition. *IEEE Transactions on Signal Processing*, 39, 563–570.

Torgersen, E. N. & Szakay, A. (2012). An investigation of speech rhythm in London English. *Lingua*, 122, 822–840.

Trudgill, P. (1974). *The Social Differentiation of English in Norwich (Vol. 13)*. Cambridge University Press Archive.

Wilcox, K. A. & Horii, Y. (1980). Age and changes in vocal jitter. *Journal of Gerontology*, 35, 194–198.

Wormald, J. (2016). *Regional Variation in Panjabi-English*. Unpublished doctoral thesis, University of York.

Wretling, P. & Eriksson, A. (1998). Is articulatory timing speaker specific? Evidence from imitated voices. In: P. Branderund & H. Traunmüller (eds) *Proceedings of FONETIK '98* (pp. 48–51). Stockholm: Stockholm University.

Xiang, B. & Berger, T. (2003). Efficient text-independent speaker verification with structural Gaussian mixture models and neural network. *IEEE Transactions on Speech and Audio Processing*, 11, 447–456.

Xue, S. A. & Hao, G. J. (2003). Changes in the human vocal tract due to aging and the acoustic correlates of speech production: a pilot study. *Journal of Speech, Language, and Hearing Research*, 46, 689–701.

Xue, S. A. & Hao, J. G. (2006). Normative standards for vocal tract dimensions by race as measured by acoustic pharyngometry. *Journal of Voice*, 20, 391–400.

Yu, K., Mason, J., & Oglesby, J. (1995). Speaker recognition using hidden Markov models, dynamic time warping and vector quantisation. *IEEE Proceedings–Vision, Image and Signal Processing*, 142, 313–318.

Zhang, C., van de Weijer, J., & Cui, J. (2006). Intra- and inter-speaker variations of formant pattern for lateral syllables in Standard Chinese. *Forensic Science International*, 158, 117–124.

Zilovic, M., Ramachandran, R., & Mammone, R. (1998). Speaker identification based on the use of robust cepstral features obtained from pole-zero transfer functions. *IEEE Transactions on Speech and Audio Processing*, 6, 260–267.

PART VII

....

CLINICAL
DISORDERS

....

CHAPTER 37

IMPAIRMENTS IN DECODING VOCAL EMOTION IN SCHIZOPHRENIA AND BIPOLAR DISORDER

DAVID I. LEITMAN AND SARAH M. HAIGH

37.1 INTRODUCTION

PROSODY is the melodic aspect of vocal intonation modulation in which cues such as pitch, change in speech rhythm, change in decibel level, and vocal timbre can communicate affective states or intentions. In clinical psychiatric studies, prosody is seen as a vocal analogue to facial affective gestures, deficits of which have been interpreted as evidence of emotional or social cognitive impairment.

In this chapter, we review the current state of research into affective prosodic dysfunction in schizophrenia, as well as the few studies that have explored prosodic deficits in bipolar disorder. We discuss the behavioural, personality, and biological factors associated with schizophrenia and bipolar dysprosodia. More importantly, in describing how dysprosodia manifests itself in these mental illnesses, we make a number of arguments. First, we argue that dysprosodia in mental illnesses can be characterized by using an information theoretical perspective, in which prosodic abilities are the product of information processing within a distributed neural network. Consequently, there are multiple a etiopathic avenues by which dysprosodia may arise. Second, we argue that abnormalities in both perceiving and producing prosody may stem, in part, from aberrant core audio sensory and motoric functions, as well as from higher-order cognitive impairment. Third, we argue that interpreting dysprosodia as evidence of 'emotional disturbance' may be limiting and misleading. Instead, prosodic deficits in mental illnesses should be evaluated within a psycholinguistic and communication framework that appreciates prosody as both a natural signal and a linguistic coding tool for the expression and recognition of a person's intentions.

This final assertion means that current information theoretical approaches that view dysprosodia as a problem in the capacity of patients to perceive and express prosodic signals in isolation, and without the context of interpersonal communicative engagement, may incompletely model social communication impairment in mental illnesses. We will therefore advocate that future brain and behaviour studies examine vocal emotion and prosody within a more general language and communication framework, and, critically, within actual interpersonal communication.

37.2 SCHIZOPHRENIA

Schizophrenia is a mental disorder that affects roughly one in a hundred persons worldwide. As a disorder, it is characterized by negative symptoms (flat voice, unengagement, lack of conversation, etc.), disorganized thinking and speech, motor disturbances, and positive symptoms (hallucinations and/or delusions). Individuals with schizophrenia may have additional affective (mood-related) symptoms, including episodes of depression and mania, that are secondary to the other symptoms. In cases where the affective symptoms are more common than the schizophrenia symptoms, the patient may be diagnosed with bipolar disorder (see Sections 37.3 and 37.4). For any of these symptoms to be clinically relevant, they must adversely impact the individual's ability to lead a normal social and occupational life.

The onset of schizophrenia is defined by the onset of the first episode of psychosis. Psychosis is defined as a detachment from reality, and episodes of psychosis can reoccur throughout the person's lifetime. Schizophrenia onset often occurs around adolescence and early adulthood, with a later schizophrenia risk in women occurring around the age of 30 years.

Individuals with schizophrenia undergo a period preceding the first onset of psychosis in which they experience symptoms, such as social withdrawal, declining grades at school, and disorganized speech (Insel, 2010), and this is known as the prodromal period. Current research is focused on identifying which prodromal behaviours are the best predictors of who will develop psychosis and schizophrenia. At present, only a third of individuals who present with these behaviours convert to having psychosis (Cannon et al., 2008).

The cause of schizophrenia is currently unknown. There appears to be a strong genetic susceptibility for developing schizophrenia. Individuals with schizophrenia are 5.2 to 9.9 times more likely to have a parent or sibling who also has schizophrenia or bipolar disorder (Lichtenstein et al., 2009). The second and third trimesters of prenatal–neonatal development appear to be the periods of risk for the fetus. Mothers who had their third trimester during the winter were more likely to have a child who developed schizophrenia (McGrath, 1999). Infections or viruses during the second trimester also increase the likelihood of developing schizophrenia (Boksa, 2008), suggesting that an infection during this sensitive neonatal period creates an invisible lesion that predisposes to schizophrenia and other psychiatric disorders. The genetic susceptibility can be triggered by environmental components such as severe, acute stress (Read et al., 2005; Van Winkel et al., 2008). Therefore, identifying genetic, behavioural, and environmental factors that are related to schizophrenia may help improve the ability to predict who will convert to psychosis and schizophrenia.

37.3 Bipolar Disorder

Bipolar disorder is another psychiatric disease that can include episodes of psychosis. It differs from schizophrenia in that psychosis is not a critical symptom for bipolar disorder. Bipolar disorder is specifically defined by large variations in mood—extreme periods of mania and periods of depression (DSM 5). Persons who experience more mania symptoms may be diagnosed as having Bipolar I Disorder, and those with more depression symptoms may be diagnosed as having Bipolar II Disorder. During these extreme mood phases, the individual may report periods of psychotic symptoms. The distinction between bipolar disorder, schizophrenia, and other affective disorders is subtle. Thus, bipolar disorder is partially associated with schizophrenia and partially associated with mood disorders such as depression.

Symptoms of mania include excessive energy, high irritability, and happiness, often accompanied by poor decision making or risky behaviours such as excessive gambling. Symptoms of depression include crying, poor outlook on life, and an increased risk of suicidal behaviour or ideation. Again, antipsychotic medication can help, particularly for those who are experiencing psychosis, but mood stabilizers are more common and can help reduce the severity of the mood swings.

Similar to schizophrenia, there are behavioural characteristics that can precede the onset of bipolar disorder. These characteristics include social withdrawal, mood swings (not grossly affecting occupational or social functioning), risky behaviour, fighting, and falling academic grades. These behavioural signs can be with or without symptoms of psychosis. Age of onset for bipolar disorder is around 25 years (NAMI), and can follow a period of acute and severe stress (Post & Leverich, 2006). Like schizophrenia, there seems to be a genetic component (Lichtenstein et al., 1999). Hence, finding behavioural characteristics that are specific to bipolar disorder vis-à-vis schizophrenia is difficult.

37.4 Prosodic Signals: Acoustic Cues Salient to Prosodic Comprehension

We began this chapter by defining prosody as a signal in which modulations of speech intonation convey intentions or feelings of the speaker. As a signal, prosodic information is encoded in its form or properties, but what is this code?

Prosodic signals result from coordinated motoric gestures made by the vocal apparatus consisting of the lungs, vocal tract, mouth, lips, and tongue. The modulations in 'speech intonation' that are generated by these gestures reflect slow (1–2 Hz) changes in both the speech tempo and dynamics that span the segmental units of speech such as syllables and words. A temporospectral map of prosodic utterances indicates highly collinear changes in pitch, speech rate, decibel level, and spectral energy, which are linked to specific emotional distinctions. For example, pitch contour is the trajectory of the fundamental frequency (Fo) over time (Majewski & Blasdell, 1969; Pell, 1999), and a rise in Fo at the end of the sentence can indicate that a sentence is interrogative and not declarative, whereas the variability in Fo conveys affect (Banse & Scherer, 1996; Davis et al., 2000; Davitz, 1964; Juslin & Laukka, 2001; Ladd et al., 1985; Pell, 1999). Supplemental online Figure 37.1 and its accompanying sound files illustrate some typical stimuli used to test various forms of prosody.

37.5 Measuring Prosody in Schizophrenia and Bipolar Disorder

In both bipolar disorder and schizophrenia, affective prosody reception, as well as its expression, has been measured. Receptive prosody examines whether individuals can either decode or differentiate emotional prosody. Expressive prosody refers to, for our purposes, an individual's ability to perceive or detect prosodic signals, including emotion.

37.5.1 Receptive Prosody

Tasks for studying receptive prosody have, by and large, focused on categorical representations of emotions such as the basic six emotions proposed by Ekman (1976). In the discrimination task, participants are presented with pairs of prosodic utterances and asked whether they portray the same or differing emotions. In the emotion identification task, subjects are asked to identify the emotion of a prosodic stimulus from a list of emotions, in a categorical or forced-choice manner. Less often employed are tasks that require subjects to adopt a dimensional approach, asking them to rate the valence and arousal or approach versus avoidance of a prosodic stimulus on a five-, seven-, or ten-point scale.

The prosodic stimuli employed can range from a single real or nonsense word, to a sentence that is semantically neutral (no emotional expression) in terms of its word content, to vocoded or filtered speech. Most often, these studies employ 'posed' prosodic stimuli (i.e. stimuli produced by actors portraying particular emotions). Research has shown that such stimuli often may exaggerate or be prosodically overexpressive of emotions compared to stimuli abstracted from actual conversations (see Juslin & Laukka, 2001, for further discussion). Therefore, the profound deficits in prosody that are observed when actor-generated stimuli are used means that receptive prosody deficits in schizophrenia may be, if anything, underestimated (Leitman, Laukka, et al., 2010). However, the fact that most studies of receptive prosody in schizophrenia utilize actor stimuli may shed light on the relationship, or lack of one, between prosody perception and prosody production seen in this illness.

37.5.2 Expressive Prosody

Measuring affective prosodic production in individuals with schizophrenia requires analysis of their speech patterns. A subject's speech is either elicited freeform in conversation, or evoked via scripted emotional induction paradigms or instruction to echo short prosodic utterances presented by the experimenter (see Hoekert et al., 2007). In addition, some studies employ repetition paradigms in which subjects are asked to copy or mimic the prosodic emotion presented by clinical interviewers orally or via audio recording. Such repetitions are usually short sentences with semantically neural word content.

37.6 STUDIES OF PROSODY IN SCHIZOPHRENIA AND BIPOLAR DISORDER

37.6.1 Schizophrenia

Our online 'WEB OF SCIENCE' search of prosody recognition studies in schizophrenia yielded forty experimental data studies between 1956 and 2016. Results of the most recent study (Hoekert et al., 2007) indicate a large effect size of d = 1.24, based on Cohen's convention for estimating effect-size magnitude (Cohen, 1988) and perhaps slightly smaller for expressive prosody. As Hoekert and colleagues note, this effect size exceeds the average effect size (d = 0.99) observed across studies of other forms of neurocognitive impairment that include estimates of attention, executive functioning, memory, and language (see Figure 37.1 and supplemental online Table 37.1).

In schizophrenia dysprosodia there is evidence of both *misperception* and *misinterpretation* of emotional intent. By *misperception* we mean that patients are unable to detect the presence of emotion in vocal intonation modulations. This is best demonstrated using

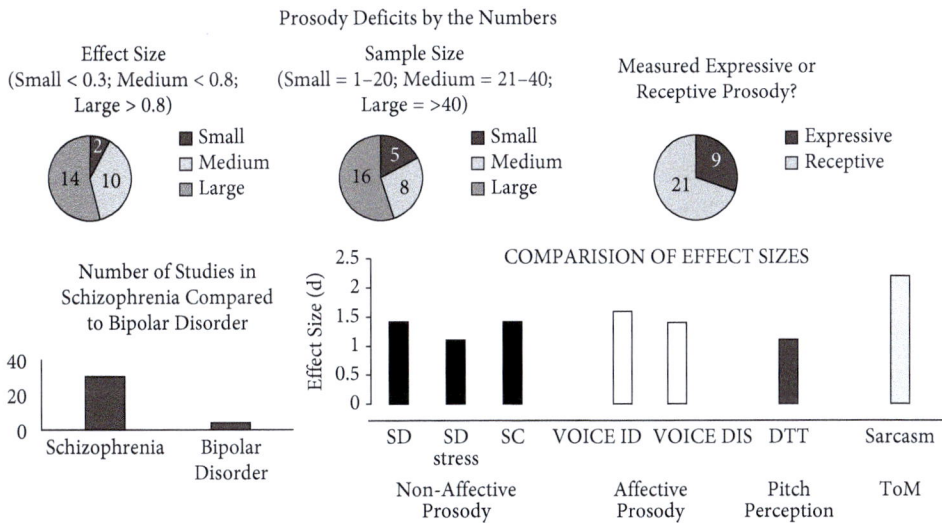

FIGURE 37.1 Prosody deficits: (top) pie charts summarizing the significant characteristics of prosody studies in schizophrenia and bipolar disorder to date; (bottom left) number of studies of prosody in bipolar disorder versus schizophrenia; (bottom right) effect-size estimates of perception deficits in schizophrenia for receptive prosody (affective and non-affective forms), pitch, and sarcasm based on studies of Leitman et al. (2005, 2006, 2007). Abbreviations: SD, SC, Sentence Discrimination and Comprehension (based on declarative versus interrogative) respectively; VOICE ID, Voice identification (emotional prosody); VOICE DIS, Voice Discrimination (emotional prosody); DTT, Distorted Tunes Test.

discrimination tasks in which subjects are presented with pairs of prosodic utterances and asked to discriminate whether they are prosodically the same or different. *Misinterpretation* refers to improperly attributing the wrong affective intent to a prosodic stimulus, such as misidentifying happy prosody as angry prosody.

Several studies have examined the attribution patterns in schizophrenia alongside categorical differences in perceiving negative versus positive emotions. These studies suggest that schizophrenia patients have greater difficulty in perceiving negative emotions and often misattribute positive affect as negative. However, there are a number of concerns that temper such conclusions. First, these studies by and large employ forced-choice categorical identification paradigms, in which happiness is the sole positive emotion in contrast to negative emotions such as fear, sadness, anger, and disgust, making sampling of impaired negative prosody much more likely and reliable. Second, given the forced-choice nature of these paradigms, misperception, in particular, (i.e. an impairment in perceiving dynamic pitch change), may be a sufficient explanation for the attribution patterns observed. For example, one study examined misattribution patterns across stimuli reflecting anger, disgust, fear, happiness, and sadness or no emotion (neutral), and employed multidimensional scaling (MDS) to calculate Euclidean distance relationships between misattribution patterns in emotion identification and the principal acoustic cues or features that differentiate them (Leitman, Laukka, et al., 2010). A significant negative emotion attribution bias in prosody identification in schizophrenia patients versus healthy participants was not observed.

However, MDS analysis revealed the following—whereas healthy subjects' attributions were significantly influenced by dynamic acoustic cues such as pitch variability (Fo_{sd}), schizophrenia patients showed no such influence. Instead, persons with schizophrenia seem to overutilize voice intensity and other secondary cues such as speech attack in discriminating emotion (Leitman, Laukka, et al., 2010). This usage may be in compensation for impaired perception of pitch change, something we address in detail later in this chapter.

Further, that study (Leitman, Laukka, et al., 2010) and another (Gold et al., 2012) demonstrated that schizophrenia patients were less able to discriminate emotional intensity across both positive and negative emotions, and that, overall, they rated emotional intensity significantly higher across all prosodic stimuli regardless of the emotional category. In conclusion, patients with schizophrenia display prosodic deficits in both discriminating prosodic tokens in pairs as well as identifying emotional intent, whether it be of positive or negative valence. Individuals with schizophrenia also display impairment in distinguishing emotional intensity. These results, as well as their identification error patterns, are most consistent with signal processing impairment and an inability to utilize particular acoustic features like pitch, and instead perhaps overutilize spectral energy or loudness (intensity) in their place (Leitman, Laukka, et al., 2010).

Several studies have shown that schizophrenia dysprosodia extends beyond emotion. Accenting or stress within sentences or even words can differentiate semantic as well as pragmatic intent. For example, when subjects are presented with sentence pairs where stress and pausing indicates 'green house' versus 'greenhouse', patients reliably fail to perceive these sentences as different (Leitman et al., 2007). Similarly, the presence of a terminal fall or rise in pitch within a sentence proves to reliably indicate a question or a statement; however, individuals with schizophrenia are considerably less capable than healthy subjects in discriminating them and identifying interrogative or declarative intent.

Patients also display profound impairment in utilizing prosody to override the meaning conveyed by words as occurs during the use of sarcasm (Leitman et al., 2006). This deficit in sarcasm or the perception of 'counterfactual intent' is linked to other forms of schizophrenia impairment in 'Theory of Mind'—or perceiving the intentions of others. Signal processing analysis indicated that impaired sarcasm in schizophrenia is the product of both reduced sensitivity (d') to counterfactual prosodic signal as well as significant bias (b") in perceiving subject speech as truthful (Leitman et al., 2006).

A comparison of the effect sizes across these differing forms of prosodic impairment indicate, overall, large effect sizes that are greatest for sarcasm perception (Leitman et al., 2006) (Figure 37.1), perhaps due to sarcasm's requirement for the individual to override the conflicting semantics contained within the words and to choose the prosodic intention.

For bipolar disorder, eleven studies were found in an equivalent 'WEB OF SCIENCE' search. Two studies directly compared schizophrenia and bipolar disorder, and one study found deficits in bipolar disorder that were significantly smaller in magnitude than in schizophrenia. The studies directly contrasting schizophrenia and bipolar disorder patients contained a small sample and observed no deficits relative to healthy subjects (see Figure 37.1 and supplemental Table 37.2).

37.6.2 Relating Expressive and Receptive Prosody

The connection between expressive and receptive prosodic abilities in schizophrenia is unclear. Analysis of prosodic cues in patients' spontaneous speech found greater impairment in prosodic expression (rather than comprehension) (Alpert et al., 2000; Andreasen et al., 1981; Fricchione et al., 1986; Haskins et al., 1995). Interestingly, several studies that compared spontaneous and receptive affective prosody found no correlation between expressive and receptive prosody (Haskins et al., 1995; Shaw, 1999; Whittaker, 1994). Together this supports the conjecture that affective vocal perception may not be a rate-limiting factor in prosodic expression, but that there may be contributions from motor-related dysfunctions (Alpert et al., 2000; Haskins et al., 1995). One of the general challenges in measuring expressive prosody in patient conversation is that patient responses to queries are often quite terse and non-discursive. This can limit one's ability to measure prosodic intonation features such as pitch variations and trajectories, and to reliably estimate expressive prosody.

These findings are limited to schizophrenia, as no expressive prosody studies have been conducted in bipolar disorder. Differences in the methods used to measure expressive and receptive prosody may explain the relatively poor association between these two forms of dysprosodia in schizophrenia.

37.7 CLINICAL RELEVANCE: THE RELATIONSHIP BETWEEN PROSODIC IMPAIRMENT, COGNITION, SYMPTOMS, AND FUNCTIONAL OUTCOME

As already noted, persons with schizophrenia and bipolar disorder have impairment in social interaction and communication. These deficits are evident even in persons with subclinical disease (Castro & Pearson, 2012), in clinical high-risk individuals with a first-degree relation with schizophrenia (Amminger et al., 2012), and when on or off medication (Hoekert et al., 2007).

In schizophrenia, prosody deficits have been reported in adolescence (Baltaxe & Simmons III, 1995), adulthood (Hoekert et al., 2007), and in the first episode of psychosis (Edwards et al., 2001), suggesting that prosodic impairment may be an illness trait (Edwards et al., 2002). This suggestion is quite provocative in light of evidence that prosodic comprehension is developmental in nature, serving as a precursor for formal language acquisition (Fernald, 1989; Homae et al., 2006). Prosodic dysfunction might therefore represent an early premorbid indicator of schizophrenia brain dysfunction. Consequently, a better understanding of schizophrenia dysprosodia could prove valuable for predictive diagnosis, provide a basis for intervention strategies, and lead to knowledge concerning the aetiology of the disease. For example, targeting schizophrenia for early intervention requires recognition of precursors that precede full symptom onset, so discovery of the neural mechanisms that underlie prosodic deficits is likely to reveal aetiological clues and, subsequently, avenues for treatment.

Neuropsychologically, schizophrenia is characterized by higher-order cognitive disturbance linked to the frontal cortex and also sizeable sensory deficits (Javitt, 2009). Abnormal functioning in glutamatergic and GABAergic systems (Lewis & Moghaddam, 2006) provide a possible unifying mechanism for this widespread dysfunction. Emerging theories suggest that the sensory and cognitive deficits are related (Javitt & Sweet, 2015), but more evidence is needed. Dysprosodia in schizophrenia is linked to both sensory-perceptual abnormalities and higher-order cognitive dysfunction and, therefore, could provide a model of how sensory-perceptual deficits impact higher-order cognition.

Abnormal processing of simple auditory stimuli is related to abnormal processing prosody (Leitman et al., 2006, 2011). At present, these findings are correlational and so it is difficult to tell whether it is the problems in processing simple stimuli that results in problems processing complex stimuli, or vice versa. There is some evidence that improving the incoming signal helps improve more complex sensory processing in schizophrenia. Sensory training methods (i.e. repeatedly being tested on discriminating between different frequency-modulated stimuli) improve sensory gating auditory responses (a positive ERP 50 ms after stimulus onset; P50; and its magnetic version M50) (Popov et al., 2011, 2012), improve N/M100 responses (negative ERP 100 ms after stimulus onset) (Dale et al., 2016), increase gamma and decrease alpha synchronization, improve sensory gating, and improve performance in global cognition and verbal learning/memory (Fisher et al., 2009; for a review, see Vinogradov et al., 2012). This suggests that improvements in sensory processing help improve sensory-related cognitive processing.

There is also evidence that poor prosody processing is related to symptom-level behaviours in schizophrenia. For example, vocal emotion recognition has been found to be correlated with measures of social functioning (Hooker & Park, 2002), and a meta-analysis found a large deficit in emotional expression which predicts social outcome (Hoekert et al., 2007). Deficits in prosody processing are associated with negative symptoms (Castagna et al., 2013; Leitman et al., 2005), positive symptoms (Ito et al., 2013), and overall symptom severity (Bozikas et al., 2004; Tseng et al., 2013). Abnormal lateralization of brain activation to emotional syllables is related to longer hospital stays and greater symptom severity (Bach et al., 2009). However, social cognition deficits are still present even in those who had no residual symptoms after medication (Bora et al., 2008), and are not significantly worse in hallucinators (McLachlan et al., 2013; Zenisek et al., 2015), suggesting that these deficits may persist longer than symptoms.

It is important to note that, although most studies have examined prosody in patients receiving medication, prosodic deficits persist in medically naïve patients as well (Hoekert et al., 2007). While there is no known correlation between medication dosage and prosodic abilities, these negative findings are not dispositive for a potential impact of medication on prosodic function (Leitman et al., 2005). Furthermore, illness chronicity and cumulative effects of medication exposure are highly entwined, complicating assessments of the putative effects of these on prosodic abilities. There is controversial evidence of a neurodegenerative impact, based on correlations linking antipsychotic medication exposure and dorsolateral prefrontal cortex structure and functional impairments. These brain regions are associated with executive functioning and attention. Therefore, diminishing affective prosodic abilities as a result of long-term antipsychotic drug exposure may likely occur. However, adjudicating the effects of medications on cognition based solely on correlations must be approached with caution, as such correlations do not imply causation.

In bipolar disorder, deficits in prosody recognition are related to social anxiety and distress (specifically in children with bipolar disorder; McClure & Nowicki, 2001). However, other studies have not found significant correlations between prosody processing and symptoms (Bozikas et al., 2007; Deveney et al., 2011), suggesting that this relationship may not be as robust in bipolar disorder as it is in schizophrenia.

37.7.1 Individual Differences in Sociality and their Relationship to Prosodic Abilities

As we have previously detailed, individuals with schizophrenia and bipolar disorder often find themselves socially isolated. Social cognitive disabilities, including deficits in prosody processing, could lead patients, either by choice or circumstance, to be isolated. There are a number of studies which examined biological mechanisms that may explain the isolation-induced changes in social behaviour. For example, in NMDAR mouse models of psychosis, social isolation leads to oxidative stress and developmentally progressive dysfunctional emotional and social hedonic behaviours, such as reward preference and nest building (Jiang et al., 2013; for reviews, see also Do et al., 2009; Schiavone et al., 2013).

Other studies identify loneliness (*perceived* isolation) as a key predictor of emotional, cognitive, and physical morbidity (Cacioppo & Patrick, 2009). These effects can be characterized as a personality trait: some individuals can live highly socially isolated lives and be happy and healthy, whereas others, despite living in large social networks, perceive themselves as being isolated. In a recent study, we found that, contrary to some stereotypes of schizophrenia, patients display not only high degrees of loneliness but also levels of desire to socially connect with others (i.e. need to belong: NTB) equivalent to those found in healthy comparison subjects (Mitchell et al., 2016).

Social connectedness refers to our desire to collaborate with others by forming interpersonal bonds and feeling a sense of belongingness to a group. Such estimates of an individual's need for positive, pleasant social contacts and acceptance, as captured by the NTB scale (Baumeister & Leary, 1995; Leary, 2012; Mellor et al., 2008), were found to positively correlate with affective prosodic detection acuity.

37.8 SUMMARY OF BEHAVIOURAL FINDINGS

In summary, loneliness and negative symptoms likely reciprocally exacerbate each other. Both loneliness and social connectedness probably play an important role in governing social interactions and social communication facility. Finally, intact social connectedness in schizophrenia patients suggests that, while they may desire to connect with others, they have difficulty decoding communicative signals because of impairments to perceptual and cognitive signal processing. Therefore, successful remediation of signal processing that improves prosodic function and social communication may ameliorate the loneliness and social isolation that individuals with schizophrenia may feel. Conversely, bipolar disorder, particularly during the depressive phase, may be mechanistically ill-suited to respond to a signal-processing enhancement approach to dysprosodia. Speculatively, bipolar depression subjects may simply lack the motive drive to connect with others and when they do communicate, they are more prone to misinterpret, rather than misperceive, prosodic and social intentions as negative. Thus, biased social communication and mood-based desires mutually reinforce each other.

37.9 NEURAL MECHANISMS FOR PROSODY IMPAIRMENT IN SCHIZOPHRENIA AND BIPOLAR DYSPROSODIA

37.9.1 Classical Theories of Prosody Dysfunction and Right Hemisphere Impairment

The history of the neurophysiological investigation of prosody is inextricably linked to observations of right-hemisphere dominance for emotion processing (Borod et al., 1998; Borod et al., 1990; Heilman et al., 1984; Heilman & Gilmore, 1998; Schirmer & Kotz, 2006). (An extended discussion of the neural mechanisms of prosody is provided by Frühholz & Ceravolo, Paulmann & Kotz, and Whitehead & Armony, this volume).

Elliot Ross (1981) identified a series of right hemispheric lesions that induced a variety of prosodic abnormalities in stroke patients. Lesions in inferior frontal and motor regions of the inferior parietal cortex resulted in impaired expressive prosody (flat affect). In contrast, lesions surrounding the angular gyrus and the temporo-parietal junction resulted in 'sensory' aprosodia, where spontaneous prosody was preserved but patients showed receptive prosody deficits. In subjects with lesions restricted to the temporal cortex, the production and expression of prosody were preserved, while comprehension was impaired. The opposite pattern was observed for subjects whose lesions were restricted to the right inferior frontal gyrus (IFG): these subjects could comprehend prosody but not produce it.

Modern neuroimaging studies indicate a role for IFG in both musical syntax, along with prosodic perception, as well as in production (George et al., 1996; Koelsch et al., 2001; Maess et al., 2001; Zatorre et al., 1994, 1992). These findings are echoed in studies of Parkinson's disease (Blonder et al., 1989; Breitenstein et al., 2001; Caekebeke et al., 1991; Critchley, 1981; Darkins et al., 1988; Pell & Leonard, 2003; Pell et al., 2006). In particular, neuroimaging and neuropsychological studies indicate that prosodic abilities involve the right temporal lobe, IFG, and right Broca's area (Ethofer et al., 2006; Friederici & Alter, 2004; Grandjean et al., 2005; Patel et al., 1998; Schirmer & Kotz, 2006; Wildgruber et al., 2005; Zatorre et al., 1992). Furthermore, right hemispheric specialization for music and melodic aspects of speech, such as prosody, have been found at the level of auditory cortex: the right hemisphere displays clear spectrally tonotopic maps, unlike its left hemisphere counterpart (Liegeois-Chauvel et al., 2001).

In summary, prosodic function is linked to auditory and language processing regions in temporal cortex, motoric processing in parietal regions, as well as frontal cortical regions classically associated with speech production and speech evaluation. As detailed in Section 37.10, schizophrenia patients have substantial information-processing deficits associated with cortical functioning in these regions. Before turning to this, a brief discussion of amygdala and limbic contributions to prosody is warranted.

37.9.2 Limbic System Abnormalities, Emotion, and Prosody

Like other auditory signals involving emotion, affective prosody is likely to involve prominent input from the amygdala (Frühholz et al., 2016). Fear-conditioning studies using sounds, for example, indicate that amygdala processing may rapidly tag incoming auditory signals to prepare for approach/avoidance responses, and afterwards contribute to more extensive, cortically-centred emotional appraisals (Armony & LeDoux, 2010). Other findings indicate that the amygdala is able to decode the emotional meaning from prosody not only when *explicitly* listening to voices (Frühholz & Grandjean, 2013; Frühholz et al., 2012), but can also *implicitly* process the emotionality of prosodic signals when emotional voices are presented outside the current focus of attention (Bach et al., 2008; Frühholz et al., 2011).

Similarly, a small number of studies has shown that contrasting frequency-modulated (FM) signals which approximate the pitch acoustic variations that typify differing emotions such as anger, fear, and happiness, generate an early (> 200 post deviance onset) preattentive evoked response—the mismatch negativity (MMN) (Kantrowitz et al., 2015; Kujala et al., 2005). This FM prosody MMN may generate response not only with auditory cortical regions, but with the insula and possibly amygdala as well. This finding would dovetail with data from both humans and animals indicating that the amygdala may rapidly process or tag incoming acoustic information in parallel with the auditory cortical regions and in a semi-autonomous fashion (Frühholz et al., 2012).

In schizophrenia, abnormal amygdala activity to vocal emotion and prosody has been demonstrated using a variety of neuroimaging approaches (Wildgruber et al., 2006). Studies indicate that the dopaminergically based reward-processing neural network, in which the amygdala interacts with the ventral tegmental area of the orbitofrontal and medial prefrontal cortex in the valuation and prediction of rewards, is severely impaired in schizophrenia (Der-Avakian & Markou, 2011; Fernando & Robbins, 2011). This finding is not surprising given the demonstrated role of dopaminergic abnormalities in schizophrenia and psychosis. Given that neuroimaging studies indicate that these systems are active during prosodic processing, it is plausible that schizophrenia dysprosodia could stem from abnormal limbic activity. However, as we will detail, these deficits fail to explain adequately the full panoply of audio-linguistic deficits including the robust impairment of non-affective prosodic processing.

37.9.3 Basal Ganglia Abnormalities in Schizophrenia

Abnormal dopaminergic transmission in schizophrenia and its role in basal ganglia function may also provide an alternative mechanism for dysprosodia. This line of evidence comes from the presence of prosodic deficits in Parkinson's disease, where aberrant dopaminergic transmission within the basal ganglia and motoric system can lead to deficits both in producing and in perceiving emotional prosody (Blonder et al., 1989; Mobes et al., 2008; Pell & Leonard 2003). Neuroimaging of prosodic impairments in Parkinson's disease has indicated abnormalities of prosody-related activity in the basal ganglia and notably in the insula (Peron et al., 2016). As abnormal prosody activity within the insula has also been observed in studies of schizophrenia prosody (Wildgruber et al., 2006), a motor system origin for schizophrenia dysprosodia is also a possibility. Importantly, as we will describe, individuals with schizophrenia display substantial audio-sensory deficits that robustly contribute to dysprosodia, and cannot be fully accounted for by motor system dysfunction alone.

In conclusion, thus far we have suggested that schizophrenia dysprosodia may be the product of aberrant frontal cortex executive functioning, limbic system activity, and/or motor system activity. However, the observation of basic audio-sensory deficits in schizophrenia, and their correlation with affective prosody abilities in healthy individuals and patients, suggest that impaired audio-sensory processing may strongly contribute to schizophrenia dysprosodia. In the following sections, we detail a series of studies that links auditory processing to affective prosodic processing in schizophrenia, the development of the prosody neural network (PNN) model in schizophrenia, and the clinical application of this model for remediation and treatment.

37.10 Audio-Sensory Perception Disturbance in Schizophrenia and its Relevance to the Prosody Model of Prosodic Appraisal

The best-studied auditory sensory deficits are those of pitch and duration. Deficits in basic pitch perception in schizophrenia manifest themselves behaviourally in simple tasks of tone matching, in which subjects discern whether pairs of pure tones separated by a short inter-stimulus interval differ in pitch. Auditory-sensory memory (ASM) stores representations of the simple physical properties of presented stimuli for periods of seconds to tens of seconds (Cowan, 1984). Using such paradigms, subjects with schizophrenia have been shown to perform extremely poorly on tests of auditory discrimination (Javitt et al., 1997; Strous et al., 1995a). However, when task difficulty was decreased by increasing pitch separation between stimuli (Δf), retention of information appeared to be unimpaired in schizophrenia (Javitt et al., 1997). This strongly suggests that ASM in schizophrenia functions similarly to that of controls, except that a reduced precision of the pitch information is retained or utilized.

Further, this deficit does not seem to reflect working memory dysfunction, as Rabinowicz et al. (2000) have shown that patients and controls show a similar rate of performance (accuracy) fall-off when tone pair sequences are interrupted by distractor noise. On average, individuals with schizophrenia need three to four times the Δf observed in healthy subjects to achieve greater than 75% tone discrimination accuracy.

37.10.1 Pitch Deficits in Schizophrenia and their Relationship to Dysprosodia

A series of studies has demonstrated that tone matching correlates significantly with affective (Leitman et al., 2005, 2006; Matsumoto et al., 2006) as well as non-affective processing (Leitman et al., 2007) deficits, and explained roughly 22% of the variance in performance of the tone-matching tasks (Gold et al., 2012) (Figure 37.2).

37.10.2 Electrophysiological Studies

The temporal resolution in electrophysiological investigations of auditory processing deficits in schizophrenia provides evidence of a distributed hierarchical pattern of dysfunction, beginning with early and pre-attentive detection of changes in the auditory environment. Event-related potentials (ERPs) of deviance detection, known as mismatch negativity (MMN), have shown that MMN (~150 ms after deviant onset) reflects pre-attentive cognitive processing of stimulus deviation. Attention and task demand also play an important

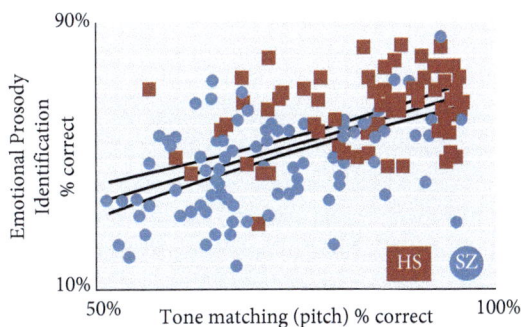

FIGURE 37.2 Correlations between tone pitch discrimination and emotional prosody in schizophrenia. Robust correlations in both healthy subjects are present and indicate that SZ tone-matching performances explain 22% of variance in emotional prosody identification.

Reproduced from Rinat Gold, Pamela Butler, Nadine Revheim, David I. Leitman, John A. Hansen, Ruben C. Gur, Joshua T. Kantrowitz, Petri Laukka, Patrik N. Juslin, Gail S. Silipo, and Daniel C. Javitt, Auditory Emotion Recognition Impairments in Schizophrenia: Relationship to Acoustic Features and Cognition, *The American Journal of Psychiatry*, 169 (4), pp. 424–432, Figure 5a, doi: 10.1176/appi.ajp.2011.11081230, Copyright © 2012, American Psychiatric Association.

role in auditory processing, and auditory selective attention is particularly impaired in schizophrenia. Leitman and colleagues contrasted healthy subjects and schizophrenia patients during both passive and active auditory oddball detection. They utilized the MMN to estimate pre-attentive detection of P300—a positive ERP ~300 ms after deviant onset—to index attention-driven detection (Leitman et al., 2007). Two stimulus conditions included deviant stimuli that were 50% Δf of the standard tones, or much more subtle deviants that were titrated to the individual subject's Δf detection threshold. A comparison of healthy subjects and patients revealed MMN deficits in the fixed 50% Δf condition, but normal MMN in the threshold condition. This result suggests that early auditory processing in schizophrenia is functional, but that pitch information is underutilized. When contrasting P300 generation to 50% Δf deviant tones and deviant tones at individual Δf thresholds, the schizophrenia P300 deficit was still substantial (Cohen's d = 0.70) (Leitman et al., 2007). Therefore, patients have both pre-attentive and attention-based deficits in detecting changes in their auditory environment. Deviance detection deficits are also evident later in the auditory hierarchy when processing deviants in patterns (Coffman et al., 2016; Haigh et al., 2016).

Studies of resting state brain activity, as well as the fluctuations in activity before and during stimulus presentation, suggest that in individuals with schizophrenia, auditory oscillatory brain rhythms and activity are intrinsically poorly orchestrated. These baseline deficits leave patients poorly predisposed to respond to incoming stimuli (Lakatos et al., 2013; Uhlhaas, 2012).

In summary, electrophysiological studies of basic auditory processing of pitch tones suggest that impaired auditory processing in schizophrenia is caused by deficits in top-down attentional modulation and deficits in the ability to utilize bottom-up information to help assess the auditory environment.

37.10.3 Neuroimaging Studies of Prosody in Healthy Subjects and Schizophrenia

As we have already detailed, the production of emotional prosody involves changing the vocal tract configuration to modulate the pitch, intensity, and spectral profile of speech in affectively salient ways. For example, modulation of fundamental frequency (perceived pitch variability: Fo_{SD}) correlates with the accuracy of fear and happiness identification, whereas anger identification improves with increasing proportions of high spectral energy (i.e. the ratio of spectral energy below and above 500 Hz: HF_{500}) (Leitman, Laukka, et al., 2010). In a series of studies, we demonstrated a linear relationship between Fo_{SD} and the ability to identify happiness and fear. This pitch emotion identification relationship is substantially weaker in individuals with schizophrenia, indicating that patients are less able to utilize pitch cues in discriminating affective intent (Leitman, Laukka, et al., 2010; Leitman, Wolf, et al., 2010; Leitman et al., 2011).

Employing functional magnetic resonance imaging (fMRI) studies in conjunction with a prosody identification paradigm, we exploited this phenomena and delineated a prosody neural network (PNN) and tested a multi-stage model (Figure 37.3) of affective prosodic processing (Leitman, Wolf, et al., 2010; Leitman et al., 2011).

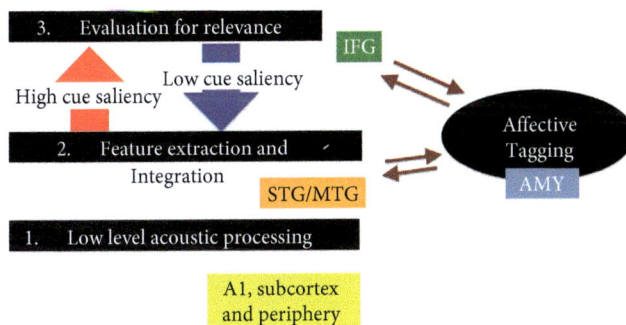

FIGURE 37.3 Cognitive model for affective prosody appraisal (based on Schirmer & Kotz, 2009; Leitman et al., 2010). Within this model, affective prosodic comprehension has been parsed into multiple stages: (1) elementary sensory processing within primary auditory cortex and below (A1); (2) temporo-spectral processing to extract salient acoustic features and integrate them into the emotional acoustic object within superior and middle temporal gyri (STG/MTG); (3) evaluation of the object for meaning and goal relevance with inferior frontal gyri (IFG); (4) fast subcortical processing of gross auditory features conducted by the amygdala to rapidly tag incoming information for fight or flight purposes. Together these processing stages comprise a circuit with reciprocal connections between nodes. Hypothetically, parametric increases in acoustic features that typify one emotion to the exclusion of all others (cue salience) mean high signal richness and predominately feedforward (bottom-up) flow of information processing within model stages (red arrow). Conversely, low cue saliences or signal ambiguity cause increased evaluation within IFG and top-down modulation of features and extraction/integration mechanisms within STG and MTG (blue arrow).

Specifically, we found a reciprocal pattern of activity in the temporal and frontal cortex as well as the amygdala. Activity in the amygdala and the superior and middle temporal gyri (STG/MTG) parametrically increased as signal richness (i.e. prosodic cue salience such as increasing pitch Fo_{SD} for happiness) became stronger, without being able to determine any amygdala–STG/MTG connectivity. In the IFG, however, *low* prosodic cue salience, leading to high perceptual ambiguity, was associated with increased activity, mirrored by higher IFG–STG/MTG functional connectivity. We concluded that increases in cue salience lead to feedforward feature extraction and integration by the amygdala and STG/MTG, whereas higher IFG activity and IFG–STG/MTG functional connectivity reflect recurrent IFG contributions to the formation of the prosodic percept. In addition to these temporal and frontal cortical regions, parametric changes in cue salience also yielded correlated activation changes in a number of additional cortical and subcortical regions including insula, presupplementary motor area, anterior and posterior cingulate, and precuneus (see Figure 37.4).

In schizophrenia, parametric increases in cue salience levels failed to produce the same identification rate increases as in healthy subjects. These deficits correlated with diminished reciprocal activation changes in superior temporal and inferior frontal gyri and reduced temporofrontal connectivity. Additionally, patient task activation also correlated with independent measures of pitch perception and negative symptom severity.

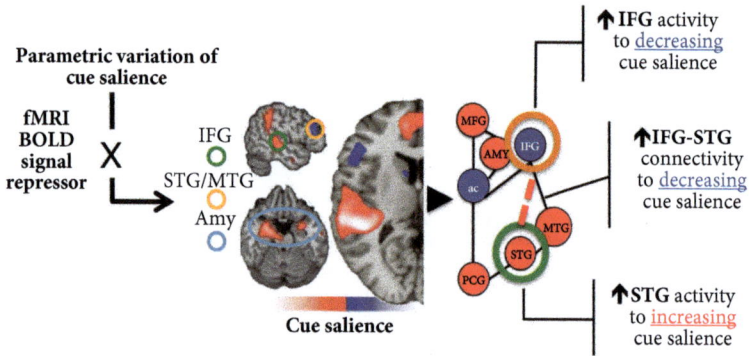

FIGURE 37.4 fMRI modelling of prosody neural network. fMRI colour maps and node schematic depict activation changes across emotions that correlated with cue salience level. Coloured rings circle a priori regions of interest (ROIs). Regressing cue salience features of the prosody with fMRI regional BOLD activity revealed how increasing cue salience correlated with activation increases in superior and middle temporal gyri and amygdala (red). Decreasing cue salience correlated with increased frontal activity within IFG and anterior cingulate gyri. Additional ROIs that displayed parametric modulations to cue salience level included posterior cingulate and precuenus (PCG) and medial frontal gyrus (MFG). Individuals with schizophrenia displayed reduced activity within all these regions as well as decreased IFG–STG connectivity as cue saliency diminished and emotion detection of prosody was difficult (red dotted line).

This PNN model integrates well with more general models of speech and language processing in which STG/MTG–IFG cross-regional communication involves dual pathways or streams (Frühholz & Grandjean, n.d.; Frühholz et al., 2015; Sammler et al., 2015). Processing communication along these pathways is effected via white-matter fibre bundles such as the dorsal superior longitudinal fasciculus and, ventrally, through fibres crossing the extreme capsule (Sammler et al., 2015; Saur et al., 2008).

Using diffusion tensor imaging (DTI), Leitman et al. (2007) found robust correlations between DTI estimates of impaired structural integrity. Moreover, schizophrenia affective prosodic identification deficits correlated specifically with estimates of the white-matter fibre pathway integrity in the fibre bundles connecting the STG and IFG (Figure 37.5).

In summary, audio-sensory perceptual impairment in pitch contributes to dysfunctions in higher-order musical perception and prosody, both of which rely heavily on pitch cues. Prosodic impairments extend beyond emotion to semantic compression, including stress prosody and the differentiation of interrogative from declarative intent. Schizophrenia deficits in pitch and prosodic processing are linked to both functional and structural impairment in both dorsal and ventral auditory-language pathways, likely reflecting a distributed and hierarchical pattern of elemental auditory processing as well as attention-based and executive impairments found in the illness. Therefore, dysprosodia in schizophrenia, rather than reflecting a right hemisphere or limbic centric-based 'emotional disturbance' per se, is better modelled from an information theoretic perspective as a malfunction in the capacity of complex signal processing.

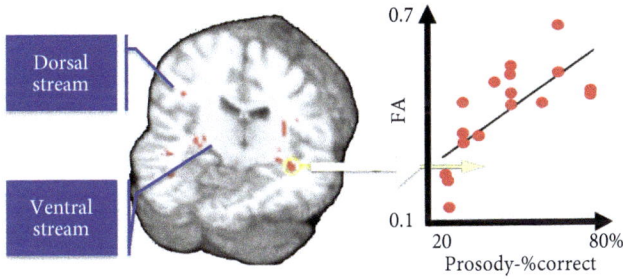

FIGURE 37.5 Three-dimensional voxel-wise correlation map for VOICEID (affective prosody) performance in schizophrenia patients, displaying correlations within the dorsal and ventral stream.

37.11 GENERAL DISCUSSION

Our aim in this chapter was to both summarize and characterize the nature and extent of vocal emotion communication impairment via prosody in individuals with schizophrenia, and, to a lesser extent, such deficits in bipolar disorder. We began by detailing two forms of affective prosody dysfunction—receptive prosody and expressive prosody—and the heterogeneous methods employed in measuring both forms. Schizophrenia studies indicate large effect-size deficits in patients for both receptive and expressive prosody (Hoekert et al., 2007).

We then detailed the ecology of prosodic disturbance in schizophrenia, in which we highlighted that schizophrenia dysprosodia takes the form of both *misperception* or the failure to detect emotional intent as well as misinterpretation, and the *misattribution* of emotional intent. In schizophrenia, misinterpretation may be due to impaired signal processing and/or the inability to utilize prosodic salient cues like pitch to decode emotional intent. In bipolar disorder, a paucity of data precludes such an extended analysis, but based on studies of negative bias in emotion perception in major depression (Luck & Dowrick, 2004; Péron et al., 2011), one might reasonably speculate that patients with depressive symptoms (such as in the depressive phase of bipolar disorder or psychotic illness) might likewise display a bias toward perceiving prosodic signals with no or low positive valence as being more negative, in comparison to healthy subjects. Such distinctions in behaviour, we argue, can in part inform the a etiopathic and mechanistic nature of the prosodic deficits (see Figure 37.6).

Indeed, as we have detailed, vocal emotion communication via prosody involves a complex distributed neural network involving limbic, audio language, and motoric/basal ganglia neural systems. Insults to any of these neural systems are sufficient to generate dysprosodia in neuropsychiatric illnesses like schizophrenia and bipolar disorder, and these multiple avenues may explain the presence of dysprosodia in a diverse range of brain disorders such as autism, learning disorders (dyslexia), Parkinson's disease, and major depression. In Figure 37.6, we outline how particular constellations of auditory processing, language, and prosodic deficits, along with measures of individual personality

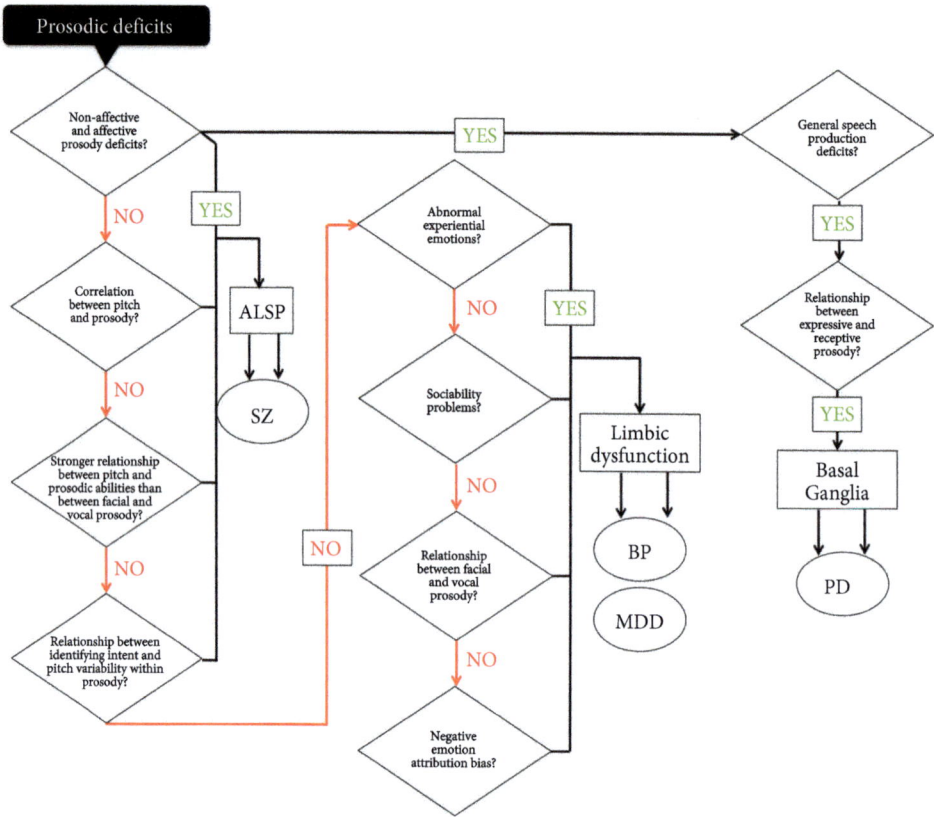

FIGURE 37.6 A decision tree model displaying how differing patterns of prosodic abilities support differing neural models and illness.

differences in sociality, can be used to selectively differentiate the best cognitive neuroscience model for dysprosodia.

37.11.1 Audio-Linguistic Signal Processing Model of Schizophrenia Dysprosodia

In schizophrenia, we argue for the audio-linguistic signal processing (ALSP) model that focuses on deficiencies in encoding incoming auditory signals. These deficits begin at early and pre-attentive stages of auditory processing and combine with higher-order cognitive impairments to critically hamper the ability of prosodic neural networks to extract and integrate acoustic prosodic features into a coherent emotional percept, as well as to evaluate it for meaning and goal relevance. We believe it is the ALSP model which best explains the data, while offering clear theoretical predictions as well as avenues for remediation.

In Figure 37.6 we summarize the impairment characteristics that we believe support the ALSP model as the best-fitting model to explain schizophrenia dysprosodia. Characteristic indicators that would support the two alternative models are also detailed—namely, impaired limbic function and motoric basal ganglia-based impairment. The dearth of comparative information regarding prosody disturbance in bipolar disorder, combined with other affective science findings, suggest that dysprosodia in bipolar disorder may be, on balance, more compatible with the limbic model, although more data is needed to fully support such a conclusion.

37.11.2 Implications of the Audio-Linguistic Signal Processing Model

37.11.2.1 *Treatment: Cognitive Remediation of Pitch Deficits*

Intact motivation to connect with others (as seen by the aforementioned NTB study), coupled with pitch-driven prosody deficits, suggests that cognitive remediation of pitch perception or targeted behavioural approaches that examine sensitivity to prosodic contours may be potential beneficial avenues for remediating prosodic dysfunction in schizophrenia. However, illnesses in which dysprosodia is symptomatic of a generalized reduction in motivation to connect with others or of diminished reward salience of social communication, which has been hypothesized to be the case in autism (Chevallier et al., 2012), may not benefit.

Signal processing remediation might also fail in mood disorders such as depression, in which prosodic deficits are more likely to be reflective of motoric and/or limbic abnormalities, and where receptive prosodic deficits manifest themselves more as misinterpretation rather than misperception. This may be the case in bipolar disorder, but a paucity of studies makes this assertion largely a matter of conjecture at this point.

37.11.2.2 *Treatment: Neurostimulation*

Linking pitch and prosody deficits to common mechanistic impairment in auditory sensory processing suggests that neurostimulation approaches may be able to enhance prosodic performance in patients. For example, two studies by Schaal and colleagues demonstrated the potential for non-invasive brain stimulation to alter auditory pitch perception. In the first study, the authors demonstrated enhanced pitch memory performance in amusia patients during online transcranial alternating current stimulation (tACS) (Schaal et al., 2015). In the second study, they observed that anodal transcranial direct stimulation (tDCS) of the supramarginal gyrus (SMG) improved subsequent (*offline*) pitch memory performance in healthy subjects (Schaal et al., 2013).

Filmer et al. (2014) recently hypothesized that excitatory/inhibitory (E/I) imbalances could be restored to homeostatic conditions with tDCS: tDCS may shift the glutamatergic balance due to changes of glutamate/GABA concentration. This notion dovetails nicely with the role of E/I balance in generating coordinated responses in pyramidal assemblies that are the principal sources for the impaired auditory electrophysiological impairments previously detailed, as well as the putative molecular mechanism for schizophrenia pathology (Lewis & Moghaddam, 2006).

37.11.2.3 *Translation*

The ALSP model and the nature of the electrophysiological deficits observed in schizophrenia suggest that it is possible to develop a framework based on 'neural oscillations' that can mechanistically explain how the perception of simple tone sequences and more complex prosodic utterances are both dependent on an individual's ability to align his/her internal brain activity to regularities in the external auditory signal. This lends ecological validity to granular studies in animals focusing on linking molecular mechanisms such as homeostatic E/I imbalances in glutamate/GABA concentrations and the brain responses to sounds, as the processing of simple 'beeps' and 'boops' is now intrinsically related to more complex signal processing of speech prosody. By conducting experiments that link pitch perception to affective prosody, through shared oscillatory mechanics, one may be able in the future to build on such studies and extend vocal emotion communication research to ecologically valid studies examining prosody in turn-taking dynamics, thereby examining oscillatory entrainment across multiple phenomenological scales. Indeed, the last couple of years has seen a strong push in developing a cognitive neuroscience framework for measuring brain activity associated with interpersonal communication (see Wilson, 2005).

37.11.2.4 *Development*

Whereas the ability for audio-sensory processing of core acoustic features such as pitch and intensity reaches maturity during childhood, social, cognitive, and communication abilities continue to mature during adolescence and early adulthood. However, only a handful of studies has examined prosody development. Moreover, clinically, psychosis most frequently emerges during adolescence. Studying the relationship between brain change, auditory processing, and social communication abilities (prosody) therefore has great clinical relevance. The ALSP model would predict that prosodic development be neutrally associated with the consolidation of both functional and structural connections in frontal and temporal cortical as well as limbic and subcortical processing hubs. It would further predict that developmental prosodic processing enhancements might be largely due to an increased capacity for top-down modulation of temporal cortical brain regions tasked with the extraction and integration of emotionally salient auditory features, leading to increased sensitivity in detecting emotional signals.

37.11.3 Feedforward and Top-Down Mechanisms: Audio-Linguistic Signal Processing (ALSP) Model

The genesis of the ALSP model for schizophrenia dysprosodia lies in observations of its strong link to more elemental auditory processing deficits. However, generalized assessments of executive function, such as perseveration rates on the Wisconsin Carts Sorting Task (WCST), also account for substantial contributions to prosodic comprehension abilities that are independent from the elemental pitch perception deficits. These data suggest that ALSP dysfunction is likely the product of both feedforward as well as more general top-down processing (Leitman et al., 2007).

37.12 BEYOND THE INFORMATION THEORETIC PERSPECTIVE: EXPLORING VOCAL EMOTION EXPRESSIONS AS COMMUNICATIVE ACTS

In his book *The Nature of Facial and Vocal Expressions in Man and Animals*, Darwin suggests that vocal emotional expression may convey internal emotional arousal states or actively *communicate* an emotional message (Darwin, 1865). This distinction between the vocal expression as portraying the inner emotional state of oneself versus a communicative tool is a crucial one, and it is of critical importance to the study of impaired emotional expressivity in psychiatric illness. As we will discuss, our primary interest is the communicative function.

In cataloguing the multiple ways we can express emotion, we can classify these expressions, as Wharton does (2003), as being '*signs* in which the sign as an object provides *evidence* of an emotional state or intention' and '*signals* in which the information is encoded within the signal form itself'. Figure 37.7 details the taxonomy of vocal emotional expressions that are delineated within this framework.

37.12.1 Prosody Utilization Within a Situational and Linguistic Context

Thus far, we have detailed the benefits of the ALSP information theoretic model by describing both its explanation of the behavioural manifestation of dysprosodia and its utility in building cognitive neuroscience models of this pathology in schizophrenia. However, it is massively self-evident that prosodic expressions are employed naturally within a context. Globally, this context is in relation to current and past conditions or actions that the individual has experienced, and, more specifically, within an interpersonal interaction such as a conversation. Such interactions utilize language, and prosody is deployed as a semi-channel of communication to the words and sentences that make up speech.

The overall majority of prosody studies have not examined receptive prosody in context in schizophrenia. Nevertheless, clinical studies of both schizophrenia and bipolar disorder demonstrate that patients often react in socially or emotionally inappropriate ways during conversational interactions. Indeed, such inappropriate responses (e.g. expressing joy in scenarios such as a funeral where sadness or grief may be more appropriate) are often prominent in bipolar mania and psychosis. In such cases, one implicitly acknowledges that it is the sad context (e.g. the funeral) that marks these 'odd' gestures as incongruent, and we judge the prosody as emotionally and socially inappropriate not only because the signal (joy) seems to be incongruent with both our own feelings (grief) and the context (funeral), but also because we judge the (subject with schizophrenia) person's intentions to prosodically share happiness in these situations to be incompatible with creating a shared conceptual common

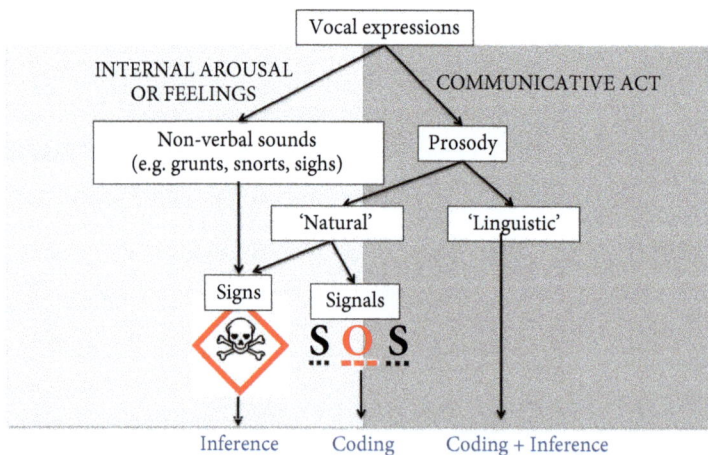

FIGURE 37.7 The taxonomy of vocal emotion expression (based in part on Wilson & Wharton, 2006). Natural signs and signals are those whose form are thought to be intrinsically connotative of affective feeling and do not necessarily rely on some preconceived linguistic code. Sighing or uttering 'ow' are non-verbal examples and, similarly, the intonations and sound profile of prosodic conveniences of surprise or anger may also convey those emotions by being intrinsically unpleasant or unexpected. For signs, meaning is inferred: thus, a sigh is not decoded as signalling tiredness, but rather as *evidence* of fatigue and *inference* of tiredness. In contrast, natural signals contain coded communicative information. Signals on the other hand do not merely infer a state or an intention but contain coded information of intention or state and are directly communicative in nature. Melodic variations in intonation that change melody or increase voice quality or harshness in tone may, like pitch dissonance, be intrinsically unpleasant. Such prosodic signals could be thought of as prosodically echomimetic, equivalent to onomatopoeic words such as 'buzz' or 'chirp' whose meaning are acoustically 'built in'. The degree of 'naturalness' of signs or signals may vary—strongly natural ones are more likely to be universally perceived regardless of language and evolutionarily preserved across species. In contrast, prosodic signals might also rely on *linguistic* coding that requires, by nature, an agreed upon and shared understanding of meaning. In summary, prosody signals that communicate emotion may prove communicative, either as signs that provide evidence of intention, or as coded signals that convey the informational intent. Such distinctions have clear clinical implications in characterizing as well as treating social cognitive and emotional dysfunction in both schizophrenia and bipolar disorder.

ground within the funeral context. (That is, as a receiver, I am thinking to myself 'even if you are happy, why would you share that or react with me that way here and now?')

In their 1967 book entitled *The Pragmatics of Human Communication*, Watzlawick et al. emphasize the importance of viewing prosody, and verbal and non-verbal communication like prosody, not merely as *monadic* impairment in one's ability to express or receive prosodic signals, but as a dysfunctional *dyadic* interaction in which the relationship between members, or lack of one, is a function of communication or its impairment (Watzlawick et al., 1967). Thus, communicatory signals such as prosody have a function and intention. Communication researchers such as Clark (Clark & Wilkes-Gibbs, 1986) and Grice (1975) argue that this function is to build common conceptual ground.

Developmental psychologists such as Tomasello argue that such communication is part of our evolutionary fitness as a species, whose survival depends on collaborative actions (Tomasello, 2010). Perhaps for this reason we, as humans, enjoy the 'communing' aspect of language and communication, which is a means to a collaborative end and also an end in and of itself (Locke, 2001). This evolutionary wiring means that we are intended to be communicative and, as Watzlawick et al. (1967) argue, it may be impossible not to communicate, as silence itself can often speak volumes. Confronted by an inability to perceive communication signals within an interpersonal interaction, it is easy to understand how individuals with these mental illnesses might find such interactions less rewarding than healthy individuals do, and even downright puzzling, and in the end seek to withdraw from social interactions completely.

37.12.2 Dyadic Communication Perspective—Additional Dimensions and Ramifications to the Study of Vocal Emotion and Prosody, and its Significance in Mental Disorders

Within dyadic communication, two or more individuals engage in a series of coordinated interactions to share their intentions and information with one another, and together build common conceptual ground. Within conversations such communication involves visual and audio-linguistic gestures. If one of the interlocutors has schizophrenia or bipolar disorder, it may very well be that internal biological factors lead the subject to either misperceive prosodic signals or misinterpret them. However, dyadic interactions and their behavioural sequelae, including the expression and perception of prosody, are the product of the dynamic interactions and mutual influence that each interlocutor exerts on the other. This means that the frame of reference for impairment is on the dyadic interaction, which is the synergistic product of communicative actions, executed by the individual with the brain disorder, as well as his interactive partner. One ramification is that the ecological manifestations of prosody and the neural network activity occurring during dyadic interactions may be quite different to what has been reported thus far, using single subjects and audio recordings.

Finally, prosody is naturally employed alongside other communicatory channels such as the semantic content of speech (words), their structural organization and phrasing (syntax), and their effects on behaviour (pragmatics). Therefore, future studies should explore prosody and its dysfunction within conversation, investigating its putative relationship to the syntactical, semantic, and pragmatic changes in both patients', as well as their healthy interlocutors', speech content and context. Pragmatic aspects should be of particular interest to research in schizophrenia and bipolar disorder given the prominent role that social, cognitive, and communication dysfunctions play in the functional outcome of patients with these illnesses.

37.13 CONCLUSION

In summary, vocal emotion involves a complex and distributed neural network, utilizing aspects of auditory-linguistic limbic and motoric systems. This complexity makes identifying particular mechanisms for dysprosodia challenging. Schizophrenia and bipolar disorder manifest a heterogeneous pattern of symptoms and a wide array of neurocognitive disabilities. By focusing on basic perception, one is able to build an information theoretic approach to schizophrenia dysprosodia that demonstrates how dysprosodia may have both basic perceptual as well as higher-order cognitive impairment. This approach also suggests that cognitive remediation of pitch perception and neurostimulation may be fruitful avenues of treatment for schizophrenia dysprosodia. Ultimately, however, future work must focus on how prosodic abilities develop and mature, and must employ communication science perspectives that examine prosody within interpersonal interactions.

REFERENCES

Alpert, M., Rosenberg, S. D., Pouget, E. R., & Shaw, R. J. (2000). Prosody and lexical accuracy in flat affect schizophrenia. *Psychiatry Research*, 97, 107–118.

Amminger, G. P., Schäfer, M. R., Klier, C. M., Schlögelhofer, M., Mossaheb, N., Thompson, A., ... Nelson, B. (2012a). Facial and vocal affect perception in people at ultra-high risk of psychosis, first-episode schizophrenia and healthy controls. *Early Intervention in Psychosis*, 6, 450–454. https://doi.org/10.1111/j.1751-7893.2012.00362.x

Amminger, G. P., Schäfer, M. R., Papageorgiou, K., Klier, C. M., Schlögelhofer, M., Mossaheb, N., ... McGorry, P. D. (2012b). Emotion recognition in individuals at clinical high-risk for schizophrenia. *Schizophrenia Bulletin*, 38, 1030–1039. https://doi.org/10.1093/schbul/sbr015

Andreasen, N. C., Alpert, M., & Martz, M. J. (1981). Acoustic analysis: an objective measure of affective flattening. *Archives of General Psychiatry*, 38, 281–285.

Armony, J. L. & LeDoux, J. E. (2010). Emotional responses to auditory stimuli. In: *The Oxford Handbook of Auditory Science: The Auditory Brain*. doi:10.1093/oxfordhb/9780199233281.013.0019

Bach, D. R., Buxtorf, K., Grandjean, D., & Strik, W. K. (2009). The influence of emotion clarity on emotional prosody identification in paranoid schizophrenia. *Psychological Medicine*, 39, 927–938. https://doi.org/10.1017/S0033291708004704

Bach, D. R., Grandjean, D., Sander, D., Herdener, M., Strik, W. K., & Seifritz, E. (2008). The effect of appraisal level on processing of emotional prosody in meaningless speech. *NeuroImage*, 42(2), 919–927. doi: S1053-8119(08)00658-7[pii]10.1016/j.neuroimage.2008.05.034

Baltaxe, C. A. & Simmons III, J. Q. (1995). Speech and language disorders in children and adolescents with schizophrenia. *Schizophrenia Bulletin*, 21(4), 677–692.

Banse, R. & Scherer, K. R. (1996). Acoustic profiles in vocal emotion expression. *Journal of Personality and Social Psychology*, 70, 614–636.

Baumeister, R. F. & Leary, M. R. (1995). The need to belong: desire for interpersonal attachments as a fundamental human motivation. *Psychology Bulletin*, 117(3), 497–529.

Blonder, L. X., Gur, R. E., & Gur, R. C. (1989). The effects of right and left hemiparkinsonism on prosody. *Brain and Language*, 36(2), 193–207.

Boksa, P. (2008). Maternal infection during pregnancy and schizophrenia. *Journal of Psychiatry and Neuroscience*, 33, 183–185.

Bora, E., Gökçen, S., Kayahan, B., & Veznedaroglu, B. (2008). Deficits of social-cognitive and social-perceptual aspects of theory of mind in remitted patients with schizophrenia: effect of residual symptoms. *Journal of Nervous and Mental Disease*, 196(2), 95–99.

Borod, J. C., Alpert, M., Brozgold, A., Martin, C., Welkowitz, J., Diller, L., ... Lieberman, A. (1989). A preliminary comparison of flat affect schizophrenics and brain-damaged patients on measures of affective processing. *Journal of Communication Disorders*, 22, 93–104.

Borod, J. C., Cicero, B. A., Obler, L. K., Welkowitz, J., Erhan, H. M., Santschi, C., ... Whalen, J. R. (1998). Right hemisphere emotional perception: evidence across multiple channels. *Neuropsychology*, 12, 446–458.

Borod, J. C., Welkowitz, J., Alpert, M., Brozgold, A. Z., Martin, C., Peselow, E., Diller, L. (1990). Parameters of emotional processing in neuropsychiatric disorders: conceptual issues and a battery of tests. *Journal of Communication Disorders*, 23, 247–271. https://doi.org/10.1016/0021-9924(90)90003-H

Bozikas, V. P., Kosmidis, M. H., Anezoulaki, D., Giannakou, M., & Karavatos, A. (2004). Relationship of affect recognition with psychopathology and cognitive performance in schizophrenia. *Journal of the International Neuropsychology Society*, 10, 549–558.

Bozikas, V. P., Kosmidis, M. H., Tonia, T., Andreou, C., Focas, K., & Karavatos, A. (2007). Impaired perception of affective prosody in remitted patients with bipolar disorder. *Journal of Neuropsychogy: Clinical Neuroscience*, 19, 436–440. https://doi.org/10.1176/appi.neuropsych.19.4.436

Brazo, P., Beaucousin, V., Lecardeur, L., Razafimandimby, A., & Dollfus, S. (2014). Social cognition in schizophrenic patients: the effect of semantic content and emotional prosody in the comprehension of emotional discourse. *Frontiers in Psychiatry*, 5. https://doi.org/10.3389/fpsyt.2014.00120

Breitenstein, C., Van Lancker, D., Daum, I., & Waters, C. H. (2001). Impaired perception of vocal emotions in Parkinson's disease: influence of speech time processing and executive functioning. *Brain and Cognition*, 45, 277–314. https://doi.org/10.1006/brcg.2000.1246

Cacioppo, J. T. & William, P. (2009). *Loneliness: Human Nature and the Need for Social Connection*. New York, NY: W. W. Norton & Company.

Caekebeke, J. F., Jennekens-Schinkel, A., van der Linden, M. E., Buruma, O. J., & Roos, R. A. (1991). The interpretation of dysprosody in patients with Parkinson's disease. *Journal of Neurology, Neurosurgery and Psychiatry*, 54, 145–148.

Cannon, T. D. et al. (2008). Prediction of psychosis in youth at high clinical risk: A multisite longitudinal study in North America. *Archives of General Psychiatry*, 65(1), 28–37.

Castagna, F., Montemagni, C., Maria Milani, A., Rocca, G., Rocca, P., Casacchia, M., & Bogetto, F. (2013). Prosody recognition and audiovisual emotion matching in schizophrenia: the contribution of cognition and psychopathology. *Psychiatry Research*, 205, 192–198. https://doi.org/10.1016/j.psychres.2012.08.038

Castro, A. & Pearson, R. (2011). Lateralisation of language and emotion in schizotypal personality: evidence from dichotic listening. *Personality and Individual Differences*, 51, 726–731. https://doi.org/10.1016/j.paid.2011.06.017

Chevallier, C., Kohls, G., Troiani, V., Brodkin, E. S., & Schultz, R. T. (2012). The social motivation theory of autism. *Trends in Cognitive Science*, 16(4), 231–239. doi: 10.1016/j.tics.2012.02.007

Clark, H. H. & Wilkes-Gibbs, D. (1986). Referring as a collaborative process. *Cognition* 22, 1–39.

Coffman, B. A., Haigh, S. M., Murphy, T. K., & Salisbury, D. F. (2016). Event-related potentials demonstrate deficits in acoustic segmentation in schizophrenia. *Schizophrenia Research*, 173, 109–115. https://doi.org/10.1016/j.schres.2016.03.012

Cohen, J. (1988). *Statistical Power Analysis for the Behavioral Sciences* (2nd edn). Hillsdale, NJ: Lawrence Erlbaum Assoc.

Cowan, N. (1984). On short and long auditory stores. *Psychology Bulletin*, 96, 341–370.

Critchley, E. M. (1981). Speech disorders of Parkinsonism: a review. *Journal of Neurology, Neurosurgery and Psychiatry*, 44, 751–758.

Dale, C. L., Brown, E. G., Fisher, M., Herman, A. B., Dowling, A. F., Hinkley, L. B., … Vinogradov, S. (2016). Auditory cortical plasticity drives training-induced cognitive changes in schizophrenia. *Schizophrenia Bulletin*, 42, 220–228. https://doi.org/10.1093/schbul/sbv087

Darkins, A. W., Fromkin, V. A., & Benson, D. F. (1988). A characterization of the prosodic loss in Parkinson's disease. *Brain and Language*, 34, 315–327.

Darwin, C. (1865). *The Expression of Emotion in Man and Animals* (1948 edn.). London, England: Watts and Co.

Davis, B. L., MacNeilage, P. F., Matyear, C. L., & Powell, J. K. (2000). Prosodic correlates of stress in babbling: an acoustical study. *Child Development*, 71(5), 1258–1270.

Davitz, J. (1964). *The Communication of Emotional Meaning*. Westport CN: Greenwood Press.

Der-Avakian, A. & Markou, A. (2011). The neurobiology of anhedonia and other reward-related deficits. *Trends in Neuroscience*, 35(1), 68–77. doi: 10.1016/j.tins.2011.11.005

Deveney, C. M., Brotman, M. A., Decker, A. M., Pine, D. S., & Leibenluft, E. (2011). Affective prosody labeling in youths with bipolar disorder or severe mood dysregulation. *Journal of Child Psychology and Psychiatry*, 53, 262–270. https://doi.org/10.1111/j.14697610.2011.02482.x

Do, K. Q., Cabungcal, J. H., Frank, A., Steullet, P., & Cuenod, M. (2009). Redox dysregulation, neurodevelopment, and schizophrenia. *Current Opinion in Neurobiology*, 19(2), 220–230. doi: 10.1016/j.conb.2009.05.001

Edwards, J., Jackson, H. J., & Pattison, P. E. (2002). Emotion recognition via facial expression and affective prosody in schizophrenia: a methodological review. *Clinical Psychology Review*, 22(6), 789–832. https://dx.doi.org/10.1016/S0272-7358(02)00130-7

Edwards, J., Pattison, P. E., Jackson, H. J., & Wales, R. J. (2001). Facial affect and affective prosody recognition in first-episode schizophrenia. *Schizophrenia Research*, 48(2–3), 235–253.

Ekman, P. (1976). *Pictures of Facial Affect*. Palo Alto, CA: Consulting Psychologists Press.

Ekman, P. & Friesen, W. V. (1971). Constants across cultures in the face and emotion. *Journal of Personality and Social Psychology*, 17, 124–129. https://doi.org/10.1037/h0030377

Ethofer, T., Anders, S., Erb, M., Herbert, C., Wiethoff, S., Kissler, J., Grodd, W., & Wildgruber, D. (2006). Cerebral pathways in processing of affective prosody: a dynamic causal modeling study. *NeuroImage*, 30, 580–587. https://doi.org/10.1016/j.neuroimage.2005.09.059

Fernald, A. (1989). Intonation and communicative intent in mothers' speech to infants: is the melody the message? *Child Development*, 60(6), 1497–1510.

Fernando, A. B. P. & Robbins, T. W. (2011). Animal models of neuropsychiatric disorders. *Annual Review of Clinical Psychology*, 7(April), 39–61. doi: 10.1146/annurev-clinpsy-032210-104454

Filmer, H. L., Dux, P. E., & Mattingley, J. B. (2014). Applications of transcranial direct current stimulation for understanding brain function. *Trends in Neuroscience*, 37(12), 742–753. doi: 10.1016/j.tins.2014.08.003

Fisher, M., Holland, C., Merzenich, M. M., & Vinogradov, S. (2009). Using neuroplasticity-based auditory training to improve verbal memory in schizophrenia. *American Journal of Psychiatry*, 166, 805–811. https://doi.org/10.1176/ appi.ajp.2009.08050757

Fisher, M., Holland, C., Subramaniam, K., & Vinogradov, S. (2010). Neuroplasticity-based cognitive training in schizophrenia: an interim report on the effects 6 months later. *Schizophrenia Bulletin*, 36, 869–879. https://doi.org/10.1093/schbul/sbn170

Fricchione, G., Sedler, M. J., & Shukla, S. (1986). Aprosodia in eight schizophrenic patients. *American Journal of Psychiatry*, 143, 1457–1459.

Friederici, A. D. & Alter, K. (2004). Lateralization of auditory language functions: a dynamic dual pathway model. *Brain and Language*, 89, 267–276. https://doi.org/10.1016/S0093-934X(03)00351-1

Frijda, N. H. & Philipszoon, E. (1963). Dimensions of recognition of expression. *Journal of Abnormal Social Psychology*, 66, 45–51. https://doi.org/10.1037/h0042578

Frühholz, S., Ceravolo, L., & Grandjean, D. (2012). Specific brain networks during explicit and implicit decoding of emotional prosody. *Cerebral Cortex*, 22(5), 1107–1117. doi: 10.1093/cercor/bhr184

Frühholz, S. & Grandjean, D. (2013). Amygdala subregions differentially respond and rapidly adapt to threatening voices. *Cortex*, 49(5), 1394–1403. doi: 10.1016/j.cortex.2012.08.003

Frühholz, S. & Grandjean, D. (n.d.) Towards a fronto-temporal neural network for the decoding of emotional vocal expressions. *Cerebral Cortex*.

Frühholz, S., Gschwind, M., & Grandjean, D. (2015). Bilateral dorsal and ventral fiber pathways for the processing of affective prosody identified by probabilistic fiber tracking. *NeuroImage*, 109(April), 27–34. doi: 10.1016/j.neuroimage.2015.01.016

Frühholz, S., Trost, W., & Kotz, S. A. (2016). The sound of emotions—towards a unifying neural network perspective of affective sound processing. *Neuroscience and Biobehavioural Review*, 68, 96–110. doi: 10.1016/j.neubiorev.2016.05.002

George, M. S., Parekh, P. I., Rosinsky, N., Ketter, T. A., Kimbrell, T. A., Heilman, K. M., Herscovitch, P., & Post, R. M. (1996). Understanding emotional prosody activates right hemisphere regions. *Archives of Neurology*, 53(7), 665–670.

Gold, R., Butler, P., Revheim, N., Leitman, D. I., Hansen, J. A., Gur, R. C. et al. (2012). Auditory emotion recognition impairments in schizophrenia: relationship to acoustic features and cognition. *American Journal of Psychiatry*, 169(4), 424–432. doi: 10.1176/appi.ajp.2011.11081230

Grandjean, D., Sander, D., Pourtois, G., Schwartz, S., Seghier, M. L., Scherer, K. R., & Vuilleumier, P. (2005). The voices of wrath: brain responses to angry prosody in meaningless speech. *Nature Neuroscience*, 8, 145–146. https://doi.org/10.1038/nn1392

Grice, H. P. (1975). Logic and conversation. In: P. Cole & J. L. Morgan (eds) *Syntax and Semantics. Volume 3: Speech Acts* (pp. 41–58). New York, NY: Elsevier.

Haigh, S. M., Coffman, B. A., Murphy, T. K., Butera, C. D., & Salisbury, D. F. (2016). Abnormal auditory pattern perception in schizophrenia. *Schizophrenia Research*, 176, 473–479. https://doi.org/10.1016/j.schres.2016.07.007

Haskins, B., Shutty, M. S., & Kellogg, E. (1995). Affect processing in chronically psychotic patients: development of a reliable assessment tool. *Schizophrenia Research*, 15, 291–297.

Heilman, K. M., Bowers, D., Speedie, L., & Coslett, H. B. (1984). Comprehension of affective and nonaffective prosody. *Neurology*, 34, 917–921.

Heilman, K. M. & Gilmore, R. L. (1998). Cortical influences in emotion. *Journal of Clinical Neurophysiology*, 15, 409–423. https://doi.org/10.1097/00004691-199809000-00005

Hoekert, M., Kahn, R. S., Pijnenborg, M., & Aleman, A. (2007). Impaired recognition and expression of emotional prosody in schizophrenia: review and meta-analysis. *Schizophrenia Research*, 96(1–3), 135–145.

Hoertnagl, C. M., Yalcin-Siedentopf, N., Baumgartner, S., Biedermann, F., Deisenhammer, E. A., Hausmann, A., … Hofer, A. (2014). Affective prosody perception in symptomatically remitted patients with schizophrenia and bipolar disorder. *Schizophrenia Research*, 158, 100–104. https://doi.org/10.1016/j.schres.2014.07.019

Homae, F., Watanabe, H., Nakano, T., Asakawa, K., & Taga, G. (2006). The right hemisphere of sleeping infant perceives sentential prosody. *Neuroscience Research*, 54(4), 276–280. doi: S0168-0102(05)00328-7[pii]10.1016/j.neures.2005.12.006.

Hooker, C. & Park, S. (2002). Emotion processing and its relationship to social functioning in schizophrenia patients. *Psychiatry Research*, 112, 41–50.

Huang, J., Chan, R. C. K., Lu, X., & Tong, Z. (2009). Emotion categorization perception in schizophrenia in conversations with different social contexts. *Australia and New Zealand Journal of Psychiatry*, 43, 438–445. https://doi.org/10.1080/00048670902817646

Insel, T. R. (2010). Rethinking schizophrenia. *Nature*, 468, 187–193. https://doi.org/10.1038/nature09552

Ito, F., Matsumoto, K., Miyakoshi, T., Ohmuro, N., Uchida, T., & Matsuoka, H. (2013). Emotional processing during speech communication and positive symptoms in schizophrenia. *Psychiatry and Clinical Neurosciences*, 67, 526–531. https://doi.org/10.1111/pcn.12103

Izard, C. E. (1971). *The Face of Emotion*. New York: Appelton-Century-Crofts.

James, W. (1890). *The Principles of Psychology* (1950 edn). New York: Dover Publications.

Javitt, D. C. (2009). When doors of perception close: bottom-up models of disrupted cognition in schizophrenia. *Annual Review of Clinical Psychology*, 5, 249–275. doi: 10.1146/annurev.clinpsy.032408.153502

Javitt, D. C., Strous, R. D., Grochowski, S., Ritter, W., & Cowan, N. (1997). Impaired precision, but normal retention, of auditory sensory ('echoic') memory information in schizophrenia. *Journal of Abnormal Psychology*, 106, 315–324.

Javitt, D. C. & Sweet, R. A. (2015). Auditory dysfunction in schizophrenia: integrating clinical and basic features. *Nature Reviews Neuroscience*, 16, 535–550. https://doi.org/10.1038/nrn4002

Jiang, Z., Rompala, G. R., Zhang, S., Cowell, R. M., & Nakazawa, K. (2013). Social isolation exacerbates schizophrenia-like phenotypes via oxidative stress in cortical interneurons. *Biological Psychiatry*, 73(10), 1024–1034. doi: 10.1016/j.biopsych.2012.12.004.

Juslin, P. N. & Laukka, P. (2001). Impact of intended emotion intensity on cue utilization and decoding accuracy in vocal expression of emotion. *Emotion*, 1, 381–412. https://doi.org/10.1037//1528-3542.1.4.381

Juslin, P. N. & Laukka, P. (2003). Communication of emotions in vocal expression and music performance: different channels, same code? *Psychology Bulletin*, 129, 770–814.

Kantrowitz, J. T., Hoptman, M. J., Leitman, D. I., Moreno-Ortega, M., Lehrfeld, J. M., Dias, E., ... Javitt, D. C. (2015). Neural substrates of auditory emotion recognition deficits in schizophrenia. *Journal of Neuroscience*, 35(44), 14909–21. doi: 10.1523/JNEUROSCI.4603-14.2015

Koelsch, S., Gunter, T. C., Schroger, E., Tervaniemi, M., Sammler, D., & Friederici, A.D. (2001a). Differentiating ERAN and MMN: an ERP study. *NeuroReport*, 12, 1385–1389.

Koelsch, S., Maess, B., Gunter, T. C., & Friederici, A. D. (2001b). Neapolitan chords activate the area of Broca. A magnetoencephalographic study. *Annals of the New York Academy of Sciences*, 930, 420–421.

Kujala, T., Lepistö, T., Nieminen von Wendt, T., Näätänen, P., & Näätänen, R. (2005). Neurophysiological evidence for cortical discrimination impairment of prosody in Asperger syndrome. *Neuroscience Letters*, 383(3), 260–65. doi: 10.1016/j.neulet.2005.04.048

Ladd, D. R., Silverman, K., Tolkmitt, F. T., Bergmann, G., & Scherer, K. R. (1985). Evidence for the independent function of intonation, contour type, voice quality, and Fo range in signalling speaker affect. *Journal of the Acoustical Society of America*, 78(2), 435–444.

Lakatos, P., Schroeder, C. E., Leitman, D. I., & Javitt, D. C. (2013). Predictive suppression of cortical excitability and its deficit in schizophrenia. *Journal of Neuroscience*, 33(28), 11692–702. doi: 10.1523/JNEUROSCI.0010-13.2013

Leary, M. R., Kelly, K. M., Cottrell, C. A., & Schreindorfer, L. S. (2013). Construct validity of the need to belong scale: mapping the nomological network. *Journal of Personality Assessment*, 95, 610–24. https://doi.org/10.1080/00223891.2013.819511

Leentjens, A. F., Wielaert, S. M., van Harskamp, F., & Wilmink, F. W. (1998). Disturbances of affective prosody in patients with schizophrenia; a cross sectional study. *Journal of Neurology, Neurosurgery and Psychiatry*, 64(3), 375–378.

Leitman, D. I., Hoptman, M. J., Foxe, J. J., Saccente, E., Wylie, G. R., Nierenberg, J., ... Javitt, D. C. (2007). The neural substrates of impaired prosodic detection in schizophrenia and its sensorial antecedents. *American Journal of Psychiatry*, 164(3), 474–82. doi: 10.1176/appi.ajp.164.3.474

Leitman, D. I., Foxe, J. J., Butler, P. D., Saperstein, A., Revheim, N., & Javitt, D. C. (2005). Sensory contributions to impaired prosodic processing in schizophrenia. *Biological Psychiatry*, 58(1), 56–61. doi: http://dx.doi.org/10.1016/j.biopsych.2005.02.034

Leitman, D. I., Laukka, P., Juslin, P. N., Saccente, E., Butler, P., & Javitt, D. C. (2010). Getting the cue: sensory contributions to auditory emotion recognition impairments in schizophrenia. *Schizophrenia Bulletin*, 36(3), 545–56. doi: 10.1093/schbul/sbn115

Leitman, D. I., Wolf, D. H., Laukka, P., Ragland, J. D., Valdez, J. N., Turetsky, B. I., Gur, R. E., & Gur, R. C. (2011). Not pitch perfect: sensory contributions to affective communication impairment in schizophrenia. *Biological Psychiatry*, 70(7), 611–18. doi: 10.1016/j.biopsych.2011.05.032

Leitman, D. I., Wolf, D. H., Ragland, D., Laukka, P., Loughead, J., Valdez, D. et al. (2010). It's not what you say, but how you say it: a reciprocal temporo-frontal network for affective prosody. *Frontiers in Human Neuroscience*, 4(19), 1–13. doi: 10.3389/fnhum.2010.00019

Leitman, D. I., Ziwich, R., Pasternak, R., & Javitt, J. C. (2006). Theory of Mind (ToM) and counterfactuality deficits in schizophrenia: misperception or misinterpretation? *Psychological Medicine*, 36(8), 1075–83. doi: 10.1017/S0033291706007653

Levin, S., Hall, J. A., Knight, R. A., & Alpert, M. (1985). Verbal and nonverbal expression of affect in speech of schizophrenic and depressed patients. *Journal of Abnormal Psychology*, 94(4), 487–497. https://doi.org/10.1037/0021-843X.94.4.487

Lewis, D. A. & Moghaddam, B. (2006). Cognitive dysfunction in schizophrenia: convergence of gamma-aminobutyric acid and glutamate alterations. *Archives of Neurology*, 63(10), 1372–76. doi: 10.1001/archneur.63.10.1372

Lichtenstein, P., Yip, B. H., Björk, C., Pawitan, Y., Cannon, T. D., Sullivan, P. F., & Hultman, C. M. (2009). Common genetic determinants of schizophrenia and bipolar disorder in Swedish families: a population-based study. *Lancet*, 373, 234–239. https://doi.org/10.1016/S0140-6736(09)60072-6

Liégeois-Chauvel, C., Giraud, K., Badier, J. M., Marquis, P., & Chauvel, P. (2001). Intracerebral evoked potentials in pitch perception reveal a functional asymmetry of the human auditory cortex. *Annals of the New York Academy of Sciences*, 930, 117–132.

Locke, J. L. (2001). First communion: the emergence of vocal relationships. *Social Development*, 10(3), 294–308.

Luck, P. & Dowrick, C. F. (2004). 'Don't look at me in that tone of voice!' Disturbances in the perception of emotion in facial expression and vocal intonation by depressed patients. *Primary Care Mental Health*, 2(2), 99–106.

Maess, B., Koelsch, S., Gunter, T. C., & Friederici, A. D. (2001). Musical syntax is processed in Broca's area: an MEG study. *Nature Neuroscience*, 4(5), 540–545.

Majewski, W. & Blasdell, R. (1969). Influence of fundamental frequency cues on the perception of some synthetic intonation contours. *Journal of the Acoustical Society of America*, 45, 450–457. https://doi.org/10.1121/1.1911394

Matsumoto, K., Samson, G. T., O'Daly, O. D., Tracy, D. K., Patel, A. D., & Shergill, S. S. (2006). Prosodic discrimination in patients with schizophrenia. *British Journal of Psychology*, 189, 180–81.

McClure, E. B. & Nowicki, S. (2001). Associations between social anxiety and nonverbal processing skill in preadolescent boys and girls. *Journal of Nonverbal Behavior*, 25, 3–19. https://doi.org/10.1023/A:1006753006870

McGrath, J. (1999). Hypothesis: is low prenatal vitamin D a risk-modifying factor for schizophrenia? *Schizophrenia Research*, 40, 173–177.

McLachlan, N. M., Phillips, D. S., Rossell, S. L., & Wilson, S. J. (2013). Auditory processing and hallucinations in schizophrenia. *Schizophrenia Research*, 150, 380–385. https://doi.org/10.1016/j.schres.2013.08.039

Mellor, D., Stokes, M., Firth, L., Hayashi, Y., & Cummins, R. (2008). Need for belonging, relationship satisfaction, loneliness, and life satisfaction. *Personality and Individual Differences*, 45(3), 213–18. doi: 10.1016/j.paid.2008.03.020

Mitchell, R., Gamez, K., Kohler, C., Calkins, M. E., Turetsky, B. I., & Leitman, D. I. (2016). Influence of desire to belong and feelings of loneliness on emotional prosody perception in schizophrenia. *bioRxiv*. doi: https://doi.org/10.1101/092080

Mobes, J., Joppich, G., Stiebritz, F., Dengler, R., & Schroder, C. (2008). Emotional speech in Parkinson's disease. *Movement Disorders*, 23(6), 824–29. doi: 10.1002/mds.21940

Murphy, D. & Cutting, J. (1990). Prosodic comprehension and expression in schizophrenia. *Journal of Neurology, Neurosurgery and Psychiatry*, 53, 727–730.

NAMI. (2017). Bipolar Disorder. https://nami.org/learn-more/mental-health-conditions/bipolar-disorder

Patel, A. D., Peretz, I., Tramo, M., & Labreque, R. (1998). Processing prosodic and musical patterns: a neuropsychological investigation. *Brain and Language*, 61, 123–144.

Pell, M. D. (1999). Fundamental frequency encoding of linguistic and emotional prosody by right hemisphere-damaged speakers. *Brain and Language*, 69, 161–192.

Pell, M. D., Cheang, H. S., & Leonard, C. L. (2006). The impact of Parkinson's disease on vocal-prosodic communication from the perspective of listeners. *Brain and Language*, 97, 123–34. https://doi.org/10.1016/j.bandl.2005.08.010

Pell, M. D. & Leonard, C. L. (2003). Processing emotional tone from speech in Parkinson's disease: a role for the basal ganglia. *Cognitive, Affective, and Behavioral Neuroscience*, 3(4), 275–88.

Péron, J., Frühholz, S., Ceravolo, L., & Grandjean, D. (2016). Structural and functional connectivity of the subthalamic nucleus during vocal emotion decoding. *Social, Cognitive, and Affective Neuroscience*, 11(2), 349–56. doi: 10.1093/scan/nsv118

Péron, J., El Tamer, S., Grandjean, D., Leray, E., Travers, D., Drapier, D., Vérin, M., & Millet, B. (2011). Major depressive disorder skews the recognition of emotional prosody. *Prog in Neuro-Psychopharmacology and Biological Psychiatry*, 35(4), 987–96. doi: 10.1016/j.pnpbp.2011.01.019

Popov, T., Jordanov, T., Rockstroh, B., Elbert, T., Merzenich, M. M., & Miller, G. A. (2011). Specific cognitive training normalizes auditory sensory gating in schizophrenia: a randomized trial. *Biological Psychiatry*, 69, 465–471. https://doi.org/10.1016/j.biopsych.2010.09.028

Popov, T., Rockstroh, B., Weisz, N., Elbert, T., & Miller, G. A. (2012). Adjusting brain dynamics in schizophrenia by means of perceptual and cognitive training. *PLoS One*, 7, e39051. https://doi.org/10.1371/journal.pone.0039051

Post, R. M. & Leverich, G. S. (2006). The role of psychosocial stress in the onset and progression of bipolar disorder and its comorbidities: the need for earlier and alternative modes of therapeutic intervention. *Developmental Psychopathology*, 18, 1181–1211. https://doi.org/10.1017/S0954579406060573

Rabinowicz, E. F., Silipo, G., Goldman, R., & Javitt, D.C. (2000). Auditory sensory dysfunction in schizophrenia: imprecision or distractibility? *Archives of General Psychiatry*, 57, 1149–1155.

Read, J., van Os, J., Morrison, A. P., & Ross, C. A. (2005). Childhood trauma, psychosis and schizophrenia: a literature review with theoretical and clinical implications. *Acta Psychiatrica Scandinavica*, 112, 330–350. https://doi.org/10.1111/j.16000447.2005.00634.x

Ross, E. D. (1981). The aprosodias. Functional-anatomic organization of the affective components of language in the right hemisphere. *Archives of Neurology*, 38(9), 561–69.

Rossell, S. L., Van Rheenen, T. E., Groot, C., Gogos, A., O'Regan, A., & Joshua, N. R. (2013). Investigating affective prosody in psychosis: a study using the Comprehensive Affective Testing System. *Psychiatry Research*, 210, 896–900. https://doi.org/10.1016/j.psychres.2013.07.037

Roux, P., Christophe, A., & Passerieux, C. (2010). The emotional paradox: dissociation between explicit and implicit processing of emotional prosody in schizophrenia. *Neuropsychologia*, 48, 3642–3649. https://doi.org/10.1016/j.neuropsychologia.2010.08.021

Sammler, D., Grosbras, M.-H., Anwander, A., Bestelmeyer, P. E. G., & Belin, P. (2015). Dorsal and ventral pathways for prosody. *Current Biology*, November, 1–7. doi: 10.1016/j.cub.2015.10.009

Saur, D., Kreher, B. W., Schnell, S., Kummerer, D., Kellmeyer, P., Vry, M.-S. et al. (2008). Ventral and dorsal pathways for language. *Proceedings of the National Academy of Sciences of the United States of America*, 105(46), 18035–40. doi: 10.1073/pnas.0805234105

Schaal, N. K., Pfeifer, J., Krause, V., & Pollok, B. (2015). From amusic to musical? Improving pitch memory in congenital amusia with transcranial alternating current stimulation. *Behavioual Brain Research*, 294, 141–48. doi: 10.1016/j.bbr.2015.08.003

Schaal, N. K., Williamson, V. J., & Banissy, M. J. (2013). Anodal transcranial direct current stimulation over the supramarginal gyrus facilitates pitch memory. *European Journal of Neuroscience*, 38(10), 3513–18. doi: 10.1111/ejn.12344

Schiavone, S., Jaquet, V., Trabace, L., & Krause, K.-H. (2013). Severe life stress and oxidative stress in the brain: from animal models to human pathology. *Antioxidants & Redox Signaling*, 18(12), 1475–90. doi: 10.1089/ars.2012.4720

Schirmer, A. & Kotz, S.A. (2006). Beyond the right hemisphere: brain mechanisms mediating vocal emotional processing. *Trends in Cognitive Sciences*, 10, 24–30. https://doi.org/10.1016/j.tics.2005.11.009

Scholten, M. R. M., Aleman, A., & Kahn, R. S. (2008). The processing of emotional prosody and semantics in schizophrenia: relationship to gender and IQ. *Psychological Medicine*, 38, 887–898. https://doi.org/10.1017/S0033291707001742

Shaw, R. J., Dong, M., Lim, K. O., Faustman, W. O., Pouget, E. R., & Alpert, M. (1999). The relationship between affect expression and affect recognition in schizophrenia. *Schizophrenia Research*, 37, 245–250.

Simpson, C., Pinkham, A. E., Kelsven, S., & Sasson, N. J. (2013). Emotion recognition abilities across stimulus modalities in schizophrenia and the role of visual attention. *Schizophrenia Research*, 151, 102–106. https://doi.org/http://dx.doi.org/10.1016/j.schres.2013.09.026

Strous, R. D., Cowan, N., Ritter, W., & Javitt, D. C. (1995). Auditory sensory ('echoic') memory dysfunction in schizophrenia. *American Journal of Psychology*, 152(10), 1517–1519.

Tomasello, M. (2010). *Origins of Human Communication*. Cambridge, MA: MIT Press.

Tseng, H.-H., Chen, S.-H., Liu, C.-M., Howes, O., Huang, Y.-L., Hsieh, M. H., ... Hwu, H.-G. (2013). Facial and prosodic emotion recognition deficits associate with specific clusters of psychotic symptoms in schizophrenia. *PLoS One* 8, e66571. https://doi.org/10.1371/journal.pone.0066571

Uhlhaas, P. J. (2012). Dysconnectivity, large-scale networks and neuronal dynamics in schizophrenia. *Current Opinion in Neurobiology*, December, 1–8. doi: 10.1016/j.conb.2012.11.004

Van Rheenen, T. E. & Rossell, S. L. (2013). Auditory-prosodic processing in bipolar disorder; from sensory perception to emotion. *Journal of Affective Disorders*, 151, 1102–1107. https://doi.org/10.1016/j.jad.2013.08.039

van Winkel, R., Stefanis, N. C., & Myin-Germeys, I. (2008). Psychosocial stress and psychosis. A review of the neurobiological mechanisms and the evidence for gene-stress interaction. *Schizophrenia Bulletin*, 34, 1095–1105. https://doi.org/10.1093/schbul/sbn101

Vinogradov, S., Fisher, M., & de Villers-Sidani, E. (2012). Cognitive training for impaired neural systems in neuropsychiatric illness. *Neuropsychopharmacology*, 37, 43–76. https://doi.org/10.1038/npp.2011.251

Vogel, B., Brück, C., Jacob, H., Eberle, M., & Wildgruber, D. (2016). Integration of verbal and nonverbal emotional signals in patients with schizophrenia: Decreased nonverbal dominance. *Psychology Research*, 241, 98–103. https://doi.org/http://dx.doi.org/ 10.1016/j.psychres.2016.03.050

Vogel, B. D., Brück, C., Jacob, H., Eberle, M., & Wildgruber, D. (2016). Effects of cue modality and emotional category on recognition of nonverbal emotional signals in schizophrenia. *BMC Psychiatry*, 16, 218. https://doi.org/10.1186/s12888-016-0913-7

Wan, M. W., Penketh, V., Salmon, M. P., & Abel, K. M. (2008). Content and style of speech from mothers with schizophrenia towards their infants. *Psychiatry Research*, 159, 109–114. https://doi.org/10.1016/j.psychres.2007.05.012

Watzlawick, P., Beavin, J., & Jackson, D. D. (1967). *Pragmatics of Human Communication: A Study of Interactional Patterns, Pathologies, and Paradoxes*. New York, NY: W. W. Norton & Company.

Whittaker, J. F., Connell, J., & Deakin, J. F. (1994). Receptive and expressive social communication in schizophrenia. *Psychopathology*, 27, 262–267. https://doi.org/10.1159/000284880

Wildgruber, D., Ackermann, H., Kreifelts, B., & Ethofer, T. (2006). Cerebral processing of linguistic and emotional prosody: fMRI studies. *Progress in Brain Research*, 156, 249–68. doi:10.1016/ S0079-6123(06)56013-3

Wildgruber, D., Riecker, A., Hertrich, I., Erb, M., Grodd, W., Ethofer, T., & Ackermann, H. (2005). Identification of emotional intonation evaluated by fMRI. *NeuroImage*, 24, 1233–1241. https://doi.org/10.1016/j.neuroimage.2004.10.034

Wilson, M. (2005). An oscillator model of the timing of turn-taking. *Cognition*, 12(6), 957–68.

Zatorre, R. J., Evans, A. C., & Meyer, E. (1994). Neural mechanisms underlying melodic perception and memory for pitch. *Journal of Neuroscience*, 14(4), 1908–1919.

Zatorre, R. J., Evans, A. C., Meyer, E., & Gjedde, A. (1992). Lateralization of phonetic and pitch discrimination in speech processing. *Science*, 256, 846–849.

Zenisek, R., Thaler, N. S., Sutton, G. P., Ringdahl, E. N., Snyder, J. S., & Allen, D. N. (2015). Auditory processing deficits in bipolar disorder with and without a history of psychotic features. *Bipolar Disorder*, 17, 769–780. https://doi.org/10.1111/bdi.12333

CHAPTER 38

PERCEPTION OF VOICES
THAT DO NOT EXIST
*Neuronal Mechanisms in Clinical
and Non-Clinical Hallucinations*

KRISTIINA KOMPUS AND KENNETH HUGDAHL

38.1 DEFINITION AND PHENOMENOLOGY OF AUDITORY VERBAL HALLUCINATIONS

AUDITORY hallucinations are the subjective experience of hearing a 'sound' in the absence of an external acoustic source. Auditory hallucinations occur in many psychiatric and neurological conditions, but may also occur in otherwise healthy persons (Johns & Van Os, 2001; Nayani & David, 1996; Shergill et al., 1998; Sommer, Daalman, et al., 2010; Sommer et al., 2008). Auditory hallucinations take on a wide range of forms, and can cause a variety of subjectively experienced phenomena, meaning that the content will vary substantially between individuals. The experience may be as subtle as intrusive and vivid auditory imagery, or be experienced as a 'real'-sounding percept with clear and distinct acoustic quality. The experience of hallucinations is different from auditory illusions, which represent a misperception of a real sound. In the case of hallucinations, the subjective experience of perceptually experiencing an external sound is independent of any external sensory stimulation.

The most common type of auditory hallucinations are auditory verbal hallucinations (AVH), consisting of hearing 'voices' which speak to the individual. A striking aspect of AVH is their phenomenological variety, in the sense that the 'voices' take many forms, with multiple, distinct identities and extensive, varied content (Jones & Fernyhough, 2007; Stephane et al., 2001). The perceived sounds may take the form of indistinct mumbles, repetitive words or sentences, or fully-formed discourse with the 'voice' (Bentall, 2004). Patients frequently experience commanding and commenting voices, but also utterances which resemble memories of previously heard real speech (McCarthy-Jones et al., 2014).

The voice may be perceived as originating from the outside space (either near or far from the ear), or from the inside of the head. While in some psychiatric traditions only the external voices have been considered to be 'true' hallucinations, distinct from internal-space 'pseudo-hallucinations' (see Jaspers, 1962), the perceived location in outer or inner space does not appear to have predictive value for the clinical outcome of the voice-hearer (Copolov et al., 2004). External voices typically have a fixed location in external space which does not move around during a hallucinatory episode and maintains the relative distance to the ear: moving 'closer' to the perceived external voice source does not lead to a change in the perceived loudness of the voice (Nayani & David, 1996). The perceived location of the hallucination as external or internal appears to be a stable characteristic of the 'voice', and has been reported to remain consistent over several years (Plaze et al., 2009).

Despite this variety in content and form, it is notable that AVH are typically meaningful utterances, rather than nonsensical or non-verbal voices. This indicates that AVH are closely connected to speech and language processing (Hugdahl, 2015; Hugdahl, Løberg, & Nygård, 2009) and that, consequently, the neural correlates of AVH are likely related to the neural correlates of speech, and in particular to speech perception (Hugdahl, Løberg, & Nygård, 2009). It is therefore not surprising that research has focused on the properties of the auditory cortex and its relationship with other language-related cognitive and neural processes in order to understand the mechanisms which elicit and maintain AVH (e.g. Badcock & Hugdahl, 2014; Dierks et al., 1999; Green et al., 1994; McGuire et al., 1995, 1993; Silbersweig et al., 1995; Waters et al., 2006; Woodruff et al., 1997).

38.2 THEORETICAL MODELS OF AUDITORY VERBAL HALLUCINATIONS

Theoretical models of AVH emphasize the relationship between the hallucinated voices and the processing of real speech and verbal information. One category of models focuses on the role of the inner speech and failure of self-monitoring in the generation of the hallucinated voices (Frith & Done, 1988; Jones, 2010). According to such models, AVH are proposed to be inner speech which is misperceived as non-self-generated speech due to dysfunctional source monitoring. These models emphasize the importance of speech production, localized to the inferior frontal cortex, and the relationship between the auditory cortex and production of inner speech.

One mechanism which may interfere with the ability to correctly recognize inner speech is proposed to be dysfunctional corollary discharge, preventing the inhibition to attenuate the activation to self-generated sounds from reaching the auditory cortex (Ford & Mathalon, 2005). More specifically (for reviews, see Blakemore, 2003; Frith et al., 2000; Jones & Fernyhough, 2007), an inner-speech model assumes that an AVH is the result of a mismatch between a self-initiated motor command (such as an utterance) and the self-awareness of such a motor action, which causes the attribution of the phenomenological experience of a 'voice' to an 'alien' other (Frith et al., 2000). Whenever a motor command is to be executed, the brain creates a prediction template of what is 'going to happen' before it happens, and the sensory feedback from the actual motor execution is then matched against such a template. The inner-speech model for AVH now assumes that this feedback mechanism is distorted or deviant in the case of an AVH such that a self-initiated movement is not properly fed back to the brain, but instead experienced as coming from an external source.

An alternative model sees AVH as representing fragmented auditory memories that are involuntarily reactivated and not cognitively inhibited (Badcock et al., 2007; Michie et al., 2005; Waters et al., 2006). Mitchie et al. (2005) suggest that patients with AVH fail to suppress irrelevant previous memories which intrude into the stream of consciousness and are phenomenologically experienced as coming from someone else. To quote Mitchie et al. (2005):

> These findings suggest that AH are related to a failure to inhibit memory traces that are no longer relevant to ongoing reality. In other words, it seems that AH arise as the result of a intrusion of strongly activated representations previously acquired in memory. (p. 126)

Still another approach considers AVH as a predominantly perceptual phenomenon, resulting from activation in the auditory areas, which may be caused either by stronger bottom-up activation in the temporal lobe or insufficient top-down inhibition from the superior frontal regions (Hugdahl, 2009; Hugdahl, 2015; Hugdahl, Løberg, & Nygård, 2009; Kompus et al., 2011). Using data from a verbal dichotic listening task with instructions to selectively focus attention to either the right or left side in auditory space, Hugdahl and colleagues (Hugdahl, Løberg, & Nygård, 2009; see also Hugdahl, 2009) made a distinction between bottom-up perceptual processes and top-down cognitive processes in AVH, where bottom-up processes represent the initial perception of a 'voice' and top-down processes represent the subsequent action taken upon the perceptual experience. More specifically, they argued that:

> … auditory hallucinations and 'hearing voices' is presented that regards such phenomena as perceptual processes, originating from speech perception areas in the left temporal lobe. Healthy individuals 'hearing voices' are, however, often aware that the experience comes from inner thought processes, which is not reported by hallucinating patients. A perceptual model can therefore, not alone explain the difference in the phenomenology of how the 'voices heard' are attributed to either an inner or outer cause. An expanded model is thus presented which takes into account top-down cognitive control, localized to prefrontal cortical areas, to inhibit and re-attribute the perceptual mis-representations. (p. 553)

It is possible that these theoretical models and approaches are not mutually exclusive and may in fact be complementary in explaining the wide variety of hallucinatory experiences. However, despite the variety in form and content, AVH have a common feature in that they are perceived as being 'heard', emphasizing the involvement of auditory perception processes.

38.3 Auditory Verbal Hallucinations in Clinical and Non-Clinical Groups

AVH are most commonly associated with schizophrenia patients due to the high frequency of hallucinations in schizophrenia. Approximately 70–80% of schizophrenia patients experience AVH (Nayani & David, 1996; Shergill et al., 1998), with varying frequency and severity.

However, it is evident and increasingly acknowledged that AVH cut across psychiatric diagnostic categories. They are found in many clinical groups such as patients with borderline personality disorder and post-traumatic stress disorder, but also in non-clinical individuals (e.g. Ford, Morris, et al., 2014). This has led to suggestions of viewing AVH as a continuum of risk in the general population (Johns et al., 2014) (see also Badcock & Hugdahl, 2014; Cuthbert & Insel, 2013), with the need for psychiatric care determined by other factors such as accompanying delusional thinking or emotional distress leading to reduced quality of life (Johns et al., 2014; Kaymaz & van Os, 2010).

The fact that AVH typically coexist with other symptoms of psychosis, such as delusions (Wallwork et al., 2012), complicates attempts to pinpoint the specific cognitive and neural features that characterize individuals with AVH. Although AVH occur in various psychiatric and neurological disorders and diseases, the bulk of research on AVH comes from patients with schizophrenia, where multiple confounding factors exist. Other psychotic symptoms, medication, pathological or degenerative processes which deepen over the course of the illness, as well as social and emotional burden due to a stigmatizing diagnosis, may all contribute to differences found between patients and healthy controls. To control for this, several approaches have been suggested to achieve a better characterization of the features that are unique for individuals with AVH. For instance, patients within the same diagnostic category but differing in hallucination status may be compared, considering hallucination severity as either a categorical or continuous variable (Larøi et al., 2012).

Recently, several studies have concentrated on non-clinical hallucinations in individuals who experience AVH but do not have the need for psychiatric care (Sommer, Daalman, et al., 2010). The experience of AVH in non-clinical individuals is phenomenologically similar to AVH experienced by clinical populations, thus the commonalities across clinical and non-clinical individuals with AVH may represent their true signature. It must be noted, however, that non-clinical individuals with AVH often also experience other subclinical psychotic experiences such as formal thought disorder (Sommer, Derwort, et al., 2010).

38.4 AUDITORY VERBAL HALLUCINATIONS AND PERCEPTION: EVIDENCE FROM BEHAVIOURAL EXPERIMENTS ·

The auditory functioning in individuals with AVH has been examined using a variety of behavioural paradigms. Most subjects in these studies have been patients with schizophrenia, which complicates the interpretation of results with more complex and cognitively demanding experimental paradigms, because impairment of higher-order cognitive functions may interfere with task performance. However, paradigms with relatively simple stimuli and response requirements have provided an insight into auditory functioning in patients with AVH.

Hallucinating patients are impaired in simple perceptual discrimination tasks such as pitch discrimination (McLachlan et al., 2013) and duration discrimination (Davalos et al., 2003). These difficulties are not restricted to patients but also found in relatives of hallucinating schizophrenia patients (Tucker et al., 2013), indicating that such relatively subtle perceptual abnormalities are not a confound of medication or illness-caused degeneration, but represent an integral part of the aetiology of AVH. Affected basic auditory processing has also been reported in non-clinical AVH subjects (Kompus et al., 2013).

Using a battery of auditory tests, McKay et al. (2000) found that hallucinating compared to non-hallucinating patients had specific deficits in tests that were sensitive to interhemispheric integration, suggestive of either altered interhemispheric pathways or dysfunction in the right-hemisphere auditory association cortex. The purpose of the McKay et al. (2000) study was to investigate whether hallucinating individuals have deficits in central auditory processing, and they consequently designed a study with behavioural tests typically used in standard audiological examinations for signs of perception and central auditory processing deficits. These tests included monaural filtered speech, binaural fusion, rapidly alternating speech perception, monaural speech discrimination in ipsilateral competition, monaural frequency tone patterns, staggered spondaic word test, competing environmental sounds, and dichotic listening to consonant-vowel syllables.

The affected interhemispheric communication between auditory processing areas in individuals with AVH is also evident in dichotic listening tasks. In such tasks, two auditory stimuli are presented simultaneously, and the subjects should report the stimulus they consciously perceive. Using speech syllables such as /ba/ and /pa/, there is a hemispheric dominance effect: syllables presented to the right ear (for left-hemisphere dominant individuals) are reported with higher accuracy (Hugdahl et al., 1995; Kimura, 1961). This can be explained with the structural model suggested by Kimura (1967) which states that the contralateral auditory projections are stronger and more preponderant, resulting in a dominant representation of auditory information in the hemisphere opposite to the ear where it originates. Speech information from the right ear therefore has a stronger representation in the speech-processing areas of the left hemisphere, whereas the input from the left ear has to transfer across the corpus callosum, via the interhemispheric pathways, before it can be processed in the left hemisphere. This gives an advantage to the right-ear input, resulting in the behaviourally observed tendency to correctly report more syllables from the right ear. Alterations from the expected right-ear advantage in the report of the stimuli indicate an altered hemispheric specialization in the auditory cortex (Hugdahl, Westerhausen, et al., 2009).

The performance of schizophrenia patients on the consonant-vowel dichotic listening task shows a consistent and striking pattern: patients with frequent and severe AVH do not show the expected right-ear advantage, whereas this deviation is not present in non-hallucinating patients to the same degree (Green et al., 1994; Hugdahl et al., 2012; Løberg et al., 1999; see also Ocklenburg et al., 2013). This finding cannot be explained by other factors such as attentional bias towards the left-ear stimulus in AVH patients, since this has been controlled for by using instructions of shifting attention between the ears (Løberg et al., 2004).

The reduction of the right-ear advantage is also correlated with hallucination frequency and severity using scores on the hallucinatory behaviour item from the Positive and Negative Syndrome Scale (PANSS) (Hugdahl et al., 2012, 2008; Kay et al., 1987). This means that the normal hemispheric dominance pattern in the auditory cortex is affected in hallucinating patients, which in turn could indicate degeneration of left-hemisphere speech-processing areas or affected interhemispheric communication.

Such difficulties in basic auditory perception and auditory processing, which persist independently of attentional processes, may contribute to more complex dysfunctions in auditory processing, and thereby either act as causal factors in the development of hallucinations or mediate impairment of daily functioning and social cognition (see Linszen et al., 2015). Difficulties in voice-identity recognition or affective prosody have also been shown in patients with AVH, and these deficits may build on lower-level auditory processing problems (Alba-Ferrara, Fernyhough, et al., 2012; Alba-Ferrara, Weis, et al., 2012).

38.5 FINDINGS FROM BRAIN STRUCTURAL AND FUNCTIONAL STUDIES

38.5.1 Brain Structural Characteristics

As reviewed in the previous section, AVH are subjectively experienced as an auditory percept, and individuals with AVH demonstrate altered performance on auditory tasks. These observations have motivated research into structural and functional properties of the primary and secondary auditory cortex. Post-mortem studies of brain tissue give detailed information on regional volumes, as well as histological information on particular cortical layers, but these studies, by necessity, have small sample sizes with variable demographic background. The advent of neuroimaging has enabled the characterization of the neural functioning and structural integrity in larger samples where demographic information and AVH features may be considered in more detail.

38.5.1.1 *Post-mortem Studies*

Examination of the auditory cortex in post-mortem samples of schizophrenia patients has concentrated on identifying the changes in patients relative to non-psychiatric controls; unfortunately, the hallucination status is typically not considered in these reports. Nonetheless, these examinations provide a valuable comparison for information provided by structural neuroimaging where the resolution is relatively limited. For instance, post-mortem studies enable the characterization of neurons in specific cortical layers, and examining whether lower grey-matter volume represents loss of neurons or rather loss of surrounding tissue (neuropil) without reduction in the number of neurons themselves. Thus, although the following overview contains studies that did not separate the patients depending on the AVH status, it gives an important perspective on the subsequently reviewed structural neuroimaging studies.

A consistent finding in post-mortem brains of patients with schizophrenia is reduced volume of the grey matter in the superior temporal gyrus (STG) (Chance et al., 2008). Within the planum temporale portion of the STG, Smiley et al. (2009) found that there was slight cortical thinning in the upper layers of the planum temporale but neither neuron densities nor neuron size were altered (suggesting slight loss in the number of neurons) in schizophrenia patients.

Within the Heschl's gyrus (HG) portion, the grey-matter volume, neuron density, or number is not reduced in schizophrenia compared to non-psychiatric samples (Chance et al., 2008; Cotter et al., 2004; Smiley et al., 2013). However, histological studies have found changes to the pyramidal cells in layer III of the primary auditory cortex. Patients with schizophrenia have lower density of dendritic spines in layer III, whereas the total number of the pyramidal neurons is not changed (Dorph-Petersen et al., 2009), suggesting a reduction in the number of spines for each pyramidal neuron. The dendritic spines of the pyramidal neurons are the recipients of excitatory inputs, consequently a reduction in the spine density would lead to reduction of the flow of information within and forward from the auditory cortex (Javitt & Sweet, 2015). Unfortunately, it is not clear whether these alterations are directly related to likelihood of experiencing AVH, or whether they represent a more general deficit in individuals with schizophrenia.

38.5.1.2 *Magnetic Resonance Structural Studies*

In vivo measurements of the grey matter in the auditory cortex in individuals experiencing AVH may be performed using magnetic resonance imaging (MRI) (for overview, see Allen & Modinos, 2012). T1-weighted images provide a whole-brain structural image with a good contrast between grey and white matter, and have a spatial resolution on the millimetre scale. There are many approaches to the quantification of regional grey matter in the resulting images. One frequently used approach is voxel-based morphometry (VBM) (Ashburner & Friston, 2000), where either the absolute volume or the relative concentration of grey and white matter in each voxel of the brain can be compared between different groups, or examined for a relationship with symptom severity. The advantage of VBM studies is that it allows analyses that are observer-independent with regard to the definition of the auditory cortex. By contrast, manual or automatized segmentation studies delineate the auditory cortex based on anatomical landmarks, and proceed to estimate the area and thickness of grey matter in the defined region of interest (Fischl, 2012).

VBM studies indicate that the auditory cortex is implicated in AVH (Gaser et al., 2004; Neckelmann et al., 2006; Williams, 2008) (for a meta-analysis, see also Modinos et al., 2013). These and other studies have consistently reported a relationship between AVH in schizophrenia patients and reduction of grey matter in the left STG and HG, with also possible reduction in the right STG (Karabay et al., 2015; Modinos et al., 2013; Palaniyappan et al., 2012). Figure 38.1 shows an example of grey-matter reduction in AVH patients (from Neckelmann et al., 2006). There are, however, also inconsistencies in the literature, in particular regarding the HG, and the possibility that grey-matter abnormalities found in the VBM studies represent illness severity rather than any hallucination-specific process cannot be excluded (van Tol et al., 2014).

Similarly to the VBM studies, region-of-interest (ROI) studies, which are based on segmentation of grey-matter volume in the auditory cortex, have demonstrated reduction of posterior STG volume and cortical thickness, with emphasis on the left hemisphere (Oertel-Knöchel et al., 2013; Sun et al., 2009; van Swam et al., 2012). There are also findings of alterations in the HG (Allen & Modinos, 2012), with severity of AVH related to reduced volume (Sumich et al., 2005), reduced cortical thickness (Chen et al., 2015), and attenuated laterality of HG volume in hallucinating patients (Hubl et al., 2010). However, similar to VBM studies, the alterations in the HG appear less consistent than the findings in the STG.

The inconsistencies found in structural imaging results, and in particular in VBM studies, could at least partly be explained by the age of the subjects in the different studies, since it has been shown that illness duration, and hence age, plays a role in cortical volume

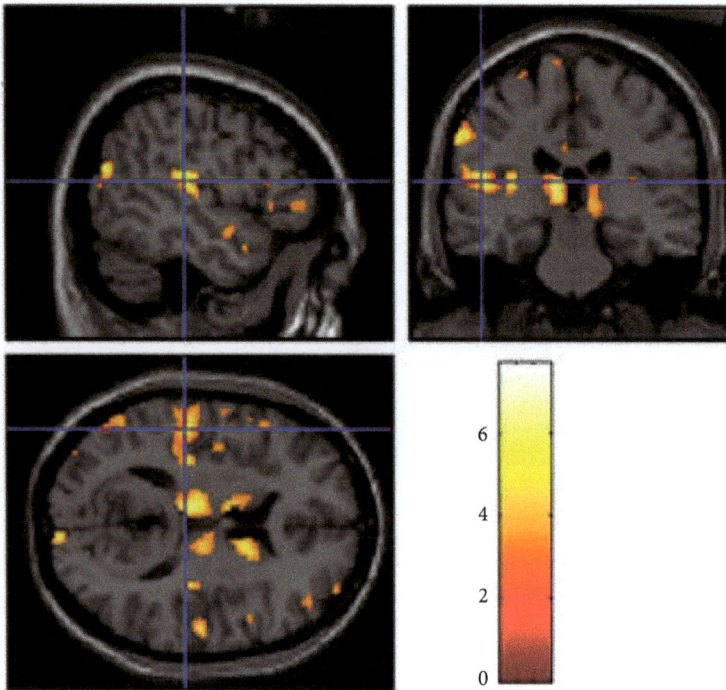

FIGURE 38.1 Example of grey-matter reduction in cortical and subcortical areas (orange areas) in AVH patients compared to healthy control subjects.

Reproduced from Neckelmann G. et al., 'MR morphometry analysis of grey matter volume reduction in schizophrenia: association with hallucinations', *International Journal of Neuroscience*, Volume 116, Issue 1, pp. 9–23, Copyright © 2006, doi: 10.1080/00207450690962244, reprinted by permission of the publisher (Taylor & Francis Ltd, http://www.tandfonline.com).

changes found in schizophrenia patients (Ho et al., 2011). Another explanation is that the VBM measure does not distinguish between cortical area and cortical thickness, since it is a measure based on voxel volume. This is possibly an important distinction, and Mørch-Johnsen et al. (2018) found that frequency and severity of AVH, as indicated from PANSS scores, correlated with cortical thickness but not with cortical area in the critical brain regions. Thus, it is currently unclear what implication can be made from structural imaging studies.

The question whether structural magnetic resonance changes in the auditory cortex are specific to AVH or represent general pathophysiology related to a diagnosis of schizophrenia could be resolved by examining non-clinical subjects with AVH, but unfortunately the literature on the structural properties of the auditory cortex in non-clinical individuals is currently very sparse. Only one structural study has reported on this issue, and the authors did not find a difference in STG cortical thickness between a non-clinical AVH group and control group (van Lutterveld, Van Den Heuvel, et al., 2014).

Structural findings do not support a link between structural properties of the auditory cortex and qualitative aspects of hallucinations, such as spatial location or attribution of voice agency. Instead, surrounding regions such as the temporo-parietal junction are implicated (Plaze et al., 2015). However, the link between the qualitative features of the AVH and neural properties of the auditory areas is, to date, an under-researched topic.

Another MRI-based technique—diffusion tensor imaging (DTI) for quantification and visualization of white-matter (WM) tract density—may be used to examine the structural connections between brain regions by examining the white-matter tracts which cross the brain. DTI is based on observing the directionality of diffusion of water molecules in the brain, and inferring thereby the path of the white-matter tracts (Le Bihan et al., 2001). One main tract of interest in connection to AVH is the arcuate fasciculus, which connects the language-relevant areas in the temporal and inferior parietal lobes with the inferior frontal cortex. Figure 38.2 shows the DTI-tracked arcuate fasciculus in a healthy subject. The interest in this connection derives from models of AVH that emphasize the importance of speech production in generating AVH. Aberrant structural connections between the speech-production areas in the frontal lobe and corresponding speech-perception areas in the auditory cortex could lead to generation of increased neuronal activity in the auditory areas without sufficient constraint from the speech-production areas to indicate that the speech representation is self-generated.

There are moderate-sized structural changes in the left arcuate fasciculus in hallucinating schizophrenia patients compared to healthy control subjects (for a meta-analysis, see Geoffroy et al., 2014), and the degree of reduced structural integrity co-varies with the severity of AVH (Curcic-Blake et al., 2015). Further, reduced structural integrity in the arcuate fasciculus appears to be specific to AVH as opposed to hallucinations in other sensory modalities (McCarthy-Jones et al., 2015). Remarkably, the arcuate fasciculus in non-clinical hallucinating individuals is affected in a similar way as for the patients, albeit to possibly a milder degree (de Weijer et al., 2013). It must be noted, however, that there are also studies which do not find a difference in the arcuate fasciculus with hallucinations, or even report stronger integrity of this tract in hallucinating patients (Hubl et al., 2004; Rotarska-Jagiela et al., 2009).

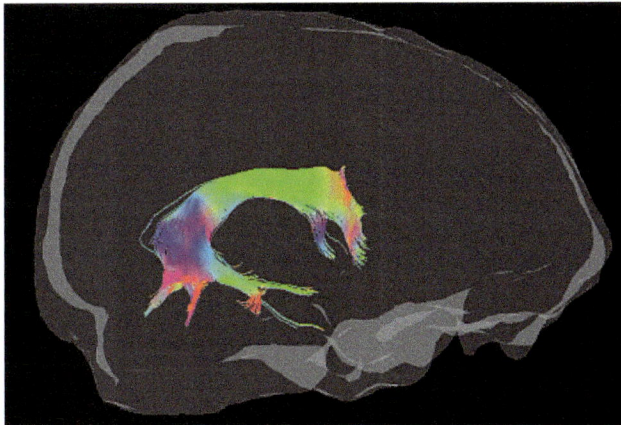

FIGURE 38.2 A DTI image of the arcuate fasciculus of a healthy subject, visualized with tractography analysis.

Data from the Bergen fMRI Group, University of Bergen, Norway.

Another neural pathway that has been examined in connection with AVH is the interhemispheric white-matter connection between the auditory cortices via the posterior corpus callosum. Many studies have found alterations in DTI measures of interhemispheric auditory pathways. However, there is disagreement in the literature regarding the direction of the difference between hallucinating and non-hallucinating patients. Both increased and decreased white-matter integrity have been reported in hallucinating compared to non-hallucinating patients (Curcic-Blake et al., 2015; Knöchel et al., 2012; Mulert et al., 2012; Rotarska-Jagiela et al., 2008; Wigand et al., 2015). The reason for the conflicting results may be due to multiple methodological issues in the analyses of the DTI images, or differences between the patient groups (e.g. differences in illness duration).

Another white-matter pathway connecting the temporal areas that has been suggested to be involved in AVH is the inferior occipito-frontal fasciculus, which is a connection involved in the hypothesized 'ventral stream' of language, relating the auditory information with the conceptual and semantic knowledge (Hickok & Poeppel, 2004). This tract has been found to be altered in hallucinating schizophrenia patients, in particular in its temporal and frontal segments (Curcic-Blake et al., 2015; Oestreich et al., 2015).

38.5.1.3 *Brain Functional Characteristics*

Attempts to characterize the functional neural correlates of AVH using neuroimaging techniques have a relatively long history (e.g. Cleghorn et al., 1992; Suzuki et al., 1993) (for reviews, see also Aleman & Vercammen, 2012: Allen et al., 2007).

There are two main approaches to attempts of understanding the neuronal mechanisms underlying AVH using functional neuroimaging (fMRI or PET). Similar to studies of structural characteristics, a common approach is to collect data on frequency, severity, and other characteristics of AVH, in separate assessments, and then correlate such data with fMRI or PET data of brain activation which is acquired during passive resting or active task processing while in the scanner (for meta-analyses, see Jardri et al., 2011; Kompus et al., 2011). Alternatively, one can identify periods of ongoing AVH during a neuroimaging session, and compare brain activation during such periods with periods when the same individual was not hallucinating. The distinction between these two approaches to functional imaging is commonly referred to as 'state-' versus 'trait-' imaging studies (cf. Kompus et al., 2011; Kühn & Gallinat, 2010).

38.5.1.4 *State Effects*

Acquiring brain-activation data on state effects is challenging due to many reasons. AVH are by their nature unpredictable and uncontrollable, and periods between episodes may be much longer than the feasible time to have a continuous neuroimaging session. In addition, the subjects must be able to correctly report when they experience AVH, in order to be able to compare brain activation during active AVH and passive rest states. The task of monitoring and reporting of AVH episodes during scanning may produce artefacts in the activations caused by motor- and attention-related processes (van Lutterveld et al., 2013). This may be mitigated by using a control task which has similar attention and monitoring demands. Despite the methodological challenges, there is an increasing body of literature describing state effects of AVH (see Jardri et al., 2011; Kompus et al., 2011; Kühn & Gallinat, 2010), and these activation patterns tend to be reproducible and reliable (Diederen, Charbonnier, et al., 2013).

fMRI studies of state effects have, in general, reported increased activation in the speech-perception areas in the left STG (Jardri et al., 2011; Kompus et al., 2011). Figure 38.3 shows state-effect fMRI activations in the left STG (data from Kompus et al., 2011). Interestingly, this activation pattern appears similar for clinical and non-clinical AVH individuals (Diederen et al., 2012), which is also consistent with phenomenological reports from non-clinical AVH individuals who report that the experienced 'voices' sound clear, salient, and 'real', just like in phenomenological reports from clinical AVH individuals.

HG activation is also frequently observed in state studies (Kompus et al., 2011); however, the consistency of this across studies appears lower than the STG activations. Studies which have looked at hallucinating patients individually have shown that HG activation during AVH episodes tends to be present in most individuals (Dierks et al., 1999), although

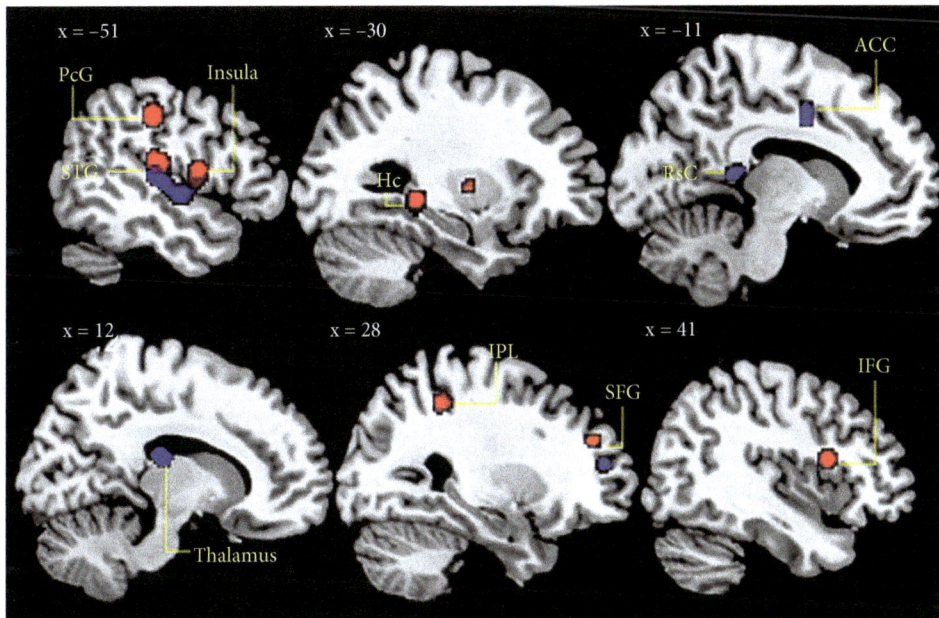

FIGURE 38.3 A meta-analysis of neuroimaging studies shows increased activation in the superior temporal gyrus in AVH patients during AVH in the absence of an external task, and reduced activations during an external task.

Abbreviations: superior temporal gyrus (STG), post-central gyrus (PcG), hippocampus (Hc), inferior parietal lobule (IPL), superior frontal gyrus (SFG), inferior frontal gyrus (IFG), anterior cingulate cortex (ACC), retrosplenial cortex (RsC).

Reprinted from *Neuropsychologia*, Volume 49, Issue 12, Kompus K., Westerhausen R., & Hugdahl K., 'The 'paradoxical' engagement of the primary auditory cortex in patients with auditory verbal hallucinations: A meta-analysis of functional neuroimaging studies', pp. 3361–9, Copyright © 2011 Elsevier Ltd., with permission from Elsevier, http://www.sciencedirect.com/science/article/pii/S0028393211003897?via%3Dihub

there is interindividual variance (Silbersweig et al., 1995). It is possible that that HG activation during an AVH episode co-varies with the perceptual intensity of the experience, since subjects who reported more vivid AVH have increased activation in the primary auditory cortex (Jardri et al., 2013). This has led to the suggestion that when HG activation is observed during ongoing hallucinations (i.e. observed as a state effect), this represents a response to back-propagation of excitatory activity from higher-level auditory areas, similar to the mechanism proposed to operate in the primary sensory cortex during retrieval from episodic memory (Jardri et al., 2013). Other characteristics may, however, also be represented in these activations. For example, the spatial location of an AVH may be determined from the activation pattern observed in the planum temporale, as this has been shown to be activated more in patients currently experiencing external-space compared to internal-space AVH (Looijestijn et al., 2013). Thus, fMRI state studies support the view that AVH are perceptual phenomena which may have a neuronal origin in the speech areas in the auditory cortex, and that this goes together with subjective reports of the qualities of experienced AVH.

Similarly to PET and fMRI studies, electrophysiological methods (EEG, MEG) have been used to examine activation patterns in the temporal lobes and the relationship to an AVH state (e.g. Ford, Mathalon, et al., 2014). EEG and MEG recordings have the advantage over fMRI in that they enable measurements to be conducted in silence, avoiding the noise caused by the gradient coils in an MR scanner, which consequently avoids the concern that the AVH-related activations would be perturbed by scanner noise. An AVH state study using EEG found increased alpha-band interhemispheric coherence between the bilateral STG (Sritharan et al., 2005). MEG studies have found increases in theta and beta activity in the left STG (Ishii et al., 2000; Reulbach et al., 2007; Ropohl et al., 2004), while one study found, by contrast, a decrease in the beta band in that region during AVH states (van Lutterveld et al., 2012).

Taken together, the electrophysiological studies are in agreement with the fMRI and PET studies showing that an AVH state leads to activation in auditory cortex regions, including the speech-perception areas of the HG and the planum temporale.

38.5.1.5 *Trait Effects*

Studies focusing on trait effects have probed the functional properties of the auditory cortex and speech-perception areas with various stimuli. With the recent developments of functional neuroimaging methods, the focus of interest has shifted from activations of a single area in the auditory cortex to characterizing the functioning of the auditory cortex in a network of interconnected brain regions, often called 'from blobology to network connectivity' (for an overview of connectivity, see Sporns, 2012). Such functional connectivity studies, either during passive rest or during task performance, aim to characterize the patterns of co-varying activations between brain regions which are not immediately adjacent but are assumed to belong to the same functional network based on the correlation of their signal time courses (Sporns et al., 2005). The evidence in the literature suggests altered functional connectivity in the auditory cortex resulting from the experience of AVH, although there are inconsistencies across studies which may be attributable to variations between methods and data-analysis procedures (for examples of the network approach to AVH, see Northoff, 2014; Northoff & Qin, 2011).

Functional connectivity between the left and right auditory areas is of interest due to the possibility that the connectivity within the auditory network, and its relationship to other networks such as the default mode network (DMN) (Raichle et al., 2001) or extrinsic mode network (EMN) (Hugdahl et al., 2015), may be related to the vulnerability to AVH (cf. Northoff & Qin, 2011). It has been reported that the bilateral resting-state connectivity in temporal lobe areas is increased in individuals who experience AVH (Diederen, Neggers, et al., 2013; Sommer et al., 2012). The left STG has also been found to act as a 'hub' for the flow of neuronal information to other brain regions in hallucinating compared to non-hallucinating patients (van Lutterveld, Diederen, et al., 2014). These findings, however, contrast with reports showing decreased resting-state interhemispheric connectivity between the bilateral primary as well as secondary auditory cortices for AVH compared to non-AVH patients (Gavrilescu et al., 2010); also no alteration to the resting-state connectivity in AVH patients has been reported (Rotarska-Jagiela et al., 2010).

There has also been considerable interest in resting-state connectivity between superior temporal lobe areas and subcortical structures. Interestingly, increased connectivity between regions in the striatum (putamen, nucleus accumbens) and bilateral STG have been reported in AVH compared to non-AVH patients, and in comparison with patients with audiovisual hallucinations (Hoffman et al., 2011; Rolland et al., 2014). This opens up the possibility of increased neuronal excitation due to increased dopaminergic links with the striatum. Reduced connectivity between the left STG and the subiculum of the hippocampus has also been reported; this was related to hallucination severity (Sommer et al., 2012).

Resting-state connectivity has, moreover, been studied with respect to phenomenological aspects of AVH. It has been found that the subjective 'reality' of hallucinations is related to increased resting-state coupling between the inferior frontal gyrus and bilateral supratemporal auditory cortices, in particular the HG (Raij et al., 2009). This suggests that connectivity between the auditory cortex and the speech-production regions in the frontal lobe may be responsible for the engagement of the primary auditory cortex during AVH.

Functional neuroimaging studies which have used external auditory stimulation with verbal and non-verbal stimuli, have in general shown reduced activation in the auditory cortex in individuals with AVH compared to non-AVH individuals (David et al., 1996; Hugdahl, Løberg, & Nygård, 2009; Woodruff et al., 1997). This is in line with behavioural studies (e.g. dichotic listening studies) which also have found impaired recognition of speech-sound stimuli (David et al., 1996; Green et al., 1994; Hugdahl, Løberg, & Nygård, 2009; Løberg et al., 1999; Woodruff et al., 1997). Meta-analyses have shown that such reduced activation is located in the left STG as well as in the left HG (Kompus et al., 2011; Kühn & Gallinat, 2010), and has been observed even for as simple stimuli as pure tones (Ford et al., 2009). Reduced activation to external stimulation has also been observed (although only in the right HG) in non-clinical AVH individuals (Kompus et al., 2013). It is, however, not clear whether there is a linear relationship between this reduced response to stimulation and hallucination severity. Moreover, caution is advised in extending this observation to encompass all populations who are prone to AVH. There are reports of non-clinical individuals with a proneness for hallucinations during sleep and hypnosis where no differences in the auditory areas were found between groups, or even increased activation was found (Lewis-Hanna et al., 2011; Szechtman et al., 1998).

Methodologically, it is important to be aware that the interpretation of activation patterns in fMRI studies occurs against a background of the scanner noise, which may change the baseline level of activation. Even though individuals with AVH and controls are equally exposed to the scanner noise, it could present a confound in that individuals with and without AVH would differ in their ability to habituate to the repetitive noise, and to separate the target stimuli from background noise.

Electrophysiological studies, on the other hand, allow for the characterization of auditory processing in the absence of background noise. Several studies have concentrated on the N1 (or N100) auditory-evoked potential, which is generated in the primary auditory cortex to external auditory stimuli, and shows sensitivity both to bottom-up features of the stimuli as well as top-down modulation by cognitive factors (Näätänen & Picton, 1987). N1-amplitude reduction has been consistently found in schizophrenia patients; however, there does not appear to be systematic significant correlations between the N1 amplitude and presence or severity of AVH (Rosburg et al., 2008, Salisbury et al., 2009). However, studies focusing on the N1 amplitude in more complex experimental situations support the observation from functional imaging studies regarding the engagement of the auditory cortex during active AVH. When tones are presented during ongoing AVH, the N1 has been shown to be delayed or attenuated (Hubl et al., 2007; Tiihonen et al., 1992), an effect similar to masking by real sounds, rather than modulation by attention (Tiihonen et al., 1992). Source-localization analyses have shown that reduction of the N1 amplitude during ongoing AVH can be attributed to reduced activity in the left temporal lobe (Hubl et al., 2007).

Furthermore, N1 latency has been used to test hypotheses of aberrant connectivity of the auditory cortex. Regarding interhemispheric connectivity as previously discussed, interhemispheric transfer time for speech stimuli to lateralized auditory stimuli has been shown to be affected in patients with AVH (Henshall, 2012). Interestingly, the interhemispheric transfer time for pure tones was not altered, indicating that the pathways connecting secondary, but not primary, auditory cortices are primarily affected in hallucinating patients. Also, structural connectivity along the arcuate fasciculus has been shown to be related to an N1 speech-suppression effect, lending support to the hypothesis that the arcuate fasciculus is relevant for the modulation of activity in the auditory cortex (Whitford et al., 2011).

Another component of interest is mismatch negativity (MMN)—a negative deflection following an unpredictable stimulus (e.g. a change in pitch) in a train of standard stimuli. The most commonly used deviant in MMN paradigms is a frequency alteration, but MMN is elicited by a wide variety of deviants (duration, intensity), as well as the omission of a stimulus, and is even elicited by changes in higher-order abstract patterns (Näätänen, 2003). The generation of MMN depends on temporal and frontal neuronal sources (Javitt et al., 1996). Multiple psychiatric and neurological conditions lead to a reduction in the MMN amplitude (Michie, 2001; Näätänen et al., 2015), and robust attenuation in schizophrenia has been shown (Umbricht & Krljes, 2005). Also, it has been shown that the reduction of grey-matter volume in the auditory cortex is correlated with a reduction of MMN amplitude over the course of illness in schizophrenia patients (Salisbury et al., 2007). However, similarly to the N1 component, there is no strong evidence for alteration of the MMN in relation to hallucinations (Umbricht & Krljes, 2005), nor have MMN alterations been found in non-clinical AVH individuals (van Lutterveld et al., 2010). However, it is possible that MMN that is elicited by duration deviants may be more sensitive to the presence of hallucinations (Fisher et al., 2008), possibly due to increased reliance on more extensive brain networks (Phillips et al., 2015).

Steady-state responses which represent the synchronization of the auditory cortex signals to externally presented trains of click sounds have been shown to be altered in AVH individuals. A paradoxical outcome is that while the auditory steady-state response in the gamma band in the left hemisphere, and synchronization across the hemispheres, is generally reduced in schizophrenia patients, these indexes are positively correlated to occurrence of AVH. Patients with more severe AVH show increased gamma-band synchronization in the left primary auditory cortex, and stronger interhemispheric synchronization (Mulert et al., 2011; Spencer et al., 2008, 2009).

38.6 SUMMARY

AVH may be experienced not only by various patient groups but also individuals who do not fulfil diagnostic criteria for any psychiatric or neurological disorder. Phenomenologically, AVH may take many forms, but it is always subjectively experienced as a perceptual event: the individual can hear 'voices' which may be indistinguishable from physically existing voices.

The behavioural and neuroimaging studies support the subjective reports by showing that individuals with AVH have alterations in auditory functioning and in brain networks that support the processing of speech. Pinpointing the neural mechanisms of AVH is challenging due to various confounds, but an increasing body of literature examining individuals with a well-characterized profile of AVH supports the view that AVH are perceptual phenomena generated by altered functional and structural connectivity between the perceptual regions in the temporal lobes and the top-down control from the frontal lobes. However, although we have emphasized a model of AVH as failure of top-down control of a bottom-up, perceptually-driven abnormality, and reviewed corresponding brain-imaging data, there is no consensus in the literature as to which cortical pathways are more important or have greater explanatory value, be it the auditory–auditory, auditory–subcortical, or auditory–frontal pathways. This should be sorted out in future research.

Future research should also aim at an increasingly fine-grained description by the subjectively experienced profile of the AVH, improving the experience-sampling methods from clinical evaluation scales to patient-controlled, mobile, and continuous assessment approaches.

REFERENCES

Alba-Ferrara, L., Fernyhough, C., Weis, S., Mitchell, R. L., & Hausmann, M. (2012). Contributions of emotional prosody comprehension deficits to the formation of auditory verbal hallucinations in schizophrenia. *Clinical Psychology Review, 32,* 244–50.

Alba-Ferrara, L., Weis, S., Damjanovic, L., Rowett, M., & Hausmann, M. (2012). Voice identity recognition failure in patients with schizophrenia. *Journal of Nervous and Mental Disease,* 200, 784–90.

Aleman, A. & Vercammen, A. (2012). Functional neuroimaging of hallucinations. In: J. D. Blom & I. E. C. Sommer (eds) *Hallucinations.* New York: Springer.

Allen, P., Aleman, A., & Mcguire, P. K. (2007). Inner speech models of auditory verbal hallucinations: evidence from behavioural and neuroimaging studies. *International Review of Psychiatry*, 19, 407–415.

Allen, P. & Modinos, G. (2012). Structural neuroimaging in psychotic patients with auditory verbal hallucinations. In: J. D. Blom & I. E. C. Sommer (eds) *Hallucinations*. New York: Springer.

Ashburner, J. & Friston, K. J. (2000). Voxel-based morphometry—the methods. *NeuroImage*, 11, 805–821.

Badcock, J. C. & Hugdahl, K. (2014). A synthesis of evidence on inhibitory control and auditory hallucinations based on the Research Domain Criteria (RDoC) framework. *Frontiers in Human Neuroscience*, 8, 180.

Badcock, J. C., Waters, F. A. V., & Maybery, M. (2007). On keeping (intrusive) thoughts to one's self: testing a cognitive model of auditory hallucinations. *Cognitive Neuropsychology*, 12, 78–89.

Bentall, R. P. (2004). *Madness Explained: Psychosis and Human Nature*. UK: Penguin Books.

Blakemore, S-J. & Frith, C. D. (2003). Self-awareness and action. *Current Opinion in Neurobiology*, 13, 219–224.

Chance, S. A., Casanova, M. F., Switala, A. E., & Crow, T. J. (2008). Auditory cortex asymmetry, altered minicolumn spacing and absence of ageing effects in schizophrenia. *Brain*, 131, 3178–3192.

Chen, X., Liang, S., Pu, W., Song, Y., Mwansisya, T. E., Yang, Q., . . . Xue, Z. (2015). Reduced cortical thickness in right Heschl's gyrus associated with auditory verbal hallucinations severity in first-episode schizophrenia. *BMC Psychiatry*, 15, 152.

Cleghorn, J. M., Franco, S., Szechtman, B., Kaplan, R. D., Szechtman, H., Brown, G. M., Nahmias, C., & Garnett, E. S. (1992). Toward a brain map of auditory hallucinations. *American Journal of Psychiatry*, 149, 1062–1069.

Copolov, D., Trauer, T., & Mackinnon, A. (2004). On the non-significance of internal versus external auditory hallucinations. *Schizophrenia Research*, 69, 1–6.

Cotter, D., Mackay, D., Frangou, S., Hudson, L., & Landau, S. (2004). Cell density and cortical thickness in Heschl's gyrus in schizophrenia, major depression and bipolar disorder. *British Journal of Psychiatry*, 185, 258–259.

Curcic-Blake, B., Nanetti, L., Van Der Meer, L., Cerliani, L., Renken, R., Pijnenborg, G. H., & Aleman, A. (2015). Not on speaking terms: hallucinations and structural network disconnectivity in schizophrenia. *Brain Structure and Function*, 220, 407–18.

Cuthbert, B. N. & Insel, T. R. (2013). Toward the future of psychiatric diagnosis: the seven pillars of RDoC. *BMC Medicine*, 11, 8.

Davalos, D. B., Kisley, M. A., & Ross, R. G. (2003). Effects of interval duration on temporal processing in schizophrenia. *Brain and Cognition*, 52, 295–301.

David, A. S., Woodruff, P. W., Howard, R., Mellers, J. D., Brammer, M., Bullmore, E., . . . Williams, S. C. (1996). Auditory hallucinations inhibit exogenous activation of auditory association cortex. *NeuroReport*, 7, 932–936.

De Weijer, A. D., Neggers, S. F. W., Diederen, K. M. S., Mandl, R. C. W., Kahn, R. S., Hulshoff Pol, H. E., & Sommer, I. E. (2013). Aberrations in the arcuate fasciculus are associated with auditory verbal hallucinations in psychotic and in non-psychotic individuals. *Human Brain Mapping*, 34, 626–634.

Diederen, K. M., Charbonnier, L., Neggers, S. F., Van Lutterveld, R., Daalman, K., Slotema, C. W., Kahn, R. S., & Sommer, I. E. (2013). Reproducibility of brain activation during auditory verbal hallucinations. *Schizophrenia Research*, 146, 320–5.

Diederen, K. M., Daalman, K., De Weijer, A. D., Neggers, S. F., Van Gastel, W., Blom, J. D., Kahn, R. S., & Sommer, I. E. (2012). Auditory hallucinations elicit similar brain activation in psychotic and nonpsychotic individuals. *Schizophrenia Bulletin, 38*, 1074–82.

Diederen, K. M., Neggers, S., De Weijer, A., Van Lutterveld, R., Daalman, K., Eickhoff, S., ... Sommer, I. (2013). Aberrant resting-state connectivity in non-psychotic individuals with auditory hallucinations. *Psychological Medicine, 43*, 1685–1696.

Dierks, T., Linden, D. E., Jandl, M., Formisano, E., Goebel, R., Lanfermann, H., & Singer, W. (1999). Activation of Heschl's gyrus during auditory hallucinations. *Neuron, 22*, 615–621.

Dorph-Petersen, K. A., Delevich, K. M., Marcsisin, M. J., Zhang, W., Sampson, A. R., Gundersen, H. J., Lewis, D. A., & Sweet, R. A. (2009). Pyramidal neuron number in layer 3 of primary auditory cortex of subjects with schizophrenia. *Brain Research, 1285*, 42–57.

Fischl, B. (2012). FreeSurfer. *NeuroImage, 62*, 774–781.

Fisher, D. J., Labelle, A., & Knott, V. J. (2008). The right profile: mismatch negativity in schizophrenia with and without auditory hallucinations as measured by a multi-feature paradigm. *Clinical Neurophysiology, 119*, 909–21.

Ford, J. M. & Mathalon, D. H. (2005). Corollary discharge dysfunction in schizophrenia: can it explain auditory hallucinations? *International Journal of Psychophysiology, 58*, 179–189.

Ford, J. M., Mathalon, D. H., Heinks, T., Kalba, S., Faustman, W. O., & Roth, W. T. (2014). Neurophysiological evidence of corollary discharge dysfunction in schizophrenia. *American Journal of Psychiatry, 158*, 2069–2071.

Ford, J. M., Morris, S. E., Hoffman, R. E., Sommer, I., Waters, F., Mccarthy-Jones, S., ... Badcock, J. C. (2014). Studying hallucinations within the NIMH RDoC framework. *Schizophrenia Bulletin, 40*, S295–S304

Ford, J. M., Roach, B. J., Jorgensen, K. W., Turner, J. A., Brown, G. G., Notestine, R., ... Lauriello, J. (2009). Tuning in to the voices: a multisite FMRI study of auditory hallucinations. *Schizophrenia Bulletin, 35*, 58–66.

Frith, C. D., Blakemore, S-J., & Wolpert, D. M. (2000). Explaining the symptoms of schizophrenia: abnormalities in the awareness of action. *Brain Research Reviews, 31*, 357–363.

Frith, C. D. & Done, D. J. (1988). Towards a neuropsychology of schizophrenia. *British Journal of Psychiatry, 153*, 437–443.

Gaser, C., Nenadic, I., Volz, H.-P., Büchel, C., & Sauer, H. (2004). Neuroanatomy of 'hearing voices': a frontotemporal brain structural abnormality associated with auditory hallucinations in schizophrenia. *Cerebral Cortex, 14*, 91–96.

Gavrilescu, M., Rossell, S., Stuart, G., Shea, T., Innes-Brown, H., Henshall, K., ... Egan, G. (2010). Reduced connectivity of the auditory cortex in patients with auditory hallucinations: a resting state functional magnetic resonance imaging study. *Psychological Medicine, 40*, 1149–1158.

Geoffroy, P. A., Houenou, J., Duhamel, A., Amad, A., De Weijer, A. D., Curcic-Blake, B., ... Jardri, R. (2014). The arcuate fasciculus in auditory-verbal hallucinations: a meta-analysis of diffusion-tensor-imaging studies. *Schizophrenia Research, 159*, 234–7.

Green, M. F., Hugdahl, K., & Mitchell, S. (1994). Dichotic listening during auditory hallucinations in patients with schizophrenia. *American Journal of Psychiatry, 151*, 357.

Henshall, K. R., Sergejew, A. A., McKay, C. M., Rance, G., Shea, T. L., Hayden, M. J., Innes-Brown, H., & Copolov, D. L. (2012). Interhemispheric transfer time in patients with auditory hallucinations: an auditory event-related potential study. *International Journal of Psychophysiology, 84*, 130–139.

Hickok, G. & Poeppel, D. (2004). Dorsal and ventral streams: a framework for understanding aspects of the functional anatomy of language. *Cognition, 92*, 67–99.

Ho, B.-C., Andreasen, N.C., Ziebell, S.,Pierson, R., & Magnotta, V. (2011). Long-term anti-psychotic treatment and brain volumes: a longitudinal study of first-episode schizophrenia. *Archives of General Psychiatry*, 68,128–137.

Hoffman, R. E., Fernandez, T., Pittman, B., & Hampson, M. (2011). Elevated functional con-nectivity along a corticostriatal loop and the mechanism of auditory/verbal hallucinations in patients with schizophrenia. *Biological Psychiatry*, 69, 407–414.

Hubl, D., Dougoud-Chauvin, V., Zeller, M., Federspiel, A., Boesch, C., Strik, W., Dierks, T., & Koenig, T. (2010). Structural analysis of Heschl's gyrus in schizophrenia patients with audi-tory hallucinations. *Neuropsychobiology*, 61, 1–9.

Hubl, D., Koenig, T., Strik, W., Federspiel, A., Kreis, R., Boesch, C., … Dierks, T. (2004). Pathways that make voices: white matter changes in auditory hallucinations. *Archives of General Psychiatry*, 61, 658–668.

Hubl, D., Koenig, T., Strik, W. K., Garcia, L. M., & Dierks, T. (2007). Competition for neur-onal resources: how hallucinations make themselves heard. *British Journal of Psychiatry*, 190, 57–62.

Hugdahl, K. (2009). 'Hearing voices': Auditory hallucinations as failure of top-down control of bottom-up perceptual processes. *Scandinavian Journal of Psychology*, 50, 553–560.

Hugdahl, K. (2015). Auditory hallucinations: a review of the ERC 'VOICE' project. *World Journal of Psychiatry*, 5, 193.

Hugdahl, K., Davidson, R., & Hugdahl, K. (1995). Dichotic listening: probing temporal lobe functional integrity. *Brain Asymmetry*, 1, 123–56.

Hugdahl, K., Loberg, E. M., Falkenberg, L. E., Johnsen, E., Kompus, K., Kroken, R. A., … Özgören, M. (2012). Auditory verbal hallucinations in schizophrenia as aberrant lateralized speech perception: evidence from dichotic listening. *Schizophrenia Research*, 140, 59–64.

Hugdahl, K., Loberg, E. M., Jorgensen, H. A., Lundervold, A., Lund, A., Green, M. F., & Rund, B. (2008). Left hemisphere lateralisation of auditory hallucinations in schizophrenia: a di-chotic listening study. *Cognitive Neuropsychiatry*, 13, 166–79.

Hugdahl, K., Løberg, E.-M., & Nygård, M. (2009). Left temporal lobe structural and functional abnormality underlying auditory hallucinations in schizophrenia. *Frontiers in Human Neuroscience*, 3, 34.

Hugdahl, K., Raichle, M. E., Mitra, A., & Specht, K. (2015). On the existence of a generalized non-specific task-dependent network. *Frontiers in Human Neuroscience*, 9, 430.

Hugdahl, K., Westerhausen, R., Alho, K., Medvedev, S., Laine, M., & Hämäläinen, H. (2009). Attention and cognitive control: unfolding the dichotic listening story. *Scandinavian Journal of Psychology*, 50, 11–22.

Ishii, R., Shinosaki, K., Ikejiri, Y., Ukai, S., Yamashita, K., Iwase, M., … Takeda, M. (2000). Theta rhythm increases in left superior temporal cortex during auditory hallucinations in schizophrenia: a case report. *NeuroReport*, 11, 3283–7.

Jardri, R., Pouchet, A., Pins, D., & Thomas, P. (2011). Cortical activations during auditory verbal hallucinations in schizophrenia: a coordinate-based meta-analysis. *American Journal of Psychiatry*, 168, 73–81.

Jardri, R., Thomas, P., Delmaire, C., Delion, P., & Pins, D. (2013). The neurodynamic organiza-tion of modality-dependent hallucinations. *Cerebral Cortex*, 23, 1108–1117.

Jaspers, K. (1962). *General Psychopathology*. Manchester University Press.

Javitt, D. C., Steinschneider, M., Schroeder, C. E., & Arezzo, J. C. (1996). Role of cortical N-methyl-D-aspartate receptors in auditory sensory memory and mismatch negativity generation: implications for schizophrenia. *Proceedings of the National Academy of Sciences of the USA*, 93(21), 11962–11967.

Javitt, D. C. & Sweet, R. A. (2015). Auditory dysfunction in schizophrenia: integrating clinical and basic features. *Nature Reviews Neuroscience*, 16, 535–550.

Johns, L. C., Kompus, K., Connell, M., Humpston, C., Lincoln, T. M., Longden, E., … Cella, M. (2014). Auditory verbal hallucinations in persons with and without a need for care. *Schizophrenia Bulletin*, 40, S255–S264.

Johns, L. C. & Van Os, J. (2001). The continuity of psychotic experiences in the general population. *Clinical Psychology Review*, 21, 1125–1141.

Jones, S. R. (2010). Do we need multiple models of auditory verbal hallucinations? Examining the phenomenological fit of cognitive and neurological models. *Schizophrenia Bulletin*, 36, 566–575.

Jones, S. R. & Fernyhough, C. (2007). Neural correlates of inner speech and auditory verbal hallucinations: a critical review and theoretical integration. *Clinical Psychology Review*, 27, 140–154.

Karabay, N., Öniz, A., Taşlıca, S., Alptekin, K., Hugdahl, K., & Özgören, M. (2015). Brain morphometry and electrophysiological recordings in relation to illness duration in schizophrenia. *Neuroscience Letters*, 593, 118–123.

Kay, S. R., Flszbein, A., & Opfer, L. A. (1987). The positive and negative syndrome scale (PANSS) for schizophrenia. *Schizophrenia Bulletin*, 13, 261.

Kaymaz, N. & Van Os, J. (2010). Extended psychosis phenotype—yes: single continuum— unlikely. *Psychological Medicine*, 40, 1963–1966.

Kimura, D. (1961). Cerebral dominance and the perception of verbal stimuli. *Canadian Journal of Psychology/Revue canadienne de psychologie*, 15, 166.

Kimura, D. (1967). Functional asymmetry of the brain in dichotic listening. *Cortex*, 3. doi:10.1016/S0010-9452(67)80010-8

Knöchel, C., Oertel-Knöchel, V., Schönmeyer, R., Rotarska-Jagiela, A., Van De Ven, V., Prvulovic, D., … Hampel, H. (2012). Interhemispheric hypoconnectivity in schizophrenia: fiber integrity and volume differences of the corpus callosum in patients and unaffected relatives. *NeuroImage*, 59, 926–934.

Kompus, K., Falkenberg, L. E., Bless, J. J., Johnsen, E., Kroken, R. A., Kråkvik, B., … Westerhausen, R. (2013). The role of the primary auditory cortex in the neural mechanism of auditory verbal hallucinations. *Frontiers in Human Neuroscience*, 7, 144.

Kompus, K., Westerhausen, R., & Hugdahl, K. (2011). The 'paradoxical' engagement of the primary auditory cortex in patients with auditory verbal hallucinations: a meta-analysis of functional neuroimaging studies. *Neuropsychologia*, 49, 3361–3369.

Kühn, S. & Gallinat, J. (2010). Quantitative meta-analysis on state and trait aspects of auditory verbal hallucinations in schizophrenia. *Schizophrenia Bulletin*, 38, 779–786.

Larøi, F., Sommer, I. E., Blom, J. D., Fernyhough, C., Hugdahl, K., Johns, L. C., … Slotema, C. W. (2012). The characteristic features of auditory verbal hallucinations in clinical and nonclinical groups: state-of-the-art overview and future directions. *Schizophrenia Bulletin*, 38, 724–733.

Le Bihan, D., Mangin, J. F., Poupon, C., Clark, C. A., Pappata, S., Molko, N., & Chabriat, H. (2001). Diffusion tensor imaging: concepts and applications. *Journal of Magnetic Resonance Imaging*, 13, 534–546.

Lewis-Hanna, L. L., Hunter, M. D., Farrow, T. F., Wilkinson, I. D., & Woodruff, P. W. (2011). Enhanced cortical effects of auditory stimulation and auditory attention in healthy individuals prone to auditory hallucinations during partial wakefulness. *NeuroImage*, 57, 1154–1161.

Linszen, M. M., Brouwer, R. M., Heringa, S. M., & Sommer, I. E. (2015). Increased risk of psychosis in patients with hearing impairment: review and meta-analyses. *Neuroscience & Biobehavioral Reviews*, 62, 1–20.

Løberg, E.-M., Hugdahl, K., & Green, M. F. (1999). Hemispheric asymmetry in schizophrenia: a 'dual deficits' model. *Biological Psychiatry*, 45, 76–81.

Løberg, E.-M., Jørgensen, H. A., & Hugdahl, K. (2004). Dichotic listening in schizophrenic patients: effects of previous vs. ongoing auditory hallucinations. *Psychiatry Research*, 128, 167–174.

Looijestijn, J., Diederen, K. M., Goekoop, R., Sommer, I. E., Daalman, K., Kahn, R. S., Hoek, H. W., & Blom, J. D. (2013). The auditory dorsal stream plays a crucial role in projecting hallucinated voices into external space. *Schizophrenia Research*, 146, 314–9.

Mccarthy-Jones, S., Oestreich, L. K., & Whitford, T. J. (2015). Reduced integrity of the left arcuate fasciculus is specifically associated with auditory verbal hallucinations in schizophrenia. *Schizophrenia Research*, 162, 1–6.

Mccarthy-Jones, S., Trauer, T., Mackinnon, A., Sims, E., Thomas, N., & Copolov, D. L. (2014). A new phenomenological survey of auditory hallucinations: evidence for subtypes and implications for theory and practice. *Schizophrenia Bulletin*, 40, 231–235.

Mcguire, P., David, A., Murray, R., Frackowiak, R., Frith, C., Wright, I., & Silbersweig, D. (1995). Abnormal monitoring of inner speech: a physiological basis for auditory hallucinations. *The Lancet*, 346, 596–600.

Mcguire, P. K., Murray, R., & Shah, G. (1993). Increased blood flow in Broca's area during auditory hallucinations in schizophrenia. *The Lancet*, 342, 703–706.

McKay, C. M., Headlam, D. M., & Copolov, D. L. (2000). Central auditory processing in patients with auditory hallucinations. *American Journal of Psychiatry*, 157, 759–766.

Mclachlan, N. M., Phillips, D. S., Rossell, S. L., & Wilson, S. J. (2013). Auditory processing and hallucinations in schizophrenia. *Schizophrenia Research*, 150, 380–5.

Michie, P. T. (2001). What has MMN revealed about the auditory system in schizophrenia? *International Journal of Psychophysiology*, 42, 177–194.

Michie, P. T., Badcock, J. C., Waters, F. A., & Mayberry, M. T. (2005). Auditory hallucinations: failure to inhibit irrelevant memories. *Cognitive Neuropsychiatry*, 10, 125–136.

Modinos, G., Costafreda, S. G., Van Tol, M.-J., Mcguire, P. K., Aleman, A., & Allen, P. (2013). Neuroanatomy of auditory verbal hallucinations in schizophrenia: a quantitative meta-analysis of voxel-based morphometry studies. *Cortex*, 49, 1046–1055.

Mørch-Johnsen, L., Nerland, S., Jørgensen, K. N., Osnes, K., Hartberg, C. B., Andreassen, O. A., ... Agartz, I. (2018). Cortical thickness abnormalities in bipolar disorder patients with a lifetime history of auditory hallucinations. *Bipolar Disorder*. doi: 10.1111/bdi.12627

Mulert, C., Kirsch, V., Pascual-Marqui, R., Mccarley, R. W., & Spencer, K. M. (2011). Long-range synchrony of gamma oscillations and auditory hallucination symptoms in schizophrenia. *International Journal of Psychophysiology*, 79, 55–63.

Mulert, C., Kirsch, V., Whitford, T. J., Alvarado, J., Pelavin, P., Mccarley, R. W., ... Shenton, M. E. (2012). Hearing voices: a role of interhemispheric auditory connectivity? *The World Journal of Biological Psychiatry*, 13, 153–158.

Nayani, T. H. & David, A. S. (1996). The auditory hallucination: a phenomenological survey. *Psychological Medicine*, 26, 177–189.

Neckelmann, G., Specht, K., Lund, A., Ersland, L., Smievoll, A. I., Neckelmann, D., & Hugdahl, K. (2006). MR morphometry analysis of grey matter volume reduction in schizophrenia: association with hallucinations. *International Journal of Neuroscience*, 116, 9–23.

Northoff, G. (2014). Are auditory hallucinations related to the brain's resting state activity? A 'neurophenomenal resting state hypothesis'. *Clinical Psychopharmacology and Neuroscience*, 12, 189–195.

Northoff, G. & Qin, P. (2011). How can the brain's resting state activity generate hallucinations? A 'resting state hypothesis' of auditory verbal hallucinations. *Schizophrenia Research*, 127, 202–214.

Näätänen, R. (2003). Mismatch negativity: clinical research and possible applications. *International Journal of Psychophysiology*, 48, 179–188.

Näätänen, R. & Picton, T. (1987). The N1 wave of the human electric and magnetic response to sound: a review and an analysis of the component structure. *Psychophysiology*, 24, 375–425.

Näätänen, R., Shiga, T., Asano, S., & Yabe, H. (2015). Mismatch negativity (MMN) deficiency: a break-through biomarker in predicting psychosis onset. *International Journal of Psychophysiology*, 95, 338–344.

Ocklenburg, S., Westerhausen, R., Hirnstein, M., & Hugdahl, K. (2013). Auditory hallucinations and reduced language lateralization in schizophrenia: a meta-analysis of dichotic listening studies. *Journal of the International Neuropsychological Society*, 19, 410–418.

Oertel-Knöchel, V., Knöchel, C., Rotarska-Jagiela, A., Reinke, B., Prvulovic, D., Haenschel, C., Hampel, H., & Linden, D. E. (2013). Association between psychotic symptoms and cortical thickness reduction across the schizophrenia spectrum. *Cerebral Cortex*, 23, 61–70.

Oestreich, L. K., Mccarthy-Jones, S., & Whitford, T. J. (2015). Decreased integrity of the fronto-temporal fibers of the left inferior occipito-frontal fasciculus associated with auditory verbal hallucinations in schizophrenia. *Brain Imaging and Behavior*, 1–10.

Palaniyappan, L., Balain, V., Radua, J., & Liddle, P. F. (2012). Structural correlates of auditory hallucinations in schizophrenia: a meta-analysis. *Schizophrenia Research*, 137, 169–173.

Phillips, H. N., Blenkmann, A., Hughes, L. E., Bekinschtein, T. A., & Rowe, J. B. (2015). Hierarchical organization of frontotemporal networks for the prediction of stimuli across multiple dimensions. *The Journal of Neuroscience*, 35, 9255–9264.

Plaze, M., Mangin, J. F., Paillere-Martinot, M. L., Artiges, E., Olie, J. P., Krebs, M. O., ... Cachia, A. (2015). 'Who is talking to me?'— self-other attribution of auditory hallucinations and sulcation of the right temporoparietal junction. *Schizophrenia Research*, 169, 95–100.

Plaze, M., Paillère-Martinot, M.-L., Penttilä, J., Januel, D., De Beaurepaire, R., Bellivier, F., ... Artiges, E. (2009). 'Where do auditory hallucinations come from?'—a brain morphometry study of schizophrenia patients with inner or outer space hallucinations. *Schizophrenia Bulletin*, sbp081.

Raichle, M. E., Macleod, A. M., Snyder, A. Z., Powers, W. J., Gusnard, D. A., & Shulman, G. L. (2001). A default mode of brain function. *Proceedings of the National Academy of Sciences*, 98, 676–682.

Raij, T. T., Valkonen-Korhonen, M., Holi, M., Therman, S., Lehtonen, J., & Hari, R. (2009). Reality of auditory verbal hallucinations. *Brain*, 132, 2994–3001.

Reulbach, U., Bleich, S., Maihöfner, C., Kornhuber, J., & Sperling, W. (2007). Specific and unspecific auditory hallucinations in patients with schizophrenia. *Neuropsychobiology*, 55, 89–95.

Rolland, B., Amad, A., Poulet, E., Bordet, R., Vignaud, A., Bation, R., … Jardri, R. (2014). Resting-state functional connectivity of the nucleus accumbens in auditory and visual hallucinations in schizophrenia. *Schizophrenia Bulletin*, sbu097.

Ropohl, A., Sperling, W., Elstner, S., Tomandl, B., Reulbach, U., Kaltenhäuser, M., Kornhuber, J., & Maihöfner, C. (2004). Cortical activity associated with auditory hallucinations. *NeuroReport*, 15, 523–526.

Rosburg, T., Boutros, N. N., & Ford, J. M. (2008). Reduced auditory evoked potential component N100 in schizophrenia—a critical review. *Psychiatry Research*, 161, 259–274.

Rotarska-Jagiela, A., Oertel-Knoechel, V., Demartino, F., Van De Ven, V., Formisano, E., Roebroeck, A., … Hendler, T. (2009). Anatomical brain connectivity and positive symptoms of schizophrenia: a diffusion tensor imaging study. *Psychiatry Research: Neuroimaging*, 174, 9–16.

Rotarska-Jagiela, A., Schönmeyer, R., Oertel, V., Haenschel, C., Vogeley, K., & Linden, D. E. (2008). The corpus callosum in schizophrenia-volume and connectivity changes affect specific regions. *NeuroImage*, 39, 1522–1532.

Rotarska-Jagiela, A., Van De Ven, V., Oertel-Knöchel, V., Uhlhaas, P. J., Vogeley, K., & Linden, D. E. (2010). Resting-state functional network correlates of psychotic symptoms in schizophrenia. *Schizophrenia Research*, 117, 21–30.

Salisbury, D. F., Collins, K., & Mccarley, R. W. (2009). Reductions in the N1 and P2 auditory event-related potentials in first-hospitalized and chronic schizophrenia. *Schizophrenia Bulletin*, 36, 991–1000.

Salisbury, D. F., Kuroki, N., Kasai, K., Shenton, M. E., & Mccarley, R. W. (2007). Progressive and interrelated functional and structural evidence of post-onset brain reduction in schizophrenia. *Archives of General Psychiatry*, 64, 521–529.

Shergill, S. S., Murray, R. M., & Mcguire, P. K. (1998). Auditory hallucinations: a review of psychological treatments. *Schizophrenia Research*, 32, 137–150.

Silbersweig, D., Stern, E., Frith, C., Cahill, C., Holmes, A., Grootoonk, S., … Schnorr, L. (1995). A functional neuroanatomy of hallucinations in schizophrenia. *Nature*, 176–179.

Smiley, J. F., Hackett, T. A., Preuss, T. M., Bleiwas, C., Figarsky, K., Mann, J. J., … Dwork, A. J. (2013). Hemispheric asymmetry of primary auditory cortex and Heschl's gyrus in schizophrenia and nonpsychiatric brains. *Psychiatry Research*, 214, 435–43.

Smiley, J. F., Rosoklija, G., Mancevski, B., Mann, J. J., Dwork, A. J., & Javitt, D. C. (2009). Altered volume and hemispheric asymmetry of the superficial cortical layers in the schizophrenia planum temporale. *European Journal of Neuroscience*, 30, 449–463.

Sommer, I. E., Clos, M., Meijering, A. L., Diederen, K. M., & Eickhoff, S. B. (2012). Resting state functional connectivity in patients with chronic hallucinations. *PLoS One*, 7, e43516.

Sommer, I. E., Daalman, K., Rietkerk, T., Diederen, K. M., Bakker, S., Wijkstra, J., & Boks, M. P. (2010). Healthy individuals with auditory verbal hallucinations; who are they? Psychiatric assessments of a selected sample of 103 subjects. *Schizophrenia Bulletin*, 36, 633–641.

Sommer, I. E., Derwort, A. M., Daalman, K., De Weijer, A. D., Liddle, P. F., & Boks, M. P. (2010). Formal thought disorder in non-clinical individuals with auditory verbal hallucinations. *Schizophrenia Research*, 118, 140–145.

Sommer, I. E., Diederen, K. M., Blom, J.-D., Willems, A., Kushan, L., Slotema, K., … Neggers, S. F. (2008). Auditory verbal hallucinations predominantly activate the right inferior frontal area. *Brain*, 131, 3169–3177.

Spencer, K. M., Niznikiewicz, M. A., Nestor, P. G., Shenton, M. E., & Mccarley, R. W. (2009). Left auditory cortex gamma synchronization and auditory hallucination symptoms in schizophrenia. *BMC Neuroscience*, 10, 85.

Spencer, K. M., Salisbury, D. F., Shenton, M. E., & Mccarley, R. W. (2008). Gamma-band auditory steady-state responses are impaired in first episode psychosis. *Biological Psychiatry, 64,* 369–75.

Sporns, O. (2012). From simple graphs to the connectome: networks in neuroimaging. *NeuroImage, 62,* 881–886.

Sporns, O., Tononi, G., & Kötter, R. (2005). The human connectome: a structural description of the human brain. *PLoS Computational Biology, 1,* e42.

Sritharan, A., Line, P., Sergejew, A., Silberstein, R., Egan, G., & Copolov, D. (2005). EEG coherence measures during auditory hallucinations in schizophrenia. *Psychiatry Research, 136,* 189–200.

Stephane, M., Barton, S., & Boutros, N. (2001). Auditory verbal hallucinations and dysfunction of the neural substrates of speech. *Schizophrenia Research, 50,* 61–78.

Sumich, A., Chitnis, X. A., Fannon, D. G., O'ceallaigh, S., Doku, V. C., Faldrowicz, A., & Sharma, T. (2005). Unreality symptoms and volumetric measures of Heschl's gyrus and planum temporal in first-episode psychosis. *Biological Psychiatry, 57,* 947–950.

Sun, J., Maller, J. J., Guo, L., & Fitzgerald, P. B. (2009). Superior temporal gyrus volume change in schizophrenia: a review on region of interest volumetric studies. *Brain Research Reviews, 61,* 14–32.

Suzuki, M., Yuasa, S., Minabe, Y., Murata, M., & Kurachi, M. (1993). Left superior temporal blood flow increases in schizophrenic and schizophreniform patients with auditory hallucination: a longitudinal case study using 123I-IMP SPECT. *European Archives of Psychiatry and Clinical Neuroscience, 242,* 257–261.

Szechtman, H., Woody, E., Bowers, K. S., & Nahmias, C. (1998). Where the imaginal appears real: a positron emission tomography study of auditory hallucinations. *Proceedings of the National Academy of Sciences, 95,* 1956–1960.

Tiihonen, J., Hari, R., Naukkarinen, H., Rimon, R., Jousmaki, V., & Kajola, M. (1992). Modified activity of the human auditory cortex during auditory hallucinations. *American Journal of Psychiatry, 149,* 255–7.

Tucker, R., Farhall, J., Thomas, N., Groot, C., & Rossell, S. L. (2013). An examination of auditory processing and affective prosody in relatives of patients with auditory hallucinations. *Frontiers in Human Neuroscience, 7,* 531.

Umbricht, D. & Krljes, S. (2005). Mismatch negativity in schizophrenia: a meta-analysis. *Schizophrenia Research, 76,* 1–23.

Van Lutterveld, R., Diederen, K. M., Otte, W. M., & Sommer, I. E. (2014). Network analysis of auditory hallucinations in nonpsychotic individuals. *Human Brain Mapping, 35,* 1436–1445.

Van Lutterveld, R., Diederen, K., Schutte, M., Bakker, R., Zandbelt, B., & Sommer, I. (2013). Brain correlates of auditory hallucinations: stimulus detection is a potential confounder. *Schizophrenia Research, 1,* 319–320.

Van Lutterveld, R., Hillebrand, A., Diederen, K., Daalman, K., Kahn, R. S., Stam, C. J., & Sommer, I. E. (2012). Oscillatory cortical network involved in auditory verbal hallucinations in schizophrenia. *PLoS One, 7,* e41149.

Van Lutterveld, R., Oranje, B., Kemner, C., Abramovic, L., Willems, A. E., Boks, M. P., … Sommer, I. E. (2010). Increased psychophysiological parameters of attention in nonpsychotic individuals with auditory verbal hallucinations. *Schizophrenia Research, 121,* 153–159.

Van Lutterveld, R., Van Den Heuvel, M. P., Diederen, K. M., De Weijer, A. D., Begemann, M. J., Brouwer, R. M., … Sommer, I. E. (2014). Cortical thickness in individuals with non-clinical and clinical psychotic symptoms. *Brain, 137,* 2664–2669.

Van Swam, C., Federspiel, A., Hubl, D., Wiest, R., Boesch, C., Vermathen, P., ... Dierks, T. (2012). Possible dysregulation of cortical plasticity in auditory verbal hallucinations—a cortical thickness study in schizophrenia. *Journal of Psychiatric Research, 46,* 1015–1023.

Van Tol, M. J., Van Der Meer, L., Bruggeman, R., Modinos, G., Knegtering, H., & Aleman, A. (2014). Voxel-based gray and white matter morphometry correlates of hallucinations in schizophrenia: the superior temporal gyrus does not stand alone. *NeuroImage Clinical, 4,* 249–57.

Wallwork, R., Fortgang, R., Hashimoto, R., Weinberger, D., & Dickinson, D. (2012). Searching for a consensus five-factor model of the Positive and Negative Syndrome Scale for schizophrenia. *Schizophrenia Research, 137,* 246–250.

Waters, F., Badcock, J., Michie, P., & Maybery, M. (2006). Auditory hallucinations in schizophrenia: intrusive thoughts and forgotten memories. *Cognitive Neuropsychiatry, 11,* 65–83.

Whitford, T., Mathalon, D., Shenton, M., Roach, B., Bammer, R., Adcock, R., ... Rausch, A. (2011). Electrophysiological and diffusion tensor imaging evidence of delayed corollary discharges in patients with schizophrenia. *Psychological Medicine, 41,* 959–969.

Wigand, M., Kubicki, M., Clemm Von Hohenberg, C., Leicht, G., Karch, S., Eckbo, R., ... Bouix, S. (2015). Auditory verbal hallucinations and the interhemispheric auditory pathway in chronic schizophrenia. *The World Journal of Biological Psychiatry, 16,* 31–44.

Williams, L. M. (2008). Voxel-based morphometry in schizophrenia: implications for neurodevelopmental connectivity models, cognition and affect. *Expert Review of Neurotherapeutics, 8,* 1049–1065.

Woodruff, P. W., Wright, I. C., Bullmore, E. T., Brammer, M., Howard, R. J., Williams, S. C., ... Mcguire, P. K. (1997). Auditory hallucinations and the temporal cortical response to speech in schizophrenia: a functional magnetic resonance imaging study. *American Journal of Psychiatry, 154,* 1676–1682.

....

CHAPTER 39

DEFICITS IN VOICE-IDENTITY PROCESSING
Acquired and Developmental Phonagnosia

....

CLAUDIA ROSWANDOWITZ*,
CORRINA MAGUINNESS*,
AND KATHARINA VON KRIEGSTEIN

39.1 INTRODUCTION

....

RECOGNIZING a person by voice is a skill, which humans master with ease. However, for some people this skill can be impaired. This deficit is termed 'phonagnosia' (Van Lancker & Canter, 1982), originating from the Greek words 'φώνημα' or 'phone', meaning voice or sound, and the term 'agnosia' (αγνώσις). Agnosia is commonly used for conditions in which the recognition of stimuli is disturbed (Freud, 1891; Lissauer, 1890). In phonagnosia, the ability to process other vocal information (e.g. gender, age, and emotion) as well as speech, music, and facial information, is largely preserved (Garrido et al., 2009; Neuner & Schweinberger, 2000; Roswandowitz et al., 2014). Phonagnosia can occur after brain damage (i.e. *acquired phonagnosia*) (Assal et al., 1976; Neuner & Schweinberger, 2000; Van Lancker & Canter, 1982) or in the absence of brain insult (i.e. *developmental phonagnosia*) (Garrido et al., 2009; Roswandowitz et al., 2014).

The disorder has currently two major subclassifications: apperceptive and associative phonagnosia. In apperceptive phonagnosia, the deficit lies in the perceptual analysis of voice features, whereas the association of semantic information to a voice is intact (Hailstone et al.,

* Both authors contributed equally to this work.

2011; Roswandowitz et al., 2014; Xu et al., 2015). Associative phonagnosia is understood as a failure to recognize a voice as familiar (familiarity decision) and to associate semantic information to a voice (semantic processing), though the perception of the voice is unaffected (Hailstone et al., 2010, 2011; Roswandowitz et al., 2014).

Though phonagnosia may offer a unique instance to study auditory person recognition, the number of scientific investigations so far has been limited. This might be due to the following factors: (i) Phonagnosia has been under scientific investigation for a rather short time. The first study on acquired phonagnosia was published in 1976 (Assal et al., 1976) and on developmental phonagnosia in 2009 (Garrido et al., 2009). (ii) Testing of voice-recognition deficits is relatively difficult, as standard tests are not readily available and are often language-dependent (but see Aglieri et al., 2017). (iii) Cases of phonagnosia are rare, although this perceived rarity may be more related to a low self-awareness, rather than a low prevalence rate, of voice-identity processing disorders (Roswandowitz et al., 2014).

In this chapter, we provide a systematic overview of investigations on phonagnosia and how they relate to current models of voice-identity processing. We begin by introducing a neurocognitive model of voice-identity processing and provide an overview of the behavioural tests which are used to assess cases and subtypes of phonagnosia. We then review clinical studies, which documented cases of acquired phonagnosia, before turning to focus on recently reported cases of developmental phonagnosia. We discuss the reviewed findings within the context of current voice-identity processing models and conclude with proposing future research directions.

39.2 MODEL OF VOICE-IDENTITY PROCESSING

Recognizing voices at the individual level is a challenge for the perceptual and cognitive system. Each voice that we hear shares the same basic perceptual features across individuals (acoustic parameters such as pitch and timbre) (Lavner et al., 2001; López et al., 2013), and thus the brain is tasked with representing a unique voice in memory, by perceiving and representing often subtle differences in these features across individuals (Belin et al., 2004, 2011). Furthermore, it is not sufficient that we simply recognize a voice as familiar. Rather, successful voice recognition also involves linking the familiar voice to stored knowledge, or semantics, including where we know the voice from, what the person looks like, and whether they are a friend or a foe. Thus, voice recognition can be conceived as a *multistage* process, which begins with the encoding of the incoming vocal signal and ends in successful identification of the voice at the level of a specific individual identity. In Figure 39.1A, we present a cognitive model of voice-identity processing, and highlight candidate brain regions in Figure 39.1B which may support this multistage process. We also outline how subtypes of phonagnosia, apperceptive and associative, may arise due to dysfunction at different *stages* of voice-identity processing.

According to the model (Figure 39.1A), the vocal sound undergoes an initial general processing phase. This processing may be partly shared and partly independent from the processing of other sound sources, including object sounds or music. After this initial phase, voice-identity processing begins. In the following, we describe these processing stages in detail.

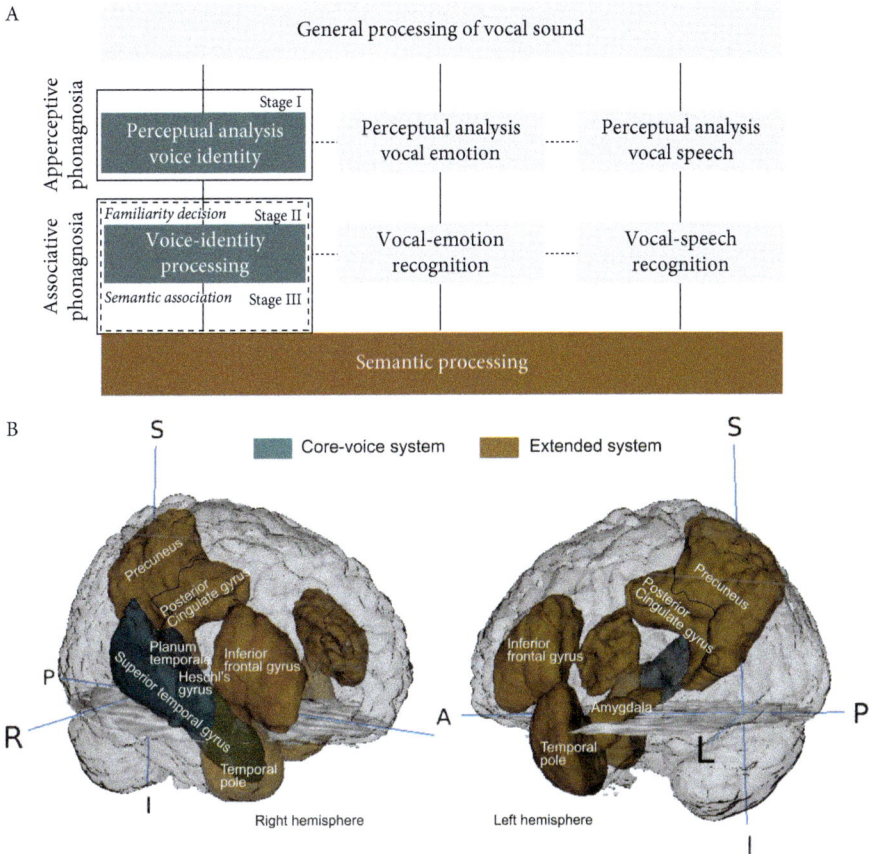

FIGURE 39.1 Neurocognitive model of voice processing. (A) Model (adapted from Ellis et al., 1997; Belin et al., 2004; Blank et al., 2014; Neuner & Schweinberger, 2000) based on a seminal model of face processing outlined by Bruce and Young (1986) which describes the cognitive processes involved in voice-identity processing. (B) Overview of potential brain structures supporting voice-identity processing, as evidenced in neuroimaging studies with neurotypical participants. (R= right; L = left; S = superior; I = inferior; A = anterior; P = posterior)

(A) Adapted from Ellis H.D., Jones D.M., & Modsell N., 'Intra- and inter-modal repetition priming of familiar faces and voices', *British Journal of Psychology*, Volume 88, Issue 1, pp. 143–56, Copyright © 1997 The British Psychological Society, doi: 10.1111/j.2044-8295.1997.tb02625.x, by permission of John Wiley and Sons; *Trends in Cognitive Sciences*, Volume 8, Issue 3, Belin P., Fecteau S, & Bédard C., 'Thinking the voice: neural correlates of voice perception', pp. 129–35, Copyright © 2004 Elsevier Ltd, with permission from Elsevier, http://www.sciencedirect.com/science/article/pii/S1364661304000257;

Blank H., Kiebel S.J., & von Kriegstein K., 'How the human brain exchanges information across sensory modalities to recognize other people', *Human Brain Mapping*, Volume 36, Issue 1, pp. 324–39, Copyright © 2014 Wiley Periodicals, Inc., doi: 10.1002/hbm.22631, by permission of John Wiley and Sons; and *Brain and Cognition*, Volume 44, Issue 3, Neuner F. & Schweinberger S.R., 'Neuropsychological Impairments in the Recognition of Faces, Voices, and Personal Names', pp. 342–66, Copyright © 2000 Academic Press, with permission from Elsevier, http://www.sciencedirect.com/science/article/pii/S027826269991196X.

39.2.1 Stage I: Perceptual Analysis of Voice Identity

Here, the perceptual system analyses complex spectrotemporal acoustical properties of the incoming vocal sound which support identity processing. This stage encompasses 'structural encoding' (e.g. Neuner & Schweinberger, 2000), where invariant properties of the voice (i.e. vocal properties which remain constant across different speech utterances or changes in prosody) are extracted. These properties are merged to create a coherent voice percept. The merged voice properties may be contrasted against a 'prototype' voice (Andics et al., 2010; Lavner et al., 2001; see Latinus & Zäske, this volume; Latinus et al., 2013; for review, see Maguinness et al., 2018). The prototype voice may represent an average approximation of the voices the listener has encountered or it may reflect a 'very common voice' (Lavner et al., 2001). The computed acoustical differences between the voice percept and the prototype voice can be passed on for analysis to support identity recognition at later stages of processing. Other features of the vocal sound, which support vocal emotion and speech processing, are also analysed at this stage but are argued to be processed in partly independent but interacting systems (Kreitewolf et al., 2014; von Kriegstein et al., 2010).

Stage I of processing is suggested to be supported by brain regions of a core-voice system. Potential candidate brain regions are the posterior and mid regions of the superior temporal gyrus/sulcus (STG/S) (e.g. Belin et al., 2000; Pernet et al., 2015; Roswandowitz, Kappes, et al., 2018; von Kriegstein & Giraud, 2004; Warren et al., 2006) and auditory regions such as the planum temporale (von Kriegstein, Warren, et al., 2006; Warren et al., 2006) and Heschl's gyrus (Bonte et al., 2014; Formisano et al., 2008), predominantly in the right hemisphere (Figure 39.1B). Apperceptive phonagnosia may emerge due to dysfunction at this early stage of processing (Figure 39.1A, Stage I).

Poor perceptual analysis of the voice may result in a weak representation of the voice-individuating features, which may impact negatively on later stages of processing (voice-identity recognition).

39.2.2 Stage II: Voice-Identity Recognition

At the stage of voice-identity recognition, a sense of familiarity is generated if the computed voice percept closely resembles a stored voice representation. These voice representations may be stored as relatively unique 'reference patterns' for each known voice identity (see Lavner at al., 2001). This process is likely supported by anterior and mid regions of the STG/S including parts of the anterior temporal lobe (most likely the superior lateral part) (e.g. Belin & Zatorre, 2003; von Kriegstein et al., 2003) in the core-voice system, while more posterior regions are concerned with perceptual voice analysis (Andics et al., 2013; Belin & Zatorre, 2003; Latinus et al., 2013; Schall et al., 2015; von Kriegstein et al., 2003). A deficit at this stage would give rise to deficient familiarity decisions, despite a successfully analysed vocal percept. We will call this 'familiarity-associative phonagnosia' (Figure 39.1A, Stage II). Disrupted access to the stored voice-identity representations constrains the ability to judge whether the voice has been encountered before.

39.2.3 Stage III: Semantic Processing

After the voice has been recognized as familiar, it is linked to stored multimodal semantic information characterizing the person's identity. This multimodal information
is processed in an extended system (semantic processing), which is proposed to share
connections with the core-voice system. Regions concerned with vocal emotion and
speech recognition may also share connections with this extended system. Potential
brain candidates for the extended system include supra-modal regions encompassing
discrete regions of the temporal pole, precuneus/posterior cingulate, amygdala, and
inferior frontal gyrus (Andics et al., 2010; Latinus et al., 2011; Shah et al., 2001; von
Kriegstein & Giraud, 2006; for review, see Blank et al., 2014). Dysfunction at this stage of
processing (i.e. poor connectivity between the core-voice and extended system) (Figure
39.1A, Stage III) may underpin cases of semantic-associative phonagnosia which are
characterized by a deficit in associating semantic information to a voice which has been
successfully perceived and categorized as familiar[1]. Note that we focus here on the auditory modality (for reviews on how voice information is linked to face representations at
several stages of processing, see Blank et al., 2014; Maguinness & von Kriegstein, 2017;
von Kriegstein, 2011).

39.3 Tests of Voice-Identity Processing

Given the theoretical framework proposed in Figure 39.1A, tests for phonagnosia need to
be designed to address the multistage nature of voice-identity processing. Currently employed voice-processing tests (summarized in Table 39.1) include measures which can
evaluate: (1) the perceptual analysis of the vocal signal, achieved through means of unfamiliar voice-discrimination and unfamiliar speaker-change detection tests which can reveal apperceptive impairments; (2) a sense of familiarity with the encoded familiar vocal

---

[1] The classification of subtypes of phonagnosia is informed by the visual agnosia literature (De Renzi
et al., 1991; Lissauer, 1890). There, an 'apperceptive' agnosia is consistently categorized as a perceptual
processing deficit (i.e. Figure 39.1A, Stage I) (De Renzi, 1986; De Renzi et al., 1991; Warrington, 1975).
However, there is much discrepancy regarding the definition of 'associative' agnosia, specifically
within the realm of prosopagnosia ('face blindness'), a visual disorder to parallel phonagnosia.
Classically, associative (prosop)agnosia has been defined as a failure to link an analysed percept to
stored multimodal semantic information (i.e. Figure 39.1A, Stage III) (Warrington, 1975; Warrington
& Shallice, 1984). However, others have stated that this poor semantic association should be labelled
'amnestic' prosopagnosia and that 'associative' prosopagnosia rather reflects a failure to link the
analysed percept to a stored facial representation (i.e. impaired familiarity decisions; Figure 39.1A,
Stage II) (Avidan & Behrmann, 2014; Fox et al., 2008; Stollhoff et al., 2011). Here, we propose to
resolve the discrepancy by adopting the general label of 'associative phonagnosia' as a deficit, which
encompasses a failure to attribute meaning to the successfully analysed vocal percept. This may arise
due to either impaired familiarity decisions or impaired semantic association to the vocal identity. To
avoid confusion, we will call the first, 'familiarity-associative phonagnosia', and the second, 'semantic-
associative phonagnosia'.

Table 39.1 Overview of the tasks and stimuli used for assessing apperceptive (upper section) and associative (lower section) voice–identity processing

Design	Stimuli		Paradigm	Reference
	Voice familiarity	Test stimuli		

Apperceptive voice–identity processing

Design	Voice familiarity	Test stimuli	Paradigm	Reference
Voice discrimination	Unfamiliar voices	3-word sentences Test 1: 2 male, 2 female, 2 child speakers Test 2: 5 females speaking English, German, Spanish, Italian, Japanese Test 3: 5 young female French speakers	Presentation of 30 pairs of sentences Same–different speaker judgement Pairs of sentences had either same or different word content	Assal et al., 1976
	Unfamiliar voices	Sentences Test 1: Male, female, child speakers Test 2: French female speakers Test 3: Hebrew female speakers	Presentation of 40 pairs of sentences Same–different speaker judgement	Assal et al., 1981
	Unfamiliar voices	Sentences 10 male speakers	Presentation of 26 pairs of sentences Same–different speaker judgement Pairs of sentences same content; if same speaker presented, different tokens used	Van Lancker et al., 1987, 1988, 1989
	Unfamiliar voices	Sentences (2 sec. long) Unfamiliar speakers	Presentation of 54 pairs of sentences Same–different speaker judgement Pairs of sentences different content, same gender	Neuner & Schweinberger, 2000
	Unfamiliar voices	Sentences with 3 key words 6 female speakers	Presentation of sentence pairs in 4 different SNRs: −6, 0, 6, or 12 dB (24 sentence pairs per SNR) Same–different speaker judgement	Garrido et al., 2009
	Unfamiliar voices	Sentences 21 female speakers	Presentation of NV sentence pairs with 6, 16, or 48 frequency channels (24 sentence pairs per frequency–channel level) Same–different speaker judgement	Garrido et al., 2009

	Unfamiliar voices	2-word sentences 3 male speakers	Brief familiarization with the voice identities (passive listening), followed by: Presentation of 54 pairs of sentences Same-different speaker judgement	Roswandowitz et al., 2014
	Unfamiliar voices	Sentences 5 female speakers	Presentation of target voice, followed by: (i) 5, 10, or 20 sec. interval, and (ii) presentation of 2 test voices (40 trials per interval duration) 2 AFC speaker-matching task	Xu et al., 2015
Speaker change detection	Unfamiliar voices	4 min.-long text	Text included 24 speaker changes Speaker-change detection	Assal et al., 1981
	Unfamiliar voices	High frequent words (names of weekdays and months) Female speakers	Sequences of words including speaker changes: - 24 trials of weekdays - 24 trials of months Speaker-change detection	Hailstone et al., 2010
	Unfamiliar voices	High frequent words (names of weekdays) Female speakers Test 1: Naturalistic stimuli Test 2: Fixed F0 (220 Hz)	Sequences of words including speaker changes Test 1: 28 trials Test 2: 12 trials Speaker-change detection	Hailstone et al., 2011

Associative voice–identity processing

Familiar voice recognition	Famous voices	7 celebrity voices Male speaker	For each voice, cross-modal matching on 4-choice response array (voice–face/name) (*semantic association*)	Van Lancker et al., 1982
	Famous voices	25 celebrity voices Male speaker 4 sec.-long samples	For each voice, cross-modal matching on 4-choice response array (voice–face/name) (*semantic association*) Debriefing of subjective familiarity with celebrities (van Lancker et al., 1989)	Van Lancker et al., 1987, 1988, 1989
	Famous and unfamiliar voices	32 celebrity voices 32 unfamiliar voices Female and male speaker 2 sec.-long samples	After voice presentation, (i) familiarity judgement (*familiarity decision*), (ii) if familiar, voice naming (*semantic association*)	Neuner & Schweinberger, 2000

(continued)

Table 39.1 Continued

Design	Stimuli		Paradigm	Reference
	Voice familiarity	Test stimuli		
	Personally familiar and unfamiliar voices	Per participant: 1 familiar voice, 5 unfamiliar voices Voice samples consisted of vowels, CVC syllables, words, and sentences	After voice presentation, familiarity judgement (*familiarity decision*)	Lang et al., 2009
	Famous and unfamiliar voices	48 celebrity voices 48 unfamiliar voices 7 sec.-long samples	After voice presentation, (i) familiarity judgement (*familiarity decision*), (ii) if familiar, voice identification (provide name or other biographical detail) (*semantic association*)	Garrido et al., 2009
	Famous and unfamiliar voices	24 celebrity voices Female and male voices	After voice presentation, familiarity judgement (*familiarity decision*)	Hailstone et al., 2010, 2011
	Famous and unfamiliar voices	24 celebrity voices (same as above)	After voice presentation, (i) voice identification (provide name or other biographical detail) (ii) cross-modal matching on a response array (voice–face/name) (*semantic association*)	Hailstone et al., 2010, 2011
	Famous and unfamiliar voices	42 celebrity voices 20 unfamiliar voices Female and male voices 5 sec.-long samples	After voice presentation, (i) familiarity judgement (*familiarity decision*) (ii) if familiar, voice identification (provide name or other biographical detail; Roswandowitz et al., 2014), cross-modal matching on a response array (voice–face/name; Roswandowitz et al. in press) (*semantic association*) Debriefing of subjective voice familiarity of celebrities	Roswandowitz et al., 2014; Roswandowitz, Kappes, et al., 2018

Famous and unfamiliar voices	100 celebrity voices 100 unfamiliar voices 6–8 sec.-long samples	Celebrity face–name composite displayed (1,2, or 4 identity composites), followed by 2 voice samples, then: (i) indicate which of the voices is a celebrity (*familiarity decision*) (ii) cross-modal matching of famous voice to face/name composite (1, 2, or 4 options) (*semantic association*)	Xu et al., 2014; see also Herald et al., 2014
Newly-learned voice recognition Newly-learned voices	6 unfamiliar female speakers Sentences with 3 key words	Cross-modal learning: name and voice, followed by: (i) Voice-recognition task (is the voice the same as the target speaker?) (ii) Voice-recognition task (what name matches the voice identity? 6 options) (iii) Old/new task (is the voice new or has it been heard before i.e. old?)	Garrido et al., 2009
Newly-learned voices	3 male and 3 female unfamiliar speakers per test (voice-name/voice-face test)	Voice-name test: Cross-modal learning: simultaneous voice–name presentation Testing: voice–name matching Voice-face test: same paradigm, just with voice–face associations	Roswandowitz et al., 2014; Roswandowitz, Kappes, et al., 2018

SNR = signal-to-noise ratio, NV = noise-vocoded, AFC = alternative forced choice

percept (i.e. familiarity decision); and (3) the ability to link the encoded familiar vocal percept to identity-specific person knowledge (i.e. semantic association). Familiar voice-recognition tests are commonly used to examine both familiarity decisions and semantic association. These tests often assess both associative abilities. Thus, listeners first indicate a sense of familiarity towards a voice and then associate semantic knowledge to the familiar voice. Voices presented in those tests may involve famous, personally familiar, or newly-learned speakers' voices.

39.4 ACQUIRED PHONAGNOSIA

Lesion studies on phonagnosia allow a strong interpretation about brain regions required to identify voices. In the following, we review brain lesion studies which aimed to characterize the cognitive and neural mechanisms supporting voice-identity processing. The term 'phonagnosia' implies a modality-specific deficit requiring many different control tests. However, the number of control tests or self-reports assessing other-person recognition or speech-processing abilities varies across clinical studies. Thus, whether the reported cases of acquired phonagnosia are also associated with other impairments often remains unclear, in particular in those studies that do not include a systematic investigation of control abilities. For an overview of the reviewed lesion studies on voice-identity processing, see Table 39.2.

39.4.1 Apperceptive Voice-Identity Processing in Acquired Phonagnosia

Although the term 'phonagnosia' was first mentioned in 1982 by van Lancker and Canter, examinations on voice-identity processes had begun almost a decade previously. These first studies addressed mainly *perceptual* aspects of voice-identity processing (e.g. unfamiliar voice discrimination). In 1976, the Swiss neurosurgeon Par G. Assal and his colleagues (Assal et al., 1976) published the first study on acquired phonagnosia. They investigated forty-seven patients with unilateral brain lesions, including twenty-five patients with lesions in the right hemisphere (right brain-damaged or RBD) and twenty-two patients with lesions in the left hemisphere (left brain-damaged or LBD), as well as twenty-nine healthy age- and handedness-matched controls. This study was centred on three main questions: (i) Does a deficit in voice discrimination after brain damage exist? (ii) Is the voice-discrimination deficit associated with right hemispheric lesions? (iii) Are voice-identity and language processes dissociable mechanisms? The authors showed that patients with brain lesions performed significantly worse than healthy controls on discrimination tasks with unfamiliar voices. Participants were tested on discrimination between unfamiliar adult male, female, and children's voices, as well as on discrimination among only unfamiliar female voices either speaking different languages or the same language (i.e. French) (Table 39.1). RBD patients performed significantly below controls on all three tests (i.e. based on Tuckey-Hayes statistics), whereas LBD patients only performed worse than controls when discriminating female voices speaking different languages. A direct statistical patient group comparison however was not conducted.

Table 39.2 Overview of lesion studies on voice–identity processing

Study	Subjects				Lesion		Brain imaging	Behavioural findings			Brain–behaviour findings
	n	Age	MSO	Hearing	Type	Location		Voice	Face	Speech	
Assal et al., 1976	47 patients 22 LBD 25 RBD 29 controls	45 46 43	N/A	Normal hearing (self-reports)	Vascular diseases (12), tumour/abscess (7), TBI (3)	LH RH	N/A	RBD: impaired unfamiliar voice DISCR Acquired voice DISCR deficit exist	N/A	LBD: aphasia no affect on voice DISCR (= independent)	RH = voice DISCR deficit
Assal et al., 1981	76 patients 40 LBD 36 RBD 35 controls	N/A	N/A	N/A	N/A	LH RH	N/A	RBD: impaired unfamiliar voice DISCR	N/A	LBD: aphasia no affect on voice DISCR (= independent)	RH = voice DISCR deficit
	52 patients 28 LBD 24 RBD 11 controls	N/A	N/A	N/A	N/A	LH RH	N/A	RBD: impaired speaker-change detection	N/A	N/A	RH = speaker-change detection deficit
	Case RB	45	N/A	Normal hearing	Vascular diseases	Bilateral anterior TL, settling after 6 months in left TL	N/A	Impaired familiar voice REC Moderately impaired unfamiliar voice DISCR (Amusic)	Intact (self report)	N/A	TL = voice REC deficit
Van Lancker et al., 1982	30 patients 21 LBD 9 RBD	62 52	8.9 (mean) 2 (mean)	Hearing sufficient for speech perception	Cerebral vascular diseases, TBI	LH RH	Neurological evaluation, CAT scans	RBD: impaired familiar voice REC	RBD: impaired familiar face REC	All LBD aphasic	RH = voice and face REC deficit = Voice and face REC tend to co-occur (termed phonagnosia)

(continued)

Table 39.2 Continued

Study	Subjects				Lesion		Brain imaging	Behavioural findings			Brain-behaviour findings
	n	Age	MSO	Hearing	Type	Location		Voice	Face	Speech	
Van Lancker et al., 1987	32 patients 15 LBD 11 RBD 6 BBD 48 controls	61 59 69 64	2–24 2–12 1–24	Normal hearing	Stroke (40), craniotomies (2), haemorrhage (1), meningioma (1), tumour (1)	LH RH Both Hs	CAT scans, EEGs, neurological evaluations	RBD: impaired familiar voice REC and unfamiliar voice DISCR LBD: impaired unfamiliar voice DISCR, intact familiar voice REC in 14 patients dissociation between familiar voice REC and unfamiliar voice DISCR	Intact face recognition in 4 patients	All LBD aphasic	RH = voice REC deficit, LH + RH = voice DISCR deficit
Van Lancker et al, 1988	6 case reports 2 LBD 1 RBD 3 BBD 30 controls	65 (52– 82) 50–85	N/A	Normal hearing reported for 2 cases	Stroke (5) Haemorrhage (1)	Mainly temporal, parietal, frontal lobe	CTs	4 BBD: impaired unfamiliar voice DISCR 3 RBD: impaired familiar voice REC 1 RBD: impaired in both tasks In 5 patients dissociation between familiar voice REC and unfamiliar voice DISCR	N/A	4 LBD with aphasia and voice DISCR deficit	Right PL = voice REC deficit Bilateral TL = voice DISCR deficit
Van Lancker et al., 1989	56 patients 25 LBD 25 RBD 6 BBD 48 controls	61 63 71 64	N/A	N/A	Cerebral infarction	Lesions classified in parietal, temporal, and temporo-parietal lesions	CTs	BBD: impaired unfamiliar voice DISCR RBD: impaired familiar voice REC	N/A	All LBD aphasic	Quantitative evidence for: Right PL = voice REC deficit Bilateral TL = voice DISCR deficit

Study	Participants	Age	Duration	Hearing	Aetiology	Lesion	Assessment	Voice findings	Face findings	Aphasia	Conclusion
Neuner & Schweinberger, 2000	36 patients 16 LBD 13 RBD 7 BBD 20 controls	48 44	8.2 (mean)	N/A	Anaemic infarct (10), haemorrhage (10), subarachnoid haemorrhage (5), TBI (5), hypoxia (2), TBI with hypoxia (1), encephalitis (2), tumour (1)	LH RH Both Hs	Surgery reports, CTs, or MRI scans	4 patients: selective voice REC deficit (intact face, name, and sound REC), 2 RBD, 1 LBD: impaired in familiar voice REC 1 RBD: impaired in familiar voice REC and unfamiliar voice DISCR	In 4 patients intact face-identity processing	N/A	RH = voice REC deficit
Lang et al., 2009	20 patients 11 LBD 9 RBD 17 controls	66 64 64	3.1 (mean) 1.6 (mean)	N/A	Ischaemic infarcts	LH: MCA (6), PCA (2), LSA (3) RH: MCA (9), PCA (1)	N/A	RBD: impaired familiar voice REC LBD: intact familiar voice REC	N/A	All LH aphasic and intact voice REC	RH = voice REC deficit
Hailstone et al., 2010	Case QR	61	N/A	Normal hearing	Behavioural variant fronto-temporal dementia	Right anterior TL extending to TL (STG)	MRI scans	Impaired familiarity and REC of familiar voices Intact unfamiliar voice DISCR (impaired music-instrument processing)	Impaired familiarity, moderately impaired REC of familiar faces Intact unfamiliar face DISCR	N/A	Right anterior TL and STG = voice REC deficit (associative phonagnosia)
	Case KL 24 controls	72	N/A	Normal hearing	Fronto-temporal lobar degeneration	Bilateral anterior TL atrophy extending to inferior temporal cortices (incl. FFA)	MRI scans	Impaired familiarity and REC of familiar voices Intact unfamiliar voice DISCR	Impaired familiarity and REC of familiar faces Intact unfamiliar face DISCR	N/A	Bilateral anterior TL = multimodal person REC deficit (voice, face, name)

(continued)

Table 39.2 Continued

Study	Subjects				Lesion		Brain imaging	Behavioural findings			Speech	Brain-behaviour findings
	n	Age	MSO	Hearing	Type	Location		Voice	Face			
Hailstone et al., 2011	36 patients 14 FTLD 22 Alzheimer's 35 controls	64 67 64	N/A N/A	Normal hearing	Fronto-temporal lobar degeneration Alzheimer's disease	Bilateral anterior TL atrophy (14) hippocampal atrophy (16), generalized cerebral atrophy (4)	MRI scans (11 FTLD, 18 Alzheimer's)	FTLD: impaired familiarity, REC of familiar voices, intact unfamiliar voice DISCR Alzheimer's: impaired familiarity, REC of familiar voices, impaired unfamiliar voice DISCR	FTLD + Alzheimer's: impaired familiar face familiarity, REC, and apperceptive face processing		N/A	*VBM analysis* Right anterior TL = voice, name, and face REC Right inferior PL (angular gyrus) = unfamiliar voice DISCR
Roswandowitz, Kappes, et al., 2018	58 patients focal brain lesions 31 RBD 27LBD	48	46 (mean)	Normal hearing (covariate in VLSM analysis)	ischaemic stroke (34), intracerebral haemorrhage (6), subarachnoid haemorrhage (6), TBI (7), tumour (4)	Bilateral TL and right inferior PL well covered by lesions	MRI scans (56), CT scans (2)	Worse performance in voice-name test in patients compared to controls (Roswandowitz et al., 2014) RBD worse in voice REC of recently familiarized voices than LBD 9% of patients report poor voice REC after lesion onset	5% of patients report poor face REC after lesion onset		No severe aphasia	*VLSM analysis* Right mid/ posterior TL = selective voice REC deficit Right inferior PL = impaired voice-face integration

All brain-behaviour findings rely on descriptive brain-behaviour associations if not stated otherwise.

MSO = months since onset, LBD = left-brain-damaged patients, RBD = right-brain-damaged patients, BBD = bilateral-brain-damaged patients, N/A = not available, TBI = traumatic brain injury, LH = left hemisphere, RH = right hemisphere, DISCR = discrimination, REC = recognition, TL = temporal lobe, PL = parietal lobe, STS/G = superior temporal sulcus/gyrus, FFA = fusiform face area, FTLD = fronto-temporal lobar degeneration, VBM = voxel-based morphometry, VLSM = voxel-based lesion-symptom mapping

This was the first indication that impaired apperceptive voice-identity processing exists after brain damage and that it might be predominantly a function of the right hemisphere. Although no information about precise lesion locations was available, the authors attempted to localize right hemispheric lesions relevant for voice discrimination with a dichotic listening test. RBD patients performed worse in voice discrimination if voices were presented to the left in comparison to the right ear. The authors speculated that voice discrimination may be assigned to the right temporal lobe.

Further, addressing the relation between voice-identity and language processes, the authors directly compared voice-discrimination abilities between LBD patients with and without aphasia (i.e. speech and language disorder caused by brain damage predominantly to the language-dominant left hemisphere). Performance in the voice-discrimination tests was similar for aphasic and non-aphasic LBD patients. This was a first indication of the separability of voice-identity processing from language abilities. In RBD patients, language abilities were not considered, probably because it is unlikely that aphasia occurs in RBD patients. However, in RBD patients, visual abilities were tested. This was done with a visual figure/ground discrimination task (Poppelreuter test) and a visual-spatial memory task. Results showed that unfamiliar voice-discrimination performance was significantly worse in RBD patients with impaired visual processing than in RBD patients with intact visual processing. Whether the RBD patients with intact visual processing had, nevertheless, voice-discrimination difficulties in contrast to healthy controls was not tested.

Five years later, Assal and colleagues (1981) elaborated on their pioneering study by assessing apperceptive voice mechanisms by testing voice-discrimination abilities alongside the ability to *detect* a change in speaker identity (Table 39.1). This time, Assal et al. investigated unfamiliar voice discrimination in a sample of seventy-six patients (forty LBD, thirty-six RBD) and thirty-five healthy controls, and unfamiliar speaker-change detection in fifty-two patients (twenty-eight LBD, twenty-four RBD) and eleven healthy controls. The authors replicated their previous findings: (i) They found a right hemispheric dominance for apperceptive voice-identity processing. This time, the authors showed that RBD patients were impaired on *both* apperceptive voice tasks (i.e. unfamiliar voice discrimination *and* unfamiliar speaker change detection). Importantly, in contrast to the previous study, this time a direct statistical group comparison between RBD and LBD patients on voice discrimination yielded a significant group difference (ANOVA at α = 0.05): RBD patients performed worse than LBD patients. (ii) Based on the dichotic listening results, the authors again suggested an important role of the right temporal lobe (this time more specifically of the temporo-parietal region) during voice discrimination. (iii) Again they noted that dissociation between speech and voice-identity processing was evident in this cohort; voice-discrimination performance was not different between aphasic and non-aphasic LBD patients.

39.4.2 The First Case Report of Acquired Phonagnosia: The Case of RB

Assal et al. (1981) also reported the first case study of acquired phonagnosia—the case of 'RB'. RB was a 45-year-old male, managing director, had musical training, and normal hearing abilities. After brain injury resulting from vascular disease, RB reported difficulties in music and irony perception, voice recognition, as well as speech and sound perception. While RB recovered from the latter two difficulties one month after lesion onset, he continued to evidence a strong deficit in recognizing familiar voices and a moderate deficit in discriminating voices compared to controls which was based on numerical group-difference inspection. Unfortunately, details on the test designs were not reported. Interestingly, face recognition was tested and intact. A brain scan (not specified by the authors, but likely a CT scan) originally revealed bilateral cortico-subcortical lesions in the anterior temporal lobe, initially more pronounced in the right hemisphere, that after six weeks resolved into a lesion predominantly in the left temporal lobe.

This first case report on acquired phonagnosia implicated a role for the temporal lobe in voice-identity processing and showed that voice-identity processing can be impaired while leaving face-identity processing intact. Further, the case report gave a first indication that voice recognition (associative voice-identity processing) and voice discrimination (apperceptive voice-identity processing) might be dissociable mechanisms.

In our view, it is remarkable that in these first studies Assal and colleagues asked questions that have shaped all future studies on voice-identity processing. However, to date, these studies are relatively unknown in the field, probably because they are reported in French only.

39.4.3 Apperceptive and Associative Voice-Identity Processing in Acquired Phonagnosia

Van Lancker and colleagues took research on phonagnosia a decisive step further. Van Lancker and Canter (1982) investigated *associative* voice-identity processing in thirty patients with focal brain lesions (twenty-one LBD, nine RBD) with a familiar voice-recognition test (Table 39.1). All LBD patients had aphasia. One aim of the study was to assess whether familiar voice recognition is primarily assigned to the right hemisphere, as found in the prosopagnosia (i.e. face-identity processing deficit) literature (Damasio et al., 1990; De Renzi, 1986; De Renzi et al., 1991). Further, van Lancker and Canter were interested in the relation between voice- and face-identity processing. Therefore, patients were tested on their voice- and face-recognition abilities. In both tasks, patients were asked to match a celebrity voice/face to a written name (Table 39.1). A deficit in the voice- and face-recognition task was more prevalent in RBD than in LBD patients. Four out of nine RBD patients were impaired on familiar voice recognition. Only in one RBD patient was this deficit selective to voice recognition; the remaining three RBD patients also had a deficit in face recognition. In contrast, only one out of twenty-one LBD patients had impaired familiar voice recognition and another one had impaired familiar face recognition. The authors concluded that associative voice-identity processing can be assigned to the right hemisphere.

Further, the authors suggested that voice- and face-recognition deficits tend to co-occur and that both may rely on neuronal mechanisms within the right hemisphere. Finally, the authors concluded that voice recognition might be dissociable from left-hemisphere language functions as twenty of twenty-one aphasic LBD patients had intact voice recognition. Interestingly, there were two cases (one RBD, one LBD) in which voice-recognition impairments seemed to be selectively impaired (i.e. with intact face recognition). The behavioural profile of these two patients might be indicative of specific neural mechanisms for familiar voice recognition that can be dissociated from those supporting language and face-recognition abilities.

Next, Van Lancker and Kreiman (1987) directly compared the relation between apperceptive and associative voice-identity processing by testing unfamiliar voice discrimination and familiar voice recognition in the same patients. Although both abilities were located in the right hemisphere in previous studies (Assal et al., 1976, 1981; Van Lancker & Canter, 1982), the case of RB had indicated a potential dissociation between both mechanisms (Assal et al., 1981). Van Lancker and colleagues tested thirty-two patients (fifteen LBD, eleven RBD, six bilateral brain-damaged—BBD) and healthy age- and education-matched controls (n = 48) on both unfamiliar voice discrimination *and* familiar voice recognition. All LBD patients had aphasia. In contrast to previous findings, patients with lesions in the left or right hemisphere were similarly impaired (relative to the control group; two-way repeated measure ANOVA at α = 0.01) in the unfamiliar voice-discrimination task. In contrast, only RBD patients showed impaired familiar voice recognition, as compared to controls (Van Lancker & Kreiman, 1987). LBD patients' familiar voice-recognition performance was similar to controls.

Looking at the cases individually, fourteen of the thirty-two patients showed dissociable behavioural performances in the unfamiliar voice-discrimination and familiar voice-recognition task (one RBD, six LBD, and three BBD; no lesion lateralization on the remaining four patients was reported). They had impaired voice discrimination and intact voice recognition or vice versa. Of the ten patients for whom they reported individual results, worse voice discrimination was associated with LBD and worse voice recognition with RBD. BBD patients had both worse voice discrimination and voice recognition. Moreover, there was no correlation between the discrimination and recognition performance in patients.

Taken together, these results suggested that both apperceptive and associative voice-identity processing might be underpinned by dissociable cognitive and neuroanatomical mechanisms. To assess the selectivity of a given voice-identity processing deficit, four patients with a severe deficit in either voice discrimination or voice recognition were also tested on their face-recognition and face-discrimination abilities as well as environmental sound processing. A voice-specific deficit pattern emerged: face and sound processing was intact in those patients, suggesting a fairly selective phonagnosia.

To reveal which anatomical regions within the respective hemisphere subserve apperceptive and associative voice-identity processing, van Lancker and colleagues (1988) studied six brain-lesioned cases for which CT scans were available. Patients were tested on both unfamiliar voice discrimination (apperceptive voice-identity processing) and familiar voice recognition (associative voice-identity processing) (Table 39.1). Patients' performance was compared to thirty healthy, age-matched control participants. Five of the six patients showed a clear discrepancy between the ability to discriminate unfamiliar voices and to recognize familiar voices (i.e. more than two standard deviations away from the controls' mean difference in test scores). Van Lancker et al. noted that the three patients who were exclusively impaired on unfamiliar voice discrimination had a lesion overlap in the temporal lobe of either the left or the right hemisphere (i.e. including anterior, mid, and posterior regions) and were aphasic.

In contrast, the two patients with *selectively* impaired familiar voice recognition had, in common, lesions which were located exclusively in the right hemisphere, including the posterior part of the temporal and parietal lobe structures such as the superior portion of the angular gyrus and the posterior supramarginal gyrus. The one patient who did not show dissociation between voice discrimination and recognition, being impaired on both tasks, had a lesion in the right mid/posterior temporal lobe and the right parietal lobe, including the superior angular gyrus and the supramarginal gyrus. The authors (Van Lancker et al., 1988) discuss a relevant role of the bilateral temporal lobe for unfamiliar voice discrimination (apperceptive voice-identity processing) and of the lateral parietal lobe in the right hemisphere for familiar voice recognition (associative voice-identity processing) (Figure 39.2). This study provided supporting evidence for distinct mechanisms underlying apperceptive and associative voice-identity processing.

In a follow-up study, Van Lancker et al. (1989) aimed to quantitatively confirm the descriptive behavioural and neuroanatomical dissociation between apperceptive and associative voice-identity processing. To allow a quantitative brain-behaviour analysis, they tested a large sample of fifty-six brain-damaged patients. Forty-four patients (twenty-three LBD, fifteen RBD, six BBD) were tested on both an unfamiliar voice-discrimination and familiar voice-recognition task (Table 39.1). Twelve patients (two LBD, ten RBD) were tested only on familiar voice recognition. All LBD patients were aphasic. Results were compared between lesion groups and forty-eight healthy age- and education-matched control participants. Behavioural results showed that both LBD and RBD patients performed worse on the unfamiliar voice-discrimination task compared to controls (two-way repeated measure ANOVA at α = 0.05). On the familiar voice-recognition task, only RBD patients were

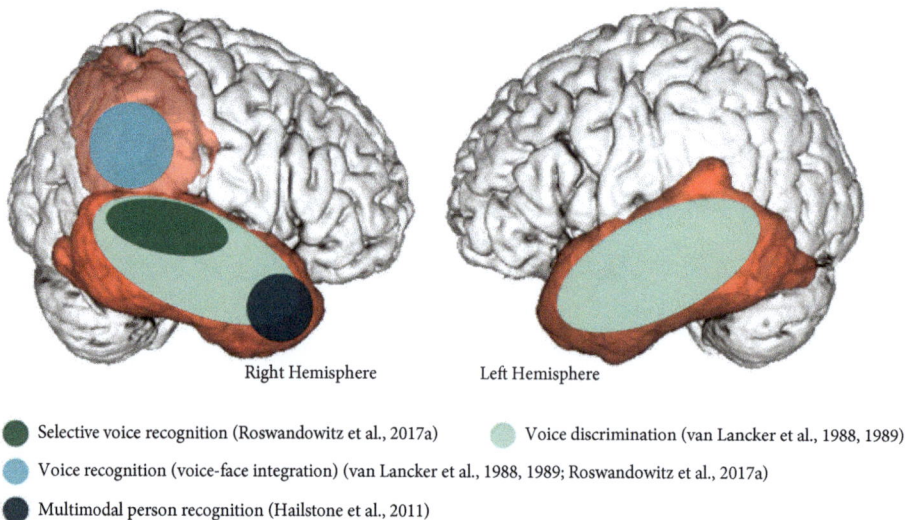

Right Hemisphere   Left Hemisphere

● Selective voice recognition (Roswandowitz et al., 2017a)   ○ Voice discrimination (van Lancker et al., 1988, 1989)

● Voice recognition (voice-face integration) (van Lancker et al., 1988, 1989; Roswandowitz et al., 2017a)

● Multimodal person recognition (Hailstone et al., 2011)

FIGURE 39.2 Schematic overview of studies reporting lesion locations associated with the respective voice-identity processing and multimodal person-recognition deficit. The temporal lobe is indicated by the dark red map and the right inferior parietal lobe by the light red map.

impaired, relative to controls. In line with previous findings (Van Lancker & Kreiman, 1987; Van Lancker et al., 1988), unfamiliar voice discrimination (apperceptive voice-identity processing) was assigned to lesions in both the *left or right* hemispheres, and familiar voice recognition (associative voice-identity processing) only to lesions in the *right* hemisphere.

Next, they investigated the neuroanatomic substrates underlying this behavioural pattern. Based on forty-three available CT scans, lesions were classified according to the lobe with the largest extent of the lesion. According to their hypothesis, a lesion in the right parietal lobe was significantly associated with a deficit in associative voice-identity processing (familiar voice-recognition task). All nine patients with a right parietal lobe lesion showed impaired familiar voice recognition, as did seven of forty-three patients having the lesion elsewhere. Unfortunately, the authors did not report the lesion location of those seven patients. It would have been interesting to observe whether lesions in these additional seven cases were located adjacent to the right parietal lobe or in other regions such as the temporal lobe, as suggested by Assal et al. (1981) and by neuroimaging findings (Figure 39.1 B).

The analysis of apperceptive voice-identity processing was based on twenty-five CT scans. Confirming the authors' hypothesis, thirteen patients with a lesion in either the left or right temporal lobe performed worse in discriminating unfamiliar voices compared to controls. There were also four patients with temporal lobe lesions and preserved task performance. These patients had lesions exclusively in the left hemisphere, indicating a higher relevance of the right hemisphere during unfamiliar voice discrimination. Of the patients with lesions outside the temporal lobe, nine had high and four had low scores on the discrimination task. Of these four patients with impaired voice discrimination, lesions were adjacent to the temporal lobe.

In summary, van Lancker and colleagues provided quantitative evidence that lesions in the right parietal lobe were associated with associative voice-identity processing, and lesions in either the left or right temporal lobe with apperceptive voice-identity processing (Figure 39.2).

39.4.4 Group Evidence for Selective Voice-Identity Processing Impairments

Previous studies were not conclusive as to whether phonagnosia may reflect a modality-specific disorder. For example, while the case of RB (Assal et al., 1981) and the six patients in van Lancker et al.'s studies (Van Lancker & Canter, 1982; Van Lancker & Kreiman, 1987) suggested dissociation between voice- and face-identity processing, the patient group reported by van Lancker and Canter (1982) showed that voice- and face-identity deficits can co-occur. The same diversity emerged when considering the relation between voice-identity processing and other auditory processing abilities, such as speech, sound, emotion, and music processing (e.g. case of RB in Assal et al., 1981; and the four cases in Van Lancker & Kreiman, 1987).

To systematically assess the relation between voice-identity processing and identity processing of other sensory modalities as well as other auditory processes, Neuner and Schweinberger (2000) developed a comprehensive behavioural test battery. They studied thirty-six brain-lesioned patients (sixteen LBD, thirteen RBD, and seven BBD) for whom brain-surgery reports, CT scans, or MRI scans were available, and twenty healthy controls (matched in age, gender, and education). The test battery assessed apperceptive (discrimination tasks) and associative (familiarity decision and semantic association tasks) abilities for persons' voices, faces, and names (Table 39.1). In addition, the test battery included control tests on word, picture, and sound recognition to investigate the specificity of a given person-recognition deficit.

In thirteen out of thirty-six patients, familiar voice recognition assessed by a familiarity decision task was significantly worse compared to controls' performance (cut-off for impairment: patient scores below the control mean at α = 0.05 and 0.01). However, only four of the thirteen patients showed a selective form of phonagnosia, with impaired familiar voice recognition but intact sound, face, and name recognition. Unfortunately, for these cases, semantic association scores were not reported. One of these four patients also showed an overlapping impairment in voice discrimination; the lesion was located in the right hemisphere (Table 39.1). Two of the four patients with selective familiar voice-recognition deficits had a lesion located in the right hemisphere and one in the left hemisphere.

Neuner and Schweinberger (2000) made large strides in investigating the specificity of phonagnosia. Their systematic investigation attested that phonagnosia can be witnessed as a specific deficit, independent of non-verbal sound, face, and name recognition.

A study by Lang and colleagues (2009) specifically examined the relation between voice-identity and speech processing. In this study, familiar voice recognition was assessed (Table 39.1). The study included twenty brain-damaged patients (eleven LBD, nine RBD) and seventeen healthy age-matched controls. The two groups were matched for lesion location and extent. Left-brain-damaged patients were tested for aphasia (Aachen Aphasia Test). The results yielded a familiar voice-recognition deficit in RBD relative to performance in LBD patients and controls (one-factorial ANOVA at α = 0.05). In contrast, LBD patients and healthy controls performed equally well on familiar voice recognition. The authors concluded that in LBD patients, aphasia (five amnestic, five Wernicke's, one Broca's aphasia) was not associated with familiar voice-recognition deficits. However, whether there is a double dissociation between voice-identity and speech processing remains open as language abilities were not assessed in RBD patients. Lesions in the right hemisphere were mostly confined to the supply areas of the middle cerebral artery, and similar lesions in the left hemisphere did not affect familiar voice recognition. Unfortunately, more exact lesion locations were not reported.

39.4.5 Case Report Evidence for Selective Voice-Identity Processing Impairments

Hailstone et al. (2010) comprehensively evaluated voice-identity processing and several control tasks in two patients with neurodegenerative diseases (fronto-temporal dementia) and twenty-four healthy age-matched controls. The authors assessed apperceptive (unfamiliar speaker-change detection) and associative (familiarity decision and semantic association) voice-identity processing as well as face, name, music, and sound processing (Table 39.1). Patient QR, 61 years old, had bilateral fronto-temporal atrophy, accentuated in the right anterior temporal lobe but extending posteriorly within the temporal lobe. Patient KL, 72 years old, had bilateral predominantly anterior temporal lobe atrophy, which was more marked in the right hemisphere and in the inferior temporal cortices including the fusiform gyrus. In both patients, processing of familiar voices (familiarity decision, semantic association) was severely impaired in contrast to controls (modified *t*-test for single case studies at α = 0.05; Crawford & Howell, 1998). In addition, both patients, as compared to controls, were impaired in familiar face and name processing. However, QR's face and name abilities were superior to KL's. This indicates a more selective phonagnosia in QR and a rather multimodal person-identity processing deficit in KL. The person-identity processing deficits observed in QR and KL seemed to be restricted to associative processes. Apperceptive processing of voices (including perceptual processing of vocal-identity, vocal-gender, and speaker-size information) and faces was preserved in both. Hence, the authors classify the patients' deficits as associative agnosias. Both patients also showed intact vocal-emotion recognition abilities. However, processing of musical instruments in an auditory and visual task design was affected in QR and KL.

The authors suggested that the bilateral anterior temporal lobe is involved in supporting multiple aspects of person knowledge including voices, faces, and names, with a right hemispheric dominance for aspects of non-verbal person knowledge.

39.4.6 Statistical Brain Lesion–Behaviour Relation: Multimodal Person-Recognition Deficit

In the past decade, sophisticated statistical approaches have been developed for high-resolution structural MRI group studies to afford more robust and objective associations between brain structure and behavioural performance (voxel-based morphometry (VBM): Ashburner & Friston, 2000; voxel-based lesion-symptom mapping (VLSM): Bates et al., 2003). The first study assessing a statistical voxel-wise association between brain structure and voice-identity processing was published in 2011 by Hailstone and colleagues (Hailstone et al., 2011). Thirty-six patients with neurodegenerative diseases (fourteen fronto-temporal lobar degeneration (FTLD), twenty-two Alzheimer's disease) and thirty-five healthy controls (matched in age, gender, handedness, and education) were tested on a comprehensive behavioural test battery. For all sixteen FTLD and twenty Alzheimer's disease patients, a high-resolution structural MRI scan was available. FTLD patients had atrophy in the anterior temporal lobes of both hemispheres. Of the Alzheimer's disease patients, sixteen had hippocampal atrophy and four had generalized cerebral atrophy.

Participants were tested on apperceptive (unfamiliar speaker-change detection) and associative (familiarity decision and semantic association) voice-identity processing (see Table 39.1). To assess the selectivity of a given voice-identity processing deficit, within and across modalities, the test battery included tests on other measures of vocal processing (including speaker-size and vocal-gender information) as well as tests on face and name processing. In the associative voice tasks, both disease groups performed significantly worse compared to controls (z-tests and 95% Wald-type confidence intervals at α = 0.05 and 0.001). However, the deficits were more profound in the FTLD than the Alzheimer's patients. A more heterogeneous pattern emerged for the apperceptive tests. During speaker-change detection and vocal-gender perception, only Alzheimer's patients were impaired. However, apperceptive face processing was impaired in both disease groups.

By applying voxel-based morphometry, the authors presented neuroanatomical evidence that the anterior temporal lobe (predominantly of the right hemisphere), as well as the right fusiform gyrus, plays an important role in associative person recognition across different modalities, including voices, faces, and names (Figure 39.2). This is consistent with previous reports of associative person-recognition deficits with anterior temporal lobe lesions in neurodegenerative disease (Gainotti et al., 2003, 2008; Hailstone et al., 2010). For apperceptive voice-identity processing (speaker-change detection), the right inferior parietal lobe (i.e. angular gyrus) was found to be relevant (Figure 39.2). In light of the previous findings (Van Lancker et al., 1988, 1989), association of the parietal lobe with apperceptive voice processing is unexpected. However, based on patients' atrophy descriptions, lesions in the Hailstone et al. (2011) study covered mostly the anterior temporal lobes and, thus, results on parietal lobes might have to be interpreted with caution.

39.4.7 Statistical Brain Lesion–Behaviour Relation: Selective Voice-Identity Recognition Deficit

In a recent study, Roswandowitz et al. (Roswandowitz, Kappes, et al., 2018) aimed to identify which lesion locations may cause a selective deficit in person-identity processing, which is confined to the auditory domain (i.e. to voice-identity recognition). The authors were, in particular, interested in examining the contribution of the right inferior parietal lobe and the temporal lobe to voice-identity recognition (Figure 39.1B, Stage II). Based on the acquired phonagnosia cases already described in Section 39.4.3, the right inferior parietal lobe is crucial for voice-identity recognition. Conversely, neuroimaging studies on neurotypicals have consistently identified recruitment of the temporal lobe during voice-identity recognition tasks (see Section 39.2). To resolve this discrepancy of regions critical for voice-identity recognition, Roswandowitz et al. conducted a voxel-based lesion-behaviour mapping study in a cohort of fifty-eight patients with unselected unilateral focal brain lesions (thirty-one RBD, twenty-seven LBD patients) and high-resolution structural brain images. The study included a comprehensive behavioural test battery including recognition tasks of recently-familiarized (i.e. newly-learned) voices (voice-name, voice-face association learning) and familiar voices (famous voice recognition), as well as visual (face-identity recognition) and acoustic control tests (vocal-pitch and vocal-timbre discrimination).

VLSM analyses revealed a strong association between lesions in the right mid/posterior temporal lobe and right inferior parietal lobe and the recognition of both recently-familiarized and familiar voices. However, a selective voice-recognition deficit, that was independent of face-identity processing *and* acoustical analyses of voice-identity features such as pitch and timbre, was associated only with lesions in the right mid/posterior *temporal lobe*. This finding implicated an obligatory function for the temporal lobe in voice-identity processing, making it the most likely key structure of the core-voice system. In contrast, lesions in the right inferior parietal lobe were associated with reduced voice-identity recognition when voices were associated with a face. This finding is similar to the earlier van Lancker studies where lesions in the right inferior parietal lobe were associated with reduced performances in tasks where patients had to match a famous voice to a display of faces (and their names) (Van Lancker et al., 1988, 1989). Thus, the right inferior parietal lobe might have a facultative role during voice-identity processing only when additional face information is available.

The study by Roswandowitz et al. is the first to provide group evidence for an association between spatially well-defined brain lesions and selective voice-identity processing impairments (Figure 39.2).

39.5 Developmental Phonagnosia

Developmental phonagnosia has been discovered only recently (Garrido et al., 2009; Herald et al., 2014; Roswandowitz et al., 2014; Xu et al., 2015). Current prevalence estimates suggest that anywhere within the range of 0.2% (Roswandowitz et al., 2014) to 1% (Xu et al., 2015) to 3.2% (Shilowich & Biederman, 2016) of the population may have this deficit. While the precise aetiology of the deficit is unknown, it is possible that phonagnosia may have a heritable component, as has been observed in developmental prosopagnosia (Duchaine et al., 2007; Grueter et al., 2007; Lee et al., 2010; Schmalzl et al., 2008). Here, we review the first documented cases of developmental phonagnosia, which have allowed for an examination of the nature and specificity of this developmental deficit.

39.5.1 The Case of KH

Garrido and colleagues reported the first case of developmental phonagnosia—the case of KH (Garrido et al., 2009). KH was a 60-year-old female who worked as a successful manager. She presented with a lifelong impairment in voice recognition and reported that she failed to even recognize her daughter's voice on the phone. To confirm and assess the specificity of her self-report deficit, KH and a group of age-matched controls ($n = 8$) undertook a detailed behavioural battery of vocal-, visual-, and auditory-processing tests. As suspected, compared to controls, KH was significantly impaired in familiar voice-identity recognition. Specifically, her ability to judge whether a voice was famous or not was close to chance. This indicated weak feelings of familiarity towards known voice identities (i.e. impaired familiarity association). In addition, her retrieval of names for the famous voices was negligible; KH could only accurately recall the name of one of the forty-eight presented famous identities, indicating impaired semantic association.

Her poor performance could not simply be explained by a lack of exposure to the vocal identities in everyday life[2]. When exposure to voices was explicitly controlled in a task, which required the learning of new, unfamiliar speakers' voices with their corresponding name, KH's performance remained significantly poorer than age-matched controls ($n = 8$) for both naming and judging the familiarity (old/new judgement) of the speakers. Interestingly, KH's ability to discriminate between unfamiliar voices, that is to say whether two voice samples

---

[2] In a post-test, KH was asked to indicate if she had significant exposure in daily life to the voices which she failed to name during testing. Taking this assessment into account, KH named only 3.85% (i.e. one of twenty-six) of the identities which she stated she had significant exposure to.

were articulated by the same or a different speaker, was similar to controls under optimal listening conditions (task as described in Neuner & Schweinberger, 2000; see Table 39.1). However, she was impaired in discriminating between identities when the task was made more difficult through the inclusion of auditory noise. When examining KH's performance across tasks, the authors found no statistical evidence for dissociation between familiar voice recognition (associative voice-identity processing) and unfamiliar voice discrimination (apperceptive voice-identity processing).

Garrido and colleagues also examined whether KH's voice-identity processing impairment could be mediated by a higher-order multimodal person-recognition deficit, and/or a general deficit in vocal or auditory processing. Interestingly, KH's memory for faces was either superior to, or within the normal range of, controls. Her recognition and processing of general auditory information, including environmental sounds and musical excerpts, was normal, as was her ability to extrapolate vocal cues to support gender and emotion categorization. In terms of speech processing, KH's performance was within the control range on a number of tasks, including vowel identification and the matching of verbal content to a visual target image.

However, her performance under more challenging listening conditions was less clear. KH was impaired, relative to controls, in perceiving speech which was embedded in auditory noise, although this impairment was not consistent across all levels of auditory noise. For example, KH's speech perception was impaired relative to controls for intermediate noise levels (SNR −3 dB, SNR 3 dB), while her performance at the highest (SNR −6 dB) and lowest (SNR 6 dB) levels of auditory noise appeared normal. The authors attributed this poor performance to possible testing fatigue.

The case of KH suggested that developmental phonagnosia could represent a deficit in the processing of vocal identity, which was mediated *neither* by a general deficit in the processing of auditory information *nor* by a higher-level multimodal deficit affecting identity recognition across the visual and auditory domain. However, evidence for a possible dissociation between voice and speech processing, as well as voice recognition and voice discrimination, would become clearer in the following years as more cases of developmental phonagnosia came to the attention of researchers (Roswandowitz, Schelinski, & von Kriegstein, 2017; Roswandowitz et al., 2014).

39.5.2 The Case of AN

AN was a 20-year-old female university student who presented with a deficit in familiar voice recognition (Herald et al., 2014; Xu et al., 2015). Intriguingly, AN stated that she was not particularly aware of her deficit growing up, as she had not thought that people could recognize an individual without seeing their face. Indeed, AN's face recognition was normal, as she obtained high scores on tests of familiar face recognition and naming (Xu et al., 2015).

Xu et al. (2015) and Herald et al. (2014) formally tested AN's familiar voice-recognition performance through a web-based experiment. In each trial, participants listened to samples of two voices—one celebrity and one non-celebrity voice. In parallel, one, two, or four celebrity face-name composites were presented. Participants first decided which of the two voices was the celebrity voice (i.e. familiarity decision), and then they indicated which celebrity face-name composite matched the familiar-rated voice. Relative to controls (*n* = 21, age range = 19–73 years), AN was markedly impaired in her ability to match the voices which she classified as familiar with the correct celebrity face and name. However, it was not explicitly reported whether her familiarity judgements towards the famous voices were also impaired.

Conversely, AN's accuracy was similar to age-matched controls (n = 9) when the task was to choose which of two unfamiliar voice samples matched a target voice. The target and test samples contained different verbal content. Given the dissociation between deficient familiar voice recognition and intact unfamiliar voice matching, her behavioural profile is most likely indicative of an associative voice-identity processing impairment. Unfortunately, AN's abilities in other auditory tasks such as speech, emotion, and music processing were not formally assessed, leaving open the possibility of additional impairments in other aspects of auditory processing.

The authors also examined the neuronal mechanisms underlying AN's voice-recognition deficit using two functional imaging experiments (Xu et al., 2015). They employed (i) a standard functional localizer known to elicit voice-sensitive responses in the temporal voice areas (TVAs) of the STS/G (Belin et al., 2000; see also Belin, this volume) and (ii) a voice-imagery task. The study included AN and nine controls (22–31 years). Functional imaging during the first experiment of passive listening to vocal as compared to non-vocal sounds (Belin et al., 2000) demonstrated typical responses in AN in the TVAs, located bilaterally along the temporal lobes (Xu et al., 2015).

The second fMRI experiment assessed functional responses during voice imagery. Here, participants were presented with pictures of familiar persons' faces and names, and non-human object pictures, and were asked to imagine the corresponding voice or sound after each image presentation. In a similar web-based test design, AN showed impaired imagery for famous voices, in comparison to non-voice sounds[3]. Reduced blood oxygen level dependency (BOLD) responses were found in the ventromedial prefrontal cortex (vmPFC), left precuneus, and left cuneus in AN during voice, as compared to non-voice, imagery. The authors speculate that it is a dysfunction of the vmPFC, possibly driven by impaired fibre connections conveying voice information from the anterior temporal lobe to this region, that can explain AN's phonagnosia. However, unfortunately, functional connectivity analyses have not been carried out for AN.

A recent meta-analysis of neuroimaging studies on person recognition has revealed vmPFC involvement in famous person-identity processing independent of input modality (i.e. voice, face, and name), but not in identity processing of personally familiar or recently learned persons (Blank et al., 2014). In our view, it is possible that atypical responses in the vmPFC may not fully explain AN's associative voice-identity processing for both personally familiar (based on a self-report) and famous voices. We speculate that the reduction of vmPFC responses in AN might be associated with her inability to imagine celebrities' voices, but may not be causal for her phonagnosia.

---

[3] Xu and colleagues noted a similar pattern of low voice-imagery ratings for KH and also for SR, a 49-year-old male who also presented with poor voice-recognition abilities (a full characterization of the specificity of SR's phonagnosia was not reported). Interestingly, KH was not only impaired in voice imagery but also in non-voice imagery. However, the neurological underpinnings of KH's and SR's behavioural deficits were not examined.

AN's case suggested that typical responses in TVAs of the STG/S for passive listening to voices (i.e. vocal versus non-vocal sounds) may be observed in developmental phonagnosia. AN's intact matching of unfamiliar voices may have been supported by preserved TVA responses. Yet, the integrity of the connectivity profile between the core-voice and extended system was not assessed in the case of AN, making it difficult to fully characterize the neural mechanisms of her associative voice-identity processing deficit. However, examination of two novel cases of developmental phonagnosia, reported by Roswandowitz et al. (2014), give rise to a more concrete understanding of how the core-voice and extended system may interact during voice-identity processing (Roswandowitz, Schelinski, & von Kriegstein, 2017).

39.5.3 The Cases of AS and SP

Cases of developmental phonagnosia seem to be rare and have often come to the attention of researchers serendipitously (Herald et al., 2014). Using a different approach, which involved large-scale web-based testing of voice-recognition performance in about a thousand volunteers, Roswandowitz et al. (2014) identified two novel cases of developmental phonagnosia—AS and SP, both successful academics.

AS was a 32-year-old female, with no history of brain injury, who reported a distinct difficulty in voice-identity processing. For example, AS stated that she found it difficult to discriminate the voice of her daughter from her daughter's friend, when they were playing in a nearby room. SP was a 32-year-old male who, like AS, reported a deficit in recognizing speaker identity from the voice alone. Interestingly, SP only became explicitly aware that his voice processing was atypical when his friend pointed out that a voice-over artist from their favourite show, which they watched together, had been replaced by a new vocal identity. This suggests that SP, unlike his friend, may have relied on compensatory strategies such as the use of current context, which remained unchanged in the case of the television show, to infer the identity of a voice.

Both AS and SP scored poorly on the original online web-based test designed to detect cases of phonagnosia (see Figure 39.3 for an illustration of the web- and laboratory-based screening measures used). This test assessed the ability to learn voice-name pairings for unfamiliar identities and to subsequently recognize the learned voice by name. In a large comprehensive behavioural test battery, Roswandowitz et al. (2014) noted that this impaired association of vocal identities with additional semantic information was not limited to voice-name associations. Rather, relative to controls, both AS (controls $n = 11$) and SP (controls $n = 10$) scored poorly on tasks requiring the association of an unfamiliar voice with a colour or a facial identity. Interestingly, AS's performance on the unfamiliar voice-face learning task showed only a trend for impaired performance. Thus, AS may have had some preserved ability to use additional facial information to enhance the representation of the vocal percept. Both AS and SP showed normal face-recognition performance as assessed by the Cambridge Face Memory Test (Duchaine & Nakayama, 2006), a standardized test used to detect cases of prosopagnosia and a novel unfamiliar face-name learning test (Roswandowitz et al., 2014).

AS and SP's familiar voice recognition was also examined. Here, they were exposed to a series of famous and non-famous vocal identities. Following each voice sample, they were

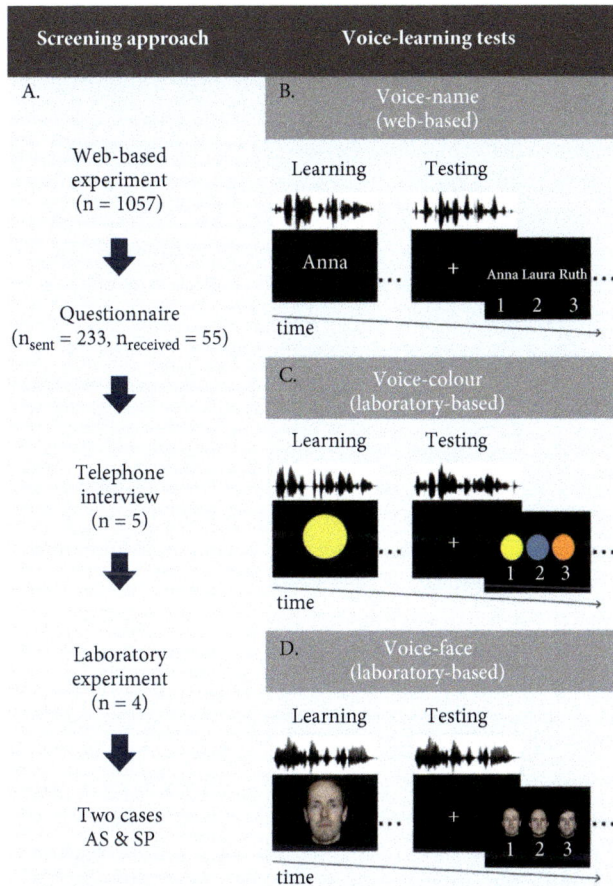

FIGURE 39.3   An overview of the web-based screening approach (A) and the voice-recognition tests (B–D) which were used to identify two unique cases of developmental phonagnosia, AS and SP (Roswandowitz et al., 2014).

asked to indicate their familiarity with the voice and to provide a name or any uniquely identifying information pertaining to the vocal identity. Both phonagnosics showed atypical response strategies when classifying voices as familiar or unfamiliar (e.g. conservative (in AS) or liberal (in SP) rules). In contrast, only AS showed poor accuracy (d') in categorizing voices as familiar. Yet interestingly, she performed well in providing unique semantic information for the voices which she successfully categorized as familiar. This pattern suggested that her voice-identity processing deficit was unlikely to be mediated by deficits at the level of semantic association. On the other hand, SP was poorer than controls in naming identities which he classified as familiar to him, suggesting he may have an associative (semantic association) form of phonagnosia. This pattern was confirmed in an additional examination of unfamiliar voice discrimination where only AS, and not SP, was significantly impaired relative to controls. As such, Roswandowitz and colleagues were the first to find evidence for a double dissociation between voice discrimination (apperceptive voice-identity processing) and recognition (associative voice-identity processing) in two cases of developmental phonagnosia.

Both phonagnosics had normal hearing levels across a range of frequencies and both performed within the normal range on tests of speech processing in noise, music, and vocal-emotion recognition. Hence, their voice-identity processing impairments could not be attributed to a general deficit in auditory processing. However, both AS and SP were impaired on vocal-pitch perception. This impairment appeared to be voice-specific, as neither phonagnosics were impaired on tests examining music pitch perception.

In a follow-up study, Roswandowitz and colleagues (Roswandowitz, Schelinski, & von Kriegstein, 2017) examined the neural mechanisms underlying both AS and SP's discrete voice-identity processing deficits. They firstly examined AS and SP's functional response profile in the core-voice system (see Figure 39.1A,B) using a vocal-sound experiment, where participants were exposed to a series of vocal and non-vocal sounds (Belin et al., 2000). For SP, BOLD responses in the core-voice system were comparable to his controls ($n = 16$). This was in accordance with his associative phonagnosia where perceptual voice processing is intact. In contrast, AS's behavioural profile of poor perceptual voice processing (apperceptive phonagnosia) was mirrored in the reduced response in the core-voice system, specifically in the Heschl's gyrus, compared to her controls ($n = 14$).

Secondly, the authors examined functional responses in AS and SP in a voice-identity recognition experiment. In this experiment, participants either performed a speaker- or a speech-recognition task on sentences spoken by different speakers (adapted from von Kriegstein et al., 2003; Blank et al., 2011; Schelinski, Borowiak, & von Kriegstein, 2016). The authors observed that for the contrast speaker versus speech task, AS showed reduced functional responses, relative to controls ($n = 16$), in regions of the core-voice system including the right anterolateral Heschl's gyrus and planum temporale and extending to the right posterior STS/G. This finding is consistent with her apperceptive deficit. Conversely, AS had increased functional responses, relative to controls ($n = 16$), in the right temporal pole and the right laterobasal amygdala—all proposed regions for the extended system (see Figure 39.1A,B). Interestingly, there was also a trend to significance for increased responses in the fusiform face area (FFA) in AS, which matches well with her relatively preserved ability to link voices with facial-identity information (voice-face learning test). Thus, it is likely that AS uses additional facial information to enhance her weak perceptual processing of voices. Responses in the FFA are likely reflective of this cross-modal compensation (von Kriegstein, Kleinschmidt, & Giraud, 2006; von Kriegstein et al., 2008).

In contrast, in SP, connectivity *between* the core-voice and extended system was altered. As such, his deficit in voice-identity processing was likely to arise within the context of poor connectivity, rather than dysfunctional recruitment of the core-voice or extended system. In addition, SP showed increased response in, and increased functional connectivity within, the core-voice system during speaker (in contrast to speech) recognition. The authors propose that SP may rely more on the perceptual analysis of the voice to compensate for his associative phonagnosia. Enhanced recruitment of the core-voice system may be reflective of this.

The findings of Roswandowitz and colleagues (Roswandowitz, Schelinski, & von Kriegstein, 2017) were the first to show that responses in and connectivity between distinct brain regions can be associated with discrete behavioural subtypes of phonagnosia. Their findings demonstrated that cases of phonagnosia, which are associative in nature, may be marked by poor propagation of signals *from* the (intact) core-voice *to* the extended system (case of SP). Additionally, cases of apperceptive phonagnosia may be characterized by atypical functioning within the core-voice system itself (case of AS).

39.6 IDENTIFYING CASES OF DEVELOPMENTAL PHONAGNOSIA: CURRENTLY AVAILABLE METHODOLOGY

Identifying cases of developmental phonagnosia can prove challenging. For example, the implementation of *standardized* screening tools for developmental phonagnosia, in comparison to prosopagnosia (e.g. Duchaine & Nakayama, 2006; Duchaine et al., 2007), is difficult. Unlike tests for face processing, tests for voice-identity processing are often constrained by the language of the listener, making testing beyond a geographical language location with the same vocal stimuli difficult.

Recently, attempts have been made to overcome such language constraints with the launch of the Glasgow Voice Memory Test (GVMT; Aglieri et al., 2017), a brief test which examines voice-identity processing. Specifically, in this test, listeners are exposed to a series of unfamiliar vocal identities uttering a single vowel and a series of unique bell sounds. Listeners must then immediately decide if these learned vocal identities, presented among a series of category-matched distractor sounds, were present during the learning stage. The strength of this test is that the vocal stimuli are delivered as vowels, rendering language-dependency minimal. Moreover, the bell condition permits for an assessment of the specificity of a voice-identity processing deficit. Aglieri et al. (2017) noted that the GVMT was sensitive in characterizing KH as phonagnosic. Specifically, KH's scores for voice, rather than bell, recognition were significantly poorer than controls.

However, as mentioned throughout, findings from the acquired and developmental literature highlight voice-identity processing as a multistage process. Abnormalities arising during different stages of processing likely characterize the heterogeneity and subtypes of phonagnosia (Roswandowitz, Schelinski, & von Kriegstein, 2017; Roswandowitz et al., 2014) (see Figure 39.1A). Thus, while the GVMT may offer a promising, globally available screening tool for voice processing, it only assesses whether a general sense of familiarity is present for recently learned vocal identities. For example, we noted that SP, characterized by Roswandowitz et al. (2014) as a semantic-associative developmental phonagnosic, performed within the normal range on the GVMT for both voice and bell recognition. Indeed, Roswandowitz and colleagues had previously noted that SP's sensitivity towards voice familiarities was relatively unimpaired. Rather, he was poor at associating the familiar voice with identity-specific semantic information. However, AS, an apperceptive developmental phonagnosic, was significantly impaired on both the voice- and the bell-recognition task (see Figure 39.4).

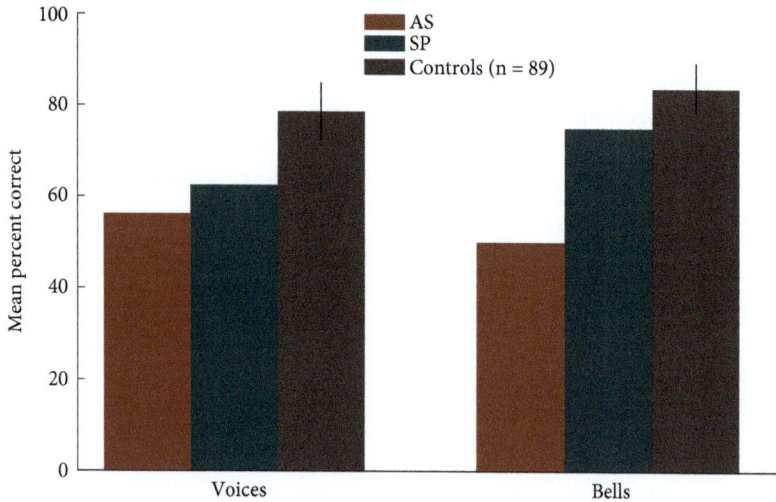

FIGURE 39.4 Plot showing AS and SP's voice- and bell-recognition performance on the GVMT, in relation to the eighty-nine controls (31–40 years old), published by Aglieri et al. (2017). AS's voice and bell recognition were statistically different from controls; SP's performance on both tasks was comparable to controls (AS—voice: p = 0.04, bell: p = 0.002; SP—voice: p = 0.14, bell: p = 0.40). Statistical differences were assessed by comparing AS and SP's scores to control participants using a modified t-test (Crawford & Howell, 1998); p values are reported based on two-tailed probability, however the same pattern is evident for a one-tailed probability analysis. Error bars show one standard deviation of the mean.

Notwithstanding the challenge of differences in language, it is important that tests for phonagnosia are designed to address the multistage nature of voice processing—tackling voice perception, familiarity decision, and semantic association (see Figure 39.1A and Table 39.1). It is possible that standardizing the test design and testing procedure may allow for comparison across study findings for phonagnosia. Furthermore, it may also allow for a deeper insight into individual differences in voice-identity processing, at multiple stages, in the general population.

39.7 PHONAGNOSIA IN RELATION TO CURRENT VOICE-IDENTITY PROCESSING MODELS

39.7.1 Voice-Identity Processing as a Multistage Process: Supporting Role of Core-Voice and Extended System

Findings from neurotypical populations (Belin et al., 2000; Bestelmeyer et al., 2011; Pernet et al., 2015; von Kriegstein et al., 2003) and the acquired and developmental phonagnosia cases reviewed throughout this chapter support the temporal lobe as a key structure in the core-voice system implicated in the stage of perceptual voice-identity analysis and voice-identity recognition. For instance, lesions in the mid/posterior temporal lobe are associated with a selective impairment in voice-identity recognition (Roswandowitz, Kappes, et al., 2018).

What brain regions support specific stages of the voice-identity processing model? Lesions in the temporal lobe of the core-voice system, predominantly in the right hemisphere, have been consistently associated with impaired apperceptive voice-identity processing abilities (Assal et al., 1976, 1981; Van Lancker et al., 1988, 1989). Unfortunately, detailed lesion descriptions were not reported in these cases. In the case of AS, a developmental apperceptive phonagnosic, atypical responses in the auditory cortex (Heschl's gyrus) and posterior part of the temporal lobe (STG) were found (Roswandowitz, Schelinski, & von Kriegstein, 2017). Together, these findings highlight the importance of the temporal lobe, in particular the posterior part, and the auditory cortex, in supporting the perceptual analysis of the voice (Figure 39.1A, Stage I; Figure 39.1B).

Based on findings in neurotypical populations, the next stage of voice-identity processing (i.e. voice-identity recognition) (Figure 39.1A, Stage II) is likely supported by the anterior/mid part of the right temporal lobe (Andics et al., 2010; Belin & Zatorre, 2003; von Kriegstein & Giraud, 2004; von Kriegstein et al., 2003) within the core-voice system. The two lesion studies which have assessed familiarity decision confirm right-hemispheric involvement in familiarity decisions, but unfortunately do not provide detailed lesion descriptions (Lang et al., 2009; Neuner & Schweinberger, 2000).

The subsequent stage of associative voice-identity processing (i.e. semantic association) may be supported by interactions between the core-voice and the extended system (Figure 39.1A, Stage III). Studies on acquired and developmental phonagnosia support the view that the anterior temporal lobe (Hailstone et al., 2010, 2011; Roswandowitz, Schelinski, & von Kriegstein, 2017), the amygdala (Roswandowitz, Schelinski, & von Kriegstein, 2017), and the vmPFC (Xu et al., 2015) may serve as potential candidates of the extended system (for review, see Blank et al., 2014). Currently, the evidence that semantic-associative phonagnosia may result from dysfunctional connections between the core-voice and extended system rests on the fMRI findings from the case of SP (Roswandowitz, Schelinski, & von Kriegstein, 2017). No other study has, to date, assessed the structural integrity or functional connectivity between these systems in phonagnosia cases. Note that direct damage to the extended system, rather than altered connectivity *between* the core-voice and extended system, would likely result in a multimodal (i.e. non-voice selective) person-recognition disorder.

39.7.2 Dissociations Between Stages of the Voice-Identity Processing Model

Findings from patients suffering brain damage (Van Lancker & Kreiman, 1987; Van Lancker et al., 1988) and neurodegenerative diseases (Hailstone et al., 2010, 2011), from individuals with ASD (Schelinski, Roswandowitz, & von Kriegstein, 2016), and from cases of developmental phonagnosia (Roswandowitz, Schelinski, & von Kriegstein, 2017; Roswandowitz et al., 2014) suggest a double dissociation between apperceptive and associative voice-identity processing abilities. There are reports on intact perceptual voice-identity analysis

(Figure 39.1A, Stage I, apperceptive processing) and impaired familiarity decision and semantic association (Figure 39.1A, Stage II, III, associative processing) and vice versa. Also, different lesion locations have been associated with impaired apperceptive and associative processes, respectively.

In contrast, there is to date only limited evidence for a double dissociation between the two stages of associative voice-identity processing—familiarity decision (Figure 39.1A, Stage II) and semantic association (Figure 39.1A, Stage III). Only a few studies compared both abilities intra-individually in cases with presumed associative voice-identity processing deficits (Garrido et al., 2009; Hailstone et al., 2010, 2011; Roswandowitz et al., 2014). Most of these cases showed marked overlapping impairments in familiarity decision and semantic association (Garrido et al., 2009; Hailstone et al., 2010, 2011; but see case SP, Roswandowitz et al., 2014).

39.7.3 Phonagnosia: Modality-Specific and Cross-Modal Interactions

Acquired and developmental cases of phonagnosia confirm dissociable processing streams for person identification by voices, face, and names (Assal et al., 1981; Van Lancker & Kreiman, 1987; Neuner & Schweinberger, 2000; Roswandowitz, Kappes, 2018). However, *interacting* mechanisms, primarily between voice and face identity, have been found as well. For instance, in acquired phonagnosia, a deficit in voice- and face-identity processing tends to co-occur (Hailstone et al., 2010, 2011; Van Lancker & Canter, 1982). This could either suggest that the lesions commonly affect regions that process voice and face information independently, or alternatively it could suggest that there is a possible overlap in the neuroanatomical mechanisms which support face and voice processing. Interestingly, cross-modal interactions between the face and voice regions have been observed in neurotypical populations (e.g. Blank et al., 2011; von Kriegstein et al., 2008). These interactions appear to be behaviourally relevant as voice recognition is often enhanced when the speaker has been previously learned by face (O'Mahony & Newell, 2012; Schall et al., 2013; Schweinberger et al., 2007; von Kriegstein & Giraud, 2006).

Taken together, these findings suggest that phonagnosia can be modality-specific. However, for potentially facilitating purposes, some degree of overlap of, and/or interaction between, the processing of faces and voices, in both the typical and atypical brain, is evident (for review, see Maguinness & von Kriegstein, 2017).

39.7.4 Phonagnosia: Relations Within the Auditory Modality

Phonagnosia findings also confirm separate pathways within the auditory modality. Cases of acquired and developmental phonagnosia have been described with intact speech and vocal-emotion recognition (Assal et al., 1976, 1981; Garrido et al., 2009; Hailstone et al., 2010; Lang et al., 2009; Roswandowitz et al., 2014). However, although such cases have been identified, the findings are far from homogeneous. For example, in lesion studies, LBD patients with aphasia showed both intact (Assal et al., 1976, 1981; Lang et al., 2009) and impaired (Van Lancker & Kreiman, 1987; Van Lancker et al., 1988, 1989) voice-identity processing. Also, in developmental phonagnosia, cases with impaired (Garrido et al., 2009) and intact (Roswandowitz et al., 2014) speech processing have been described.

In neurotypical populations, interacting mechanisms between voice-identity and speech processing have been proposed. For example, voice-identity processing is facilitated when the speaker's language is familiar, rather than unfamiliar, to the listener (Bregman et al., 2012; Fleming et al., 2014; Perrachione et al., 2011). Also, speech content is more easily recognized when the speaker is familiar, rather than unfamiliar, to the listener (Levi et al., 2011; Nygaard & Pisoni, 1998). Currently whether, in phonagnosia, voice-identity and speech mechanisms do interact or are dissociable remains somewhat unclear.

Anecdotal reports of phonagnosic participants suggest that they can rely on the way of speaking and speech content to recognize voice identity. We speculate that in phonagnosia, for instance, information about the speech content (e.g. reference to a past common situation) could help with recognizing a speaker's voice identity. On the other hand, the facilitative effect of voice familiarity for speech recognition might not be available and could potentially explain difficulties with speech recognition in phonagnosia in certain cases (e.g. in KH for speech in noise) (Garrido et al., 2009). Such interactions would be in accordance with recent suggestions on potential neural mechanisms for interaction between speech and voice processing (Kreitewolf et al., 2014; von Kriegstein et al., 2010).

39.8 CONCLUSION

In sum, this chapter suggests that voice-identity processing may represent a unique cognitive process or, more aptly, processes, which can be selectively impaired. These processes appear to be supported by an interactive brain network. Disturbances arising at different stages of processing along this network, either due to brain insult or atypical development, may give rise to distinct impairments in the *apperception* and *association* of vocal identities. This heterogeneous behavioural profile emphasizes the need for standardized behavioural testing, which takes into consideration the multistage nature of voice-identity processing and the resulting subtypes of phonagnosia. Furthermore, this multistage framework highlights that imaging studies should strive to address the integrity of connectivity *between* regions of the voice-processing network, as well as responses within the regions themselves. We propose that the present classification of test designs (Table 39.1) could become a useful guide for future studies investigating voice-identity processing.

Recent findings from the field of face processing suggest that both typical (Wilmer et al., 2010; Zhu et al., 2010) and atypical (developmental prosopagnosia) (Duchaine et al., 2007; Grueter et al., 2007; Lee et al., 2010) face-identity processing may share a heritable component. These findings have been propelled by the availability of standardized testing designs for face perception and recognition. Using this same approach, it is possible that the coming years will provide insight into individual differences in voice-identity processing and their aetiology.

REFERENCES

Aglieri, V., Watson, R., Pernet, C., Latinus, M., Garrido, L., & Belin, P. (2017). The Glasgow Voice Memory Test: assessing the ability to memorize and recognize unfamiliar voices. *Behavior Research Methods*, 49(1), 97–110. doi: 10.3758/s13428-015-0689-6

Andics, A., McQueen, J. M., & Petersson, K. M. (2013). Mean-based neural coding of voices. *NeuroImage*, 79, 351–360.

Andics, A., McQueen, J. M., Petersson, K. M., Gal, V., Rudas, G., & Vidnyanszky, Z. (2010). Neural mechanisms for voice recognition. *NeuroImage*, 52(4), 1528–1540.

Ashburner, J. & Friston, K. J. (2000). Voxel-based morphometry—the methods. *NeuroImage*, 11(6 Pt 1), 805–821.

Assal, G., Aubert, C., & Buttet, J. (1981). Asymetrie cerebrale et reconnaissance de la voix. *Review Neurology (Paris)*, 137(4), 255–268.

Assal, G., Zander, E., Kremin, H., & Buttet, J. (1976). Discrimination des voix lors des lesions du cortex cerebral. *Archives Suisses de Neurologie, Neurochirurgie et de Psychiatrie*, 119(2), 307–315.

Avidan, G. & Behrmann, M. (2014). Impairment of the face processing network in congenital prosopagnosia. *Frontiers in Bioscience*, 6, 236–257.

Bates, E., Wilson, S. M., Saygin, A. P., Dick, F., Sereno, M. I., Knight, R. T. et al. (2003). Voxel-based lesion-symptom mapping. *Nature Neuroscience*, 6(5), 448–450.

Belin, P., Bestelmeyer, P. E. G., Latinus, M., & Watson, R. (2011). Understanding voice perception. *British Journal of Psychology*, 102(4), 711–725.

Belin, P., Fecteau, S., & Bedard, C. (2004). Thinking the voice: neural correlates of voice perception. *Trends in Cognitive Sciences*, 8(3), 129–135.

Belin, P. & Zatorre, R. J. (2003). Adaptation to speaker's voice in right anterior temporal lobe. *NeuroReport*, 14(16), 2105–2109.

Belin, P., Zatorre, R. J., Lafaille, P., Ahad, P., & Pike, B. (2000). Voice-selective areas in human auditory cortex. *Nature*, 403(6767), 309–312.

Bestelmeyer, P. E., Belin, P., & Grosbras, M. H. (2011). Right temporal TMS impairs voice detection. *Current Biology*, 21(20), R838–839.

Blank, H., Anwander, A., & von Kriegstein, K. (2011). Direct structural connections between voice-and face-recognition areas. *Journal of Neuroscience*, 31(36), 12906–12915.

Blank, H., Kiebel, S. J., & von Kriegstein, K. (2014). How the human brain exchanges information across sensory modalities to recognize other people. *Human Brain Mapping*, 36(1), 324–339.

Bonte, M., Hausfeld, L., Scharke, W., Valente, G., & Formisano, E. (2014). Task-dependent decoding of speaker and vowel identity from auditory cortical response patterns. *Journal of Neuroscience*, 34(13), 4548–4557.

Bregman, M. R. & Creel, S. C. (2012). Learning to recognize unfamiliar voices: the role of language familiarity and music experience. *Proceedings of the Annual Meeting of the Cognitive Science Society*, 34(34).

Crawford, J. R. & Howell, D. C. (1998). Comparing an individual's test score against norms derived from small samples. *The Clinical Neuropsychologist*, 12(4), 482–486.

Damasio, A. R., Tranel, D., & Damasio, H. (1990). Face agnosia and the neural substrates of memory. *Annual Reviews in Neuroscience*, 13, 89–109.

De Renzi, E. (1986). Prosopagnosia in two patients with CT scan evidence of damage confined to the right hemisphere. *Neuropsychologia*, 24(3), 385–389.

De Renzi, E., Faglioni, P., Grossi, D., & Nichelli, P. (1991). Apperceptive and associative forms of prosopagnosia. *Cortex*, 27(2), 213–221.

Duchaine, B., Germine, L., & Nakayama, K. (2007). Family resemblance: ten family members with prosopagnosia and within-class object agnosia. *Cognitive Neuropsychology*, 24(4), 419–430.

Duchaine, B. & Nakayama, K. (2006). The Cambridge Face Memory Test: results for neurologically intact individuals and an investigation of its validity using inverted face stimuli and prosopagnosic participants. *Neuropsychologia*, 44(4), 576–585.

Fleming, D., Giordano, B. L., Caldara, R., & Belin, P. (2014). A language-familiarity effect for speaker discrimination without comprehension. *Proceedings of the National Academy of Sciences of the United States of America*, 111(38), 13795–13798.

Formisano, E., De Martino, F., Bonte, M., & Goebel, R. (2008). 'Who' is saying 'what'? Brain-based decoding of human voice and speech. *Science*, 322(5903), 970–973.

Fox, C. J., Iaria, G., & Barton, J. J. S. (2008). Disconnection in prosopagnosia and face processing. *Cortex*, 44(8), 996–1009.

Freud, S. (1891). *Zur Auffassung der Aphasien—Eine Kritische Studie*. Wien: Fischer Taschenbuch.

Gainotti, G., Barbier, A., & Marra, C. (2003). Slowly progressive defect in recognition of familiar people in a patient with right anterior temporal atrophy. *Brain*, 126(Pt 4), 792–803.

Gainotti, G., Ferraccioli, M., Quaranta, D., & Marra, C. (2008). Cross- modal recognition disorders for persons and other unique entities in a patient with right fronto-temporal degeneration. *Cortex*, 44(3), 238–248.

Garrido, L., Eisner, F., McGettigan, C., Stewart, L., Sauter, D., Hanley, J. R. et al. (2009). Developmental phonagnosia: a selective deficit of vocal identity recognition. *Neuropsychologia*, 47(1), 123–131.

Grueter, M., Grueter, T., Bell, V., Horst, J., & Laskowski, W. (2007). Hereditary prosopagnosia: the first case series. *Cortex*, 43, 734–749.

Hailstone, J. C., Crutch, S. J., Vestergaard, M. D., Patterson, R. D., & Warren, J. D. (2010). Progressive associative phonagnosia: a neuropsychological analysis. *Neuropsychologia*, 48(4), 1104–1114.

Hailstone, J. C., Ridgway, G. R., Bartlett, J. W., Goll, J. C., Buckley, A. H., Crutch, S. J. et al. (2011). Voice processing in dementia: a neuropsychological and neuroanatomical analysis. *Brain*, 134(9), 2535–2547.

Herald, S. B., Xu, X., Biederman, I., Amir, O., & Shilowich, B. E. (2014). Phonagnosia: a voice homologue to prosopagnosia. *Visual Cognition*, 22(8), 1031–1033.

Kreitewolf, J., Gaudrain, E., & von Kriegstein, K. (2014). A neural mechanism for recognizing speech spoken by different speakers. *NeuroImage*, 91, 375–385.

Lang, C. J., Kneidl, O., Hielscher-Fastabend, M., & Heckmann, J. G. (2009). Voice recognition in aphasic and non-aphasic stroke patients. *Journal of Neurology*, 256(8), 1303–1306.

Latinus, M., Crabbe, F., & Belin, P. (2011). Learning-induced changes in the cerebral processing of voice identity. *Cerebral Cortex*, 21(12), 2820–2828.

Latinus, M., McAleer, P., Bestelmeyer, P. E., & Belin, P. (2013). Norm-based coding of voice identity in human auditory cortex. *Current Biology*, 23(12), 1075–1080.

Lavner, Y., Rosenhouse, J., & Gath, I. (2001). The prototype model in speaker identification by human listeners. *International Journal of Speech Technology*, 4(1), 63–74.

Lee, Y., Duchaine, B., Wilson, H. R., & Nakayama, K. (2010). Three cases of developmental prosopagnosia from one family: detailed neuropsychological and psychophysical investigation of face processing. *Cortex*, 46(8), 949–964.

Levi, S. V., Winters, S. J., & Pisoni, D. B. (2011). Effects of cross-language voice training on speech perception: whose familiar voices are more intelligible? *Journal of the Acoustical Society of America*, 130(6), 4053–4062.

Lissauer, H. (1890). Ein fall von seelenblindheit nebst einem beitrage zur theorie derselben. *Archiv fur Psychiatrie*, 21(2), 222–270.

López, S., Riera, P., Assaneo, M. F., Eguía, M., Sigman, M., & Trevisana, M. A. (2013). Vocal caricatures reveal signatures of speaker identity. *Scientific Reports*, 3, 3407.

Maguinness, C., Roswandowitz, C., & von Kriegstein, K. (2018). Understanding the mechanisms of familiar voice recognition in the human brain. *Neuropsychologia*, S0028-3932(18), 30140-30144. doi: 10.1016/j.neuropsychologia2018.03.039

Maguinness, C. & von Kriegstein, K. (2017). Cross-modal processing of voices and faces in developmental prosopagnosia and developmental phonagnosia. *Visual Cognition*, 25(4–6), 644–657.

Neuner, F. & Schweinberger, S. R. (2000). Neuropsychological impairments in the recognition of faces, voices, and personal names. *Brain Cognition*, 44(3), 342–366.

Nygaard, L. C. & Pisoni, D. B. (1998). Talker-specific learning in speech perception. *Attention, Perception & Psychophysics*, 60(3), 355–376.

O'Mahony, C. & Newell, F. N. (2012). Integration of faces and voices, but not faces and names, in person recognition. *British Journal of Psychology*, 103(1), 73–82.

Pernet, C. R., McAleer, P., Latinus, M., Gorgolewski, K. J., Charest, I., Bestelmeyer, P. E. et al. (2015). The human voice areas: spatial organization and inter-individual variability in temporal and extra- temporal cortices. *NeuroImage*, 119, 164–174.

Perrachione, T. K., Del Tufo, S. N., & Gabrieli, J. D. (2011). Human voice recognition depends on language ability. *Science*, 333(6042), 595.

Roswandowitz, C., Kappes, C., Obrig, H., & von Kriegstein, K. (2018). Obligatory and facultative brain regions for voice-identity recognition. *Brain*, 141(1), 234–247.

Roswandowitz, C., Mathias Samuel, R., Hintz, F., Kreitewolf, J., Schelinski, S., & von Kriegstein, K. (2014). Two cases of selective developmental voice-recognition impairments. *Current Biology*, 24(19), 2348–2353.

Roswandowitz, C., Schelinski, S., & von Kriegstein, K. (2017). Developmental phonagnosia: linking neural mechanisms with the behavioural phenotype. *NeuroImage*, 155, 97–112.

Schall, S., Kiebel, S. J., Maess, B., & von Kriegstein, K. (2013). Early auditory sensory processing of voices is facilitated by visual mechanisms. *NeuroImage*, 77, 237–245.

Schall, S., Kiebel, S. J., Maess, B., & von Kriegstein, K. (2015). Voice identity recognition: functional division of the right STS and its behavioral relevance. *Journal of Cognitive Neuroscience*, 27(2), 280–291.

Schelinski, S., Borowiak, K., & von Kriegstein, K. (2016). Temporal voice areas exist in autism spectrum disorder but are dysfunctional for voice identity recognition. *Social, Cognitive, and Affective Neuroscience*, 11(11), 1812–1822.

Schelinski, S., Roswandowitz, C., & von Kriegstein, K. (2016). Voice identity processing in autism spectrum disorder. *Autism Research*, 10(1), 155–168.

Schmalzl, L., Palermo, R., & Coltheart, M. (2008). Cognitive heterogeneity in genetically based prosopagnosia: a family study. *Journal of Neuropsychology*, 2(1), 99–117.

Schweinberger, S. R., Robertson, D., & Kaufmann, J. M. (2007). Hearing facial identities. *Quarterly Journal of Experimental Psychology*, 60(10), 1446–1456.

Shah, N. J., Marshall, J. C., Zafiris, O., Schwab, A., Zilles, K., & Markowitsch, H. J. et al. (2001). The neural correlates of person familiarity. A functional magnetic resonance imaging study with clinical implications. *Brain*, 124(Pt 4), 804–815.

Shilowich, B. E. & Biederman, I. (2016). An estimate of the prevalence of developmental phonagnosia. *Brain and Language*, 159, 84–91.

Stollhoff, R., Jost, J., Elze, T., & Kennerknecht, I. (2011). Deficits in long-term recognition memory reveal dissociated subtypes in congenital prosopagnosia. *PLoS One*, 6(1), e15702

Van Lancker, D. & Kreiman, J. (1987). Voice discrimination and recognition are separate abilities. *Neuropsychologia*, 25(5), 829–834.

Van Lancker, D. R. & Canter, G. J. (1982). Impairment of voice and face recognition in patients with hemispheric damage. *Brain and Cognition*, 1(2), 185–195.

Van Lancker, D. R., Cummings, J. L., Kreiman, J., & Dobkin, B. H. (1988). Phonagnosia: a dissociation between familiar and unfamiliar voices. *Cortex*, 24, 195–209.

Van Lancker, D. R., Kreiman, J., & Cummings, J. (1989). Voice perception deficits: neuroanatomical correlates of phonagnosia. *Journal of Clinical and Experimental Neuropsychology*, 11(5), 665–674.

von Kriegstein, K. (2011). A multisensory perspective on human auditory communication. In: M. M. Murray & M. T. Wallace (eds) *The Neural Bases of Multisensory Processes* (pp. 683–700). Boca Raton: Taylor & Francis.

von Kriegstein, K., Dogan, O., Gruter, M., Giraud, A. L., Kell, C. A., Gruter, T. et al. (2008). Simulation of talking faces in the human brain improves auditory speech recognition. *Proceedings of the National Academy of Sciences of the United States of America*, 105(18), 6747–6752.

von Kriegstein, K., Eger, E., Kleinschmidt, A., & Giraud, A. L. (2003). Modulation of neural responses to speech by directing attention to voices or verbal content. *Brain Research: Cognitive Brain Research*, 17(1), 48–55.

von Kriegstein, K. & Giraud, A. L. (2004). Distinct functional substrates along the right superior temporal sulcus for the processing of voices. *NeuroImage*, 22(2), 948–955.

von Kriegstein, K. & Giraud, A. L. (2006). Implicit multisensory associations influence voice recognition. *PLoS Biology*, 4(10).

von Kriegstein, K., Kleinschmidt, A., & Giraud A. L. (2006). Voice recognition and cross-modal responses to familiar speakers' voices in prosopagnosia. *Cerebral Cortex*, 16(9), 1314–1322.

von Kriegstein, K., Smith, D. R., Patterson, R. D., Kiebel, S. J., & Griffiths, T. D. (2010). How the human brain recognizes speech in the context of changing speakers. *Journal of Neuroscience*, 30(2), 629–638.

von Kriegstein, K., Warren, J. D., Ives, D. T., Patterson, R. D., & Griffiths, T. D. (2006). Processing the acoustic effect of size in speech sounds. *NeuroImage*, 32(1), 368–375.

Warren, J., Scott, S., Price, C., & Griffiths, T. (2006). Human brain mechanisms for the early analysis of voices. *NeuroImage*, 31(3), 1389–1397.

Warrington, E. K. (1975). The selective impairment of semantic memory. *Quarterly Journal of Experimental Psychology*, 27, 635–657.

Warrington, E. K. & Shallice, T. (1984). Category specific semantic impairments. *Brain*, 107, 829–854.

Wilmer, J. B., Germine, L., Chabris, C. F., Chatterjee, G., Williams, M., Loken, E. et al. (2010). Human face recognition ability is specific and highly heritable. *Proceedings of the National Academy of Sciences*, 107(11), 5238–5241.

Xu, X., Biederman, I., Shilowich, B. E., Herald, S. B., Amir, O., & Allen, N. E. (2015). Developmental phonagnosia: neural correlates and a behavioral marker. *Brain and Language*, 149, 106–117.

Zhu, Q., Song, Y., Hu, S., Li, X., Tian, M., Zhen, Z. et al. (2010). Heritability of the specific cognitive ability of face perception. *Current Biology*, 20(2), 137–142.

CHAPTER 40

VOICE PROCESSING IN DEMENTIA

JENNIFER L. AGUSTUS, JULIA C. HAILSTONE, AND JASON D. WARREN

40.1 OVERVIEW

In this chapter we summarize the clinical features, cognitive mechanisms, and neuroanatomical substrates of voice-processing disorders associated with the major dementias. Although disturbances of voice processing are rarely the leading feature of these diseases, impaired perception or recognition of voice identity and non-verbal vocal signals contribute to daily-life disability in the dementias and constitute a significant source of distress for patients and caregivers. The major neurodegenerative dementias are underpinned by the deposition of pathogenic proteins in neural tissue: these proteins spread through specific, large-scale brain networks that encompass temporal, frontal, and parietal cortical areas and their subcortical projections (Warren, Rohrer, & Rossor, 2013; Warren et al., 2012, 2013). The brain networks targeted by proteinopathies provide a substrate for the characteristic clinico-anatomical phenotypes that define different dementias, and more particularly, for the development of voice-processing deficits, as the networks overlap closely those implicated in the processing of voices in the healthy brain (Hanley, 2014; Warren et al., 2006; see Parts I, IV, and V, this volume).

We firstly review key clinical and neuroanatomical characteristics of common dementias that affect voice processing, and consider the challenges of assessing voice processing in these diseases. We then outline a taxonomy of voice-processing symptoms and deficits in the dementias, related to the perception and recognition of voices as complex 'auditory objects' that signal speaker identity as well as much other paralinguistic information (in particular, prosody and accent). We consider the extent to which deficits may be selective for voice attributes versus other domains of non-verbal sound and person knowledge, and the demands of integrating vocal with other sensory (in particular, visual) information. We survey the neuroanatomical correlates of disordered voice processing in neurodegenerative syndromes. Based on the available evidence, we conclude by proposing a framework for understanding voice processing in the dementias and indicate directions for future work.

40.2 Important Dementias Associated with Impaired Voice Processing

40.2.1 Alzheimer's Disease

Alzheimer's disease (AD) is the most common form of dementia and is defined histo-pathologically by deposition of abnormal proteins in the form of plaques (containing beta-amyloid) and neurofibrillary tangles (containing phosphorylated tau). AD typically presents with deficits of episodic memory affecting autobiographical and topographical material but deficits of visuospatial awareness, executive functions, and other cognitive domains generally supervene. This phenotype is underpinned by dysfunction and atrophy of a core temporo-parietal network including hippocampi, the posterior cingulate, and parietal cortices, previously implicated in stimulus-independent thought and monitoring of self in relation to the external environment (Warren et al., 2012).

There are several important clinical variants of AD, including posterior cortical atrophy (led by visuoperceptual, visuospatial, and other parietal lobe deficits) and logopenic aphasia (led by word-finding difficulty, speech errors, and impaired verbal working memory) associated with dominant hemispheric temporo-parietal atrophy (Warren et al., 2012).

40.2.2 Fronto-temporal Dementias

The fronto-temporal dementias (fronto-temporal lobar degenerations) are a complex and heterogeneous group of diseases collectively characterized by relatively selective atrophy of frontal and temporal lobes (Warren et al., 2013). These diseases constitute a leading cause of dementia in people before the age of 65 years and genetic forms account for a substantial proportion of cases, usually attributable to a pathogenic mutation in one of three major genes (progranulin [GRN], microtubule-associated protein tau [MAPT], or open reading frame 72 on chromosome 9 [C9orf72]). Histopathological associations are diverse but the majority of cases have abnormal deposition of protein TDP-43 or phosphorylated tau.

The clinical picture is generally dominated by progressive behavioural or language disturbances, comprising one of three canonical clinico-anatomical syndromes. The syndrome of behavioural variant fronto-temporal dementia is led by alterations of inter-personal behaviour and executive dysfunction: this syndrome is underpinned by disintegration of distributed fronto-temporal networks that process salient emotional and social signals, model contingencies, and programme contextually appropriate behavioural responses, often with marked involvement of the right cerebral hemisphere.

The syndrome of semantic dementia usually presents with loss of vocabulary and word-finding difficulty as part of a more widespread and ultimately profound impairment of semantic memory that degrades knowledge of sensory objects as well as language; this syndrome is characteristically associated with asymmetric involvement of anterior temporal lobe semantic networks, more severe in the left (dominant) hemisphere. Impaired knowledge about familiar people may be a prominent feature in both behavioural variant fronto-temporal dementia and semantic dementia; progressive prosopagnosia (affecting face recognition) is usually the most salient clinical deficit in such cases.

The syndrome of progressive non-fluent aphasia is led by impaired language output, with prominent speech sound and/or grammatical errors. It is associated with asymmetric involvement of language networks surrounding the Sylvian fissure, more marked in the left hemisphere.

The fronto-temporal dementia spectrum overlaps with parkinsonian disorders (including progressive supranuclear palsy) and motor neuron disease.

40.2.3 Parkinson's Disease and Lewy Body Dementia

Dementia is a common issue in Parkinson's disease and may dominate the clinical presentation (also designated 'Lewy body dementia' on account of the characteristic histopathological deposits containing abnormal protein synuclein). Executive deficits and hallucinations are typically prominent features, and abnormalities of visual processing, memory, and other cognitive domains are also common (Weil et al., 2016). These deficits and associated extrapyramidal motor features are underpinned by involvement of cortico-subcortical circuitry including the basal ganglia.

40.2.4 Huntington's Disease

Though uncommon, Huntington's disease is an important genetic cause of cognitive and behavioural decline. It is caused by pathogenic expansions in the huntingtin gene, leading to degeneration of striato-cortical networks. In addition to the characteristic choreiform movement disorder, dysexecutive, affective, and other neuropsychiatric features develop early in its course (Papoutsi et al., 2014).

40.3 CHALLENGES OF ASSESSING VOICE PROCESSING IN DEMENTIA

Defining deficits of voice processing in dementia is challenging, on a number of levels. Until comparatively recently, neuropsychological and neuroanatomical frameworks for understanding voice-processing deficits had been much less well worked out than for other complex cognitive functions (notably, the processing of faces). Symptoms of altered voice perception and recognition do not form part of routine clinical history taking and may not be volunteered by patients or caregivers, particularly where other symptoms dominate the presentation or other sensory (e.g. visual) cues mask the patient's difficulty with voices; this may only be exposed in particular situations, such as when using the telephone. Even if such symptoms are acknowledged, there is a dearth of standardized neuropsychological instruments for assessing voice perception and recognition. Tests to probe these capacities generally remain research tools. Moreover, tests of voice processing may be difficult to interpret in the context of other cognitive deficits; associated aphasia may preclude the use of procedures that rely on verbal labelling, while executive and working-memory deficits may confound procedures that depend on serial matching or discrimination between vocal exemplars.

Some neuropsychological tests that have been used in research settings to assess different aspects of voice processing in patients with dementia are summarized in Table 40.1. These include the Queen Square Tests of Auditory Cognition incorporating sub-batteries to assess voice perception and recognition, vocal emotion, prosody, and accent processing, based, where feasible, on simple forced-choice and matching procedures that do not rely on verbal skills (Fletcher et al., 2013; Hailstone et al., 2010, 2011, 2012; Hardy et al, 2016; Rohrer et al., 2012). Most of these tests of voice processing have yet to be normed in healthy older people.

Not uncommonly in the dementias, disorders of voice processing are accompanied by other deficits of non-verbal sound processing (for a recent review, see Hardy et al., 2016): even if impaired voice processing is the most salient auditory symptom, this need not imply that auditory impairment is voice-selective, since voices play a much more direct role in interpersonal communication than most other sounds.

40.4 Voice Perception and Recognition

It is commonplace to analogize voices as 'auditory faces'. Following this analogy, the processing of voice identity can be approached as a hierarchically organized series of cognitive operations, broadly entailing the initial encoding of vocal features, construction of a percept of the individual voice (vocal apperceptive processing), and linking of this vocal percept with other knowledge about the person (vocal semantic processing) (Hailstone et al., 2010, 2011). The analogy with faces might be extended to predict some dissociation of mechanisms for processing voice identity versus other kinds of information conveyed by the voice. This cognitive scheme is in line with models proposed for the processing of other auditory objects as well as faces (Goll et al., 2010); it is relevant to the symptoms exhibited by patients with dementia and has motivated the design of neuropsychological experiments (see Table 40.1). However, it should be emphasized that it remains unclear how far models of face (and other sensory object) processing translate to voices (Hailstone et al., 2010). This is difficult to resolve by studying patients with dementia, since neurodegenerative pathologies often involve several different processing stages and cognitive modules conjointly.

40.4.1 Early Encoding of Vocal Features

In daily life, voices must generally be distinguished from other noises in the acoustic background before other speaker attributes can be processed. This is a particular instance of auditory scene analysis, whereby acoustic features belonging to a given sound source are grouped and different sound sources are segregated from one another using information derived from previously stored sound object schemas; the 'cocktail party' scenario is the classical

Table 40.1 Some neuropsychological tests used to assess aspects of voice
processing in patients with dementia

Function	Procedure	Reference
Voice identity		
Parsing of voices from acoustic background	Detection of name spoken against babble	Golden et al., 2015
Feature encoding	Vocal size[a], gender discrimination	Hailstone et al., 2010, 2011
Apperception	Unfamiliar speaker discrimination	
Familiarity	Familiarity decision on famous voices vs unfamiliar foils	
Recognition	Naming of famous voices Supply other biographical information about famous voices Cross-modal matching to famous faces	
Non-verbal emotion		
Recognition	Matching of vocal emotions to emotion labels[b]	Keane et al., 2002 Hailstone et al., 2010 Omar et al., 2011
Prosody		
Acoustic	Discrimination (in syllable, phrase pairs) of pitch, duration, intensity variation	Rohrer et al., 2012
Emotional	Discrimination of emotional prosodic contours Matching of emotional prosodic contours (in sentences, syllable strings) to emotion labels[b]	Testa et al., 2001 Rohrer et al., 2012
Linguistic	Identification of stressed syllable in spoken phrase Discrimination of statement vs question	Rohrer et al., 2012
Sarcasm	Distinction of sincere vs sarcastic (simple [opposite meaning], paradoxical [context-dependent]) exchanges in video vignettes[c]	Kipps et al., 2009
Accents		
Comprehension	Comprehension of questions spoken in native vs non-native accent Verification of single words spoken in native vs non-native accent	Hailstone et al., 2012
Apperception	Accent discrimination (independent of speaker identity)	Fletcher et al., 2013
Recognition	Matching of accents to written labels or maps	Hailstone et al., 2012 Fletcher et al., 2013

The table summarizes tests used to assess particular stages and dimensions of voice processing in dementia syndromes. These tests have generally been developed in the research setting to address specific experimental questions, and most have not been normed in healthy age-matched populations. Details of voice-processing tests and analogous tests to assess corresponding processes for faces, other environmental sounds, speech signals, and related general neuropsychological functions (e.g. semantic memory) are described in the studies referenced.

a: vocal tract length; b: 'universal' emotions (happiness, anger, disgust, fear, sadness, surprise);
c: the Awareness of Social Inference Test (published norms available)

illustration of the process in action. Auditory scene analysis is a computationally demanding process that is potentially vulnerable to neurodegenerative pathologies, and deficits of the process (including the parsing of speaker information from background) have been documented in AD (Golden et al., 2015; Goll et al., 2012).

There is currently little information available concerning the encoding of generic vocal features such as speaker size (vocal tract length), age, and gender in patients with dementia. Perception of vocal size has been shown to be intact in patients with AD and semantic dementia, while perception of vocal gender may be retained in semantic dementia but variably affected in AD (Hailstone et al., 2011).

40.4.2 Perception of Voice Identity

Identification of particular voices relies on accurate discrimination between individuals as well as a robust percept of the individual voice under varying listening conditions which might include a changing acoustic environment, changes in the verbal message delivered by the voice, or changes in vocal characteristics per se (such as speaking over the telephone or with a heavy cold). Clinical experience suggests that perception of voice identity may present difficulties for some patients with dementia. Although the neuropsychological evidence remains rather slight, discrimination of unfamiliar voices has been shown to be impaired in patients with AD but intact in patients with semantic dementia (Hailstone et al., 2011). In Hailstone et al.'s (2011) study, the task was to determine whether the speaker changed or remained the same over the course of a short phrase (a changing sequence of phonemes). This evidence suggests that patients with AD have a group-level deficit of vocal 'apperceptive' processing: impaired ability to abstract a constant percept of the voice as a sensory object from the set of constituent features that together define individual vocal identity.

40.4.3 Recognition of Familiar Voices

Impaired ability to recognize familiar voices, or 'phonagnosia', is the auditory equivalent of prosopagnosia (inability to recognize faces) but substantially less commonly volunteered as a symptom of dementia. It remains unclear whether this discrepancy simply reflects the circumstances under which we typically encounter other people, a bias in clinical history taking, or some more fundamental characteristic of the brain mechanisms that represent familiar faces and voices. Nevertheless, phonagnosia typically supervenes in patients presenting with progressive prosopagnosia (Fletcher et al., 2013; Gainotti et al., 2003, 2008; Gentileschi et al., 2001; Hailstone et al., 2010) and is occasionally itself a dominant presenting feature of dementia (Hailstone et al., 2010).

At group level, deficits of voice recognition have been demonstrated in AD but are more severe in semantic dementia, in line with the more marked and pervasive, multimodal impairment of person knowledge in that condition (Hailstone et al., 2011; Luzzi et al., 2017). Impaired voice recognition in these patients has been demonstrated using various neuropsychological procedures, including explicit identification (naming), cross-modal (face) matching, and familiarity decisions (whether or not a given voice belongs to a famous person), after controlling for potentially confounding perceptual and semantic attributes.

Deficits of voice recognition have been documented, despite intact voice discrimination, in individual patients with behavioural variant fronto-temporal dementia, progressive non-fluent aphasia, and semantic dementia (Fletcher et al., 2013; Hailstone et al., 2010) and do not correlate closely with discrimination accuracy at group level (Hailstone et al., 2011), suggesting that phonagnosia in these cases is 'associative' in nature, reflecting impaired semantic memory for voices. Furthermore, patients who are unable to recognize individual voices may still recognize vocal emotions normally (Hailstone et al., 2010), arguing that the semantic mechanisms for processing vocal identity and emotion are differentially vulnerable in at least some cases of dementia. Taken together, this evidence is in line with the previously proposed modular organization of voice cognition (Hanley, 2014) and suggests that the brain may contain a 'lexicon' of familiar voices analogous to those for words, faces, and other sensory objects, that can be similarly targeted by neurodegenerative pathologies.

40.4.4 Processing of Own Voice

One's own voice is a privileged vocal signal that has certain unique attributes. Our own voices (unlike other voices) are generally subject to the acoustic filtering effect of bone conduction. In addition, one's own vocalizations normally entail an 'efference copy' of the motor command that is used to predict vocal output and detect feedback errors. On-line monitoring of own vocalizations plays a fundamental role in normal speech and may be targeted by certain dementias, as suggested by the disruptive effect of delayed auditory feedback closely simulating progressive aphasia in some healthy people (Maruta et al., 2014; Warren et al., 2005). Moreover, one's voice belongs to that peculiar class of sensory signals that originates not from the environment but from one's own internal milieu. Such signals are potentially vulnerable to dementias that disrupt the representation of the self and its boundaries, and there is some evidence that patients with AD have a selective relative deficit in retrieving information conveyed by own voice versus other, unfamiliar voices (Bond et al., 2016).

40.4.5 Processing of Voices Versus Other Sensory Objects

In patients with dementia, recognition of voices may dissociate from recognition of other sounds, faces, and names. In a detailed study of two patients with phonagnosia in the setting of fronto-temporal dementia (Hailstone et al., 2010), recognition of environmental sounds was intact in both cases, and recognition of familiar faces and names was also preserved in one case. Interestingly, this patient had impaired recognition of musical instrument timbres: this finding raises the possibility that phonagnosia reflects a more general impairment in the processing of highly differentiated sound categories or alternatively, that instrumental 'voices' have co-opted brain mechanisms attuned to biological vocalizations.

40.5 VOCAL PARALINGUISTIC INFORMATION

Voices carry a variety of information apart from (and independently of) speaker identity. Typically this 'paralinguistic' information amplifies or modifies a spoken verbal message. Processing of vocal paralinguistic signals is also vulnerable to the effects of dementia.

40.5.1 Non-verbal Vocal Emotion

The auditory equivalents of universal emotions can be transmitted by non-verbal vocal sounds (laughter, retching, screams, sobbing, etc). In this elementary form, recognition of vocal emotions has been shown to be impaired in patients with semantic dementia, behavioural variant fronto-temporal dementia, progressive supranuclear palsy, and Huntington's disease (Ghosh et al., 2012; Henley et al., 2012; Keane et al., 2002; Omar et al., 2011; Rees et al., 2014; Snowden et al., 2008). In general, deficits are more severe for recognition of 'negative' vocal emotions such as anger, disgust, and fear than 'positive' emotions (joy and mirth), with the caveat that our labelling of negative emotions is more precise. The available evidence suggests shared vulnerability of brain mechanisms for processing emotions from the voice and from other sensory channels (notably, facial expressions) in these diseases. Less secure, however, is any claim to specific vulnerability of particular emotions, with little consistency across studies and the suggestion of an interaction between emotion and stimulus modality that would be difficult to predict a priori (Henley et al., 2012; Rees et al., 2014).

40.5.2 Prosody

The prosody of a verbal message (the pattern of variations in vocal pitch, timing, and intensity in the speech signal) may have emotional or semantic significance. Acoustic features (such as pitch and loudness variations) of the prosody used by caregivers have been shown to influence the overall quality of communication with patients with dementia (Small et al., 2009).

40.5.2.1 *Emotional Prosody*

Processing of emotional prosody has been studied more widely than the processing of non-verbal vocal emotional sounds in dementia. Impaired comprehension of emotional prosody occurs with AD, albeit not consistently, suggesting this may become more evident as the disease evolves (Bucks & Radford, 2004; Cadieux & Greve, 1997; Horley et al., 2010; Koff et al., 1999; Roberts et al., 1996; Taler et al., 2008; Testa et al., 2001). Moreover, prosody deficits can be demonstrated after neutralizing verbal semantic content (Testa et al., 2001).

Deficits of emotional prosody comprehension have been documented in the logopenic aphasia variant of AD and progressive non-fluent aphasia (Rohrer et al., 2012), in behavioural variant fronto-temporal dementia (Dara et al., 2013; Perry et al., 2001; Rankin et al., 2009; Shany-Ur et al., 2012), and motor neuron disease (Andrews et al., 2017). In both AD and fronto-temporal dementia syndromes, performance in processing emotional prosody may dissociate both from verbal language skills and from processing of other emotion modalities (such as facial expressions) (Cadieux & Grieve 1997; Dara et al., 2013; Drapeau et al., 2009; Koff et al., 1999; Rohrer et al., 2012; Testa et al., 2001); recognition of particular emotions may interact with stimulus modality, though data on this remains limited (Rohrer et al., 2012).

Difficulty comprehending emotional prosody may be a relatively early signal of reduced social functioning in Huntington's disease (Speedie et al., 1990; Sprengelmeyer et al., 1996) and Parkinson's disease/Lewy body dementia (Breitenstein et al., 2001; Buxton et al., 2013; Dara et al., 2008; Ventura et al., 2012). At least in Parkinson's disease, there may be an effect from valence (comprehension of negative more severely affected than positive vocal emotions), though auditory working memory and acoustic perceptual factors may modulate performance (Breitenstein et al., 2001; Dara et al., 2008; Lima et al., 2013; Peron et al., 2015).

40.5.2.2 *Linguistic Prosody*

Deficits of processing linguistic prosody (the intonational or stress contours used to disambiguate verbal messages or pose a question) have been demonstrated in AD, logopenic aphasia, progressive non-fluent aphasia, and progressive aphasia associated with *GRN* mutations and in Huntington's disease (Cadieux & Greve, 1997; Rohrer et al., 2012; Speedie et al., 1990; Taler et al., 2008). Processing of prosodic contours extending over several syllables appears to present more difficulty than the processing of simple (monosyllabic) acoustic cues based on pitch, intensity, or duration (Rohrer et al., 2012). This is not attributable simply to reduced working-memory capacity per se. The cognitive mechanisms that process linguistic and emotional prosody may be differentially vulnerable in AD (Testa et al., 2001).

40.5.2.3 *Output Prosody*

Patients with dementia may have altered voice quality, most often due to involvement of motor effector pathways. However, in some neurodegenerative disease settings, the prosody of patients' speech may change due to disturbed trafficking of paralinguistic signals, perhaps reflecting the close relationship between speech production and feedback processing of spoken output (Warren et al., 2005). Patients with behavioural variant fronto-temporal dementia may have sometimes strikingly impaired ability to convey vocal as well as facial emotions (Nevler et al., 2017). This is in line with an inability to recognize emotional prosody in this syndrome (Dara et al., 2013), though it may occasionally manifest as an isolated disturbance in producing emotional expressions (Ghacibeh & Heilman, 2003).

Studies in AD suggest that generation of prosodic emotions may be affected in this condition, too. Though spontaneous dysprosody is not generally a prominent clinical feature, at least earlier in the disease (Horley et al., 2010; Roberts et al., 1996; Testa et al., 2001), more quantitative analysis suggests that expression of negative vocal emotions may be attenuated in AD from a relatively early stage (Han et al., 2014). There has been some interest in using prosodic signatures to assist dementia diagnosis (Kato et al., 2013; Nevler et al., 2017).

40.5.3 Accents

Accents are an important meta-linguistic attribute of speech signals, encompassing a range of phonatory, articulatory, and prosodic features that together constitute the characteristic, stable vocal patterns we perceive as a particular accent. The processing of accents involves several different cognitive computations. Comprehension of verbal messages spoken with an unfamiliar accent entails the recognition of non-canonical phonemes: the auditory brain is presented with an 'unusual view' of the constituent auditory (phonemic) objects and decoding these objects engages auditory apperceptive mechanisms. In addition, accents carry non-verbal semantic information about the speaker's geographical and sociocultural origins.

Patients with progressive non-fluent aphasia and AD may have particular difficulty comprehending speech delivered in a non-native accent (Burda et al., 2004; Hailstone et al., 2012); while progressive non-fluent aphasia, AD, and semantic dementia may impair recognition of accents (Fletcher et al., 2013; Hailstone et al., 2012). Accent-processing deficits are most consistently observed and most severe in progressive non-fluent aphasia, and accent agnosia may occasionally dominate the presentation in these patients (Fletcher et al., 2013). Progressive non-fluent aphasia and AD are associated with impaired analysis of perceptual features of accents, at single-word and phrasal level, respectively. The ability to discriminate accents may be lost despite preserved discrimination of voices and phonemes (Fletcher et al., 2013), arguing for at least some selectivity in the apperceptive processing of these different kinds of vocal information. In contrast, semantic dementia may affect the recognition or semantic processing of accents as higher-order auditory 'objects' with geographical and cultural associations. It remains to be established whether the semantic analysis of accents and other paralinguistic signals dissociates from voice identification in patients with dementia.

40.5.4 Sarcasm

Sarcasm is a special case of paralinguistic communication at the interface between semantic, emotional, and social-signal processing. Accurate comprehension of sarcasm requires decoding of a mismatch between the literal content of a verbal message and the speaker's true meaning, which typically carries humorous or hostile connotations. Processing of this mismatch in turn requires a correct inference about the speaker's mental workspace. While detection of sarcasm depends on accurate processing of prosodic features (Shany-Ur et al., 2012), sarcasm therefore probes additional, multimodal processes of social cognition and 'theory of mind' (judgements about others' feelings and beliefs).

Impaired comprehension of sarcasm accompanies a more pervasive disorder of social-signal decoding in behavioural variant fronto-temporal dementia, semantic dementia, and progressive supranuclear palsy (Downey et al., 2015; Ghosh et al., 2012; Kipps et al., 2009; Kosmidis et al., 2008; Rankin et al., 2009; Shany-Ur et al., 2012) and may track clinical evolution in fronto-temporal dementia, Huntington's disease, and parkinsonian syndromes (Kumfor et al., 2014; Larsen et al., 2016; Pell et al., 2014; Philpott et al., 2016; Shany-Ur et al., 2012). Abnormalities of sarcasm processing have also been documented in motor neuron disease (Staios et al., 2013). However, the cognitive mechanism of impaired sarcasm processing is likely to differ between dementia syndromes; for example, patients with behavioural variant fronto-temporal dementia may have particular difficulty in using additional, contextual (including facial expression and gestural) information when decoding sarcastic intent (Rankin et al., 2009). Patients with AD typically remain relatively sensitive to sarcasm, though this may decline later in the course (Kumfor et al., 2014; Shany-Ur et al., 2012).

As the most widely used test of sarcasm processing (the Awareness of Social Inference Test: Kipps et al., 2009) employs audiovisual video vignettes, it remains unclear to what extent impaired sarcasm awareness in dementia can be considered specific to vocal-signal decoding.

40.6 COMBINING VOICES WITH VISION

Under everyday listening conditions, information from the voice must often be integrated with other sensory (typically visual) information. This cross-modal processing may assist in deciphering vocal information under challenging listening conditions, such as a noisy room. Our normal reliance on coherent cross-modal audiovisual cues is exposed by certain experimental paradigms, such as the classical McGurk effect (McGurk & Macdonald, 1976), whereby presentation of a spoken phoneme (e.g. 'ba') while viewing lip movements corresponding to a conflicting phoneme (e.g. 'ga') creates the percept of an illusory composite phoneme ('da'). Patients with AD are less susceptible to this audiovisual illusion, perhaps reflecting impaired mechanisms for cross-modal integration of vocal with visual stimuli (Delbeuck et al., 2007). However, our clinical experience suggests that patients with AD and behavioural variant fronto-temporal dementia retain some ability to use visual cues to help disambiguate degraded vocal targets (e.g. in the well-known 'cocktail party' scenario in which a name is overheard against background babble).

40.7 HALLUCINATIONS OF VOICES

Hearing voices is less common than other (visual and non-verbal auditory) hallucinations in dementia. However, between 1% and around 30% of patients with dementia are reported to have experienced vocal (auditory verbal) hallucinations across published series (Bassiony & Lyketsos, 2003; Laroi & Sommer, 2012). Associated auditory (particularly musical) hallucinations are common (Golden & Josephs, 2015).

The frequency and phenomenology of vocal hallucinations varies between dementia syndromes and pathologies. In Parkinson's disease, hallucinated voices are often 'muffled' (not uncommonly, the patient will have sought the source of the voice in the next room or outside the house) and tend to occur without psychotic elaboration (Laroi & Sommer, 2012). In contrast, patients with behavioural variant fronto-temporal dementia due to C9orf72 mutations may experience well-formed, second-person vocal hallucinations as part of an elaborate delusional system (Sommerlad et al., 2014). Patients with these mutations appear to be at higher risk of hallucinations and other psychotic symptoms than are those with sporadic forms of fronto-temporal dementia (Kertesz et al., 2013).

40.8 Neuroanatomical Correlates of Voice Processing in Dementia

There remains relatively little information about the neuroanatomical bases of voice-processing deficits in the dementias. As these are network-based diseases, it is generally not possible to establish neuroanatomical substrates based on single case studies alone. Most correlative studies have used voxel-based morphometry to establish structural grey-matter associations of performance on voice-processing tasks, chiefly in patient cohorts with AD or fronto-temporal dementia syndromes. This neuroanatomical perspective has recently been extended using diffusion tensor tractography and functional MRI. Together, these studies in the dementias have implicated extensive temporo-parietal and prefrontal networks, in line with neuroanatomical evidence in the healthy brain (Kreitewolf et al., 2014; Nakamura et al., 2001; Warren et al., 2006; Wildgruber et al., 2006).

40.8.1 Voice-Identity Processing

Impaired discrimination of voices in AD has been linked to atrophy of the right inferior parietal lobe, consistent with a role for this region in vocal apperceptive processing (Hailstone et al., 2011). Associative phonagnosia in semantic dementia and AD cohorts has been correlated with grey-matter loss and hypometabolism in right antero-medial temporal structures (Hailstone et al., 2011; Luzzi et al., 2017): impaired recognition of voices and other modalities of person knowledge (faces and names) was associated with atrophy of the temporal pole and anterior fusiform gyrus, while impaired recognition of voices was specifically correlated with additional atrophy of the amygdala and hippocampus (Hailstone et al., 2011). These group-level correlates corroborate single case studies suggesting that phonagnosia and other impairments of person knowledge are clinically prominent in patients with focal right temporal lobe atrophy (Fletcher et al., 2013; Gainotti et al., 2003, 2008; Gentileschi et al., 2001; Hailstone et al., 2010; see Figure 40.1) and are consistent with studies of voice-identity processing in the healthy brain (Warren et al., 2006).

40.8.2 Paralinguistic Information Processing

Impaired processing of non-verbal vocal emotional sounds in patients with progressive supranuclear palsy has been correlated, using voxel-based morphometry, with regional atrophy of the right inferior frontal cortex (Ghosh et al., 2012); and in one functional MRI study, processing of laughter and crying was associated with reduced activation of the left anterior and posterior superior temporal sulcus in patients with behavioural variant fronto-temporal dementia compared with healthy, older individuals (Agustus et al., 2015).

Reduced recognition of emotional prosody (for negative emotions of fear, disgust, or sadness) in patients with non-fluent progressive aphasias has been associated with grey-matter loss in a distributed bi-hemispheric network including dorsolateral and inferior frontal, cingulate, insular, antero-mesial temporal, and temporo-parietal areas (Rohrer et al., 2012). In that study, impaired processing of linguistic prosody was correlated with atrophy of an

Phonagnosia   Accent agnosia

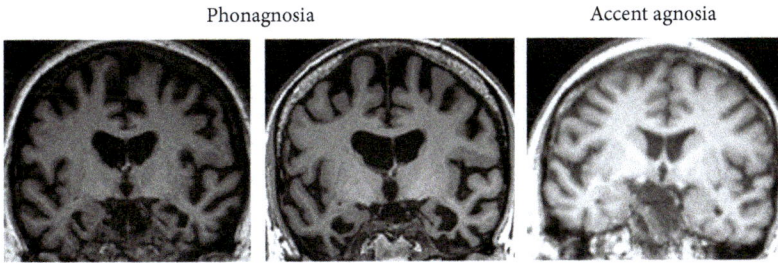

FIGURE 40.1 Brain-imaging findings in patients with dementia and prominent voice-processing deficits. The figure shows coronal T1-weighted MRI brain sections from patients with clinically prominent disorders of voice processing (the right hemisphere is displayed on the right in each case): (**left panel**) asymmetric (more prominently right-sided) anterior superior temporal and peri-Sylvian atrophy in a patient presenting with behavioural variant fronto-temporal dementia accompanied by associative phonagnosia; (**middle panel**) asymmetric (predominantly right-sided) antero-mesial temporal lobe atrophy in a patient presenting with progressive prosopagnosia and phonagnosia; (**right panel**) asymmetric (more prominently left sided) peri-Sylvian atrophy in a patient presenting with progressive non-fluent aphasia and apperceptive agnosia for accents (impaired accent discrimination).

overlapping, predominantly left-lateralized cortical network. Another study, in patients with AD, identified grey-matter correlates of non-native accent comprehension in the left anterior superior temporal cortex and accent recognition in the right anterior temporal cortex (Hailstone et al., 2012). This is consistent with individual neuroimaging findings in progressive non-fluent aphasia associated with prominent accent agnosia (see Figure 40.1).

The cerebral networks collectively demonstrated by these studies include areas previously implicated in the analysis of paralinguistic information as well as more generic operations of auditory working memory and attention in the healthy brain (Hardy et al., 2016; Kreitewolf et al., 2014).

The cerebral correlates of sarcasm processing have been studied somewhat more systematically than other aspects of voice processing in patients with dementia. Impaired comprehension of sarcasm is associated with grey-matter loss in the anterior medial prefrontal cortex in progressive supranuclear palsy (Ghosh et al., 2012); with atrophy of the right amygdala, right temporal pole, and orbitofrontal cortex in behavioural variant fronto-temporal dementia and semantic dementia (Downey et al., 2015; Kipps et al., 2009); and with atrophy of a fronto-temporal network including the right temporal pole, right medial frontal pole, and bilateral parahippocampal gyri across neurodegenerative syndromes (Rankin et al., 2009). Using diffusion tensor tractography, correlates of impaired sarcasm processing have been identified in the uncinate fasciculus (a key fronto-temporal white-matter tract) in patients with behavioural variant fronto-temporal dementia and semantic dementia (Downey et al., 2015).

These neuroanatomical correlates of sarcasm processing in the dementias align with findings in the healthy brain that implicate distributed mechanisms engaged in the analysis of acoustic features, affective evaluation, social conceptual knowledge, and decoding of the speaker's intentions ('theory of mind') during sarcastic communication (Matsui et al., 2016; Uchiyama et al., 2012).

Studying patients with neurodegenerative diseases may sometimes yield unique insights into the cerebral organization of voice processing that would not otherwise be available. One example of this is the modulatory effect of deep brain stimulation on emotional prosody perception observed in patients with Parkinson's disease. Stimulation of the subthalamic nucleus has been shown to bias patients' ratings of the intensity of particular vocal emotions, and this effect has been correlated with altered use of acoustic voice parameters (Peron et al., 2015). The findings argue for a role of basal ganglia structures in coordinating the cerebral networks that bind sensory features with semantic and affective information during voice processing. Disturbance of this modulatory or facilitatory influence from the basal ganglia might also account for the emergence of difficulties processing higher-order vocal social signals (such as sarcasm) relatively early in the course of Parkinson's disease (Pell et al., 2014).

40.8.3 Vocal Hallucinations

There remains little direct evidence for the cerebral substrate of verbal and other auditory hallucinations in the dementias. The relative prominence of hallucinations and related neuropsychiatric symptoms in patients with *C9orf72* mutations may reflect involvement of a cortico-thalamo-cerebellar network previously implicated in mediating disordered representations of the self in relation to other people and the wider sensory environment (Downey et al., 2014; Marshall et al., 2016).

40.9 CONCLUSIONS

Although conclusions must remain tentative, given the relatively small numbers of cases assessed, neuropsychological and neuroanatomical studies have together outlined a coherent framework for understanding voice processing in the dementias. This framework is summarized in Figures 40.2 and 40.3. While many details remain to be worked out, the emerging picture is broadly in accord with hierarchical, fractionated cognitive and neuroanatomical models proposed for the processing of other kinds of sounds and other aspects of person knowledge (in particular, human faces) in the dementias (Goll et al., 2010; Hanley, 2014; Hardy et al., 2016).

Although associated deficits are common, detailed analysis of voice-processing impairments in individual patients and in patient cohorts representing a range of dementia syndromes indicate that voice recognition is at least partly dissociable from the perceptual encoding and discrimination of voices, from recognition of non-verbal vocal emotions and from other domains of person knowledge (in particular, face recognition) (Fletcher et al., 2013; Hailstone et al., 2010, 2011, 2012; Rees et al., 2014; Rohrer et al., 2012). In addition, there is some evidence that deficits of paralinguistic (prosody and accent) processing may dissociate from linguistic functions in these diseases (Dara et al., 2013; Fletcher et al., 2013; Testa et al., 2001).

The initial parsing of voices from the acoustic background and perceptual analysis of voice features implicates posterior auditory association and temporo-parietal cortices, while recognition of familiar voices depends on semantic mechanisms instantiated in the

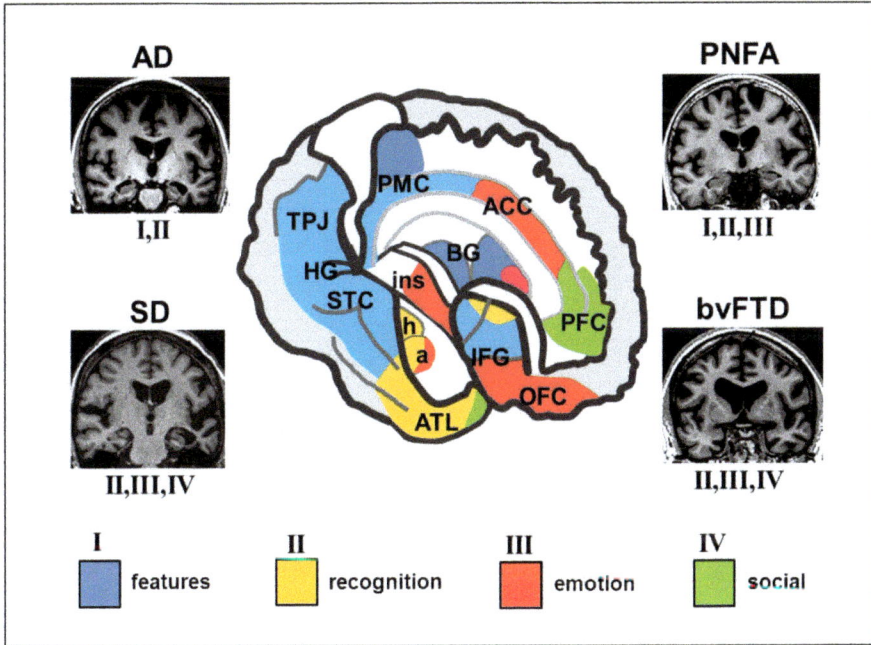

FIGURE 40.2 Neuroanatomical substrates for voice-processing operations affected by dementias. The cut-away brain schematic (centre) shows cerebral networks that mediate key cognitive operations in voice processing, coded I to IV (below) and based on clinical and normal functional neuroanatomical evidence (see text). 'Features' (I, blue) here subsumes brain substrates for detection and analysis of vocal acoustic features to the level of voices as 'objects' corresponding to different speakers; 'recognition' (II, gold) corresponds to substrates for semantic processing of familiar voices; 'emotion' (III, red) corresponds to substrates for processing vocal emotions and affective valuation of voices; 'social' (IV, green) corresponds to substrates of social inference and 'theory of mind'. The right cerebral hemisphere is projected forward in the schematic; however, neuroanatomical substrates of voice processing are bi-hemispherically distributed, principally including: a, amygdala; ACC, anterior cingulate cortex; ATL, anterior temporal lobe; BG, basal ganglia; h, hippocampus; HG, Heschl's gyrus (containing primary auditory cortex); IFG, inferior frontal gyrus/frontal operculum; ins, insula; OFC, orbitofrontal cortex; PFC, medial prefrontal cortex; PMC, posterior medial cortex (posterior cingulate, precuneus); STC, superior temporal cortex (gyrus/sulcus); TPJ, temporo-parietal junction. Side panels show characteristic profiles of regional cerebral atrophy (coronal MRI sections, left hemisphere displayed on right) and voice-processing operations chiefly affected in selected dementias: typical Alzheimer's disease (AD), bilateral symmetrical mesial temporal and more diffuse (especially posterior) cerebral atrophy; behavioural variant fronto-temporal dementia (bvFTD), predominant bifrontal atrophy; progressive non-fluent aphasia (PNFA), predominantly left-sided peri-Sylvian atrophy; and semantic dementia (SD), asymmetric (predominantly left-sided) anterior temporal lobe atrophy.

anterior (especially non-dominant) temporal lobe. Paralinguistic attributes of vocal signals are processed partly in parallel to voice identity, with partly overlapping brain substrates in the auditory association cortex (engaged in the perceptual analysis of paralinguistic signals) and more distributed prefrontal and limbic circuitry (engaged in assigning affective and

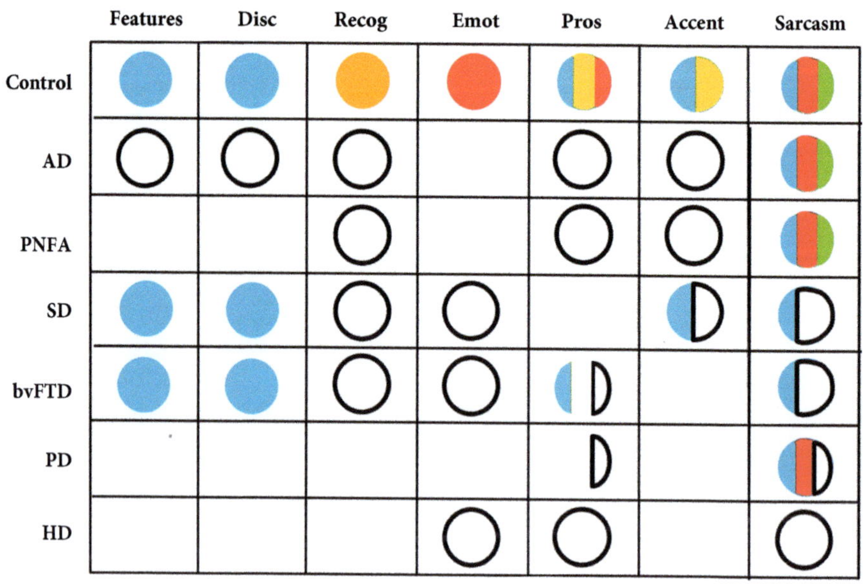

	Features	Disc	Recog	Emot	Pros	Accent	Sarcasm

FIGURE 40.3 Voice-processing phenotypes of some important dementias. This scheme summarizes current evidence from group and single-case neuropsychological studies of voice processing in representative dementia syndromes. Here, coloured circles code the general cognitive operations involved in particular aspects of voice processing, following the conventions used to delineate brain substrates of these operations in Figure 40.2: blue signifies perceptual analysis of voice information; gold, semantic processing; red, emotion processing and affective valuation; green, social inference and 'theory of mind'. Unfilled circles or segments indicate impairment of the relevant process in that dementia syndrome; empty squares or 'gaps' indicate the relevant process has not been adequately assessed in that syndrome. AD, typical Alzheimer's disease; bvFTD, behavioural variant fronto-temporal dementia; Control, healthy reference performance profile; Disc, discrimination of speakers (vocal apperceptive processing); Emot, vocal emotion processing; Features, encoding of generic perceptual characteristics of voices including speaker size (vocal tract length), gender; HD, Huntington's disease; PD, Parkinson's disease/Lewy body dementia; PNFA, progressive non-fluent aphasia; Pros, prosody perception and comprehension (emotional and linguistic); Recog, recognition of familiar speaker (vocal semantic processing); SD, semantic dementia.

semantic value to these signals). The processing of more complex vocal signals with high social salience (notably sarcasm) engages additional specific mechanisms of social cognition and theory of mind.

The 'voice phenotypes' of major dementias (summarized in Figure 40.3) largely follow this framework. AD is characteristically associated with impaired apperceptive processing of voice-identity and paralinguistic signals, as predicted from the temporo-parietal emphasis of AD pathology. A primary perceptual deficit might, in turn, impact on the semantic processing of voice signals in AD, though retained ability to use contextual cues may modulate performance on certain tasks (such as detection of sarcasm), perhaps accounting for the somewhat variable profile of voice-processing deficits observed across studies in AD (Luzzi et al., 2017).

The clinically and pathologically heterogeneous spectrum of fronto-temporal dementias is associated with a correspondingly diverse array of voice-processing deficits. Recognition of voices and vocal feeling states are characteristically impaired in the semantic and primary behavioural syndromes, as predicted from involvement of bifronto-temporal networks in these syndromes; while comprehension of paralinguistic information in prosody and accents is characteristically impaired in progressive non-fluent aphasia, as predicted from involvement of dominant peri-Sylvian cortices in this syndrome.

Other disorders, such as Parkinson's disease and Huntington's disease, give rise to particular difficulties processing emotional signals from voices, perhaps reflecting impaired modulation or biasing of the mechanisms that decode such signals due to heavy involvement of subcortical networks (Pell et al., 2014; Peron et al., 2015).

There is much further work to be done. Future studies should assess the dimensions of voice processing in tandem, systematically and longitudinally, in larger cohorts of patients representing a broad range of neurodegenerative pathologies and with neuroanatomical and histopathological correlation. An accurate picture of voice processing in the dementias will depend on closing the remaining substantial 'gaps' in neuropsychological data across major syndromes and diseases (see Figure 40.3). Comparing AD-variant syndromes may be particularly pertinent to disambiguate the effects of disease topography versus underlying proteinopathy on voice-processing mechanisms.

As intrinsically network-based diseases, the dementias pose both challenges and opportunities. On the one hand, it is not straightforward to assess voice-processing functions and to interpret regional neuroanatomical associations in the setting of diffuse disease; on the other hand, these diseases might potentially help define the critical roles played by large-scale neural systems and pathogenic proteins in analysing vocal signals (Warren et al., 2013). Realising this potential will require functional neuroanatomical and electrophysiological studies that can measure changes in connectivity and the temporal signature of vocal information processing across the cerebral networks targeted by neurodegenerative pathologies.

From a clinical perspective, the ultimate goal of this enterprise is therapy. Simple strategies such as ensuring that the speaker's lips are visible and maximizing facial and other cross-modal cues to speaker identity can be effective in managing voice-processing deficits in daily life (Hardy et al., 2016). Improved understanding of how and why these deficits develop in particular dementias might advance diagnosis and disease tracking (Kumfor et al., 2014) and enable the design of more sophisticated, principled interventions targeting specific aspects of vocal signal analysis and modifying communication accordingly (Small et al., 2009).

ACKNOWLEDGEMENTS

This work is supported by the Alzheimer's Society and the NIHR UCLH Biomedical Research Centre.

REFERENCES

Agustus, J. L., Mahoney, C. J., Downey, L. E., Omar, R., Cohen, M., White, M. J., ... Warren, J. D. (2015). Functional MRI of music emotion processing in frontotemporal dementia. *Annals of the New York Academy of Sciences*, 1337, 232–240.

Andrews, S. C., Staios, M., Howe, J., Reardon, K., & Fisher, F. (2017). Multimodal emotion processing deficits are present in amyotrophic lateral sclerosis. *Neuropsychology*, 31, 304–310.

Bassiony, M. M. & Lyketsos, C. G. (2003). Delusions and hallucinations in Alzheimer's disease: review of the brain decade. *Psychosomatics*, 44, 388–401.

Bond, R. L., Downey, L. E., Weston, P. S., Slattery, C. F., Clark, C. N., Macpherson, K., Mummery, C. J., & Warren, J. D. (2016). Processing of self versus non-self in Alzheimer's disease. *Frontiers in Human Neuroscience*, 10, 97.

Breitenstein, C., Van Lancker, D., Daum, I., & Waters, C. H. (2001). Impaired perception of vocal emotions in Parkinson's disease: influence of speech time processing and executive functioning. *Brain and Cognition*, 45, 277–314.

Bucks, R. S. & Radford, S. A. (2004). Emotion processing in Alzheimer's disease. *Aging and Mental Health*, 8(3), 222–232.

Burda, A. N., Hageman, C. F., Brousard, K. T., & Miller, A. L. (2004). Dementia and identification of words and sentences produced by native and nonnative English speakers. *Perceptual and Motor Skills*, 98, 1359–1362.

Buxton, S. L., MacDonald, L., & Tippett, L. J. (2013). Impaired recognition of prosody and subtle emotional facial expressions in Parkinson's disease. *Behavioral Neuroscience*, 127, 193–203.

Cadieux, N. L. & Greve, K. W. (1997). Emotion processing in Alzheimer's disease. *Journal of the International Neuropsychological Society*, 3(5), 411–419.

Dara, C., Kirsch-Darrow, L., Ochfeld, E., Slenz, J., Agranovich, A., Vasconcellos-Faria, A., … Kortte, K. B. (2013). Impaired emotion processing from vocal and facial cues in frontotemporal dementia compared to right hemisphere stroke. *Neurocase*, 19(6), 521–529.

Dara, C., Monetta, L., & Pell, M. D. (2008). Vocal emotion processing in Parkinson's disease: reduced sensitivity to negative emotions. *Brain Research*, 1188, 100–11.

Delbeuck, X., Collette, F., & Van der Linden, M. (2007). Is Alzheimer's disease a disconnection syndrome? Evidence from a crossmodal audio-visual illusory experiment. *Neuropsychologia*, 45(14), 3315–3323.

Downey, L. E., Fletcher, P. D., Golden, H. L., Mahoney, C. J., Agustus, J. L., Schott, J. M., … Warren, J. D. (2014). Altered body schema processing in frontotemporal dementia with C9ORF72 mutations. *Journal of Neurology, Neurosurgery and Psychiatry*, 85, 1016–1023.

Downey, L. E., Mahoney, C. J., Buckley, A. H., Golden, H. L., Henley, S. M., Schmitz, N., … Warren, J. D. (2015). White matter tract signatures of impaired social cognition in frontotemporal lobar degeneration. *NeuroImage Clinical*, 8, 640–651.

Drapeau, J., Gosselin, N., Gagnon, L., Peretz, I., & Lorrain, D. (2009). Emotional recognition from face, voice, and music in dementia of the Alzheimer type. *Annals of the New York Academy of Sciences*, 1169, 342–345.

Fletcher, P. D., Downey, L. E., Agustus, J. L., Hailstone, J. C., Tyndall, M. H., Cifelli, A., … Warren, J. D. (2013). Agnosia for accents in primary progressive aphasia. *Neuropsychologia*, 51(9), 1709–1715.

Gainotti, G., Barbier, A., & Marra, C. (2003). Slowly progressive defect in recognition of familiar people in a patient with right anterior temporal atrophy. *Brain*, 126, 792–803.

Gainotti, G., Ferraccioli, M., Quaranta, D., & Marra, C. (2008). Cross-modal recognition disorders for persons and other unique entities in a patient with right fronto-temporal degeneration. *Cortex*, 44(3), 238–248.

Gentileschi, V., Sperber, S., & Spinnler, H. (2001). Crossmodal agnosia for familiar people as a consequence of right infero-polar temporal atrophy. *Cognitive Neuropsychology*, 18, 439–463.

Ghacibeh, G.A. & Heilman, K. M. (2003). Progressive affective aprosodia and prosoplegia. *Neurology*, 60, 1192–1194.

Ghosh, B., Calder, A. J., Peers, P. V., Lawrence, A. D., Acosta-Cabronero, J., Pereira, J. M., Hodges, J. R., & Rowe, J. B. (2012). Social cognitive deficits and their neural correlates in progressive supranuclear palsy. *Brain*, 135, 2089–2102.

Golden, E. C. & Josephs, K. A. (2015). Minds on replay: musical hallucinations and their relationship to neurological disease. *Brain*, 138, 3793–3802.

Golden, H. L., Agustus, J. L., Goll, J. C., Downey, L. E., Mummery, C. J., Schott, J. M., Crutch, S. J., & Warren, J. D. (2015). Functional neuroanatomy of auditory scene analysis in Alzheimer's disease. *NeuroImage Clinical*, 7, 699–708.

Goll, J. C., Crutch, S. J., & Warren, J. D. (2010). Central auditory disorders: toward a neuropsychology of auditory objects. *Current Opinion in Neurology*, 23, 617–627.

Goll, J. C., Kim, L. G., Ridgway, G. R., Hailstone, J. C., Lehmann, M., Buckley, A. H., Crutch, S. J., & Warren, J. D. (2012). Impairments of auditory scene analysis in Alzheimer's disease. *Brain*, 135(1), 190–200.

Hailstone, J. C., Crutch, S. J., Vestergaard, M. D., Patterson, R. D., & Warren, J. D. (2010). Progressive associative phonagnosia: a neuropsychological analysis. *Neuropsychologia*, 48(4), 1104–1114.

Hailstone, J. C., Ridgway, G. R., Bartlett, J. W., Goll, J. C., Buckley, A. H., Crutch, S. J., & Warren, J. D. (2011). Voice processing in dementia: a neuropsychological and neuroanatomical analysis. *Brain*, 134(9), 2535–2547.

Hailstone, J. C., Ridgway, G. R., Bartlett, J. W., Goll, J. C., Crutch, S. J., & Warren, J. D. (2012). Accent processing in dementia. *Neuropsychologia*, 50(9), 2233–2244.

Han, K. H., Zaytseva, Y., Bao, Y., Pöppel, E., Chung, S. Y., Kim, J. W., & Kim, H. T. (2014). Impairment of vocal expression of negative emotions in patients with Alzheimer's disease. *Frontiers of Aging Neuroscience*, 6, 101.

Hanley, J. R. (2014). Accessing stored knowledge of familiar people from faces, names and voices: a review. *Frontiers in Bioscience*, 6, 198–207.

Hardy, C .J., Marshall, C. R., Golden, H. L., Clark, C. N., Mummery, C. J., Griffiths, T. D., Bamiou, D. E., & Warren, J. D. (2016). Hearing and dementia. *Journal of Neurology*, 263(11), 2339–2354.

Henley, S. M., Novak, M. J., Frost, C., King, J., Tabrizi, S. J., & Warren, J. D. (2012). Emotion recognition in Huntington's disease: a systematic review. *Neuroscience and Biobehavioral Reviews*, 36, 237–253.

Horley, K., Reid, A., & Burnham, D. (2010). Emotional prosody perception and production in dementia of the Alzheimer's type. *Journal of Speech Language and Hearing Research*, 53(5), 1132–1146.

Kato, S., Endo, H., Homma, A., Sakuma, T., & Watanabe, K. (2013). Early detection of cognitive impairment in the elderly based on Bayesian mining using speech prosody and cerebral blood flow activation. *Conference Proceedings of the IEEE Engineering in Medicine and Biology Society*, pp. 5813–5816.

Keane, J., Calder, A. J., Hodges, J. R., & Young, A. W. (2002). Face and emotion processing in frontal variant frontotemporal dementia. *Neuropsychologia*, 40, 655–665.

Kertesz, A., Ang, L. C., Jesso, S., MacKinley, J., Baker, M., Brown, P., ... Finger, E. C. (2013). Psychosis and hallucinations in frontotemporal dementia with the C9ORF72 mutation: a detailed clinical cohort. *Cognitive and Behavioral Neurology*, 26, 146–154.

Kipps, C. M., Nestor, P. J., Acosta-Cabronero, J., Arnold, R., & Hodges, J. R. (2009). Understanding social dysfunction in the behavioural variant of frontotemporal dementia: the role of emotion and sarcasm processing. *Brain*, 132, 592–603.

Koff, E., Zaitchik, D., Montepare, J., & Albert, M. S. (1999). Emotion processing in the visual and auditory domains by patients with Alzheimer's disease. *Journal of the International Neuropsychological Society*, 5(1), 32–40.

Kosmidis, M. H., Aretouli, E., Bozikas, V. P., Giannakou, M., & Ioannidis, P. (2008). Studying social cognition in patients with schizophrenia and patients with frontotemporal dementia: theory of mind and the perception of sarcasm. *Behavioral Neurology*, 19, 65–69.

Kreitewolf, J., Friederici, A. D., & von Kriegstein, K. (2014). Hemispheric lateralization of linguistic prosody recognition in comparison to speech and speaker recognition. *NeuroImage*, 102, 332–344.

Kumfor, F., Irish, M., Leyton, C., Miller, L., Lah, S., Devenney, E., Hodges, J. R., & Piguet, O. (2014). Tracking the progression of social cognition in neurodegenerative disorders. *Journal of Neurology, Neurosurgery and Psychiatry*, 85, 1076–1083.

Larøi, F. & Sommer, I. E. (2012). The characteristic features of auditory verbal hallucinations in clinical and nonclinical groups: state-of-the-art overview and future directions. *Schizophrenia Bulletin*, 38, 724–733.

Larsen, I. U., Vinther-Jensen, T., Gade, A., Nielsen, J. E., & Vogel, A. (2016). Do I misconstrue? Sarcasm detection, emotion recognition, and theory of mind in Huntington disease. *Neuropsychology*, 30, 181–189.

Lima, C. F., Garrett, C., & Castro, S. L. (2013). Not all sounds sound the same: Parkinson's disease affects differently emotion processing in music and in speech prosody. *Journal of Clinical and Expermental Neuropsychology*, 35, 373–392.

Luzzi, S., Baldinelli, S., Ranaldi, V., Fabi, K., Cafazzo, V., Fringuelli, F., ... Gainotti, G. (2017). Famous faces and voices: Differential profiles in early right and left semantic dementia and in Alzheimer's disease. *Neuropsychologia*, 94, 118–128.

Marshall, C. R., Bocchetta, M., Rohrer, J. D., & Warren, J. D. (2016). C9orf72 mutations and the puzzle of cerebro-cerebellar network degeneration. *Brain*, 139(8), e44. doi: 10.1093/brain/aww103

Maruta, C., Makhmood, S., Downey, L. E., Golden, H. L., Fletcher, P. D., Witoonpanich, P., Rohrer, J. D., & Warren, J. D. (2014). Delayed auditory feedback simulates features of nonfluent primary progressive aphasia. *Journal of the Neurological Sciences*, 347, 345–348.

Matsui, T., Nakamura, T., Utsumi, A., Sasaki, A. T., Koike, T., Yoshida, Y., ... Sadato, N. (2016). The role of prosody and context in sarcasm comprehension: behavioral and fMRI evidence. *Neuropsychologia*, 87, 74–84.

McGurk, H. & MacDonald, J. (1976). Hearing lips and seeing voices. *Nature*, 264, 746–748.

Nakamura, K., Kawashima, R., Sugiura, M., Kato, T., Nakamura, A., Hatano, K., ... Kojima, S. (2001). Neural substrates for recognition of familiar voices: a PET study. *Neuropsychologia*, 39(10), 1047–1054.

Nevler, N., Ash, S., Jester, C., Irwin, D. J., Liberman, M., & Grossman, M. (2017). Automatic measurement of prosody in behavioral variant FTD. *Neurology*, 89, 650–656.

Omar, R., Henley, S. M., Bartlett, J. W., Hailstone, J. C., Gordon, E., Sauter, D. A., ... Warren, J. D. (2011). The structural neuroanatomy of music emotion recognition: evidence from frontotemporal lobar degeneration. *NeuroImage*, 56, 1814–1821.

Papoutsi, M., Labuschagne, I., Tabrizi, S. J., & Stout, J. C. (2014). The cognitive burden in Huntington's disease: pathology, phenotype, and mechanisms of compensation. *Movement Disorders*, 29, 673–683.

Pell, M. D., Monetta, L., Rothermich, K., Kotz, S. A., Cheang, H. S., & McDonald, S. (2014). Social perception in adults with Parkinson's disease. *Neuropsychology,* 28, 905–916.

Péron, J., Cekic, S., Haegelen, C., Sauleau, P., Patel, S., Drapier, D., Vérin, M., & Grandjean, D. (2015). Sensory contribution to vocal emotion deficit in Parkinson's disease after subthalamic stimulation. *Cortex,* 63, 172–183.

Perry, R. J., Rosen, H. R., Kramer, J. H., Beer, J. S., Levenson, R. L., & Miller, B. L. (2001). Hemispheric dominance for emotions, empathy and social behaviour: evidence from right and left handers with frontotemporal dementia. *Neurocase,* 7(2), 145–160.

Philpott, A. L., Andrews, S. C., Staios, M., Churchyard, A., & Fisher, F. (2016). Emotion evaluation and social inference impairments in Huntington's disease. *Journal of Huntington's Disease,* 5, 175–183.

Rankin, K. P., Salazar, A., Gorno-Tempini, M. L., Sollberger, M., Wilson, S. M., Pavlic, D., ... Miller, B. L. (2009). Detecting sarcasm from paralinguistic cues: anatomic and cognitive correlates in neurodegenerative disease. *NeuroImage,* 47(4), 2005–2015.

Rees, E. M., Farmer, R., Cole, J. H., Henley, S. M., Sprengelmeyer, R., Frost, C., ... Tabrizi, S. J. (2014). Inconsistent emotion recognition deficits across stimulus modalities in Huntington's disease. *Neuropsychologia,* 64, 99–104.

Roberts, V. J., Ingram, S. M., Lamar, M., & Green, R. C. (1996). Prosody impairment and associated affective and behavioral disturbances in Alzheimer's disease. *Neurology,* 47(6), 1482–1488.

Rohrer, J. D., Sauter, D., Scott, S., Rossor, M. N., & Warren, J. D. (2012). Receptive prosody in nonfluent primary progressive aphasias. *Cortex,* 48(3), 308–316.

Shany-Ur, T., Poorzand, P., Grossman, S. N., Growdon, M. E., Jang, J. Y., Ketelle, R. S., Miller, B. L., & Rankin, K. P. (2012). Comprehension of insincere communication in neurodegenerative disease: lies, sarcasm, and theory of mind. *Cortex,* 48, 1329–1341.

Small, J. A., Huxtable, A., & Walsh, M. (2009). The role of caregiver prosody in conversations with persons who have Alzheimer's disease. *American Journal of Alzheimer's Disease and Other Dementias,* 24(6), 469–475.

Snowden, J. S., Austin, N. A., Sembi, S., Thompson, J. C., Craufurd, D., & Neary, D. (2008). Emotion recognition in Huntington's disease and frontotemporal dementia. *Neuropsychologia,* 46, 2638–2649.

Sommerlad, A., Lee, J., Warren J. D., & Price, G. (2014). Neurodegenerative disorder masquerading as psychosis in a forensic psychiatry setting. *BMJ Case Reports.* doi: 10.1136/bcr-2013-203458

Speedie, L. J., Brake, N., Folstein, S. E., Bowers, D., & Heilman, K. M. (1990). Comprehension of prosody in Huntington's disease. *Journal of Neurology, Neurosurgery and Psychiatry,* 53, 607–610.

Sprengelmeyer, R., Young, A. W., Calder, A. J., Karnat, A., Lange, H., Hömberg, V., Perrett, D. I., & Rowland, D. (1996). Loss of disgust—perception of faces and emotions in Huntington's disease. *Brain,* 119, 1647–1665.

Staios, M., Fisher, F., Lindell, A. K., Ong, B., Howe, J., & Reardon, K. (2013). Exploring sarcasm detection in amyotrophic lateral sclerosis using ecologically valid measures. *Frontiers in Human Neuroscience,* 7, 178.

Taler, V., Baum, S. R., Chertkow, H., & Saumier, D. (2008). Comprehension of grammatical and emotional prosody is impaired in Alzheimer's disease. *Neuropsychology,* 22(2), 188–195.

Testa, J. A., Beatty, W. W., Gleason, A. C., Orbelo, D. M., & Ross, E. D. (2001). Impaired affective prosody in AD: relationship to aphasic deficits and emotional behaviors. *Neurology,* 57(8), 1474–1481.

Uchiyama, H. T., Saito, D. N., Tanabe, H. C., Harada, T., Seki, A., Ohno, K., Koeda, T., & Sadato, N. (2012). Distinction between the literal and intended meanings of sentences: a functional magnetic resonance imaging study of metaphor and sarcasm. *Cortex, 48,* 563–583.

Ventura, M. I., Baynes, K., Sigvardt, K. A., Unruh, A. M., Acklin, S. S., Kirsch, H. E., & Disbrow, E. A. (2012). Hemispheric asymmetries and prosodic emotion recognition deficits in Parkinson's disease. *Neuropsychologia, 50,* 1936–1945.

Warren, J. D., Fletcher, P. D., & Golden, H. L. (2012). The paradox of syndromic diversity in Alzheimer disease. *Nature Reviews Neurology, 8,* 451–464.

Warren, J. D., Rohrer, J. D., & Rossor, M. N. (2013). Clinical review. Frontotemporal dementia. *British Medical Journal, 347,* f4827. doi: https://doi.org/10.1136/bmj.f4827

Warren, J. D., Rohrer, J. D., Schott, J. M., Fox, N. C., Hardy, J., & Rossor, M. N. (2013). Molecular nexopathies: a new paradigm of neurodegenerative disease. *Trends in Neurosciences, 36,* 561–569.

Warren, J. D., Scott, S. K., Price, C. J., & Griffiths, T. D. (2006). Human brain mechanisms for the early analysis of voices. *NeuroImage, 31,* 1389–1397.

Warren, J. E., Wise, R. J., & Warren, J. D. (2005). Sounds do-able: auditory-motor transformations and the posterior temporal plane. *Trends in Neurosciences, 28,* 636–643.

Weil, R. S., Schrag, A., Warren, J. D., Crutch, S. J., Lees, A. J., & Morris, H. R. (2016). Visual dysfunction in Parkinson's disease. *Brain,* 139(11), 2827–2843.

Wildgruber, D., Ackermann, H., Kreifelts, B., & Ethofer, T. (2006). Cerebral processing of linguistic and emotional prosody: fMRI studies. *Progress in Brain Research, 156,* 249–268.

INDEX